Biology of Bladder Cancer

Margaret A. Knowles • Lars Dyrskjøt
Editors

Biology of Bladder Cancer

From Molecular Insights to Clinical Strategies

Springer

Editors
Margaret A. Knowles
Division of Molecular Medicine,
Leeds Institute of Medical Research
at St James's
St James's University Hospital
Leeds, UK

Lars Dyrskjøt
Department of Clinical Medicine
Aarhus University
Aarhus, Denmark

ISBN 978-3-031-68507-1 ISBN 978-3-031-68505-7 (eBook)
https://doi.org/10.1007/978-3-031-68505-7

This Springer imprint is published by the registered company Springer Nature Switzerland AG
The registered company address is: Gewerbestrasse 11, 6330 Cham, Switzerland

Preface

The field of bladder cancer research and treatment has seen great progress in recent years, influenced by rapid advancements in medical technologies and a deeper understanding of underlying molecular biology. "Biology of Bladder Cancer: From Molecular Insights to Clinical Strategies" is designed to serve as an essential resource for healthcare professionals, researchers, and students in the field of oncology, particularly those focusing on bladder cancer. Its aim is to synthesize the wealth of current knowledge and the latest advancements in bladder cancer research and management and to address possibilities and challenges in translating research into effective clinical practice.

The structure of the book is designed to provide a thorough exploration of bladder cancer, beginning with fundamental aspects, such as epidemiology, genetic predisposition, the biology of the normal urothelium, and current standard treatments, followed by molecular genetics and pathogenesis. It guides the reader through understanding microenvironment dynamics, the various molecular and histological subtypes, and the latest experimental models used in research. Subsequent sections discuss biomarkers for diagnosis and treatment, outline the latest therapeutic strategies based on molecular insights, and conclude with a vision for future research directions. This comprehensive approach ensures coverage of each aspect of bladder cancer, from basic science to clinical and therapeutic strategies, making it an indispensable resource for all involved in bladder cancer management and research.

We extend our deepest gratitude to all the authors who have contributed to this book. Their expertise and dedication have been instrumental in creating a resource that not only advances our understanding of disease biology and its application in developing better treatments but also serves as a practical guide for clinical practitioners and researchers. Their collective effort has made this comprehensive insight into bladder cancer biology and clinical strategies possible. We recognize the challenges of dedicating time to write a book chapter in a busy research and clinical environment. For that, we are immensely thankful. We are confident that their expert knowledge and this multidisciplinary approach will inspire continued research and advance the quality of care for bladder cancer patients.

Leeds, UK — Margaret A. Knowles
Aarhus, Denmark — Lars Dyrskjøt
June 2024

Contents

About the Editors

Margaret (Maggie) Knowles, PhD is Emeritus Professor of Experimental Cancer Research at the University of Leeds in the UK. She has worked on bladder cancer for more than forty years with the goal of improving disease management through molecular studies. Her work has included identification of key genes involved in the development of bladder cancer, sub-classification of non-invasive tumors through genomic and transcriptional analyses, and development of in vitro models for preclinical validation of potential therapeutic targets and improved understanding of gene function. Her extensive publications and leadership roles have played an important part in shaping bladder cancer research over the past two decades.

Lars Dyrskjøt, PhD is a Professor of Molecular Medicine at Aarhus University in Denmark, where he leads a team focused on translational bladder cancer research. His work has greatly enhanced understanding of the disease's molecular pathogenesis, especially through the identification of prognostic and predictive biomarkers in early-stage bladder cancer, and the innovative use of liquid biopsies for monitoring and guiding treatment in advanced bladder cancer. Prof. Dyrskjøt's numerous publications and leadership in international cancer research initiatives make him a key contributor to the global advancement of bladder cancer research.

Part I

Fundamentals of Bladder Cancer

1 Epidemiology of Bladder Cancer

Ali A. Nasrallah and Stephen B. Williams

Abstract

Bladder cancer (BC) is the tenth most incident malignancy globally, with substantial morbidity and mortality. Although fourfold more likely to present in males, females have worse oncologic outcomes even when controlling for other known predictors of adverse outcomes such as smoking and delay to treatment. African-American race is also an independent risk factor for advanced disease when diagnosed, as is lower socioeconomic status. Many modifiable risk factors have been associated with BC risk, with tobacco smoking being the leading risk factor and accounting for an estimated 50% of BC cases. Occupational exposures account for 5–10% of BC cases, due to chemicals such as aromatic amines and polycyclic aromatic hydrocarbons. Environmental exposures such as arsenic-containing drinking water, Agent Orange (AO), and residential exposure to hydrocarbons from oil refineries may also increase risk of BC incidence and mortality. Mediterranean diets and fish consumption are among potential protective dietary factors. Genetics also plays a role, with germline mutations in mismatch repair genes and a range of single-nucleotide polymorphisms identified as risk factors (see Chap. 2). In this chapter, we outline the main demographic trends of BC and identify emerging risk factors for incidence, morbidity, and mortality.

Keywords

Bladder cancer · Epidemiology · Risk factors · Smoking · Environmental carcinogens · Occupational exposure · Diet

A. A. Nasrallah · S. B. Williams (✉)
Department of Surgery, Division of Urology, The University of Texas Medical Branch, Galveston, TX, USA
e-mail: alnasral@utmb.edu; stbwilli@utmb.edu

1.1 Incidence and Mortality

In 2020, there were over 573,000 new cases of bladder cancer (BC) globally, thereby giving BC the tenth highest incidence rate of all cancers, second only to prostate cancer within urologic malignancies (Sung et al. 2021). Differences in age, sex, and geography exist as well. BC incidence in males is almost four times that of females with age-standardized rates (ASRs) of 9.5 to 2.4 per 100,000 individuals, respectively, with overall ASR of 5.6. Geographically, the highest age-standardized incidence rates were seen in Southern Europe (15.3) which included Greece, Spain, and Italy. This is followed by Western Europe and North America. South-Central Asia and Middle Africa recorded the lowest ASRs (Sung et al. 2021) (Fig. 1.1).

M. A. Knowles, L. Dyrskjøt (eds.), *Biology of Bladder Cancer*,
https://doi.org/10.1007/978-3-031-68505-7_1

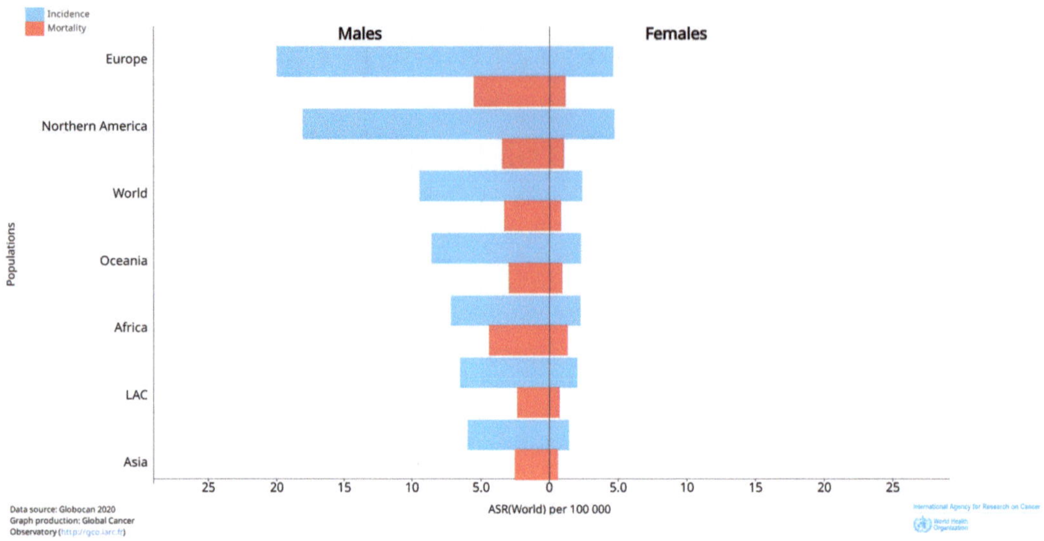

Fig. 1.1 Estimated age-standardized worldwide bladder cancer incidence and mortality rates. © International Agency for Research on Cancer. Date accessed 1/28/2024

There were 212,536 deaths attributed to BC globally in 2020 (Sung et al. 2021), placing it 13th among all cancer mortalities. When stratified by sex, 158,785 (74.7%) deaths occurred among male patients. Among geographic regions, North Africa recorded the highest mortality ASR of 5.2 per 100,000, followed by Southern and Western Europe. The lowest mortality ASRs were seen in Central America and Middle Africa (Sung et al. 2021). However, comparisons of BC mortality rates internationally carry limitations, as variations in reporting mortality directly attributable to BC exist. It is also important to note that such population-level data does not incorporate or account for tumor-specific factors such as stage, grade, and treatment. This is particularly important in BC epidemiology due to the significant difference in patient prognosis with muscle-invasive versus non-muscle-invasive BCs (MIBC vs. NMIBC) (Cumberbatch et al. 2018). Given that NMIBC represents the dominant proportion of BC (Nielsen et al. 2014) and is associated with more favorable prognosis versus MIBC, BC mortality rates provide the best marker of disease control and a useful tool for geographic comparisons and temporal trends (Antoni et al. 2017).

Many factors, both modifiable and non-modifiable, have been cited as potential predictors for the variation in BC incidence and mortality rates (Tables 1.1 and 1.2). Such factors include tobacco smoking, socioeconomic status (SES) (income/education/poverty), environmental or occupational exposures, and the parasitic infection schistosomiasis. Recent reports have demonstrated that countries of higher economic development tend to have higher BC incidence with lower mortality rates (Wong et al. 2018; Teoh et al. 2020). This suggests that improved national economic status may be associated with higher rates of early disease detection, improved public health awareness, enhanced oncologic treatment, and therefore reduced mortality rates. For example, more economically developed countries have increased access to a variety of therapeutic modalities which can influence mortality rates, such as transurethral endoscopic resection, perioperative intravesical chemotherapy, intravesical immunotherapy, radiation therapy, and robotic surgery. Exceptions to this include countries undergoing rapid economic transition such as Eastern/Central/Southern European countries, the Baltic region, and Central/South America (Sung et al. 2021). On the other hand, the economically developing Asian

Table 1.1 Modifiable risk factors and summary of their risks

Modifiable risk factors	Summary of risks	References
Tobacco	Contributes to 50% of BC cases	Burger et al. (2013)
	Threefold odds of BC for smokers	van Osch et al. (2016)
	Dose-response relationship between smoking and BC	van Osch et al. (2016)
	Increases risk of recurrence in NMIBC	Lammers et al. (2011) Ślusarczyk et al. (2022)
	Increases risk of progression in NMIBC	Rink et al. (2013)
	Increases risk of overall mortality, disease-specific mortality, and disease recurrence in MIBC	Cacciamani et al. (2020)
	Increases risk of incomplete response to NAC	Cacciamani et al. (2020) Boeri et al. (2019)
	Higher risk of recurrence after RC in MIBC	Boeri et al. (2019)
	Higher risk of metastasis	Cumberbatch et al. (2016)
	Higher risk of complications after RC	Nasrallah et al. (2021)
Electronic cigarettes	Contain carcinogens with established BC links	Bjurlin et al. (2021)
	Development of urothelial hyperplasia	Tang et al. (2019)
Occupational exposures	Contribute to 10% of BC in the United States	Doll and Peto (1981)
	Contribute to 5.3% of BC in Britain	Rushton et al. (2010)
	Aromatic amine and PAH exposure occupations had highest risk of BC	Cumberbatch et al. (2015) Daniels et al. (2014) Stec et al. (2018)
	Heavy metal or PAH exposure had highest BC-specific mortality	Cumberbatch et al. (2015)
Environmental exposures	Arsenic exposure from drinking water increases BC risk	Baris et al. (2016) Huang et al. (2008)
	Arsenic and BC risk have a dose-response relationship	Di Giovanni et al. (2020) Boffetta and Borron (2019)
	Chlorinated drinking water long-term and high-level consumption may increase BC risk	Villanueva et al. (2003) Costet et al. (2011)
	Nitrogen-containing compounds in water have inconsistent findings	Picetti et al. (2022)
	Personal hair dye use had no association with BC	Zhang et al. (2020) Turati et al. (2014)
	AO high level of exposure had a twofold increased risk of BC in Korean veterans	Yi and Ohrr (2014)
	AO exposure caused a slight increased risk of developing NMIBC in US veterans	Williams et al. (2023)
	Air pollution did not increase risk in European study	Pedersen et al. (2018)
	Residence proximity to oil refineries increased risk	Williams et al. (2020)
Dietary habits	Mediterranean diet is protective	Witlox et al. (2020) Dianatinasab et al. (2022a)
	Western diet is risk factor in males	Dianatinasab et al. (2020) Dianatinasab et al. (2022a)
	MUFAs are protective in females; higher cholesterol intake is a risk factor in males	Dianatinasab et al. (2022b)
	Red meat consumption is a risk factor; fish consumption is protective in males	Dianatinasab et al. (2021)
	Vegetable consumption is protective in females	Yu et al. (2021)
	Increased fiber and whole grain intake is protective	Yu et al. (2020)
	Conflicting evidence regarding B vitamins	Boot et al. (2022)
	Conflicting evidence regarding dairy products	Acham et al. (2020)
	Coffee consumption is a risk factor	Yu et al. (2019)
	Alcohol consumption is a risk factor	Lao et al. (2021)

BC bladder cancer, *NMIBC* non-muscle-invasive bladder cancer, *RC* radical cystectomy, *PAH* polycyclic aromatic hydrocarbons, *AO* Agent Orange, *MUFAs* monounsaturated fatty acids

Table 1.2 Non-modifiable risk factors and medical conditions/therapies and summary of their risks

Non-modifiable risk factors and medical conditions/therapies	Summary of risks	References
Sex	Males have fourfold incidence	Sung et al. (2021)
	Oncologic outcomes are worse in females even after controlling for treatment delay	Uhlig et al. (2018a) Uhlig et al. (2018b) Scosyrev et al. (2009) Wang et al. (2020), Radkiewicz et al. (2020)
	Sex-related discrepancy exists despite controlling for tobacco	Hartge et al. (1990) Hemelt et al. (2009)
	Androgens are linked to carcinogen metabolism and increased risk	Imaoka et al. (2001) Bertram and Craig (1972) Mäkelä et al. (2018) Zhang (2013) Izumi et al. (2013) Dobruch et al. (2016)
	Estrogen receptors are linked to increased BC aggressiveness	George et al. (2013) Kashiwagi et al. (2016)
	X chromosome is protective	Kaneko and Li (2018)
	Y chromosome is a risk factor	Fadl-Elmula et al. (2000)
Race and SES	Black race is associated with more advanced stage at diagnosis	Weiner et al. (2018)
	Black patients have worse overall survival	Gild et al. (2018)
	Black patients have increased expression of genes related to muscle invasion and drug resistance	You et al. (2022)
	Black patients have less lymph nodes removed during PLND, longer wait time to RC after NAC, and longer hospital stays and are less likely to undergo PLND	Gild et al. (2018) Williams et al. (2017)
	Low SES, no insurance, and Medicaid insurance are risk factors for more advanced disease at diagnosis and worse oncologic outcomes	Nazemi et al. (2019)
Diabetes mellitus (DM)	DM may increase risk in males and females	Xu et al. (2017) Fang et al. (2013)
	DM increases recurrence, progression, ACM, and CSM	Lu and Tao (2021)
	Conflicting evidence on metformin protective effect	van Hattum et al. (2022) Liu et al. (2022)
	Pioglitazone may increase risk and has FDA black box warning, although with some conflicting evidence	Tang et al. (2018) Mehtälä et al. (2019) Yan et al. (2018) Adil et al. (2018) Filipova et al. (2017) Pai and Kshirsagar (2016)
	Conflicting evidence regarding SGLT2 inhibitors increasing risk	Tang et al. (2017) Dicembrini et al. (2019)
Chronic bladder inflammation	Chronic UTI status increases risk	Akhtar et al. (2018)
	Chronic urinary catheters increase risk	Ho et al. (2015)
Radiation therapy (RT)	Adjuvant RT for gynecologic cancers more than doubled the risk of BC	Wen et al. (2022)
	RT for prostate cancer increased risk of BC by 1.6x	Zhao et al. (2019)
Cyclophosphamide (CYC)	CYC increases risk of BC by 4.5x in NHL patients	Travis et al. (1995)
	CYC-induced BC may be dose-dependent	Travis et al. (1995)
	CYC increases risk of MIBC and high-grade pathology	Chou et al. (2021)

(continued)

Table 1.2 (continued)

Non-modifiable risk factors and medical conditions/therapies	Summary of risks	References
Schistosomiasis	*Schistosoma haematobium* is associated with SCC	Efared et al. (2022)
	Significant presence in Africa	Efared et al. (2022)
Viruses	Polyomavirus is linked to BC in both immunocompetent and immunocompromised patients	Weinreb et al. (2006) Starrett et al. (2023)
	HPV increases risk of BC in Asia	Khatami et al. (2022)
Solid organ transplant	Renal transplant recipients have threefold increased risk	Wang et al. (2018)
	Higher risk among Asian vs. European recipients	Yan et al. (2014)

PLND pelvic lymph node dissection, *RC* radical cystectomy, *NAC* neoadjuvant chemotherapy, *SES* socioeconomic status, *ACM* all-cause mortality, *CSM* cancer-specific mortality, *UTI* urinary tract infection, *HPV* human papillomavirus

nations have witnessed reduced incidence rate, although with an increase in male BC mortality rates (Teoh et al. 2020).

1.2 Risk Factors

1.2.1 Tobacco

Tobacco usage continues to be a leading risk factor for BC. Over several decades, concentrated research has been conducted to identify the chemical compounds present in tobacco, with over 9500 different compounds identified in a 2013 study (Rodgman and Perfetti 2013). The carcinogens found in tobacco include compounds such as N-nitrosamines, polycyclic aromatic hydrocarbons (PAH), aromatic amines, ethers, and halogenated compounds (Li and Hecht 2022). These carcinogens, as well as reactive oxygen species, can cause DNA damage to urothelial cells via a multitude of pathways such as single- and double-strand DNA breaks, DNA bulky adducts, and base modifications (Stern et al. 2009).

Clinical evidence that tobacco is a principal risk factor for BC development is robust, with an estimated 50% of bladder cancers attributable to smoking (Burger et al. 2013). A recent meta-analysis of 89 observational studies spanning over 57,000 patients with BC showed that present smokers had over threefold increased odds of having BC versus never smokers (van Osch et al. 2016). Even former smokers were at a significantly increased risk with almost double the odds of developing BC relative to never smokers. In addition to smoking status, the quantity of tobacco smoked was shown to be directly associated with BC risk. A dose-response analysis showed a gradual increase in BC incidence with increasing pack-years, plateauing at 15 cigarettes per day and 50 pack-years (van Osch et al. 2016). Furthermore, a recent pooled analysis showed that for a fixed pack-years total, smoking for a longer time span at a lower intensity was more harmful than smoking at a higher intensity for a shorter duration; thus, the relationship of BC risk and tobacco smoking is complex and multifactorial (van Osch et al. 2019). Moreover, patients who started smoking at a younger age were at higher risk. Although smoking cessation can help reduce the risk of BC, data has shown that even after smoking cessation for 20 years, former smokers continue to have almost double the risk of BC versus never smokers (van Osch et al. 2016).

Not only is tobacco smoking a risk factor for the development of BC, but it is also a risk factor for recurrence and progression of NMIBC (Lammers et al. 2011; Rink et al. 2013; Ślusarczyk et al. 2022). A prospective study comparing the recurrence-free survival (RFS) of nonsmokers with present and ex-smokers showed that both present and ex-smokers had a significantly shorter RFS (Lammers et al. 2011). A recent meta-analysis of 28 studies with over 7800 patients with NMIBC provided robust evidence that present and former smokers had a significantly higher risk of cancer recurrence versus never smokers (OR = 1.68; 95% CI 1.34–2.09; $P < 0.0001$), with present smokers at higher risk than former smokers (OR = 1.24; 95% CI 1.02–1.50; $P = 0.03$) (Ślusarczyk et al. 2022). Smoking status was also shown to increase the risk of disease progression, and survival from NMIBC was significantly reduced in smokers (Rink et al. 2013).

Tobacco consumption also has detrimental effects in MIBC patients. A meta-analysis of 17 studies and over 13,000 patients showed that present smokers had significantly increased risk of overall mortality (HR 1.21, 95% CI 1.08–1.36), disease-specific mortality (HR 1.24, 95% CI 1.13–1.36), and disease recurrence (HR 1.24, 95% CI 1.12–1.38) (Cacciamani et al. 2020). Response to treatment is also impaired in MIBC due to smoking, as smoking status in patients with MIBC undergoing neoadjuvant chemotherapy (NAC) followed by radical cystectomy (RC) was a significant risk factor for incomplete response to NAC (Cacciamani et al. 2020). A multivariable analysis showed that former and present smokers had twofold and fourfold increased odds of having no response to cisplatin-based NAC, respectively, and present smoking status was shown to be an independent risk factor for recurrence (HR 2.14; $p = 0.03$) after RC (Boeri et al. 2019). Furthermore, smoking was also associated with a higher risk of developing metastatic disease and mortality from BC (Cumberbatch et al. 2016). Risk of postoperative complications is also increased in smokers. Patients with history of smoking undergoing RC were at significantly higher risk of wound dehiscence (OR = 1.8, $p < 0.001$) in a recent multivariable analysis of over 11,000 patients (Nasrallah et al. 2021).

1.2.2 Electronic Cigarettes

Recent investigations into the role of electronic cigarettes (e-cigarettes) have gained traction as the use of e-cigarettes has increased, though the long-term impact on health remains unclear. A systematic review showed that e-cigarette users had a significantly higher urine concentration of carcinogen biomarkers and metabolites, several of which have established links to BC (Bjurlin et al. 2021). A study comparing mice exposed to e-cigarettes versus air showed that e-cigarettes led to the development of bladder urothelial hyperplasia and hence a potential risk for BC (Tang et al. 2019). Further investigation with long-term follow-up of e-cigarette smokers is necessary to better quantify the risk of BC development, recurrence, progression, and survival; however, preliminary evidence suggests a similar pathologic relationship.

1.2.3 Occupational Exposures

The second most significant risk factor for BC is exposure to carcinogens during occupational tasks. Studies show increased risk with exposure to compounds such as aromatic amines (2-napthylamine, 4-aminobiphenyl, 4,4′-methylenebis[2-chloroaniline]), benzidine, polycyclic aromatic hydrocarbons (PAH), toluene, and perchloroethylene (Pesch et al. 2013; Porru et al. 2014). In 1981, it was estimated that occupational exposure contributed to the incidence of 10% of BC in the United States (Doll and Peto 1981). More recent data from Britain suggests that 5.3% of all BC incidence is attributable to occupational exposures (Rushton et al. 2010). One systematic review and meta-analysis of 263 studies showed that the highest BC occupational exposure risk was related to aromatic amines and PAH (Cumberbatch et al. 2015). Occupations most exposed to aromatic amines include tobacco, dye, rubber, and leather workers, as well as hairdressers and printers (Cumberbatch et al. 2015). Occupations with known high exposure to PAH included nurses, waiters, chimney sweeps, aluminum workers, and oil/petroleum workers (Cumberbatch et al. 2015). Other occupations with emerging links to BC include firefighters (Daniels et al. 2014) due to their exposure to PAH and other combustion products (Stec et al. 2018), as well as occupations with exposure to diesel combustion such as bus/truck drivers and engine mechanics (Koutros et al. 2020). The highest BC-specific mortality risk was associated with occupations with exposure to heavy metals or PAH (Cumberbatch et al. 2015).

Occupational carcinogens linked to BC have been classified by the International Agency for Research on Cancer (IARC), with compounds having sufficient evidence of carcinogenicity to humans being categorized as group 1 (Samet et al. 2020). The use of and exposure to these group 1 compounds has become better controlled; present occupational exposure is likely to be to lower-risk compounds with less evidence for carcinogenic properties.

1.2.4 Environmental Exposures

1.2.4.1 Drinking Water

Drinking water can be a medium for transmission of environmental carcinogens, and several compounds present in drinking water have links to BC. Arsenic is one such chemical. Population-level data from the United States showed that cumulative arsenic exposure was associated with a higher risk of BC (Baris et al. 2016; Huang et al. 2008). Private wells, particularly shallow wells, dug in areas where arsenic-containing pesticide use was widespread were noted to be a significant source of arsenic-containing drinking water (Baris et al. 2016).

Arsenic metabolites found in urine are significantly associated with BC risk, as shown in a systematic review and meta-analysis. Metabolites were categorized into monomethylated metabolites (MMA), demethylated metabolites (DMA), and inorganic arsenic (IA). Increased urine levels of IA and MMA were associated with increased risk of BC development, with a 50% increase in BC risk with extreme levels of MMA (Di Giovanni et al. 2020). This observation is supported by molecular studies demonstrating the genotoxic attributes of MMA, which caused DNA damage or degradation (Mass et al. 2001). Conversely, recent data in the form of a systematic review and meta-analysis examining the association of low-dose arsenic exposure (defined as concentrations no greater than 150 µg/L) in drinking water with risk of BC showed no increased risk (Boffetta and Borron 2019), suggesting a dose-response relationship between arsenic exposure and BC risk.

Chlorinated drinking water is another potential risk factor for BC development, particularly via chlorination byproducts such as chloroform and trihalomethanes (THMs) (Villanueva et al. 2003; Costet et al. 2011). A meta-analysis of eight observational studies conducted in North America and Europe showed that long-term consumption of chlorinated drinking water may be associated with an increased risk of BC (OR 1.4, 95% CI 1.2–1.7), with the association being more pronounced in males (Villanueva et al. 2003). A subsequent meta-analysis of European studies showed that the risk of BC significantly increased when the exposure level of THMs was above 25 µg/L and for periods >30 years (Costet et al. 2011). A recent European study estimated that the average population-weighted level of exposure to THMs in 28 European countries was 11.7 µg/L (Evlampidou et al. 2020), which is well below the 25 µg/L observed cutoff level (Costet et al. 2011) and hence lower than the level previously shown to increase BC risk.

Nitrogen-containing compounds present in drinking water due to the common use of nitrogen-containing fertilizers and pesticides have been studied as a potential risk factor for cancer development; however, the data is inconsistent. A systematic review and meta-analysis of 60 studies examining the potential association of nitrates and nitrites present in drinking water with cancer showed no overall increased risk specifically of BC (Picetti et al. 2022). Eight of these 60 studies measured the association of nitrates in drinking water with BC. Although the meta-analysis of two cohort studies demonstrated an increased risk of BC with a 10 mg/mL increase in water nitrate concentration (RR 1.31, 95% CI 1.03–1.66), the pooled analysis of all eight studies (four case-control, three cohort, and one cross-sectional) showed no association (Picetti et al. 2022).

1.2.4.2 Personal Hair Dye Use

Personal hair dye use was studied as a potential risk factor for BC development, likely due to the known increased risk of BC development in occupational exposure to hair dyes in the hairdresser profession (Cumberbatch et al. 2015). The IARC classified occupational exposure to hair dyes as a probable carcinogen (group 2A), whereas personal use carcinogenicity was unclassified (group 3) (Humans 2010). Thus, this exposure was studied in a large cohort of over 117,000 female nurses who reported personal use of permanent hair dyes, and the participants were followed for 36 years; no significant positive association linking personal permanent hair dye use and BC was found (Zhang et al. 2020). This result supported the previous null hypothesis made by a meta-analysis of 17 observational studies of over 600,000 persons. The association between personal hair dye use and risk of BC remains uncertain (Turati et al. 2014).

1.2.4.3 Agent Orange

Agent Orange (AO) was one of the herbicides utilized by the US military between 1961 and 1971 in the Vietnam War with the purpose of defoliating mangroves and forests (Stellman and Stellman 2018). AO contained a compound called 2,3,7,8-tetrachlorodibenzo-p-dioxin (TCDD), which is classified as a group 1 human carcinogen (Steenland et al. 1999). So far, only limited data exists showing an association between AO and BC risk or mortality (Committee to Review the Health Effects in Vietnam Veterans of Exposure to Herbicides 2016; Mossanen et al. 2017; Chang et al. 2017; Yi and Ohrr 2014; Yi et al. 2014; Matic et al. 2014; Kogevinas et al. 1997; Steenland et al. 1999).

Initial studies and data proposing an association between TCDD and BC incidence (Steenland et al. 1999; Yi and Ohrr 2014) and mortality (Breslin et al. 1988) were limited. However, a subsequent large population-based study in 2014 from South Korea analyzing over 177,000 Korean Vietnam veterans showed that veterans with high exposure to TCDD/AO were associated with a twofold increase in risk of BC (Yi et al. 2014). This doubling in risk is inconsistent with older studies, possibly due to BC exhibiting a long latency period between time of carcinogen exposure and cancer detection (Chang et al. 2017). More recently, a large matched cohort study of 2.5 million male US Veterans who served in Vietnam showed that AO exposure was significantly associated with an increased risk of BC (HR = 1.04, 95% CI 1.02–1.06) albeit with a modest hazard ratio. Interestingly, these patients were more likely to develop NMIBC versus MIBC (Williams et al. 2023). This area remains a high priority for research, and further high-quality studies are needed. In fact, the relationship of AO exposure with BC risk and mortality has been designated as an area requiring further research by the Institute of Medicine (Committee to Review the Health Effects in Vietnam Veterans of Exposure to Herbicides 2016). Due to this designation and the aforementioned data, the Veterans Affairs (VA) has categorized AO as a cause of BC (Committee to Review the Health Effects in Vietnam Veterans of Exposure to Herbicides 2016).

1.2.4.4 Air Pollution

Exposure to pollutants and carcinogens via ambient air can occur continuously, both outdoors and indoors. Several carcinogens may be transmitted via ambient air pollution, including compounds such as fossil fuel combustion products, PAHs, and metals (Humans 2016). Among air pollutants, diesel engine exhaust has been classified as a group 1 carcinogen by the IARC, while gasoline engine exhaust was classified as group 2B (Humans 2016). The potential association between ambient air pollution and risk of BC was evaluated in a meta-analysis of 15 European cohorts with over 300,000 participants exposed to varying levels of nitrogen oxides and particulate matter; no association between BC incidence and exposure to outdoor air pollution at places of residence was found (Pedersen et al. 2018). Although a large population was analyzed, this study did not account for lifetime air pollutant exposures. Oil refineries can be a significant source of air pollutants such as benzene and toluene. Hence, residence proximity to oil refineries and risk of BC was assessed in over six million

Texas residents. It was found that residence within 0–16 km of an oil refinery increased BC risk (RR 1.07, 95% CI 1.00–1.14), and living within 0–16 vs. 34–48 km from an oil refinery relatively increased the risk of BC (RR 1.30, 95% CI 1.02–1.65) (Williams et al. 2020).

1.2.5 Dietary Habits

Dietary habits are a well-studied risk factor for many cancers, but the data and findings for BC may be inconsistent and biased, with other risk factors such as sex, occupation, and environmental exposures acting as potential confounders. Investigations into the role of nutrition as a risk factor for BC were more limited prior to the establishment of the BC Epidemiology and Nutritional Determinants (BLEND) international study in 2016 (Goossens et al. 2016). Twenty-four observational studies including over 11,000 BC cases with over 675,000 controls from different nations and continents were pooled together, and individual data was collected, creating a large database with enhanced statistical power (Goossens et al. 2016).

Dietary patterns, rather than individual dietary components, have been studied as potential risk factors for BC, with scholars arguing that this approach may provide valuable information regarding BC carcinogenesis (Witlox et al. 2020). The Mediterranean diet was deemed to be a protective factor with respect to BC development, as data from a BLEND analysis of 13 studies showed an inverse relationship between a higher Mediterranean diet score and BC incidence (HR 0.85, 95% CI 0.77–0.93) (Witlox et al. 2020). On the contrary, BLEND data analyzing the association of a Western diet with BC demonstrated a strong link, albeit only for male patients (HR 1.72, 95% CI 1.51–1.96) (Dianatinasab et al. 2020). A systematic review and meta-analysis of 12 studies confirmed these findings, showing that a Mediterranean diet was overall protective against BC incidence (RR 0.93, 95% CI 0.88–0.97), while a Western diet was a significant risk factor for developing BC (RR 1.52, 95% CI 1.36–1.67) (Dianatinasab et al. 2022a).

Individual dietary components have also been studied. Monounsaturated fatty acids (MUFAs) were found to be protective and had an inverse relationship with risk of NMIBC in females (Dianatinasab et al. 2022b). On the other hand, higher cholesterol intake was associated with a significant increase in BC risk in males only (HR 1.37, 95% CI 1.16–1.61) (Dianatinasab et al. 2022b). Red meat consumption was also examined as a potential risk factor, and a high intake of red meat was linked to BC development (HR 1.18, 95% CI 1.03–1.36) (Dianatinasab et al. 2021). Fish intake was found to be a protective factor for BC in males only (HR 0.79, 95% CI 0.65–0.97) (Dianatinasab et al. 2021). Vegetable consumption, both total and non-starchy, was shown to decrease risk of BC incidence in females only (Yu et al. 2021).

Whole grains and dietary fibers have been linked to several health benefits and lower risks of systemic inflammation, and an increased intake of dietary fibers and whole grains was associated with a decreased risk of BC (Yu et al. 2020). Many food items contain the B group vitamin complex, some of which play a role in energy metabolism (Depeint et al. 2006), while others are involved in reducing oxidative stress and therefore have a protective effect on DNA stability (Zhang et al. 2013). However, vitamins B1 and B2 and those needed for energy metabolism were associated with a higher risk of BC in males (Boot et al. 2022). Conversely, a high intake of all B vitamins was associated with a reduced risk of BC in females (Boot et al. 2022). Dairy products, another staple food item, were also studied; no relationship with overall dairy intake was found, though moderate to high consumption of yogurt was linked to reduced BC risk (Acham et al. 2020). Coffee, another highly consumed item, was shown to increase risk of BC both absolutely and in a dose-response manner (Yu et al. 2019). Alcohol was investigated in a meta-analysis of nine cohort studies and 1.9 million individuals; liquor and spirits significantly increased BC risk, and a dose-response relationship between alcohol and BC risk was found to affect males (Lao et al. 2021).

1.2.6 Demographics

1.2.6.1 Sex

While the incidence of BC in males is fourfold that in females (Sung et al. 2021), oncologic outcomes are poorer in females (Uhlig et al. 2018b). This observation has been amply investigated, with studies suggesting that the discrepancies in incidence and oncologic outcomes are multifactorial. Temporally, the rate of BC diagnosis between 1998 and 2008 was 25% higher in males (Jemal et al. 2008). Many theories have been investigated to explain this discrepancy, with explanations including disparities in occupational exposures, roles of sex hormones, or sex discrepancies in diagnostic workup. However, it has been noted that females diagnosed with BC tend to present with more locally advanced malignancy (Scosyrev et al. 2009). Moreover, females have worse outcomes in terms of BC recurrence (Uhlig et al. 2018b; Kluth et al. 2013), disease progression, and mortality after treatment (Uhlig et al. 2018a; Wang et al. 2020; Radkiewicz et al. 2020) even after controlling for delay to treatment (Krimphove et al. 2021; Williams et al. 2017a).

Exposure to carcinogens such as tobacco was evaluated as a potential cause of BC incidence differences, and the sex-related risk persisted even in the absence of exposure to tobacco (Hartge et al. 1990). Meta-analysis showed that tobacco smoking may only partially explain the sex discrepancy (Hemelt et al. 2009). More research is required to provide higher level evidence with regard to carcinogen exposure and the sex-related risk of BC.

Recent investigations into the sex-related differences of BC risk have focused on the roles of hormones, sex chromosomes, and tumor genetics (Koti et al. 2020). At a hormonal level, carcinogen metabolism may hold sex-related differences and thus impact BC risk. N-hydroxylation of aromatic amines by cytochrome P450 enzymes is considered a key step in their mutagenic activation; one such enzyme, CYP4B1, is found at higher levels in male bladders in rats, and expression was related to androgen exposure (Imaoka et al. 2001). Prior evidence supported this notion, as castration of male mice led to a reduction of BC incidence (Bertram and Craig 1972). A cohort study of over 10,000 Finnish males diagnosed with BC showed that 5α-reductase inhibitor use in the treatment of benign prostatic hyperplasia was associated with a lower risk of BC-specific mortality (HR 0.84, 95% CI 0.73–0.97) (Mäkelä et al. 2018). Estrogen receptors (ER) may play a role in BC aggressiveness and carcinogen-induced tumorigenesis, as a mouse-model study showed a decreased incidence of MIBC with tamoxifen chemoprevention when exposed to N-butyl-N-(4-hydroxybutyl) nitrosamine (BBN) (George et al. 2013). Moreover, ERα and progesterone receptors (PR) have been associated with increased BC-specific mortality (Kashiwagi et al. 2016). Such enzymes are also present in the liver, and sex hormones may play a regulatory effect there, resulting in sex-related differences in urothelial exposure to carcinogens (Dobruch et al. 2016). The enzyme uridine 5′-diphosphoglucuronosyltransferase (UGT) is an example of a hepatic enzyme involved in aromatic amine metabolism, and its expression is regulated by androgen receptor signaling (Zhang 2013; Izumi et al. 2013). These studies and findings provide evidence for the role of sex hormones in influencing sex discrepancies in BC.

The role of sex chromosomes in BC has been shown to be potentially independent from that of sex hormones, as an innovative study showed that the X chromosome was protective against BC in mice exposed to BBN with over double the risk in XY vs. XX mice regardless of gonadal status (HR 2.549, 95% CI 1.55–4.28) (Kaneko and Li 2018). The effect of male sex hormones on BC (HR 4.714, 95% CI 2.77–8.28) was markedly increased when combined with male sex chromosomes (HR 12.390, 95% CI 5.54–31.36) (Kaneko and Li 2018); thus, sex hormones and chromosomes independently and synergistically influence the sex-related BC disparities. The X chromosome's BC tumor suppressor qualities were linked to the *Kdm6a* gene, which escapes X chromosome inactivation (XCI) and is expressed at higher levels in female mice. The conditional knockout of *Kdm6a* from female mouse urothelium exposed to BBN resulted in a significant rise in detected BC (100% vs. 50%) and overall mortality within 40 weeks (85.7% vs. 30.4%) (Kaneko and Li 2018). Conversely, the Y chromosome may hold oncogenic activity, as it is found to be frequently lost in BC samples (Fadl-Elmula et al. 2000).

1.2.6.2 Race and Socioeconomic Status

Race is a well-studied factor influencing oncologic outcomes of BC, specifically when comparing White and African-American patients (Scosyrev et al. 2009; Cole et al. 2019; Mahran et al. 2022; Weiner et al. 2018). Black race is associated with more advanced disease stage at diagnosis (HR 1.10, 95% CI 1.04–1.18) (Weiner et al. 2018). One potential factor influencing the association of race with BC risk is discrepancies in access to healthcare (Cole et al. 2019). Black patients were found to be more commonly treated at hospitals and by surgeons that see lower case volumes, thereby indicating a difference in treatment quality (Barocas et al. 2014). Clinical outcomes also differ between Black and White patients, where Black patients are less likely to receive pelvic lymph node dissection (PLND) (OR 0.70, 95% CI 0.55–0.91), have less lymph nodes removed even when PLND is performed, have a longer wait time to undergo radical cystectomy after neoadjuvant therapy, and have a longer hospital stay (Gild et al. 2018; Williams et al. 2017b). Oncologic outcomes show that Black patients have lower overall survival rates (HR 0.87, 95% CI 0.79–0.97) (Gild et al. 2018). Biologically, there is evidence showing that Black patients may have a higher rate of expression of genes which increase the risk of progression to muscle invasion, mitomycin C resistance, and BCG durability (You et al. 2022). Race is often investigated with SES, and both have been shown to be independent BC prognostic factors after adjusting for other patient characteristics (Sung et al. 2019). SES and medical insurance status or subtype tend to be linked, and evidence showed that patients with low SES, no insurance, or Medicaid insurance were at higher risk of being diagnosed with a more advanced tumor (Nazemi et al. 2019). Moreover, lower SES, no insurance, and Medicaid insurance were all associated with worse oncologic outcomes, even when adjusting for tumor stage (Nazemi et al. 2019).

1.2.7 Medical Comorbidities and Treatment-Related Effects

1.2.7.1 Diabetes Mellitus

Diabetes mellitus (DM) is a medical condition associated with countless consequences and complications. Several studies have investigated its role in BC, with varying results. One such study was a meta-analysis showing an increased risk of BC specifically in males with DM (RR 1.23, 95% CI 1.06–1.42) (Xu et al. 2017). Conversely, another meta-analysis found that diabetes increased the risk of BC in females only (RR 1.23, 95% CI 1.02–1.49) (Fang et al. 2013). Diabetic patients were also found to have higher risks of BC recurrence, disease progression, all-cause mortality, and cancer-specific mortality (Lu and Tao 2021).

DM medications have been investigated as potential protective or risk factors for BC incidence. Some studies suggest that metformin, one of the most common oral medications used for treatment of type II DM, has potential anticancer effects (Pollak 2012; Vancura et al. 2018). However, meta-analysis of 13 studies did not demonstrate an association between metformin use and reduced BC incidence or oncologic outcomes (van Hattum et al. 2022). A more recent meta-analysis found that BC incidence risk was almost halved with metformin use (OR 0.45, 95% CI 0.37–0.56) (Liu et al. 2022). Another common DM medication class are thiazolidinediones, such as pioglitazone. Several meta-analyses have shown a significantly increased risk of BC with usage of pioglitazone (Tang et al. 2018; Mehtälä et al. 2019; Yan et al. 2018; Adil et al. 2018), and a dose-response effect was also demonstrated (Yan et al. 2018; Adil et al. 2018). However, it should be noted that widely heterogeneous data was being used, thus resulting in biased estimations (Ripamonti et al. 2019). Inconsistency also existed as another meta-analysis did not find a statistically significantly increased risk of BC with pioglitazone use (Filipova et al. 2017). Ultimately, the US Food and Drug Administration added a black box warning for increased BC risk (Pai and Kshirsagar 2016). On the other hand, French regulators completely withdrew the drug from the market (Pai and Kshirsagar 2016). Following the pioglitazone investigations, sodium-glucose cotransporter 2 (SGLT2) inhibitors were also studied as a potential BC risk factor. A meta-analysis in 2017 showed almost a fourfold increased risk of BC with SGLT2 inhibitor usage (OR 3.87, 95% CI 1.48–10.08), particularly empagliflozin (OR 4.49, 95% CI 1.21–16.73) (Tang et al. 2017). Conversely, another meta-analysis in 2019 found no significant association between SGLT2 inhibitors and BC risk (Dicembrini et al. 2019).

1.2.7.2 Chronic Bladder Inflammation

Inflammation is a well-studied host response to insult, be it physical, chemical, or biological; its chronicity may contribute to tumorigenesis (Leibovici et al. 2005). Chronic bladder inflammation due to recurrent UTIs has been investigated as a potential risk factor, and a meta-analysis showed that chronic UTI status was an independent risk factor among case-control (OR 2.33, 95% CI 1.86–2.92) and cohort studies (RR 2.88, 95% CI 1.20–6.89) (Akhtar et al. 2018). Another cause of chronic bladder inflammation is chronic urinary catheter use, which has been shown to significantly increase the risk of BC (Ho et al. 2015).

1.2.7.3 Radiation Therapy

Radiation therapy (RT) is a mainstay of treatment of multiple pelvic malignancies, in neoadjuvant, adjuvant, and primary therapy roles. RT has been associated with several treatment morbidities, and one studied risk is that of secondary malignancies. Radiation therapy damages the genome of the targeted cells, thereby causing radiation-induced genetic alterations (Baskar et al. 2014). A study of over 120,000 patients with a gynecologic cancer diagnosis investigated the risk of secondary BC after radiation therapy (Wen et al. 2022). It was found that the risk of developing secondary BC was more than doubled in patients receiving adjuvant RT in both external beam radiotherapy (HR 2.81, 95% CI 2.34–3.43) and brachytherapy (HR 2.17, 95% CI 1.67–2.82) subgroups (Wen et al. 2022). A meta-analysis of over 600,000 prostate cancer patients in 15 studies also found that RT was significantly associated with an increased risk of secondary BC overall (HR 1.6, 95% CI 1.33–1.92) (Zhao et al. 2019).

1.2.7.4 Cyclophosphamide

Cyclophosphamide (CYC) is a chemotherapeutic and immunosuppressive agent used for a multitude of indications ranging from solid organ and hematologic malignancy to immunosuppression for solid organ and bone marrow transplant (Emadi et al. 2009). A systematic review in 2021 evaluating CYC-associated BC found 122 studies, of which 61% were case reports of individual patients (Chou et al. 2021). Urothelial carcinoma was the most common pathology (74%), followed by leiomyosarcoma (9%); almost half (48%) of the cases were MIBC at diagnosis, and the majority (58%) of cases were high grade (Chou et al. 2021). In a cohort study of non-Hodgkin lymphoma patients, BC risk was higher for patients who underwent CYC treatment (HR 4.5, 95% CI 1.5–13.6). This relationship was dose-dependent as patients had sixfold and 14.5-fold the risk when exposed to a cumulative dose of 20–49 g or >50 g of CYC, respectively (Travis et al. 1995).

1.2.7.5 Schistosomiasis

Schistosomiasis is a public health burden, particularly in developing countries, with a significant presence in Africa (Efared et al. 2022), and it is the most prevalent parasitic infection in humans. *Schistosoma haematobium* is the species commonly associated with urogenital schistosomiasis (Lai et al. 2015) and squamous cell carcinoma (SCC) of the bladder (Efared et al. 2022). However, the histopathologic presentation may be changing; a retrospective analysis of over 1900 patients in Egypt showed an increasing proportion of urothelial carcinoma and decreased presentations of SCC over time, likely due to improved *Schistosoma* control (Salem and Mahfouz 2012).

1.2.7.6 Viruses

Viral infections have been estimated to contribute to 15–20% of all cancers (McLaughlin-Drubin and Munger 2008). Polyomavirus (PV) presence detected by polymerase chain reaction (PCR) was significantly higher in the bladders of 32 patients with primary BC versus 20 controls (Fioriti et al. 2003). Another study evaluated 133 immunocompetent individuals with diagnosed PV infection, and 15.8% of patients were found to have BC (Weinreb et al. 2006). Among a cohort of 43 immunocompromised transplant recipients, 21% of BC patients harbored PV (Starrett et al. 2023).

A meta-analysis of 27 datasets and 2954 BC patients showed that the pooled HPV infection prevalence among BC patients was 14.3% (95% CI 8.9–22.2), with the high-risk subtypes having the highest prevalence (Khatami et al. 2022). However, no overall association between HPV infection and BC was found (OR 2.077, 95% CI 0.940–4.587) (Khatami et al. 2022). A geographical subgroup analysis did yield a significant association between HPV and BC in Asia (OR 6.289, 95% CI 2.167–18.250) (Khatami et al. 2022).

1.2.7.7 Solid Organ Transplant

Although the incidence rates of BC in transplant patients taking immunosuppressive drugs are quite low, there may be a significantly increased risk when compared to the general population (Buzzeo et al. 1997; Ehdaie et al. 2009). A meta-analysis of 11 prospective studies and over 79,000 renal transplant patients found a higher risk of developing numerous cancers, with over a threefold increase in risk of BC (SIR 3.52 95% CI 1.48–8.37) (Wang et al. 2018). Another meta-analysis also found a threefold risk increase, with stratification by ethnicity showing a much higher risk in Asian (SIR 14.74, 95% CI 3.66–59.35) than in European (SIR 2.00, 95% CI 1.51–2.65) transplant recipients (Yan et al. 2014). The presentation of BC following solid organ transplant seems to be variable, as one study investigated 2925 renal and 2761 liver transplant patients and identified 11 (0.2%) cases of BC incidence following transplantation, with presentations ranging from low-grade, stage T1 urothelial carcinoma to unresectable MIBC requiring urinary diversion and palliative RT (Tomaszewski et al. 2011).

References

Acham M, Wesselius A, van Osch FHM, Yu EY, van den Brandt PA, White E, Adami HO, Weiderpass E, Brinkman M, Giles GG, Milne RL, Zeegers MP (2020) Intake of milk and other dairy products and the risk of bladder cancer: a pooled analysis of 13 cohort studies. Eur J Clin Nutr 74(1):28–35. https://doi.org/10.1038/s41430-019-0453-6

Adil M, Khan RA, Ghosh P, Venkata SK, Kandhare AD, Sharma M (2018) Pioglitazone and risk of bladder cancer in type 2 diabetes mellitus patients: a systematic literature review and meta-analysis of observational studies using real-world data. Clin Epidemiol Glob Health 6(2):61–68. https://doi.org/10.1016/j.cegh.2017.08.002

Akhtar S, Al-Shammari A, Al-Abkal J (2018) Chronic urinary tract infection and bladder carcinoma risk: a meta-analysis of case-control and cohort studies. World J Urol 36(6):839–848. https://doi.org/10.1007/s00345-018-2206-x

Antoni S, Ferlay J, Soerjomataram I, Znaor A, Jemal A, Bray F (2017) Bladder cancer incidence and mortality: a global overview and recent trends. Eur Urol 71(1):96–108. https://doi.org/10.1016/j.eururo.2016.06.010

Baris D, Waddell R, Beane Freeman LE, Schwenn M, Colt JS, Ayotte JD, Ward MH, Nuckols J, Schned A, Jackson B, Clerkin C, Rothman N, Moore LE, Taylor A, Robinson G, Hosain GM, Armenti KR, McCoy R, Samanic C, Hoover RN, Fraumeni JF Jr, Johnson A, Karagas MR, Silverman DT (2016) Elevated bladder cancer in Northern New England: the role of drinking water and arsenic. J Natl Cancer Inst 108(9). https://doi.org/10.1093/jnci/djw099

Barocas DA, Alvarez J, Koyama T, Anderson CB, Gray DT, Fowke JH, You C, Chang SS, Cookson MS, Smith JA Jr, Penson DF (2014) Racial variation in the quality of surgical care for bladder cancer. Cancer 120(7):1018–1025. https://doi.org/10.1002/cncr.28520

Baskar R, Dai J, Wenlong N, Yeo R, Yeoh KW (2014) Biological response of cancer cells to radiation treatment. Front Mol Biosci 1:24. https://doi.org/10.3389/fmolb.2014.00024

Bertram JS, Craig AW (1972) Specific induction of bladder cancer in mice by butyl-(4-hydroxybutyl)-nitrosamine and the effects of hormonal modifications on the sex difference in response. Eur J Cancer (1965) 8(6):587–594. https://doi.org/10.1016/0014-2964(72)90137-5

Bjurlin MA, Matulewicz RS, Roberts TR, Dearing BA, Schatz D, Sherman S, Gordon T, Shahawy OE

(2021) Carcinogen biomarkers in the urine of electronic cigarette users and implications for the development of bladder cancer: a systematic review. Eur Urol Oncol 4(5):766–783. https://doi.org/10.1016/j.euo.2020.02.004
Boeri L, Soligo M, Frank I, Boorjian SA, Thompson RH, Tollefson M, Quevedo FJ, Cheville JC, Karnes RJ (2019) Cigarette smoking is associated with adverse pathological response and increased disease recurrence amongst patients with muscle-invasive bladder cancer treated with cisplatin-based neoadjuvant chemotherapy and radical cystectomy: a single-Centre experience. BJU Int 123(6):1011–1019. https://doi.org/10.1111/bju.14612
Boffetta P, Borron C (2019) Low-level exposure to arsenic in drinking water and risk of lung and bladder cancer: a systematic review and dose-response meta-analysis. Dose Response 17(3):1559325819863634. https://doi.org/10.1177/1559325819863634
Boot IWA, Wesselius A, Yu EYW, Brinkman M, van den Brandt P, Grant EJ, White E, Weiderpass E, Ferrari P, Schulze MB, Bueno-de-Mesquita B, Jose-Sanchez M, Gylling B, Zeegers MP (2022) Dietary B group vitamin intake and the bladder cancer risk: a pooled analysis of prospective cohort studies. Eur J Nutr 61(5):2397–2416. https://doi.org/10.1007/s00394-022-02805-2
Breslin P, Kang HK, Lee Y, Burt V, Shepard BM (1988) Proportionate mortality study of US Army and US marine corps veterans of the Vietnam war. J Occup Med 30(5):412–419. https://doi.org/10.1097/00043764-198805000-00007
Burger M, Catto JW, Dalbagni G, Grossman HB, Herr H, Karakiewicz P, Kassouf W, Kiemeney LA, La Vecchia C, Shariat S, Lotan Y (2013) Epidemiology and risk factors of urothelial bladder cancer. Eur Urol 63(2):234–241. https://doi.org/10.1016/j.eururo.2012.07.033
Buzzeo BD, Heisey DM, Messing EM (1997) Bladder cancer in renal transplant recipients. Urology 50(4):525–528. https://doi.org/10.1016/s0090-4295(97)00305-1
Cacciamani GE, Ghodoussipour S, Mari A, Gill KS, Desai M, Artibani W, Gill PS, Shariat SF, Gill IS, Djaladat H (2020) Association between smoking exposure, neoadjuvant chemotherapy response and survival outcomes following radical cystectomy: systematic review and meta-analysis. J Urol 204(4):649–660. https://doi.org/10.1097/ju.0000000000000813
Chang C, Benson M, Fam MM (2017) A review of Agent Orange and its associated oncologic risk of genitourinary cancers. Urol Oncol 35(11):633–639. https://doi.org/10.1016/j.urolonc.2017.08.029
Chou WH, McGregor B, Schmidt A, Carvalho FLF, Hirsch MS, Chang SL, Kibel A, Mossanen M (2021) Cyclophosphamide-associated bladder cancers and considerations for survivorship care: a systematic review. Urol Oncol 39(10):678–685. https://doi.org/10.1016/j.urolonc.2021.05.017
Cole AP, Fletcher SA, Berg S, Nabi J, Mahal BA, Sonpavde GP, Nguyen PL, Lipsitz SR, Sun M, Choueiri TK, Preston MA, Kibel AS, Trinh QD (2019) Impact of tumor, treatment, and access on outcomes in bladder cancer: can equal access overcome race-based differences in survival? Cancer 125(8):1319–1329. https://doi.org/10.1002/cncr.31926
Committee to Review the Health Effects in Vietnam Veterans of Exposure to H, Board on the Health of Select P, Institute of M, National Academies of Sciences E, Medicine (2016). In: Veterans and Agent Orange: Update 2014. National Academies Press (US) Copyright 2016 by the National Academy of Sciences. All rights reserved., Washington, DC. https://doi.org/10.17226/21845
Costet N, Villanueva CM, Jaakkola JJ, Kogevinas M, Cantor KP, King WD, Lynch CF, Nieuwenhuijsen MJ, Cordier S (2011) Water disinfection by-products and bladder cancer: is there a European specificity? A pooled and meta-analysis of European case-control studies. Occup Environ Med 68(5):379–385. https://doi.org/10.1136/oem.2010.062703
Cumberbatch MG, Cox A, Teare D, Catto JW (2015) Contemporary occupational carcinogen exposure and bladder cancer: a systematic review and meta-analysis. JAMA Oncol 1(9):1282–1290. https://doi.org/10.1001/jamaoncol.2015.3209
Cumberbatch MG, Rota M, Catto JW, La Vecchia C (2016) The role of tobacco smoke in bladder and kidney carcinogenesis: a comparison of exposures and meta-analysis of incidence and mortality risks. Eur Urol 70(3):458–466. https://doi.org/10.1016/j.eururo.2015.06.042
Cumberbatch MGK, Jubber I, Black PC, Esperto F, Figueroa JD, Kamat AM, Kiemeney L, Lotan Y, Pang K, Silverman DT, Znaor A, Catto JWF (2018) Epidemiology of bladder cancer: a systematic review and contemporary update of risk factors in 2018. Eur Urol 74(6):784–795. https://doi.org/10.1016/j.eururo.2018.09.001
Daniels RD, Kubale TL, Yiin JH, Dahm MM, Hales TR, Baris D, Zahm SH, Beaumont JJ, Waters KM, Pinkerton LE (2014) Mortality and cancer incidence in a pooled cohort of US firefighters from San Francisco, Chicago and Philadelphia (1950-2009). Occup Environ Med 71(6):388–397. https://doi.org/10.1136/oemed-2013-101662
Depeint F, Bruce WR, Shangari N, Mehta R, O'Brien PJ (2006) Mitochondrial function and toxicity: role of the B vitamin family on mitochondrial energy metabolism. Chem Biol Interact 163(1–2):94–112. https://doi.org/10.1016/j.cbi.2006.04.014
Di Giovanni P, Di Martino G, Scampoli P, Cedrone F, Meo F, Lucisano G, Romano F, Staniscia T (2020) Arsenic exposure and risk of urothelial cancer: systematic review and meta-analysis. Int J Environ Res Public Health 17(9). https://doi.org/10.3390/ijerph17093105
Dianatinasab M, Wesselius A, Salehi-Abargouei A, Yu EYW, Brinkman M, Fararouei M, van den Brandt P,

White E, Weiderpass E, Le Calvez-Kelm F, Gunter M, Huybrechts I, Liedberg F, Skeie G, Tjonneland A, Riboli E, Giles GG, Milne RL, Zeegers MP (2020) Adherence to a Western dietary pattern and risk of bladder cancer: a pooled analysis of 13 cohort studies of the bladder cancer epidemiology and nutritional determinants international study. Int J Cancer 147(12):3394–3403. https://doi.org/10.1002/ijc.33173

Dianatinasab M, Wesselius A, de Loeij T, Salehi-Abargouei A, Yu EYW, Fararouei M, Brinkman M, van den Brandt P, White E, Weiderpass E, Le Calvez-Kelm F, Gunter MJ, Huybrechts I, Liedberg F, Skeie G, Tjonneland A, Riboli E, Zeegers MP (2021) The association between meat and fish consumption and bladder cancer risk: a pooled analysis of 11 cohort studies. Eur J Epidemiol 36(8):781–792. https://doi.org/10.1007/s10654-021-00762-4

Dianatinasab M, Forozani E, Akbari A, Azmi N, Bastam D, Fararouei M, Wesselius A, Zeegres MP (2022a) Dietary patterns and risk of bladder cancer: a systematic review and meta-analysis. BMC Public Health 22(1):73. https://doi.org/10.1186/s12889-022-12516-2

Dianatinasab M, Wesselius A, Salehi-Abargouei A, Yu EYW, Fararouei M, Brinkman M, van den Brandt P, White E, Weiderpass E, Le Calvez-Kelm F, Gunter MJ, Huybrechts I, Zeegers MP (2022b) Dietary fats and their sources in association with the risk of bladder cancer: a pooled analysis of 11 prospective cohort studies. Int J Cancer 151(1):44–55. https://doi.org/10.1002/ijc.33970

Dicembrini I, Nreu B, Mannucci E, Monami M (2019) Sodium-glucose co-transporter-2 (SGLT-2) inhibitors and cancer: a meta-analysis of randomized controlled trials. Diabetes Obes Metab 21(8):1871–1877. https://doi.org/10.1111/dom.13745

Dobruch J, Daneshmand S, Fisch M, Lotan Y, Noon AP, Resnick MJ, Shariat SF, Zlotta AR, Boorjian SA (2016) Gender and bladder cancer: a collaborative review of etiology, biology, and outcomes. Eur Urol 69(2):300–310. https://doi.org/10.1016/j.eururo.2015.08.037

Doll R, Peto R (1981) The causes of cancer: quantitative estimates of avoidable risks of cancer in the United States today. J Natl Cancer Inst 66(6):1191–1308

Efared B, Bako ABA, Idrissa B, Alhousseini D, Boureima HS, Sodé HC, Nouhou H (2022) Urinary bladder Schistosoma haematobium-related squamous cell carcinoma: a report of two fatal cases and literature review. Trop Dis Travel Med Vaccines 8(1):3. https://doi.org/10.1186/s40794-022-00161-x

Ehdaie B, Stukenborg GJ, Theodorescu D (2009) Renal transplant recipients and patients with end stage renal disease present with more advanced bladder cancer. J Urol 182(4):1482–1487. https://doi.org/10.1016/j.juro.2009.06.043

Emadi A, Jones RJ, Brodsky RA (2009) Cyclophosphamide and cancer: golden anniversary. Nat Rev Clin Oncol 6(11):638–647. https://doi.org/10.1038/nrclinonc.2009.146

Evlampidou I, Font-Ribera L, Rojas-Rueda D, Gracia-Lavedan E, Costet N, Pearce N, Vineis P, Jaakkola JJK, Delloye F, Makris KC, Stephanou EG, Kargaki S, Kozisek F, Sigsgaard T, Hansen B, Schullehner J, Nahkur R, Galey C, Zwiener C, Vargha M, Righi E, Aggazzotti G, Kalnina G, Grazuleviciene R, Polanska K, Gubkova D, Bitenc K, Goslan EH, Kogevinas M, Villanueva CM (2020) Trihalomethanes in drinking water and bladder cancer burden in the European Union. Environ Health Perspect 128(1):17001. https://doi.org/10.1289/ehp4495

Fadl-Elmula I, Gorunova L, Mandahl N, Elfving P, Lundgren R, Mitelman F, Heim S (2000) Karyotypic characterization of urinary bladder transitional cell carcinomas. Genes Chromosomes Cancer 29(3):256–265

Fang H, Yao B, Yan Y, Xu H, Liu Y, Tang H, Zhou J, Cao L, Wang W, Zhang J, Zhao L, Chen X, Zhang F, Zhao Y (2013) Diabetes mellitus increases the risk of bladder cancer: an updated meta-analysis of observational studies. Diabetes Technol Ther 15(11):914–922. https://doi.org/10.1089/dia.2013.0131

Filipova E, Uzunova K, Kalinov K, Vekov T (2017) Pioglitazone and the risk of bladder cancer: a meta-analysis. Diabetes Ther 8(4):705–726. https://doi.org/10.1007/s13300-017-0273-4

Fioriti D, Pietropaolo V, Dal Forno S, Laurenti C, Chiarini F, Degener AM (2003) Urothelial bladder carcinoma and viral infections: different association with human polyomaviruses and papillomaviruses. Int J Immunopathol Pharmacol 16(3):283–288. https://doi.org/10.1177/039463200301600315

George SK, Tovar-Sepulveda V, Shen SS, Jian W, Zhang Y, Hilsenbeck SG, Lerner SP, Smith CL (2013) Chemoprevention of BBN-induced bladder carcinogenesis by the selective estrogen receptor modulator tamoxifen. Transl Oncol 6(3):244–255. https://doi.org/10.1593/tlo.13247

Gild P, Wankowicz SA, Sood A, von Landenberg N, Friedlander DF, Alanee S, Chun FKH, Fisch M, Menon M, Trinh QD, Bellmunt J, Abdollah F (2018) Racial disparity in quality of care and overall survival among black vs. white patients with muscle-invasive bladder cancer treated with radical cystectomy: a national cancer database analysis. Urol Oncol 36(10):469.e461–469.e411. https://doi.org/10.1016/j.urolonc.2018.07.012

Goossens ME, Isa F, Brinkman M, Mak D, Reulen R, Wesselius A, Benhamou S, Bosetti C, Bueno-de-Mesquita B, Carta A, Allam MF, Golka K, Grant EJ, Jiang X, Johnson KC, Karagas MR, Kellen E, La Vecchia C, Lu CM, Marshall J, Moysich K, Pohlabeln H, Porru S, Steineck G, Stern MC, Tang L, Taylor JA, van den Brandt P, Villeneuve PJ, Wakai K, Weiderpass E, White E, Wolk A, Zhang ZF, Buntinx F, Zeegers MP (2016) International pooled study on diet and bladder cancer: the bladder cancer, epidemiology and nutritional determinants (BLEND) study: design and baseline characteristics. Arch Public Health 74:30. https://doi.org/10.1186/s13690-016-0140-1

Hartge P, Harvey EB, Linehan WM, Silverman DT, Sullivan JW, Hoover RN, Fraumeni JF Jr (1990) Unexplained excess risk of bladder cancer in men. J Natl Cancer Inst 82(20):1636–1640. https://doi.org/10.1093/jnci/82.20.1636

Hemelt M, Yamamoto H, Cheng KK, Zeegers MP (2009) The effect of smoking on the male excess of bladder cancer: a meta-analysis and geographical analyses. Int J Cancer 124(2):412–419. https://doi.org/10.1002/ijc.23856

Ho CH, Sung KC, Lim SW, Liao CH, Liang FW, Wang JJ, Wu CC (2015) Chronic indwelling urinary catheter increase the risk of bladder cancer, even in patients without spinal cord injury. Medicine (Baltimore) 94(43):e1736. https://doi.org/10.1097/md.0000000000001736

Huang YK, Huang YL, Hsueh YM, Yang MH, Wu MM, Chen SY, Hsu LI, Chen CJ (2008) Arsenic exposure, urinary arsenic speciation, and the incidence of urothelial carcinoma: a twelve-year follow-up study. Cancer Causes Control 19(8):829–839. https://doi.org/10.1007/s10552-008-9146-5

IARC (2010) Some aromatic amines, organic dyes, and related exposures. IARC Monogr Eval Carcinog Risks Hum 99:1–658

IARC (2016) Outdoor air pollution. IARC Monogr Eval Carcinog Risks Hum 109:9–444

Imaoka S, Yoneda Y, Sugimoto T, Ikemoto S, Hiroi T, Yamamoto K, Nakatani T, Funae Y (2001) Androgen regulation of CYP4B1 responsible for mutagenic activation of bladder carcinogens in the rat bladder: detection of CYP4B1 mRNA by competitive reverse transcription-polymerase chain reaction. Cancer Lett 166(2):119–123. https://doi.org/10.1016/s0304-3835(00)00572-3

Izumi K, Zheng Y, Hsu JW, Chang C, Miyamoto H (2013) Androgen receptor signals regulate UDP-glucuronosyltransferases in the urinary bladder: a potential mechanism of androgen-induced bladder carcinogenesis. Mol Carcinog 52(2):94–102. https://doi.org/10.1002/mc.21833

Jemal A, Siegel R, Ward E, Hao Y, Xu J, Murray T, Thun MJ (2008) Cancer statistics, 2008. CA Cancer J Clin 58(2):71–96. https://doi.org/10.3322/ca.2007.0010

Kaneko S, Li X (2018) X chromosome protects against bladder cancer in females via a KDM6A-dependent epigenetic mechanism. Sci Adv 4(6):eaar5598. https://doi.org/10.1126/sciadv.aar5598

Kashiwagi E, Fujita K, Yamaguchi S, Fushimi H, Ide H, Inoue S, Mizushima T, Reis LO, Sharma R, Netto GJ, Nonomura N, Miyamoto H (2016) Expression of steroid hormone receptors and its prognostic significance in urothelial carcinoma of the upper urinary tract. Cancer Biol Ther 17(11):1188–1196. https://doi.org/10.1080/15384047.2016.1235667

Khatami A, Salavatiha Z, Razizadeh MH (2022) Bladder cancer and human papillomavirus association: a systematic review and meta-analysis. Infect Agent Cancer 17(1):3. https://doi.org/10.1186/s13027-022-00415-5

Kluth LA, Fajkovic H, Xylinas E, Crivelli JJ, Passoni N, Rouprêt M, Becker A, Comploj E, Pycha A, Holmang S, Gupta A, Lotan Y, Karakiewicz PI, Gontero P, Chun FK, Fisch M, Scherr DS, Shariat SF (2013) Female gender is associated with higher risk of disease recurrence in patients with primary T1 high-grade urothelial carcinoma of the bladder. World J Urol 31(5):1029–1036. https://doi.org/10.1007/s00345-012-0996-9

Kogevinas M, Becher H, Benn T, Bertazzi PA, Boffetta P, Bueno-de-Mesquita HB, Coggon D, Colin D, Flesch-Janys D, Fingerhut M, Green L, Kauppinen T, Littorin M, Lynge E, Mathews JD, Neuberger M, Pearce N, Saracci R (1997) Cancer mortality in workers exposed to phenoxy herbicides, chlorophenols, and dioxins. An expanded and updated international cohort study. Am J Epidemiol 145(12):1061–1075. https://doi.org/10.1093/oxfordjournals.aje.a009069

Koti M, Ingersoll MA, Gupta S, Lam CM, Li X, Kamat AM, Black PC, Siemens DR (2020) Sex differences in bladder cancer immunobiology and outcomes: a collaborative review with implications for treatment. Eur Urol Oncol 3(5):622–630. https://doi.org/10.1016/j.euo.2020.08.013

Koutros S, Kogevinas M, Friesen MC, Stewart PA, Baris D, Karagas MR, Schwenn M, Johnson A, Monawar Hosain GM, Serra C, Tardon A, Carrato A, Garcia-Closas R, Moore LE, Nickerson ML, Hewitt SM, Lenz P, Schned AR, Lloreta J, Allory Y, Zhang H, Chatterjee N, Garcia-Closas M, Rothman N, Malats N, Silverman DT (2020) Diesel exhaust and bladder cancer risk by pathologic stage and grade subtypes. Environ Int 135:105346. https://doi.org/10.1016/j.envint.2019.105346

Krimphove MJ, Szymaniak J, Marchese M, Tully KH, D'Andrea D, Mossanen M, Lipsitz SR, Kilbridge K, Kibel AS, Kluth LA, Shariat SF, Trinh QD (2021) Sex-specific differences in the quality of treatment of muscle-invasive bladder cancer do not explain the overall survival discrepancy. Eur Urol Focus 7(1):124–131. https://doi.org/10.1016/j.euf.2019.06.001

Lai YS, Biedermann P, Ekpo UF, Garba A, Mathieu E, Midzi N, Mwinzi P, N'Goran EK, Raso G, Assaré RK, Sacko M, Schur N, Talla I, Tchuenté LA, Touré S, Winkler MS, Utzinger J, Vounatsou P (2015) Spatial distribution of schistosomiasis and treatment needs in sub-Saharan Africa: a systematic review and geostatistical analysis. Lancet Infect Dis 15(8):927–940. https://doi.org/10.1016/s1473-3099(15)00066-3

Lammers RJ, Witjes WP, Hendricksen K, Caris CT, Janzing-Pastors MH, Witjes JA (2011) Smoking status is a risk factor for recurrence after transurethral resection of non-muscle-invasive bladder cancer. Eur Urol 60(4):713–720. https://doi.org/10.1016/j.eururo.2011.07.010

Lao Y, Li X, He L, Guan X, Li R, Wang Y, Li Y, Wang Y, Li X, Liu S, Dong Z (2021) Association between alcohol consumption and risk of bladder cancer: a dose-response meta-analysis of prospective cohort studies. Front Oncol 11:696676. https://doi.org/10.3389/fonc.2021.696676

Leibovici D, Grossman HB, Dinney CP, Millikan RE, Lerner S, Wang Y, Gu J, Dong Q, Wu X (2005) Polymorphisms in inflammation genes and bladder cancer: from initiation to recurrence, progression, and survival. J Clin Oncol 23(24):5746–5756. https://doi.org/10.1200/jco.2005.01.598

Li Y, Hecht SS (2022) Carcinogenic components of tobacco and tobacco smoke: a 2022 update. Food Chem Toxicol 165:113179. https://doi.org/10.1016/j.fct.2022.113179

Liu CQ, Sun JX, Xu JZ, Qian XY, Hong SY, Xu MY, An Y, Xia QD, Hu J, Wang SG (2022) Metformin use on incidence and oncologic outcomes of bladder cancer patients with T2DM: An updated meta-analysis. Front Pharmacol 13:865988. https://doi.org/10.3389/fphar.2022.865988

Lu Y, Tao J (2021) Diabetes mellitus and obesity as risk factors for bladder cancer prognosis: a systematic review and meta-analysis. Front Endocrinol (Lausanne) 12:699732. https://doi.org/10.3389/fendo.2021.699732

Mahran A, Miller A, Calaway A, Prunty M, Arenas-Gallo C, Isali I, Ginsburg KB, Ponsky L, Markt S, Schumacher F, Bukavina L (2022) The impact of race and sex on metastatic bladder cancer survival. Urology 165:98–105. https://doi.org/10.1016/j.urology.2021.08.049

Mäkelä VJ, Kotsar A, Tammela TLJ, Murtola TJ (2018) Bladder cancer survival of men receiving 5α-reductase inhibitors. J Urol 200(4):743–748. https://doi.org/10.1016/j.juro.2018.04.082

Mass MJ, Tennant A, Roop BC, Cullen WR, Styblo M, Thomas DJ, Kligerman AD (2001) Methylated trivalent arsenic species are genotoxic. Chem Res Toxicol 14(4):355–361. https://doi.org/10.1021/tx000251l

Matic MG, Coric VM, Savic-Radojevic AR, Bulat PV, Pljesa-Ercegovac MS, Dragicevic DP, Djukic TI, Simic TP, Pekmezovic TD (2014) Does occupational exposure to solvents and pesticides in association with glutathione S-transferase A1, M1, P1, and T1 polymorphisms increase the risk of bladder cancer? The Belgrade case-control study. PLoS One 9(6):e99448. https://doi.org/10.1371/journal.pone.0099448

McLaughlin-Drubin ME, Munger K (2008) Viruses associated with human cancer. Biochim Biophys Acta 1782(3):127–150. https://doi.org/10.1016/j.bbadis.2007.12.005

Mehtälä J, Khanfir H, Bennett D, Ye Y, Korhonen P, Hoti F (2019) Pioglitazone use and risk of bladder cancer: a systematic literature review and meta-analysis of observational studies. Diabetol Int 10(1):24–36. https://doi.org/10.1007/s13340-018-0360-4

Mossanen M, Kibel AS, Goldman RH (2017) Exploring exposure to agent Orange and increased mortality due to bladder cancer. Urol Oncol 35(11):627–632. https://doi.org/10.1016/j.urolonc.2017.07.030

Nasrallah AA, Mansour M, Abou Heidar NF, Ayoub C, Najdi JA, Tamim H, El Hajj A (2021) Risk factors for wound dehiscence following radical cystectomy: a prediction model. Ther Adv Urol 13:17562872211060570. https://doi.org/10.1177/17562872211060570

Nazemi A, Ghodoussipour S, Pearce S, Bhanvadia S, Daneshmand S (2019) Socioeconomic and insurance status are independent prognostic indicators of higher disease stage and worse prognosis in bladder cancer. Urol Oncol 37(10):784–790. https://doi.org/10.1016/j.urolonc.2019.04.021

Nielsen ME, Smith AB, Meyer AM, Kuo TM, Tyree S, Kim WY, Milowsky MI, Pruthi RS, Millikan RC (2014) Trends in stage-specific incidence rates for urothelial carcinoma of the bladder in the United States: 1988 to 2006. Cancer 120(1):86–95. https://doi.org/10.1002/cncr.28397

Pai SA, Kshirsagar NA (2016) Pioglitazone utilization, efficacy & safety in Indian type 2 diabetic patients: a systematic review & comparison with European medicines agency assessment report. Indian J Med Res 144(5):672–681. https://doi.org/10.4103/ijmr.IJMR_650_15

Pedersen M, Stafoggia M, Weinmayr G, Andersen ZJ, Galassi C, Sommar J, Forsberg B, Olsson D, Oftedal B, Krog NH, Aamodt G, Pyko A, Pershagen G, Korek M, De Faire U, Pedersen NL, Östenson CG, Fratiglioni L, Sørensen M, Eriksen KT, Tjønneland A, Peeters PH, Bueno-de-Mesquita B, Vermeulen R, Eeftens M, Plusquin M, Key TJ, Jaensch A, Nagel G, Concin H, Wang M, Tsai MY, Grioni S, Marcon A, Krogh V, Ricceri F, Sacerdote C, Ranzi A, Cesaroni G, Forastiere F, Tamayo I, Amiano P, Dorronsoro M, Stayner LT, Kogevinas M, Nieuwenhuijsen MJ, Sokhi R, de Hoogh K, Beelen R, Vineis P, Brunekreef B, Hoek G, Raaschou-Nielsen O (2018) Is there an association between ambient air pollution and bladder cancer incidence? Analysis of 15 European cohorts. Eur Urol Focus 4(1):113–120. https://doi.org/10.1016/j.euf.2016.11.008

Pesch B, Gawrych K, Rabstein S, Weiss T, Casjens S, Rihs HP, Ding H, Angerer J, Illig T, Klopp N, Bueno-de-Mesquita B, Ros MM, Kaaks R, Chang-Claude J, Roswall N, Tjønneland A, Overvad K, Clavel-Chapelon F, Boutron-Ruault MC, Dossus L, Boeing H, Weikert S, Trichopoulos D, Palli D, Sieri S, Tumino R, Panico S, Quirós JR, González C, Sánchez MJ, Dorronsoro M, Navarro C, Barricarte A, Ljungberg B, Johansson M, Ulmert D, Ehrnström R, Khaw KT, Wareham N, Key TJ, Ferrari P, Romieu I, Riboli E, Brüning T, Vineis P (2013) N-acetyltransferase 2 phenotype, occupation, and bladder cancer risk: results from the EPIC cohort. Cancer Epidemiol Biomarkers Prev 22(11):2055–2065. https://doi.org/10.1158/1055-9965.Epi-13-0119-t

Picetti R, Deeney M, Pastorino S, Miller MR, Shah A, Leon DA, Dangour AD, Green R (2022) Nitrate and nitrite contamination in drinking water and cancer risk: a systematic review with meta-analysis. Environ Res 210:112988. https://doi.org/10.1016/j.envres.2022.112988

Pollak MN (2012) Investigating metformin for cancer prevention and treatment: the end of the beginning. Cancer Discov 2(9):778–790. https://doi.org/10.1158/2159-8290.Cd-12-0263

Porru S, Pavanello S, Carta A, Arici C, Simeone C, Izzotti A, Mastrangelo G (2014) Complex relationships between occupation, environment, DNA adducts, genetic polymorphisms and bladder cancer in a case-control study using a structural equation modeling. PLoS One 9(4):e94566. https://doi.org/10.1371/journal.pone.0094566

Radkiewicz C, Edgren G, Johansson ALV, Jahnson S, Häggström C, Akre O, Lambe M, Dickman PW (2020) Sex differences in urothelial bladder cancer survival. Clin Genitourin Cancer 18(1):26–34.e26. https://doi.org/10.1016/j.clgc.2019.10.020

Rink M, Furberg H, Zabor EC, Xylinas E, Babjuk M, Pycha A, Lotan Y, Karakiewicz PI, Novara G, Robinson BD, Montorsi F, Chun FK, Scherr DS, Shariat SF (2013) Impact of smoking and smoking cessation on oncologic outcomes in primary non-muscle-invasive bladder cancer. Eur Urol 63(4):724–732. https://doi.org/10.1016/j.eururo.2012.08.025

Ripamonti E, Azoulay L, Abrahamowicz M, Platt RW, Suissa S (2019) A systematic review of observational studies of the association between pioglitazone use and bladder cancer. Diabet Med 36(1):22–35. https://doi.org/10.1111/dme.13854

Rodgman A, Perfetti TA (2013) The chemical components of tobacco and tobacco smoke. CRC Press

Rushton L, Bagga S, Bevan R, Brown TP, Cherrie JW, Holmes P, Fortunato L, Slack R, Van Tongeren M, Young C, Hutchings SJ (2010) Occupation and cancer in Britain. Br J Cancer 102(9):1428–1437. https://doi.org/10.1038/sj.bjc.6605637

Salem HK, Mahfouz S (2012) Changing patterns (age, incidence, and pathologic types) of schistosoma-associated bladder cancer in Egypt in the past decade. Urology 79(2):379–383. https://doi.org/10.1016/j.urology.2011.08.072

Samet JM, Chiu WA, Cogliano V, Jinot J, Kriebel D, Lunn RM, Beland FA, Bero L, Browne P, Fritschi L, Kanno J, Lachenmeier DW, Lan Q, Lasfargues G, Le Curieux F, Peters S, Shubat P, Sone H, White MC, Williamson J, Yakubovskaya M, Siemiatycki J, White PA, Guyton KZ, Schubauer-Berigan MK, Hall AL, Grosse Y, Bouvard V, Benbrahim-Tallaa L, El Ghissassi F, Lauby-Secretan B, Armstrong B, Saracci R, Zavadil J, Straif K, Wild CP (2020) The IARC monographs: updated procedures for modern and transparent evidence synthesis in cancer hazard identification. J Natl Cancer Inst 112(1):30–37. https://doi.org/10.1093/jnci/djz169

Scosyrev E, Noyes K, Feng C, Messing E (2009) Sex and racial differences in bladder cancer presentation and mortality in the US. Cancer 115(1):68–74. https://doi.org/10.1002/cncr.23986

Ślusarczyk A, Zapała P, Zapała Ł, Radziszewski P (2022) The impact of smoking on recurrence and progression of non-muscle invasive bladder cancer: a systematic review and meta-analysis. J Cancer Res Clin Oncol 149:2673. https://doi.org/10.1007/s00432-022-04464-6

Starrett GJ, Yu K, Golubeva Y, Lenz P, Piaskowski ML, Petersen D, Dean M, Israni A, Hernandez BY, Tucker TC, Cheng I, Gonsalves L, Morris CR, Hussain SK, Lynch CF, Harris RS, Prokunina-Olsson L, Meltzer PS, Buck CB, Engels EA (2023) Evidence for virus-mediated oncogenesis in bladder cancers arising in solid organ transplant recipients. elife 12. https://doi.org/10.7554/eLife.82690

Stec AA, Dickens KE, Salden M, Hewitt FE, Watts DP, Houldsworth PE, Martin FL (2018) Occupational exposure to polycyclic aromatic hydrocarbons and elevated cancer incidence in firefighters. Sci Rep 8(1):2476. https://doi.org/10.1038/s41598-018-20616-6

Steenland K, Piacitelli L, Deddens J, Fingerhut M, Chang LI (1999) Cancer, heart disease, and diabetes in workers exposed to 2,3,7,8-tetrachlorodibenzo-p-dioxin. J Natl Cancer Inst 91(9):779–786. https://doi.org/10.1093/jnci/91.9.779

Stellman JM, Stellman SD (2018) Agent orange during the Vietnam war: the lingering issue of its civilian and military health impact. Am J Public Health 108(6):726–728. https://doi.org/10.2105/ajph.2018.304426

Stern MC, Lin J, Figueroa JD, Kelsey KT, Kiltie AE, Yuan JM, Matullo G, Fletcher T, Benhamou S, Taylor JA, Placidi D, Zhang ZF, Steineck G, Rothman N, Kogevinas M, Silverman D, Malats N, Chanock S, Wu X, Karagas MR, Andrew AS, Nelson HH, Bishop DT, Sak SC, Choudhury A, Barrett JH, Elliot F, Corral R, Joshi AD, Gago-Dominguez M, Cortessis VK, Xiang YB, Gao YT, Vineis P, Sacerdote C, Guarrera S, Polidoro S, Allione A, Gurzau E, Koppova K, Kumar R, Rudnai P, Porru S, Carta A, Campagna M, Arici C, Park SS, Garcia-Closas M (2009) Polymorphisms in DNA repair genes, smoking, and bladder cancer risk: findings from the international consortium of bladder cancer. Cancer Res 69(17):6857–6864. https://doi.org/10.1158/0008-5472.Can-09-1091

Sung JM, Martin JW, Jefferson FA, Sidhom DA, Piranviseh K, Huang M, Nguyen N, Chang J, Ziogas A, Anton-Culver H, Youssef RF (2019) Racial and socioeconomic disparities in bladder cancer survival: analysis of the California cancer registry. Clin Genitourin Cancer 17(5):e995–e1002. https://doi.org/10.1016/j.clgc.2019.05.008

Sung H, Ferlay J, Siegel RL, Laversanne M, Soerjomataram I, Jemal A, Bray F (2021) Global cancer statistics 2020: GLOBOCAN estimates of incidence and mortality worldwide for 36 cancers in 185 countries. CA Cancer J Clin 71(3):209–249. https://doi.org/10.3322/caac.21660

Tang H, Dai Q, Shi W, Zhai S, Song Y, Han J (2017) SGLT2 inhibitors and risk of cancer in type 2 diabetes: a systematic review and meta-analysis of randomised controlled trials. Diabetologia 60(10):1862–1872. https://doi.org/10.1007/s00125-017-4370-8

Tang H, Shi W, Fu S, Wang T, Zhai S, Song Y, Han J (2018) Pioglitazone and bladder cancer risk: a systematic review and meta-analysis. Cancer Med 7(4):1070–1080. https://doi.org/10.1002/cam4.1354

Tang MS, Wu XR, Lee HW, Xia Y, Deng FM, Moreira AL, Chen LC, Huang WC, Lepor H (2019) Electronic-cigarette smoke induces lung adenocarcinoma and bladder urothelial hyperplasia in mice. Proc Natl Acad Sci USA 116(43):21727–21731. https://doi.org/10.1073/pnas.1911321116

Teoh JY, Huang J, Ko WY, Lok V, Choi P, Ng CF, Sengupta S, Mostafid H, Kamat AM, Black PC, Shariat S, Babjuk M, Wong MC (2020) Global trends of bladder cancer incidence and mortality, and their associations with tobacco use and gross domestic product per capita. Eur Urol 78(6):893–906. https://doi.org/10.1016/j.eururo.2020.09.006

Tomaszewski JJ, Larson JA, Smaldone MC, Hayn MH, Jackman SV (2011) Management of bladder cancer following solid organ transplantation. Adv Urol 2011:256985. https://doi.org/10.1155/2011/256985

Travis LB, Curtis RE, Glimelius B, Holowaty EJ, Van Leeuwen FE, Lynch CF, Hagenbeek A, Stovall M, Banks PM, Adami J et al (1995) Bladder and kidney cancer following cyclophosphamide therapy for non-Hodgkin's lymphoma. J Natl Cancer Inst 87(7):524–530. https://doi.org/10.1093/jnci/87.7.524

Turati F, Pelucchi C, Galeone C, Decarli A, La Vecchia C (2014) Personal hair dye use and bladder cancer: a meta-analysis. Ann Epidemiol 24(2):151–159. https://doi.org/10.1016/j.annepidem.2013.11.003

Uhlig A, Seif Amir Hosseini A, Simon J, Lotz J, Trojan L, Schmid M, Uhlig J (2018a) Gender specific differences in disease-free, cancer specific and overall survival after radical cystectomy for bladder cancer: a systematic review and meta-analysis. J Urol 200(1):48–60. https://doi.org/10.1016/j.juro.2017.11.150

Uhlig A, Strauss A, Seif Amir Hosseini A, Lotz J, Trojan L, Schmid M, Uhlig J (2018b) Gender-specific differences in recurrence of non-muscle-invasive bladder cancer: a systematic review and meta-analysis. Eur Urol Focus 4(6):924–936. https://doi.org/10.1016/j.euf.2017.08.007

van Hattum JW, de Ruiter BM, Oddens JR, de Reijke TM, Wilmink JW, Molenaar RJ (2022) The effect of metformin on bladder cancer incidence and outcomes: a systematic review and meta-analysis. Bladder Cancer 8:211–228. https://doi.org/10.3233/BLC-211653

van Osch FH, Jochems SH, van Schooten FJ, Bryan RT, Zeegers MP (2016) Quantified relations between exposure to tobacco smoking and bladder cancer risk: a meta-analysis of 89 observational studies. Int J Epidemiol 45(3):857–870. https://doi.org/10.1093/ije/dyw044

van Osch FHM, Vlaanderen J, Jochems SHJ, Bosetti C, Polesel J, Porru S, Carta A, Golka K, Jiang X, Stern MC, Zhong WD, Kellen E, Pohlabeln H, Tang L, Marshall J, Steineck G, Karagas MR, Johnson KC, Zhang ZF, Taylor JA, La Vecchia C, Bryan RT, van Schooten FJ, Wesselius A, Zeegers MP (2019) Modeling the complex exposure history of smoking in predicting bladder cancer: a pooled analysis of 15 case-control studies. Epidemiology 30(3):458–465. https://doi.org/10.1097/ede.0000000000000964

Vancura A, Bu P, Bhagwat M, Zeng J, Vancurova I (2018) Metformin as an anticancer agent. Trends Pharmacol Sci 39(10):867–878. https://doi.org/10.1016/j.tips.2018.07.006

Villanueva CM, Fernández F, Malats N, Grimalt JO, Kogevinas M (2003) Meta-analysis of studies on individual consumption of chlorinated drinking water and bladder cancer. J Epidemiol Community Health 57(3):166–173. https://doi.org/10.1136/jech.57.3.166

Wang Y, Lan GB, Peng FH, Xie XB (2018) Cancer risks in recipients of renal transplants: a meta-analysis of cohort studies. Oncotarget 9(20):15375–15385. https://doi.org/10.18632/oncotarget.23841

Wang PF, Song HF, Zhang Q, Yan CX (2020) Pan-cancer immunogenomic analyses reveal sex disparity in the efficacy of cancer immunotherapy. Eur J Cancer 126:136–138. https://doi.org/10.1016/j.ejca.2019.12.008

Weiner AB, Keeter MK, Manjunath A, Meeks JJ (2018) Discrepancies in staging, treatment, and delays to treatment may explain disparities in bladder cancer outcomes: An update from the National Cancer Data Base (2004-2013). Urol Oncol 36(5):237.e239–237.e217. https://doi.org/10.1016/j.urolonc.2017.12.015

Weinreb DB, Desman GT, Amolat-Apiado MJ, Burstein DE, Godbold JH Jr, Johnson EM (2006) Polyoma virus infection is a prominent risk factor for bladder carcinoma in immunocompetent individuals. Diagn Cytopathol 34(3):201–203. https://doi.org/10.1002/dc.20429

Wen L, Zhong G, Zhang Y, Zhong M (2022) Risk and prognosis of secondary bladder cancer after post-operative radiotherapy for gynecological cancer. Bosn J Basic Med Sci 22(3):471–480. https://doi.org/10.17305/bjbms.2021.6338

Williams SB, Huo J, Dafashy TJ, Ghaffary CK, Baillargeon JG, Morales EE, Kim SP, Kuo YF, Orihuela E, Tyler DS, Freedland SJ, Kamat AM (2017a) Survival differences among patients with bladder cancer according to sex: critical evaluation of radical cystectomy use and delay to treatment. Urol Oncol 35(10):602.e601–602.e609. https://doi.org/10.1016/j.urolonc.2017.05.022

Williams SB, Huo J, Kosarek CD, Chamie K, Rogers SO Jr, Williams MA, Giordano SH, Kim SP, Kamat AM (2017b) Population-based assessment of racial/ethnic differences in utilization of radical cystectomy for patients diagnosed with bladder cancer. Cancer Causes Control 28(7):755–766. https://doi.org/10.1007/s10552-017-0902-2

Williams SB, Shan Y, Jazzar U, Kerr PS, Okereke I, Klimberg VS, Tyler DS, Putluri N, Lopez DS, Prochaska JD, Elferink C, Baillargeon JG, Kuo YF, Mehta HB (2020) Proximity to oil refineries and risk of cancer: a population-based analysis. JNCI Cancer Spectr 4(6):pkaa088. https://doi.org/10.1093/jncics/pkaa088

Williams SB, Janes JL, Howard LE, Yang R, De Hoedt AM, Baillargeon JG, Kuo YF, Tyler DS, Terris MK, Freedland SJ (2023) Exposure to agent orange and risk of bladder cancer among US veterans. JAMA

Netw Open 6(6):e2320593. https://doi.org/10.1001/jamanetworkopen.2023.20593

Witlox WJA, van Osch FHM, Brinkman M, Jochems S, Goossens ME, Weiderpass E, White E, van den Brandt PA, Giles GG, Milne RL, Huybrechts I, Adami HO, Bueno-de-Mesquita B, Wesselius A, Zeegers MP (2020) An inverse association between the Mediterranean diet and bladder cancer risk: a pooled analysis of 13 cohort studies. Eur J Nutr 59(1):287–296. https://doi.org/10.1007/s00394-019-01907-8

Wong MCS, Fung FDH, Leung C, Cheung WWL, Goggins WB, Ng CF (2018) The global epidemiology of bladder cancer: a joinpoint regression analysis of its incidence and mortality trends and projection. Sci Rep 8(1):1129. https://doi.org/10.1038/s41598-018-19199-z

Xu Y, Huo R, Chen X, Yu X (2017) Diabetes mellitus and the risk of bladder cancer: a PRISMA-compliant meta-analysis of cohort studies. Medicine (Baltimore) 96(46):e8588. https://doi.org/10.1097/md.0000000000008588

Yan L, Chen P, Chen EZ, Gu A, Jiang ZY (2014) Risk of bladder cancer in renal transplant recipients: a meta-analysis. Br J Cancer 110(7):1871–1877. https://doi.org/10.1038/bjc.2014.44

Yan H, Xie H, Ying Y, Li J, Wang X, Xu X, Zheng X (2018) Pioglitazone use in patients with diabetes and risk of bladder cancer: a systematic review and meta-analysis. Cancer Manag Res 10:1627–1638. https://doi.org/10.2147/cmar.S164840

Yi SW, Ohrr H (2014) Agent Orange exposure and cancer incidence in Korean Vietnam veterans: a prospective cohort study. Cancer 120(23):3699–3706. https://doi.org/10.1002/cncr.28961

Yi SW, Ryu SY, Ohrr H, Hong JS (2014) Agent Orange exposure and risk of death in Korean Vietnam veterans: Korean Veterans Health Study. Int J Epidemiol 43(6):1825–1834. https://doi.org/10.1093/ije/dyu183

You S, Kim M, Widen S, Yu A, Galvan GC, Choi-Kuaea Y, Eyzaguirre EJ, Dyrskjøt L, McConkey DJ, Choi W, Theodorescu D, Chan KS, Shan Y, Tyler DS, De Hoedt AM, Freedland SJ, Williams SB (2022) Characterizing molecular subtypes of high-risk non-muscle-invasive bladder cancer in African American patients. Urol Oncol 40(9):410.e419–410.e427. https://doi.org/10.1016/j.urolonc.2022.04.013

Yu EY, Wesselius A, van Osch F, Stern MC, Jiang X, Kellen E, Lu CM, Pohlabeln H, Steineck G, Marshall J, Allam MF, La Vecchia C, Johnson KC, Benhamou S, Zhang ZF, Bosetti C, Taylor JA, Zeegers MP (2019) The association between coffee consumption and bladder cancer in the bladder cancer epidemiology and nutritional determinants (BLEND) international pooled study. Cancer Causes Control 30(8):859–870. https://doi.org/10.1007/s10552-019-01191-1

Yu EYW, Wesselius A, Mehrkanoon S, Brinkman M, van den Brandt P, White E, Weiderpass E, Le Calvez-Kelm F, Gunter M, Huybrechts I, Liedberg F, Skeie G, Tjonneland A, Riboli E, Giles GG, Milne RL, Zeegers MP (2020) Grain and dietary fiber intake and bladder cancer risk: a pooled analysis of prospective cohort studies. Am J Clin Nutr 112(5):1252–1266. https://doi.org/10.1093/ajcn/nqaa215

Yu EY, Wesselius A, Mehrkanoon S, Goosens M, Brinkman M, van den Brandt P, Grant EJ, White E, Weiderpass E, Le Calvez-Kelm F, Gunter MJ, Huybrechts I, Riboli E, Tjonneland A, Masala G, Giles GG, Milne RL, Zeegers MP (2021) Vegetable intake and the risk of bladder cancer in the BLadder Cancer Epidemiology and Nutritional Determinants (BLEND) international study. BMC Med 19(1):56. https://doi.org/10.1186/s12916-021-01931-8

Zhang Y (2013) Understanding the gender disparity in bladder cancer risk: the impact of sex hormones and liver on bladder susceptibility to carcinogens. J Environ Sci Health C Environ Carcinog Ecotoxicol Rev 31(4):287–304. https://doi.org/10.1080/10590501.2013.844755

Zhang XH, Ma J, Smith-Warner SA, Lee JE, Giovannucci E (2013) Vitamin B6 and colorectal cancer: current evidence and future directions. World J Gastroenterol 19(7):1005–1010. https://doi.org/10.3748/wjg.v19.i7.1005

Zhang Y, Birmann BM, Han J, Giovannucci EL, Speizer FE, Stampfer MJ, Rosner BA, Schernhammer ES (2020) Personal use of permanent hair dyes and cancer risk and mortality in US women: prospective cohort study. BMJ 370:m2942. https://doi.org/10.1136/bmj.m2942

Zhao S, Xie Q, Yang R, Wang J, Zhang C, Luo L, Zhu Z, Liu Y, Li E, Zhao Z (2019) High prevalence of secondary bladder cancer in men on radiotherapy for prostate cancer: evidence from a meta-analysis. Cancer Manag Res 11:587–598. https://doi.org/10.2147/cmar.S185867

Genetic Predisposition to Bladder Cancer

2

Lambertus A. Kiemeney, Nathaniel Rothman, Stella Koutros, Ludmila Prokunina-Olsson, Gerald Verhaegh, and Sita H. Vermeulen

Abstract

Cancer may be caused by a combination of factors, including random mutations introduced during cell division, mutations caused by extrinsic lifestyle or environmental exposures (see Chap. 1), or intrinsic characteristics that speed up or slow down the mutational processes. One of the most important intrinsic characteristics is aging, which causes (1) decreased efficiency of DNA repair mechanisms, (2) accumulation of DNA errors in cells, (3) conversion of protective mechanisms in early life (such as senescence) into risk factors later in life (i.e., antagonistic pleiotropy), and (4) immune senescence. The other important characteristic is germline DNA variation which can prevent or support the initiation and promotion of somatic mutagenesis through variation in several pathways such as DNA repair, immune response, detoxification of carcinogens, or susceptibility to risk factors such as smoking, alcohol, or obesity.

It is estimated that 5–10% of all cancers are caused by a strong genetic predisposition in which high-penetrance rare alleles in a single or few genes affect susceptibility. Usually, such a strong predisposition can be suspected based on the familial clustering of cancers. Clinical geneticists frequently consult families on the risk of breast, ovarian, colorectal, and many other cancers. This is not the case for bladder cancer (BC), for which familial clustering due to high-penetrance germline mutations is extremely rare. However, lower-penetrance germline DNA variations play an important role. Many such variants have been discovered through genome-wide association studies (GWAS) using high-resolution genome-wide DNA variation chips and imputation. This has also been augmented by targeted sequencing of panels of higher-penetrance candidate genes (see Fig. 2.2). Meta-analyses of multiple GWAS and targeted studies help to refine the map of low-penetrance DNA variation. Ongoing efforts aim to identify genetic variation that influences BC prognosis directly or

L. A. Kiemeney
IQ Health Science Department, Radboud University Medical Center, Nijmegen, The Netherlands

Department of Urology, Radboud University Medical Center, Nijmegen, The Netherlands

N. Rothman · S. Koutros · L. Prokunina-Olsson
Division of Cancer Epidemiology and Genetics, National Cancer Institute, National Institutes of Health, Bethesda, MD, USA

G. Verhaegh
Department of Urology, Radboud University Medical Center, Nijmegen, The Netherlands

S. H. Vermeulen (✉)
IQ Health Science Department, Radboud University Medical Center, Nijmegen, The Netherlands
e-mail: sita.vermeulen@radboudumc.nl

M. A. Knowles, L. Dyrskjøt (eds.), *Biology of Bladder Cancer*,
https://doi.org/10.1007/978-3-031-68505-7_2

through modification of treatment effects. This chapter will summarize the evidence on the genetic predisposition of BC and BC prognosis, from early case reports to recent sequencing studies.

Keywords

Genetic susceptibility · Germline DNA · Gene · Sequencing · Genome-wide association study (GWAS) · Risk factors

2.1 Familial Clustering

2.1.1 Case Reports of High-Risk Families

The first anecdotal indication of an inherited form of BC came from a German paper in 1957 in which identical male twins were described with "urothelial papillomas" (Thelen and Schaeuble 1957). Ten years later, Fraumeni and Thomas reported a father and three of his five sons being affected by BC, with relatively young ages at diagnosis between 54 and 64 (Fraumeni and Thomas 1967). One of the sons had squamous cell carcinoma of the bladder. In a later report on this striking family, one of two sisters was also reported to have BC at the age of 70. Two of the brothers with BC were later diagnosed with lung cancer. A paternal niece also had a combination of bladder (age 66) and lung cancer (Mueller et al. 2008).

The family with the strongest clustering of BC was reported by McCullough et al. in 1975 (Fig. 2.1). Six relatives were affected in this two-generation family of Western-European descent. Four affected relatives were diagnosed before the age of 50, two of them even before age 40. The tumors were partly low-grade non-muscle-invasive bladder cancers (NMIBC), partly metastatic cancers. Two of the patients also developed upper urinary tract (UUT) tumors. Other cancers diagnosed in the same family were prostate, stomach, breast, cervix, ovarian, brain, and skin cancers, plus leukemia and metastasis to the lung of unknown origin (McCullough et al. 1975). Multiple other case reports have been published since then (Aben et al. 2001; Benton and Henderson 1973; Brown et al. 2014; Egilsson et al. 1993; Ilic et al. 2011; Kenet et al. 1995; Kiemeney et al. 2006; Leklem and Brown 1976; Lynch et al. 1979; Mahboubi et al. 1981; Marchetto et al. 1983; Mueller et al. 2008; Purtilo et al. 1979; Schoenberg et al. 1996; Sharma et al. 1976). In the case report by Schoenberg et al., a 29-year-old man with BC and renal pelvis cancer had a mother who died at the age of 65 from metastatic BC. The father died at the age of 68 from prostate cancer and a brother from melanoma at the age of 27. Triggered by a history of mul-

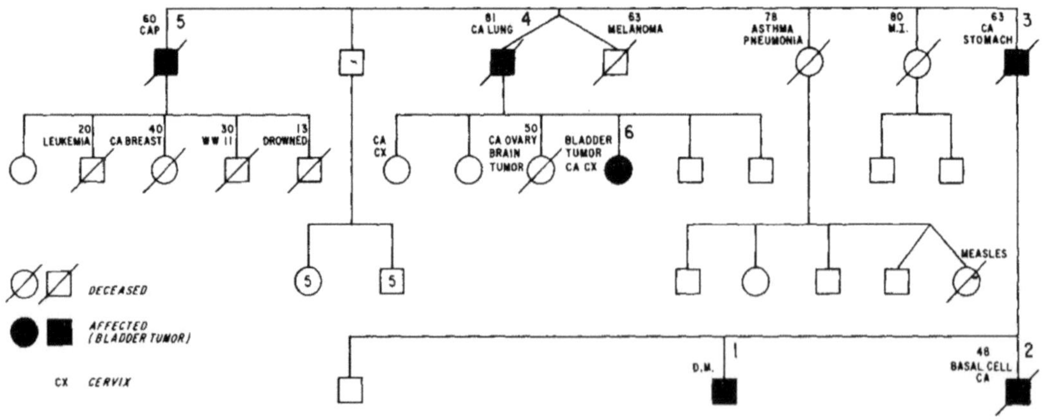

Fig. 2.1 The most striking pedigree reported in the literature with six BC patients in two generations. Source: (McCullough et al. 1975)

tiple miscarriages by his wife, this 29-year-old BC patient was karyotyped. A balanced germline translocation 46,XY,t(5;20)(p15;q11) was found. Analyses of the breakpoints revealed *CDC91L1* at 20q11 as the only gene whose expression was affected by the translocation (Schoenberg et al. 1996). It is still unclear, however, whether this gene plays a role in the development of BC and, if so, how (Guo et al. 2004; Schultz et al. 2005; Shen et al. 2008).

Except for the few families mentioned in more detail above, in all of the other families, the clustering was limited to two or three cases among the first-degree relatives. A striking clustering with other cancers, such as in Lynch syndrome families, was not observed in these case reports. A more systematic and larger-scale study on such clustering was performed in the Utah Population Database (Hanson et al. 2020). Kidney and prostate cancers were most commonly enriched in more than 1000 families with a significantly higher BC rate than in population controls (i.e., "familial" BC). Laryngeal, lung, stomach, acute lymphocytic leukemia, Hodgkin disease, soft tissue carcinoma, esophageal, breast, lung, uterine, thyroid, and melanoma cancers were the other cancer types with increased incidence in these BC families.

Especially in the earlier case reports, most affected individuals smoked, and many had occupations with exposures to bladder carcinogens. Although the observed familial clustering could be purely by chance, several case reports, especially on patients with very early ages at the onset of BC, suggest the existence of a genetic component in BC susceptibility.

2.1.2 Familial Risk Quantified by Epidemiological Studies

Many epidemiological studies evaluated family history as a potential risk factor for BC (reviewed in Mueller et al. 2008). Most of these studies had a case-control design in which patients with BC, as well as some types of controls, were simply asked about the occurrence of BC in first-degree and sometimes second-degree relatives. The disadvantage of this approach is that (usually) the family composition (size, ages, types of relatives), as well as environmental risk factors shared among family members, is not taken into account. Generally, only risk factors among the cases and controls are controlled for when estimating the effect of family history. Also, there may be some misclassification of family history, especially in second-degree relatives, because patients and controls are frequently not aware of the exact medical history of their relatives (Flint et al. 2021). Overall, the estimated risk of BC is increased approximately twofold with a first-degree relative with BC (Mueller et al. 2008). Other, more optimal studies used a cohort design in which the relatives of BC patients were identified, either by questioning the participants or by using genealogy registers, and subsequently the occurrence of BC in this cohort of relatives was examined, e.g., by linking the cohort of relatives to a population-based cancer registry. This occurrence is compared with the occurrence in the general population or in a cohort of relatives of controls (see Table 2.1). Overall, the relative risks for relatives of BC patients seem similar but a little bit weaker than those estimated from case-control studies, without a clear pattern between family degrees and ages at diagnosis of the probands. The studies from the Swedish Family-Cancer Database do report a higher risk among siblings than among offspring of cancer patients (Bermejo et al. 2009; Dong and Hemminki 2001; Plna and Hemminki 2001).

2.1.3 Heritability

Even though some of the case-control and familial cohort studies tried to adjust the familial risk estimates for nongenetic factors, it is difficult to assess the cause of the familial clustering, which may be due to shared germline genetic as well as shared environmental factors. Other study designs are more suited to differentiate these two. In a study from the Nordic countries, Lichtenstein and colleagues reported an almost four times higher relative risk of BC among monozygotic twins, who share 100% of their genes (RR = 6.6;

95% CI: 2.6–16.9) than among dizygotic twins, who share only 50% (RR = 1.7; 95% CI: 0.4–6.9) (Lichtenstein et al. 2000). If the correlation of environmental factors is similarly strong among monozygotic and dizygotic twin pairs, this finding suggests that the clustering among twins is at least partly genetic. According to the study, 31% (95% CI: 0–45%) of the variance in the occurrence of BC among twins can be explained by heritable factors, although this should be interpreted with caution considering the arbitrary finding that 0% was caused by shared environmental causes. In a later paper by the same group, now also including Norway, 18 concordant and 471 discordant monozygotic twins (RR = 9.9; 95% CI: 6.2–15.5) and 13 concordant and 870 discordant dizygotic twins (RR = 5.5; 95% CI: 3.1–9.7) were reported (Mucci et al. 2016). The proportion of variance explained by heritable factors was now 30%, still with 0% explained by shared environment.

The studies that used the Swedish Family-Cancer Database (Bermejo et al. 2009; Dong and Hemminki 2001; Plna and Hemminki 2001) reported higher risks for siblings than for offspring of BC patients and considered this as a suggestion for a recessive or X-linked transmission model. However, ascertainment bias due to cohort effects, such as diagnostic procedures and data quality, may also result in higher risks for siblings. The same holds for a higher correlation in environmental exposures between siblings compared with parents and offspring (Kiemeney 2008). In a later study by the same group, a more formal attempt was made to dissect genetic from nongenetic causes of familial clustering (Czene et al. 2002). Structural equation modeling was used, in which correlations between different pairs of relatives for shared environmental, childhood environmental, non-shared environmental, and genetic effects were set to fixed values according to their degree of genetic and environmental relationship. It was estimated that 7% of the occurrence of BC is due to genetic effects, 12% to shared environmental effects, 4% to childhood environmental effects, and 77% to non-shared environmental effects (Czene et al. 2002). Note that both estimation and interpretation of heritability estimates are not straightforward. They are study-specific, and interactions among genes and environmental factors are difficult to account for (Lu and Bourrat 2022).

In summary, the abovementioned studies indicate moderate effects of germline DNA variation on BC susceptibility. The limited familial clustering and abundance of sporadic (i.e., nonfamilial) BC patients suggest a limited role for rare, high-penetrance alleles and a more complex genetic etiology with the contribution of multiple rare to common alleles with low to moderate penetrance. This is supported by a Dutch cohort study by Aben et al. (see Table 2.1). Here, the segregation pattern of BC within 1193 families of probands with urothelial cancer (UC) was evaluated. There was no strong evidence for a Mendelian inheritance pattern through a single major gene. The sporadic model seemed to be the most parsimonious one, although none of the Mendelian models could be rejected. In other words, a major gene may segregate in some families, but this effect might be masked in a background of high sporadic incidence. A drawback of this study is that the families consisted of first-degree relatives only, which results in low power for segregation analyses (Aben et al. 2006).

2.2 Bladder Cancer Predisposition Genes and Pathways

2.2.1 Bladder Cancer in Known Cancer Syndromes

Many studies suggest that the risk of BC is increased in specific cancer syndromes that are caused by high-penetrance germline mutations in the *RB1*, *HRAS*, or mismatch repair (MMR) genes.

2.2.1.1 Retinoblastoma *(RB1)*

Retinoblastomas are rare intraocular malignancies that are predominantly present in children. They can occur unilaterally or bilaterally. In 1971, Alfred Knudson hypothesized that retino-

Table 2.1 Cohort studies on family history of bladder cancer

Source	Population	Comparison	Adjustments	Results	Comments
(Lynch et al. 1987), United States	First- and second-degree relatives of 49 BC patients	The cumulative risk in the Third National Cancer Survey	Age, sex, smoking	RR = 1.63	Of all living first- and second-degree relatives, only 4.8% and 9.8%, respectively, returned a questionnaire 61.5% of cancers among relatives could be verified
(Kramer et al. 1991), United States	1619 first-degree relatives of 319 male BC patients	1773 first-degree relatives of 319 controls	Sex, smoking	O/E = 1.9 (95% CI: 1.1–2.7)	Cancer occurrence was obtained by linkage to the New York State Tumor Registry. No significant difference between smoking and nonsmoking relatives.
(Goldgar et al. 1994), United States	First-degree relatives of 1452 BC patients	The cumulative risk in the Utah Population Database	Age, sex	RR = 1.53 (95% CI: 0.98–2.20)	Based on 48 BC patients among relatives RR = 5.07 (95% CI: 0.97–12.5) among relatives of BC patients <60 years of age at dx
(Kiemeney et al. 1997), Iceland	1238 first- to third-degree relatives of 190 patients with BC and ureter or renal pelvis cancer	Population-based rates according to the Icelandic Cancer Registry	Age, sex	O/E = 1.24 (95% CI: 0.90–1.67)	First degree: O/E = 0.96 Second degree: O/E = 1.38 Third degree: O/E = 1.27
(Plna and Hemminki 2001), Sweden	Offspring of approx. 27,000 BC patients	General population BC rates according to the Swedish Cancer Registry	Age, sex	O/E = 1.59 (95% CI: 1.23–2.00)	O/E in sons = 1.35 O/E in daughters = 2.27 O/E in siblings = 2.96
(Dong and Hemminki 2001), Sweden	5,520,756 offspring and their parents from 2,112,616 nuclear families	Risk of cancer among offspring with and without a parent or sibling with BC	Age, sex	SIR = 1.53 (95% CI: 1.16–1.99) for offspring with a parent with BC SIR = 3.30 (95% CI: 1.70–5.78) for offspring with a sibling with BC	The higher risk among siblings than among offspring is considered a suggestion for an X-linked or recessive etiology

(continued)

Table 2.1 (continued)

Source	Population	Comparison	Adjustments	Results	Comments
(Aben et al. 2002), the Netherlands	First-degree relatives (excluding offspring) of 1193 patients with UC of the bladder, ureter, renal pelvis, or urethra	First-degree relatives (excluding offspring) of 853 partners of the patients	Age, sex, and smoking	HR = 1.8 (95% CI: 1.3–2.7)	No difference in risk among relatives of bladder and UUT cancer patients Stronger risks among nonsmoking and female relatives
(Bermejo et al. 2009), Sweden	Relatives of parents or siblings with BC	Population-based risks according to the Swedish Cancer Registry	Age, sex, socioeconomic index, region, calendar year	Relatives of parents with BC: SIR = 1.78 (95% CI: 1.58–2.01) Relatives of siblings with BC: 2.41 (95% CI: 1.70–3.42)	Risks also increased for relatives of parents with kidney or thyroid cancer and for relatives of siblings with stomach, laryngeal, endometrial, and kidney cancer and leukemias
(Martin et al. 2018), United States	229,251 first- and second-degree relatives plus first cousins of BC patients and 1,197,552 relatives of matched control	1,197,552 relatives of matched controls	Age, sex, and smoking	First degree: HR = 1.69 (95% CI: 1.47–1.95) Second degree: HR = 1.35 (95% CI: 1.20–1.50)	Risks for lung (HR = 1.34), kidney (HR = 1.30), and cervical (HR = 1.25) cancers are also increased Risks are not clearly different for relatives of younger and older probands
(Hidaka et al. 2020), Japan	228 relatives of patients with BC	103,479 relatives of controls	Age, sex, BMI, smoking, alcohol, physical activity, diabetes, and medical examination within the past year	HR = 6.06 (95% CI: 2.49–14.74)	Based on five BC diagnoses among the relatives of BC patients (and 413 among relatives of controls)

BC, bladder cancer; UC, urothelial cancer; RR, relative risk or risk ratio; O/E, observed-expected ratio; SIR, standardized incidence ratio; HR, hazard ratio; CI, confidence interval; UUT, upper urinary tract; the Swedish studies all report about the Swedish Family-Cancer Database which means that the results are not independent

blastomas are caused by two independent mutational events in the same cell, of which one can be inherited (Knudson 1971). In 1983, these mutations were identified to be in the *RB1* gene, which would turn out to be the first recognized tumor suppressor gene (Berry et al. 2019), which encodes the pRB protein involved in various cellular processes (i.e., proliferation, DNA replication and repair, and checkpoint control of the cell cycle). pRB has also been linked to the development of secondary carcinomas, such as lung, bone, breast, and BC (Cote et al. 1998; Fletcher et al. 2004; Mitra et al. 2007). In retinoblastoma survivors, these secondary malignancies are known to be the main cause of death (Ohan et al. 2020).

Several case reports on secondary BC in retinoblastoma survivors have been published in recent decades (Bleoo et al. 2003; Cao et al. 2021; Doddamani et al. 2015; Leinwand et al. 2019; Liang et al. 2001; Minagawa et al. 2008; Parekh et al. 2002; Ramirez Sevilla et al. 2018; Tanguay et al. 2003; Venkatraman et al. 2003). The patients mentioned in the reports range in age from 16 to 65 years, which is extremely young in comparison with the median age of 73 in the general BC population. Remarkably, almost all secondary BC are leiomyosarcomas (i.e., originating from the smooth muscle fibers in the bladder wall instead of the urothelium), while only 1% of all BC in the population have leiomyosarcoma histology (Fakhoury et al. 2016).

Three of the largest cohorts of "hereditary retinoblastoma" survivors ("hereditary" defined based on verified germline *RB1* mutation status, bilateral retinoblastoma, or unilateral retinoblastoma with a positive family history of retinoblastoma) are from the United States, the United Kingdom, and the Netherlands. The most recent report on the UK cohort by MacCarthy and colleagues observed eight BC cases in 806 retinoblastoma survivors with a standardized incidence ratio (SIR) of 83.0 (95% CI: 35.8–163.5) (MacCarthy et al. 2013). The latest paper on the US cohort found only one BC case in 1128 retinoblastoma survivors but did not report a SIR (Schonfeld et al. 2021). Similarly, only four BC cases were diagnosed among 199 retinoblastoma survivors in the latest report on the Dutch cohort (Dommering et al. 2012). Earlier reports on the US and the Dutch cohorts reported SIRs of 6.15 (95% CI: 0.7–22) and 124 (95% CI: 34.0–319), respectively (Kleinerman et al. 2005; Marees et al. 2008). Comparable to the case reports, the UK cohort observed mainly leiomyosarcomas of the bladder ($N = 5$). One of the three other patients had a rhabdomyosarcoma, and the remaining two had epithelial carcinomas of the bladder. The five patients in the US and NL cohorts all had epithelial BC.

Even though hereditary retinoblastoma survivors appear to have an increased risk of secondary BC, argued by the young ages at diagnosis as well as the high SIRs, there are a few caveats to these findings. None of the mentioned studies included any data on smoking behavior and (occupational) exposure to carcinogens. Furthermore, there are now four more cohorts of hereditary retinoblastoma patients from France (N = 160), Germany (N = 648), Argentina ($N = 311$), and Denmark ($N = 133$) in which not a single BC case was observed (Chaussade et al. 2019; Gregersen et al. 2020; Temming et al. 2017; Villanueva et al. 2022).

2.2.1.2 Costello Syndrome (*HRAS*)

Costello syndrome (CS) is a very rare congenital multiple abnormality disorder caused by activating mutations in the *HRAS* proto-oncogene (Gripp et al. 2019). The disorder, first described by Costello in 1971, is autosomal dominantly inherited, with a prevalence of about 1 in 380,000 live births in the United Kingdom (Costello 1971; Giannoulatou et al. 2013). CS affects multiple organ systems since the *HRAS* proto-oncogene protein product is associated with the Ras/mitogen-activated protein kinase (Ras/MAPK) pathway, which is primarily involved in the regulation of cell division throughout the body (Gripp and Lin 2012; Gripp et al. 2006). Even though CS is classified as an overgrowth syndrome due to high birth weight and macrocephaly, patients' phenotypes include failure to thrive (i.e., short stature), intellectual disability, wartlike skin lesions, coarse facial appearance, and various cardiac problems (Gripp and Lin 2012; White et al. 2005). Overgrowth syndromes such as CS also have a risk of developing malignant carcinomas (Brioude et al. 2019; Gripp 2005). Tumors that occur most often in CS patients are rhabdomyosarcomas, neuroblastomas, and BC (Gripp 2005; Zhang and Zhang 2015).

The association between CS and BC originates from case reports on BC development in CS patients at a very young age. A literature review by Kratz and colleagues found 268 CS patients, of which four were case reports of CS patients diagnosed with BC at an extremely young mean age of 13.5 years (Franceschini et al. 1999; Gripp et al. 2000; Kratz et al. 2011; Sovik et al. 2007; Urakami et al. 2002). Three additional reported cases of BC in CS patients were diagnosed at 2.5, 17, and 25 years (Gripp et al. 2002; Gripp et al. 2006; White et al. 2005). Five of the seven patients had urothelial carcinoma, and one rhabdomyosarcoma, while the histological type of one patient was not specified.

Recently, a systematic review of 234 studies and subsequent meta-analysis on cancer development in 573 CS patients from 35 countries was published (Astiazaran-Symonds et al. 2023). In addition to 30 rhabdomyosarcomas, five neuroblastomas, and some other malignancies, 13 patients developed BC. Using US cancer incidence rates as reported by the Surveillance, Epidemiology, and End Results program as a reference, this corresponds with an extremely high SIR of 1971 (95% CI: 1050–3372). The mean age at diagnosis was 16, in line with the case reports. There was some suggestion that the most common *HRAS*-p.Gly12Ser mutation carried a lower risk of cancer compared to all other variants in *HRAS*.

Interestingly, in a study from the Netherlands, somatic mutations in *FGFR3, PIK3CA*, and *HRAS* were compared in BC patients under vs. above 20 years of age. A relatively high frequency of four *HRAS* mutations (1 p.Gly12Ala, 2 p.Gly12Ser, and 1 p.Gln61Arg) was observed among the 14 young patients, compared with nine mutations in 146 patients above 20 years; only one of these nine mutations was a p.Gly12Ser mutation. A 29-year-old patient with a p.Gly12Ala mutation was known as a Costello syndrome patient. Because the normal tissue (stroma) of a 16-year-old boy with a p.Gly12Ala *HRAS* mutation in his bladder tumor also displayed this *HRAS* mutation, the authors suggest that this patient might be mosaic, and such mosaicism may be a BC risk factor (Beukers et al. 2014).

2.2.1.3 Lynch Syndrome (MMR Genes)

Lynch syndrome is an autosomal dominant disorder, previously known as hereditary nonpolyposis colorectal cancer, caused by germline mutations in one of the DNA mismatch repair (MMR) genes *MSH2, MSH6, MLH1*, and *PMS2* or deletion of the *EPCAM* gene (Nassour et al. 2023). In contrast to retinoblastoma and Costello syndrome, Lynch syndrome is a fairly common disorder with an estimated incidence between 1:2000 and 1:660 (de la Chapelle 2005). The MMR genes play a major role in detecting and correcting mistakes made during DNA replication (Martin-Lopez and Fishel 2013). Therefore, loss of this function may lead to the development of cancer. Along with a chance of developing colorectal cancer of up to 80%, individuals with Lynch syndrome also appear to have an increased risk of acquiring several other primary carcinomas at a relatively young age, such as endometrial, brain, pancreatic, ovarian, and urothelial cancers of the upper and lower urinary tract (Bhattacharya and McHugh 2023; van der Post et al. 2010).

The relative risk of developing BC in Lynch mutation carriers has been estimated in a systematic review and meta-analysis. Compared to the general population, the RR of BC was found to be 7.48 (95% CI: 3.70–15.13) (Nassour et al. 2023). The four included studies in the meta-analysis were selected based on strict inclusion and exclusion criteria, including the requirement of genetic testing of all participants (Engel et al. 2012; Pande et al. 2012; Win et al. 2012; Wischhusen et al. 2020). The combined number of Lynch syndrome patients in the four studies totaled 6760, with mean ages at BC diagnosis ranging from 57 to 64 years. However, smoking behavior was not taken into account (Nassour et al. 2023).

Notwithstanding the clearly increased risk of BC occurrence in Lynch syndrome patients in the abovementioned meta-analysis, no distinction was made between the effects of different MMR genes on BC risk. In 130 UK families with mutations in MMR genes, BC was observed in 14 families, resulting in a RR of 1.9. Since ten of the 14 families had an *MSH2* mutation, a higher RR of 3.6 was established for patients with a mutation in *MSH2* (Geary et al. 2008). Similar results were observed in a Dutch study among 95 Lynch syndrome families (van der Post et al. 2010). Twenty-one individuals from 19 families were found to have BC with an average age at diagnosis of 60 years; the vast majority (71%) had an *MSH2* mutation. The RR for carriers of any of the MMR mutations was 4.2 (95% CI: 2.2–7.2) for men and 2.2 (95% CI: 0.3–8.0) for women, while the RR for *MSH2* carriers was 7.0 (95% CI: 3.4–13.0) for men and 5.8 (95% CI: 0.5–16.1) for women. No data on smoking behavior was present in either study.

Several other studies support an increased risk of BC among Lynch syndrome mutation carriers

(Bermejo et al. 2005; Joost et al. 2015; Skeldon et al. 2013) and more specifically among *MSH2* mutation carriers (Barrow et al. 2013; Joost et al. 2015; Moller et al. 2018; Saita et al. 2018; Skeldon et al. 2013). The average age (54–64 years) at BC diagnosis in Lynch syndrome patients is fairly consistent across studies. In the study by van der Post et al., the cumulative risk of BC before 70 years in MMR gene carriers was approximately 7.5% (95% CI: 3.1–11.9%) for men and 1.0% (95% CI: 0–2.4%) for women, compared to 1.8% and 0.5% in the general Dutch population (van der Post et al. 2010).

In a recent update of the Dutch study, the cancer risk among 1745 individuals with Lynch syndrome from 457 families was evaluated (Elze et al. 2023). The SIR for BC was 4.0 (95% CI: 2.8–5.6), based on 54 cases of BC (of which 11, 23, 18, and 2 were diagnosed among *MLH1, MSH2/EPCAM, MSH6*, and *PMS2* carriers, respectively). More than half (18 of 34) of bladder tumors for which tissue was available appeared to be MMR-deficient (dMMR), causing microsatellite instability (MSI-H). This may have direct clinical relevance since MSI-H/dMMR tumors are known to respond very well to immune checkpoint inhibitors (Maio et al. 2022).

2.2.2 Sequencing Studies and Rare Germline Pathogenic DNA Variants

Many studies have applied next-generation (targeted) sequencing techniques to tumor DNA of BC patients to identify and describe somatic, non-germline mutations in driver genes. To date, a smaller number of sequencing studies have reported on germline mutations in BC patients. In contrast to genome-wide association studies (see Sect. 2.2.3), these studies mostly analyzed selected sets of a few to a few hundred known cancer predisposition genes (CPGs), including DNA damage response and repair (DDR) genes Fig. (2.2). Generally, only germline variant alleles that are designated as pathogenic (P) or likely pathogenic (LP) according to accepted criteria [e.g., American College of Medical Genetics and Genomics (ACMG) guidelines (Richards et al. 2015)] and annotation tools [e.g., PathoMAN (Ravichandran et al. 2019)] and that are absent or observed at very low frequencies in control populations [e.g., gnomAD (Chen et al. 2022)] are considered relevant and are reported. Reporting

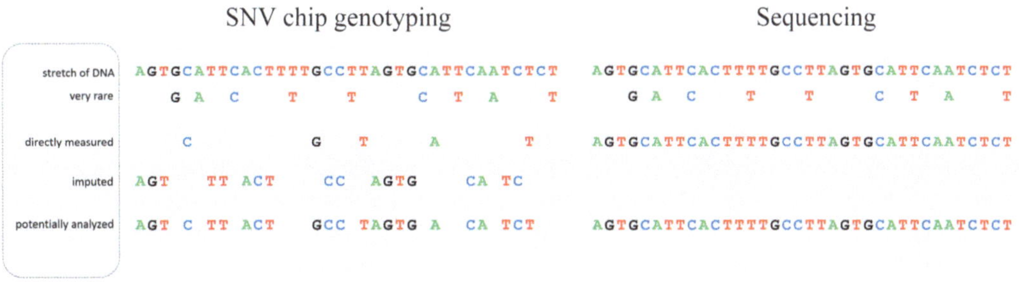

Fig. 2.2 Differences in measurement of germline DNA variation via single-nucleotide variant chip genotyping and via sequencing. This figure illustrates the difference between the measurement and analysis of germline DNA variation based on application of single-nucleotide variant (SNV) chip genotyping versus application of sequencing. A short stretch of (single-stranded) DNA is visualized on the first row; the second row indicates which of the positions contain a very-low-frequency allele. Left plot: in SNV chip genotyping, direct measurement of a set of low-frequency to common germline DNA variants is followed by imputation of alleles at unmeasured low-frequency to common variants. In imputation, existing and known allelic correlation (linkage disequilibrium, LD) patterns among variants in the human genome are used to estimate the alleles at unmeasured positions. Given the low correlation between alleles of low-frequency to common variants and (very) rare allele variants, these (very) rare alleles are not or only poorly imputed. These therefore remain unmeasured and cannot be analyzed for association to a disease trait of interest by application of (genome-wide) SNV chip genotyping. Right plot: in contrast, by application of sequencing techniques, alleles at all variants, including very rare alleles, are directly measured and can be analyzed for association with a disease trait

is often done on the gene level in which P/LP variants in a single gene are aggregated.

An overview of the genes for which multiple studies suggest carriership of germline P/LP variant alleles in BC patients is given in Table 2.2. The table includes eight genes which all belong to the DDR pathway and of which seven are actionable for a related cancer phenotype according to ACMG guidelines (Miller et al. 2022). Observed gene carrier rates are low, and rate estimates differ between studies, which may be due, among other reasons, to sampling variation, differences in inclusion of types of DNA variants (i.e., single-nucleotide variants [SNV] only versus inclusion of larger variants), and differences in the genetic background of the studied population. A relatively high P/LP variant carrier rate of around 2% was found in some studies for *CHEK2* (Mian et al. 2023; Pemov et al. 2021; Stadler et al. 2021), *MUTYH* (mono- and biallelic) (Gerald et al. 2023; Mian et al. 2023), *MSH2*, and *BRCA1/2* (Carlo et al. 2020). Also, studies that included patients with a high suspicion of heritable pathogenic variants showed specifically high carrier rates (4–6% for *BRCA1/2* and *MSH2*) (Mossanen et al. 2022; Nassar et al. 2020).

Only a subset of studies has performed statistical analyses in which the difference in frequency of P/LP variants is compared between BC patients and a control population. A systematic review of reports of statistically significant associations for rare germline variant alleles and BC risk (Mian et al. 2023) identified eight studies (Carlo et al. 2020; Chen et al. 2004; Na et al. 2018; Nassar et al. 2020; Vogt et al. 2009; Win et al. 2016; Zeng et al. 2022; Zlowocka et al. 2008), and for nine genes a statistically significant association was found in at least one of the eight studies: *ATM*, *BRCA2*, *CHEK2*, *ERCC5*, *MLH1*, *MSH2*, *MSH6*, *MUTYH*, and *TGFB1*. Differentiation between patients with urothelial carcinoma of the bladder and that of the upper urinary tract indicates that Lynch syndrome-related germline DNA mismatch repair (MMR) gene mutations (*MLH1*, *MSH2*, *MSH6*) and MSI-H/dMMR in tumor tissue are observed mainly in upper urinary tract carcinoma (Carlo et al. 2020; Nassar et al. 2020). P/LP variant alleles in other non-MMR DDR genes are mainly found in BC, and in a proportion of carriers this is accompanied by loss of heterozygosity/somatic mutation in the tumor (Carlo et al. 2020). Mian and colleagues studied associations with BC risk for the genes that were identified in their systematic review (i.e., *ATM*, *BRCA2*, *CHEK2*, *ERCC5*, *MLH1*, *MSH2*, *MSH6*, *MUTYH*, and *TGFB1*) in 1695 BC patients and 186,271 controls with whole-exome sequencing data from the UK Biobank (UKB) and confirmed statistical significant associations for *ATM*, *BRCA2*, and *CHEK2*, all breast cancer genes; suggestive evidence of association was found for *MLH1* and *MSH2* (Mian et al. 2023). Carrier frequencies in BC patients for these genes in the UKB ranged from 0.06% (*MSH2*) to 2.01% (*CHEK2*), and reported point estimates of the odds ratios (ORs) for BC risk ranged from 1.6 to 4.9, suggesting low to moderate penetrance. The latter is in line with ORs of 1.5 to 4.6 for *ATM*, *BRCA*1/2, and *MSH2* in an extended cohort of urothelial carcinoma patients (Carlo et al. 2020); Nassar et al. reported higher ORs (Nassar et al. 2020).

Estimates of the percentage of BC patients that carry at least one P/LP variant allele in candidate (cancer predisposing) genes vary from 5% in a study of 50 known cancer syndrome genes in $n = 966$ stage 1–4 BC patients (Gerald et al. 2023) to 34% in a study of 2–83 candidate genes among $n = 80$ BC patients with suspicion for cancer predisposition (Mossanen et al. 2022). Most studies included mainly muscle-invasive and metastatic BC patients. However, Pietzak et al. specifically studied the rate of P/LP germline variants in 214 patients initially diagnosed with non-muscle-invasive bladder cancer (NMIBC) and found that 10% carried at least one P/LP germline variant allele in an analyzed set of 76 known CPGs (Pietzak et al. 2022). Two-thirds of variant alleles were found in DDR genes, including *ATM*, *BRCA1*, *CHEK2*, *ERCC2*, *ERCC3*, and *RAD50*. Non-DDR CPGs in which P/LP variant alleles were found were *APC* (p.Ile1307Lys, a low-penetrance colorectal cancer allele which is common among Ashkenazi Jews), *FH*, and *SDHA*. Of note, all P/LP variants were observed in the

Table 2.2 Genes for which presence of germline pathogenic/likely pathogenic allelic variants is reported in multiple bladder cancer series

Gene	Pathway	Related cancer phenotype	Actionable?[a]	Sources (geographical background bladder cancer patients)
ATM	DDR	Breast cancer	No	(Mian et al. (2023), UK (Pietzak et al. 2022), US (Nassar et al. 2020), US (Yap et al. 2022), US (Carlo et al. 2020), US (Pemov et al. 2021), US (Huang et al. 2018), mainly US (Mossanen et al. 2022), US (Gerald et al. 2023), US (Stadler et al. 2021), US
BRCA1	DDR: HRR	Hereditary breast and/or ovarian cancer	Yes	(Pietzak et al. 2022), US (Nassar et al. 2020), US (Carlo et al. 2020), US (Stadler et al. 2021), US (Yap et al. 2022), US (Mossanen et al. 2022), US (Gerald et al. 2023), US (Tang et al. 2022), China
BRCA2	DDR: HRR	Hereditary breast and/or ovarian cancer	Yes	(Mian et al. 2023), UK (Nassar et al. 2020), US (Carlo et al. 2020), US (Yap et al. 2022), US (Pemov et al. 2021), US (Mossanen et al. 2022), US (Gerald et al. 2023), US (Tang et al. 2022), China (Stadler et al. 2021), US (Vosoughi et al. 2020), US
CHEK2	DDR	Breast cancer, colorectal cancer	No	(Mian et al. 2023), UK (Pietzak et al. 2022), US (Nassar et al. 2020), US (Na et al. 2018), China (Zlowocka et al. 2008), Poland (Carlo et al. 2020), US (Naslund-Koch et al. 2016), Denmark (Pemov et al. 2021), US (Yap et al. 2022), US (Huang et al. 2018), mainly US (Mossanen et al. 2022), US (Gerald et al. 2023), US (Tang et al. 2022), China (Stadler et al. 2021), US
MLH1	DDR: MMR	Lynch syndrome	Yes	(Mian et al. 2023), UK (Nassar et al. 2020), US (Pemov et al. 2021), US (Stadler et al. 2021), US (Na et al. 2018), China (Yap et al. 2022), US (Mossanen et al. 2022), US

(continued)

Table 2.2 (continued)

Gene	Pathway	Related cancer phenotype	Actionable?[a]	Sources (geographical background bladder cancer patients)
MSH2	DDR: MMR	Lynch syndrome	Yes	(Mian et al. 2023), UK (Nassar et al. 2020), US (Pemov et al. 2021), US (Yap et al. 2022), US (Carlo et al. 2020, US (Mossanen et al. 2022), US (Stadler et al. 2021), US
MSH6	DDR: MMR	Lynch syndrome	Yes	(Zeng et al. 2022, US/UK (Yap et al. 2022), US (Gerald et al. 2023), US (Stadler et al. 2021), US
MUTYH[b]	DDR: BER	MUTYH-associated polyposis/ colorectal cancer	Yes	(Nassar et al. 2020), US (Vogt et al. 2009), Europe (Win et al. 2016), US (Yap et al. 2022), US (Carlo et al. 2020), US (Pemov et al. 2021), US (Mossanen et al. 2022), US (Gerald et al. 2023), US

BER base excision repair, *DDR* DNA damage repair, *FA* Fanconi anemia, *HRR* homologous recombination repair, *MMR* mismatch repair, *UK* United Kingdom, *US* United States

[a]Medically actionable gene in case of presence of pathogenic or likely pathogenic allele according to guidelines of American College of Medical Genetics and Genomics (ACMG) for phenotype that is indicated in column "Related cancer phenotype" (Miller et al. 2022)

[b]Presumed autosomal recessive inheritance but both monoallelic and biallelic carriers included

high-grade NMIBC patients (n = 163) and none in the low-grade NMIBC patients (n = 46), suggesting different underlying mechanisms. In contrast, the proportion of patients with a P/LP germline variant for high-grade NMIBC was similar to that observed in patients initially diagnosed with muscle-invasive or de novo metastatic BC (n = 169), both overall (13% vs. 12%) and in DDR genes specifically (9.2% vs. 11%). Unfortunately, differentiation between low- and high-grade NMIBC is lacking in other studies. P/LP variants are found more commonly in BC patients diagnosed at a relatively early age (Carlo et al. 2020; Mossanen et al. 2022; Na et al. 2018) but not consistent across all studies (Nassar et al. 2020). Data on the relation between germline P/LP variants and prognostic outcomes and response to therapy in BC are very scarce. Pietzak et al. observed no relationship between P/LP variants in DDR genes and recurrence and progression-free survival in 148 BCG-treated NMIBC patients (Pietzak et al. 2022).

2.2.3 Candidate Gene and Genome-Wide Association Studies (GWAS) for Common Germline DNA Variants

Early candidate gene studies for BC, initially based on single biochemical phenotype assays using drug probes (Rothman et al. 2007) and then by DNA-based assays of either single polymorphisms or a group of polymorphisms related to the function of one gene, reported associations for common germline polymorphisms in carcinogen detoxification enzymes. *N*-acetylation by N-acetyltransferase 2 (NAT2) is a major route of biotransformation of aromatic amine compounds (Hein 2002), and glutathione S-transferase mu 1 (*GSTM1*) plays a role in the detoxification of benzo[a]pyrene and other polycyclic aromatic hydrocarbons (Hayes and Strange 2000), important carcinogens in tobacco smoke. Early pre-GWAS meta-analyses showed strong evidence for an association between polymorphisms in *NAT2* and *GSTM1* (Engel et al. 2002; Garcia-Closas et al. 2005; Moore et al. 2011; Rothman et al. 2007), with *NAT2* slow acetylation phenotypes (measured biochemically or by genotyping most or all functional variants) and homozygous deletion of *GSTM1* resulting in significantly increased risks for BC in studies conducted in the general population in many countries (NAT2 slow acetylation phenotype/genotype: OR = 1.37 [95% CI: 1.24–1.52], $p = 1.17 \times 10^{-9}$, cases = 7961; *GSTM1* null genotype: OR = 1.5 [95% CI: 1.3–1.6], $p = 9 \times 10^{-15}$, cases = 5108) (Engel et al. 2002; Garcia-Closas et al. 2005; Moore et al. 2011). Unequivocal evidence of a gene-environment interaction between the NAT2 slow acetylation phenotype/genotype and tobacco use was also demonstrated and thought to be based on detoxification of aryl monoamines such as 4-aminobiphenyl and 2-naphthylamine (Garcia-Closas et al. 2005; Marcus et al. 2000; Moore et al. 2011). In addition, NAT2 slow acetylation has been associated with increased BC risk in industry-based studies where workers were exposed to mixed aromatic amines (Cartwright et al. 1982). Conversely, rapid NAT2 acetylation phenotype/genotype was associated with increased risk of BC among workers exposed to benzidine, an aryldiamine, consistent with evidence that N-acetylation represents an activation rather than a detoxification step for this compound (Carreon et al. 2006; Hein 2002). In contrast, the evidence for a gene-environment interaction for *GSTM1* null genotype with tobacco (Engel et al. 2002; Garcia-Closas et al. 2005) is somewhat weaker and dependent on the statistical interaction model that is used.

These early findings for germline variation in *NAT2* and *GSTM1* and BC risk have been subsequently confirmed in several large-scale GWAS (Figueroa et al. 2014, 2016; Garcia-Closas et al. 2011a, b; Kiemeney et al. 2010; Kiemeney et al. 2008; Koutros et al. 2016; Rafnar et al. 2014; Rafnar et al. 2011; Rothman et al. 2010; Wang et al. 2016b; Wu et al. 2009). An overview of all common DNA variants for which a genome-wide statistically significant association with BC risk was found is given in Table 2.3. This table includes common variants in additional carcinogen metabolizing enzymes, specifically genetic variants at *UGT1A6* (Rothman et al. 2010; Tang et al. 2012) and *CYP1A2* (Matsuda et al. 2015). In addition, several markers associated with BC risk have been identified in or near oncogenes or tumor suppressor genes (*MYC*, *CCNE1*, *TP63*, *FGFR3*) and DNA maintenance genes (*TERC*, *TERT-CLPTML1*). As further elaborated in Sect. 2.2.4, studies of molecular mechanisms underlying GWAS signals have also provided insights into the biology of several identified BC loci identified within/near: *PSCA* (Fu et al. 2012; Kohaar et al. 2013; Wu et al. 2009), *UGT1A6* (Tang et al. 2012), *CCNE1* (Fu et al. 2014), *SCL14A1* (Koutros et al. 2013), and *FGFR3* (Figueroa et al. 2015; Koutros et al. 2023).

Other germline susceptibility loci identified appear in regions with known somatic alterations in tumors, particularly those related to cell cycle regulation (6p22 and 9q21.3) and the RAS–MAPK pathway (4p16.3). The role of other GWAS signals remains to be explored.

The majority of patients that were included in BC GWASs were diagnosed with low-risk NMIBC, reflecting the distribution of BC stage and grade in the general population. Often, initial GWAS findings were followed by evaluation of the DNA variant associations in strata of (low-grade or high-grade) NMIBC or MIBC. Indications for heterogeneity of effects were reported by some, including strongest associations for low-grade NMIBC for the *TACC3/FGFR3* locus (Koutros et al. 2023) and *MYC* locus (Kiemeney et al. 2008) and a stronger signal for MIBC for the 20p12.2 locus (Figueroa et al. 2016). However, these stratified analyses were limited to a selected set of DNA variants and lack solid replication. Also, thus far, most of the GWAS efforts have been conducted only in individuals of European ancestry. In the future, there is a need to conduct larger, diverse GWAS that will enable cross-ancestry identification of additional common susceptibility variants for BC as well as further define the genetic architecture of BC, how it relates to environmental exposures that drive BC risk, and if and how these risk factors can be used to prevent BC or conduct early disease screening among the highest risk groups (Garcia-Closas et al. 2013; Koutros et al. 2023).

Table 2.3 Common germline DNA variants associated with BC risk in GWAS or fine-mapping studies

SNP	Chromosome band	Position (hg19)	Gene region	Effect allele frequency[a]	Effect allele odds ratio
GSTM1	1p13.3	110229772	*GSTM1*	0.70[b]	1.27[b]
rs17863783	2q37.1	234602277	*UGT1A* cluster	0.98	1.75
rs10936599	3q26.2	169492101	*MYNN, TERC*	0.75	1.10
rs710521	3q28	189645933	*TP63*	0.74	1.15
rs2896518	4p16.3	1757559	*TACC3, FGFR3*	0.21	1.17
rs2242652	5p15.33	1280028	*CLPTM1L, TERT*	0.8	1.18
rs6910215	6p22.3	20783394	*CDKAL1*	0.57	1.10
rs72826305	6p22.3	21826729	*CASC15/LOC105374970*	0.34	1.12
rs2125484	7q36.3	155759638	*LOC389602*	0.58	1.11
rs1495741	8p22	18272881	*NAT2*	0.60^	1.19[c]
rs5003154	8q21.13	81986953	*PAG1*	0.51	1.11
rs10094872	8q24.21	128719884	*CASC11, MYC*	0.38	1.24
rs2294008	8q24.3	143761931	*PSCA*	0.45	1.14
rs1414253	9p21.3	21755630	*LOC107987026, MTAP/CDKN2A*	0.42	1.14[d]
rs4743687	9q31.1	106856910	*SMC2*	0.44	1.10
rs7076867	10q22.1	71582996	*COL13A1*	0.95	1.31
rs907611	11p15.5	1874072	*TNNT3, LSP1*	0.32	1.11
rs7937265	11p15.5	1947800	*TNNT3, LSP1*	0.19	1.13
rs4907479	13q34	113659108	*MCF2L*	0.27	1.10
rs10853535	18q12.3	43317547	*SLC14A1*	0.44	1.14
rs8102137	19q12	30296853	*CCNE1*	0.33	1.12
rs411482	19q13.33	49103447	*SULT2B1-FAM83E*	0.61	1.13
rs62185668	20p12.2	10961935	Gene desert	0.25	1.11
rs1014971	22q13.1	39332623	*APOBEC3A*	0.65	1.12

Source: S. Koutros, L.A. Kiemeney, P. Pal Choudhury et al., Genome-wide Association Study of Bladder Cancer Reveals New Biological and Translational Insights, Eur Urol (2023), https://doi.org/10.1016/j.eururo.2023.04.020)

[a] Allele frequency observed in controls

[b] Frequency and odds ratio for GSTM1 null genotype

[c] Frequency and odds ratio for NAT2 slow acetylation phenotype/genotype

[d] Odds ratio for subgroup of ever smokers

In addition, more insight into common germline DNA variants that affect BC outcomes is warranted. Candidate gene studies into recurrence, progression, and survival in BC have been plentiful but are hampered by small sample sizes and lack of validation studies, reflecting the scarcity of BC cohorts with both germline DNA variation and demographic, tumor, and clinical follow-up data. Lipunova and colleagues identified a total of 81 reported associations for common germline DNA variants and recurrence, 24 for progression, and 54 for death in a set of 112 articles that were published until late 2018 (Lipunova et al. 2019b). Unfortunately, without proper replication studies, the validity of these associations is unknown. Indeed, an earlier validation study was able to replicate only six out of 114 reported associations for BC prognosis and treatment response: rs1799793 (*ERCC2*) and rs187238 (*IL18*) for recurrence among patients treated with BCG, rs6678136 (*RGS4*) and rs11585883 (*RGS5*) for NMIBC progression, and rs12035879 (*RGS5*) and rs2075786 (*TERT*) for overall survival in MIBC (Grotenhuis et al. 2016). No additional replicated findings in candidate gene studies have been reported in recent years. The first meta-GWAS for NMIBC recurrence and progression in 3400 newly diagnosed patients identified several novel candidate germline loci; five genes showed substantial evidence for association with either recurrence (*SCFD1*) or progression (*IFT140*, *UBE2I*, *FAHD1*, and

NME3) (Galesloot et al. 2022). Published GWAS on BCG response and NMIBC aggressiveness were underpowered and lacking thorough validation (Lenfant et al. 2021; Lipunova et al. 2019a; Nagakawa et al. 2021), and GWAS for outcome and therapy response in muscle-invasive and metastatic BC are lacking. Given the known relevance of germline genetics for a patient's cancer-immune phenotype (Lim et al. 2018), such studies may however shed light on factors that underlie differential response to therapy (Khan et al. 2020).

2.2.4 Mechanisms of Action of Germline Variants Associated with BC Risk

Sequencing studies have revealed carriership of pathogenic variants in DDR genes in a substantial proportion of BC patients, and GWAS have identified a number of common low-penetrance genetic variants (referred to as GWAS signals) that are statistically significantly associated with BC susceptibility. Although some of the GWAS signals or their proxies are protein-coding or transcribed, most are located within non-coding regions and thus could be regulatory. In silico analyses, including expression quantitative trait loci (eQTL) analysis, demonstrated that some of the GWAS signals might regulate gene expression at the transcriptional level. Other analyses, such as GARFIELD (i.e., GWAS Analysis of Regulatory or Functional Information Enrichment with Linkage Disequilibrium (LD) correction), identified the enrichment of GWAS signals in regions with putative regulatory characteristics (Koutros et al. 2023). Pathway analyses show the enrichment of the GWAS signals in genes responsible for critical cellular processes, such as xenobiotic detoxification, cell cycle regulation, chromosome and telomere maintenance, gene regulation, and signal transduction. Detailed fine-mapping and functional investigations of several individual GWAS regions have uncovered the underlying molecular mechanisms and likely causal variants.

2.2.4.1 In silico Analyses

eQTL analyses for BC GWAS signals are predominantly based on the data from The Cancer Genome Atlas (TCGA) that represent muscle-invasive bladder cancer (MIBC) (Cancer Genome Atlas Research 2014). eQTL evaluations are usually integrated into regional functional analyses of associated regions to generate plausible hypotheses on biological mechanisms underlying these associations; these results will be discussed in the corresponding sections below. However, the eQTL analyses in TCGA could be affected by the genomic changes that occur in tumors, such as somatic alterations and copy number changes that need to be taken into account as they can mask relatively weak effects of genetic variants. The Genotype-Tissue Expression (GTEx) project includes tissue samples from multiple non-cancer donors, but the resource for bladder tissue is limited by only 21 samples, which is insufficient for meaningful eQTL analyses (Consortium 2015).

Genome-wide analyses of regulatory elements, such as through GARFIELD (Iotchkova et al. 2019), help to annotate the genomic landscapes of the associated genetic variants using functional features from ENCODE, GENCODE, and Roadmap Epigenomics projects, including chromatin states, genic annotations, histone modifications, DNase I hypersensitive sites, and transcription factor binding sites, in publicly available cell lines. GARFIELD analysis of BC GWAS signals showed the enrichment of genome-wide significant variants within promoter flanks and transcriptionally repressed regions, characterized by chromatin marks of tri-methylation of lysine 27 on histone H3 protein (H3K27me3) (Koutros et al. 2023).

2.2.4.2 Pathways and Functional Studies

Germline genetic risk variants for BC have been identified in genes that are crucial for various cellular processes such as detoxification of xenobiotics (*GSTM1*, *NAT2*, *UGT1A6*), DNA damage response (DDR genes), regulation of the cell cycle (*CCNE1*), maintenance of chromosomes and telomeres (*SMC2*, *TERC*, *TERT*), gene regulation (*TP63*), and signal transduction (*FGFR3*).

Thus, dysfunction in these processes may contribute to the development of BC. In addition, GWAS has detected variations in genes involved in the regulation of global somatic mutagenesis (through the activity of APOBEC3B enzyme). Pathways associated with other GWAS signals, often located in gene deserts and intergenic regions, are yet to be annotated. Follow-up studies of GWAS signals have shed light on the underlying molecular mechanisms (Beane Freeman et al. 2022; Dudek et al. 2018; Fu et al. 2012, 2014; Garcia-Closas et al. 2005; Killedar et al. 2015; Kohaar et al. 2013; Koutros et al. 2013; Middlebrooks et al. 2016; Pattison et al. 2016; Saeki et al. 2015; Tang et al. 2012; Toupance et al. 2020; Wang et al. 2016b; Wu et al. 2009). Functional analyses have demonstrated the causality of several GWAS signals (Table 2.4 and Fig. 2.3): APOBEC-rs1014971 (Middlebrooks et al. 2016), CCNE1-rs8102137 and rs7257330 (Fu et al. 2014; Pattison et al. 2016), PSCA-rs2294008 and rs2978974 (Fu et al. 2012; Kohaar et al. 2013; Saeki et al. 2015; Wu et al. 2009), SLC14A1-rs10775480/rs10853535 (Koutros et al. 2013), TERC/MYNN-rs10936599 (Toupance et al. 2020), TERT-10069690 (Killedar et al. 2015), TP63-rs710521/rs35592567 (Dudek et al. 2018; Wang et al. 2016a), UGT1A6-rs17863783 (Tang et al. 2012), and LSP1-rs907611 (Beane Freeman et al. 2022). The detoxification and DDR pathways and functional studies of the abovementioned variants will be discussed in more detail below.

2.2.4.3 Phase II Carcinogen Detoxification System: *GSTM1-null, NAT2-slow,* and *UGT1A6*

The most compelling evidence for the relationship between genetic variations and increased BC risk has been found for variants affecting genes responsible for phase II carcinogen detoxification: GSTM1-null genotype (Garcia-Closas et al. 2005), NAT2-slow acetylation (tagged by

Table 2.4 Regional functional analyses of GWAS signals

GWAS variants (→ functional variants)	Gene regions	Location	Molecular mechanisms	References
rs36209093—proxy	*GSTM1*	Intronic	Loss of GSTM1 enzyme	Garcia-Closas et al. (2005)
rs1495741—proxy	*NAT2*	Intergenic	Slower metabolizing activity	Garcia-Closas et al. (2005)
rs11892031 → rs17863783	*UGT1A* cluster	Intronic, exonic	Splicing, carcinogen removal	Tang et al. (2012)
rs1014971 → rs1014971	*APOBEC3B*	Enhancer for *APOBEC3B*	*APOBEC3B* expression, APOBEC-type somatic mutagenesis	Middlebrooks et al. (2016)
rs8102137 → rs7257330, rs200996365	*CCNE1/ C19orf12*	Intergenic, intronic, promoter	Transcription (*CCNE1*, *KLF5*)	Fu et al. 2014; Pattison et al. (2016)
rs2294008 → rs2294008, rs2978974	*PSCA*	Exonic, 5'UTR, or enhancer	Transcription, alternative start site	Fu et al. (2012), Kohaar et al. (2013), Saeki et al. (2015), Wu et al. (2009)
rs10853535/rs10775480	*SLC14A1*	Intronic	Urea transport	Koutros et al. (2013)
rs10936599 (not explored)	*TERC/ MYNN*	Exonic, MYNN	Longer telomeres	Toupance et al. (2020)
rs2242652/rs10069690	*TERT/ CLPTM1L*	Intronic	Alt. splicing (exon 4)	Killedar et al. (2015)
rs710521 → rs4687103	*TP63/ LEPREL1*	Intergenic	Enhancer, miRNA binding	Dudek et al. (2018), Wang et al. (2016b)
rs907611 (not explored)	*LSP1*	Promoter	Inflammation	Beane Freeman et al. (2022)

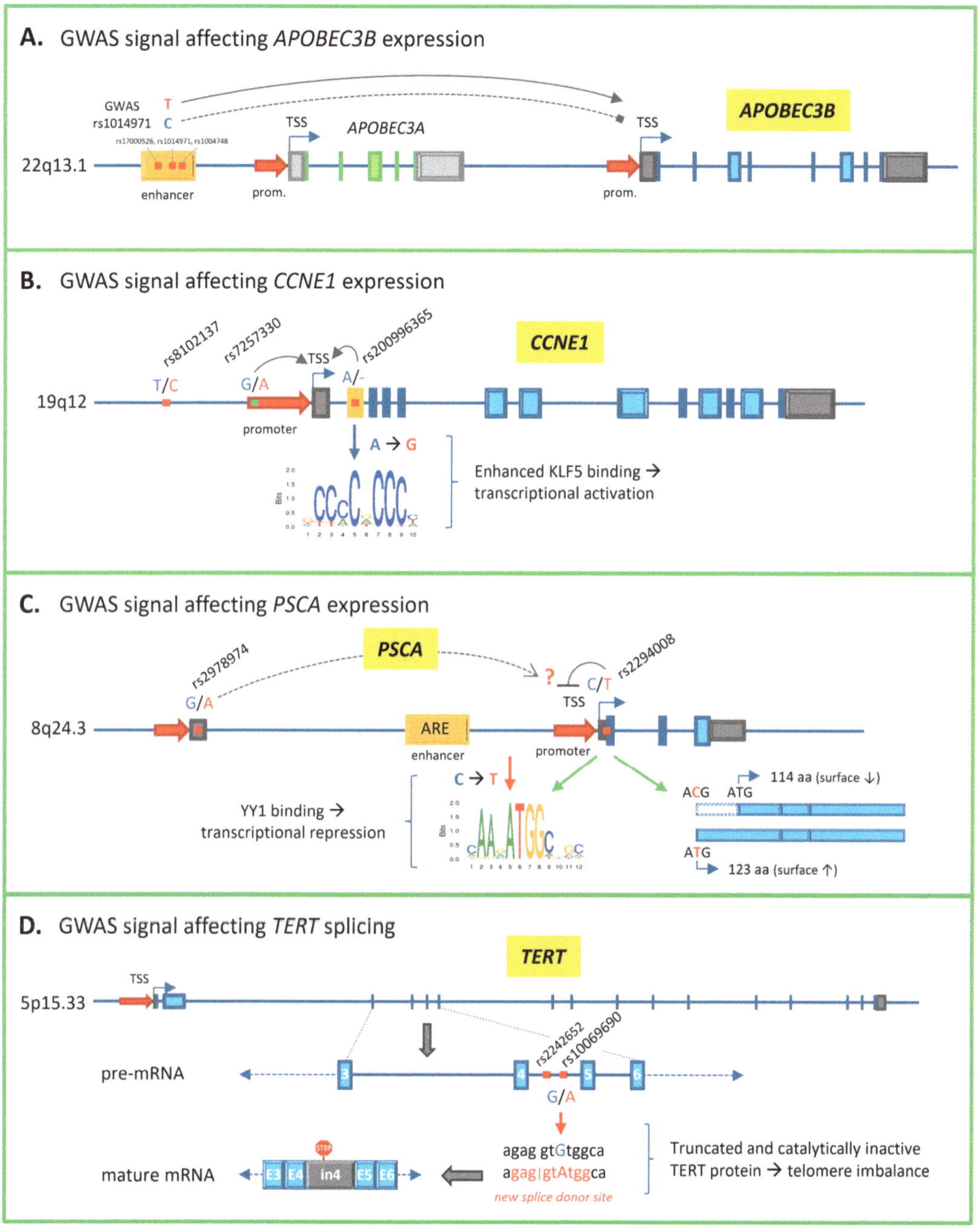

Fig. 2.3 The structure of four selected genes and functional variants. The functional implications of the best characterized GWAS signals in four different gene loci are depicted: (**a**) rs1014971 in *APOBEC3A*/*APOBEC3B*, (**b**) rs8102137, rs7257330, and rs200996365 in *CCNE1*, (**c**) rs2294008 and rs2978974 in *PSCA*, and (**d**) rs2242652 and rs10069690 in *TERT*. Grey boxes, noncoding exons; blue/green boxes, coding exons; small red or green squares, the variant locations; red arrows, gene promoter; orange boxes, enhancers; TSS, transcription start site. Transcription factor binding profiles in B and C are from JASPAR (note the antiparallel orientation of the TF profile and the SNP sequence). Drawings are not to scale. For further details, see text

rs1495741-A), and UGT1A6-rs17863783-G allele. BC is caused by environmental factors such as tobacco smoking (which contains both aromatic amines and polycyclic aromatic hydrocarbons), occupational exposure to aromatic amines (e.g., benzidine, 4-aminobiphenyl, 2-naphthylamine), and water disinfection by-products. N-acetyltransferase 2 (NAT2) protein in the liver can N-acetylate such amines, which transforms some into less reactive intermediates, providing a detoxification step for monoarylamines such as 4-aminobiphenyl and 2-naphthylamine but an activation step for benzidine, an aryldiamine (Hein 2002). On the other hand, cytochrome P450 1A2 (CYP1A2) can N-hydroxylate these amines, leading to the formation of hydroxylamines. Nonconjugated hydroxylamine molecules can be transported to the bladder and undergo O-acetylation by NAT1 to form a highly reactive species that can form DNA adducts.

Phase II detoxification involves additional mechanisms mediated by UGT and SULT enzymes. UDP-glucuronosyltransferases (UGT) catalyze the transfer of the glucuronic acid from UDP-glucuronic acid to 4-aminobiphenyl and its N-hydroxy metabolite. On the other hand, sulfotransferases (SULT) catalyze the sulfate conjugation of aromatic amines such as 4-aminobiphenyl (Glatt and Meinl 2004). These glucuronidated amines become more water-soluble, allowing for easier excretion by the kidneys. It is important to note that certain conjugated amines can be rapidly hydrolyzed in acidic urine, leading to further metabolic activation by NAT1 and the formation of DNA adducts in the urothelium. Notably, a consistently acidic urine pH $\leq$6.0 has been linked to an increased risk of BC among smokers (Alguacil et al. 2011). Through fine-mapping of the rs11892031 GWAS signal within the *UGT1A* gene locus, an uncommon synonymous variant, rs17863783-(Val209Val), was discovered and found to improve the GWAS association in this region (Tang et al. 2012). Importantly, rs17863783 is located within the functional *UGT1A6.1* splicing form, which is highly expressed in the bladder. The protective T allele of rs17863783 has been associated with increased mRNA expression of *UGT1A6.1*, as demonstrated by in vitro exon-trap assays (Tang et al. 2012). This finding suggests that rs17863783 may confer protection against BC by enhancing the removal of carcinogens from the bladder epithelium through the action of the UGT1A6.1 enzyme.

2.2.4.4 DNA Damage Response

Aromatic amines undergo complex metabolic changes, leading to the formation of reactive metabolites that interact with DNA, RNA, and proteins. For instance, 4-aminobiphenyl can covalently bind to DNA, forming adducts such as highly mutagenic and carcinogenic guanine-C8 adducts (Hatcher and Swaminathan 2002; Kadlubar 1994). Moreover, other types of DNA lesions are formed depending on the specific carcinogens and metabolites involved. Nucleotide excision repair (NER) is thought to be the primary mechanism for repairing DNA damage caused by 4-aminobiphenyl. Additionally, various other DNA repair pathways, such as base excision repair (BER), mismatch repair (MMR), and homology-directed repair (HDR), are used based on the type of DNA lesion to be repaired (reviewed in Chatterjee and Walker 2017). The NER pathway recognizes and removes damaged DNA segments containing, for example, C8-guanine-C-8 lesions. BER, on the other hand, specifically recognizes and removes a modified base. MMR primarily corrects errors that arise during DNA replication and recombination. While MMR does not directly repair adducts, it can detect and remove adduct-induced mismatches or insertions/deletions, ensuring accurate DNA repair. Finally, HDR is used to repair DNA double-strand breaks (DSBs) using a homologous DNA template as a guide. DSBs can occur due to various factors such as radiation, chemicals, or errors during DNA replication.

Several factors can influence the repair of carcinogen-induced DNA lesions, including the extent of DNA damage, the availability of repair enzymes, and the efficiency of the repair pathways. Therefore, BC risk-associated pathogenic (P) or likely pathogenic (LP) variants in DNA damage response genes, such as *ATM, BRCA1, BRCA2, CHEK2*, and *RAD50* (HRR), *ERCC2,*

ERCC3, and *ERCC5* (NER), *MUTYH* (BER), and *MLH1, MSH2,* and *MSH6* (MRR), can impact the repair efficiency of DNA adducts/lesions in bladder urothelium. Insufficient or overwhelmed repair mechanisms can result in persistent DNA damage and genomic instability and potentially contribute to mutagenesis and carcinogenesis.

2.2.4.5 *APOBEC3B* (rs1014971)

Somatic mutations of C to T or C to G substitutions in TCA or TCT motifs have been described in bladder tumors and are attributed to the activity of cytidine deaminases belonging to the apolipoprotein B mRNA-editing enzyme, catalytic polypeptide-like (APOBEC) family (Swanton et al. 2015). APOBEC-signature mutagenesis contributes up to 70% of the observed mutations in bladder tumors (Cancer Genome Atlas Research 2014; Robertson et al. 2017). Fine-mapping analysis of a common germline variant, rs1014971, in the *APOBEC3* gene cluster showed that three SNPs, rs1014971, rs1004748, and rs17000526, were strongly associated with BC risk (Middlebrooks et al. 2016). These SNPs are located within a 2 kb genomic region, 20 kb upstream of *APOBEC3B*, in a putative long-distance enhancer region (Fig. 2.3a). Of these equally associated variants, only the rs1014971-T risk allele was exclusively bound by nuclear factors from BC cell lines and linked to elevated *APOBEC3B* expression and genome-wide APOBEC-signature mutations in bladder tumors (Middlebrooks et al. 2016). In BC cell lines, *APOBEC3B* expression was predominantly induced by treatment with DNA-damaging drugs, implying a potential role of environmental oncogenic triggers in individuals with risk rs1014971-T allele.

2.2.4.6 *CCNE1* (rs8102137, rs7257330, and rs200996365)

A GWAS signal, rs8102137, was identified 6 kb upstream of the *CCNE1* gene, which encodes the cell cycle protein cyclin E1. Further genetic fine-mapping analysis showed that rs8102137-C allele is part of a group of 47 linked variants associated with increased BC risk. Among these, a functional promoter variant rs7257330 was strongly associated with aggressive BC (Fu et al. 2014). Nuclear proteins in several cell lines showed strong allele-specific binding to rs7257330, and expression of the CCNE1 gene and protein was found to be increased in cell lines and tumors carrying the rs7257330-A risk allele (Fu et al. 2014). A novel enhancer element was identified within the first intron of *CCNE1* that binds Kruppel-like factor 5 (KLF5). rs200996365, a SNP in high linkage disequilibrium with rs8102137, was found to alter KLF5 binding to this genomic region, thereby regulating *CCNE1* transcription (Pattison et al. 2016) (Fig. 2.3b). Overexpression of cyclin E in cell lines caused a significant acceleration of the cell cycle (Fu et al. 2014), and subtle enhancement of CCNE1 expression from higher risk variants in non-transformed cells could lead to enhanced cell proliferation or genomic instability, predisposing individuals to BC.

2.2.4.7 *PSCA* (rs2294008 and rs2978974)

Prostate stem cell antigen (*PSCA*) gene has been consistently associated with BC risk through a GWAS signal, rs2294008 (Wu et al. 2009). Further analysis of this region revealed another variant, rs2978974, located 10 kb upstream of rs2294008 in an alternative untranslated first exon of *PSCA* (Fu et al. 2012). The risk rs2294008-T allele, which creates an alternative start codon, reduces PSCA promoter activity in vitro (Wu et al. 2009). Paradoxically, the T allele is associated with increased PSCA mRNA and protein expression in bladder tumors (Fu et al. 2012; Kohaar et al. 2013). The non-risk allele of rs2978974 shows strong binding with nuclear proteins (Fu et al. 2012). Therefore, both SNPs may play a role in BC susceptibility through different mechanisms that affect the control of *PSCA* mRNA expression. By creating an alternative start codon, the risk allele rs2294008-T produces protein with longer leader peptide, resulting in surface expression of PSCA (Kohaar et al. 2013) (Fig. 2.3c). In contrast, the BC non-risk rs2294008-C allele is associated with an increased risk of gastric cancer. In gastric cancer cell lines, the rs2294008-T allele suppresses *PSCA* expression by recruiting the polycomb group transcription factor Yin Yang 1 (YY1) to its promoter (Saeki et al. 2015). Immunotherapy against PSCA may be a promising therapeutic strategy for BC patients with high tumor cell surface PSCA expression, which is determined by the BC risk allele rs2294008-T (Kohaar et al. 2013).

2.2.4.8 *SLC14A1* (rs10775480/rs10853535)

Variants rs10775480/rs10853535 are located within the solute carrier family 14, member 1 (*SLC14A1*) gene, which is responsible for urine concentration in the kidney. The association between rs10775480 and urine concentration was measured by determining urinary specific gravity (USG) on overnight urine samples. Each copy of the risk rs10775480 -T allele was associated with decreased USG, with a significant difference between CC and TT genotypes (Koutros et al. 2013). Further analysis revealed high expression of *SLC14A1* mRNA and the absence of *SLC14A2* in bladder tissue, while both transporters were expressed in the kidney (Koutros et al. 2013). These results suggest that the molecular phenotype of this GWAS finding is the genotype-specific biological activity of *SLC14A1* in bladder tissue.

2.2.4.9 *TERC/MYNN* (rs10936599) and *TERT* (rs2242652/rs10069690)

Telomeres play a crucial role in protecting the ends of linear chromosomes from being detected as DNA double-strand breaks, but they become shorter with each round of cell division. Once telomeres reach a critical length, normal human somatic cells enter permanent cell cycle arrest and become senescent. In tumor cells, telomere shortening can impair chromosomal integrity. However, telomerase activity can counteract telomere shortening by adding new telomeric repeat sequences to each end of the chromosomes. Telomerase comprises two subunits: a telomerase reverse transcriptase (TERT) catalytic subunit and a telomerase RNA component (*TERC*). Two GWAS signals associated with BC have been identified within regions for both telomerase subunits, TERC/MYNN-rs10936599 and TERT-rs2242652/rs10096690. Functional in vitro studies have shown that the non-risk TERT-rs10069690-A allele creates a new splice donor site within intron 4 of *TERT* (Fig. 2.3d), leading to alternative splicing of the *TERT* transcript. The resulting truncated isoform includes an in-frame stop codon, causing premature translation termination, yielding a catalytically inactive protein (Killedar et al. 2015). The exonic variant MYNN-rs10936599-C was associated with increased leukocyte telomere length (Toupance et al. 2020). Neither variant is associated with mRNA expression of any genes in TCGA-BLCA dataset, and their functional impact in BC-relevant cell types or tissues is yet to be established.

2.2.4.10 *TP63* (rs710521 and rs35592567)

Tumor protein 63 (TP63, a.k.a. p63), a member of the p53 family of tumor suppressors, plays a vital role in regulating cell growth and differentiation. The GWAS variant rs710521 is located in the intergenic region between the *TP63* and *P3H2* (*LEPREL1*) genes. Fine-mapping studies have identified 20 additional SNPs, including rs4687103, with a stronger association with BC risk than risk rs710521-T allele (Dudek et al. 2018). These TP63 variants are located within active enhancer elements downstream of the *TP63* gene. Biochemical and genetic studies have revealed that the risk allele of rs4687103 is linked to increased expression of *ΔNTP63* and activation of *NOTCH1*. Another SNP, rs35592567, identified in a Han Chinese cohort through fine-mapping of the rs710521 signal, is located in the 3′ untranslated region (UTR) of TP63 (Wang et al. 2016a). Biochemical assays have demonstrated that the non-risk rs35592567-T allele reduces posttranscriptional levels of *TP63* by interfering with the binding efficiency of miR-140-5p (Wang et al. 2016a). Both studies have also revealed that tampering with *TP63* levels, either by CRISPR-Cas9-mediated enhancer knockout or by miR-

140-5p expression, reduces cancer cell survival.

2.2.4.11 *LSP1* (rs907611)

In two case-control studies, a GWAS variant within the promoter of the lymphocyte-specific protein 1 (LSP1) has been associated with BC risk in individuals exposed to disinfection by-products in drinking water. Surprisingly, the GWAS rs907611-A risk allele was protective from BC in individuals with the highest exposure to disinfection by-products. Because LSP1-rs907611-A has been associated with reduced lymphocyte counts, it might be increasing BC risk due to chronic inflammation. On the other hand, in individuals exposed to carcinogenic disinfection by-products, increased lymphocyte infiltration would facilitate more efficient immune surveillance, potentially preventing tumor initiation and development. Thus, this GWAS signal provides a suggestive example of gene-environment interaction on BC risk (Beane Freeman et al. 2022).

2.3 Relevance for Public Health and Bladder Cancer Patients

2.3.1 Screening of Patients and Relatives

The risk of BC for relatives of a BC patient seems to be increased by 1.5- to twofold. This means that the absolute risk of developing BC within the next 10 years for a 50- or 60-year-old female in the United States is still below 1%, even including nonaggressive Ta tumors (Richters et al. 2020). For males, this absolute risk is somewhat higher (about 1.5%), but the difference with females is caused at least partly by a higher historical smoking prevalence among males. Such small absolute risks do not suggest that screening of relatives of a BC patient is useful. Because of the rarity of families with two or more BC patients in the first-degree relatives, it is unclear whether screening of unaffected relatives in such families should be performed. However, whether or not such screening is efficient, high-risk families may consult healthcare providers. In that case, there is no standardized screening protocol yet (see Chap. 18). A recommendation could be to start screening 5 years before the earliest age at diagnosis in the family with a cystoscopy or an ultrasound if the cystoscopy is considered too invasive, together with a urinary biomarker such as the Xpert Bladder Cancer Monitor or the Bladder EpiCheck methylation test. Thereafter, the urinary biomarker test could be repeated annually or even more frequently. The same protocol could be used in known carriers of a high-penetrance mutation in *MSH2*, but, given the increased risk for upper tract urothelial carcinoma in particular, screening should include proper evaluation of the ureters via, for example, a CT urogram. This screening protocol could also be applied in carriers of other P/LP variant alleles (Table 2.2) and *HRAS*, although the absolute risk of BC for these carriers is probably still very small. Identification of these germline P/LP variants in BC patients, either directly via germline sequencing or triggered by results of tumor sequencing, may however warrant screening of BC patients and carriers among relatives for other types of cancer (Table 2.2) (Lincoln et al. 2020; Mandelker et al. 2019). Increased understanding of actionable germline variants underlying BC and their potential interaction with somatic mutations and a reduction in the cost of genetic testing may pave the way toward a clinical cancer genetic approach with improved cancer screening in BC patients and family members (Vlachostergios et al. 2020).

2.3.2 Polygenic Risk Scores and Population Screening

The effects of germline susceptibility variants along with those of environmental factors can be combined into a polygenic risk score (PRS). This was recently done by Koutros and colleagues using data on smoking and 24 genetic markers identified from GWAS (Fig. 2.4) (Koutros et al. 2023). Individuals in the highest risk decile had a fourfold higher risk than those in the lowest decile in each of the three smoking categories

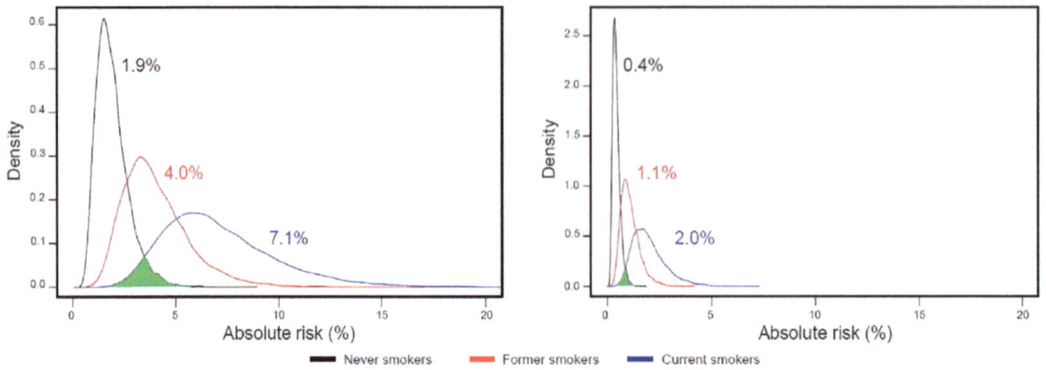

Fig. 2.4 Example of PRS for BC risk among white non-Hispanic males (L) and females (R). Population density plots of the entire absolute risk distributions for male (Left) and female (Right) never, former, and current smokers. Green shading depicts the overlap in absolute risk distribution for never and current smokers, indicating that some proportion of never smokers at high genetic risk have the same absolute risk of BC as current smokers at low genetic risk (Source: S. Koutros, L.A. Kiemeney, P. Pal Choudhury et al., Genome-wide Association Study of Bladder Cancer Reveals New Biological and Translational Insights, Eur Urol (2023), https://doi.org/10.1016/j.eururo.2023.04.020)

(never, former, current). For never-smoking males, the lifetime risk of BC ranged from 0.9% to 3.5% in the lowest to highest PRS deciles. For currently smoking males, the lifetime risk ranged from 3.4% to 13.0% by PRS deciles. The ranges in never-smoking and currently smoking females were 0.2% to 0.8% and 0.9% to 3.7%, respectively. The lifetime risk for the highest one percentile smoking men and women was 18% and 5.3%, respectively. This suggests that the PRS might be used to select high-risk groups for future more intensive screening or other preventative interventions. However, the current PRS would need to be based on larger GWAS that fully characterize the genetic architecture of BC and include all important lifestyle, occupational, and environmental risk factors before it would be ready for evaluation in the clinical setting and/or public health. The efficacy of applying prevention modalities in subgroups at higher risk of developing BC would need to be tested in controlled trials before they could be implemented.

2.3.3 Therapy and Future Outlook

Identification of germline mutations and predisposition variants for BC and the functional characterization of GWAS signals for BC risk has provided a significant advance in our understanding of this disease. It has shed light on the underlying genes, pathways, and mechanisms, thus offering crucial knowledge regarding BC initiation and development. These novel insights could lead to the implementation of novel preventative strategies for disease management or the development of targeted therapies to treat BC. For specific patient groups, this may already be the case (Waarts et al. 2022). If and when selection of treatment on germline P/LP (or somatic) variants in BC is relevant is presently unclear. Available studies in BC are focused on somatic variants and limited to small phase II studies and case reports. For P/LP DDR variants and poly-(ADP-ribose)-polymerase (PARP)-inhibitors, such as olaparib and rucaparib, these show inconsistent and inconclusive results (Crabb et al. 2023; Grivas et al. 2021; Powles et al. 2021; Rosenberg et al. 2023; Sweis et al. 2018). Patients with germline P/LP variant alleles in MMR genes and (resulting) MSI-H/dMMR, high TMB, and high tumor neoantigen production may show improved response to immune checkpoint inhibitors such as pembrolizumab (Le et al. 2017; Le et al. 2015; Marcus et al. 2019; Shah et al. 2022) although this is not supported by presently available data for durvalumab and BC (Powles et al. 2021).

Progress has been made in identification of common germline DNA variants that affect drug response and treatment-related toxicities in cancer and hence warrant dose reduction or close monitoring of patients during treatment. The Table of Pharmacogenetic Associations that is published and maintained by the US Food and Drug Administration (FDA) contains an overview of relevant pharmacogenetic associations which includes the advice to monitor erdafitinib-treated patients who are poor metabolizers based on germline *CYP2C9* genotype for adverse reactions (Table of Pharmacogenetic Associations | FDA). Future studies into therapy response and toxicity in the field of BC, for example, the study from Khan et al. that showed that a PRS for dermatological autoimmunity impacts immune-related adverse effects of the skin and overall survival of BC patients treated with atezolizumab in comparison with chemotherapy, may lead to novel BC pharmacogenetic associations.

References

Aben KK, Macville MV, Smeets DF, Schoenberg MP, Witjes JA, Kiemeney LA (2001) Absence of karyotype abnormalities in patients with familial urothelial cell carcinoma. Urology 57(2):266–269. https://doi.org/10.1016/s0090-4295(00)00905-5

Aben KK, Witjes JA, Schoenberg MP, Hulsbergen-van de Kaa C, Verbeek AL, Kiemeney LA (2002) Familial aggregation of urothelial cell carcinoma. Int J Cancer 98(2):274–278. https://doi.org/10.1002/ijc.10191

Aben KK, Baglietto L, Baffoe-Bonnie A, Coebergh JW, Bailey-Wilson JE, Trink B, Verbeek AL, Schoenberg MP, Alfred Witjes J, Kiemeney LA (2006) Segregation analysis of urothelial cell carcinoma. Eur J Cancer 42(10):1428–1433. https://doi.org/10.1016/j.ejca.2005.07.039

Alguacil J, Kogevinas M, Silverman DT, Malats N, Real FX, Garcia-Closas M, Tardon A, Rivas M, Tora M, Garcia-Closas R, Serra C, Carrato A, Pfeiffer RM, Fortuny J, Samanic C, Rothman N (2011) Urinary pH, cigarette smoking and bladder cancer risk. Carcinogenesis 32(6):843–847. https://doi.org/10.1093/carcin/bgr048

Astiazaran-Symonds E, Ney GM, Higgs C, Oba L, Srivastava R, Livinski AA, Rosenberg PS, Stewart DR (2023) Cancer in Costello syndrome: a systematic review and meta-analysis. Br J Cancer 128:2089. https://doi.org/10.1038/s41416-023-02229-7

Barrow PJ, Ingham S, O'Hara C, Green K, McIntyre I, Lalloo F, Hill J, Evans DG (2013) The spectrum of urological malignancy in Lynch syndrome. Fam Cancer 12(1):57–63. https://doi.org/10.1007/s10689-012-9573-z

Beane Freeman LE, Kogevinas M, Cantor KP, Villanueva CM, Prokunina-Olsson L, Florez-Vargas O, Figueroa JD, Ward MH, Koutros S, Baris D, Garcia-Closas M, Schwenn M, Johnson A, Serra C, Tardon A, Garcia-Closas R, Carrato A, Malats N, Karagas MR, Silverman DT et al (2022) Disinfection by-products in drinking water and bladder cancer: evaluation of risk modification by common genetic polymorphisms in two case-control studies. Environ Health Perspect 130(5):57006. https://doi.org/10.1289/EHP9895

Benton B, Henderson BE (1973) Environmental exposure and bladder cancer in young males. J Natl Cancer Inst 51(1):269–270. https://doi.org/10.1093/jnci/51.1.269

Bermejo JL, Eng C, Hemminki K (2005) Cancer characteristics in Swedish families fulfilling criteria for hereditary nonpolyposis colorectal cancer. Gastroenterology 129(6):1889–1899. https://doi.org/10.1053/j.gastro.2005.09.012

Bermejo JL, Sundquist J, Hemminki K (2009) Sex-specific familial risks of urinary bladder cancer and associated neoplasms in Sweden. Int J Cancer 124(9):2166–2171. https://doi.org/10.1002/ijc.24178

Berry JL, Polski A, Cavenee WK, Dryja TP, Murphree AL, Gallie BL (2019) The RB1 story: characterization and cloning of the first tumor suppressor gene. Genes (Basel) 10(11). https://doi.org/10.3390/genes10110879

Beukers W, Hercegovac A, Zwarthoff EC (2014) HRAS mutations in bladder cancer at an early age and the possible association with the Costello syndrome. Eur J Hum Genet 22(6):837–839. https://doi.org/10.1038/ejhg.2013.251

Bhattacharya P, McHugh TW (2023) Lynch syndrome. In StatPearls. https://www.ncbi.nlm.nih.gov/pubmed/28613748

Bleoo SL, Godbout R, Rayner D, Tamimi Y, Moore RB (2003) Leiomyosarcoma of the bladder in a retinoblastoma patient. Urol Int 71(1):118–121. https://doi.org/10.1159/000071109

Brioude F, Toutain A, Giabicani E, Cottereau E, Cormier-Daire V, Netchine I (2019) Overgrowth syndromes - clinical and molecular aspects and tumour risk. Nat Rev Endocrinol 15(5):299–311. https://doi.org/10.1038/s41574-019-0180-z

Brown R, Donnelly DE, Allen D, Loughrey MB, Morrison PJ (2014) Familial urothelial cell carcinoma of the bladder with autosomal dominant inheritance and late onset phenotype. Springerplus 3:281. https://doi.org/10.1186/2193-1801-3-281

Cancer Genome Atlas Research, N (2014) Comprehensive molecular characterization of urothelial bladder carcinoma. Nature 507(7492):315–322. https://doi.org/10.1038/nature12965

Cao C, Fu Z, Liu Y, Zhou A, Wang J, Shou J (2021) A muscle-invasive bladder cancer patient with high tumor mutational burden and RB1 mutation achieved bladder preservation following chemotherapy combined with immunotherapy: a case report. Front Immunol 12:684879. https://doi.org/10.3389/fimmu.2021.684879

Carlo MI, Ravichandran V, Srinavasan P, Bandlamudi C, Kemel Y, Ceyhan-Birsoy O, Mukherjee S, Mandelker D, Chaim J, Knezevic A, Rana S, Fnu Z, Breen K, Arnold AG, Khurram A, Tkachuk K, Cipolla CK, Regazzi A, Hakimi AA, Offit K et al (2020) Cancer susceptibility mutations in patients with urothelial malignancies. J Clin Oncol 38(5):406–414. https://doi.org/10.1200/JCO.19.01395

Carreon T, Ruder AM, Schulte PA, Hayes RB, Rothman N, Waters M, Grant DJ, Boissy R, Bell DA, Kadlubar FF, Hemstreet GP 3rd, Yin S, LeMasters GK (2006) NAT2 slow acetylation and bladder cancer in workers exposed to benzidine. Int J Cancer 118(1):161–168. https://doi.org/10.1002/ijc.21308

Cartwright RA, Glashan RW, Rogers HJ, Ahmad RA, Barham-Hall D, Higgins E, Kahn MA (1982) Role of N-acetyltransferase phenotypes in bladder carcinogenesis: a pharmacogenetic epidemiological approach to bladder cancer. Lancet 2(8303):842–845. https://doi.org/10.1016/s0140-6736(82)90810-8

Chatterjee N, Walker GC (2017) Mechanisms of DNA damage, repair, and mutagenesis. Environ Mol Mutagen 58(5):235–263. https://doi.org/10.1002/em.22087

Chaussade A, Millot G, Wells C, Brisse H, Lae M, Savignoni A, Desjardins L, Dendale R, Doz F, Aerts I, Jimenez I, Cassoux N, Stoppa Lyonnet D, Gauthier Villars M, Houdayer C (2019) Correlation between RB1germline mutations and second primary malignancies in hereditary retinoblastoma patients treated with external beam radiotherapy. Eur J Med Genet 62(3):217–223. https://doi.org/10.1016/j.ejmg.2018.07.017

Chen T, Jackson C, Costello B, Singer N, Colligan B, Douglass L, Pemberton J, Deddens J, Graff JR, Carter JH (2004) An intronic variant of the TGFBR1 gene is associated with carcinomas of the kidney and bladder. Int J Cancer 112(3):420–425. https://doi.org/10.1002/ijc.20419

Chen S, Francioli LC, Goodrich JK, Collins RL, Kanai M, Wang Q, Alföldi J, Watts NA, Vittal C, Gauthier LD, Poterba T, Wilson MW, Tarasova Y, Phu W, Yohannes MT, Koenig Z, Farjoun Y, Banks E, Donnelly S, Karczewski KJ et al (2022) A genome-wide mutational constraint map quantified from variation in 76,156 human genomes. bioRxiv 2022.2003.2020.485034. https://doi.org/10.1101/2022.03.20.485034

Consortium, G. T (2015) Human genomics. The genotype-tissue expression (GTEx) pilot analysis: multitissue gene regulation in humans. Science 348(6235):648–660. https://doi.org/10.1126/science.1262110

Costello JM (1971) New syndrome. N Z Med J 74(475): 397-&. <Go to ISI>://WOS:A1971L587900034

Cote RJ, Dunn MD, Chatterjee SJ, Stein JP, Shi SR, Tran QC, Hu SX, Xu HJ, Groshen S, Taylor CR, Skinner DG, Benedict WF (1998) Elevated and absent pRb expression is associated with bladder cancer progression and has cooperative effects with p53. Cancer Res 58(6):1090–1094. https://www.ncbi.nlm.nih.gov/pubmed/9515785

Crabb SJ, Hussain S, Soulis E, Hinsley S, Dempsey L, Trevethan A, Song Y, Barber J, Frew J, Gale J, Faust G, Brock S, McGovern U, Parikh O, Enting D, Sundar S, Ratnayake G, Lees K, Birtle AJ, Jones RJ et al (2023) A randomized, double-blind, biomarker-selected, phase II clinical trial of maintenance poly ADP-ribose polymerase inhibition with Rucaparib following chemotherapy for metastatic urothelial carcinoma. J Clin Oncol 41(1):54–64. https://doi.org/10.1200/JCO.22.00405

Czene K, Lichtenstein P, Hemminki K (2002) Environmental and heritable causes of cancer among 9.6 million individuals in the Swedish family-cancer database. Int J Cancer 99(2):260–266. https://doi.org/10.1002/ijc.10332

de la Chapelle A (2005) The incidence of Lynch syndrome. Fam Cancer 4(3):233–237. https://doi.org/10.1007/s10689-004-5811-3

Doddamani SC, Bhat S, Jacob A (2015) Urinary bladder leiomyosarcoma following radiotherapy in a patient with bilateral retinoblastoma: a case report. Indian J Urol 31(4):366–368. https://doi.org/10.4103/0970-1591.166471

Dommering CJ, Marees T, van der Hout AH, Imhof SM, Meijers-Heijboer H, Ringens PJ, van Leeuwen FE, Moll AC (2012) RB1 mutations and second primary malignancies after hereditary retinoblastoma. Fam Cancer 11(2):225–233. https://doi.org/10.1007/s10689-011-9505-3

Dong C, Hemminki K (2001) Modification of cancer risks in offspring by sibling and parental cancers from 2,112,616 nuclear families. Int J Cancer 92(1):144–150. https://www.ncbi.nlm.nih.gov/pubmed/11279618

Dudek AM, Vermeulen SH, Kolev D, Grotenhuis AJ, Kiemeney L, Verhaegh GW (2018) Identification of an enhancer region within the TP63/LEPREL1 locus containing genetic variants associated with bladder cancer risk. Cell Oncol (Dordr) 41(5):555–568. https://doi.org/10.1007/s13402-018-0393-5

Egilsson V, Einarsson GV, Thorhallsson P, Ingvarsson S (1993) Urinary system tumours in a family. Eur J Cancer 29A(16):2335–2336. https://doi.org/10.1016/0959-8049(93)90233-6

Elze L, van der Post RS, Vos JR, Mensenkamp AR, de Hullu MSC, Nagtegaal ID, Hoogerbrugge N, de Voer RM, Ligtenberg MJL (2023) Microsatellite instability in non-colorectal and non-endometrial malignancies in patients with Lynch syndrome. J Natl Cancer Inst 115:853. https://doi.org/10.1093/jnci/djad063

Engel LS, Taioli E, Pfeiffer R, Garcia-Closas M, Marcus PM, Lan Q, Boffetta P, Vineis P, Autrup H, Bell DA, Branch RA, Brockmoller J, Daly AK, Heckbert SR, Kalina I, Kang D, Katoh T, Lafuente A, Lin HJ, Rothman N et al (2002) Pooled analysis and meta-analysis of glutathione S-transferase M1 and bladder cancer: a HuGE review. Am J Epidemiol 156(2):95–109. https://doi.org/10.1093/aje/kwf018

Engel C, Loeffler M, Steinke V, Rahner N, Holinski-Feder E, Dietmaier W, Schackert HK, Goergens H, von Knebel Doeberitz M, Goecke TO, Schmiegel W, Buettner R, Moeslein G, Letteboer TG, Gomez Garcia E, Hes FJ, Hoogerbrugge N, Menko FH, van Os TA, Vasen HF et al (2012) Risks of less common cancers in proven mutation carriers with lynch syndrome. J Clin Oncol 30(35):4409–4415. https://doi.org/10.1200/JCO.2012.43.2278

Fakhoury M, Hwang RR, Silletti J, Bjurlin MA (2016) Bladder Leiomyosarcoma: A rare, but aggressive diagnosis. Curr Urol 9(3):166–168. https://doi.org/10.1159/000447135

FDA. Table of pharmacogenetic associations. Retrieved May 15, 2023 from fda.gov/medical-devices/precision-medicine/table-pharmacogenetic-associations

Figueroa JD, Han SS, Garcia-Closas M, Baris D, Jacobs EJ, Kogevinas M, Schwenn M, Malats N, Johnson A, Purdue MP, Caporaso N, Landi MT, Prokunina-Olsson L, Wang ZM, Hutchinson A, Burdette L, Wheeler W, Vineis P, Siddiq A, Silverman DT et al (2014) Genome-wide interaction study of smoking and bladder cancer risk. Carcinogenesis 35(8):1737–1744. https://doi.org/10.1093/carcin/bgu064

Figueroa JD, Koutros S, Colt JS, Kogevinas M, Garcia-Closas M, Real FX, Friesen MC, Baris D, Stewart P, Schwenn M, Johnson A, Karagas MR, Armenti KR, Moore LE, Schned A, Lenz P, Prokunina Olsson L, Banday AR, Paquin A, Silverman DT et al (2015) Modification of occupational exposures on bladder cancer risk by common genetic polymorphisms. J Natl Cancer Inst 107(11):djv223. https://doi.org/10.1093/jnci/djv223

Figueroa JD, Middlebrooks CD, Banday AR, Ye Y, Garcia-Closas M, Chatterjee N, Koutros S, Kiemeney LA, Rafnar T, Bishop T, Furberg H, Matullo G, Golka K, Gago-Dominguez M, Taylor JA, Fletcher T, Siddiq A, Cortessis VK, Kooperberg C, Rothman N et al (2016) Identification of a novel susceptibility locus at 13q34 and refinement of the 20p12.2 region as a multi-signal locus associated with bladder cancer risk in individuals of European ancestry. Hum Mol Genet 25(6):1203–1214. https://doi.org/10.1093/hmg/ddv492

Fletcher O, Easton D, Anderson K, Gilham C, Jay M, Peto J (2004) Lifetime risks of common cancers among retinoblastoma survivors. J Natl Cancer Inst 96(5):357–363. https://doi.org/10.1093/jnci/djh058

Flint ND, Bishop MD, Smart TC, Strunck JL, Boucher KM, Grossman D, Secrest AM (2021) Low accuracy of self-reported family history of melanoma in high-risk patients. Fam Cancer 20(1):41–48. https://doi.org/10.1007/s10689-020-00187-0

Franceschini P, Licata D, Di Cara G, Guala A, Bianchi M, Ingrosso G, Franceschini D (1999) Bladder carcinoma in Costello syndrome: report on a patient born to consanguineous parents and review. Am J Med Genet 86(2):174–179. https://www.ncbi.nlm.nih.gov/pubmed/10449656

Fraumeni JF Jr, Thomas LB (1967) Malignant bladder tumors in a man and his three sons. JAMA 201(7):507–509

Fu YP, Kohaar I, Rothman N, Earl J, Figueroa JD, Ye Y, Malats N, Tang W, Liu L, Garcia-Closas M, Muchmore B, Chatterjee N, Tarway M, Kogevinas M, Porter-Gill P, Baris D, Mumy A, Albanes D, Purdue MP, Prokunina-Olsson L et al (2012) Common genetic variants in the PSCA gene influence gene expression and bladder cancer risk. Proc Natl Acad Sci USA 109(13):4974–4979. https://doi.org/10.1073/pnas.1202189109

Fu YP, Kohaar I, Moore LE, Lenz P, Figueroa JD, Tang W, Porter-Gill P, Chatterjee N, Scott-Johnson A, Garcia-Closas M, Muchmore B, Baris D, Paquin A, Ylaya K, Schwenn M, Apolo AB, Karagas MR, Tarway M, Johnson A, Prokunina-Olsson L et al (2014) The 19q12 bladder cancer GWAS signal: association with cyclin E function and aggressive disease. Cancer Res 74(20):5808–5818. https://doi.org/10.1158/0008-5472.CAN-14-1531

Galesloot TE, Grotenhuis AJ, Kolev D, Aben KK, Bryan RT, Catto JWF, Cheng KK, Conroy S, Dyrskjot L, Fleshner NE, James ND, Lamy P, Lindskrog SV, Malats N, Mengual L, Verhaegh G, Zeegers MP, Kiemeney L, Vermeulen SH (2022) Genome-wide meta-analysis identifies novel genes associated with recurrence and progression in non-muscle-invasive bladder cancer. Eur Urol Oncol 5(1):70–83. https://doi.org/10.1016/j.euo.2021.07.001

Garcia-Closas M, Malats N, Silverman D, Dosemeci M, Kogevinas M, Hein DW, Tardon A, Serra C, Carrato A, Garcia-Closas R, Lloreta J, Castano-Vinyals G, Yeager M, Welch R, Chanock S, Chatterjee N, Wacholder S, Samanic C, Tora M, Rothman N et al (2005) NAT2 slow acetylation, GSTM1 null genotype, and risk of bladder cancer: results from the Spanish bladder cancer study and meta-analyses. Lancet 366(9486):649–659. https://doi.org/10.1016/S0140-6736(05)67137-1

Garcia-Closas M, Hein DW, Silverman D, Malats N, Yeager M, Jacobs K, Doll MA, Figueroa JD, Baris D, Schwenn M, Kogevinas M, Johnson A, Chatterjee N, Moore LE, Moeller T, Real FX, Chanock S, Rothman N (2011a) A single nucleotide polymorphism tags variation in the arylamine N-acetyltransferase 2 phenotype in populations of European background. Pharmacogenet Genomics 21(4):231–236. https://doi.org/10.1097/FPC.0b013e32833e1b54

Garcia-Closas M, Ye YQ, Rothman N, Figueroa JD, Malats N, Dinney CP, Chatterjee N, Prokunina-Olsson L, Wang ZM, Lin J, Real FX, Jacobs KB, Baris D, Thun M, De Vivo I, Albanes D, Purdue MP, Kogevinas

M, Kamat AM, Wu XF et al (2011b) A genome-wide association study of bladder cancer identifies a new susceptibility locus within SLC14A1, a urea transporter gene on chromosome 18q12.3. Hum Mol Genet 20(21):4282–4289. https://doi.org/10.1093/hmg/ddr342

Garcia-Closas M, Rothman N, Figueroa JD, Prokunina-Olsson L, Han SS, Baris D, Jacobs EJ, Malats N, De Vivo I, Albanes D, Purdue MP, Sharma S, Fu YP, Kogevinas M, Wang Z, Tang W, Tardon A, Serra C, Carrato A, Chatterjee N et al (2013) Common genetic polymorphisms modify the effect of smoking on absolute risk of bladder cancer. Cancer Res 73(7):2211–2220. https://doi.org/10.1158/0008-5472.Can-12-2388

Geary J, Sasieni P, Houlston R, Izatt L, Eeles R, Payne SJ, Fisher S, Hodgson SV (2008) Gene-related cancer spectrum in families with hereditary non-polyposis colorectal cancer (HNPCC). Fam Cancer 7(2):163–172. https://doi.org/10.1007/s10689-007-9164-6

Gerald T, Margulis V, Meng X, Bagrodia A, Cole S, Qin Q, Call SG, Mauer E, Lotan Y, Woldu SL (2023) Actionable genomic landscapes from a real-world cohort of urothelial carcinoma patients. Urol Oncol 41(3):148 e117–148 e124. https://doi.org/10.1016/j.urolonc.2022.12.008

Giannoulatou E, McVean G, Taylor IB, McGowan SJ, Maher GJ, Iqbal Z, Pfeifer SP, Turner I, Burkitt Wright EM, Shorto J, Itani A, Turner K, Gregory L, Buck D, Rajpert-De Meyts E, Looijenga LH, Kerr B, Wilkie AO, Goriely A (2013) Contributions of intrinsic mutation rate and selfish selection to levels of de novo HRAS mutations in the paternal germline. Proc Natl Acad Sci USA 110(50):20152–20157. https://doi.org/10.1073/pnas.1311381110

Glatt H, Meinl W (2004) Pharmacogenetics of soluble sulfotransferases (SULTs). Naunyn Schmiedeberg's Arch Pharmacol 369(1):55–68. https://doi.org/10.1007/s00210-003-0826-0

Goldgar DE, Easton DF, Cannon-Albright LA, Skolnick MH (1994) Systematic population-based assessment of cancer risk in first-degree relatives of cancer probands. J Natl Cancer Inst 86(21):1600–1608. https://doi.org/10.1093/jnci/86.21.1600

Gregersen PA, Olsen MH, Urbak SF, Funding M, Dalton SO, Overgaard J, Alsner J (2020) Incidence and mortality of second primary cancers in Danish patients with retinoblastoma, 1943-2013. JAMA Netw Open 3(10):e2022126. https://doi.org/10.1001/jamanetworkopen.2020.22126

Gripp KW (2005) Tumor predisposition in Costello syndrome. Am J Med Genet C Semin Med Genet 137C(1):72–77. https://doi.org/10.1002/ajmg.c.30065

Gripp KW, Lin AE (2012) Costello syndrome: a Ras/mitogen activated protein kinase pathway syndrome (rasopathy) resulting from HRAS germline mutations. Genet Med 14(3):285–292. https://doi.org/10.1038/gim.0b013e31822dd91f

Gripp KW, Scott CI Jr, Nicholson L, Figueroa TE (2000) Second case of bladder carcinoma in a patient with Costello syndrome. Am J Med Genet 90(3):256–259. https://doi.org/10.1002/(sici)1096--8628(20000131)90:3<256::aid-ajmg16>3.0.co;2-d

Gripp KW, Scott CI Jr, Nicholson L, McDonald-McGinn DM, Ozeran JD, Jones MC, Lin AE, Zackai EH (2002) Five additional Costello syndrome patients with rhabdomyosarcoma: proposal for a tumor screening protocol. Am J Med Genet 108(1):80–87. https://doi.org/10.1002/ajmg.10241

Gripp KW, Stabley DL, Nicholson L, Hoffman JD, Sol-Church K (2006) Somatic mosaicism for an HRAS mutation causes Costello syndrome. Am J Med Genet A 140(20):2163–2169. https://doi.org/10.1002/ajmg.a.31456

Gripp KW, Morse LA, Axelrad M, Chatfield KC, Chidekel A, Dobyns W, Doyle D, Kerr B, Lin AE, Schwartz DD, Sibbles BJ, Siegel D, Shankar SP, Stevenson DA, Thacker MM, Weaver KN, White SM, Rauen KA (2019) Costello syndrome: clinical phenotype, genotype, and management guidelines. Am J Med Genet A 179(9):1725–1744. https://doi.org/10.1002/ajmg.a.61270

Grivas P, Loriot Y, Morales-Barrera R, Teo MY, Zakharia Y, Feyerabend S, Vogelzang NJ, Grande E, Adra N, Alva A, Necchi A, Rodriguez-Vida A, Gupta S, Josephs DH, Srinivas S, Wride K, Thomas D, Simmons A, Loehr A, Chowdhury S et al (2021) Efficacy and safety of rucaparib in previously treated, locally advanced or metastatic urothelial carcinoma from a phase 2, open-label trial (ATLAS). BMC Cancer 21(1):593. https://doi.org/10.1186/s12885-021-08085-z

Grotenhuis AJ, Dudek AM, Verhaegh GW, Aben KK, Witjes JA, Kiemeney LA, Vermeulen SH (2016) Independent replication of published germline polymorphisms associated with urinary bladder cancer prognosis and treatment response. Bladder Cancer 2(1):77–89. https://doi.org/10.3233/BLC-150027

Guo Z, Linn JF, Wu G, Anzick SL, Eisenberger CF, Halachmi S, Cohen Y, Fomenkov A, Hoque MO, Okami K, Steiner G, Engles JM, Osada M, Moon C, Ratovitski E, Trent JM, Meltzer PS, Westra WH, Kiemeney LA, Trink B et al (2004) CDC91L1 (PIG-U) is a newly discovered oncogene in human bladder cancer. Nat Med 10(4):374–381. https://doi.org/10.1038/nm1010

Hanson HA, Leiser CL, O'Neil B, Martin C, Gupta S, Smith KR, Dechet C, Lowrance WT, Madsen MJ, Camp NJ (2020) Harnessing population pedigree data and machine learning methods to identify patterns of familial bladder cancer risk. Cancer Epidemiol Biomarkers Prev 29(5):918–926. https://doi.org/10.1158/1055-9965.EPI-19-0681

Hatcher JF, Swaminathan S (2002) Identification of N-(deoxyguanosin-8-yl)-4-azobiphenyl by (32) P-postlabeling analyses of DNA in human uroepithelial cells exposed to proximate metabolites of the environmental carcinogen 4-aminobiphenyl. Environ

Mol Mutagen 39(4):314–322. https://doi.org/10.1002/em.10079
Hayes JD, Strange RC (2000) Glutathione S-transferase polymorphisms and their biological consequences. Pharmacology 61(3):154–166. https://doi.org/10.1159/000028396
Hein DW (2002) Molecular genetics and function of NAT1 and NAT2: role in aromatic amine metabolism and carcinogenesis. Mutat Res 506-507:65–77. https://doi.org/10.1016/s0027-5107(02)00153-7
Hidaka A, Sawada N, Svensson T, Goto A, Yamaji T, Shimazu T, Iwasaki M, Inoue M, Tsugane S, Group, J. S (2020) Family history of cancer and subsequent risk of cancer: a large-scale population-based prospective study in Japan. Int J Cancer 147(2):331–337. https://doi.org/10.1002/ijc.32724
Huang KL, Mashl RJ, Wu Y, Ritter DI, Wang J, Oh C, Paczkowska M, Reynolds S, Wyczalkowski MA, Oak N, Scott AD, Krassowski M, Cherniack AD, Houlahan KE, Jayasinghe R, Wang LB, Zhou DC, Liu D, Cao S, Ding L et al (2018) Pathogenic germline variants in 10,389 adult cancers. Cell 173(2):355–370 e314. https://doi.org/10.1016/j.cell.2018.03.039
Ilic M, Stojadinovic M, Milosavljevic Z (2011) Familial aggregation of bladder cancer. Vojnosanit Pregl 68(5):447–451. https://doi.org/10.2298/vsp1105447i
Iotchkova V, Ritchie GRS, Geihs M, Morganella S, Min JL, Walter K, Timpson NJ, Consortium, U. K, Dunham I, Birney E, Soranzo N (2019) GARFIELD classifies disease-relevant genomic features through integration of functional annotations with association signals. Nat Genet 51(2):343–353. https://doi.org/10.1038/s41588-018-0322-6
Joost P, Therkildsen C, Dominguez-Valentin M, Jonsson M, Nilbert M (2015) Urinary tract cancer in Lynch syndrome; increased risk in carriers of MSH2 mutations. Urology 86(6):1212–1217. https://doi.org/10.1016/j.urology.2015.08.018
Kadlubar FF (1994) DNA adducts of carcinogenic aromatic amines. IARC Sci Publ(125), 199–216. https://www.ncbi.nlm.nih.gov/pubmed/7806313
Kenet G, Mandel M, Mor Y, Toren A, Jonas P, Kende G, Rechavi G, Neumann Y (1995) Genetic predisposition and cyclophosphamide treatment in a girl with bladder carcinoma? Med Pediatr Oncol 24(4):269–270. https://doi.org/10.1002/mpo.2950240411
Khan Z, Di Nucci F, Kwan A, Hammer C, Mariathasan S, Rouilly V, Carroll J, Fontes M, Ley Acosta S, Guardino E, Chen-Harris H, Bhangale T, Mellman I, Rosenberg J, Powles T, Hunkapiller J, Chandler GS, Albert ML (2020) Polygenic risk for skin autoimmunity impacts immune checkpoint blockade in bladder cancer. Proc Natl Acad Sci USA 117(22):12288–12294. https://doi.org/10.1073/pnas.1922867117
Kiemeney LA (2008) Hereditary bladder cancer. Scand J Urol Nephrol Suppl(218):110–115. https://doi.org/10.1080/03008880802283755
Kiemeney LA, Moret NC, Witjes JA, Schoenberg MP, Tulinius H (1997) Familial transitional cell carcinoma among the population of Iceland. J Urol 157(5):1649–1651. https://www.ncbi.nlm.nih.gov/pubmed/9112497
Kiemeney LA, Kuiper RP, Pfundt R, van Reijmersdal S, Schoenberg MP, Aben KK, Niermeijer MF, Witjes JA, Schoenmakers EF (2006) No evidence for large-scale germline genomic aberrations in hereditary bladder cancer patients with high-resolution array-based comparative genomic hybridization. Cancer Epidemiol Biomarkers Prev 15(1):180–183. https://doi.org/10.1158/1055-9965.EPI-05-0714
Kiemeney LA, Thorlacius S, Sulem P, Geller F, Aben KKH, Stacey SN, Gudmundsson J, Jakobsdottir M, Bergthorsson JT, Sigurdsson A, Blondal T, Witjes JA, Vermeulen SH, Hulsbergen-van de Kaa CA, Swinkels DW, Ploeg M, Cornel EB, Vergunst H, Thorgeirsson TE, Stefansson K et al (2008) Sequence variant on 8q24 confers susceptibility to urinary bladder cancer. Nat Genet 40(11):1307–1312. https://doi.org/10.1038/ng.229
Kiemeney LA, Sulem P, Besenbacher S, Vermeulen SH, Sigurdsson A, Thorleifsson G, Gudbjartsson DF, Stacey SN, Zanon C, Kostic J, Masson G, Bjarnason H, Palsson ST, Skarphedinsson OB, Gudjonsson SA, Witjes JA, Grotenhuis AJ, Verhaegh GW, Bishop DT, Stefansson K et al (2010) A sequence variant at 4p16.3 confers susceptibility to urinary bladder cancer. Nat Genet 42(5):415–U467. https://doi.org/10.1038/ng.558
Killedar A, Stutz MD, Sobinoff AP, Tomlinson CG, Bryan TM, Beesley J, Chenevix-Trench G, Reddel RR, Pickett HA (2015) A common cancer risk-associated allele in the hTERT locus encodes a dominant negative inhibitor of telomerase. PLoS Genet 11(6):e1005286. https://doi.org/10.1371/journal.pgen.1005286
Kleinerman RA, Tucker MA, Tarone RE, Abramson DH, Seddon JM, Stovall M, Li FP, Fraumeni JF Jr (2005) Risk of new cancers after radiotherapy in long-term survivors of retinoblastoma: an extended follow-up. J Clin Oncol 23(10):2272–2279. https://doi.org/10.1200/JCO.2005.05.054
Knudson AG Jr (1971) Mutation and cancer: statistical study of retinoblastoma. Proc Natl Acad Sci USA 68(4):820–823. https://doi.org/10.1073/pnas.68.4.820
Kohaar I, Porter-Gill P, Lenz P, Fu YP, Mumy A, Tang W, Apolo AB, Rothman N, Baris D, Schned AR, Ylaya K, Schwenn M, Johnson A, Jones M, Kida M, Silverman DT, Hewitt SM, Moore LE, Prokunina-Olsson L (2013) Genetic variant as a selection marker for anti-prostate stem cell antigen immunotherapy of bladder cancer. J Natl Cancer Inst 105(1):69–73. https://doi.org/10.1093/jnci/djs458
Koutros S, Baris D, Fischer A, Tang W, Garcia-Closas M, Karagas MR, Schwenn M, Johnson A, Figueroa J, Waddell R, Prokunina-Olsson L, Rothman N, Silverman DT (2013) Differential urinary specific gravity as a molecular phenotype of the bladder cancer genetic association in the urea transporter gene, SLC14A1. Int J Cancer 133(12):3008–3013. https://doi.org/10.1002/ijc.28325

Koutros S, Kiemeney LA, Pal Choudhury P, Milne RL, Lopez de Maturana E, Ye Y, Joseph V, Florez-Vargas O, Dyrskjot L, Figueroa J, Dutta D, Giles GG, Hildebrandt MAT, Offit K, Kogevinas M, Weiderpass E, McCullough ML, Freedman ND, Albanes D, Rothman N et al (2023) Genome-wide association study of bladder cancer reveals new biological and translational insights. Eur Urol 84(1):127–137. https://doi.org/10.1016/j.eururo.2023.04.020

Kramer AA, Graham S, Burnett WS, Nasca P (1991) Familial aggregation of bladder cancer stratified by smoking status. Epidemiology 2(2):145–148. https://doi.org/10.1097/00001648-199103000-00010

Kratz CP, Rapisuwon S, Reed H, Hasle H, Rosenberg PS (2011) Cancer in Noonan, Costello, cardiofaciocutaneous and LEOPARD syndromes. Am J Med Genet C Semin Med Genet 157C(2):83–89. https://doi.org/10.1002/ajmg.c.30300

Le DT, Uram JN, Wang H, Bartlett BR, Kemberling H, Eyring AD, Skora AD, Luber BS, Azad NS, Laheru D, Biedrzycki B, Donehower RC, Zaheer A, Fisher GA, Crocenzi TS, Lee JJ, Duffy SM, Goldberg RM, de la Chapelle A, Diaz LA Jr et al (2015) PD-1 blockade in tumors with mismatch-repair deficiency. N Engl J Med 372(26):2509–2520. https://doi.org/10.1056/NEJMoa1500596

Le DT, Durham JN, Smith KN, Wang H, Bartlett BR, Aulakh LK, Lu S, Kemberling H, Wilt C, Luber BS, Wong F, Azad NS, Rucki AA, Laheru D, Donehower R, Zaheer A, Fisher GA, Crocenzi TS, Lee JJ, Diaz LA Jr et al (2017) Mismatch repair deficiency predicts response of solid tumors to PD-1 blockade. Science 357(6349):409–413. https://doi.org/10.1126/science.aan6733

Leinwand GZ, Greenberg JW, Sholl AB, Krane LS (2019) Synchronous urothelial bladder and renal malignancies. Case report and review of urologic cancers in patients with familial Rb mutations. Urology 131:89–92. https://doi.org/10.1016/j.urology.2019.05.026

Leklem JE, Brown RR (1976) Abnormal tryptophan metabolism in a family with a history of bladder cancer. J Natl Cancer Inst 56(6):1101–1104. https://doi.org/10.1093/jnci/56.6.1101

Lenfant L, Cancel-Tassin G, Gazut S, Compérat E, Rouprêt M, Cussenot O (2021) Genetic variability in 13q33 and 9q34 is linked to aggressiveness patterns and a higher risk of progression of non-muscle-invasive bladder cancer at the time of diagnosis. BJU Int 127(3):375–383. https://doi.org/10.1111/bju.15254

Liang SX, Lakshmanan Y, Woda BA, Jiang Z (2001) A high-grade primary leiomyosarcoma of the bladder in a survivor of retinoblastoma. Arch Pathol Lab Med 125(9):1231–1234. https://doi.org/10.5858/2001-125-1231-AHGPLO

Lichtenstein P, Holm NV, Verkasalo PK, Iliadou A, Kaprio J, Koskenvuo M, Pukkala E, Skytthe A, Hemminki K (2000) Environmental and heritable factors in the causation of cancer--analyses of cohorts of twins from Sweden, Denmark, and Finland. N Engl J Med 343(2):78–85. https://doi.org/10.1056/NEJM200007133430201

Lim YW, Chen-Harris H, Mayba O, Lianoglou S, Wuster A, Bhangale T, Khan Z, Mariathasan S, Daemen A, Reeder J, Haverty PM, Forrest WF, Brauer M, Mellman I, Albert ML (2018) Germline genetic polymorphisms influence tumor gene expression and immune cell infiltration. Proc Natl Acad Sci USA 115(50):E11701–e11710. https://doi.org/10.1073/pnas.1804506115

Lincoln SE, Nussbaum RL, Kurian AW, Nielsen SM, Das K, Michalski S, Yang S, Ngo N, Blanco A, Esplin ED (2020) Yield and utility of germline testing following tumor sequencing in patients with cancer. JAMA Netw Open 3(10):e2019452. https://doi.org/10.1001/jamanetworkopen.2020.19452

Lipunova N, Wesselius A, Cheng KK, van Schooten FJ, Bryan RT, Cazier JB, Galesloot TE, Kiemeney L, Zeegers MP (2019a) Genome-wide association study for tumour stage, grade, size, and age at diagnosis of non-muscle-invasive bladder cancer. Eur Urol Oncol 2(4):381–389. https://doi.org/10.1016/j.euo.2018.08.020

Lipunova N, Wesselius A, Cheng KK, van Schooten FJ, Cazier JB, Bryan RT, Zeegers MP (2019b) Systematic review: genetic associations for prognostic factors of urinary bladder cancer. Biomark Cancer 11:1179299X19897255. https://doi.org/10.1177/1179299X19897255

Lu Q, Bourrat P (2022) On the causal interpretation of heritability from a structural causal modeling perspective. Stud Hist Phil Sci 94:87–98. https://doi.org/10.1016/j.shpsa.2022.05.005

Lynch HT, Walzak MP, Fried R, Domina AH, Lynch JF (1979) Familial factors in bladder carcinoma. J Urol 122(4):458–461. https://doi.org/10.1016/s0022-5347(17)56461-7

Lynch HT, Kimberling WJ, Lynch JF, Brennan K (1987) Familial bladder cancer in an oncology clinic. Cancer Genet Cytogenet 27(1):161–165. https://doi.org/10.1016/0165-4608(87)90270-6

MacCarthy A, Bayne AM, Brownbill PA, Bunch KJ, Diggens NL, Draper GJ, Hawkins MM, Jenkinson HC, Kingston JE, Stiller CA, Vincent TJ, Murphy MF (2013) Second and subsequent tumours among 1927 retinoblastoma patients diagnosed in Britain 1951-2004. Br J Cancer 108(12):2455–2463. https://doi.org/10.1038/bjc.2013.228

Mahboubi AO, Ahlvin RC, Mahboubi EO (1981) Familial aggregation of urothelial carcinoma. J Urol 126(5):691–692. https://doi.org/10.1016/s0022-5347(17)54693-5

Maio M, Ascierto PA, Manzyuk L, Motola-Kuba D, Penel N, Cassier PA, Bariani GM, De Jesus Acosta A, Doi T, Longo F, Miller WH, Oh DY, Gottfried M, Xu L, Jin F, Norwood K, Marabelle A (2022) Pembrolizumab in microsatellite instability high or mismatch repair deficient cancers: updated analysis from the phase II KEYNOTE-158 study. Ann Oncol 33(9):929–938. https://doi.org/10.1016/j.annonc.2022.05.519

Mandelker D, Donoghue M, Talukdar S, Bandlamudi C, Srinivasan P, Vivek M, Jezdic S, Hanson H, Snape K, Kulkarni A, Hawkes L, Douillard JY, Wallace SE, Rial-Sebbag E, Meric-Bersntam F, George A, Chubb D, Loveday C, Ladanyi M, Turnbull C et al (2019) Germline-focussed analysis of tumour-only sequencing: recommendations from the ESMO precision medicine working group. Ann Oncol 30(8):1221–1231. https://doi.org/10.1093/annonc/mdz136

Marchetto D, Li FP, Henson DE (1983) Familial carcinoma of ureters and other genitourinary organs. J Urol 130(4):772–773. https://doi.org/10.1016/s0022-5347(17)51452-4

Marcus PM, Hayes RB, Vineis P, Garcia-Closas M, Caporaso NE, Autrup H, Branch RA, Brockmoller J, Ishizaki T, Karakaya AE, Ladero JM, Mommsen S, Okkels H, Romkes M, Roots I, Rothman N (2000) Cigarette smoking, N-acetyltransferase 2 acetylation status, and bladder cancer risk: a case-series meta-analysis of a gene-environment interaction. Cancer Epidemiol Biomarkers Prev 9(5):461–467. https://www.ncbi.nlm.nih.gov/pubmed/10815690

Marcus L, Lemery SJ, Keegan P, Pazdur R (2019) FDA approval summary: Pembrolizumab for the treatment of microsatellite instability-high solid tumors. Clin Cancer Res 25(13):3753–3758. https://doi.org/10.1158/1078-0432.CCR-18-4070

Marees T, Moll AC, Imhof SM, de Boer MR, Ringens PJ, van Leeuwen FE (2008) Risk of second malignancies in survivors of retinoblastoma: more than 40 years of follow-up. J Natl Cancer Inst 100(24):1771–1779. https://doi.org/10.1093/jnci/djn394

Martin C, Leiser CL, O'Neil B, Gupta S, Lowrance WT, Kohlmann W, Greenberg S, Pathak P, Smith KR, Hanson HA (2018) Familial cancer clustering in urothelial cancer: a population-based case-control study. J Natl Cancer Inst 110(5):527–533. https://doi.org/10.1093/jnci/djx237

Martin-Lopez JV, Fishel R (2013) The mechanism of mismatch repair and the functional analysis of mismatch repair defects in Lynch syndrome. Fam Cancer 12(2):159–168. https://doi.org/10.1007/s10689-013-9635-x

Matsuda K, Takahashi A, Middlebrooks CD, Obara W, Nasu Y, Inoue K, Tamura K, Yamasaki I, Naya Y, Tanikawa C, Cui R, Figueroa JD, Silverman DT, Rothman N, Namiki M, Tomita Y, Nishiyama H, Kohri K, Deguchi T, Shuin T et al (2015) Genome-wide association study identified SNP on 15q24 associated with bladder cancer risk in Japanese population. Hum Mol Genet 24(4):1177–1184. https://doi.org/10.1093/hmg/ddu512

McCullough DL, Lamm DL, McLaughlin AP 3rd, Gittes RF (1975) Familial transitional cell carcinoma of the bladder. J Urol 113(5):629–635. https://doi.org/10.1016/s0022-5347(17)59540-3

Mian A, Wei J, Shi Z, Rifkin AS, Zheng SL, Glaser AP, Kearns JT, Helfand BT, Xu J (2023) Systematic review of reported association studies of monogenic genes and bladder cancer risk and confirmation analysis in a large population cohort. BJUI Compass 4(2):156–163. https://doi.org/10.1002/bco2.206

Middlebrooks CD, Banday AR, Matsuda K, Udquim KI, Onabajo OO, Paquin A, Figueroa JD, Zhu B, Koutros S, Kubo M, Shuin T, Freedman ND, Kogevinas M, Malats N, Chanock SJ, Garcia-Closas M, Silverman DT, Rothman N, Prokunina-Olsson L (2016) Association of germline variants in the APOBEC3 region with cancer risk and enrichment with APOBEC-signature mutations in tumors. Nat Genet 48(11):1330–1338. https://doi.org/10.1038/ng.3670

Miller DT, Lee K, Abul-Husn NS, Amendola LM, Brothers K, Chung WK, Gollob MH, Gordon AS, Harrison SM, Hershberger RE, Klein TE, Richards CS, Stewart DR, Martin CL, documents@acmg.net, A. S. F. W. G. E. a (2022) ACMG SF v3.1 list for reporting of secondary findings in clinical exome and genome sequencing: A policy statement of the American College of Medical Genetics and Genomics (ACMG). Genet Med 24(7):1407–1414. https://doi.org/10.1016/j.gim.2022.04.006

Minagawa T, Okaneya T, Kamigaito M, Nishizawa S, Ogawa T, Kawakami M, Nakayama T, Imamura T, Kato H, Nishizawa O (2008) Leiomyosarcoma of the urinary bladder in a patient with bilateral retinoblastoma. Int J Urol 15(6):548–550. https://doi.org/10.1111/j.1442-2042.2008.02024.x

Mitra AP, Birkhahn M, Cote RJ (2007) p53 and retinoblastoma pathways in bladder cancer. World J Urol 25(6):563–571. https://doi.org/10.1007/s00345-007-0197-0

Moller P, Seppala TT, Bernstein I, Holinski-Feder E, Sala P, Gareth Evans D, Lindblom A, Macrae F, Blanco I, Sijmons RH, Jeffries J, Vasen HFA, Burn J, Nakken S, Hovig E, Rodland EA, Tharmaratnam K, de Vos Tot Nederveen Cappel WH, Hill J, Mallorca G et al (2018) Cancer risk and survival in path_MMR carriers by gene and gender up to 75 years of age: a report from the prospective Lynch syndrome database. Gut 67(7):1306–1316. https://doi.org/10.1136/gutjnl-2017-314057

Moore LE, Baris DR, Figueroa JD, Garcia-Closas M, Karagas MR, Schwenn MR, Johnson AT, Lubin JH, Hein DW, Dagnall CL, Colt JS, Kida M, Jones MA, Schned AR, Cherala SS, Chanock SJ, Cantor KP, Silverman DT, Rothman N (2011) GSTM1 null and NAT2 slow acetylation genotypes, smoking intensity and bladder cancer risk: results from the New England bladder cancer study and NAT2 meta-analysis. Carcinogenesis 32(2):182–189. https://doi.org/10.1093/carcin/bgq223

Mossanen M, Nassar AH, Stokes SM, Martinez-Chanza N, Kumar V, Nuzzo PV, Kwiatkowski DJ, Garber JE, Curran C, Freeman D, Preston M, Mouw KW, Kibel A, Choueiri TK, Sonpavde G, Rana HQ (2022) Incidence of germline variants in familial bladder cancer and among patients with cancer predisposition syndromes. Clin Genitourin Cancer 20(6):568–574. https://doi.org/10.1016/j.clgc.2022.08.009

Mucci LA, Hjelmborg JB, Harris JR, Czene K, Havelick DJ, Scheike T, Graff RE, Holst K, Moller S, Unger RH, McIntosh C, Nuttall E, Brandt I, Penney KL, Hartman M, Kraft P, Parmigiani G, Christensen K, Koskenvuo M, Nordic Twin Study of Cancer, C et al (2016) Familial risk and heritability of cancer among twins in nordic countries. JAMA 315(1):68–76. https://doi.org/10.1001/jama.2015.17703

Mueller CM, Caporaso N, Greene MH (2008) Familial and genetic risk of transitional cell carcinoma of the urinary tract. Urol Oncol 26(5):451–464. https://doi.org/10.1016/j.urolonc.2008.02.016

Na R, Wu Y, Jiang G, Yu H, Lin X, Wang M, Conran CA, Fantus RJ, Zhang N, Liu S, Helfand BT, Zheng SL, Isaacs WB, Ding Q, Shen Z, Xu J (2018) Germline mutations in DNA repair genes are associated with bladder cancer risk and unfavourable prognosis. BJU Int 122(5):808–813. https://doi.org/10.1111/bju.14370

Nagakawa S, Shiota M, Fujimoto N, Yamamoto Y, Blas L, Tsukahara S, Matsumoto T, Kashiwagi E, Takeuchi A, Inokuchi J, Uchiumi T, Matsuyama H, Eto M (2021) The impact of single-nucleotide polymorphisms on intravesical recurrence after bacillus Calmette-Guérin therapy for non-muscle invasive bladder cancer in a genome-wide association study. Urol Oncol 39(10):733.e717–733.e724. https://doi.org/10.1016/j.urolonc.2021.05.034

Naslund-Koch C, Nordestgaard BG, Bojesen SE (2016) Increased risk for other cancers in addition to breast cancer for CHEK2*1100delC heterozygotes estimated from the Copenhagen general population study. J Clin Oncol 34(11):1208–1216. https://doi.org/10.1200/JCO.2015.63.3594

Nassar AH, Abou Alaiwi S, AlDubayan SH, Moore N, Mouw KW, Kwiatkowski DJ, Choueiri TK, Curran C, Berchuck JE, Harshman LC, Nuzzo PV, Chanza NM, Van Allen E, Esplin ED, Yang S, Callis T, Garber JE, Rana HQ, Sonpavde G (2020) Prevalence of pathogenic germline cancer risk variants in high-risk urothelial carcinoma. Genet Med 22(4):709–718. https://doi.org/10.1038/s41436-019-0720-x

Nassour AJ, Jain A, Hui N, Siopis G, Symons J, Woo H (2023) Relative risk of bladder and kidney cancer in Lynch syndrome: systematic review and meta-analysis. Cancers (Basel) 15(2). https://doi.org/10.3390/cancers15020506

Ohan H, Minassian G, Minassian H, Farooq T, Zdilla MJ (2020) Retinoblastoma in infancy with subsequent bladder leiomyosarcoma in adulthood: genomic considerations. Urology 140:38–40. https://doi.org/10.1016/j.urology.2020.03.010

Pande M, Wei C, Chen J, Amos CI, Lynch PM, Lu KH, Lucio LA, Boyd-Rogers SG, Bannon SA, Mork ME, Frazier ML (2012) Cancer spectrum in DNA mismatch repair gene mutation carriers: results from a hospital based Lynch syndrome registry. Fam Cancer 11(3):441–447. https://doi.org/10.1007/s10689-012-9534-6

Parekh DJ, Jung C, O'Conner J, Dutta S, Smith ER Jr (2002) Leiomyosarcoma in urinary bladder after cyclophosphamide therapy for retinoblastoma and review of bladder sarcomas. Urology 60(1):164. https://doi.org/10.1016/s0090-4295(02)01701-6

Pattison JM, Posternak V, Cole MD (2016) Transcription factor KLF5 binds a cyclin E1 polymorphic intronic enhancer to confer increased bladder cancer risk. Mol Cancer Res 14(11):1078–1086. https://doi.org/10.1158/1541-7786.MCR-16-0123

Pemov A, Wegman-Ostrosky T, Kim J, Koutros S, Douthitt B, Jones K, Zhu B, Baris D, Schwenn M, Johnson A, Karagas MR, Carter BD, McCullough ML, Landi MT, Freedman ND, Albanes D, Silverman DT, Rothman N, Caporaso NE, Stewart DR et al (2021) Identification of genetic risk factors for familial urinary bladder cancer: an exome sequencing study. JCO Precis Oncol 5. https://doi.org/10.1200/PO.21.00115

Pietzak EJ, Whiting K, Srinivasan P, Bandlamudi C, Khurram A, Joseph V, Walasek A, Bochner E, Clinton T, Almassi N, Truong H, de Jesus Escano MR, Wiseman M, Mandelker D, Kemel Y, Zhang L, Walsh MF, Cadoo KA, Coleman JA, Bochner BH et al (2022) Inherited germline cancer susceptibility gene variants in individuals with non-muscle-invasive bladder cancer. Clin Cancer Res 28(19):4267–4277. https://doi.org/10.1158/1078-0432.CCR-22-1006

Plna K, Hemminki K (2001) Familial bladder cancer in the National Swedish Family Cancer Database. J Urol 166(6):2129–2133. https://www.ncbi.nlm.nih.gov/pubmed/11696721

Powles T, Carroll D, Chowdhury S, Gravis G, Joly F, Carles J, Flechon A, Maroto P, Petrylak D, Rolland F, Cook N, Balar AV, Sridhar SS, Galsky MD, Grivas P, Ravaud A, Jones R, Cosaert J, Hodgson D, Landers D et al (2021) An adaptive, biomarker-directed platform study of durvalumab in combination with targeted therapies in advanced urothelial cancer. Nat Med 27(5):793–801. https://doi.org/10.1038/s41591-021-01317-6

Purtilo DT, McCarthy B, Yang JP, Friedell GH (1979) Familial urinary bladder cancer. Semin Oncol 6(2):254–256. https://www.ncbi.nlm.nih.gov/pubmed/482963

Rafnar T, Vermeulen SH, Sulem P, Thorleifsson G, Aben KK, Witjes JA, Grotenhuis AJ, Verhaegh GW, Hulsbergen-van de Kaa CA, Besenbacher S, Gudbjartsson D, Stacey SN, Gudmundsson J, Johannsdottir H, Bjarnason H, Zanon C, Helgadottir H, Jonasson JG, Tryggvadottir L, Kiemeney LA et al (2011) European genome-wide association study identifies SLC14A1 as a new urinary bladder cancer susceptibility gene. Hum Mol Genet 20(21):4268–4281. https://doi.org/10.1093/hmg/ddr303

Rafnar T, Sulem P, Thorleifsson G, Vermeulen SH, Helgason H, Saemundsdottir J, Gudjonsson SA, Sigurdsson A, Stacey SN, Gudmundsson J, Johannsdottir H, Alexiusdottir K, Petursdottir V, Nikulasson S, Geirsson G, Jonsson T, Aben KK,

Grotenhuis AJ, Verhaegh GW, Stefansson K et al (2014) Genome-wide association study yields variants at 20p12.2 that associate with urinary bladder cancer. Hum Mol Genet 23(20):5545–5557. https://doi.org/10.1093/hmg/ddu264

Ramirez Sevilla C, Admella-Salvador C, Romero-Martin JA, Llopis-Manzanera J, Barranco-Sanz MA (2018) Bladder leiomyosarcoma 25 years after treatment with cyclophosphamide in patient with history of retinoblastoma. Urol Int 100(1):119–121. https://doi.org/10.1159/000437442

Ravichandran V, Shameer Z, Kemel Y, Walsh M, Cadoo K, Lipkin S, Mandelker D, Zhang L, Stadler Z, Robson M, Offit K, Vijai J (2019) Toward automation of germline variant curation in clinical cancer genetics. Genet Med 21(9):2116–2125. https://doi.org/10.1038/s41436-019-0463-8

Richards S, Aziz N, Bale S, Bick D, Das S, Gastier-Foster J, Grody WW, Hegde M, Lyon E, Spector E, Voelkerding K, Rehm HL, Committee ALQA (2015) Standards and guidelines for the interpretation of sequence variants: a joint consensus recommendation of the American College of Medical Genetics and Genomics and the Association for Molecular Pathology. Genet Med 17(5):405–424. https://doi.org/10.1038/gim.2015.30

Richters A, Aben KKH, Kiemeney L (2020) The global burden of urinary bladder cancer: an update. World J Urol 38(8):1895–1904. https://doi.org/10.1007/s00345-019-02984-4

Robertson AG, Kim J, Al-Ahmadie H, Bellmunt J, Guo G, Cherniack AD, Hinoue T, Laird PW, Hoadley KA, Akbani R, Castro MAA, Gibb EA, Kanchi RS, Gordenin DA, Shukla SA, Sanchez-Vega F, Hansel DE, Czerniak BA, Reuter VE, Lerner SP et al (2017) Comprehensive molecular characterization of muscle-invasive bladder cancer. Cell 171(3):540–556 e525. https://doi.org/10.1016/j.cell.2017.09.007

Rosenberg JE, Park SH, Kozlov V, Dao TV, Castellano D, Li JR, Mukherjee SD, Howells K, Dry H, Lanasa MC, Stewart R, Bajorin DF (2023) Durvalumab plus olaparib in previously untreated, platinum-ineligible patients with metastatic urothelial carcinoma: a multicenter, randomized, phase II trial (BAYOU). J Clin Oncol 41(1):43–53. https://doi.org/10.1200/JCO.22.00205

Rothman N, Garcia-Closas M, Hein DW (2007) Commentary: reflections on G. M. Lower and colleagues' 1979 study associating slow acetylator phenotype with urinary bladder cancer: meta-analysis, historical refinements of the hypothesis, and lessons learned. Int J Epidemiol 36(1):23–28. https://doi.org/10.1093/ije/dym026

Rothman N, Garcia-Closas M, Chatterjee N, Malats N, Wu X, Figueroa JD, Real FX, Van Den Berg D, Matullo G, Baris D, Thun M, Kiemeney LA, Vineis P, De Vivo I, Albanes D, Purdue MP, Rafnar T, Hildebrandt MA, Kiltie AE, Chanock SJ et al (2010) A multi-stage genome-wide association study of bladder cancer identifies multiple susceptibility loci. Nat Genet 42(11):978–984. https://doi.org/10.1038/ng.687

Saeki N, Ono H, Yanagihara K, Aoyagi K, Sasaki H, Sakamoto H, Yoshida T (2015) rs2294008T, a risk allele for gastric and gallbladder cancers, suppresses the PSCA promoter by recruiting the transcription factor YY1. Genes Cells 20(5):382–391. https://doi.org/10.1111/gtc.12228

Saita C, Yamaguchi T, Horiguchi SI, Yamada R, Takao M, Iijima T, Wakaume R, Aruga T, Tabata T, Koizumi K (2018) Tumor development in Japanese patients with Lynch syndrome. PLoS One 13(4):e0195572. https://doi.org/10.1371/journal.pone.0195572

Schoenberg M, Kiemeney L, Walsh PC, Griffin CA, Sidransky D (1996) Germline translocation t(5;20)(p15;q11) and familial transitional cell carcinoma. J Urol 155(3):1035–1036. https://www.ncbi.nlm.nih.gov/pubmed/8583556

Schonfeld SJ, Kleinerman RA, Abramson DH, Seddon JM, Tucker MA, Morton LM (2021) Long-term risk of subsequent cancer incidence among hereditary and nonhereditary retinoblastoma survivors. Br J Cancer 124(7):1312–1319. https://doi.org/10.1038/s41416-020-01248-y

Schultz IJ, Kiemeney LA, Witjes JA, Schalken JA, Willems JL, Swinkels DW, de Kok JB (2005) CDC91L1 (PIG-U) mRNA expression in urothelial cell carcinomas. Int J Cancer 116(2):282–284. https://doi.org/10.1002/ijc.21040

Shah SM, Demidova EV, Lesh RW, Hall MJ, Daly MB, Meyer JE, Edelman MJ, Arora S (2022) Therapeutic implications of germline vulnerabilities in DNA repair for precision oncology. Cancer Treat Rev 104:102337. https://doi.org/10.1016/j.ctrv.2021.102337

Sharma SK, Bapna BC, Singh SM (1976) Familial profile of transitional cell carcinoma. Br J Urol 48(6):442. https://doi.org/10.1111/j.1464-410x.1976.tb06677.x

Shen YJ, Ye DW, Yao XD, Trink B, Zhou XY, Zhang SL, Dai B, Zhang HL, Zhu Y, Guo Z, Wu G, Nagpal J (2008) Overexpression of CDC91L1 (PIG-U) in bladder urothelial cell carcinoma: correlation with clinical variables and prognostic significance. BJU Int 101(1):113–119. https://doi.org/10.1111/j.1464-410X.2007.07192.x

Skeldon SC, Semotiuk K, Aronson M, Holter S, Gallinger S, Pollett A, Kuk C, van Rhijn B, Bostrom P, Cohen Z, Fleshner NE, Jewett MA, Hanna S, Shariat SF, Van Der Kwast TH, Evans A, Catto J, Bapat B, Zlotta AR (2013) Patients with Lynch syndrome mismatch repair gene mutations are at higher risk for not only upper tract urothelial cancer but also bladder cancer. Eur Urol 63(2):379–385. https://doi.org/10.1016/j.eururo.2012.07.047

Sovik O, Schubbert S, Houge G, Steine SJ, Norgard G, Engelsen B, Njolstad PR, Shannon K, Molven A (2007) De novo HRAS and KRAS mutations in two siblings with short stature and neuro-cardio-facio-cutaneous features. J Med Genet 44(7):e84. https://doi.org/10.1136/jmg.2007.049361

Stadler ZK, Maio A, Chakravarty D, Kemel Y, Sheehan M, Salo-Mullen E, Tkachuk K, Fong CJ, Nguyen B, Erakky A, Cadoo K, Liu Y, Carlo MI, Latham A, Zhang H, Kundra R, Smith S, Galle J, Aghajanian C, Robson ME et al (2021) Therapeutic implications of germline testing in patients with advanced cancers. J Clin Oncol 39(24):2698–2709. https://doi.org/10.1200/JCO.20.03661

Swanton C, McGranahan N, Starrett GJ, Harris RS (2015) APOBEC enzymes: mutagenic fuel for cancer evolution and heterogeneity. Cancer Discov 5(7):704–712. https://doi.org/10.1158/2159-8290.CD-15-0344

Sweis RF, Heiss B, Segal J, Ritterhouse L, Kadri S, Churpek JE, Allen K, Conway D, Marinier C, Smith ND, Pitroda SP, Stadler WM (2018) Clinical activity of olaparib in urothelial bladder cancer with DNA damage response gene mutations. JCO Precis Oncol 2:1–7. https://doi.org/10.1200/PO.18.00264

Tang W, Fu YP, Figueroa JD, Malats N, Garcia-Closas M, Chatterjee N, Kogevinas M, Baris D, Thun M, Hall JL, De Vivo I, Albanes D, Porter-Gill P, Purdue MP, Burdett L, Liu L, Hutchinson A, Myers T, Tardon A, Prokunina-Olsson L et al (2012) Mapping of the UGT1A locus identifies an uncommon coding variant that affects mRNA expression and protects from bladder cancer. Hum Mol Genet 21(8):1918–1930. https://doi.org/10.1093/hmg/ddr619

Tang Q, Zuo W, Wan C, Xiong S, Xu C, Yuan C, Sun Q, Zhou L, Li X (2022) Comprehensive genomic profiling of upper tract urothelial carcinoma and urothelial carcinoma of the bladder identifies distinct molecular characterizations with potential implications for targeted therapy & immunotherapy. Front Immunol 13:1097730. https://doi.org/10.3389/fimmu.2022.1097730

Tanguay C, Harvey I, Houde M, Srigley JR, Tetu B (2003) Leiomyosarcoma of urinary bladder following cyclophosphamide therapy: report of two cases. Mod Pathol 16(5):512–514. https://doi.org/10.1097/01.MP.0000068237.38715.D9

Temming P, Arendt M, Viehmann A, Eisele L, Le Guin CH, Schundeln MM, Biewald E, Astrahantseff K, Wieland R, Bornfeld N, Sauerwein W, Eggert A, Jockel KH, Lohmann DR (2017) Incidence of second cancers after radiotherapy and systemic chemotherapy in heritable retinoblastoma survivors: a report from the German reference center. Pediatr Blood Cancer 64(1):71–80. https://doi.org/10.1002/pbc.26193

Thelen A, Schaeuble J (1957) Simultaneous occurrence of bladder papilloma in uniovular twins. Z Urol 50(4):188–195. https://www.ncbi.nlm.nih.gov/pubmed/13456948 (Gleichzeitiges Vorkommen von Blasepapillomen bei eineiigen Zwillingen)

Toupance S, Stathopoulou MG, Petrelis AM, Gorenjak V, Labat C, Lai TP, Visvikis-Siest S, Benetos A (2020) TERC variants associated with short leukocyte telomeres: implication of higher early life leukocyte telomere attrition as assessed by the blood-and-muscle model. Cells 9(6):1360. https://doi.org/10.3390/cells9061360

Urakami S, Igawa M, Shiina H, Shigeno K, Kikuno N, Yoshino T (2002) Recurrent transitional cell carcinoma in a child with the Costello syndrome. J Urol 168(3):1133–1134. https://doi.org/10.1016/S0022-5347(05)64609-5

van der Post RS, Kiemeney LA, Ligtenberg MJ, Witjes JA, Hulsbergen-van de Kaa CA, Bodmer D, Schaap L, Kets CM, van Krieken JH, Hoogerbrugge N (2010) Risk of urothelial bladder cancer in Lynch syndrome is increased, in particular among MSH2 mutation carriers. J Med Genet 47(7):464–470. https://doi.org/10.1136/jmg.2010.076992

Venkatraman L, Goepel JR, Steele K, Dobbs SP, Lyness RW, McCluggage WG (2003) Soft tissue, pelvic, and urinary bladder leiomyosarcoma as second neoplasm following hereditary retinoblastoma. J Clin Pathol 56(3):233–236. https://doi.org/10.1136/jcp.56.3.233

Villanueva G, Sampor C, Moreno F, Alderete D, Moresco A, Pinto N, Szijan I, Schaiquevich P, Felice MS, Rose A, Zubizarreta P, Sgroi M, Fandino A, Chantada G (2022) Subsequent malignant neoplasms in the pediatric age in retinoblastoma survivors in Argentina. Pediatr Blood Cancer 69(8):e29710. https://doi.org/10.1002/pbc.29710

Vlachostergios PJ, Faltas BM, Carlo MI, Nassar AH, Alaiwi SA, Sonpavde G (2020) The emerging landscape of germline variants in urothelial carcinoma: implications for genetic testing. Cancer Treat Res Commun 23:100165. https://doi.org/10.1016/j.ctarc.2020.100165

Vogt S, Jones N, Christian D, Engel C, Nielsen M, Kaufmann A, Steinke V, Vasen HF, Propping P, Sampson JR, Hes FJ, Aretz S (2009) Expanded extracolonic tumor spectrum in MUTYH-associated polyposis. Gastroenterology 137(6):1976-1985 e1971-1910. https://doi.org/10.1053/j.gastro.2009.08.052

Vosoughi A, Zhang T, Shohdy KS, Vlachostergios PJ, Wilkes DC, Bhinder B, Tagawa ST, Nanus DM, Molina AM, Beltran H, Sternberg CN, Motanagh S, Robinson BD, Xiang J, Fan X, Chung WK, Rubin MA, Elemento O, Sboner A, Faltas BM et al (2020) Common germline-somatic variant interactions in advanced urothelial cancer. Nat Commun 11(1):6195. https://doi.org/10.1038/s41467-020-19971-8

Waarts MR, Stonestrom AJ, Park YC, Levine RL (2022) Targeting mutations in cancer. J Clin Invest 132(8). https://doi.org/10.1172/JCI154943

Wang M, Du M, Ma L, Chu H, Lv Q, Ye D, Guo J, Gu C, Xia G, Zhu Y, Ding Q, Yuan L, Fu G, Tong N, Qin C, Yin C, Xu J, Zhang Z (2016a) A functional variant in TP63 at 3q28 associated with bladder cancer risk by creating an miR-140-5p binding site. Int J Cancer 139(1):65–74. https://doi.org/10.1002/ijc.29978

Wang ML, Li ZQ, Chu HY, Lv Q, Ye DW, Ding Q, Xu CL, Guo JM, Du ML, Chen JH, Song ZJ, Yin CJ, Qin C, Gu CY, Zhu Y, Xia GW, Liu F, Zhang ZS, Yuan L, Zhang ZD et al (2016b) Genome-wide association study of bladder cancer in a Chinese cohort reveals a new susceptibility locus at 5q12.3. Cancer Res 76(11):3277–3284. https://doi.org/10.1158/0008-5472.Can-15-2564

White SM, Graham JM Jr, Kerr B, Gripp K, Weksberg R, Cytrynbaum C, Reeder JL, Stewart FJ, Edwards M, Wilson M, Bankier A (2005) The adult phenotype in Costello syndrome. Am J Med Genet A 136(2):128–135. https://doi.org/10.1002/ajmg.a.30747

Win AK, Young JP, Lindor NM, Tucker KM, Ahnen DJ, Young GP, Buchanan DD, Clendenning M, Giles GG, Winship I, Macrae FA, Goldblatt J, Southey MC, Arnold J, Thibodeau SN, Gunawardena SR, Bapat B, Baron JA, Casey G, Jenkins MA et al (2012) Colorectal and other cancer risks for carriers and noncarriers from families with a DNA mismatch repair gene mutation: a prospective cohort study. J Clin Oncol 30(9):958–964. https://doi.org/10.1200/JCO.2011.39.5590

Win AK, Reece JC, Dowty JG, Buchanan DD, Clendenning M, Rosty C, Southey MC, Young JP, Cleary SP, Kim H, Cotterchio M, Macrae FA, Tucker KM, Baron JA, Burnett T, Le Marchand L, Casey G, Haile RW, Newcomb PA, Jenkins MA et al (2016) Risk of extracolonic cancers for people with biallelic and monoallelic mutations in MUTYH. Int J Cancer 139(7):1557–1563. https://doi.org/10.1002/ijc.30197

Wischhusen JW, Ukaegbu C, Dhingra TG, Uno H, Kastrinos F, Syngal S, Yurgelun MB (2020) Clinical factors associated with urinary tract cancer in individuals with Lynch syndrome. Cancer Epidemiol Biomarkers Prev 29(1):193–199. https://doi.org/10.1158/1055-9965.EPI-19-0213

Wu X, Ye Y, Kiemeney LA, Sulem P, Rafnar T, Matullo G, Seminara D, Yoshida T, Saeki N, Andrew AS, Dinney CP, Czerniak B, Zhang ZF, Kiltie AE, Bishop DT, Vineis P, Porru S, Buntinx F, Kellen E, Zeegers MP, Kumar R, Rudnai P, Gurzau E, Koppova K, Mayordomo JI, Sanchez M, Saez B, Lindblom A, de Verdier P, Steineck G, Mills GB, Schned A, Guarrera S, Polidoro S, Chang SC, Lin J, Chang DW, Hale KS, Majewski T, Grossman HB, Thorlacius S, Thorsteinsdottir U, Aben KK, Witjes JA, Stefansson K, Amos CI, Karagas MR, Gu J (2009) Genetic variation in the prostate stem cell antigen gene PSCA confers susceptibility to urinary bladder cancer. Nat Genet 41(9):991–995. https://doi.org/10.1038/ng.421

Yap TA, Ashok A, Stoll J, Mauer E, Nepomuceno VM, Blackwell KL, Garber JE, Meric-Bernstam F (2022) Prevalence of germline findings among tumors from cancer types lacking hereditary testing guidelines. JAMA Netw Open 5(5):e2213070. https://doi.org/10.1001/jamanetworkopen.2022.13070

Zeng C, Bastarache LA, Tao R, Venner E, Hebbring S, Andujar JD, Bland ST, Crosslin DR, Pratap S, Cooley A, Pacheco JA, Christensen KD, Perez E, Zawatsky CLB, Witkowski L, Zouk H, Weng C, Leppig KA, Sleiman PMA, Denny JC et al (2022) Association of pathogenic variants in hereditary cancer genes with multiple diseases. JAMA Oncol 8(6):835–844. https://doi.org/10.1001/jamaoncol.2022.0373

Zhang X, Zhang Y (2015) Bladder cancer and genetic mutations. Cell Biochem Biophys 73(1):65–69. https://doi.org/10.1007/s12013-015-0574-z

Zlowocka E, Cybulski C, Gorski B, Debniak T, Slojewski M, Wokolorczyk D, Serrano-Fernandez P, Matyjasik J, van de Wetering T, Sikorski A, Scott RJ, Lubinski J (2008) Germline mutations in the CHEK2 kinase gene are associated with an increased risk of bladder cancer. Int J Cancer 122(3):583–586. https://doi.org/10.1002/ijc.23099

3 Human Urothelium

Jennifer Southgate, Jens Stahlschmidt, and Mateja Erdani Kreft

Abstract

Urothelium is the epithelium found lining the bladder and associated urinary tract. It functions as a predominantly impermeable urinary barrier even while accommodating major changes in surface area during bladder filling and voiding. Evolved for this role, urothelium displays many adaptations, exemplified in the highly specialized tight junctions and uroplakin plaques of the urine-facing superficial cells, combined with an exceptional "on-demand" capacity for repair and regeneration. Intrinsic to the specialized nature of urothelium is how proliferation and differentiation are regulated during tissue homeostasis as this can provide unique insight into the drivers, pathways, and emergent phenotypes of urothelial cancer. This chapter looks at developmental and functional features of normal human urothelium that influence its pathogenesis. It considers different experimental platforms available for investigating urothelial biology and highlights some of the differences between urothelia from human and other species. While generally of uncertain significance, these differences can confuse reports and reviews where species derivation is not made evident. Nevertheless, animal models have been instrumental in advancing knowledge as, by enabling study of genetic and molecular mechanisms involved in urothelial development, they have identified key cellular processes and signaling pathways implicated in urothelial form and function. On the other hand, limitations of cross-species comparisons, the massive expansion of human data, and, ultimately, the prize of understanding the specific biology and pathology of human urothelium all fuel interest in alternative in vitro and increasingly computational approaches aimed toward predicting biological processes and responses.

Keywords

Urothelium · Development · Differentiation · Urinary barrier · Blood/urine barrier · Tissue homeostasis · Regeneration · Cell culture · Computational models

J. Southgate (✉)
Jack Birch Unit of Molecular Carcinogenesis, Department of Biology and York Biomedical Research Institute, University of York, York, UK
e-mail: j.southgate@york.ac.uk

J. Stahlschmidt
Department of Histopathology and Molecular Pathology, St James's University Hospital, Leeds, UK
e-mail: jens.stahlschmidt@nhs.net

M. E. Kreft
Faculty of Medicine, Institute of Cell Biology, University of Ljubljana, Ljubljana, Slovenia
e-mail: mateja.erdani@mf.uni-lj.si

M. A. Knowles, L. Dyrskjøt (eds.), *Biology of Bladder Cancer*,
https://doi.org/10.1007/978-3-031-68505-7_3

3.1 The Urothelium

Although the focus of bladder cancer research is usually the cancer, the study of the normal cell and tissue counterpart can offer a unique tissue-specific perspective on the tissue homeostatic mechanisms dysregulated in cancer. This not only defines the environment behind initiation of urothelial carcinogenesis but offers insight into emergent tumor phenotypes and can help interpret the mechanisms behind drivers and suppressors of malignancy.

The urinary tract comprises the kidneys, ureters, the urinary bladder, and the urethra. After concentration in the kidneys, urine transfers from the collecting ducts by peristalsis along the ureters and into the urinary bladder, which provides a secure reservoir for the collection and temporary storage of urine. The bladder, along with other regions of the urinary tract that come into direct contact with urine, is exclusively lined by a highly specialized epithelium, the urothelium. The exception is the urethra. In the female, the proximal third has a urothelial lining, which transitions to a nonkeratinizing squamous epithelium distally. In the male, the preprostatic, prostatic, and membranous urethra are lined by urothelium, the bulbous, and the pendulous parts by a stratified columnar epithelium, and the most distal aspect is lined by a nonkeratinizing squamous epithelium.

Urothelium from different regions of the urinary tract shares a common morphology, comprising a five- to seven-cell-layered complex epithelium in humans and classified histologically as a transitional epithelium due to its morphology resembling a transition between stratified squamous and simple glandular epithelia (Wheater et al. 1990). Three structurally distinct cell zones are recognized, based on morphology, position, and differences in marker gene/protein expression (Fig. 3.1).

Basal cells constitute a single cell layer attached via hemidesmosomes to a basement membrane. The basement membrane derives from both epithelial and stromal cells (Scriven et al. 1997) and has a low turnover rate. Intermediate cells are larger than basal cells (up to 20 μm) and are the most frequent cell type in human urothelium (Castillo-Martin et al. 2010). Urothelial cells of the intermediate cell zone show variability in shape and number of layers depending on the expansion state of the bladder during the micturition cycle.

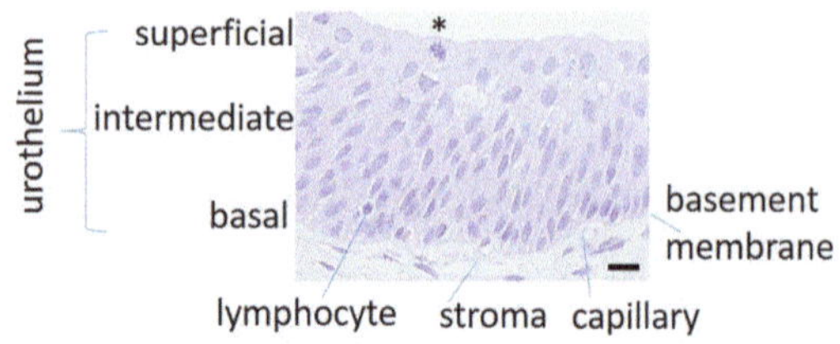

Fig. 3.1 Hematoxylin- and eosin-stained section of normal human bladder urothelium. As a transitional epithelium, urothelium is stratified into morphologically distinct basal, intermediate, and superficial cell zones. The basal cells attach to a basement membrane, while the superficial cells are uniquely specialized as the main urine-facing barrier. Note: the mitotic cell in the superficial cell layer (marked *) which, although unusual, is occasionally observed in normal human urothelium (see Sect. 3.3.2). During the micturition cycle, urothelium accommodates the large change in intraluminal surface area in part through the intermediate cell layer, which varies from three to five or more cells thick depending on bladder distention, and secondly through modifying the surface area of the apical superficial cell membrane. These features contribute to maintaining the urinary tract as a low-pressure non-refluxing system that protects the kidneys from damaging pressures and ascending bacterial infections. Scale bar 20 μm

Superficial cells, also sometimes known as "umbrella" or "facet" cells, are large, ranging from 25 to 250 μm in diameter depending on the species and bladder distension state. In the relaxed state, superficial cells form dome-shaped structures and can cover multiple underlying intermediate cells (Khandelwal et al. 2009). These are long-lived cells (estimated at ~200 days in rodents) and are highly polarized and occasionally binucleated, with a specialized apical membrane that abuts directly onto the intravesicular (luminal) space. Being in direct contact with urine, the superficial cells provide the main urine-proofing features, with highly developed intercellular tight junctions and uroplakin plaques restricting permeability across the epithelium (Lasič et al. 2015).

Although generally regarded as a true stratified epithelium, morphological studies not uncommonly describe regional pseudostratification, where intermediate and occasionally superficially positioned urothelial cells attach via a slim pedicle to the basement membrane (Jost et al. 1989). A role for the pedicled cell remains enigmatic, with suggestions including positional registration during accommodation when urothelial cells move relative to each other as the bladder fills and voids or release of factors when under physical strain during bladder filling as a signal for voiding.

3.2 The Developmental Origins of (Human) Urothelium

The placenta plays a significant role in water and electrolyte hemostasis during human intrauterine development, and the timing of urothelial development in the fetus coincides with the first production of urine. Urothelium is highly unusual in that the same epithelium arises from two embryonic germ layers, with the renal collecting ducts and ureters developing from mesoderm, while the bladder, proximal urethra, and prostatic ducts develop from the endoderm (Hicks 1975).

3.2.1 The Histology of the Epithelial Lining of the Developing Human Bladder

Gyllensten (1949) described the epithelial lining of the sinus and the caudal part of the mesonephric duct in an early gestation embryo (approximately day 35, embryo length: 5.2 mm) as uniformly one-layered. In the following 6 mm embryo, the bladder epithelium was described as "stratified" (Gyllensten 1949), and according to Felix, it is bi- or trilayered by the end of week 6 (Felix 1912). The urothelium then remains unaltered for almost 2.5 weeks being "two layered and thicker on the concave dorsal than the concave ventral surface. The one-layered epithelium occurs at the apex and the many-layered at the fundus."

By week 9, the urothelium is four to five cell layers and considered by Felix as "transitional" in form (Felix 1912). Newman and Antonakopoulos described a third cell layer in urothelium after 13 weeks and the occurrence of large, binucleated superficial cells at around 21 weeks. The latter and the ultrastructural presence of an asymmetric membrane at the same time were regarded by the authors as objective features of a differentiating transitional epithelium (Newman and Antonakopoulos 1989). The formation of rigid asymmetric plaques in the apical membrane of superficial cells was described at 26 weeks of development. However, Hoyes and colleagues observed ultrastructural features in human superficial urothelial cells, such as a thickened apical membrane in fetuses as early as 16 weeks (Hoyes et al. 1972). Using immunohistological markers, the first appearance of a transitional differentiated phenotype was observed at 10 weeks' gestation, based on cytokeratin expression profile and apical membrane expression of uroplakins (Baker et al. 2018b).

3.2.2 Urothelial Differentiation and Associated Developmental Anomalies

In brief, the interactions between the developing urothelium and its underlying mesenchyme are crucial in the development of the bladder and ureter, with disruption of the signaling pathways having consequences for the precise spatiotemporal development of the urinary tract. This accounts for congenital anomalies of the kidney and urinary tract [referred to pragmatically as CAKUT phenotypes (Knoers 2022)] in the mouse and human, including the congenital conditions of hydroureteronephrosis due to disrupted smooth-muscle differentiation (Trowe et al. 2012), hydroureter, hydronephrosis, and hypoplastic bladder (Haraguchi et al. 2007; Yu et al. 2002).

Renal tissue develops from the intermediate mesoderm or urogenital ridge that extends from the cervical to the caudal region of the embryo. Mammals develop three consecutive renal stages: the pronephros (pre-kidney), the mesonephros (original kidney), and the metanephros. The first two renal vestiges regress in utero to leave the metanephros as the permanent or true kidney (Rehman and Ahmed 2022). The pronephros develops in the fourth gestational week, with the cranial part degenerating and the caudal portion forming the Wolffian or mesonephric duct. A localized region of the mesonephros develops into a temporary excretory organ between weeks 6 and 10, until the development of the metanephros. After the mesonephric duct enters the cloaca, a second bud develops from its dorsomedial portion and grows into the metanephric blastema from the fourth gestational week. By reciprocal induction (epithelial and mesenchymal interaction), nephrons are developed up to the 32nd gestational week. Parallel to the development of the metanephric kidney, the distal part of the mesonephric duct that gives rise to the ureteric bud becomes incorporated into the urogenital sinus.

The end of the distal gut (hindgut) represents the cloaca, which gives rise to the urethra and the urinary bladder (the proximal urethra and bladder urothelium is endodermal derived; the urothelial lining of the ureters and renal pelvis are mesodermal in origin). From the fourth gestational week, the cloaca is divided by the urorectale septum into the ventral urogenital sinus (the primordial urinary bladder) and the dorsal rectum. The embryonal bladder is also called the allantois and collects primordial urine, which distends into the umbilical cord. The remainder of the allantois is the urachus or original urine conduit which occludes as term is reached.

3.2.3 The Uroplakins

The species-conserved uroplakins ("urothelial plaque-associated proteins") were discovered and characterized through painstaking biochemical, electron microscopy, immunochemistry, and, latterly, transgenic studies (Sun et al. 1996). There are four major protein species, with the UPK1A and UPK1B tetraspanins interacting respectively with the unrelated single transmembrane UPK2 and UPK3 proteins (Wu et al. 1994). The formation of uroplakins into membrane-inserted plaques is well characterized, with precise changes in glycosylation required for correct assembly in the Golgi and translocation in membrane-bound "fusiform vesicles" which open onto the superficial apical membrane to extend urothelial surface area during bladder filling (Kątnik-Prastowska et al. 2014; Kreft et al. 2022). In humans, UPK1A and UPK2 are regarded as the most urothelium-restricted of the uroplakins (Olsburgh et al. 2003).

The application of transgenic and knockout strategies has underpinned much of our understanding of how the urothelium contributes to the development, health, and pathology of the bladder and urinary tracts. The *Upk3* knockout mouse showed that Upk3 protein ablation led to overexpression, defective glycosylation, and abnormal targeting of Upklb, the partner of Upk3. The resultant Upk3-depleted urothelium was leaky with small apical plaques; structurally, the bladder showed enlarged ureteric orifices, leading to urine reflux and altered renal function due to hydronephrosis (Hu et al. 2000, 2002). Thus, loss of a single urothelium-restricted gene resulted in primary vesicoureteral reflux (VUR), a developmental condition that occurs in about 1% of human pregnancies and is a leading cause of kidney failure in infants. Similarly, *Upk2*-null mice also suffered from VUR and severe hydronephrosis (Kong et al. 2004). Although the animal studies provided promising insight for follow on human studies, the observations were not directly translatable, as neither *UPK2* (Jenkins et al. 2006) nor *UPK3* (Kelly et al. 2005) could be linked as major causes of primary VUR in humans (van Eerde et al. 2012). The idea that disruption to the uroplakins has more severe consequences for human than mouse urinary tract development is proposed to explain why congenital human *UPK* gene mutations are rare (Jenkins et al. 2005).

3.3 Form and Function

The urothelium can be considered to have evolved highly fit for purpose as a consequence of needing to survive and function at the harsh interface with urine, and, as a perspective, this provides interesting insights into the biology of urothelium.

3.3.1 The Urinary Barrier

The main function of urothelium is to provide a stable urinary barrier that retains urine from the kidneys in a concentrated state, preventing reabsorption of toxic urinary excretion products or any free exchange of water or solutes across what is often referred to as the "blood/urine barrier". During bladder filling, the urothelium extends its surface area by incorporating uroplakin plaques into the apical surface (see Sect. 3.2.2) as well as reducing the number of intermediate cell layers. By extending its surface area while retaining barrier function, the urothelium enables the bladder to store large volumes of urine under low pressure and helps to prevent urine from refluxing back into the kidneys.

The urothelium is the tightest (least permeable) epithelial tissue of the body as a result of well-developed terminal tight junctions between the superficial cells, which act to restrict the free movement of solutes between cells. Experimentally, epithelial barrier tightness is typically assessed by measuring transepithelial electrical resistance (TEER) (Rubenwolf and Southgate 2011), with in vitro differentiated human urothelium typically achieving >3000 Ω cm^2 (Cross et al. 2005; Smith et al. 2011). Claudins are the superfamily of tight junction constituent proteins that determine epithelial tightness by regulating the permeability of the paracellular pore. Here there is some controversy between human and rodent studies. In mouse urothelium in vivo and in vitro, the highly resistant tight junctions are attributed to the specific distribution of claudin 8 around superficial urothelial cells containing apical uroplakin plaques and a CK20-positive cytoskeleton (Kreft et al. 2006). As such, claudin 8 is frequently used as a specific marker for superficial urothelial cells in mice and other nonhuman species (Acharya et al. 2004; Višnjar et al. 2012). By contrast, human urothelium is reported to express claudins 3, 4, 5, and 7 (Varley et al. 2006), with claudin 3, identified by both immunolocalization and experimental studies as functionally responsible for human urothelial barrier tightness (Smith et al. 2011).

Although it is often assumed that urine is not modified in the bladder, it is worth mentioning that the expression of aquaporins and ion channels provides a physiological mechanism for urothelium to be involved in salt and water homeostasis (Rubenwolf et al. 2012). This holds particular bearing for hibernating species but is also implicated in human urinary dysfunction (McCloskey et al. 2017; Rehman and Ahmed 2022).

3.3.2 Urothelial Turnover

Unlike most epithelial tissues that display a constant turnover cycle, urothelium is essentially mitotically quiescent with one of the slowest turnover rates of all mammalian epithelia but with a high regenerative capacity in response to damage or injury (Hicks 1975). Morphometric analysis of bladders from mice pulsed via their drinking water with tritiated thymidine was important in demonstrating the long-lived quiescent but regenerative nature of normal adult urothelium. Such analysis estimated a cell cycle time of about 1 year, reducing to 15 h when urothelial cells are rapidly regenerating (Jost 1986). Other rodent studies have also been useful in detailing the regenerative response of urothelium to damage (Romih et al. 1998) and in identifying growth factors involved in regulating urothelial repair (Baskin et al. 1997).

Nevertheless, critical differences between human and rodent urothelium have been noted. Possibly of most significance is the observation that while all urothelia are mitotically quiescent, human urothelium is arrested in G0 (out of cell cycle), whereas the urothelia from rodents (both rat and mouse bladders) are arrested in G1 (Chopra et al. 2008). This biological difference may be reflective of differences in lifespan, which includes an absence of telomere restriction as a transformation block in rodent somatic cells (Calado and Dumitriu 2013; Hahn and Weinberg 2002).

The mitotically quiescent nature of urothelium is similar to the liver, where hepatocytes are mitotically quiescent but retain regenerative capacity in response to damage (Marceau 1990). This supports the concept of a tissue homeostasis program where proliferation is "on-demand" and where differentiation is not necessarily the terminal (death) event associated with other epithelial tissues that display a constitutive cell cycling and turnover program.

This raises another question: whether an on-demand regeneration program requires a progenitor stem cell population that gives rise to differentiated progeny through a hierarchical differentiation process. In urothelium at least, it is possible to speculate an alternative nonhierarchical model where individual cells are plastic and locally responsive to external cues or niche. This is supported by several observations: (1) all cells (including superficial cells; see Fig. 3.1) retain potential to proliferate in response to tissue damage (Hicks 1975), (2) separated basal and suprabasal populations isolated from normal (porcine) urothelium assume a similar proliferative phenotype in vitro—both produce progeny capable of differentiating into a functional barrier urothelium composed of distinct basal and superficial compartments (including "reverse" production of basal cells from the suprabasal-derived subpopulation) (Wezel et al. 2014)—and (3) no unequivocal stem cell has been identified or isolated from urothelium. The question whether urothelial cells (and presumptive neoplastic cells) are hierarchical or plastic is important when it comes to understanding the cellular targets of carcinogenesis from exposure to urinary carcinogens and in deciding whether particular cancer ("stem") cells should be targeted therapeutically.

3.3.3 Role in Innate Defense

Urothelium plays an important role in innate defense, producing antimicrobial peptides in response to specific pathogen-associated molecular patterns (PAMPS) to self-limit urinary tract infections. By protecting against urine reflux and ascending infections, the urinary bladder serves an essential role in preserving kidney function by protecting the delicate and non-regenerative renal tubule structures from damage.

Failure of urothelium as a barrier results in the ingress of urine into underlying tissues and symptoms of cystitis (bladder inflammation) typified by urinary urgency, pain, and nocturia. Such symptoms are commonly associated with bacterial cystitis caused by uropathogenic *E. coli* but are also typical of chronic non-resolving conditions known collectively as bladder pain syndrome. This highlights the evolutionary drive on urothelium to be regenerative and to limit inflammation; it is noteworthy that human urothelium has few resident immunocytes in its normal state (see Fig. 3.1).

The mechanics of the normal urinary tract are such that there is a powerful unidirectional expulsion of urine, preventing most bacteria and other pathogens from entering or colonizing the urinary tract. Symptomatic urinary tract infections are caused by uropathogenic *E. coli* which have pili and are flagellated, enabling them to adhere to the urothelium and move in a retrograde direction to flow. Human urothelium expresses Toll-like receptor 5 (TLR5) which, when activated by flagellin, leads via canonical NFκB signaling to the secretion of antimicrobial proteins, including β-defensin 2, resulting in direct killing of bacteria and making urinary tract infection (UTI) self-limiting in most individuals (Smith et al. 2011; Ali et al. 2017).

The signaling involved in excluding or recruiting immunocytes into the urothelium is poorly understood but is important for understanding how the urothelium interacts with the innate and adaptive immune systems for functions such as tumor surveillance. The latter is particularly relevant given the potential for immunotherapies to overcome host anergy to tumors. A recent analysis of the immune landscape of normal urothelium revealed it to express immune inhibitory factors, such as V-domain immunoglobulin suppressor of T-cell activation (VISTA) which will tend to suppress inflammation. By contrast, various exogenous stimulators including IFNγ are able to induce urothelial expression of chemokine genes critical to the recruitment of natural killer (NK) cells and other immunocytes into the urothelium (Baker et al. 2022a). These observations from studying normal human urothelium bring an additional perspective for the design of immunotherapeutic strategies, as it may be predicted that the combination targeting of VISTA and PD-L1 could enhance efficacy against urothelial cancers.

3.4 Urothelial Differentiation: Transitional Versus Squamous States

3.4.1 Cytokeratins: Markers of Differentiation

The 10 nm intermediate filament proteins of epithelial cells, the cytokeratins (CKs), provide useful markers as they show epithelial tissue-associated and differentiation stage-related expression patterns (Moll et al. 1982). Cytokeratins are obligate heteropolymers formed from pairing of type I (small, acidic) and type II (large, basic) polypeptides, with frequent coexpression and colocalization of particular isotype pairs in tissues (Fig. 3.2).

3.4.2 Squamous Changes in Benign (Metaplastic) and Malignant States

Changes in CK expression and/or distribution pattern are useful histopathologically. It is particularly notable that CK14 gain is an early marker of squamous metaplasia in urothelium (Harnden and Southgate 1997). It has long been known that squamous differentiation of bladder urothelium is a consequence of a vitamin A-deficient diet in mice (Molloy and Laskin 1988) and with implications for human pathology (El-Aaser et al. 1982). A paradigm for this benign squamous switch is found in vitro when normal human urothelial (NHU) cells cultured in serum-free medium assume a non-differentiated, CK13-CK14+ squamous phenotype that can be resolved upon supplementation of the medium with retinoids (Southgate et al. 1994).

Cancers arise as a result of escape from the growth-suppressive tissue homeostatic or regulatory pathways that maintain normal urothelial cells in check (mitotically quiescent) within the tissue. From analysis of bladder cancer transcriptomes, two major cancer subtypes have been identified (see Chaps. 13 and 14). The transcriptome of the luminal subtype reflects tumors that retain expression of genes associated with the differentiated transitional phenotype of normal urothelium. This implies an "addiction" to the highly efficient on-demand regeneration program used by normal differentiated urothelium (see Sect. 3.3.2). By contrast, basal subtype cancers are marked by the absence of urothelial differentiation-associated gene expression, a loss of CK13, and a switch to the CK14+ squamous program. This indicates that BASQ (i.e., basal/squamous (Lerner et al. 2016)) subtype tumors have "escaped" the constraints of urothelial differentiation and regressed to a more primitive squamous state.

Of note, the antibody (anti-CK5/6 clone D5/16 B4) used widely as the main immunohistopathological marker for distinguishing BASQ from luminal muscle-invasive bladder cancer (MIBC) subtypes is not ideal as, by reacting with both CK5 and CK6, it does not clearly distinguish between CK5+ transitional and CK6+ squamous epithelia. This confusion is further compounded by the original terminology of "basal" adopted from the breast cancer field to describe the BASQ subtype, as it tends to (mis)imply a phenotype based on position rather than differentiation state. To add yet further confusion, while CK14 is not expressed by human urothelium except in association with squamous metaplasia, basally positioned cells of normal mouse urothelium are CK14 positive. Thus, a basally located label-retaining CK5+ CK14+ population described in rodent urothelium (Kurzrock et al. 2008) has no equivalent in human urothelium.

3.4.3 Regulators of Differentiation and Development

Nuclear receptor ligands have been shown to play a differentiation-inductive role, with retinoids able to switch NHU cells in vitro from KRT14+

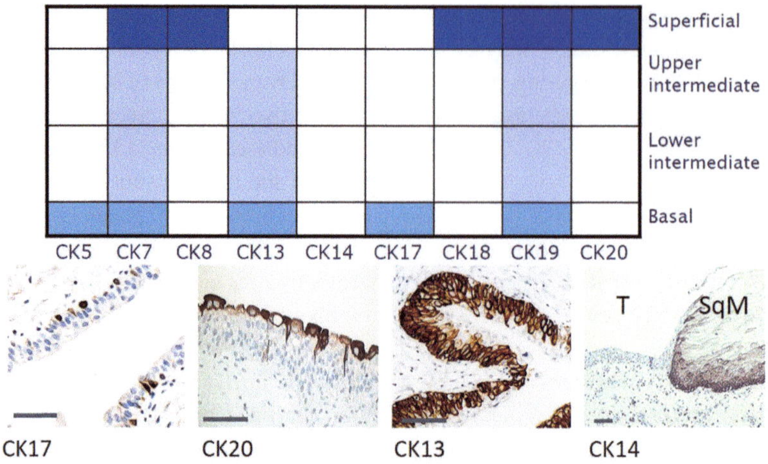

Fig. 3.2 Cytokeratin expression in human urothelium. CK7 and CK19 are present throughout the urothelium, CK5 and CK17 are found in basal and variably lower intermediate cell zones, and CK20 is restricted to superficial cells (Southgate et al. 1999; Harnden and Southgate 1997). CK13 is normally detected throughout but with specific exclusion from the superficial cell layer, which contrasts distinctly, but subtly, from non-cornified stratified squamous epithelia where CK13 is present in all but the basal cell layer. CK14 is absent from normal human urothelium (T = transitional) but is expressed in association with squamous metaplasia (SqM), where it can provide an early marker of squamous change (Harnden and Southgate 1997). Scale bar 50 μm. Figure adapted from Booth et al. (1997)

squamous to KRT13+ transitional (Southgate et al. 1994). Another key nuclear receptor is peroxisome proliferator-activated receptor gamma (PPARγ), activation of which has been shown to induce expression of genes associated with urothelial differentiation, including uroplakins, cytokeratins, and claudins (Varley et al. 2006, 2004a, b). PPARγ-induced differentiation is mediated indirectly via a network of intermediary transcription factors including FOXA1 (Varley et al. 2009), ELF3 (Böck et al. 2014), and GATA3 (Fishwick et al. 2017), which function as part of a heterarchical network. Opposing this, p63 (gene *TP63*) has emerged as an important driver of the more basal-squamous phenotype that cells adopt in cultures lacking nuclear receptor activation. In the absence of PPARγ stimulation, p63 transrepresses genes normally activated as part of the urothelial specialization program (Fishwick et al. 2017), while forced expression of PPARγ in non-urothelial (buccal epithelial) cells can partially recapitulate the urothelial differentiation program (Hustler et al. 2018).

Bladder exstrophy (BEX) is a rare developmental anomaly where failure to partition the cloacal membrane during midline closure results in an open, exposed bladder plate. In mice, where the N-terminal truncated isoform of Tp63, ΔNp63, has been linked to early bladder development, *Tp63−/−* knockout mice present with a classic BEX phenotype (Cheng et al. 2006). However, no evidence for genetic alterations of p63 has been found in BEX or the wider spectrum of human bladder exstrophy–epispadias complex (BEEC) malformations (Ching et al. 2010). While normal bladder urothelium is a mitotically quiescent barrier epithelium, histological studies of human BEX epithelia have reported squamous and proliferative changes that can persist even after surgical closure of the plate (Rubenwolf et al. 2013). Recent in vitro studies using human BEX-derived epithelial cells showed a constitutional failure to express the transcriptional regulators required to drive transitional-type differentiation by a subset of BEX cases, suggesting a developmental failure which could be either indirect (instructive/epigenetic) or intrinsic in nature (Hinley et al. 2022).

Thus, there appear strong parallels between the regulation of urothelial differentiation observed developmentally or in vitro and the groupings established by transcriptomic analysis of

MIBC. BASQ tumors depend on autocrine activation of the epidermal growth factor receptor (EGFR) for growth (Rebouissou et al. 2014) and are enriched for p63 gene expression signatures, whereas the hallmark differentiated luminal tumors have a PPARγ-activated profile (Choi et al. 2014). Of the intermediary transcription factors identified in differentiating urothelial cells (Böck et al. 2014), ELF3 has emerged as frequently mutated in its coding sequence, and these, presumed activating, mutations are associated with a luminal phenotype (Dadhania et al. 2016).

3.5 Experimental Platforms and Models for Studying the Urothelium

A wide range of species and experimental platforms have been used to study urothelial cells and tissues, and it is beyond the scope of this chapter to review them all. The following sections describe some of the approaches that have contributed to our understanding of (human) urothelium in normal/healthy and pathological states.

3.5.1 In vitro Models

The advantage of in vitro approaches is that cells/tissues can be maintained under highly controlled laboratory conditions to study their behavior, responses, and interactions. For these purposes, urothelial cells may be derived from normal, disease, and tumor tissues, originate from different species (typically human, rodent, or porcine), and be grown alone (monoculture) or combined with other cell types (coculture or organotypic cultures).

One of the challenges with studying human bladder-derived urothelial cells is the sourcing of tissue. Finite bladder NHU cell lines have been developed from deceased heart beating (DHB) brain-stem dead donors, but it has been shown that the rapid postmortem changes of the bladder affect the quality and viability of the urothelium, making tissue from deceased non-heart-beating (DNHB) donors nonviable (Garthwaite et al. 2014). An alternative source of human urothelium is discarded ureteric tissue from kidney donors or uninvolved renal cell carcinoma, but as noted above, ureteric urothelium is embryologically distinct from bladder.

Typical experimental configurations used to study urothelium include (a) monoculture of urothelial cells grown on a 2D substrate as a single or stratified multilayer (by manipulating the calcium concentration of the medium from 0.09 to 2.00 mM); (b) tissue mimetic 3D cultures where urothelial cells are combined with extracellular matrix, biocompatible scaffold, or bioprinted structures; and (c) other configurations, such as organoids and organoid-on-a-chip.

3.5.2 Bladder Urothelial 2D and 3D Cultures

Cell culture provides a tractable experimental platform for investigating mechanisms regulating proliferation, stratification, and differentiation of urothelial cells in health and disease (Varley and Southgate 2011; Baker et al. 2014). A reproducible culture system is clearly an essential prerequisite, and robust methods exist to isolate and propagate NHU cells from primary culture and through serial passages as finite (non-immortalized) cell lines (Southgate et al. 2002). NHU cell cultures are typically propagated in a modified serum-free growth medium developed for the culture of keratinocytes, and under these conditions, NHU cells adopt a CK14+ basal/squamous phenotype but can be differentiated to a CK13+ transitional (urothelial) phenotype with barrier (TEER >3000 Ω cm^2) properties (Cross et al. 2005). Unlike cancer-derived cell lines, NHU cells are finite (non-immortal) and invariably senesce in culture (Southgate et al. 1994). To overcome this, different groups have independently produced hTERT-immortalized human urothelial cell lines (Chapman et al. 2006; Georgopoulos et al. 2011). In both cases, it was reported that although immortalization occurred without major karyotypic changes, the capacity for differentiation was impaired, limiting their usefulness for studying normal urothelial cell biology. One advantage of working with finite NHU lines is that studies typically use independent lines generated from multiple individuals, which can provide important insight into genetic variance (Baker et al. 2018a, 2022a, b), absent from studies based on single established cell lines. Alternatively, starting with cells from pathological samples (Hinley et al. 2022), or by experimental manipulation [such as using retroviral infection to overexpress a transgene or dominant negative gene (Georgopoulos et al. 2010)], this approach can offer insight into human pathological processes.

Studies using finite NHU cell lines can inform on intrinsic mechanisms, such as autocrine growth regulation by EGFR ligands (Varley et al. 2005; Daher et al. 2003). It is notable that NHU cells displaying the non-differentiated, squamous phenotype have proliferation driven by autocrine activation of EGFR by amphiregulin (Varley et al. 2005; Rebouissou et al. 2014), which is also the dominant growth driver of basal/squamous MIBC (Rebouissou et al. 2014).

While there is much utility in isolating and expanding urothelial cells for characterization and experimental studies, this disrupts spatial organization and eliminates paracrine and other interactions between epithelium and stroma that are implicit in urothelial tissue biology in situ. A more physiological approach is to use an air–liquid interface to maintain urothelium intact with its stroma (Knowles et al. 1983) or reconstituted by combining cultured NHU cells with stroma (Scriven et al. 1997). Organ culture approaches simulate a more physiological tissue environment for studying cell-to-cell and cell-to-ECM interactions and have been used to maintain urothelium in a mature state for 100 days (Knowles et al. 1983), but these approaches tend only to support small-scale studies (reviewed by Varley and Southgate 2011).

3.5.3 In vitro Studies Using Animal-Derived Urothelium

The potential to expand and post-differentiate urothelial cell cultures has supported research with clinical goals, such as tissue engineering for reconstructive bladder surgery. As well as promoting NHU cell/tissue research, the need for methods for surgical delivery of in vitro-engineered tissues has driven parallel in vitro methods for normal porcine urothelial cells (Turner et al. 2008), in advance of testing in experimental surgical models (Turner et al. 2011). Cultures of normal porcine urothelial cells have also been used in basic cell biological research, as they show good equivalence to human urothelium in vitro and the tissue is available fresh and in quantity from an abattoir. Thus, subcultured normal porcine bladder urothelial cells have been used in studies of barrier repair after injury (Višnjar et al. 2012; Višnjar and Kreft 2013), leading to new insights into the relationships between cytoskeletal organization, apical endocytosis, and uroplakin expression that modulate barrier function in superficial cells (Kreft et al. 2022).

Obtaining sufficient quantities of healthy human bladder tissue remains a major obstacle preventing extensive preclinical studies of differentiated cultures of human bladder urothelium. Mouse urothelium is well characterized (Romih et al. 2005), and one study using mouse bladder tissue demonstrated the possibility of reusing explants up to ten times to generate serial outgrowths of highly differentiated urothelia. Even after ten reuses, mouse bladder urothelial outgrowths had supramolecular and ultrastructural features comparable to native urothelium or primary outgrowths, with tight junction-forming CK20+ superficial cells and p63+ basal cells, indicating sustained proliferative capacity. The same method was proposed (but not tested) for human bladder to support repeated production of highly differentiated human urothelium in vitro for experiments previously not feasible due to small amounts of donor tissue (Jerman and Kreft 2018).

While animal models clearly offer important insights, as noted above, it is important to be aware of differences between species in terms of developmental processes and timing, or variation, in anatomical or physiological features. A recent study used single-cell RNA sequencing to compare bladder cells from mouse and human in a single integrated dataset, revealing potential differences in developmental trajectories between mouse and human bladder cells (Shi et al. 2022). While this indicates the potential for these new approaches to bring insight from interspecies studies in the future, challenges remain and verification remains an absolute requirement (Ma et al. 2020).

3.5.4 Modeling of Bladder Urothelium with Computational and In silico/In virtuo Tools

Modeling takes different forms (Reyes-Aldasoro 2023), including in virtuo, which can itself extend to mathematical or computational approaches and operate at different scales to provide insight into biological processes. One interesting high-resolution application has been the use of mathematical modeling to explore stretch-induced membrane traffic in bladder umbrella cells (Moulton et al. 2016).

Computational approaches can be particularly useful where the outcome of modeling is emergent rather than fixed or programmed, as this can be used to generate or test hypotheses, including predicting experimental outcomes. A computational model called the epitheliome was used to explore how urothelial cell/cell interactions would influence the growth and size of a cell population over time (Walker et al. 2004b). Biological cells were represented by autonomous software agents interacting on a 2D substrate. Each agent had a cell cycle clock and, at each iteration, executed a set of rules in response to local feedback, similar to how the individual components of a complex social system might behave. The user-programmed cell-type parameters were based on the average cell cycle durations and migration rates observed in experimental studies with NHU cells (Southgate et al. 1994). The growth kinetics of the overall population was an emergent behavior that depended on the interactions between individual cells and the experimental setup (e.g., cell number, distribution, and calcium concentration). The model was used to explore other scenarios including the response of individual cells and the population to scratch wounding (Walker et al. 2004a) and reciprocal effects of normal and mutated (antisocial) cell/cell interactions on individual and population growth (Walker et al. 2010). Later, a multiscale model combining computational and mathematical modeling approaches was developed to explore the emergent heterogeneity resulting from the influences of intercellular signaling on individual cells within a population (Walker et al. 2008). The results from comparing in virtuo with in vitro (time-lapse) experiments predicted a novel pro-proliferation signaling pathway, later confirmed experimentally as operating through a PI3K pathway triggered in NHU cells in direct cell/cell contact (Georgopoulos et al. 2010). Together the computational approach suggested that the microenvironment, including local cell density and the presence of normal versus E-cadherin-compromised neighbors, could play a critical role in determining whether a single abnormal cell within the monolayer proliferates or remains mitotically suppressed. These predictions provide insight on the modulating effect of cell–cell contact on the tumorigenic potential of premalignant epithelial cells.

3.5.5 Artificial Intelligence (AI) for Studying Bladder Urothelium

What might the future hold for studying human urothelial cell biology in health and disease? The relatively recent switch to quantitative biology and data-driven approaches has fueled interest in using AI approaches to reveal and predict patterns in large, complex datasets. In brief, AI is a field of computer science that develops and integrates software tools to enable complex input data to be analyzed "intelligently," enabling solutions to emerge that are not pre-programmed and even self-evolving the process to learn and improve the output over multiple iterations. One field of AI is machine learning (ML), which uses approaches such as statistical algorithms or generative neural networks to find data solutions that can then be applied to unseen datasets. The important feature of ML algorithms is their data-driven approach to learning, contrasting to the rule-based models (discussed in Sect. 3.5.4) that rely on domain knowledge. A criticism of ML approaches is that they are often referred to as "black box" solutions as it can be difficult to understand exactly how the input data is manipulated to achieve the result obtained. However, the field is rapidly evolving and carries enormous potential for analyzing large multimodality datasets.

The uptake of AI and ML tools by academics and clinicians will facilitate assessment of their benefits, risks, and uncertainties, thereby increasing the likelihood of successful adoption. Already in urology practice, AI has been tested in areas such as prognostic histopathology (Wessels et al. 2022) and radiation treatment planning (Moore et al. 2023). A recent, publicly available volumetric electron microscopy dataset for urothelial cells evaluated several state-of-the-art segmentation methods and presented a novel analysis pipeline based on supervised deep learning that reduces the impact of dependencies in the input data, artifacts, and annotation errors (Žerovnik Mekuč et al. 2022). The UroCell dataset is publicly available at https://github.com/MancaZerovnikMekuc/UroCell.

By contrast, it is fair to say that AI-based studies applied to urothelial cell biology predominantly represent early pilot studies (e.g., Zhang et al. 2016), exemplifying only the potential of AI approaches. While there is hope that AI models will in the future be used to train complex multiscale models to simulate aspects of urothelial cell biology, models are only ever as good as the input data and cannot presently be used as a substitute for experimental validation. A vision of the future might be where AI integrates temporal and spatial multi-omic (genomic, epigenetic, transcriptomic, proteomic, phosphoproteomic, metabolomic) data into computational representations of urothelial cells and tissues for experimental and preclinical studies, but this ambition lies some way off.

3.6 Concluding Remarks

The essential need for a urinary barrier has led to evolution of urothelium, an epithelium that is structurally and functionally specialized for the role. Developmentally, the differentiated urothelial phenotype marked by a normal transitional cytokeratin expression profile and apical membrane expression of uroplakins can already be observed in the fetal bladder before the end of the first trimester. Urothelium provides a stable, mitotically quiescent barrier with inbuilt capacity for repair and regeneration. As well as protecting underlying tissues from urinary exposure to toxins and genotoxins, it plays a direct role in innate defense against uropathogens while potentially suppressing inflammation. The study of normal urothelial cell and tissue biology can provide insight into the mutated pathways and other regulatory mechanisms that provide selection advantage during tumorigenesis. Whereas basal (BASQ) subtype cancers escape the constraints of differentiation by assuming a primitive squamous phenotype similar to the autocrine EGFR-regulated NHU cell, it appears that luminal cancers hijack the differentiated urothelial transcriptomic program—potentially selecting those pathways that support regeneration and repair in the normal tissue. This raises interesting questions about what initiates and selects for MIBCs to follow the luminal versus BASQ routes and how different therapeutic agents might target each or be used to promote particular outcomes, including alleviation of immunosuppression.

References

Acharya P, Beckel J, Ruiz WG, Wang E, Rojas R, Birder L, Apodaca G (2004) Distribution of the tight junction proteins ZO-1, occludin, and claudin-4, −8, and −12 in bladder epithelium. Am J Physiol Renal Physiol 287:F305–F318

Ali ASM, Mowbray C, Lanz M, Stanton A, Bowen S, Varley CL, Hilton P, Brown K, Robson W, Southgate J, Aldridge PD, Tyson-Capper A, Abraham S, Pickard RS, Hall J (2017) Targeting deficiencies in the TLR5 mediated vaginal response to treat female recurrent urinary tract infection. Sci Rep 7:11039

Baker SC, Shabir S, Southgate J (2014) Biomimetic urothelial tissue models for the in vitro evaluation of barrier physiology and bladder drug efficacy. Mol Pharm 11:1964–1970

Baker SC, Arlt VM, Indra R, Joel M, Stiborová M, Eardley I, Ahmad N, Otto W, Burger M, Rubenwolf P, Phillips DH, Southgate J (2018a) Differentiation-associated urothelial cytochrome P450 oxidoreductase predicates the xenobiotic-metabolizing activity of "luminal" muscle-invasive bladder cancers. Mol Carcinog 57:606–618

Baker SC, Stahlschmidt J, Trejdosiewicz LK, Southgate J (2018b) Developmental aspects of human urothelial differentiation in vitro and in vivo. In: Lerner McConkey SP (ed) SIU-ICUD joint consultation on bladder cancer - Basic Science

Baker SC, Mason AS, Slip RG, Eriksson P, Sjödahl G, Trejdosiewicz LK, Southgate J (2022a) The urothelial transcriptomic response to interferon gamma: implications for bladder cancer prognosis and immunotherapy. Cancers (Basel) 14

Baker SC, Mason AS, Slip RG, Skinner KT, Macdonald A, Masood O, Harris RS, Fenton TR, Periyasamy M, Ali S, Southgate J (2022b) Induction of APOBEC3-mediated genomic damage in urothelium implicates BK polyomavirus (BKPyV) as a hit-and-run driver for bladder cancer. Oncogene 41:2139–2151

Baskin LS, Sutherland RS, Thomson AA, Nguyen HT, Morgan DM, Hayward SW, Hom YK, DiSandro M, Cunha GR (1997) Growth factors in bladder wound healing. J Urol 157:2388–2395

Böck M, Hinley J, Schmitt C, Wahlicht T, Kramer S, Southgate J (2014) Identification of ELF3 as an early transcriptional regulator of human urothelium. Dev Biol 386:321–330

Booth C, Harnden P, Trejdosiewicz LK, Scriven S, Selby PJ, Southgate J (1997) Stromal and vascular invasion in an human in vitro bladder cancer model. Lab Investig 76:843–857

Calado RT, Dumitriu B (2013) Telomere dynamics in mice and humans. Semin Hematol 50:165–174

Castillo-Martin M, Domingo-Domenech J, Karni-Schmidt O, Matos T, Cordon-Cardo C (2010) Molecular pathways of urothelial development and bladder tumorigenesis. Urologic Oncol 28:401–408

Chapman EJ, Hurst CD, Pitt E, Chambers P, Aveyard JS, Knowles MA (2006) Expression of hTERT immortalises normal human urothelial cells without inactivation of the p16/Rb pathway. Oncogene 25:5037–5045

Cheng W, Jacobs WB, Zhang JJ, Moro A, Park JH, Kushida M, Qiu W, Mills AA, Kim PC (2006) DeltaNp63 plays an anti-apoptotic role in ventral bladder development. Development 133:4783–4792

Ching BJ, Wittler L, Proske J, Yagnik G, Qi L, Draaken M, Reutter H, Gearhart JP, Ludwig M, Boyadjiev SA (2010) p63 (TP73L) a key player in embryonic urogenital development with significant dysregulation in human bladder exstrophy tissue. Int J Mol Med 26:861–867

Choi W, Porten S, Kim S, Willis D, Plimack ER, Hoffman-Censits J, Roth B, Cheng T, Tran M, Lee IL, Melquist J, Bondaruk J, Majewski T, Zhang S, Pretzsch S, Baggerly K, Siefker-Radtke A, Czerniak B, Dinney CP, McConkey DJ (2014) Identification of distinct basal and luminal subtypes of muscle-invasive bladder cancer with different sensitivities to frontline chemotherapy. Cancer Cell 25:152–165

Chopra B, Hinley J, Oleksiewicz MB, Southgate J (2008) Trans-species comparison of PPAR and RXR expression by rat and human urothelial tissues. Toxicol Pathol 36:485–495

Cross WR, Eardley I, Leese HJ, Southgate J (2005) A biomimetic tissue from cultured normal human urothelial cells: analysis of physiological function. Am J Physiol Renal Physiol 289:F459–F468

Dadhania V, Zhang M, Zhang L, Bondaruk J, Majewski T, Siefker-Radtke A, Guo CC, Dinney C, Cogdell DE, Zhang S, Lee S, Lee JG, Weinstein JN, Baggerly K, McConkey D, Czerniak B (2016) Meta-analysis of the luminal and basal subtypes of bladder cancer and the identification of signature immunohistochemical markers for clinical use. EBioMedicine 12:105–117

Daher A, de Boer WI, El-Marjou A, van der Kwast T, Abbou CC, Thiery JP, Radvanyi F, Chopin DK (2003) Epidermal growth factor receptor regulates normal urothelial regeneration. Lab Investig 83:1333–1341

El-Aaser AA, El-Merzabani MM, Abdel-Reheem KA, Hamza BM (1982) A study on the etiological factors of bilharzial bladder cancer in Egypt: 4. Beta-carotene and vitamin A level in serum. Tumori 68:19–22

Felix W (1912) The development of the urinogenital organs. I. The development of the excretory glands and their ducts. Manual of human embryology, pp 752–880

Fishwick C, Higgins J, Percival-Alwyn L, Hustler A, Pearson J, Bastkowski S, Moxon S, Swarbreck D, Greenman CD, Southgate J (2017) Heterarchy of transcription factors driving basal and luminal cell phenotypes in human urothelium. Cell Death Differ 24:809–818

Garthwaite M, Hinley J, Cross W, Warwick RM, Ambrose A, Hardaker H, Eardley I, Southgate J (2014) Use of donor bladder tissues for in vitro research. BJU Int 113:160–166

Georgopoulos NT, Kirkwood LA, Walker DC, Southgate J (2010) Differential regulation of growth-promoting signalling pathways by E-cadherin. PLoS One 5:e13621

Georgopoulos NT, Kirkwood LA, Varley CL, MacLaine NJ, Aziz N, Southgate J (2011) Immortalisation of normal human urothelial cells compromises differentiation capacity. Eur Urol 60:141–149

Gyllensten L (1949) Contributions to the embryology of the urinary bladder. Acta Anat (Basel) 7:305–344

Hahn WC, Weinberg RA (2002) Modelling the molecular circuitry of cancer. Nat Rev Cancer 2:331–341

Haraguchi R, Motoyama J, Sasaki H, Satoh Y, Miyagawa S, Nakagata N, Moon A, Yamada G (2007) Molecular analysis of coordinated bladder and urogenital organ formation by hedgehog signaling. Development 134:525–533

Harnden P, Southgate J (1997) Cytokeratin 14 as a marker of squamous differentiation in transitional cell carcinomas. J Clin Pathol 50:1032–1033

Hicks RM (1975) The mammalian urinary bladder: an accommodating organ. Biol Rev Camb Philos Soc 50:215–246

Hinley J, Duke R, Jinks J, Stahlschmidt J, Keene D, Cervellione RM, Mushtaq I, De Coppi P, Garriboli M, Southgate J (2022) Barrier-forming potential of epithelial cells from the exstrophic bladder. Am J Pathol 192:943–955

Hoyes AD, Ramus NI, Martin BG (1972) Fine structure of the epithelium of the human fetal bladder. J Anat 111:415–425

Hu P, Deng FM, Liang FX, Hu CM, Auerbach AB, Shapiro E, Wu XR, Kachar B, Sun TT (2000) Ablation of uroplakin III gene results in small urothelial plaques, urothelial leakage, and vesicoureteral reflux. J Cell Biol 151:961–972

Hu P, Meyers S, Liang FX, Deng FM, Kachar B, Zeidel ML, Sun TT (2002) Role of membrane proteins in permeability barrier function: uroplakin ablation elevates urothelial permeability. Am J Physiol Renal Physiol 283:F1200–F1207

Hustler A, Eardley I, Hinley J, Pearson J, Wezel F, Radvanyi F, Baker SC, Southgate J (2018) Differential transcription factor expression by human epithelial cells of buccal and urothelial derivation. Exp Cell Res 369:284–294

Jenkins D, Bitner-Glindzicz M, Malcolm S, Hu CC, Allison J, Winyard PJ, Gullett AM, Thomas DF, Belk RA, Feather SA, Sun TT, Woolf AS (2005) De novo Uroplakin IIIa heterozygous mutations cause human renal adysplasia leading to severe kidney failure. J Am Soc Nephrol 16:2141–2149

Jenkins D, Bitner-Glindzicz M, Malcolm S, Allison J, de Bruyn R, Flanagan S, Thomas DF, Belk RA, Feather SA, Bingham C, Southgate J, Woolf AS (2006) Mutation analyses of Uroplakin II in children with renal tract malformations. Nephrol Dial Transplant 21:3415–3421

Jerman UD, Kreft ME (2018) Reuse of bladder mucosa explants provides a long lasting source of urothelial cells for the establishment of differentiated urothelia. Histochem Cell Biol 150:567–574

Jost SP (1986) Renewal of normal urothelium in adult mice. Virchows Arch B Cell Pathol Incl Mol Pathol 51:65–70

Jost SP, Gosling JA, Dixon JS (1989) The morphology of normal human bladder urothelium. J Anat 167:103–115

Kątnik-Prastowska I, Lis J, Matejuk A (2014) Glycosylation of uroplakins. Implications for bladder physiopathology. Glycoconj J 31:623–636

Kelly H, Ennis S, Yoneda A, Bermingham C, Shields DC, Molony C, Green AJ, Puri P, Barton DE (2005) Uroplakin III is not a major candidate gene for primary vesicoureteral reflux. Eur J Hum Genet 13:500–502

Khandelwal P, Abraham SN, Apodaca G (2009) Cell biology and physiology of the uroepithelium. Am J Physiol Renal Physiol 297:F1477–F1501

Knoers NVAM (2022) The term CAKUT has outlived its usefulness: the case for the defense. Pediatr Nephrol 37:2793–2798

Knowles MA, Finesilver A, Harvey AE, Berry RJ, Hicks RM (1983) Long-term organ culture of normal human bladder. Cancer Res 43:374–385

Kong XT, Deng FM, Hu P, Liang FX, Zhou G, Auerbach AB, Genieser N, Nelson PK, Robbins ES, Shapiro E, Kachar B, Sun TT (2004) Roles of uroplakins in plaque formation, umbrella cell enlargement, and urinary tract diseases. J Cell Biol 167:1195–1204

Kreft ME, Sterle M, Jezernik K (2006) Distribution of junction- and differentiation-related proteins in urothelial cells at the leading edge of primary explant outgrowths. Histochem Cell Biol 125:475–485

Kreft ME, Mironov AA, Hudoklin S (2022) The Golgi complex: an organelle that determines urothelial cell biology in health and disease. Histochem Cell Biol 158:229–240

Kurzrock EA, Lieu DK, Degraffenried LA, Chan CW, Isseroff RR (2008) Label-retaining cells of the bladder: candidate urothelial stem cells. Am J Physiol Renal Physiol 294:F1415–F1421

Lasič E, Višnjar T, Kreft ME (2015) Properties of the urothelium that establish the blood-urine barrier and their implications for drug delivery. Rev Physiol Biochem Pharmacol 168:1–29

Lerner SP, McConkey DJ, Hoadley KA, Chan KS, Kim WY, Radvanyi F, Höglund M, Real FX (2016) Bladder cancer molecular taxonomy: summary from a consensus meeting. Bladder Cancer 2:37–47

Ma A, McDermaid A, Xu J, Chang Y, Ma Q (2020) Integrative methods and practical challenges for single-cell multi-omics. Trends Biotechnol 38:1007–1022

Marceau N (1990) Cell lineages and differentiation programs in epidermal, urothelial and hepatic tissues and their neoplasms. Lab Investig 63:4–20

McCloskey KD, Vahabi B, Fry CH (2017) Is electrolyte transfer across the urothelium important?: ICI-RS 2015. Neurourol Urodyn 36:863–868

Mekuč Ž, Manca CB, Boneš E, Hudoklin S, Romih R, Marolt M (2022) Automatic segmentation and reconstruction of intracellular compartments in volumetric electron microscopy data. Comput Methods Prog Biomed 223:106959

Moll R, Franke WW, Schiller DL, Geiger B, Krepler R (1982) The catalog of human cytokeratins: patterns of expression in normal epithelia, tumors and cultured cells. Cell 31:11–24

Molloy CJ, Laskin JD (1988) Effect of retinoid deficiency on keratin expression in mouse bladder. Exp Mol Pathol 49:128–140

Moore NS, McWilliam A, Aneja S (2023) Bladder cancer radiation oncology of the future: prognostic modelling, radiomics, and treatment planning with artificial intelligence. Semin Radiat Oncol 33:70–75

Moulton DE, Sulzer V, Apodaca G, Byrne HM, Waters SL (2016) Mathematical modelling of stretch-induced membrane traffic in bladder umbrella cells. J Theor Biol 409:115–132
Newman J, Antonakopoulos GN (1989) The fine structure of the human fetal urinary bladder. Development and maturation. A light, transmission and scanning electron microscopic study. J Anat 166:135–150
Olsburgh J, Harnden P, Weeks R, Smith B, Joyce A, Hall G, Poulsom R, Selby P, Southgate J (2003) Uroplakin gene expression in normal human tissues and locally advanced bladder cancer. J Pathol 199:41–49
Rebouissou S, Bernard-Pierrot I, de Reynies A, Lepage ML, Krucker C, Chapeaublanc E, Herault A, Kamoun A, Caillault A, Letouze E, Elarouci N, Neuzillet Y, Denoux Y, Molinie V, Vordos D, Laplanche A, Maille P, Soyeux P, Ofualuka K, Reyal F, Biton A, Sibony M, Paoletti X, Southgate J, Benhamou S, Lebret T, Allory Y, Radvanyi F (2014) EGFR as a potential therapeutic target for a subset of muscle-invasive bladder cancers presenting a basal-like phenotype. Sci Transl Med 6:244ra91
Rehman S, Ahmed D (2022) Embryology, kidney, bladder, and ureter. In: StatPearls [Internet]. StatPearls Publishing, Treasure Island (FL)
Reyes-Aldasoro CC (2023) Modelling the tumour microenvironment, but what exactly do we mean by “model”? Cancers 15:3796
Romih R, Jezernik K, Masera A (1998) Uroplakins and cytokeratins in the regenerating rat urothelium after sodium saccharin treatment. Histochem Cell Biol 109:263–269
Romih R, Korosec P, de Mello W, Jr., and K. Jezernik. (2005) Differentiation of epithelial cells in the urinary tract. Cell Tissue Res 320:259–268
Rubenwolf P, Southgate J (2011) Permeability of differentiated human urothelium in vitro. Methods Mol Biol 763:207–222
Rubenwolf PC, Georgopoulos NT, Kirkwood LA, Baker SC, Southgate J (2012) Aquaporin expression contributes to human transurothelial permeability in vitro and is modulated by NaCl. PLoS One 7:e45339
Rubenwolf PC, Eder F, Ebert AK, Hofstaedter F, Woodhouse CR, Roesch WH (2013) Persistent histological changes in the exstrophic bladder after primary closure-a cause for concern? J Urol 189:671–677
Scriven SD, Booth C, Thomas DF, Trejdosiewicz LK, Southgate J (1997) Reconstitution of human urothelium from monolayer cultures. J Urol 158:1147–1152
Shi B, Wu Y, Chen H, Ding J, Qi J (2022) Understanding of mouse and human bladder at single-cell resolution: integrated analysis of trajectory and cell-cell interactive networks based on multiple scRNA-seq datasets. Cell Prolif 55:e13170
Smith NJ, Varley CL, Eardley I, Feather S, Trejdosiewicz LK, Southgate J (2011) Toll-like receptor responses of normal human urothelial cells to bacterial flagellin and lipopolysaccharide. J Urol 186:1084–1092
Southgate J, Hutton KA, Thomas DF, Trejdosiewicz LK (1994) Normal human urothelial cells in vitro: proliferation and induction of stratification. Lab Investig 71:583–594
Southgate J, Harnden P, Trejdosiewicz LK (1999) Cytokeratin expression patterns in normal and malignant urothelium: a review of the biological and diagnostic implications. Histol Histopathol 14:657–664
Southgate J, Masters J, Trejdosiewicz LK (2002) Culture of human urothelium. In Freshney RI, Freshney MG (eds) Culture of epithelial cells. Wiley
Sun TT, Zhao H, Provet J, Aebi U, Wu XR (1996) Formation of asymmetric unit membrane during urothelial differentiation. Mol Biol Rep 23:3–11
Trowe MO, Airik R, Weiss AC, Farin HF, Foik AB, Bettenhausen E, Schuster-Gossler K, Taketo MM, Kispert A (2012) Canonical Wnt signaling regulates smooth muscle precursor development in the mouse ureter. Development 139:3099–3108
Turner AM, Subramaniam R, Thomas DF, Southgate J (2008) Generation of a functional, differentiated porcine urothelial tissue in vitro. Eur Urol 54:1423–1432
Turner A, Subramanian R, Thomas DF, Hinley J, Abbas SK, Stahlschmidt J, Southgate J (2011) Transplantation of autologous differentiated urothelium in an experimental model of composite cystoplasty. Eur Urol 59:447–454
van Eerde AM, Duran K, van Riel E, de Kovel CG, Koeleman BP, Knoers NV, Renkema KY, van der Horst HJ, Bökenkamp A, van Hagen JM, van den Berg LH, Wolffenbuttel KP, van den Hoek J, Feitz WF, de Jong TP, Giltay JC, Wijmenga C (2012) Genes in the ureteric budding pathway: association study on vesico-ureteral reflux patients. PLoS One 7:e31327
Varley CL, Southgate J (2011) Organotypic and 3D reconstructed cultures of the human bladder and urinary tract. Methods Mol Biol 695:197–211
Varley CL, Stahlschmidt J, Lee WC, Holder J, Diggle C, Selby PJ, Trejdosiewicz LK, Southgate J (2004a) Role of PPARgamma and EGFR signalling in the urothelial terminal differentiation programme. J Cell Sci 117:2029–2036
Varley CL, Stahlschmidt J, Smith B, Stower M, Southgate J (2004b) Activation of peroxisome proliferator-activated receptor-gamma reverses squamous metaplasia and induces transitional differentiation in normal human urothelial cells. Am J Pathol 164:1789–1798
Varley C, Hill G, Pellegrin S, Shaw NJ, Selby PJ, Trejdosiewicz LK, Southgate J (2005) Autocrine regulation of human urothelial cell proliferation and migration during regenerative responses in vitro. Exp Cell Res 306:216–229
Varley CL, Garthwaite MA, Cross W, Hinley J, Trejdosiewicz LK, Southgate J (2006) PPARgamma-regulated tight junction development during human urothelial cytodifferentiation. J Cell Physiol 208:407–417
Varley CL, Bacon EJ, Holder JC, Southgate J (2009) FOXA1 and IRF-1 intermediary transcriptional regulators of PPARgamma-induced urothelial cytodifferentiation. Cell Death Differ 16:103–114

Višnjar T, Kreft ME (2013) Air-liquid and liquid-liquid interfaces influence the formation of the urothelial permeability barrier in vitro. In Vitro Cell Dev Biol Anim 49:196–204
Višnjar T, Kocbek P, Kreft ME (2012) Hyperplasia as a mechanism for rapid resealing urothelial injuries and maintaining high transepithelial resistance. Histochem Cell Biol 137:177–186
Walker DC, Hill G, Wood SM, Smallwood RH, Southgate J (2004a) Agent-based computational modeling of wounded epithelial cell monolayers. IEEE Trans Nanobioscience 3:153–163
Walker DC, Southgate J, Hill G, Holcombe M, Hose DR, Wood SM, Mac Neil S, Smallwood RH (2004b) The epitheliome: agent-based modelling of the social behaviour of cells. Biosystems 76:89–100
Walker DC, Georgopoulos NT, Southgate J (2008) From pathway to population--a multiscale model of juxtacrine EGFR-MAPK signalling. BMC Syst Biol 2:102
Walker DC, Georgopoulos NT, Southgate J (2010) Anti-social cells: predicting the influence of E-cadherin loss on the growth of epithelial cell populations. J Theor Biol 262:425–440
Wessels F, Kuntz S, Krieghoff-Henning E, Schmitt M, Braun V, Worst TS, Neuberger M, Steeg M, Gaiser T, Fröhling S, Michel MS, Nuhn P, Brinker TJ (2022) Artificial intelligence to predict oncological outcome directly from hematoxylin and eosin-stained slides in urology. Minerva Urol Nephrol 74:538–550
Wezel F, Pearson J, Southgate J (2014) Plasticity of in vitro-generated urothelial cells for functional tissue formation. Tissue Eng Part A 20:1358–1368
Wheater P, Burkitt H, Daniels V (1990) Functional histology: a text and colour atlas. Churchhill Livingstone
Wu XR, Lin JH, Walz T, Haner M, Yu J, Aebi U, Sun TT (1994) Mammalian uroplakins. A group of highly conserved urothelial differentiation-related membrane proteins. J Biol Chem 269:13716–13724
Yu J, Carroll TJ, McMahon AP (2002) Sonic hedgehog regulates proliferation and differentiation of mesenchymal cells in the mouse metanephric kidney. Development 129:5301–5312
Zhang Z, Bedder M, Smith SL, Walker D, Shabir S, Southgate J (2016) Characterization and classification of adherent cells in monolayer culture using automated tracking and evolutionary algorithms. Biosystems 146:110–121

Bladder Cancer Pathology

4

Eva Compérat

Abstract

Many changes have been made in recent years with regard to pathological assessment of bladder cancer/urothelial carcinoma (BC/UC), and understanding of bladder carcinogenesis has evolved. This chapter describes the latest findings of the WHO (World Health Organization) 2022 classification. New approaches and developments in pathological assessment are described, emphasizing key issues, some of which lack consensus. Molecular findings play an important role in the pathological assessment of UC. With the help of this information, pathologists and clinicians have improved understanding of urothelial carcinogenesis, and this can identify the key facts to prioritize in reporting to provide optimal information to guide patient management.

This chapter focuses on several issues; first, staging approaches are described and then issues of grading. This is followed by discussion of the relevance of some BC molecular subtypes in histology and a brief insight into the importance of clinical information, especially with regard to the bladder wall. The chapter concludes by discussing rare issues such as bladder diverticulum and urachus carcinomas, the role of immunohistochemistry in diagnosis, urinary cytology using the Paris system, and the ICCR (International Collaboration on Cancer Reporting) worldwide consensus reporting scheme.

Keywords

Urothelial carcinoma · Stage · Grade · Histology · Subtypes · Divergent differentiation · Carcinoma in situ

4.1 Preneoplastic Lesions

Recognizing precancerous lesions is crucial for both clinicians and researchers. These lesions significantly influence diagnosis and, ultimately, treatment decisions, and it is essential to distinguish them from benign lesions. The precancerous lesions can be divided into three categories:

Dysplasia: The diagnosis of dysplasia remains controversial. The definition of dysplasia is not a synonym of intraepithelial neoplasia. Nevertheless, the lesion encompasses changes that are thought to be preneoplastic in nature but cytologically fall short of the diagnosis of carcinoma in situ (Cis) (Netto et al. 2022). In a general manner, Cis shows disturbed archi-

E. Compérat (✉)
Department of Pathology, Medical University, Vienna, Austria
e-mail: eva.comperat@meduniwien.ac.at

M. A. Knowles, L. Dyrskjøt (eds.), *Biology of Bladder Cancer*,
https://doi.org/10.1007/978-3-031-68505-7_4

tecture and important nuclear atypia sometimes with pseudostratification.

Reactive atypia: On the other hand, reactive atypia is an inflammatory lesion which is always benign. Differential diagnosis with Cis (without associated clinical history) can be extremely difficult, as urothelial architectural disorders, meaning that the urothelium has an irregular aspect, can exist.

Hyperplasia: Hyperplasia is an increase in urothelial thickness due to an increased number of cell layers. It is often a "shoulder lesion" of low-grade (LG) noninvasive (pTa) tumors (see below). Isolated hyperplasia is rare. The real incidence is unknown as it is asymptomatic and is termed AUP (atypical urothelial proliferation). This can be flat or "tented" (undulated). These aspects can be seen by urologists and must be reported if they exist in the histological specimen (Compérat et al. 2021, 2022a).

4.2 Staging

BC staging has not changed over many decades. Different groups of tumors are distinguished according to the 2017 pTNM staging system. Here, "p" stands for pathological. The most frequent group is pTa (noninvasive papillary) tumors, growing only in the epithelium, without any invasive features (low-grade pTa around 75%, high-grade (HG) pTa around 20%). pTis (carcinoma in situ, noninvasive) and pT1 (lamina propria invasive) carcinomas also belong to this non-muscle-invasive BC (NMIBC) group, which are mostly managed conservatively (i.e., without radical cystectomy) after the initial diagnosis (Babjuk et al. 2019) (see also Chap. 5). Muscle-invasive bladder cancer (MIBC) is treated differently (see Chap. 6), and these are subdivided into pT2 (detrusor muscle-invasive carcinomas/"a" and "b" for the inner and outer layers of the detrusor muscle), pT3 (perivesical fat-invading carcinomas/"a" microscopic invasion, "b" macroscopic invasion), and pT4 (invasion of another organ, cancers invading adjacent structures) (Table 4.1, Fig. 4.1).

The NMIBC group is heterogeneous, including noninvasive papillary urothelial neoplasm of low malignant potential (PUNLMP), noninvasive low-grade (LG) papillary urothelial carcinoma, and noninvasive high-grade (HG) papillary urothelial carcinoma. All three of these belong to the pTa tumor category. Cis, a noninvasive lesion, and pT1 carcinoma invading the lamina propria also belong to the NMIBC group. All the high-grade tumors with pTis seem to belong to the

Table 4.1 pTNM classification according to UICC 2017

T—Primary tumor		
TX	Primary tumor cannot be assessed	
T0	No evidence of primary tumor	
Ta	Noninvasive papillary carcinoma	
Tis	Carcinoma in situ: "flat tumor"	
T1	Tumor invades subepithelial connective tissue	
T2	Tumor invades muscle	
	T2a	Tumor invades superficial muscle (inner half)
	T2b	Tumor invades deep muscle (outer half)
T3	Tumor invades perivesical tissue	
	T3a	Microscopically
	T3b	Macroscopically (extravesical mass)
T4	Tumor invades any of the following: prostate stroma, seminal vesicles, uterus, vagina, pelvic wall, and abdominal wall	
	T4a	Tumor invades prostate stroma, seminal vesicles, uterus, or vagina
	T4b	Tumor invades pelvic wall or abdominal wall[a]
N—Regional lymph nodes		
NX	Regional lymph nodes cannot be assessed	
N0	No regional lymph node metastasis	
N1	Metastasis in a single lymph node in the true pelvis (hypogastric, obturator, external iliac, or presacral)	
N2	Metastasis in multiple regional lymph nodes in the true pelvis (hypogastric, obturator, external iliac, or presacral)	
N3	Metastasis in common iliac lymph node(s)	
M—Distant metastasis		
M0	No distant metastasis	
	M1a	Non-regional lymph nodes
	M1b	Other distant metastases

[a] The invasion of the rectum is not mentioned in UICC; nevertheless, in case of this, the tumor must be considered as pT4a

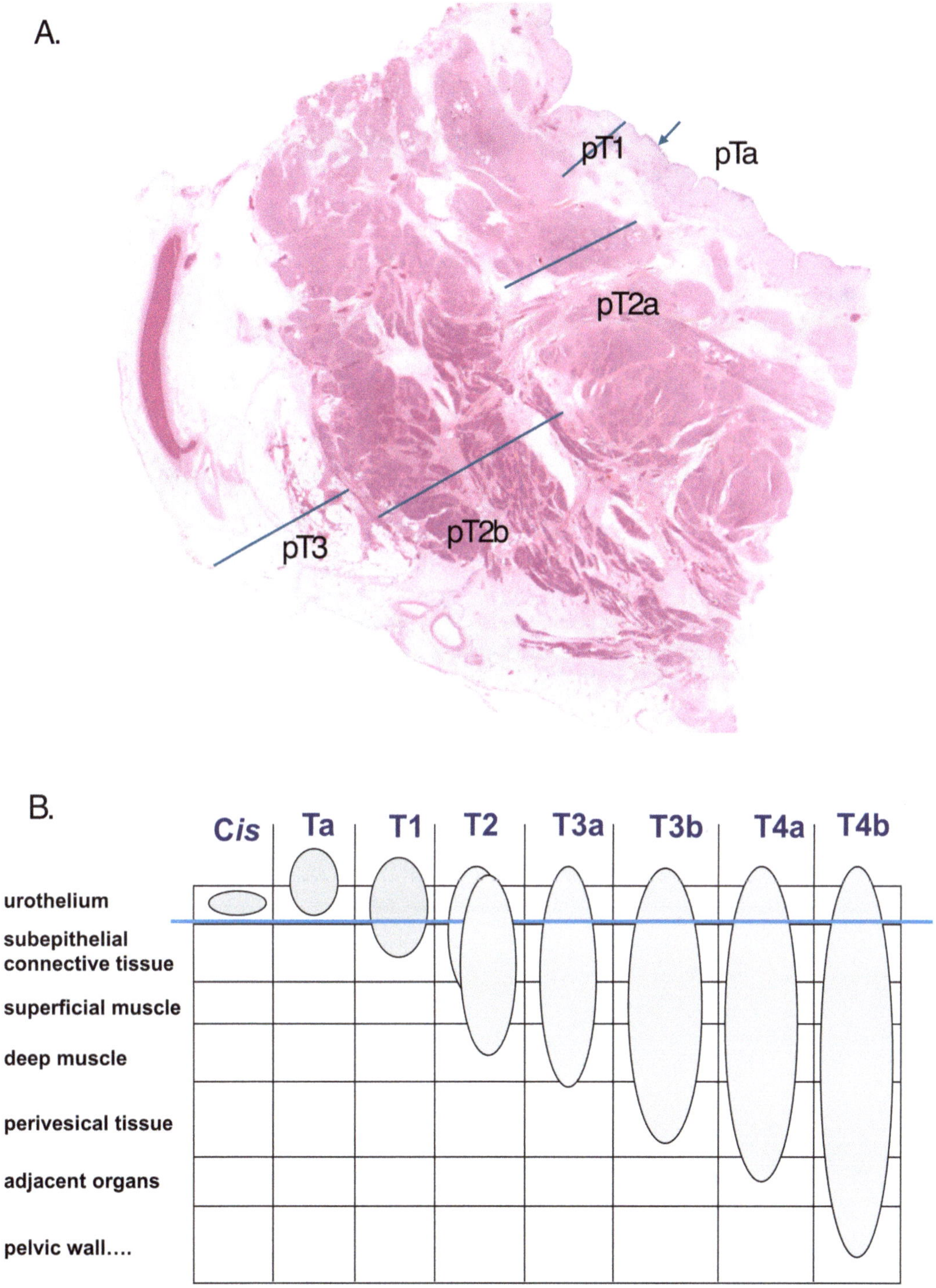

Fig. 4.1 Staging of bladder cancer. (**a**) Depth of invasion depicted on histological section of bladder wall. (**b**) Cartoon showing pTNM stage classification according to UICC 2017

same group, and high-grade tumors without Cis seem to have different molecular underpinnings (Dyrskjøt et al. 2004). During recent years, mUC (metastatic urothelial carcinoma) has been adopted as a separate category.

If the patient has been treated with neoadjuvant chemotherapy (NAC) before cystectomy, "y" pTNM is employed, to underline that this is the staging after oncological treatment. In this case, patients with tumor regression (≤pT2) following NAC have better outcomes (Witjes et al. 2020).

On biopsies or transurethral resection of the bladder tumor (TURBT), no higher stage than T2 can be given. Although adipose tissue is normally below the detrusor muscle wall, it can sometimes be seen in higher layers of the bladder wall, albeit only in small amounts. Therefore, it is strongly not recommended to give a higher stage than T2 on resection specimens (Fig. 4.2). According to the recommendations on bladder reporting, pT staging should only be done on cystectomy specimens.

4.2.1 pTa

The pTa group is heterogeneous. PUNLMP (papillary urothelial neoplasia of low malignant potential), pTa low-grade (LG), and pTa high-grade (HG) tumors are considered together (Figs. 4.3, 4.4 and 4.5). These neoplasias do not invade the lamina propria; therefore, they do not have any metastatic potential. Their recurrence and progression rates are very different, and their prognosis differs and is linked to their grading (see below), which heavily impacts prognosis. The recurrence and progression rates are 8% and 10%, respectively, for PUNLMP, 10% and 1%, respectively, for pTa low-grade, and 36% and 28%, respectively, for pTa high-grade tumors (Babjuk et al. 2019; Jones and Cheng 2006; Amin et al. 2021).

The WHO 2022 classification has also shed light on the nomenclature of tumors with inverted (endophytic) histology. These tumors are rare but always problematic from a pathological point of view. Endophytic PUNLMP, pTaLG, and pTaHG

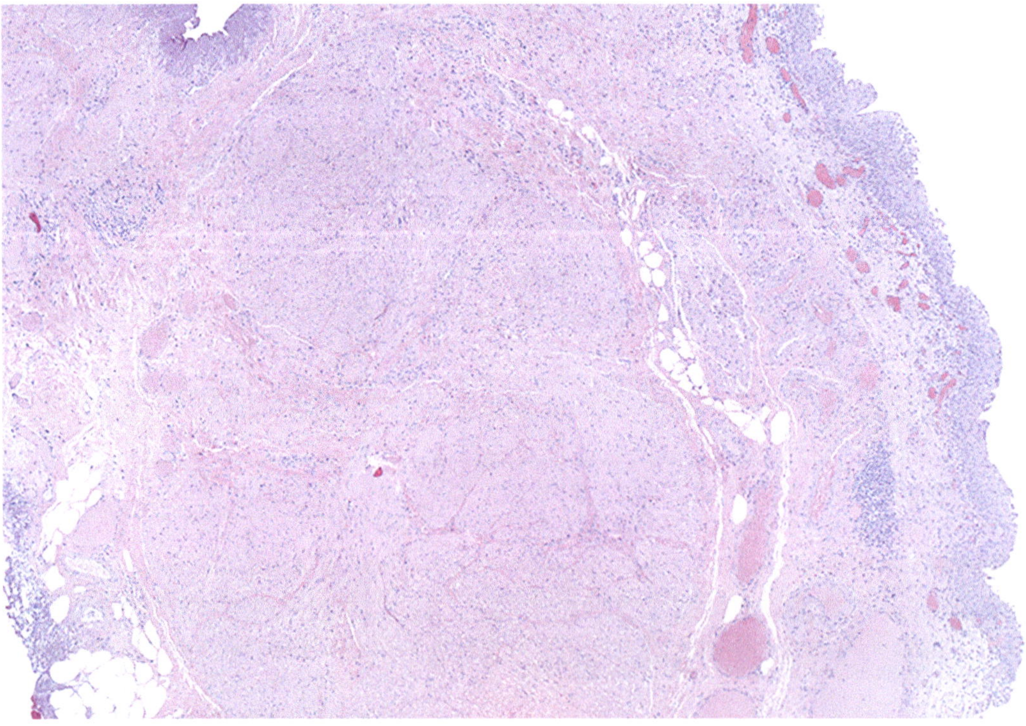

Fig. 4.2 Adipose tissue in the lamina propria, above the muscularis propria ×40

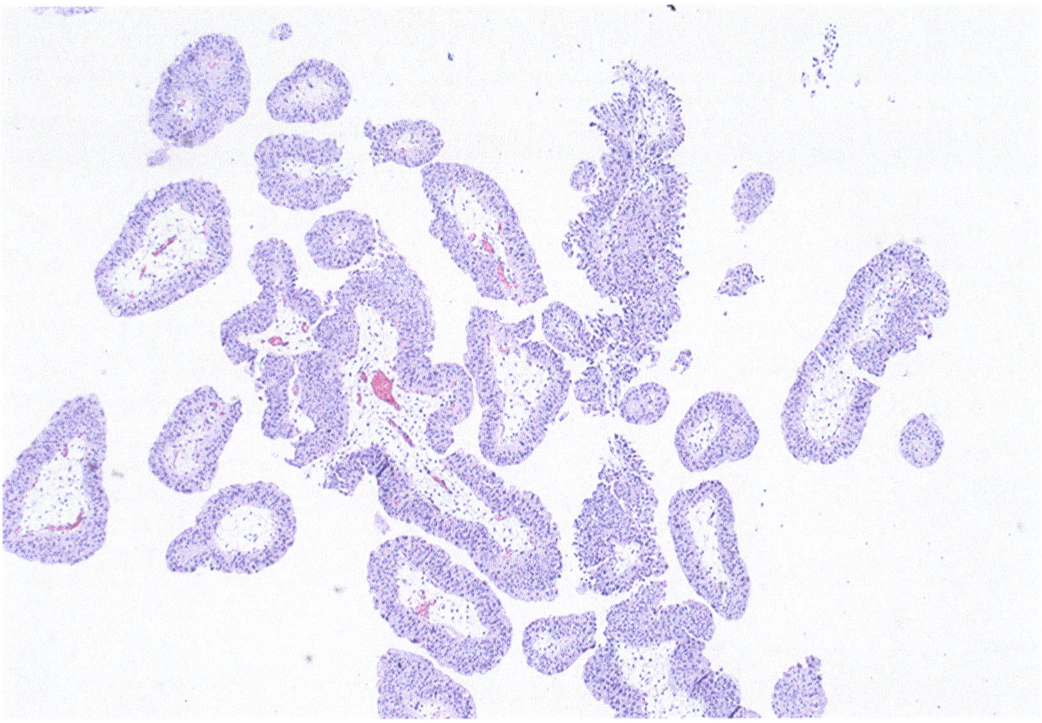

Fig. 4.3 PUNLMP (papillary urothelial neoplasm of low malignant potential) ×100

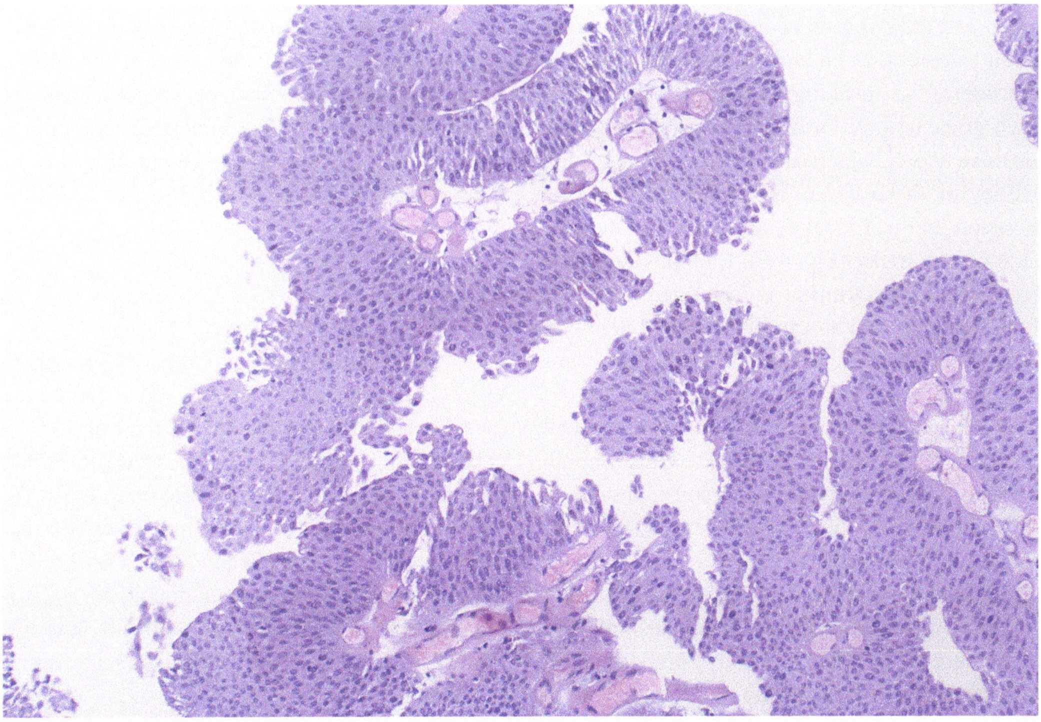

Fig. 4.4 Ta low grade (noninvasive papillary carcinoma of low grade) ×200

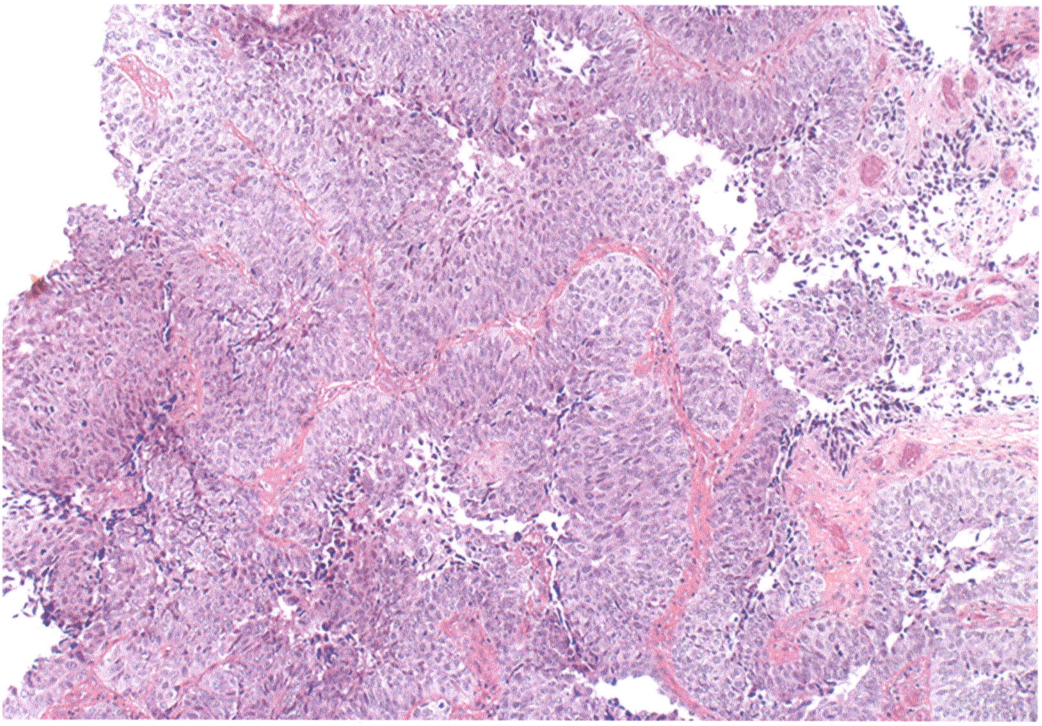

Fig. 4.5 Ta high grade (noninvasive papillary carcinoma of high grade) ×200

exist, and the question of invasion is always difficult to assess, as endophytic aspects cannot be considered as pushing borders, especially in high-grade lesions. Pushing borders show a broad invasive aspect, which can destroy the underlying tissue; in these cases, the difference between invasion and just local destruction without invasion can be tricky (Fig. 4.6). Endophytic tumors have a wide spectrum of morphologic and cytologic features, and an exophytic component may also be present. Nevertheless, like their exclusively exophytic counterpart, these tumors display branching and anastomosing cords, which most of the time are associated with smooth, expansile pushing borders. Grading should be done according to the ISUP 1998/WHO 2022 criteria (Amin et al. 2021).

Endophytic tumors may recur, but according to the few existing studies, such lesions only recur once, if the tumor displays predominantly endophytic features (>80%). The largest study known to date, which explored invasive urothelial carcinomas arising from inverted lesions, showed that 19% of patients with an invasive UC coming from an inverted lesion developed metastasis and 26% died of urothelial cancer. These data show the importance of recognizing an invasive focus and not misdiagnosing it as an inverted lesion (Netto et al. 2022).

4.2.2 pTis

Cis (carcinoma in situ) is always a high-grade lesion but not invasive. It is defined as a flat noninvasive lesion characterized by the presence of cells with atypia such as large, irregular, hyperchromatic nuclei that may be present either in the entire thickness of the epithelium or only a part of it or even only in von Brunn's nests (McKenney 2021) (Fig. 4.7). Even though diagnosis of Cis is not present in association with all invasive tumors, it is important to recognize and to report if present.

Sometimes denuded areas may exist, underlining the discohesive nature of tumor cells, and

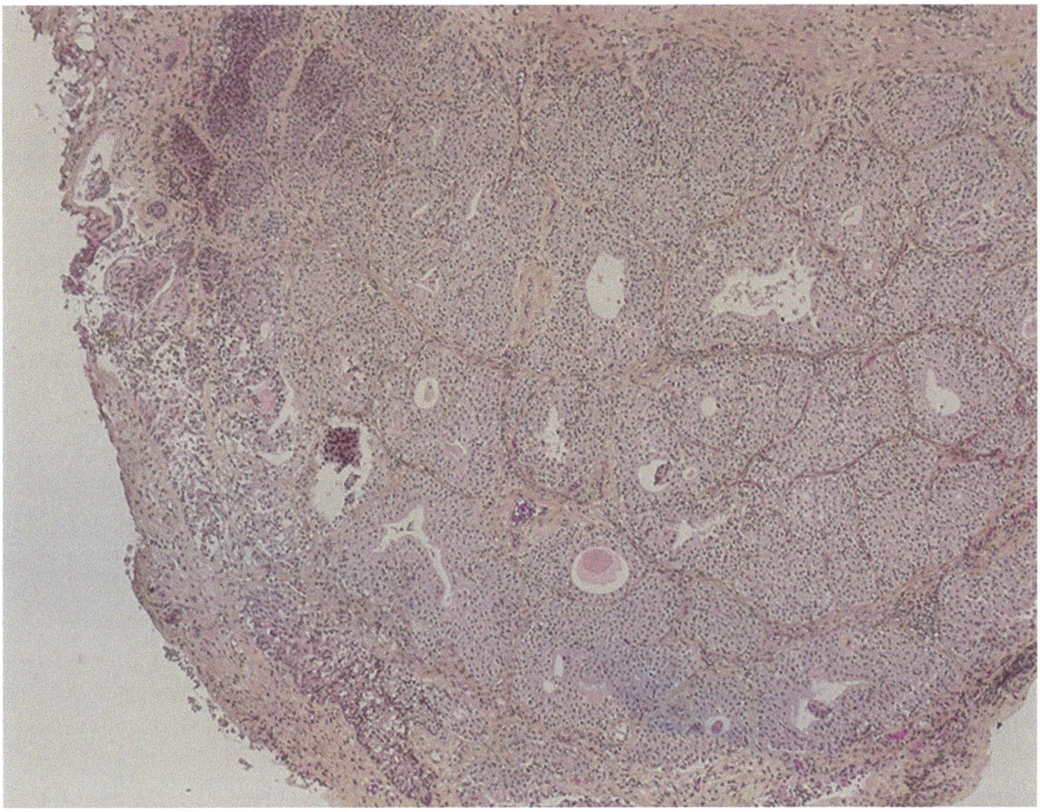

Fig. 4.6 Endophytic lesion without invasion and low-grade aspects ×100

this can further complicate diagnosis. In case of denudation, urinary cytology may be helpful in making the diagnosis (Williamson et al. 2010). Interestingly, distended small blood vessels can often be seen right underneath the basal membrane. Pathologists should be cautious in diagnosing Cis, especially in case of cautery artifacts or in anatomically confined areas (Compérat et al. 2019). Several different histological patterns of Cis exist, but it is not recommended to subclassify these aspects in the pathology report, because these different patterns do not make any difference to prognosis. Furthermore, in many cases, different patterns may coexist in the same patient (Compérat et al. 2013). In rare cases, the phenotype of Cis looks like an in situ adenocarcinoma or an in situ squamous cell carcinoma, which seem to show similar aggressiveness, although only few cases have been reported (Chan and Epstein 2001).

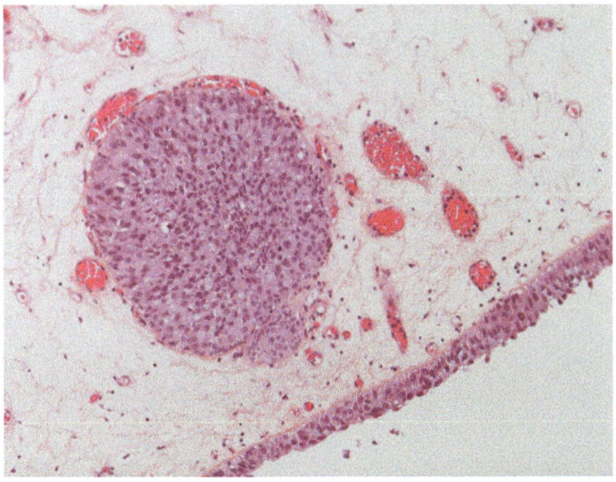

Fig. 4.7 Carcinoma in situ (Cis) on the surface and in von Brunn's nest ×200

Normally, Cis is defined as a flat lesion (Fig. 4.8), but lesions composed of very short microscopic papillae coated with urothelium with important cytological atypia can also be classified as carcinoma "in situ" (Amin et al. 2021). These criteria can be complemented

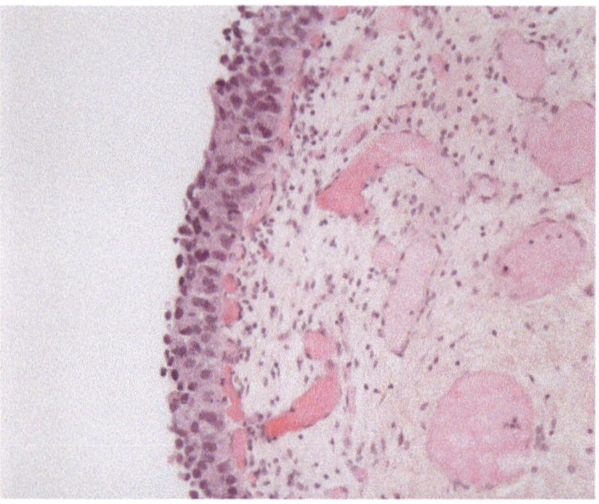

Fig. 4.8 Typical aspect of a carcinoma in situ (Cis) flat lesion with pleomorphism and loss of cellular polarity ×400

with staining using a panel of immunohistochemical antibodies (CD44, CK20, MIB-1, and p53) if necessary, to help distinguish between benign reactive/regenerative atypia and Cis (Amin et al. 2021). Sometimes, immunohistochemistry can be helpful, but diagnosis always needs to be based on morphological features, and pathologists are not allowed to diagnose Cis on the basis of immunohistochemistry only.

Rarely, Cis of the urethra may extend into underlying prostate ducts or from the renal upper urinary tract into renal collecting ducts; both of these extensions are considered as Cis (Humphrey et al. 2016). The development of true invasion into the underlying tissue is seen in 20–30% of the cases. Patients with primary Cis in any part of the urinary tract have worse prognosis (Babjuk et al. 2019; Witjes 2004).

Differential diagnosis with reactive atypia which is always a benign lesion may prove difficult. As such atypia may be induced by radiotherapy, knowledge of treatment history is essential to avoid misinterpretation. Cis may extend into von Brunn's nests or may be exclusively present in the latter. However, this does not represent microinvasion. A study by Dyrskjot et al. demonstrated that a specific Cis gene expression signature is present not only in Cis biopsies but also in the surrounding UC and histologically normal-looking urothelium adjacent to Cis. Therefore, UC with Cis may be regarded as potentially a different disease from UC without Cis (Dyrskjøt et al. 2004).

4.2.3 pT1

For a pathologist, the term "invasive UC" indicates the presence of any tumor cells/nests beneath the urothelial basal membrane, which includes invasion limited to the lamina propria (pT1) (Fig. 4.9). Some urologists still use "invasive" in their daily practice to refer only to muscle-invasive disease (pT2), but knowledge is increasing and the pathological point of view has evolved. pT1 tumors progress more frequently than their pTa counterparts, they are more aggressive, and early cystectomy, especially in the presence of some histological subtypes, may be considered (Willis et al. 2015).

According to the previous WHO 2016 version, substaging of pT1 tumors was recommended, but no specific method was suggested, and this issue is still not entirely settled (Humphrey et al. 2016). Clinicians and pathologists agree on the importance of substaging in pT1 tumors, although this is not part of the official pTNM staging. Many different systems have been tried. The two most common and relatively reproducible systems are the micrometric and the histo-anatomic approach. The former measures a microscopic (1 high-power field (HPF) ×40) versus an extensive/mul-

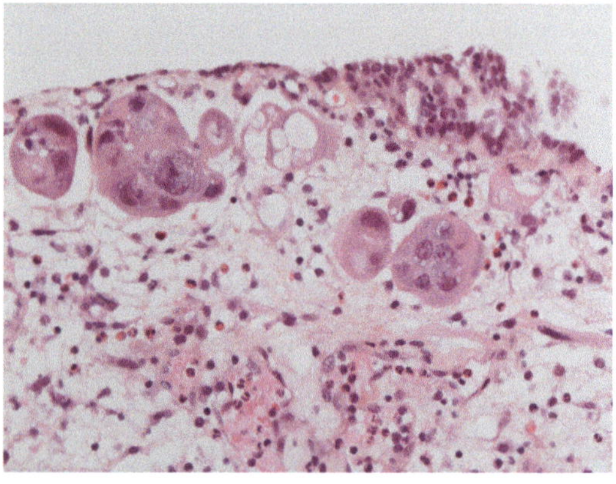

Fig. 4.9 Tumor invading the lamina propria associated with Cis on the surface; tumor remains above the plexus vascularis and the muscularis mucosae ×400

tifocal invasion (pT1m-pT1e). The latter uses landmarks such as the muscularis mucosae or the plexus vascularis of the lamina propria in order to produce substaging (pT1a-pT1b). Problems which may lead to a false evaluation include a hyperplastic appearance of the muscularis mucosae (after multiple resections or chemical treatment), a lack of orientation in the resection specimen, and the histo-anatomical variations of the bladder wall, which also have to be considered (Netto et al. 2022; Compérat et al. 2019). Although we still lack head-to-head comparisons of the different methods, pathologists are strongly encouraged to report the extent of lamina propria invasion, using and reporting any of the different proposed approaches. The micrometric method seems to be more feasible, but final proof in favor of one or the other method has not been shown (Fransen van de Putte et al. 2015).

As mentioned above, NMIBC pT1 is graded as low or high grade according to the ISUP 1998 and the latest WHO 2022 criteria. There are presently no existing criteria as to how to report a low-grade invasive T1 UC, and this entity is probably exceptional, especially as the WHO 2022 classification claims that all invasive subtypes shall be considered high grade (Netto et al. 2022). This is also true for bland-looking subtypes such as the nested, microcystic, or large nested carcinoma. If a UC contains nonclassical aspects (foci of squamous, glandular, or trophoblastic differentiation and/or variant histologies) (see below), it must be reported as "UC with X differentiation" as well as the percentage of the subtype. If only squamous or glandular features are present, the UC must be considered as a pure squamous carcinoma or pure adenocarcinoma (Netto et al. 2022).

4.2.4 pT2-4

Therapeutically, all MIBC should undergo nonconservative management. According to the EAU (European Association of Urology) guidelines, neoadjuvant chemotherapy followed by radical cystectomy is suggested (Compérat et al. 2022b) (see Chap. 6). Staging of MIBC after cystectomy is easier than that of NMIBC, as the whole bladder is at the pathologist's disposal. However, some gray zones also exist here; in particular, the distinction between pT2b (UC in the outer layer of the bladder wall) and pT3a (UC microscopically invading the perivesical fat) can be challenging. A tumor surrounding fibrotic or desmoplastic stroma may exist, sometimes even with heavy inflammation, without adipocytes, but clearly underneath the outer muscle. Particularly in these tumors, but also in all other invasive (also T1) UC, the presence of lymphovascular invasion must be reported, as it is an important clinical factor (Mathieu et al. 2016). The same is true for the concomitant presence of Cis (Compérat et al. 2019).

4.3 Grading

The tumor grade in BC is an important prognostic indicator in NMIBC and in all Ta and some rare T1 tumors. All MIBC are considered high grade (HG). Grading describes the cytological features of the tumor, including nuclear atypia and nuclear size, as well as the ratio nucleus/cytoplasm which in high-grade lesions is >0.7, reflecting the increased size of the nucleus in high-grade tumors. A grade can also be given according to disorganization of the architecture, pseudostratification of the nuclei, the presence of mitoses, and intratumoral necrosis.

Presently, two classification systems are used: The ISUP 1998/WHO2004/2016/2022 system is used worldwide and recommended by nearly all official institutions (for clarity here we refer to the ISUP 1998/WHO 2004/2022 system as "WHO 2004"). Some pathologists/urologists also use the 1973 WHO system, which divides pTa and pT1 tumors into three groups from a grading point of view. The main criticism of this system is the lack of detailed description and the heterogeneity of grade 2 in the middle (Sylvester et al. 2023).

The WHO 1973 classification defines grades 1–3 (G1-G3), and the WHO 2004 system defines low grade (LG), HG, and PUNLMP, the latter being a very rare entity. The WHO 2004 system has been used for more than 25 years and was again published as reference in WHO 2022 (Netto et al. 2022). Some authors have tried to establish a correlation between the two grading systems in order to homogenize them, but a direct correlation is not possible, and a central pathological review is required (Busch and Algaba 2002). Older schemes have shown the concordance and overlap, but the latest research results showed that PUNLMP are less frequent than shown in these schemes.

Both classifications have been criticized: The main criticism of the 1973 grading system is the lack of detailed grading criteria for each subgroup (G1–G3) which results in low interobserver reproducibility. The second major point is that G2 is a "potpourri" of different entities. Low-grade tumors, being slightly too atypical to be defined as G1, are assigned to this group, as well as high-grade tumors lacking all criteria for G3. Therefore, grade 2 is heterogeneous (McKenney 2021). The WHO 2004 classification provides a detailed description of each category but has been criticized in over-diagnosing high-grade tumors (van Rhijn et al. 2010).

When the WHO 2004 system was introduced, the authors aimed to mitigate the issues of intra- and interobserver variability, and recent literature reports an advantage of this system (Soukup et al. 2017). In 2014 a study about reproducibility and prognostic value of the WHO 1973 and WHO 2004 grading systems in Ta/T1 UC showed that neither of the grading systems were prognostically stronger than the other. Twenty-four (24.5%) of the grade 2 and 50 (98.0%) of the grade 3 tumors were reclassified as high-grade tumors, and one grade 3 downgraded to a low-grade tumor (Mangrud et al. 2014).

The WHO 2004 system overlaps well with the Paris system, which was introduced for urinary cytology (Wojcik et al. 2022), and it is also compatible with our understanding of the two distinct groups of bladder tumors (Ta LG vs. Cis, T1, and MIBC). This grading system was developed and published by pathologists, urologists, urologic oncologists, and basic research scientists with an interest in bladder neoplasia. The aim was to come up with a universally acceptable classification system for bladder neoplasia that could be used effectively by everyone, in line with the idea of an international classification.

As mentioned above, one of the limitations of all systems is observer variability, which is probably independent of any classification. Most published observer variability studies indicate that all WHO urinary bladder grading systems show discordances. The reasons for disagreement are manifold. Grading is subjective, and defining 100% definable hallmarks is complicated. Tumor heterogeneity clearly plays a role, and different/mixed features are frequent in NMIBC. The most problematic issue is cellular heterogeneity in NMIBC. The WHO 2022 system, as in previous WHO classifications, suggests a 5% cutoff in the case of heterogeneous grades in the same lesion. If more than 5% of the tumor is HG, the tumor should be classified in the HG category. Some studies demonstrate that even normal-looking urothelium can already display HG changes at a molecular level, thus leaving the question as to when to classify a tumor as HG unresolved (Downes et al. 2017). Unfortunately, only a few outcome studies with only a few cases exist, which renders it difficult to confirm whether the cutoff should be 5 or 10% (Amin et al. 2021).

The ISUP (International Society of Uropathology) has endorsed the WHO 2004 system. In North America, most pathologists use the WHO 2004 classification, which is recommended by the CAP (College of American Pathologists), the AJCC (American Joint Committee on Cancer), and the ICCR (International Collaboration on Cancer Reporting) (Varma et al. 2020). The NCCN (National Comprehensive Cancer Network) also uses LG and HG categories in order to make treatment decisions. The AUA (American Urological Association) refers to the WHO 2004 classification system. Each of these institutions recommend classifying NMIBC into Ta PUNLMP, LG, and HG tumors or T1 LG/HG. The UICC (Union for International Cancer Control) refers to grade as a prognostic factor but does not indicate which type of grading should be used. The ENCR (European Network of Cancer Registries) also refers to LG/HG (The

2022 ENCR Recommendations on recording and reporting of urothelial tumours of the urinary tract - PubMed [Internet] 2023). The WHO 2004 system is now recommended by almost all major pathology and urology organizations as the preferred grading system. The EAU Guidelines Panel recommends a slightly different system, which is a hybrid system, that divides G2 lesions into G2HG and G3HG (Sylvester et al. 2021).

Most pathologists agree that all grading systems suffer from deficiencies, but maybe in the long term, artificial intelligence will be able to assist pathologists in grading and deliver more clarity and objectivity. Presently, studies are ongoing in BC with machine learning to provide an automated prediction of invasiveness and tumor grade. Sensitivities of around 85% for invasiveness have been reported, although grading remains problematic. However, this is a quickly evolving field (Kujdowicz et al. 2023).

4.4 Histological Subtypes

One of the important points in the WHO 2022 classification is that histological characteristics remain the gold standard for the classification and diagnosis of urothelial tract tumors and, secondly, that an updated nomenclature of subtype histology is provided. The WHO 2022 has tried to avoid the term "variant" histology, which unfortunately is frequently used in the literature for other tumor types. This approach is consistent with terminology used in other sections in the WHO 5th edition since the term "variant" is more commonly used to denote genomic alterations.

Subtypes of urothelial carcinoma include nested UC, microcystic and tubular, large nested, micropapillary, lymphoepithelioma-like, plasmacytoid UC, giant cell UC, sarcomatoid, poorly differentiated, lipid rich, and clear cell UC. Although these are all of urothelial origin, prognosis and response to chemotherapy may differ (Netto et al. 2022). Urothelial carcinomas with squamous, adenocarcinomatous, and trophoblastic inflexion also exist and also pure forms of squamous cell, adeno-, and trophoblastic carcinoma. These are called "tumors with divergent differentiation" and are very rare (Netto et al. 2022).

Since molecular classifications with relationships to outcome, progression, and survival exist, an overlap between molecular classification and histomorphology has been sought. However, differences between both classifications exist. Both classifications are complementary and in some issues overlapping (Sjödahl et al. 2012; Warrick et al. 2019).

The reporting of subtypes or divergent differentiation is recommended, as these have prognostic and therapeutic implications. According to the literature, subtypes occur in more than 27% of BC cases (Ngo et al. 2020). Reporting of these subtypes can be controversial, and some subtypes, e.g., micropapillary carcinoma, are not well recognized, especially when they show non-typical features. Some studies have reported poor agreement among pathologists, which is problematic when the therapeutic approach depends on the pathology report (Sangoi et al. 2010; Cimadamore et al. 2022). Some subtypes are clearly underreported, although awareness of the importance of detailed reporting is increasing. However, some subtypes are difficult to evaluate, as they resemble normal or hyperplastic urothelium or urothelium sectioned tangentially. This can be observed frequently in the nested (Fig. 4.10), microcystic, microtubular, or large nested subtypes. Plasmacytoid UC, known to be very aggressive and invasive, can also be mistaken for inflammatory changes, and effective reporting can therefore be delayed (Song et al. 2022).

The ICCR has given very precise instructions on how to report each subtype correctly, including percentages of each recognized subtype. It must be emphasized that molecular data exist for many of these subtypes, which impact on the treatment options for these patients (see Chap. 15). One of the typical examples is the presence of a pure "large nested UC." These lesions mostly harbor *FGFR3* mutations. Therefore, recognizing these tumors as MIBC at an early stage can allow initiation of personalized treatment with an

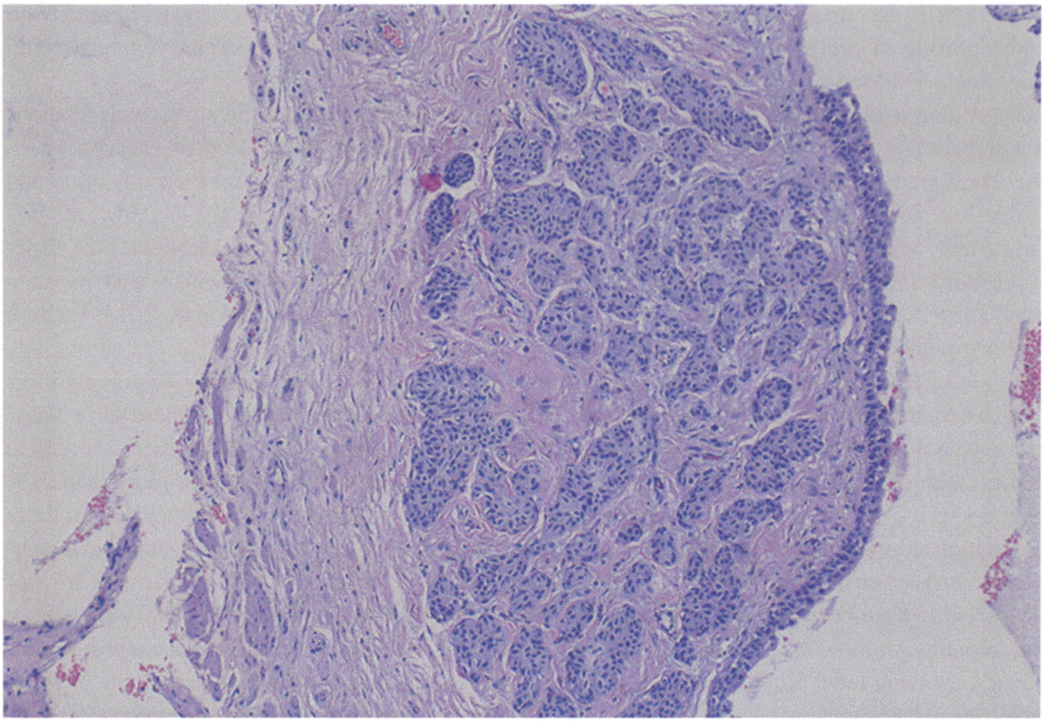

Fig. 4.10 Nested carcinoma, a subtype which can be difficult to recognize, and to be considered as invasive, differential diagnosis would be a hyperplasia of von Brunn's nests ×200

FGFR inhibitor very early in the course of the disease (Weyerer et al. 2020).

4.5 Importance of Provision of Relevant Samples and Clinical Information for Pathological Assessment

It is important for the pathologist to have relevant clinical information in order to make an accurate diagnosis. If lesions are mistaken, serious consequences for the patient can be an issue. As the bladder wall shows anatomical differences, pathologists need to know the localization of the resection/biopsy (Minardi et al. 2016). If the patient has already been treated (e.g., BCG therapy), the aspect of the bladder urothelium and wall will have changed; highly inflammatory aspects may be mistaken for Cis, which would have serious consequences on a repeat biopsy/resection. On the other hand, not recognizing Cis also heavily impacts the patient's outcome.

Ideally, both the base of the tumor and the tumor edges should be sent to the pathologist in separate containers to ensure the presence of bladder muscle in the specimen. This is essential for accurate staging. Because associated Cis has been shown to be an adverse prognostic factor, bladder biopsies should be taken from reddish, suspicious areas where present, or random biopsies from normal-looking urothelium if there is a positive cytology or a previous diagnosis of associated Cis. Similarly, biopsies from the prostatic urethra should be taken if the tumor is located at the trigone or bladder neck area or when there is no bladder tumor, and the procedure is carried out to study a positive cytology, since the tumor could be located in the urothelium lining, the prostatic urethra, or the prostatic ducts (Minardi et al. 2016). Another important piece of information is the localization of the resection/biopsy, as the bladder wall displays important differences according to the topography. Some studies have shown that tumors in the trigone and bladder neck involve a greater risk of progression, shorter recurrence-free survival, lymph node metastases, and decreased recurrence-free and cancer-specific survival (Voskuilen et al. 2020).

4.6 UC Involving Diverticula

This is a rare disease, but nevertheless most subtypes can be seen in diverticula (areas where the bladder lining bulges out through the bladder wall). The most frequent localizations are the lateral bladder wall, the dome, and the orifices of ureters (Humphrey et al. 2016). In diverticula, the risk of urinary stasis and therefore a prolonging effect of carcinogens in the diverticulum might lead to increased inflammation, infections, metaplasia (replacement of one normal tissue by another normal tissue), and calculi formation. From a histological point of view, there is no muscle layer in the wall; therefore, T2 staging cannot be done. The only possible stages are Ta, T1, and T3 (Fig. 4.11). Some authors found no differences in overall survival or metastasis-free survival between partial and radical cystectomies, thus arguing that partial cystectomy might be a good option in selected patients (Voskuilen et al. 2020).

4.7 Urachus

Urachal lesions and tumors are extremely rare. They arise from urachal remnants, and one of the most frequent localizations is the bladder dome (Humphrey et al. 2016). Their histological appearance can be diverse, and most frequently non-cystic or cystic adenocarcinomas are seen (Fig. 4.12).

In a recent paper, Maurer et al. have compared different aspects of glandular lesions in thc bladder (adenocarcinoma, urachus carcinoma, and urothelial carcinoma with glandular differentiation). The authors could demonstrate a higher proximity of urachus cancers to carcinomas of the colon on a molecular level (Maurer et al. 2020). This might explain why these patients respond better to chemotherapies administered for colorectal cancers. It is important to know that the Sheldon system should be used for staging (Sheldon et al. 1984). The most frequent metastatic site is the peritoneum (Guerin et al. 2023), and prognosis is stage dependent.

4.8 Use of Immunohistochemistry in Diagnosis and Prediction of Therapeutic Response

Staining to detect specific proteins by immunohistochemistry (IHC) can provide much additional information to morphology. However, most of the time it is not necessary to use IHC in the setting of urothelial carcinomas. No ideal marker to confirm urothelial differentiation exists, and this can be problematic especially in the metastatic setting where identification of the tissue of origin is important. A panel of different markers, including GATA3, CK7, p63, thrombomodulin, uroplakin III, CK5/6, and CK 14, can be used to identify urothelial origin, but none is specific (Paner et al. 2014; Amin et al. 2014). In addition, most UC express HMWCK (high molecular weight cytokeratin). Expression in 96% has been reported. S-100P has been described as a good marker for urothelial origin, expressed in 86% of classical UC cases according to some studies (Paner et al. 2014). Different subtypes show differential expression of proteins; S-100P is a good marker for micropapillary, nested, microcystic, and clear cell carcinomas, with expression in 96% of cases. These tumors also express GATA3 (88%), CK7 (95%), and p63 (69%). In undifferentiated carcinomas, markers typically used for the urothelium do not perform well (Paner et al. 2014).

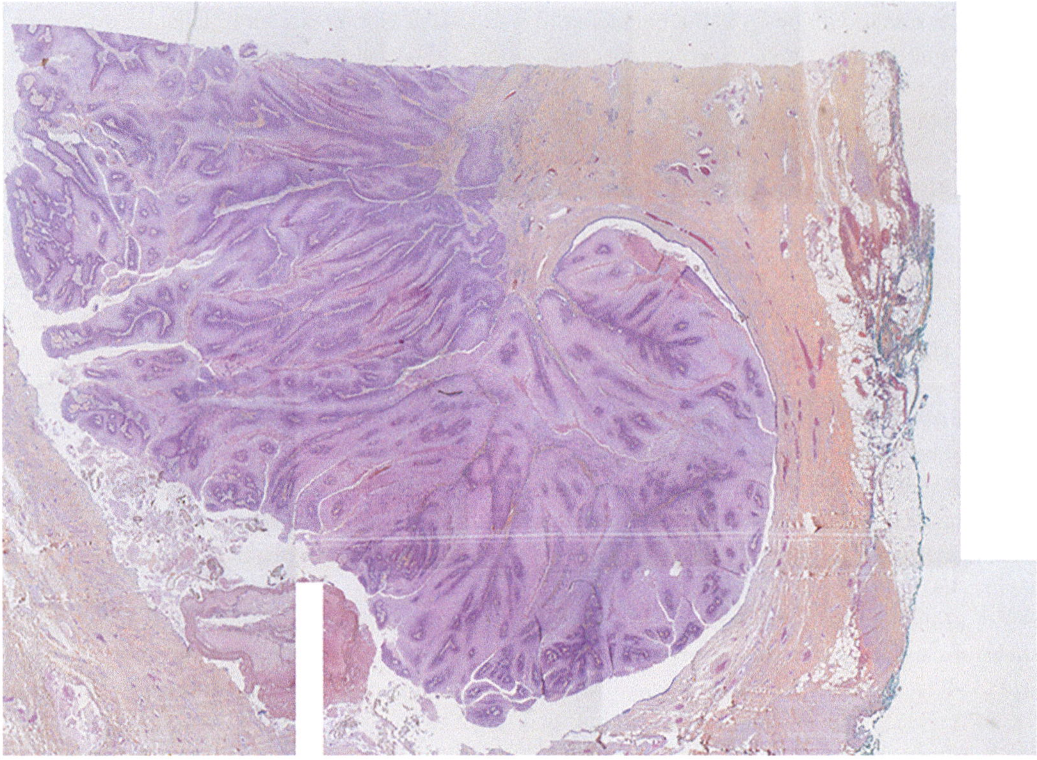

Fig. 4.11 Diverticulum with squamous cell carcinoma/verrucous carcinoma, diverticulum wall made only of fibrosis, no muscle ×25

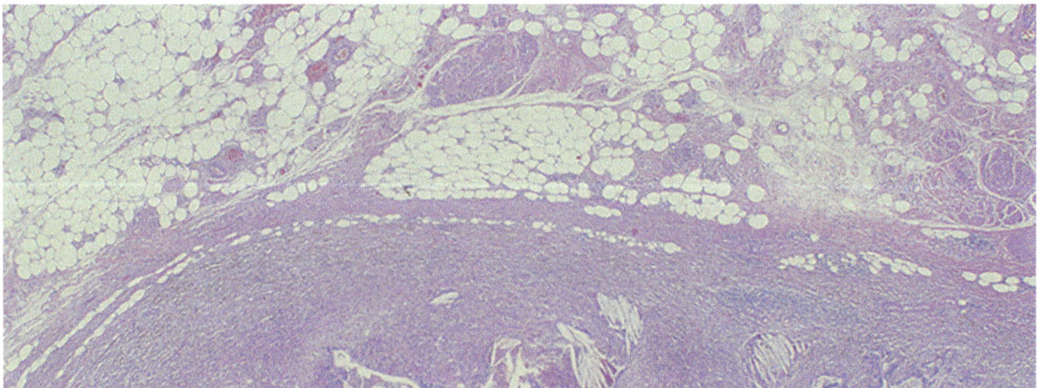

Fig. 4.12 Urachus carcinoma with adenocarcinomatous features ×25

With regard to molecular classification, we have a good understanding of molecular underpinnings and the distinction between luminal and basal molecular subtypes (see Chaps. 13 and 14). FOXA1 and GATA3 are typical luminal markers, whereas CK5/6, CK14, and p63 are markers for basal UC (Bontoux et al. 2021). Some authors have described molecular testing with a panel of proteins and have established that 13 different antibodies yield good molecular distinction in the MIBC setting (Sjödahl 2018). One of the molecular classification systems, the Lund taxonomy, has tried to align gene expression-level classification with immunohistochemical classification in order to identify cancer cell phenotypes. The authors take a systematic approach, and tumor gene expression clusters are validated by immunohistochemistry (Queipo et al. 2022; Höglund et al. 2023). Alignment of these defined molecular subtypes with histopathological assessment as described above will now be important.

In non-UC such as mesenchymatous and neuroendocrine (NE) tumors, immunohistochemistry has an important role. Neuroendocrine carcinomas, which are described in a separate chapter in the WHO 2022 classification, have a poor prognosis and can be pure or mixed. In the bladder, small-cell or large-cell NE carcinomas as well as cases admixed with a non-neuroendocrine component can be found. Around 50% of cases are mixed tumors (classical urothelial and neuroendocrine features), the presence of a neuroendocrine component having an impact on clinical management. Neuroendocrine tumors express synaptophysin and chromogranin A, cytokeratins (at lower levels), and CD56, although this marker is not very specific. Around 30–50% of NE carcinomas express TTF-1 (Fan et al. 2022).

Multiple programmed death-1 (PD1)/programmed death-ligand 1 (PD-L1) inhibitors have been approved for the treatment of locally advanced or metastatic urothelial carcinomas, and several studies have attempted to predict the patient's response to these immune checkpoint inhibitors (ICIs). For several ICI treatments, immunohistochemical PD-L1 testing is required. Several studies have demonstrated the interchangeability of different antibodies (Gevaert et al. 2021; Tretiakova et al. 2018; Torlakovic et al. 2020). It is noteworthy that different subtypes probably express PD-L1 in a different manner (Reis et al. 2019). Although PD-L1 stains are done routinely, many concerns regarding the problems with PD-L1 testing have been voiced (see also Chap. 23). The issues of interpreting and reporting of PD-L1 can be challenging with regard to tumor heterogeneity and interobserver reproducibility. For instance, expression can be heterogeneous within the same patient, especially when the tumor contains a subtype, with regions of squamous differentiation showing the highest expression and regions of plasmacytoid UC demonstrating the lowest expression (Reis et al. 2019). It is important to understand these differences and to select the tissue block accordingly and not to overlook possible positive areas, in order not to deprive a patient of the therapeutic option of ICIs. Interobserver variability is also an issue in the interpretation of PD-L1 staining. In several types of cancer, some studies have shown that digital image analysis can improve the precision of PD-L1 expression interpretation and better predict treatment response (Reis et al. 2019). Finally, a co-localization of PD-L1 expression and CD8+ T cells may indicate an adaptive immune response that might predict response to therapy (Kates et al. 2020).

4.9 Urinary Cytology

Urine cytology plays a major role in detecting BC, especially high-grade lesions. It is simple, noninvasive, and cheap. The College of American Pathologists (CAP) encourages the use of a standardized terminology in the reporting of urine cytology, following the Paris system. A negative cystoscopy together with negative cytology is a good indicator of the absence of the disease, the same being true for the opposite situation. The terminology in this system scores the following:

adequacy of urine specimens, negative for high-grade UC, atypical urothelial cells, suspicious for high-grade UC, and high-grade UC. Low-grade urothelial neoplasia is difficult to identify and is no longer scored separately from normal urothelium (Wojcik et al. 2022).

Several aims have been achieved with the Paris system, which benefits from a focus on individual cells and not on the architecture of several cells clumped together, which minimizes atypical diagnoses (McIntire et al. 2021). The system is robust and displays very good definitions for each category, which have been corroborated by several follow-up papers (McIntire et al. 2021).

4.10 Standard Reporting

Many attempts have been made to reduce the length of the pathology report, without sacrificing any relevant information. In addition to providing maximum information for clinical decision-making, comprehensive reporting can facilitate interpretation and hypothesis generation in any translational studies that are carried out. According to the ICCR, a pathology report has to contain the items listed in Table 4.2.

The CAP (Collegium of American Pathologists) also updates the reporting of BC in a regular manner (College of American Pathologists [Internet] 2023). The next update for both takes place in 2023.

Table 4.2 www.ICCR-cancer.org

Item	Recommended	Required
Clinical information	✓	✓
Specimen site	–	✓
Additional specimens submitted	–	✓
Operative procedure	–	+
Block identification key	✓ (TURBT)	✓
Histological tumor type	–	✓
Presence of invasive carcinoma	–	✓
Associated epithelial lesions (depends on operative procedure)	✓	✓
Histological grade	–	✓
Extent of invasion	–	✓
Macroscopic extent of invasion	–	✓
Microscopic extent of invasion	–	✓
Tumor focality	✓	–
Substaging T1 disease	✓	–
Lymphovascular invasion	–	✓
Only for cystectomies		
Response to neoadjuvant therapy	–	✓
Margin status	–	✓
Lymph node status	–	✓
Histologically confirmed metastasis	–	✓
Coexistent pathology	✓	–
Staging (if applicable)	✓	–

4.11 Conclusion

In recent years, knowledge of BC has evolved and changed. The molecular underpinnings identified have helped pathologists to refine their evaluation. The unification of the Paris system in cytology has also improved the diagnosis of high-grade lesions as has improved collaboration between urologists and pathologists.

At present, surgical pathology is still the gold standard for reporting urothelial lesions. Nevertheless, working hand in hand with molecular pathology has become possible and shows great promise for improving patient management.

Acknowledgments Pr. C. Magi-Galluzzi (reading proof as a pathologist)

Dr. G. Wasinger (reading proof and including the refs)

References

Amin MB, Trpkov K, Lopez-Beltran A, Grignon D (2014) Members of the ISUP immunohistochemistry in diagnostic urologic pathology group. Best practices recommendations in the application of immunohistochemistry in the bladder lesions: report from the International Society of Urologic Pathology consensus conference. Am J Surg Pathol 38(8):e20–e34

Amin MB, Comperat E, Epstein JI, True LD, Hansel D, Paner GP (2021) The genitourinary pathology society update on classification and grading of flat and papillary urothelial neoplasia with new reporting recommendations and approach to lesions with mixed and early patterns of neoplasia. Adv Anat Pathol 28(4):179–195

Babjuk M, Burger M, Compérat EM, Gontero P, Mostafid AH, Palou J (2019) European Association of Urology guidelines on non-muscle-invasive bladder cancer (TaT1 and carcinoma in situ) - 2019 update. Eur Urol 76(5):639–657

Bontoux C, Rialland T, Cussenot O, Compérat E (2021) A four-antibody immunohistochemical panel can distinguish clinico-pathological clusters of urothelial carcinoma and reveals high concordance between primary tumor and lymph node metastases. Virchows Arch 478(4):637–645

Busch C, Algaba F (2002) The WHO/ISUP 1998 and WHO 1999 systems for malignancy grading of bladder cancer. Scientific foundation and translation to one another and previous systems. Virchows Arch 441(2):105–108

Chan TY, Epstein JI (2001) In situ adenocarcinoma of the bladder. Am J Surg Pathol 25(7):892–899

Cimadamore A, Lonati C, Di Trapani E, De Cobelli O, Rink M, Zamboni S (2022) Variant histologies in bladder cancer: does the Centre have an impact in detection accuracy? Urol Oncol 40(6):273.e11–273.e20

College of American Pathologists [Internet] (2023) Cancer protocol templates. Verfügbar unter. https://www.cap.org/protocols-and-guidelines/cancer-reporting-tools/cancer-protocol-templates

Compérat E, Jacquet SF, Varinot J, Conort P, Roupret M, Chartier-Kastler E (2013) Different subtypes of carcinoma in situ of the bladder do not have a different prognosis. Virchows Arch März 462(3):343–348

Compérat E, Babjuk M, Algaba F, Amin M, Brimo F, Grignon D (2019) SIU-ICUD on bladder cancer: pathology. World J Urol 37(1):41–50

Compérat E, Amin MB, Epstein JI, Hansel DE, Paner G, Al-Ahmadie H (2021) The genitourinary pathology society update on classification of variant Histologies, T1 substaging, molecular taxonomy, and immunotherapy and PD-L1 testing implications of urothelial cancers. Adv Anat Pathol 28(4):196–208

Compérat E, Oszwald A, Wasinger G, Shariat S, Amin M (2022a) Update on flat and papillary urothelial lesions: genitourinary pathology society consensus recommendations. Surg Pathol Clin 15(4):629–640

Compérat E, Amin MB, Cathomas R, Choudhury A, De Santis M, Kamat A (2022b) Current best practice for bladder cancer: a narrative review of diagnostics and treatments. Lancet 400(10364):1712–1721

Downes MR, Weening B, van Rhijn BWG, Have CL, Treurniet KM, van der Kwast TH (2017) Analysis of papillary urothelial carcinomas of the bladder with grade heterogeneity: supportive evidence for an early role of CDKN2A deletions in the FGFR3 pathway. Histopathology 70(2):281–289

Dyrskjøt L, Kruhøffer M, Thykjaer T, Marcussen N, Jensen JL, Møller K (2004) Gene expression in the urinary bladder: a common carcinoma in situ gene expression signature exists disregarding histopathological classification. Cancer Res 64(11):4040–4048

Fan J, Li H, Zhou C, Xiong W, Villamil C, Ionescu D (2022) u. a. classifying pulmonary and urinary high-grade neuroendocrine carcinoma by CK7 immunohistochemistry. Appl Immunohistochem Mol Morphol 30(6):459–468

Fransen van de Putte EE, Behrendt MA, Pigot GLS, van der Kwast TH, van Rhijn BWG (2015) Prognostic significance of substage and WHO classification systems in T1 urothelial carcinoma of the bladder. Curr Opin Urol 25(5):427–435

Gevaert T, Cimadamore A, Montironi R, Eckstein M (2021) PD-L1 testing for urothelial carcinoma: interchangeability, reliability and future perspectives. Curr Drug Targets 22(2):162–170

Guerin M, Miran C, Colomba E, Cabart M, Herrmann T, Pericart S, u. a. (2023) Urachal carcinoma: a large retrospective multicentric study from the French Genito-Urinary Tumor Group. Front Oncologia 13:1110003

Höglund M, Bernardo C, Sjödahl G, Eriksson P, Axelson H, Liedberg F (2023) The Lund taxonomy for bladder cancer classification - from gene expression clustering to cancer cell molecular phenotypes, and back again. J Pathol 259(4):369–375

Humphrey PA, Moch H, Cubilla AL, Ulbright TM, Reuter VE (2016) The 2016 WHO classification of tumours of the urinary system and male genital organs-part B: prostate and bladder tumours. Eur Urol 70(1):106–119

Jones TD, Cheng L (2006) Papillary urothelial neoplasm of low malignant potential: evolving terminology and concepts. J Urol 175(6):1995–2003

Kates M, Matoso A, Choi W, Baras AS, Daniels MJ, Lombardo K (2020) u. a. adaptive immune resistance to intravesical BCG in non-muscle invasive bladder cancer: implications for prospective BCG-unresponsive trials. Clin Cancer Res 26(4):882–891

Kujdowicz M, Perez-Guaita D, Chlosta P, Okon K, Malek K (2023) Evaluation of grade and invasiveness of bladder urothelial carcinoma using infrared imaging and machine learning. Analyst 148(2):278–285

Mangrud OM, Waalen R, Gudlaugsson E, Dalen I, Tasdemir I, Janssen EAM (2014) Reproducibility and prognostic value of WHO1973 and WHO2004 grading systems in TaT1 urothelial carcinoma of the urinary bladder. PLoS One 9(1):e83192

Mathieu R, Lucca I, Rouprêt M, Briganti A, Shariat SF (2016) The prognostic role of lymphovascular invasion in urothelial carcinoma of the bladder. Nat Rev Urol 13(8):471–479

Maurer A, Ortiz-Bruechle N, Guricova K, Rose M, Morsch R, Garczyk S (2020) Comparative genomic

profiling of glandular bladder tumours. Virchows Arch 477(3):445–454
McIntire PJ, Kilic I, Pambuccian SE, Wojcik EM, Barkan GA (2021) The Paris system for reporting urinary cytology reduces atypia rates and does not alter the negative predictive value of urine cytology. J Am Soc Cytopathol 10(1):14–19
McKenney JK (2021) Urothelial carcinoma in situ: diagnostic update. Pathology 53(1):86–95
Minardi D, Milanese G, Parri G, Lacetera V, Muzzonigro G (2016) Non-muscle invasive high grade urothelial carcinoma of the bladder. Which factors can influence understaging at the time of radical cystectomy? Arch Ital Urol Androl 88(1):13–16
Netto GJ, Amin MB, Berney DM, Compérat EM, Gill AJ, Hartmann A (2022) The 2022 World Health Organization classification of tumors of the urinary system and male genital organs-part B: prostate and urinary tract tumors. Eur Urol 82(5):469–482
Ngo C, Cussenot O, Compérat E (2020) Transurethral resection of bladder and radical cystectomy: concordance of histology. Are we good enough? Turk J Urol 46(5):354–359
Paner GP, Annaiah C, Gulmann C, Rao P, Ro JY, Hansel DE (2014) Immunohistochemical evaluation of novel and traditional markers associated with urothelial differentiation in a spectrum of variants of urothelial carcinoma of the urinary bladder. Hum Pathol 45(7):1473–1482
Queipo FJ, Unamunzaga GM, Negro BF, Fuertes SG, Cortés MÁ, Tejedor EC (2022) Immunohistochemistry subtyping of urothelial carcinoma is feasible in the daily practice. Virchows Arch 481(2):191–200
Reis H, Serrette R, Posada J, Lu V, Chen YB, Gopalan A (2019) PD-L1 expression in urothelial carcinoma with predominant or pure variant histology: concordance among 3 commonly used and commercially available antibodies. Am J Surg Pathol 43(7):920–927
Sangoi AR, Beck AH, Amin MB, Cheng L, Epstein JI, Hansel DE (2010) Interobserver reproducibility in the diagnosis of invasive micropapillary carcinoma of the urinary tract among urologic pathologists. Am J Surg Pathol 34(9):1367–1376
Sheldon CA, Clayman RV, Gonzalez R, Williams RD, Fraley EE (1984) Malignant urachal lesions. J Urol 131(1):1–8
Sjödahl G (2018) Molecular subtype profiling of urothelial carcinoma using a subtype-specific immunohistochemistry panel. Methods Mol Biol 1655:53–64
Sjödahl G, Lauss M, Lövgren K, Chebil G, Gudjonsson S, Veerla S (2012) A molecular taxonomy for urothelial carcinoma. Clin Cancer Res 18(12):3377–3386
Song Y, Qin C, Du Y, Xu T (2022) Radical cystectomy and chemotherapy on plasmacytoid variant bladder urothelial carcinoma. World J Urol 40(9):2353–2354
Soukup V, Čapoun O, Cohen D, Hernández V, Babjuk M, Burger M (2017) Prognostic performance and reproducibility of the 1973 and 2004/2016 World Health Organization grading classification Systems in non-muscle-invasive Bladder Cancer: a European Association of Urology non-muscle invasive bladder cancer guidelines panel systematic review. Eur Urol 72(5):801–813
Sylvester RJ, Rodríguez O, Hernández V, Turturica D, Bauerová L, Bruins HM (2021) European Association of Urology (EAU) prognostic factor risk groups for non-muscle-invasive bladder cancer (NMIBC) incorporating the WHO 2004/2016 and WHO 1973 classification Systems for Grade: an update from the EAU NMIBC guidelines panel. Eur Urol 79(4):480–488
Sylvester RJ, Rodríguez O, Hernández V, Turturica D, Bauerová L, Max Bruins H (2023) Erratum to "European Association of Urology (EAU) Prognostic Factor Risk Groups for Non-muscle-invasive Bladder Cancer (NMIBC) Incorporating the WHO 2004/2016 and WHO 1973 Classification Systems for Grade: An Update from the EAU NMIBC Guidelines Panel" [Eur. Urol. 79(4) (2021) 480–488]. Eur Urol 83(5):e140–e141
The 2022 ENCR Recommendations on recording and reporting of urothelial tumours of the urinary tract - PubMed [Internet] (2023) Verfügbar unter: https://pubmed.ncbi.nlm.nih.gov/36505871/
Torlakovic E, Lim HJ, Adam J, Barnes P, Bigras G, Chan AWH (2020) "Interchangeability" of PD-L1 immunohistochemistry assays: a meta-analysis of diagnostic accuracy. Mod Pathol 33(1):4–17
Tretiakova M, Fulton R, Kocherginsky M, Long T, Ussakli C, Antic T (2018) Concordance study of PD-L1 expression in primary and metastatic bladder carcinomas: comparison of four commonly used antibodies and RNA expression. Mod Pathol 31(4):623–632
van Rhijn BWG, van Leenders GJLH, Ooms BCM, Kirkels WJ, Zlotta AR, Boevé ER (2010) The pathologist's mean grade is constant and individualizes the prognostic value of bladder cancer grading. Eur Urol 57(6):1052–1057
Varma M, Srigley JR, Brimo F, Compérat E, Delahunt B, Koch M (2020) Dataset for the reporting of urinary tract carcinoma-biopsy and transurethral resection specimen: recommendations from the international collaboration on cancer reporting (ICCR). Mod Pathol 33(4):700–712
Voskuilen CS, Seiler R, Rink M, Poyet C, Noon AP, Roghmann F (2020) u. a. urothelial carcinoma in bladder diverticula: a multicenter analysis of characteristics and clinical outcomes. Eur Urol Focus 6(6):1226–1232
Warrick JI, Sjödahl G, Kaag M, Raman JD, Merrill S, Shuman L (2019) Intratumoral heterogeneity of bladder cancer by molecular subtypes and histologic variants. Eur Urol 75(1):18–22
Weyerer V, Eckstein M, Compérat E, Juette H, Gaisa NT, Allory Y (2020) Pure large nested variant of urothelial carcinoma (LNUC) is the prototype of an FGFR3

mutated aggressive urothelial carcinoma with luminal-papillary phenotype. Cancers (Basel) 12(3):763

Williamson SR, Montironi R, Lopez-Beltran A, MacLennan GT, Davidson DD, Cheng L (2010) Diagnosis, evaluation and treatment of carcinoma in situ of the urinary bladder: the state of the art. Crit Rev Oncol Hematol 76(2):112–126

Willis DL, Fernandez MI, Dickstein RJ, Parikh S, Shah JB, Pisters LL (2015) Clinical outcomes of cT1 micropapillary bladder cancer. J Urol 193(4):1129–1134

Witjes JA (2004) Bladder carcinoma in situ in 2003: state of the art. Eur Urol 45(2):142–146

Witjes JA, Babjuk M, Bellmunt J, Bruins HM, De Reijke TM, De Santis M (2020) EAU-ESMO consensus statements on the Management of Advanced and Variant Bladder Cancer-an International Collaborative Multistakeholder Effort†: under the auspices of the EAU-ESMO guidelines committees. Eur Urol 77(2):223–250

Wojcik EM, Kurtycz DFI, Rosenthal DL, Herausgeber (2022) The Paris system for reporting urinary cytology [internet]. Springer International Publishing, Cham. Verfügbar unter: https://doi.org/10.1007/978-3-030-88686-8

Overview of Standard Therapy of Non-Muscle-Invasive Bladder Cancer

5

E. Bos, C. I. Dijkstra, and J. A. Witjes

Abstract

Bladder cancer (BC) is one of the most frequently diagnosed cancers worldwide. This chapter will focus on clinical presentation, diagnostics, and a brief recap of pathology followed by the standard treatment options and follow-up.

Painless gross hematuria is the most common presenting symptom and warrants further diagnostic procedures. The present gold standard in diagnostics is cystoscopy, complemented with urinary cytology and imaging to evaluate the upper urinary tract.

To establish both accurate pathological diagnoses and completely remove all visible lesions as part of treatment, transurethral resection of the bladder tumor (TURBT) is performed. In approximately 75% of patients, the BC is confined to the mucosa (stage Ta, CIS [carcinoma in situ]) or submucosa (stage T1), meaning the BC is non-muscle-invasive (NMIBC). Furthermore, the histological grading is established. The combination of pathological factors (stage and grading) and clinical factors determines the risk of disease recurrence and progression.

Several models have been developed to stratify patients into risk groups, which further determine the appropriate treatment schedule with intravesical installations (chemotherapy or Bacillus Calmette-Guèrin [BCG]) following the TURBT. In case of low-risk disease, a single postoperative intravesical chemotherapy is sufficient treatment, whereas for the higher risk groups treatment can consist of up to 1 year of chemotherapy or up to 3 years of BCG. In very-high-risk disease or in case of disease recurrence during BCG, this may require treatment with radical cystectomy.

Additionally, the risk group stratification determines the follow-up frequency of cystoscopy. Urinary molecular markers may play a significant role in follow-up in the future.

Keywords

Non-muscle-invasive bladder cancer · Hematuria · Cystoscopy · NMIBC risk group stratification · Intravesical chemotherapy · Intravesical BCG installations · NMIBC follow-up

E. Bos · C. I. Dijkstra · J. A. Witjes (✉)
Department of Urology, Radboud University Medical Center, Nijmegen, the Netherlands
e-mail: fred.witjes@radboudumc.nl

M. A. Knowles, L. Dyrskjøt (eds.), *Biology of Bladder Cancer*,
https://doi.org/10.1007/978-3-031-68505-7_5

5.1 Clinical Presentation and Diagnostics

5.1.1 Clinical Presentation

The most common clinical presentation of bladder cancer is painless gross hematuria or microscopic hematuria. In 85% of the cases in which bladder cancer is found, hematuria was the presenting symptom (Kirkali et al. 2005). Gross hematuria means blood is visible in the urine; the color can range from dark brown to bright red, and the urine may contain clots that could potentially obstruct the urethra (Lenis et al. 2020). Microscopic hematuria is non-visible to the patient and is found in a collected urine sample, where the urinalysis shows ≥3 red blood cells per high-power field. Microscopic hematuria also is commonly associated with benign causes, such as infection, vigorous exercise, medical renal disease, or menstruation (Lenis et al. 2020). Depending on the estimated risk of bladder cancer, repeating the urinalysis in several months or immediate further diagnostic workup can be considered. The finding of gross hematuria warrants immediate further diagnostic procedures.

Gross or visible hematuria has been associated with higher stage disease when compared to microscopic or non-visible hematuria (Ramirez et al. 2016). In patients with microscopic hematuria, the risk of bladder cancer has been found to be approximately 4%, whereas in patients with gross hematuria this risk is as high as 16.5% (Edwards et al. 2006).

Other symptoms that have been associated with bladder cancer are dysuria or irritative voiding symptoms, abdominal pain, constipation, and a medical history of urinary tract infection (Ramirez et al. 2016; Shephard et al. 2012). The symptom complex of bladder irritability, urinary frequency, urgency, and dysuria is the second most common symptom of bladder cancer and may be associated with diffuse CIS or invasive cancer (Kirkali et al. 2005). It has been found that the risk of bladder cancer is increased with multiple or repeated symptoms, although in the absence of visible hematuria or irritative voiding symptoms, the risk of finding bladder cancer was low (Shephard et al. 2012).

The evaluation of gross hematuria, and other symptoms leading to the suspicion of bladder cancer, involves visualization of the bladder through cystoscopy, microscopic evaluation of voided urine including cytology, and imaging of the urinary tract.

5.1.2 Initial Diagnostics

5.1.2.1 Cystoscopy

Cystoscopy is the present standard test in the diagnostics of bladder cancer (Trinh et al. 2018). Cystoscopy is recommended in patients presenting with suggestive symptoms as well as during surveillance and follow-up. To date, cystoscopy cannot be replaced by urinary cytology or any other noninvasive test (Babjuk et al. 2022).

Cystoscopy is generally performed in the outpatient clinic using topical intraurethral anesthetic lubricant instillation. It is recommended to use a flexible cystoscope, as, especially in men, this results with better compliance with the examination.

During cystoscopy the bladder mucosa is examined systematically. If a tumor is detected, it is advised to describe all macroscopic features of the tumor (site, size, number, and appearance) using a bladder diagram, as depicted in Fig. 5.1

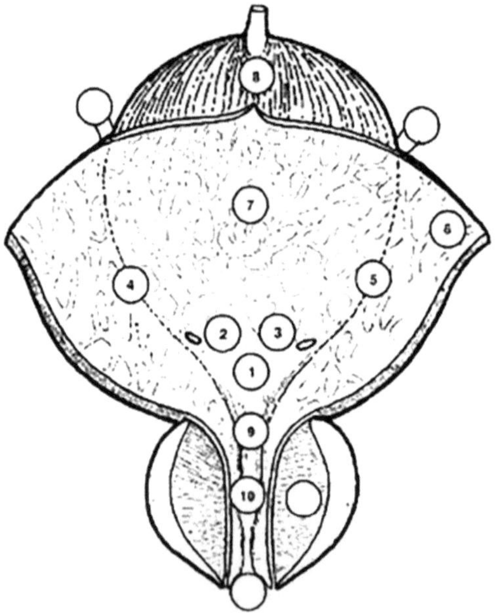

Fig. 5.1 Diagram of the bladder used to record information on tumors identified at cystoscopy. Reprinted with permission from EAU Guidelines on Non-Muscle-Invasive Bladder Cancer, 2024

(Babjuk et al. 2022). Also any mucosal abnormalities are reported in the same fashion.

1 = Trigone	6 = Anterior wall
2 = Right ureteral orifice	7 = Posterior wall
3 = Left ureteral orifice	8 = Dome
4 = Right wall	9 = Neck
5 = Left wall	10 = Posterior urethra

During cystoscopy the use of white light is standard. However, this has led to missing lesions that are present but invisible in white light. New technologies using different techniques such as fluorescence and narrowband imaging have been developed to improve the outcomes of cystoscopy. See Sect. 5.2.4 for further information about these new technologies. Furthermore, white light cystoscopy has demonstrated a lack of sensitivity for flat lesions such as CIS (Burger et al. 2013).

Cystoscopy is the present gold standard in diagnosis of bladder cancer, but research groups are working on other diagnostic methods. The main driver to do so is that cystoscopy is a costly procedure, it is uncomfortable for the patient (carrying the risk of noncompliance with follow-up schedules), and it carries a risk of infection (Burger et al. 2013).

5.1.2.2 Urine Cytology/Urinary Cytopathology

Urinary cytology (UC) is based on a cytopathologist's interpretation of changes in disaggregated cells in voided urine or following bladder irrigation and processed for light microscopy (Kirkali et al. 2005). The sensitivity of urinary cytology differs between high-grade and low-grade tumors and CIS. Sensitivity is high in high-grade tumors (84%) but low for low-grade tumors (16%) (Yafi et al. 2015). The sensitivity for CIS detection differs among studies between 28% and 100%, with a median of 48% (Têtu 2009).

The specificity of the test is user-dependent, but in experienced hands it is above 90% (Raitanen et al. 2002). The evaluation can be hampered by the presence of urinary tract infection or stones in the urinary tract. Also, a low cellular yield and intravesical instillations can make results less valid (Raitanen et al. 2002). The main advantage of using urinary cytology is that the test is noninvasive, compared to cystoscopy.

Table 5.1 The Paris System for reporting urinary cytology—2016

1. Nondiagnostic/unsatisfactory
2. Negative for high-grade urothelial carcinoma (NHGUC)
3. Atypical urothelial cells (AUC)
4. Suspicious for high-grade urothelial carcinoma (SHGUC)
5. High-grade urothelial carcinoma (HGUC)
6. Low-grade urothelial neoplasm (LGUN)
7. Others: primary and secondary malignancies and miscellaneous lesions

In 2016 the *Paris System for Reporting Urinary Cytology* was published, standardizing diagnostic categories (Nikas et al. 2022). The system has been shown to better characterize the cytology (Meilleroux et al. 2018). The Paris System comprises seven diagnostic categories, as shown in Table 5.1.

It is recommended to use voided urine cytology as an adjunct to cystoscopy to detect high-grade tumors, but cystoscopy cannot be replaced by cytology (Babjuk et al. 2022).

5.1.2.3 Urinary Molecular Marker Tests

As a result of the low sensitivity of urine cytology, urinary molecular marker tests have been developed. None of the marker tests can presently replace cystoscopy, though they can be used to enhance cystoscopy; it was found that awareness of a positive marker test significantly improves the detection rate of urothelial carcinoma using cystoscopy (van der Aa et al. 2010). Several promising urinary biomarkers assessing multiple mRNA and/or DNA targets frequently identified in bladder cancer have already been tested in prospective multicenter studies, showing a high negative predictive value and outperforming urinary cytology in follow-up of patients with previous non-muscle-invasive bladder tumors (Konety et al. 2019; Valenberg et al. 2019; D'Andrea et al. 2019) (see Chap. 18). Although these tests are not accepted as routine practice by clinical guidelines, it is hypothesized that reliable classification and differentiation between aggressive and nonaggressive tumors using marker tests may change surveillance and reduce the frequent use of cystoscopies (Maas et al. 2019). Several prospective and intervention studies with these tests in the diagnostic phase are presently being done.

5.1.2.4 Imaging

Computed Tomography (CT) Urography and Intravenous Urography

CT urography is used in the detection of papillary tumors in the urinary tract, which may be indicated by filling defects and/or hydronephrosis (Trinh et al. 2018). Particularly for bladder cancer, focal bladder wall thickening and the presence of a discrete mass or nodule in the bladder should be considered suspicious for malignancy. In several cohort studies, a high sensitivity and specificity has been reported using CT urography (alone or alongside cystoscopy) to detect bladder cancer in patients with hematuria, but the findings have not been considered sufficient to do away with the standard diagnostic tool cystoscopy (Raman and Fishman 2014). CT urography's main purpose in the initial evaluation of hematuria is the evaluation of possible causes of hematuria in the upper urinary tracts, such as malignancy and kidney stones.

The inclusion of CT urography in guidelines on follow-up has principally been to evaluate the upper urinary tract for malignancies, although the necessity is questionable due to the low incidence of significant findings (Davis et al. 2012; Palou et al. 2005). The incidence of simultaneous bladder cancer and upper urinary tract tumors (UUTT) has been found to be 1.8%. The only significant variable found to be related to UUTT was bladder cancer in the trigone. Of these tumors, 7.5% were associated with UUTT (Palou et al. 2005). Patients with multiple and high-risk tumors also have a higher risk of UUTT (Millán-Rodríguez et al. 2000). Therefore, it is recommended to incorporate CT urography in patients with the listed risk factors.

Ultrasound

In the evaluation of hematuria, ultrasound permits the visualization of intraluminal masses in the bladder as well as an evaluation of the upper urinary tract to detect renal masses and hydronephrosis (Hilton and Jones 2014). Technological advancements in radiology have increased the diagnostic accuracy of ultrasonography but cannot rule out all potential causes of hematuria. Both external factors, such as degree of bladder distension and obesity of the patient, and tumor-related factors, such as size, location, and tumor type, potentially lead to misdiagnosis (Ozden et al. 2007; Stamatiou et al. 2009). Ultrasonography of the urinary tract cannot reliably exclude urothelial carcinoma in the bladder and upper urinary tract and therefore cannot replace the use of CT urography (Babjuk et al. 2022).

Magnetic Resonance Imaging

The use of magnetic resonance imaging (MRI) scans in the diagnostics of bladder cancer is becoming more common. A standardized methodology for MRI reporting of bladder cancer has been published: the Vesical Imaging-Reporting and Data System (VI-RADS) (Panebianco et al. 2018). VI-RADS allows simplified reporting which improves communication between doctors and allows for comparison of patients. It is hypothesized that the use of MRI could contribute to better staging of bladder cancer, perhaps in the future changing the diagnostic approach and possibly even the treatment strategy. The overall accuracy of MRI for local staging of bladder cancer is superior to CT, but still only moderately accurate (Hilton and Jones 2014).

5.2 Transurethral Resection of Bladder Tumor

Transurethral resection of bladder tumor (TURBT) is a crucial procedure in the management of NMIBC. TURBT in combination with the subsequent histological evaluation is essential for diagnosis and staging. Furthermore, the other important goal of a TURBT is to remove all visible lesions with detrusor muscle in the specimen to improve prognosis (Babjuk et al. 2022). The absence of detrusor muscle, even in small tumors, is independently associated with an increased risk of early tumor recurrence and residual disease (Mariappan et al. 2010). TURBT can be performed in two ways (see below), depending on the size and location of the tumor and the experience of the surgeon.

5.2.1 Surgical Techniques of TURBT

1. Piecemeal resection in fractions: the exophytic part of the tumor, the underlying bladder wall, and the edges of the resection area are removed in separate fractions, using monopolar or bipolar resection with a U-shaped 5-mm electrical loop (Richterstetter et al. 2012). There are no differences in outcomes, including the occurrence of complications, between monopolar and bipolar resections.
2. En bloc resection: the tumor is removed in one piece. This technique is safe and reliable and can be performed with electrical (monopolar of bipolar) or laser (thulium or holmium) energy. Detrusor muscle is present in nearly 100% of specimens obtained with en bloc resection (Kramer et al. 2015).

Whatever surgical procedure is used, it is important that a high-quality TURBT is performed. A complete resection of tumor is crucial, because it decreases the rate of recurrence. The use of a surgical checklist can be helpful to improve surgical standardization and operative reporting and decreases recurrence rates (Suarez-Ibarrola et al. 2019). The following prognostic factors should be reported after TURBT: number and size of tumors, characteristics of tumors (papillary, flat, sessile, nodular), primary vs. recurrent tumor, and suspicion of the presence of CIS. Clinical staging (cTis, cTa, cT1, cT2, cT3, cT4) should also be reported (see also Chap. 4), including bimanual exam under anesthesia. The urologist should also mention whether the resection is radical (visually complete with musculus detrusor visible in the resection base) and if a complication (perforation of the bladder) is present (Anderson et al. 2016).

Several studies have shown that the quality of a TURBT depends on surgical experience. Resected specimens are more likely to contain detrusor muscle when obtained by experienced surgeons. One possible explanation is that an experienced surgeon is more confident to resect widely and deeply enough to obtain detrusor muscle without risking causing a complication. A dedicated teaching program, with an important component being the presence of a senior urologist in the operating room as a tutor, leads to a greater presence of detrusor muscle in the specimen and a reduction of complications (Mariappen et al. 2020).

5.2.2 Second TURBT

It is recommended to perform a second TURBT 2–6 weeks after the initial TURBT in case of:

- A T1 tumor.
- An incomplete initial TURBT or suspicion thereof. This suspicion may arise in case of immediate cessation of the procedure due to major bleeding or perforation or in case of a very large tumor that is difficult to reach.
- Absence of musculus detrusor in the initial TURBT specimen (Ta LG/G1 tumors and primary CIS excluded) (Babjuk et al. 2022).

The second TURBT has implications in several ways. Firstly, in case of a T1 tumor, the prevalence of residual tumor after the initial TURBT has been found to be up to 50%. Patients with a T1 tumor that received a second TURBT have higher recurrence and progression-free survival and also an overall survival advantage (Eroglu et al. 2020). Secondly, it provides more accurate staging and important prognostic information. The absence of tumor at the repeat TURBT is associated with lower recurrence rates and better progression-free survival. Consequently, it may select candidates for conservative management.

Persistent NMIBC at the second TURBT requires close follow-up, and sometimes early cystectomy may be considered because of the high risk of progression to muscle-invasive bladder cancer (MIBC) (Bishr et al. 2014). Moreover, there are patients in whom MIBC is found to be present immediately on the second TURBT and thus require more radical therapy. Lastly, it improves outcomes after bacillus Calmette-Guérin (BCG) treatment in patients with high-grade T1 tumors. This again is related to better staging and therefore earlier provision of radical therapy (Gordon et al. 2019). Details about BCG treatment can be found in Sect. 5.5.

5.2.3 Biopsies During TURBT

During TURBT it is recommended to take biopsies from abnormal-looking urothelium because CIS may be present. As mentioned, CIS can be difficult to recognize, but it is a high-grade tumor that must be detected and treated to prevent progression to MIBC. Sometimes the mucosa looks normal, but the urinary cytology or urinary molecular marker test is positive. In that case mapping biopsies should be taken (Hara et al. 2009), which involves taking biopsies from the trigone, bladder dome, and right, left, anterior, and posterior bladder wall. Fluorescence cystoscopy can be a useful tool in taking biopsies (see below). If pathology shows that there is no bladder tumor, then a biopsy of the prostatic urethra should also be taken afterward. One may also consider taking a biopsy from the prostatic urethra while taking the mapping biopsies to spare the patient a possible additional burden. The prostatic urethra should also be biopsied if it looks abnormal, in case of a bladder neck tumor or the presence or suspicion of CIS (Mungan et al. 2005).

5.2.4 Tumor Visualization During TURBT

Like cystoscopy, TURBT is usually performed using white light. Unfortunately, some lesions can easily be overlooked with white light, for example, small papillary bladder tumors or CIS. New techniques have been designed to visualize these lesions. Two techniques that are used in daily practice are described below.

5.2.4.1 Fluorescence Cystoscopy

In fluorescence cystoscopy (FC), violet light is used after hexaminolaevulinic acid (HAL) is applied intravesically. HAL is a photosensitizing drug which should be administered approximately an hour before the TURBT. This interacts with cells to cause accumulation of photoactive porphyrins. Photoactive porphyrins preferentially accumulate in neoplastic cells, which then turn bright pink under violet light (Fig. 5.2).

Several studies have shown beneficial effects of using FC. FC-guided biopsy and resection have a higher sensitivity for detection of bladder tumors, especially CIS and high-grade tumors, than white light cystoscopy (WLC) (Burger et al. 2013; Kausch et al. 2010). It provides a more complete resection, reduces recurrence, and prolongs recurrence-free survival (Mowatt et al. 2011). Although these results suggest many benefits of the usage of FC, they should be interpreted with caution given that there may have been both a performance and a publication bias (Chou et al. 2017). A disadvantage of FC is that it has low specificity. False positive results can be explained by inflammation, a recent TURBT, or BCG instillation 3 months before FC-guided biopsies or resection (Draga et al. 2010).

5.2.4.2 Narrowband Imaging

Narrowband imaging (NBI) is a technique that improves the optical image by filtering white light into two narrowbands (415 and 540 nm). These short-wavelength light beams are strongly absorbed by hemoglobin, making the capillaries in mucosa and submucosa more visible and improving the contrast between superficial tumors and normal mucosa. NBI has a higher detection rate for bladder tumors including CIS in comparison to cystoscopy with white light only. However, its clinical relevance is limited, as it does not lead to a lower recurrence rate (Ye et al. 2015).

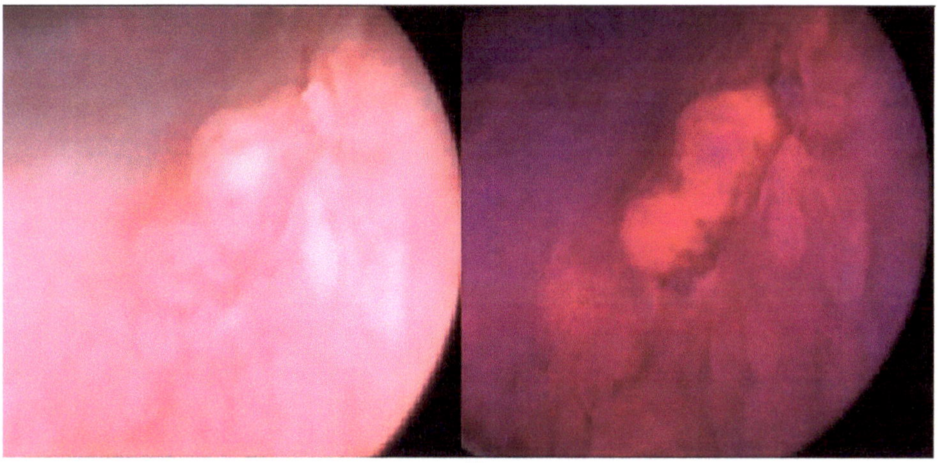

Fig. 5.2 White light cystoscopy versus fluorescence cystoscopy

5.3 Pathology

5.3.1 Tumor, Node, Metastasis (TNM) Classification

The TNM classification system (Brierley et al. 2016) and histological grading according to the WHO 1973 or 2014/2016 classification system (MacLennan et al. 2007) are used to divide bladder carcinoma into different stages. Table 5.2 shows the complete 8th edition TNM classification of the Union International Contre le Cancer (UICC). NMIBC is a group definition based on the required treatment. It includes Ta, T1, and CIS (Tis) because they can all be treated by a transurethral resection or biopsy of the tumor with or without intravesical instillations. Stage Ta means that the tumor is confined to the mucosa. This also applies for CIS, but these are flat, high-grade intraepithelial tumors. In T1 the tumor invades the lamina propria. Stage T2 and beyond are muscle-invasive forms of bladder carcinoma and are therefore not discussed in this chapter (Babjuk et al. 2022). For an overview, see Fig. 5.3 (see also Chap. 4).

T1 tumors can be further divided into two different substaging systems based on the depth (T1a-c) or extension (T1m or T1e) of lamina propria invasion. T1a tumors have invasion above

Table 5.2 Complete 8th edition TNM classification or urinary bladder cancer of the UICC

T—primary tumor
TX Primary tumor cannot be assessed
T0 No evidence of primary tumor
Ta Noninvasive papillary carcinoma
Tis Carcinoma in situ: "flat tumor"
T1 Tumor invades subepithelial connective tissue
T2 Tumor invades muscle T2a Tumor invades superficial muscle (inner half) T2b Tumor invades deep muscle (outer half)
T3 Tumor invades perivesical tissue T3a Microscopically T3b Macroscopically (extravesical mass)
T4 Tumor invades any of the following: prostate stroma, seminal vesicles, uterus, vagina pelvic wall, and abdominal wall T4a Tumor invades prostate stroma, seminal vesicles, uterus, or vagina T4b Tumor invades pelvic wall or abdominal wall
N—regional lymph nodes
NX Regional lymph nodes cannot be assessed
N0 No regional lymph node metastasis
N1 Metastasis in a single lymph node in the true pelvis (hypogastric, obturator, external iliac, or presacral)
N2 Metastasis in multiple regional lymph nodes in the true pelvis (hypogastric, obturator, external iliac, or presacral)
N3 Metastasis in common iliac lymph nodes
M—distant metastasis
M0 No distant metastasis M1a Non-regional lymph nodes M1b Other distant metastasis

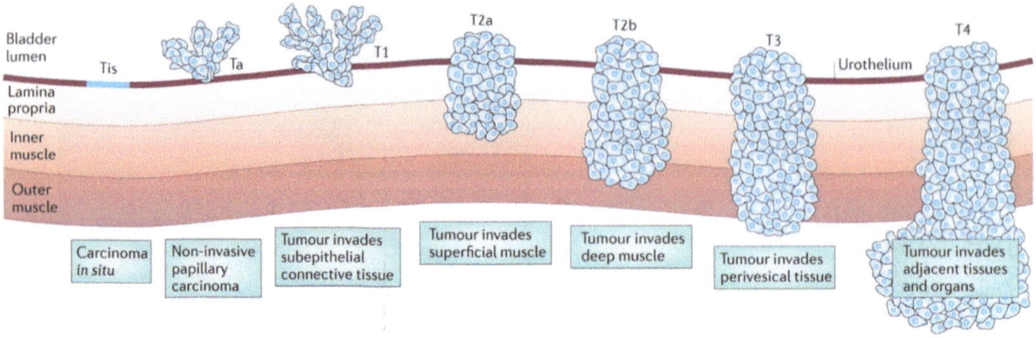

Fig. 5.3 Bladder cancer staging (Knowles and Hurst 2015)

the muscularis mucosae-vascular plexus (MM-VP), T1b tumors invade the MM-VP, and T1c tumors invade beyond the MM-VP. T1m means that there is a single focus of lamina propria invasion ≤0.5 mm (within one high-power field, objective × 40). In T1e there is a single focus of invasion ≥0.5 mm or there are multiple microinvasive areas (van Rhijn et al. 2012). T1 substaging, with one of the above systems, is recommended (Compérat et al. 2021). Among these subcategories, T1c and T1e had a significantly higher rate of recurrence and progression in comparison with T1a and T1m, respectively. The optimal classification system has yet to be determined (Asimakopoulos et al. 2021).

CIS is a unique clinical entity of NMIBC due to its high grade and aggressiveness. When left untreated, approximately 50% of urothelial CIS of the bladder may result in progression to muscle-invasive disease. CIS is a flat urothelial lesion, which can be hard to recognize with white light cystoscopy, as it may resemble the appearance of cystitis. CIS can affect the bladder but also the upper urinary tract, prostatic ducts and urethra, and penile urethra. Based on the clinical presentation, there are three types of CIS:

- Primary: CIS not associated with any past or present urothelial carcinoma
- Secondary: CIS detected during the follow-up of patient with a previous urothelial carcinoma
- Concurrent: CIS in the presence of any other urothelial carcinoma in the bladder (Akhtar et al. 2019; Lamm et al. 1998)

5.3.2 Histological Grading

The WHO published two histological classification systems for urothelial carcinomas (Netto et al. 2022). The system of 1973 contains three categories based on microscopic features:

- Grade 1 (well differentiated): only mild degrees of cytological atypia and infrequent mitotic figures
- Grade 2 (moderately differentiated): all tumors between grade 1 and grade 3
- Grade 3 (poorly differentiated): marked nuclear pleomorphism, loss of maturation from the base of the surface, and mitotic activity

The system of 2004, which was maintained in the WHO 2016 and 2022 guidelines, was created in an attempt to reduce variability and increase reproducibility. The system is based on more detailed histological criteria and also consists of three categories:

- PUNLMP: papillary urothelial neoplasm with low malignant potential. Defined as a slim papillae without atypia, no thickening of the urothelium.
- Low grade: characterized by orderly arranged papillae, with increased layers. Atypia is rare and polarity is conserved.
- High grade: characterized by nuclear atypia (nuclei have prominent nucleoli and are pleomorphic, with frequent mitosis). Major destruction of the architecture is present.

If different grades are detected in the same lesion, the tumor is graded according to the highest grade observed (Soukup et al. 2017; Compérat et al. 2019).

However, there is a shift of patients between the categories of the WHO 1973 and the WHO 2004/2016 classification system (see also Chap. 4). A subset of grade 2 patients is included into the high-grade group, and therefore this group has increased. Over time PUNLMP diagnosis substantially decreased to approximately 1–2.5% of all Ta tumors (2010–2018). It seems that pathologists nowadays classify a majority of former PUNLMPs as low-grade tumors. Ta tumors diagnosed as PUNLMP or low grade have similar prognosis. Nevertheless, PUNLMP remains a separate category in the WHO 2022 guidelines (Hentschel et al. 2020).

Both classification systems are still used, and in general pathologists agree on stage and grade in 50–60% of the cases. The WHO 2004/2016 classification did not outperform the WHO 1973 classification in prediction of progression. Reproducibility was only slightly better for the 2004/2016 classification but still too low. On the other hand, it has a major disadvantage, since it gives almost no prognostic information for T1 tumors. According to the 2004/2016 classification, almost all T1 tumors are classified as high grade, whereas the 1973 classification makes a better division of the T1 tumors into grade 2 or grade 3 (Soukup et al. 2017). Furthermore, a large prognostic factor study in 2021 showed that both classification systems are prognostic for progression but not for recurrence, and the system from 1973 was shown to be a stronger prognosticator of progression in Ta/T1 NMIBC. A combination of both systems (LG/G1, LG/G2, HG/G2, HG/G3) may be superior to either classification system alone, since the large group of G2 patients is divided into two subgroups with different prognoses (van Rhijn et al. 2021).

5.3.3 NMIBC Subtypes

Most cases of bladder cancer are urothelial carcinomas, including histological subtypes or forms of divergent differentiation. Examples of subtypes are micropapillary, plasmacytoid, or nested. Squamous, glandular, or Mullerian are forms of divergent differentiation. In the 2022 World Health Organization classification, all subtypes are considered as high grade (Lamm et al. 1998). It is important to report the percentage of subtype present in the specimen, because it has been shown to be of prognostic value (Babjuk et al. 2022). The vast majority of the subtypes are MIBC; no more than 15–30% of the subtypes are NIMBC. About 5% of bladder cancers are non-urothelial carcinomas including adenocarcinoma, small cell carcinoma, and squamous cell carcinoma (Lamm et al. 1998). For more information about pathology, see Chap. 4.

5.4 Prediction of Disease Recurrence and Progression

Depending on the pathological reports and the patient's medical history, the risk of both recurrence of disease and progression from NMIBC to MIBC can be determined. Several models have been developed according to tumor and treatment type, such as treatment with intravesical Bacillus Calmette-Guérin (BCG) or chemotherapy after TURBT or early cystectomy. It is important to note beforehand that different models have been developed for patients treated with chemotherapy versus BCG installations. The latter group will be discussed at the end of this section.

5.4.1 Stratification into Risk Groups to Predict Progression

In order to be able to facilitate treatment recommendations, it is recommended by the EAU guidelines to stratify patients with a primary bladder tumor into risk groups, according to the EAU NMIBC 2021 scoring model (Sylvester et al. 2021). The risk groups are based on their probability to progress to muscle-invasive disease. The 2021 EAU NMIBC scoring model does not determine the risk for recurrence; other models have been developed to determine this risk which will be discussed later.

Independent predictors of disease progression were found to be tumor stage, WHO 1973 and/or WHO2004/2022 grade, concomitant CIS, number of tumors, tumor size, and age. The risk groups are based on the WHO 2004/2016 or the WHO 1973 grading classification systems (Table 5.3). Only one of the two systems is required to use the table. If both are available in an individual patient, it is recommended to use the WHO 1973 system. Additional clinical risk factors are age > 70 years, the presence of multiple papillary tumors, and tumor diameter >3 cm.

The scoring model does not consider patients with primary CIS, who are always high risk, or with recurrent tumors. Furthermore, pathologic parameters are not considered. An important addition to the table is the following:

- All patients with CIS in the prostatic urethra, with subtypes of UC as mentioned in "Pathology," or with lymphovascular invasion should be included in the very-high-risk group.
- Patients with recurrent tumors should be included in the intermediate-, high-, or very-high-risk groups according to their other prognostic factors.

Table 5.3 Risk of progression for patients with NMIBC

Risk group	
Low risk	A primary, single, TaT1 LG/G1 tumor <3 cm in diameter without CIS in a patient ≤70 years A primary Ta LG/G1 tumor without CIS with at most *one* of the additional clinical risk factors
Intermediate risk	Patients without CIS who are not included in either the low-, high-, or very-high-risk groups
High risk	All T1 HG/G3 without CIS, *except* those included in the very-high-risk group All CIS patients, *except* those included in the very-high-risk group *Stage, grade with additional clinical risk factors:* Ta LG/G2 or T1G1, no CIS with all three risk factors Ta HG/G3 or T1 LG, no CIS with at least two risk factors T1G2 no CIS with at least one risk factor
Very high risk	*Stage, grade with additional clinical risk factors:* Ta Hg/G2 and CIS with all three risk factors T1G2 and CIS with at least two risk factors T1 HG/G3 and CIS with at least one risk factor T1 HG/G3 no CIS with all three risk factors

Once the individual patient is stratified in a risk group, Table 5.4 can be used to predict the probability of progression (Sylvester et al. 2021).

As mentioned above, Table 5.4 has the limitation that it cannot be used for patients treated with BCG. Different prediction models have been developed for this patient group and will be discussed later in this chapter. The consequence of the limitations mentioned above is that the EAU risk classification clearly overestimates the risk of progression if patients are treated according to present guidelines.

Several additional prognostic factors have been formulated in selected patient populations, most important of which are:

- In T1 HG/G3 tumors, female sex, age, tumor size, CIS in the prostatic urethra in men treated with an induction course of BCG, and concurrent CIS in BCG-treated patients were found to be important prognostic factors (Gontero et al. 2015).
- Patients with T1 HG/G3 tumors in bladder diverticula must be given attention because of the absence of a muscle layer in the diverticulum (Voskuilen et al. 2020).
- The finding of residual T1 disease at second TURBT in patients with primary T1 tumors is an unfavorable prognostic factor (Bishr et al. 2014).
- Recurrence at 3 months in T1G2 patients treated with TURBT was the most important predictor for progression (Palou et al. 2009).

Finally, T1 substaging has been investigated as a prognostic tool in high-risk NMIBC. As dis-

Table 5.4 Probabilities of disease progression in 1, 5, and 10 year(s) for the new EAU NMIBC risk groups (Cambier et al. 2016)

	Probability of progression and 95% confidence interval (CI)		
Risk group	1 year	5 years	10 years
New risk groups with WHO 2004/2016			
Low	0.06% (CI: 0.01–0.43%)	0.93% (CI: 0.49–1.7%)	3.7% (CI: 2.3–5.9%)
Intermediate	1.0% (CI: 0.50–2.0%)	4.9% (CI: 3.4–7.0%)	8.5% (CI: 5.6–13%)
High	3.5% (CI: 2.4–5.2%)	9.6% (CI: 7.4–12%)	14% (CI: 11–18%)
Very high	16% (CI: 10–26%)	40% (CI: 29–54%)	53% (CI: 36–73%)
New risk groups with WHO 1973			
Low	0.12% (CI: 0.02–0.82%)	0.57% (CI: 0.21–1.5%)	3.0% (CI: 1.5–6.3%)
Intermediate	0.65% (CI: 0.36–1.2%)	3.6% (CI: 2.7–4.9%)	7.4% (CI: 5.5–10%)
High	3.8% (CI: 2.6–5.7%)	11% (CI: 8.1–14%)	14% (CI: 10–19%)
Very high	20% (CI: 12–32%)	44% (CI: 30–61%)	59% (CI: 39–79%)

cussed in Sect. 5.3, T1 tumors can be further divided with two different substaging systems based on the depth (T1a-c) or extension (T1m, microinvasive, invasion <0.5 mm or T1e, extensive invasive, invasion ≥0.5 mm) of lamina propria invasion. The latter system, based on extension of lamina propria invasion, the so-called metric system, has been found to be superior in predicting progression and survival (Fransen van de Putte et al. 2018). Patients with T1e disease reportedly have significantly worse prognosis. These patients more often experience BCG failure and have worse progression-free survival compared to T1m patients (de Jong et al. 2021). T1 substaging can be used to guide treatment decisions.

5.4.2 Stratification into Risk Groups to Predict Recurrence

To determine the risk of recurrence and progression in patients with a Ta/T1 tumor not treated with BCG, the Genito-Urinary Cancer Group (GUCG) of the European Organization for Research and Treatment of Cancer (EORTC) published a scoring model in 2006, which can be used by clinicians to predict the risks of disease recurrence and progression in individual patients (Sylvester et al. 2006). The variables found of prognostic importance for recurrence are prior treatment, prior recurrence and recurrence rate, number of tumors, tumor size, T category, grade, and the presence of concomitant CIS (Sylvester et al. 2006).

Using the 2006 EORTC model, an individual patient's score can be calculated based on the listed variables. With the patient's score, the probabilities of recurrence and progression at both 1 and 5 years can be estimated. Depending on the individual patient's score, the probability of recurrence can vary between 15% and 61% at 1 year and 31% and 78% at 5 years. Probability of progression can vary between 0.2% and 17% at 1 year and 0.8% and 45% at 5 years (Sylvester et al. 2006).

5.4.3 Prediction Models in Patients Treated with BCG

Studies have found that the risk of progression in patients treated with BCG is significantly lower than suggested in the EAU NMIBC 2021 scoring model, hence the development of separate scoring models for this patient group (Sylvester et al. 2021).

5.4.3.1 Club Urologico Espanol de Tratamiento Oncologica (CUETO) Scoring Model

The CUETO scoring model predicts both the recurrence and progression risk for patients treated with BCG. The model is based on 12 doses of intravesical BCG over a 5–6-month period following TURBT (Fernandez-Gomez et al. 2009). Prognostic factors found to be of important predictive value were gender, age, prior recurrence, number of tumors, T category, associated CIS, and tumor grade (based on WHO 1973).

Again, patient's individual scores can be calculated, stratifying patients into risk groups. Depending on the individual patient's score, the probability of recurrence can vary between 8.2% and 42% at 1 year and 21% and 68% at 5 years. Probability of progression can vary between 1.2% and 3.7% at 1 year and 14% and 34% at 5 years (Fernandez-Gomez et al. 2009). Looking at these figures, it becomes apparent that the 2006 EORTC model overestimates the risk of recurrence in this specific BCG-treated patient group (Fernandez-Gomez et al. 2011).

5.4.3.2 The 2016 EORTC Scoring Model

The present European guidelines recommend a longer treatment scheme with intravesical BCG than the CUETO scoring model used. The recommendation presently is that patients are treated with 1 to 3 years of maintenance BCG, in which case the CUETO model cannot be used in predictions (Cambier et al. 2016). Based on individual patients and tumor characteristics, four prognostic groups were made for both recurrence and progression. For recurrence, the prior disease recurrence rate and number of tumors were found to be the most important prognostic factors. The best prognostic group showed a recurrence probability of 14% and 28.3% at 1 and 5 years, respectively, whereas the worst prognostic group showed a probability of 33% and 51.7% at 1 and 5 years, respectively (Cambier et al. 2016). For progression, stage and WHO 1973 grade were found to be the most important prognostic factors. The best prognostic groups had a progression probability of 1.9% and 7.1% at 1 and 5 years, respectively, and the worst prognostic groups had a probability of 11.4% and 19.8% at 1 and 5 years, respectively.

In conclusion, the 1- and 5-year chances of recurrence are around 15% and 31% in low-risk disease, 24% and 46% in intermediate-risk disease, 38% and 62% in high-risk disease, and 61% and 78% in very-high-risk disease. The 1- and 5-year chances of progression are around 0.12% and 0.57% in low-risk disease, 0.65% and 3.6% in intermediate-risk disease, 3.8% and 11% in high-risk disease, and 20% and 44% in very-high-risk disease. The chances are generally lower in patients treated with BCG.

5.4.4 Carcinoma In situ

No reliable prognostic factors have been found for CIS. However, it is important to note that without treatment, approximately 54% of patients with CIS progress to MIBC (Akhtar et al. 2019). Several studies do suggest worse prognostic outcomes in case of CIS in the prostatic urethra, CIS in concurrence with T1 tumors compared to primary CIS, and in case of extended CIS (Palou et al. 2012; Griffiths et al. 2002; Takenaka et al. 2008). Most importantly, the response to intravesical treatment with BCG or chemotherapy is an important factor for the prognosis. An estimated 10–20% of complete responders to intravesical BCG or chemotherapy progress to muscle-invasive disease, whereas more than 60% of nonresponders do so (Solsona et al. 2000; van Gils-Gielen et al. 1995).

5.5 Disease Management

5.5.1 General Considerations

TURBT is the first step in the management of NMIBC, and it can remove a Ta/T1 tumor completely. Nevertheless, adjuvant therapy should be considered in all patients, because these tumors often recur and can progress to MIBC (Babjuk et al. 2022). Reasons for recurrence are (1) regrowth of residual tumor at the resection site, (2) a residual lesion that has been overlooked, (3) suspended tumor cells at the time of the TURBT that have caused a new lesion, or (4) a neoplasm with a high aggressive biology (Brausi et al. 2002).

Required therapy depends on the EAU NMIBC risk groups (Sect. 5.4). The risk groups and thus recommendations for treatment are based on the risk of disease progression. A summary of recommended therapy for every risk group will be provided at the end of this chapter.

In addition to adjuvant treatment, all patients should be counseled to stop smoking. Recurrence and progression rates of NMIBC increase with smoking (Rink et al. 2012).

5.5.2 Single Postoperative Intravesical Instillation of Chemotherapy

After TURBT, a single instillation of chemotherapy can be administered to reduce the recurrence rate. In vitro studies show that bladder cancer cells readily adhere to the subendothelial extracellular matrix and that injury of the bladder wall results in more tumor outgrowth compared to non-traumatized bladders. TURBT causes damage to the bladder wall and releases tumor cells, making it easier for bladder cancer to reimplant (Brocks et al. 2005). Intravesical chemotherapy destroys tumor cells floating in the urine or irrigation fluid after TURBT and has an ablative effect on residual tumor cells at the resection site and on small overlooked tumors. Mitomycin and epirubicin are commonly used and are equally effective (Sylvester et al. 2016). They should be administered within 24 h after TURBT but preferably within an hour to achieve maximum effect. After 24 h, tumor cells are firmly implanted and covered by the extracellular matrix (Pode et al. 1986). The length of the instillation should be 1–2 h (Babjuk et al. 2022).

Epirubicin and mitomycin can cause severe complications when they leak outside the bladder. Therefore, it is important to avoid an immediate instillation of these agents in cases of overt or suspected bladder wall perforation or bleeding requiring bladder irrigation (Oddens et al. 2004; Elmamoun et al. 2014). It is recommended to offer postoperative water or saline continued irrigation of the bladder (for approximately 24 h) to patients who are unable to receive a single postoperative instillation of chemotherapy. Several studies have shown irrigation to be as effective as immediate chemotherapy instillations (Zhou et al. 2019).

Not all patients benefit from a single postoperative instillation with chemotherapy. Patients with a recurrence rate of more than once per year and those with an EORTC score ≥ 5 do not show a reduced recurrence rate after a single adjuvant instillation (Sylvester et al. 2016). In practice this means that a single instillation with chemotherapy is offered to:

- Patients with low-risk NMIBC. During the TURBT, likely stage and grade of the tumor(s) are assessed by the surgeon to allow immediate postoperative instillation for patients likely to be in the low-risk group. Pathology reports are necessary to determine the definitive risk group.
- Patients with a small papillary recurrence (presumably Ta LG/G1) detected more than 1 year after the previous TURBT.

In patients with a low-risk tumor, TURBT followed by a single instillation of chemotherapy is considered to be the standard and complete treatment (Babjuk et al. 2022).

5.5.3 Additional Adjuvant Intravesical Chemotherapy Instillations

For patients other than low-risk patients, TURBT followed by a single instillation of chemotherapy remains an incomplete treatment. Patients in the intermediate-, high-, or very-high-risk group have a considerable likelihood of recurrence and/or progression (Sect. 5.4). Further treatment depends on each individual prognosis.

Additional adjuvant intravesical chemotherapy has a place in the treatment of patients in the intermediate-risk group. In these patients, repeat chemotherapy instillations (with or without previous single instillation) decreases the recurrence rate and improves recurrence-free survival (Tolley et al. 1996; Huncharek et al. 2001). Many different schedules have been used for the administration of intravesical chemotherapy, varying in frequency (e.g., weekly or quarterly), duration (weeks to 3 years postoperative), and dosage. There is no consensus on the optimal schedule; however, intravesical chemotherapy instillations should not be given for more than 1 year (Sylvester et al. 2008).

Although adjuvant chemotherapy instillations have a beneficial effect, intravesical Bacillus Calmette-Guerin (BCG) maintenance treatment (see 5.5.5) is superior in reducing the risk of recurrence. Furthermore, two meta-analyses show that BCG treatment may reduce the risk of tumor progression (Böhle and Bock 2004; Sylvester and van der Ma 2002). On the other hand, BCG causes more local side effects (hematuria and drug-induced cystitis) and more systemic adverse events, for instance, fever (Sect. 5.5.6) (Shang et al. 2011). The choice between intravesical chemotherapy and BCG should depend on the individual patient's risk of recurrence and progression, as well as the efficacy and side effects of each treatment method (Tan et al. 2022).

5.5.4 Options for Improving Efficacy of Intravesical Chemotherapy

One randomized controlled trial showed that optimization of intravesical mitomycin treatment reduced the recurrence rate at 5 years after TURBT and prolonged median recurrence-free survival. Optimization, to increase the drug concentration in the urine, took place through several actions. The patients had a fluid restriction (before and during the instillation), and their bladders were emptied (<10 ml residual urine) before administration of mitomycin. Furthermore, they received an oral dose of sodium bicarbonate to alkalinize the urine, and the dose of mitomycin was 40 mg (instead of 20 mg) at a concentration of 2 mg/mL in water (instead of 0.5 mg/mL) (Au et al. 2001). Another study also showed that treatment with epirubicin has a better recurrence-free rate if the drug solution concentration is higher (Kuroda et al. 2004).

Chemohyperthermia is a relatively new approach for patients in whom standard adjuvant intravesical treatment (chemotherapy or BCG) fails. A special system allows chemotherapy to be inserted into the bladder through a catheter and delivers hyperthermia to the bladder wall via radiofrequency energy through an antenna on the catheter. Hyperthermia has a lethal effect on cancer cells by inhibiting DNA, RNA, and protein synthesis. Moreover, it provides better penetration of the chemotherapy into the bladder wall, which may improve the effect on residual cancer cells at the resected area during TURBT (Arends et al. 2014). Chemohyperthermia after previous intravesical chemotherapy or BCG improves recurrence-free survival in intermediate- and high-risk patients. Moreover, a randomized controlled trial shows that chemohyperthermia is a reliable alternative to adjuvant BCG treatment with at least the same recurrence-free survival, perhaps even better (Arends et al. 2016). Side effects of chemohyperthermia are common but are often mild and limited to the genitourinary tract. They rarely lead to discontinuation of therapy.

5.5.5 Adjuvant Intravesical Bacillus Calmette-Guèrin (BCG) Treatment

Intravesical BCG treatment is a form of immunotherapy and was first used in 1976 (Morales et al. 1976). BCG is the tuberculosis vaccine containing viable avirulent attenuated *Mycobacterium bovis*. The precise mechanism of action has not been sufficiently elucidated. The effect might be the result of an immune response activating macrophages, T lymphocytes, B lymphocytes, and natural killer cells, which ensures improved surveillance of tumor cells in the bladder (Shang et al. 2011) (see Chap. 20 for more detailed discussion).

Intravesical BCG after TURBT reduces the risk of tumor recurrence and is more effective than intravesical chemotherapy in patients with intermediate- and high-risk tumors. Several studies have compared BCG with mitomycin or epirubicin, and all show that BCG is superior in preventing recurrence (Sylvester et al. 2010; Malmström et al. 2009). There are conflicting results on the effect of BCG on the risk of progression, which may be explained by differences in duration of follow-up, patient characteristics, methodology, and statistical power. However, most studies show a reduction in the risk of progression compared to intravesical chemotherapy when a BCG maintenance treatment is administered in high- and intermediate-risk patients (Böhle and Bock 2004; Sylvester and van der Ma 2002). Furthermore, one randomized controlled trial with long-term follow-up (median follow-up time was 9.2 years) showed that BCG in comparison to epirubicin favorably influenced the occurrence of distant metastases (5 vs. 8.6%) and death due to bladder cancer (3.4 vs. 6.8%) (Morales et al. 1976). A meta-analysis comparing BCG and mitomycin could not confirm these effects (Schmidt et al. 2020).

In summary, intermediate-risk patients are recommended to be treated with BCG or chemotherapy for 1 year. Treatment with BCG for 3 years is indicated in patients with high-risk tumors. The latter regimen can also be offered to patients in the very-high-risk group if they are unwilling or unable to undergo radical cystectomy.

For optimal efficacy, the treatment regimen of BCG should consist of induction instillations followed by a maintenance schedule (Böhle et al. 2003). To date, induction instillations are given according to the empirical 6-weekly schedule introduced in 1976 (Morales et al. 1976). At least 1 year of maintenance BCG is required to obtain superiority of BCG, with several schemes described (Böhle and Bock 2004). The standard 1-year schedule consists of 6-weekly induction instillations followed by 3-weekly instillations at 3, 6, and 12 months (15 instillations in total). To determine the optimal dose and duration of BCG treatment, a study compared different schedules. The results show that patients in the intermediate-risk group should be treated according to the standard schedule for 1 year. In high-risk patients, extending therapy to 3 years (adding 3-weekly instillations at 12, 18, 24, 30, and 36 months) has a beneficial effect on recurrence but not on progression or death. Intermediate-risk patients do not benefit from an additional 2 years of BCG (Oddens et al. 2013).

5.5.6 BCG Toxicity

BCG is superior in reducing the risk of recurrence, but it is also associated with more side effects compared to intravesical chemotherapy. Local side effects occur in up to 75.2% treated with BCG and include (bacterial or BCG induced) cystitis, dysuria, frequency/urgency, hematuria, ureteral obstructions, granulomatous prostatitis, and epididymo-orchitis. Systemic side effects occur in up to 39.4% and include general malaise and chills, fever, arthralgia and/or arthritis, BCG-induced lung infection, liver toxicity, and BCG sepsis. An allergic reaction to BCG may also occur. Serious side effects (need for hospitalization or life-threatening) occur in up to <5% and can be properly treated in most cases (Babjuk et al. 2022).

The dosage and duration of BCG does not affect the occurrence of side effects. BCG-related adverse effects are generally seen during induction and the first year of maintenance therapy. Discontinuation of BCG treatment due to local or systemic adverse effects, especially in the first year of treatment, is seen in up to 20% of patients (van der Meijden et al. 2003; Brausi et al. 2014; Witjes et al. 2008).

Systemic absorption of BCG can lead to major complications. Therefore, absolute contraindications of intravesical BCG instillations are (Babjuk et al. 2022):

- During the first 2 weeks after TURBT
- Macroscopic hematuria (delay instillations until this has resolved)
- After traumatic catheterization (defer instillations for 1 week)
- Symptomatic urinary tract infection (defer instillation for 1 week or until resolution of the urinary tract infection with antibiotics)

BCG should be used with caution in patients who are immunocompromised, yet small studies have shown no difference in complications or the efficacy of BCG compared to non-immunocompromised patients (Yossepowitch et al. 2006).

5.5.7 Specific Consideration for the Treatment of Carcinoma In situ (CIS)

CIS cannot be cured by TURBT alone. The presence of CIS immediately places a patient in the high- or very-high-risk group and increases the risk of recurrence and progression. If histology shows CIS, further treatment consists of induction instillations of BCG followed by maintenance for 3 years or a radical cystectomy. BCG treatment increases the complete response rate to 72–93% compared to a rate with 48% in chemotherapy. Unfortunately, approximately 50% of patients with a complete response have a recurrence with risk of invasion and/or extravesical recurrence (Jakse et al. 2001). Furthermore, BCG also allows patients to remain disease-free longer with less risk of progression, again compared to chemotherapy (Sylvester and van der Ma 2002; Sylvester et al. 2005). Immediate radical cystectomy in patients with CIS leads to excellent tumor-specific survival rates, but a large proportion of the patients may be overtreated (Lamm 1992).

Approximately 63% of the patients with CIS develop extravesical involvement in the upper urinary tract and/or prostate. These patients have a worse survival than patients with CIS limited to the bladder (Solsona et al. 1996). For therapeutic purposes, it is important to distinguish the presence of CIS in the epithelial lining of the prostatic urethra or in the prostatic duct from tumor invasion into the prostatic stroma. Tumor invasion in the prostatic stroma is a stage T4a bladder tumor for which immediate radical cystoprostatectomy is recommended. There are insufficient data on patients with CIS in the epithelial lining of the urethra, and therefore no clear treatment recommendations can be made. Radical surgery should be considered in these patients, but intravesical BCG is an alternative treatment that preserves the bladder (Palou Redorta et al. 2006).

5.5.8 Radical Cystectomy

Radical cystectomy is not the first choice of treatment in NMIBC but may be considered because of the following reasons:

- Even if detrusor muscle is present in the specimen of the first TURBT, still 11% of the patients experience upstaging to MIBC at the second TURBT (Naselli et al. 2018).
- Patients with NMIBC can progress to muscle-invasive disease. These patients have a worse prognosis than patients who present with "primary" muscle-invasive disease (Moschini et al. 2016).
- Although treatment with BCG significantly reduces the risk of progression, still 5.3% of high-risk patients and 14.9% of very-high-risk patients experience progression to MIBC 5 years after diagnosis (Lobo et al. 2022).

Patients who are at very high risk of disease progression according to the EAU NMIBC 2021 scoring model should be counseled about an upfront radical cystectomy. For other patients, scoring models (e.g., EORTC or CUETO scoring model) can be used to predict the risk of progression. For each patient, the potential benefit of a radical cystectomy must be weighed against its risks, morbidity, and impact on quality of life. This should be discussed in a shared decision-making process.

Radical cystectomy is strongly recommended in patients with BCG-unresponsive tumors (see below). A delay in RC may lead to decreased disease-specific survival (Raj et al. 2007; Willis et al. 2015). A radical cystectomy before progression to MIBC gives a 5-year disease-free survival rate of more than 80% (Stein et al. 2001).

5.5.9 Treatment Failure

If a patient with NMBIC has a recurrence during or after intravesical chemotherapy instillations, BCG instillations can be administered. BCG with maintenance is effective in these patients for the prophylaxis of recurrence (Malmström et al. 2009).

BCG failure is defined as a high-grade disease during or after BCG therapy. This group is further divided to specify the subgroup of patients in whom additional BCG is unlikely to benefit:

- *BCG-refractory tumor*: no response to BCG at all
  - T1 HG/G3 tumor present at 3 months
  - Ta HG/G3 tumor present at 3 months and/or (after re-induction or the first maintenance) at 6 months
  - CIS (without concomitant papillary tumor) at 3 months and persists (after re-induction or the first maintenance) at 6 months
  - Any high-grade tumor during BCG maintenance therapy
- *BCG-relapsing tumor:* recurrence with a TaT1 HG/G3 tumor >6 months or CIS >12 months after completion and initial response on BCG maintenance
- *BCG-unresponsive tumor*: all BCG-refractory tumors and recurrence of a T1/Ta HG tumor within 6 months or CIS within 12 months after completion of BCG maintenance

Patients who have CIS at month 3 in BCG treatment should be offered an additional course of BCG. In >50% of cases, this additional therapy can lead to a complete response (Jakse et al. 2001).

Special consideration should be given to patients with BCG-unresponsive tumors, because they are unlikely to respond to further BCG therapy. Studies show that the 3-month clinical response is a predictor of invasive progression, which in turn leads to a higher disease-specific mortality rate. One study showed that cystectomy in patients with invasive progression reduces the disease-specific mortality but remains high (around 46%). Therefore, radical cystectomy is the standard and preferred therapy in patients with BCG-unresponsive tumors (Solsona et al. 2000; Holmang and Johansson 2002).

Bladder-preserving treatments in patients with BCG-unresponsive disease are considered oncologically inferior to radical cystectomy. Preservation strategies should be offered to the patients who are not candidates for radical cystectomy. Examples include intravesical chemohyperthermia, intravesical immunotherapy other than BCG, or systemic immunotherapy (Babjuk et al. 2022).

Low-grade recurrences during or after BCG therapy are not considered as BCG failure. Treatment decisions depend on the tumor characteristics and should be individualized.

5.5.10 Summary: Recommended Therapy by EAU NMIBC 2021 Risk Group

Low

- TURBT followed by one immediate postoperative instillation of intravesical chemotherapy. Given the negligible risk of disease progression, this is considered complete treatment.

Intermediate

- One-year full-dose BCG treatment which consists of induction with 6-weekly instillations followed by 3-weekly instillations at 3, 6, and 12 months or instillations of chemotherapy. The optimal schedule for chemotherapy instillations is not known, but the duration should not exceed 1 year.
- The choice of therapy should take into account the individual patient's risk of recurrence and progression, as well as the risk of side effects and efficacy.
- In case of a small papillary recurrence (presumably Ta LG/G1), 1 year after a previous TURBT, offer one immediate chemotherapy instillation.

High

- Full-dose intravesical BCG treatment which consists of induction with 6-weekly instillations followed by 3-weekly instillations at 3, 6, 12, 18, 24, 30, and 36 months.
- Given the high risk of disease progression in these patients, immediate radical cystectomy may be discussed with the patient. This is the safest option from an oncological point of view but is associated with quality of life impairment, risks, and overtreatment in some patients.

Very high

- Radical cystectomy is the recommended treatment because of the extremely high risk of tumor progression.
- BCG induction followed by maintenance (for 1–3 years) should be offered if radical cystectomy is not feasible or is refused by the patient.

5.6 Follow-Up of Patients with NMIBC

Considering the risk of recurrence and progression, patients with NMIBC need follow-up. The frequency and duration of both cystoscopy and imaging should reflect the individual patient's risk. The short- and long-term risks of recurrence and progression can be predicted using the EAU NMIBC prognostic factor risk groups or other models for specific patient populations as discussed above. The follow-up schedules can be adapted accordingly. It is however important to note that recommendations for follow-up have been mainly based on retrospective data. There is a lack of randomized controlled trials researching reduction of cystoscopy and imaging frequency.

The goal of planning follow-up is to ensure prompt detection of muscle-invasive and HG/G3 NMIBC. The percentage of tumors missed should be as low as possible, as delays in both diagnosis and therapy are potentially life-threatening.

The basis of follow-up in NMIBC is cystoscopy. Three months after TURBT, a cystoscopy should be performed in all patients, because it is an important prognostic indicator for both recurrence and progression (Palou et al. 2009; Holmang and Johansson 2002). The European guideline recommends, in case of a negative cystoscopy at 3 months post-TURBT in patients with low-risk tumors, that the subsequent cystoscopy should be 9 months later, followed by yearly cystoscopy for 5 years (Babjuk et al. 2022). The risk of recurrence after 5 recurrence-free years is very low in low-risk tumors, and therefore discontinuation of yearly cystoscopy can be considered or replacement with less invasive methods (Soukup et al. 2012). In patients with high risk (and with very high risk treated conservatively), negative cystoscopy at 3 months post-TURBT should be followed by repeated cystoscopy every 3 months for 2 years and every 6 months thereafter until 5 years. Recurrence in this patient group is not uncommon, and therefore it is recommended these patients have lifelong follow-up (Soukup et al. 2012). After the first 5 years with negative cystoscopy, it is recommended that patients receive a yearly cystoscopy lifelong. The follow-up in intermediate-risk patients should be done using cystoscopy as well, though there is no fixed recommendation on the frequency. It is advised that patients with intermediate-risk tumors are followed-up lifelong, the follow-up schedule adapted to the individual patient. Furthermore, regular upper tract imaging is recommended for high-risk and very-high-risk tumors (Babjuk et al. 2022).

As mentioned above, cystoscopy cannot be replaced by urine cytology or urinary molecular markers. Urine cytology can be used to enhance cystoscopy outcomes: one randomized controlled trial found that knowledge of positive cytology can improve the quality of follow-up cystoscopy (van der Aa et al. 2010). Guidelines recommend the performance of TURBT or bladder biopsies in case cystoscopy shows suspicious lesions. In case urine cytology is positive, but cystoscopy does not show any tumor in the bladder, mapping biopsies (including prostatic urethral biopsy) and CT urography are recommended (Babjuk et al. 2022). Even though, presently, no urinary marker can replace or lower the frequency of cystoscopy during follow-up, some urinary markers have shown high sensitivity in the detection of recurrence along with high negative predictive value.

References

Akhtar M, Al-Bozom IA, Ben Gashir M, Taha NM, Rashid S, Al-Nabet A (2019) Urothelial carcinoma in situ (CIS): new insights. Adv Anat Pathol 26(5):313–319. https://doi.org/10.1097/pap.0000000000000239

Anderson C, Weber R, Patel D, Lowrance W, Mellis A, Cookson M et al (2016) A 10-item checklist improves reporting of critical procedural elements during transurethral resection of bladder tumor. J Urol 196(4):1014–1020. https://doi.org/10.1016/j.juro.2016.03.151

Arends TJ, van der Heijden AG, Witjes JA (2014) Combined chemohyperthermia: 10-year single center experience in 160 patients with nonmuscle invasive bladder cancer. J Urol 192(3):708–713. https://doi.org/10.1016/j.juro.2014.03.101

Arends TJ, Nativ O, Maffezzini M, de Cobelli O, Canepa G, Verweij F et al (2016) Results of a randomised controlled trial comparing intravesical chemohyperthermia with mitomycin C versus Bacillus Calmette-Guérin for adjuvant treatment of patients with intermediate- and high-risk non-muscle-invasive bladder cancer. Eur Urol 69(6):1046–1052. https://doi.org/10.1016/j.eururo.2016.01.006

Asimakopoulos AD, Colalillo G, Telesca R, Mauriello A, Miano R, Di Stasi SM et al (2021) T1 bladder cancer: comparison of the prognostic impact of two substaging systems on disease recurrence and progression and suggestion of a novel nomogram. Front Surg 8:704902. https://doi.org/10.3389/fsurg.2021.704902

Au JL, Badalament RA, Wientjes MG, Young DC, Warner JA, Venema PL et al (2001) Methods to improve efficacy of intravesical mitomycin C: results of a randomized phase III trial. J Natl Cancer Inst 93(8):597–604. https://doi.org/10.1093/jnci/93.8.597

M. Babjuk, M. Burger, E. Compérat, Gontero FL, A. Masson-Lecomte, A.H. Mostafid, J. Palou BWGvR, M. Rouprêt, S.F. Shariat, Sylvester R, Patient Advocates: I. Benedicte Gurses RW, Guidelines Associates: O. Capoun DC, et al. 2022 EAU-Guidelines-on-Non-Muscle-Invasive-Bladder-Cancer-2022

Bishr M, Lattouf JB, Latour M, Saad F (2014) Tumour stage on re-staging transurethral resection predicts recurrence and progression-free survival of patients with high-risk non-muscle invasive bladder cancer. Can Urol Assoc J 8(5–6):E306–E310. https://doi.org/10.5489/cuaj.1514

Böhle A, Bock PR (2004) Intravesical bacillus Calmette-Guérin versus mitomycin C in superficial bladder cancer: formal meta-analysis of comparative studies on tumor progression. Urology 63(4):682–686; discussion 6-7. https://doi.org/10.1016/j.urology.2003.11.049

Böhle A, Jocham D, Bock PR (2003) Intravesical bacillus Calmette-Guerin versus mitomycin C for superficial bladder cancer: a formal meta-analysis of comparative studies on recurrence and toxicity. J Urol 169(1):90–95. https://doi.org/10.1016/s0022-5347(05)64043-8

Brausi M, Collette L, Kurth K, van der Meijden AP, Oosterlinck W, Witjes JA et al (2002) Variability in the recurrence rate at first follow-up cystoscopy after TUR in stage Ta T1 transitional cell carcinoma of the bladder: a combined analysis of seven EORTC studies. Eur Urol 41(5):523–531. https://doi.org/10.1016/s0302-2838(02)00068-4

Brausi M, Oddens J, Sylvester R, Bono A, van de Beek C, van Andel G et al (2014) Side effects of Bacillus Calmette-Guérin (BCG) in the treatment of intermediate- and high-risk Ta, T1 papillary carcinoma of the bladder: results of the EORTC genito-urinary cancers group randomised phase 3 study comparing one-third dose with full dose and 1 year with 3 years of maintenance BCG. Eur Urol 65(1):69–76. https://doi.org/10.1016/j.eururo.2013.07.021

Brierley JD, Gospodarowicz MK, Wittekind C (2016) TNM classification of malignant tumours, 8th edn. Wiley-Backwell

Brocks CP, Büttner H, Böhle A (2005) Inhibition of tumor implantation by intravesical gemcitabine in a murine model of superficial bladder cancer. J Urol 174(3):1115–1118. https://doi.org/10.1097/01.ju.0000168657.51551.49

Burger M, Grossman HB, Droller M, Schmidbauer J, Hermann G, Drăgoescu O et al (2013) Photodynamic diagnosis of non-muscle-invasive bladder cancer with hexaminolevulinate cystoscopy: a meta-analysis of detection and recurrence based on raw data. Eur Urol 64(5):846–854. https://doi.org/10.1016/j.eururo.2013.03.059

Cambier S, Sylvester RJ, Collette L, Gontero P, Brausi MA, van Andel G et al (2016) EORTC nomograms and risk groups for predicting recurrence, progression, and disease-specific and overall survival in non-muscle-invasive stage ta-T1 urothelial bladder cancer patients treated with 1-3 years of maintenance Bacillus Calmette-Guérin. Eur Urol 69(1):60–69. https://doi.org/10.1016/j.eururo.2015.06.045

Chou R, Selph S, Buckley DI, Fu R, Griffin JC, Grusing S et al (2017) Comparative effectiveness of fluorescent versus white light cystoscopy for initial diagnosis or surveillance of bladder cancer on clinical outcomes: systematic review and meta-analysis. J Urol 197(3 Pt 1):548–558. https://doi.org/10.1016/j.juro.2016.10.061

Compérat EM, Burger M, Gontero P, Mostafid AH, Palou J, Rouprêt M et al (2019) Grading of urothelial carcinoma and the new "World Health Organisation classification of tumours of the urinary system and male genital organs 2016". Eur Urol Focus 5(3):457–466. https://doi.org/10.1016/j.euf.2018.01.003

Compérat E, Amin MB, Epstein JI, Hansel DE, Paner G, Al-Ahmadie H et al (2021) The genitourinary pathology society update on classification of variant histologies, T1 substaging, molecular taxonomy, and immunotherapy and PD-L1 testing implications of urothelial cancers. Adv Anat Pathol 28(4):196–208. https://doi.org/10.1097/pap.0000000000000309

D'Andrea D, Soria F, Zehetmayer S, Gust KM, Korn S, Witjes JA et al (2019) Diagnostic accuracy, clinical utility and influence on decision-making of a methylation urine biomarker test in the surveillance of non-muscle-invasive bladder cancer. BJU Int 123(6):959–967. https://doi.org/10.1111/bju.14673

Davis R, Jones JS, Barocas DA, Castle EP, Lang EK, Leveillee RJ et al (2012) Diagnosis, evaluation and follow-up of asymptomatic microhematuria (AMH) in adults: AUA guideline. J Urol 188(6 Suppl):2473–2481. https://doi.org/10.1016/j.juro.2012.09.078

de Jong FC, Hoedemaeker RF, Kvikstad V, Mensink JTM, de Jong JJ, Boevé ER et al (2021) T1 substaging of nonmuscle invasive bladder cancer is associated with bacillus Calmette-Guérin failure and improves patient stratification at diagnosis. J Urol 205(3):701–708. https://doi.org/10.1097/ju.0000000000001422

Draga RO, Grimbergen MC, Kok ET, Jonges TN, van Swol CF, Bosch JL (2010) Photodynamic diagnosis (5-aminolevulinic acid) of transitional cell carcinoma after bacillus Calmette-Guérin immunotherapy and mitomycin C intravesical therapy. Eur Urol 57(4):655–660. https://doi.org/10.1016/j.eururo.2009.09.037

Edwards TJ, Dickinson AJ, Natale S, Gosling J, McGrath JS (2006) A prospective analysis of the diagnostic yield resulting from the attendance of 4020 patients at a protocol-driven haematuria clinic. BJU Int 97(2):301–305.; discussion 5. https://doi.org/10.1111/j.1464-410X.2006.05976.x

Elmamoun MH, Christmas TJ, Woodhouse CR (2014) Destruction of the bladder by single dose Mitomycin C for low-stage transitional cell carcinoma (TCC)—avoidance, recognition, management and consent. BJU Int 113(5b):E34–E38. https://doi.org/10.1111/bju.12340

Eroglu A, Ekin RG, Koc G, Divrik RT (2020) The prognostic value of routine second transurethral resection in patients with newly diagnosed stage pT1 non-muscle-invasive bladder cancer: results from randomized 10-year extension trial. Int J Clin Oncol 25(4):698–704. https://doi.org/10.1007/s10147-019-01581-0

Fernandez-Gomez J, Madero R, Solsona E, Unda M, Martinez-Piñeiro L, Gonzalez M et al (2009) Predicting nonmuscle invasive bladder cancer recurrence and progression in patients treated with bacillus Calmette-Guerin: the CUETO scoring model. J Urol 182(5):2195–2203. https://doi.org/10.1016/j.juro.2009.07.016

Fernandez-Gomez J, Madero R, Solsona E, Unda M, Martinez-Piñeiro L, Ojea A et al (2011) The EORTC tables overestimate the risk of recurrence and progression in patients with non-muscle-invasive bladder cancer treated with bacillus Calmette-Guérin: external validation of the EORTC risk tables. Eur Urol 60(3):423–430. https://doi.org/10.1016/j.eururo.2011.05.033

Fransen van de Putte EE, Otto W, Hartmann A, Bertz S, Mayr R, Bründl J et al (2018) Metric substage according to micro and extensive lamina propria invasion improves prognostics in T1 bladder cancer. Urol Oncol 36(8):361.e7–361e13. https://doi.org/10.1016/j.urolonc.2018.05.007

Gontero P, Sylvester R, Pisano F, Joniau S, Vander Eeckt K, Serretta V et al (2015) Prognostic factors and risk groups in T1G3 non-muscle-invasive bladder cancer patients initially treated with bacillus Calmette-Guérin: results of a retrospective multicenter study of 2451 patients. Eur Urol 67(1):74–82. https://doi.org/10.1016/j.eururo.2014.06.040

Gordon PC, Thomas F, Noon AP, Rosario DJ, Catto JWF (2019) Long-term outcomes from re-resection for high-risk non-muscle-invasive bladder cancer: a potential to rationalize use. Eur Urol Focus 5(4):650–657. https://doi.org/10.1016/j.euf.2017.10.004

Griffiths TR, Charlton M, Neal DE, Powell PH (2002) Treatment of carcinoma in situ with intravesical bacillus Calmette-Guerin without maintenance. J Urol 167(6):2408–2412

Hara T, Takahashi M, Gondo T, Nagao K, Ohmi C, Sakano S et al (2009) Risk of concomitant carcinoma in situ determining biopsy candidates among primary non-muscle-invasive bladder cancer patients: retrospective analysis of 173 Japanese cases. Int J Urol 16(3):293–298. https://doi.org/10.1111/j.1442-2042.2008.02241.x

Hentschel AE, van Rhijn BWG, Bründl J, Compérat EM, Plass K, Rodríguez O et al (2020) Papillary urothelial neoplasm of low malignant potential (PUN-LMP): still a meaningful histo-pathological grade category for Ta, noninvasive bladder tumors in 2019? Urol Oncol 38(5):440–448. https://doi.org/10.1016/j.urolonc.2019.10.002

Hilton S, Jones LP (2014) Recent advances in imaging cancer of the kidney and urinary tract. Surg Oncol Clin N Am 23(4):863–910. https://doi.org/10.1016/j.soc.2014.06.001

Holmang S, Johansson SL (2002) Stage ta-T1 bladder cancer: the relationship between findings at first follow-up cystoscopy and subsequent recurrence and progression. J Urol 167(4):1634–1637

Huncharek M, McGarry R, Kupelnick B (2001) Impact of intravesical chemotherapy on recurrence rate of recurrent superficial transitional cell carcinoma of the bladder: results of a meta-analysis. Anticancer Res 21(1b):765–769

Jakse G, Hall R, Bono A, Höltl W, Carpentier P, Spaander JP et al (2001) Intravesical BCG in patients with carcinoma in situ of the urinary bladder: long-term results of EORTC GU Group phase II protocol 30861. Eur Urol 40(2):144–150. https://doi.org/10.1159/000049765

Kausch I, Sommerauer M, Montorsi F, Stenzl A, Jacqmin D, Jichlinski P et al (2010) Photodynamic diagnosis in non-muscle-invasive bladder cancer: a systematic review and cumulative analysis of prospective studies. Eur Urol 57(4):595–606. https://doi.org/10.1016/j.eururo.2009.11.041

Kirkali Z, Chan T, Manoharan M, Algaba F, Busch C, Cheng L et al (2005) Bladder cancer: epidemiology, staging and grading, and diagnosis. Urology 66(6 Suppl 1):4–34. https://doi.org/10.1016/j.urology.2005.07.062

Knowles MA, Hurst CD (2015) Molecular biology of bladder cancer: new insights into pathogenesis and clinical diversity. Nat Rev Cancer 15(1):25–41. https://doi.org/10.1038/nrc3817

Konety B, Shore N, Kader AK, Porten S, Daneshmand S, Lough T et al (2019) Evaluation of Cxbladder and adjudication of atypical cytology and equivocal cystoscopy. Eur Urol 76(2):238–243. https://doi.org/10.1016/j.eururo.2019.04.035

Kramer MW, Rassweiler JJ, Klein J, Martov A, Baykov N, Lusuardi L et al (2015) En bloc resection of urothelium carcinoma of the bladder (EBRUC): a European multicenter study to compare safety, efficacy, and outcome of laser and electrical en bloc transurethral resection of bladder tumor. World J Urol 33(12):1937–1943. https://doi.org/10.1007/s00345-015-1568-6

Kuroda M, Niijima T, Kotake T, Akaza H, Hinotsu S (2004) Effect of prophylactic treatment with intravesical epirubicin on recurrence of superficial bladder cancer—the 6th trial of the Japanese Urological Cancer Research Group (JUCRG): a randomized trial of intravesical epirubicin at dose of 20mg/40ml, 30mg/40ml, 40mg/40ml. Eur Urol 45(5):600–605. https://doi.org/10.1016/j.eururo.2003.12.010

Lamm DL (1992) Carcinoma in situ. Urol Clin North Am 19(3):499–508

Lamm D, Herr H, Jakse G, Kuroda M, Mostofi FK, Okajima E et al (1998) Updated concepts and treatment of carcinoma in situ. Urol Oncol 4(4–5):130–138. https://doi.org/10.1016/s1078-1439(99)00020-4

Lenis AT, Lec PM, Chamie K, Mshs MD (2020) Bladder cancer: a review. JAMA 324(19):1980–1991. https://doi.org/10.1001/jama.2020.17598

Lobo N, Hensley PJ, Bree KK, Nogueras-Gonzalez GM, Navai N, Dinney CP et al (2022) Updated European Association of Urology (EAU) prognostic factor risk groups overestimate the risk of progression in patients with non-muscle-invasive bladder cancer treated with bacillus Calmette-Guérin. Eur Urol Oncol 5(1):84–91. https://doi.org/10.1016/j.euo.2021.11.006

Maas M, Bedke J, Stenzl A, Todenhöfer T (2019) Can urinary biomarkers replace cystoscopy? World J Urol 37(9):1741–1749. https://doi.org/10.1007/s00345-018-2505-2

MacLennan GT, Kirkali Z, Cheng L (2007) Histologic grading of noninvasive papillary urothelial neoplasms. Eur Urol 51(4):889–897.; discussion 97-8. https://doi.org/10.1016/j.eururo.2006.10.037

Malmström PU, Sylvester RJ, Crawford DE, Friedrich M, Krege S, Rintala E et al (2009) An individual patient data meta-analysis of the long-term outcome of randomised studies comparing intravesical mitomycin C versus bacillus Calmette-Guérin for non-muscle-invasive bladder cancer. Eur Urol 56(2):247–256. https://doi.org/10.1016/j.eururo.2009.04.038

Mariappan P, Zachou A, Grigor KM (2010) Detrusor muscle in the first, apparently complete transurethral resection of bladder tumour specimen is a surrogate marker of resection quality, predicts risk of early recurrence, and is dependent on operator experience. Eur Urol 57(5):843–849. https://doi.org/10.1016/j.eururo.2009.05.047

Mariappen P, Johnston A, Padovani L, Clark E, Trail M, Hamid S et al (2020) Enhanced quality and effectiveness of transurethral resection of bladder tumour in non-muscle-invasive bladder cancer: a multicentre real-world experience from Scotland's quality performance indicators programme. Eur Urol 78(4):520–530. https://doi.org/10.1016/j.eururo.2020.06.051

Meilleroux J, Daniel G, Aziza J, d'Aure DM, Quintyn-Ranty ML, Basset CM et al (2018) One year of experience using the Paris system for reporting urinary cytology. Cancer Cytopathol 126(6):430–436. https://doi.org/10.1002/cncy.21999

Millán-Rodríguez F, Chéchile-Toniolo G, Salvador-Bayarri J, Huguet-Pérez J, Vicente-Rodríguez J (2000) Upper urinary tract tumors after primary superficial bladder tumors: prognostic factors and risk groups. J Urol 164(4):1183–1187

Morales A, Eidinger D, Bruce AW (1976) Intracavitary Bacillus Calmette-Guerin in the treatment of superficial bladder tumors. J Urol 116(2):180–183. https://doi.org/10.1016/s0022-5347(17)58737-6

Moschini M, Sharma V, Dell'oglio P, Cucchiara V, Gandaglia G, Cantiello F et al (2016) Comparing long-term outcomes of primary and progressive carcinoma invading bladder muscle after radical cystectomy. BJU Int 117(4):604–610. https://doi.org/10.1111/bju.13146

Mowatt G, N'Dow J, Vale L, Nabi G, Boachie C, Cook JA et al (2011) Photodynamic diagnosis of bladder cancer compared with white light cystoscopy: systematic review and meta-analysis. Int J Technol Assess Health Care 27(1):3–10. https://doi.org/10.1017/s0266462310001364

Mungan MU, Canda AE, Tuzel E, Yorukoglu K, Kirkali Z (2005) Risk factors for mucosal prostatic urethral involvement in superficial transitional cell carcinoma of the bladder. Eur Urol 48(5):760–763. https://doi.org/10.1016/j.eururo.2005.05.021

Naselli A, Hurle R, Paparella S, Buffi NM, Lughezzani G, Lista G et al (2018) Role of restaging transurethral resection for T1 non-muscle invasive bladder cancer: a systematic review and meta-analysis. Eur Urol Focus 4(4):558–567. https://doi.org/10.1016/j.euf.2016.12.011

Netto GJ, Amin MB, Berney DM, Compérat EM, Gill AJ, Hartmann A et al (2022) The 2022 World Health

Organization classification of tumors of the urinary system and male genital organs-part B: prostate and urinary tract tumors. Eur Urol 82(5):469–482. https://doi.org/10.1016/j.eururo.2022.07.002

Nikas IP, Seide S, Proctor T, Kleinaki Z, Kleinaki M, Reynolds JP (2022) The Paris system for reporting urinary cytology: a meta-analysis. J Pers Med 12(2). https://doi.org/10.3390/jpm12020170

Oddens JR, van der Meijden AP, Sylvester R (2004) One immediate postoperative instillation of chemotherapy in low risk Ta, T1 bladder cancer patients. Is it always safe? Eur Urol 46(3):336–338. https://doi.org/10.1016/j.eururo.2004.05.003

Oddens J, Brausi M, Sylvester R, Bono A, van de Beek C, van Andel G et al (2013) Final results of an EORTC-GU cancers group randomized study of maintenance bacillus Calmette-Guérin in intermediate- and high-risk Ta, T1 papillary carcinoma of the urinary bladder: one-third dose versus full dose and 1 year versus 3 years of maintenance. Eur Urol 63(3):462–472. https://doi.org/10.1016/j.eururo.2012.10.039

Ozden E, Turgut AT, Turkolmez K, Resorlu B, Safak M (2007) Effect of bladder carcinoma location on detection rates by ultrasonography and computed tomography. Urology 69(5):889–892. https://doi.org/10.1016/j.urology.2007.01.077

Palou Redorta J, Schatteman P, Huguet Pérez J, Segarra Tomás J, Rosales Bordes A, Algaba F et al (2006) Intravesical instillations with bacillus calmette-guérin for the treatment of carcinoma in situ involving prostatic ducts. Eur Urol 49(5):834–838; discussion 8. https://doi.org/10.1016/j.eururo.2005.12.019

Palou J, Rodríguez-Rubio F, Huguet J, Segarra J, Ribal MJ, Alcaraz A et al (2005) Multivariate analysis of clinical parameters of synchronous primary superficial bladder cancer and upper urinary tract tumor. J Urol 174(3):859–861; discussion 61. https://doi.org/10.1097/01.ju.0000169424.79702.6d

Palou J, Rodríguez-Rubio F, Millán F, Algaba F, Rodríguez-Faba O, Huguet J et al (2009) Recurrence at three months and high-grade recurrence as prognostic factor of progression in multivariate analysis of T1G2 bladder tumors. Urology 73(6):1313–1317. https://doi.org/10.1016/j.urology.2008.12.047

Palou J, Sylvester RJ, Faba OR, Parada R, Peña JA, Algaba F et al (2012) Female gender and carcinoma in situ in the prostatic urethra are prognostic factors for recurrence, progression, and disease-specific mortality in T1G3 bladder cancer patients treated with bacillus Calmette-Guérin. Eur Urol 62(1):118–125. https://doi.org/10.1016/j.eururo.2011.10.029

Panebianco V, Narumi Y, Altun E, Bochner BH, Efstathiou JA, Hafeez S et al (2018) Multiparametric magnetic resonance imaging for bladder cancer: development of VI-RADS (vesical imaging-reporting and data system). Eur Urol 74(3):294–306. https://doi.org/10.1016/j.eururo.2018.04.029

Pode D, Alon Y, Horowitz AT, Vlodavsky I, Biran S (1986) The mechanism of human bladder tumor implantation in an in vitro model. J Urol 136(2):482–486. https://doi.org/10.1016/s0022-5347(17)44926-3

Raitanen MP, Aine R, Rintala E, Kallio J, Rajala P, Juusela H et al (2002) Differences between local and review urinary cytology in diagnosis of bladder cancer. An interobserver multicenter analysis. Eur Urol 41(3):284–289. https://doi.org/10.1016/s0302-2838(02)00006-4

Raj GV, Herr H, Serio AM, Donat SM, Bochner BH, Vickers AJ et al (2007) Treatment paradigm shift may improve survival of patients with high risk superficial bladder cancer. J Urol 177(4):1283–1286; discussion 6. https://doi.org/10.1016/j.juro.2006.11.090

Raman SP, Fishman EK (2014) Bladder malignancies on CT: the underrated role of CT in diagnosis. AJR Am J Roentgenol 203(2):347–354. https://doi.org/10.2214/ajr.13.12021

Ramirez D, Gupta A, Canter D, Harrow B, Dobbs RW, Kucherov V et al (2016) Microscopic haematuria at time of diagnosis is associated with lower disease stage in patients with newly diagnosed bladder cancer. BJU Int 117(5):783–786. https://doi.org/10.1111/bju.13345

Richterstetter M, Wullich B, Amann K, Haeberle L, Engehausen DG, Goebell PJ et al (2012) The value of extended transurethral resection of bladder tumour (TURBT) in the treatment of bladder cancer. BJU Int 110(2 Pt 2):E76–E79. https://doi.org/10.1111/j.1464-410X.2011.10904.x

Rink M, Xylinas E, Babjuk M, Hansen J, Pycha A, Comploj E et al (2012) Impact of smoking on outcomes of patients with a history of recurrent nonmuscle invasive bladder cancer. J Urol 188(6):2120–2127. https://doi.org/10.1016/j.juro.2012.08.029

Schmidt S, Kunath F, Coles B, Draeger DL, Krabbe LM, Dersch R et al (2020) Intravesical Bacillus Calmette-Guérin versus mitomycin C for Ta and T1 bladder cancer. Cochrane Database Syst Rev 1(1):Cd011935. https://doi.org/10.1002/14651858.CD011935.pub2

Shang PF, Kwong J, Wang ZP, Tian J, Jiang L, Yang K et al (2011) Intravesical Bacillus Calmette-Guérin versus epirubicin for Ta and T1 bladder cancer. Cochrane Database Syst Rev (5):Cd006885. https://doi.org/10.1002/14651858.CD006885.pub2

Shephard EA, Stapley S, Neal RD, Rose P, Walter FM, Hamilton WT (2012) Clinical features of bladder cancer in primary care. Br J Gen Pract 62(602):e598–e604. https://doi.org/10.3399/bjgp12X654560

Solsona E, Iborra I, Ricós JV, Monrós JL, Dumont R, Almenar S (1996) Extravesical involvement in patients with bladder carcinoma in situ: biological and therapy implications. J Urol 155(3):895–899.; discussion 9-900. https://doi.org/10.1016/s0022-5347(01)66338-9

Solsona E, Iborra I, Dumont R, Rubio-Briones J, Casanova J, Almenar S (2000) The 3-month clinical response to intravesical therapy as a predictive factor for progression in patients with high risk superficial bladder cancer. J Urol 164(3 Pt 1):685–689. https://doi.org/10.1097/00005392-200009010-00016

Soukup V, Babjuk M, Bellmunt J, Dalbagni G, Giannarini G, Hakenberg OW et al (2012) Follow-up after surgical treatment of bladder cancer: a critical analysis of the literature. Eur Urol 62(2):290–302. https://doi.org/10.1016/j.eururo.2012.05.008

Soukup V, Čapoun O, Cohen D, Hernández V, Babjuk M, Burger M et al (2017) Prognostic performance and reproducibility of the 1973 and 2004/2016 World Health Organization grading classification Systems in non-muscle-invasive Bladder Cancer: a European Association of Urology non-muscle invasive bladder cancer guidelines panel systematic review. Eur Urol 72(5):801–813. https://doi.org/10.1016/j.eururo.2017.04.015

Stamatiou K, Papadoliopoulos I, Dahanis S, Zafiropoulos G, Polizois K (2009) The accuracy of ultrasonography in the diagnosis of superficial bladder tumors in patients presenting with hematuria. Ann Saudi Med 29(2):134–137. https://doi.org/10.4103/0256-4947.51802

Stein JP, Lieskovsky G, Cote R, Groshen S, Feng AC, Boyd S et al (2001) Radical cystectomy in the treatment of invasive bladder cancer: long-term results in 1,054 patients. J Clin Oncol 19(3):666–675. https://doi.org/10.1200/jco.2001.19.3.666

Suarez-Ibarrola R, Soria F, Abufaraj M, D'Andrea D, Preto M, Gust KM et al (2019) Surgical checklist impact on recurrence-free survival of patients with non-muscle-invasive bladder cancer undergoing transurethral resection of bladder tumour. BJU Int 123(4):646–650. https://doi.org/10.1111/bju.14557

Sylvester RJ, van der Ma LDL (2002) Intravesical bacillus Calmette-Guerin reduces the risk of progression in patients with superficial bladder cancer: a meta-analysis of the published results of randomized clinical trials. J Urol 168(5):1964–1970. https://doi.org/10.1016/s0022-5347(05)64273-5

Sylvester RJ, van der Meijden AP, Witjes JA, Kurth K (2005) Bacillus calmette-guerin versus chemotherapy for the intravesical treatment of patients with carcinoma in situ of the bladder: a meta-analysis of the published results of randomized clinical trials. J Urol 174(1):86–91.; discussion –2. https://doi.org/10.1097/01.ju.0000162059.64886.1c

Sylvester RJ, van der Meijden AP, Oosterlinck W, Witjes JA, Bouffioux C, Denis L et al (2006) Predicting recurrence and progression in individual patients with stage Ta T1 bladder cancer using EORTC risk tables: a combined analysis of 2596 patients from seven EORTC trials. Eur Urol 49(3):466–465.; discussion 75-7. https://doi.org/10.1016/j.eururo.2005.12.031

Sylvester RJ, Oosterlinck W, Witjes JA (2008) The schedule and duration of intravesical chemotherapy in patients with non-muscle-invasive bladder cancer: a systematic review of the published results of randomized clinical trials. Eur Urol 53(4):709–719. https://doi.org/10.1016/j.eururo.2008.01.015

Sylvester RJ, Brausi MA, Kirkels WJ, Hoeltl W, Calais Da Silva F, Powell PH et al (2010) Long-term efficacy results of EORTC genito-urinary group randomized phase 3 study 30911 comparing intravesical instillations of epirubicin, bacillus Calmette-Guérin, and bacillus Calmette-Guérin plus isoniazid in patients with intermediate- and high-risk stage Ta T1 urothelial carcinoma of the bladder. Eur Urol 57(5):766–773. https://doi.org/10.1016/j.eururo.2009.12.024

Sylvester RJ, Oosterlinck W, Holmang S, Sydes MR, Birtle A, Gudjonsson S et al (2016) Systematic review and individual patient data meta-analysis of randomized trials comparing a single immediate instillation of chemotherapy after transurethral resection with transurethral resection alone in patients with stage pTa-pT1 urothelial carcinoma of the bladder: which patients benefit from the instillation? Eur Urol 69(2):231–244. https://doi.org/10.1016/j.eururo.2015.05.050

Sylvester RJ, Rodríguez O, Hernández V, Turturica D, Bauerová L, Bruins HM et al (2021) European Association of Urology (EAU) prognostic factor risk groups for non-muscle-invasive bladder cancer (NMIBC) incorporating the WHO 2004/2016 and WHO 1973 classification Systems for Grade: an update from the EAU NMIBC guidelines panel. Eur Urol 79(4):480–488. https://doi.org/10.1016/j.eururo.2020.12.033

Takenaka A, Yamada Y, Miyake H, Hara I, Fujisawa M (2008) Clinical outcomes of bacillus Calmette-Guérin instillation therapy for carcinoma in situ of urinary bladder. Int J Urol 15(4):309–313. https://doi.org/10.1111/j.1442-2042.2008.02012.x

Tan WS, Steinberg G, Witjes JA, Li R, Shariat SF, Roupret M et al (2022) Intermediate-risk non-muscle-invasive bladder cancer: updated consensus definition and management recommendations from the international bladder cancer group. Eur Urol Oncol. 5(5):505–516. https://doi.org/10.1016/j.euo.2022.05.005

Têtu B (2009) Diagnosis of urothelial carcinoma from urine. Mod Pathol 22(Suppl 2):S53–S59. https://doi.org/10.1038/modpathol.2008.193

Tolley DA, Parmar MK, Grigor KM, Lallemand G, Benyon LL, Fellows J et al (1996) The effect of intravesical mitomycin C on recurrence of newly diagnosed superficial bladder cancer: a further report with 7 years of follow up. J Urol 155(4):1233–1238

Trinh TW, Glazer DI, Sadow CA, Sahni VA, Geller NL, Silverman SG (2018) Bladder cancer diagnosis with CT urography: test characteristics and reasons for false-positive and false-negative results. Abdom Radiol (NY) 43(3):663–671. https://doi.org/10.1007/s00261-017-1249-6

Valenberg F, Hiar AM, Wallace E, Bridge JA, Mayne DJ, Beqaj S et al (2019) Prospective validation of an mRNA-based urine test for surveillance of patients with bladder cancer. Eur Urol 75(5):853–860. https://doi.org/10.1016/j.eururo.2018.11.055

van der Aa MN, Steyerberg EW, Bangma C, van Rhijn BW, Zwarthoff EC, van der Kwast TH (2010) Cystoscopy revisited as the gold standard for detecting bladder cancer recurrence: diagnostic review bias in the randomized, prospective CEFUB trial. J Urol 183(1):76–80. https://doi.org/10.1016/j.juro.2009.08.150

van der Meijden AP, Sylvester RJ, Oosterlinck W, Hoeltl W, Bono AV (2003) Maintenance Bacillus Calmette-Guerin for Ta T1 bladder tumors is not associated with increased toxicity: results from a European Organisation for Research and Treatment of Cancer Genito-Urinary Group Phase III Trial. Eur Urol 44(4):429–434. https://doi.org/10.1016/s0302-2838(03)00357-9

van Gils-Gielen RJ, Witjes WP, Caris CT, Debruyne FM, Witjes JA, Oosterhof GO (1995) Risk factors in carcinoma in situ of the urinary bladder. Dutch South East Cooperative Urological Group. Urology 45(4):581–586. https://doi.org/10.1016/s0090-4295(99)80047-8

van Rhijn BW, van der Kwast TH, Alkhateeb SS, Fleshner NE, van Leenders GJ, Bostrom PJ et al (2012) A new and highly prognostic system to discern T1 bladder cancer substage. Eur Urol 61(2):378–384. https://doi.org/10.1016/j.eururo.2011.10.026

van Rhijn BWG, Hentschel AE, Bründl J, Compérat EM, Hernández V, Čapoun O et al (2021) Prognostic value of the WHO1973 and WHO2004/2016 classification Systems for Grade in primary ta/T1 non-muscle-invasive bladder cancer: a multicenter European Association of Urology non-muscle-invasive bladder cancer guidelines panel study. Eur Urol Oncol 4(2):182–191. https://doi.org/10.1016/j.euo.2020.12.002

Voskuilen CS, Seiler R, Rink M, Poyet C, Noon AP, Roghmann F et al (2020) Urothelial carcinoma in bladder diverticula: a multicenter analysis of characteristics and clinical outcomes. Eur Urol Focus 6(6):1226–1232. https://doi.org/10.1016/j.euf.2018.12.002

Willis DL, Fernandez MI, Dickstein RJ, Parikh S, Shah JB, Pisters LL et al (2015) Clinical outcomes of cT1 micropapillary bladder cancer. J Urol 193(4):1129–1134. https://doi.org/10.1016/j.juro.2014.09.092

Witjes JA, Palou J, Soloway M, Lamm D, Brausi M, Spermon JR et al (2008) Clinical practice recommendations for the prevention and management of intravesical therapy-associated adverse events. Eur Urol Suppl 7(10):667–674. https://doi.org/10.1016/j.eursup.2008.08.001

Yafi FA, Brimo F, Steinberg J, Aprikian AG, Tanguay S, Kassouf W (2015) Prospective analysis of sensitivity and specificity of urinary cytology and other urinary biomarkers for bladder cancer. Urol Oncol 33(2):66.e25–31. https://doi.org/10.1016/j.urolonc.2014.06.008

Ye Z, Hu J, Song X, Li F, Zhao X, Chen S et al (2015) A comparison of NBI and WLI cystoscopy in detecting non-muscle-invasive bladder cancer: a prospective, randomized and multi-center study. Sci Rep 5:10905. https://doi.org/10.1038/srep10905

Yossepowitch O, Eggener SE, Bochner BH, Donat SM, Herr HW, Dalbagni G (2006) Safety and efficacy of intravesical bacillus Calmette-Guerin instillations in steroid treated and immunocompromised patients. J Urol 176(2):482–485. https://doi.org/10.1016/j.juro.2006.03.066

Zhou Z, Zhao S, Lu Y, Wu J, Li Y, Gao Z et al (2019) Meta-analysis of efficacy and safety of continuous saline bladder irrigation compared with intravesical chemotherapy after transurethral resection of bladder tumors. World J Urol 37(6):1075–1084. https://doi.org/10.1007/s00345-019-02628-7

Overview of Standard Therapy of Muscle-Invasive Bladder Cancer

6

Laura Mertens, Eva Schaake, and Michiel S. van der Heijden

Abstract

Treatment of muscle-invasive and metastatic bladder cancer requires a multidisciplinary approach, in which the urologist, radiation oncologist, and medical oncologist closely work together and counsel the patient to determine the most appropriate treatment. The main components of treatment are surgical resection, radiotherapy, and systemic therapy, traditionally involving chemotherapy. In recent years, major advances have been made in the treatment of bladder cancer, particularly in systemic treatment. New treatment modalities include immune checkpoint inhibitors, antibody drug conjugates, and targeted therapy. While these advancements have primarily been applied to the treatment of advanced urothelial cancer, it is likely that these novel treatments will enter the nonmetastatic bladder cancer space. Additionally, bladder-preserving therapy has gained attention and is a frequent wish of patients, given the major impact of removal of the bladder on quality of life. These new developments will require even better multidisciplinary collaboration by the specialists involved in bladder cancer treatment and will hopefully lead to significant improvements in survival and quality of life for patients with bladder cancer.

Keywords

Cystectomy · Radiotherapy · Immunotherapy · Chemotherapy · Targeted therapy · Antibody-drug conjugate

6.1 Introduction

Treatment of muscle-invasive and metastatic bladder cancer requires a multidisciplinary approach, in which the urologist, radiation oncologist, and medical oncologist work closely together and counsel the patient to determine the most appropriate treatment. In this chapter, the main treatment modalities are discussed (summarized in Table 6.1). Further discussion of the evidence for these approaches and ongoing studies of new approaches can be found in Chaps. 22 and 23.

L. Mertens
Department of Surgical Oncology (urology), Netherlands Cancer Institute, Amsterdam, The Netherlands

E. Schaake
Department of Radiotherapy, Netherlands Cancer Institute, Amsterdam, The Netherlands

M. S. van der Heijden (✉)
Department of Medical Oncology, Netherlands Cancer Institute, Amsterdam, The Netherlands
e-mail: ms.vd.heijden@nki.nl

M. A. Knowles, L. Dyrskjøt (eds.), *Biology of Bladder Cancer*,
https://doi.org/10.1007/978-3-031-68505-7_6

Table 6.1 Summary of recommended treatments for muscle-invasive and advanced bladder cancer

Treatment setting	Commonly used therapeutic options
Localized muscle-invasive urothelial cancer	
Resection (cT2-4aN0–1)	Radical cystectomy with pelvic lymph node dissection
Bladder preservation (cT2-4aN0)	Chemoradiotherapy
Neoadjuvant	ddMVAC or cisplatin-gemcitabine
Adjuvant	Nivolumab (only patients having PDL1+ tumors in EU)
	ddMVAC or cisplatin-gemcitabine
Advanced urothelial cancer	
First line	Platinum-based chemotherapy
	Enfortumab vedotin + pembrolizumab
Maintenance therapy after chemo response	Avelumab
Second line	Pembrolizumab[a]
Third line	Enfortumab vedotin
	Erdafitinib in *FGFR*-mutated cancers
Other options in therapy-refractory disease	Chemotherapy (vinflunine, taxanes)
	Sacituzumab govitecan

[a] Preferred over other immune checkpoint inhibitors as randomized data is available

6.2 Surgical Therapy

Radical cystectomy (RC) with pelvic lymph node dissection (PLND) is the standard treatment for nonmetastatic muscle-invasive bladder cancer (Witjes et al. 2024). In men, standard RC includes removal of the bladder, prostate, seminal vesicles, distal ureters, and regional lymph nodes. Prostate cancer is incidentally found in approximately a quarter of male RC patients (Fahmy et al. 2017). Prostate-sparing, capsule-sparing, seminal vesical-sparing, and nerve-sparing techniques can lead to better sexual outcomes than standard RC (Hernandez et al. 2017). Postoperative potency has been found to be significantly better in patients who underwent any type of sexuality-preserving RC compared to standard RC. However, the overall quality of evidence is moderate, and no consensus exists on the best approach; hence, if a sexuality-preserving RC is offered, patients must be carefully selected, counseled, and monitored.

In women, standard RC involves the removal of the bladder, urethra, anterior vaginal wall, uterus with the ovaries, and regional lymph nodes (Witjes et al. 2024). This procedure has been associated with pelvic floor disorders and sexual and voiding dysfunction. Pelvic organ-preserving techniques, which involve preserving the neurovascular bundle, vagina, uterus, ovaries, or variations of these techniques, have been developed to mitigate these adverse effects. Retention of the ovaries in premenopausal women can help maintain hormonal homeostasis and reduce the risk of cognitive impairment, cardiovascular diseases, and loss of bone density. Removal of the uterus can lead to anterior or posterior vaginal prolapse, but in the case of an existing uterine prolapse, uterus removal can be beneficial. Also, preservation of the uterus and vagina can provide crucial support for a neobladder, decreasing the incidence of urinary retention. Resection of the vaginal wall will shorten the vagina, impairing sexual function and satisfaction. Based on a systematic review of low-quality retrospective data, preservation of the female reproductive organs during RC appears to be oncologically safe and improves functional outcomes (Veskimae et al. 2017).

6.2.1 Lymph Node Dissection

The optimal extent of lymph node dissection (LND) for muscle-invasive bladder cancer remains uncertain. Standard LND involves removal of lymph nodes up to the common iliac bifurcation, including the internal iliac, presacral, obturator fossa, and external iliac nodes. Extended LND extends cranially to the region of the aortic bifurcation or even to the level of the inferior mesenteric artery (Witjes et al. 2024). The clinical importance of LND is controversial, as it is unclear whether it is primarily a staging tool, a therapeutic procedure, or both. Lymph node mapping studies have demonstrated that approximately 25% of muscle-invasive bladder cancer patients have lymph-node-positive disease, with over 40% of these patients having positive lymph nodes cranial to the iliac bifurcation, but skip metastases (metastases which skip over adjacent lymph nodes and spread to nodes farther along the lymphatic chain) were very rare (1%) (Jensen et al. 2010; Leissner et al. 2004). Based solely on staging considerations, the results of these studies indicate that a standard LND may be adequate for detecting almost all patients with node-positive disease.

Two recent prospective randomized trials (the LEA trial and the SWOG 1011 trial) indeed failed to demonstrate a significant advantage of extended LND over limited LND in terms of survival, while extended LND was associated with an elevated risk of morbidity.

6.2.2 Robot-Assisted Cystectomy

Multiple systematic reviews that compared open RC and robot-assisted RC have reported similar findings: robot-assisted RC is associated with a slightly shorter hospital stay (by approximately 1 day) and lower blood loss but a longer operative time (Khetrapal et al. 2023). The rates of complications appear to be similar for both approaches. Older patients in particular tend to have markedly shorter hospital stays. The complication rates appear to be similar for both approaches. Limited evidence suggests that robot-assisted RC and open RC have comparable recurrence-free survival, cancer-specific survival, and overall survival (Khetrapal et al. 2023).

Recently, a randomized controlled trial was performed to compare open RC with robot-assisted RC. The study reported a median of 82 and 80 days alive and out of the hospital within 90 days of surgery, for robot-assisted versus open RC, respectively (Catto et al. 2022). Robotic surgery was associated with lower rates of thromboembolic and wound complications. At a median follow-up of 18 months, there were no statistically significant differences in cancer recurrence or overall mortality between the groups. In another study that compared open RC and robot-assisted RC, it was found that both mean healthcare costs and societal costs per patient were significantly higher for robot-assisted RC, with almost no increase in quality-adjusted life-years (Wijburg et al. 2021).

Presently, it is recommended to inform the patient of the advantages and disadvantages of open RC and robot-assisted RC to allow selection of the proper procedure. Surgeons' experience and institutional volume may be considered the key factor for outcome, rather than the specific technique.

6.2.3 Urinary Diversion

Various segments of the intestinal tract, such as the ileum, colon, and appendix, can be utilized for reconstructing the urinary tract. The ileum is the most commonly used segment. There are several different types of urinary diversions. The ileal conduit, characterized by the isolation of an ileal section, connection of the ureters to this segment, and the creation of a stoma, is the most common choice for urinary diversion. A ureteral diversion, characterized by externalization of the ureter to the abdominal wall (ureterocutaneostomy), is a simple form of a urinary diversion, particularly suitable for frail patients with a solitary kidney. An orthotopic bladder substitution, referred to as a "neobladder," involves the isolation of an extended intestinal segment, which is then folded and connected to both the ureters. In this procedure, the reservoir is anastomosed to the urethra and requires abdominal straining and sphincter relaxation. This reservoir is used in 10–20% of male and female patients and can be constructed using several techniques, aiming for upper urinary tract reflux protection. Finally, continent cutaneous urinary diversions, reservoirs that can be catheterized through the abdominal wall, are rarely used techniques nowadays, because of the high complication rates.

When selecting a urinary diversion method, factors such as comorbidities, cardiac and pulmonary function, cognitive ability, social support, and patient preference should be taken into consideration. The advantages and disadvantages of different urinary diversions, in terms of quality of life, sexual function, urinary continence, and body image, have been studied, although not in randomized controlled trials. It is important that patients are well informed about the different urinary diversions prior to making a decision. The type of urinary diversion does not affect oncological outcome (Witjes et al. 2024).

For patients aged over 80, neobladder reconstruction is generally not recommended. Also, an orthotopic bladder substitute diversion should not be offered to patients who have an invasive tumor in the urethra or at the level of the urethral dissection. In women, localization of the primary tumor at the bladder neck is associated with concomitant urethral malignancy (Stein et al. 2007; Roth et al. 2019). Therefore, it is important to take bladder neck biopsies in women scheduled for a neobladder. Other contraindications to a neobladder include severe neurological and psychiatric illnesses, limited life expectancy, and severe impaired liver or renal function. High-dose preoperative radiotherapy, complex urethral strictures, and severe incontinence are not ideal situations and, while not strictly impossible, are considered relative contraindications.

6.2.4 Morbidity and Mortality

The rates of mortality during the perioperative period following RC are reported to be in the range of 2.1% to 3.2% at 30 days and 3.4% to 8.0% at 90 days (Bochner et al. 2015; Mossanen et al. 2019). The reported rates of morbidity differ significantly based on the methodology used for reporting. In studies in which the Clavien-Dindo classification system was used, the overall complication rates ranged from 50% to 88%, with severe complications ranging from 30% to 42% (grade III or higher) (Cicione et al. 2020; Demaegd et al. 2020). Lower rates of morbidity and perioperative mortality have been observed in surgeons and hospitals with a higher volume of cases (Bruins et al. 2020; Richters et al. 2021). Hence, it seems reasonable to recommend to perform at least ten RCs per center annually and preferably more than 20 (Witjes et al. 2024).

6.3 Organ-Preservation Therapy

Organ-preservation therapy for MIBC is an attractive option for patients seeking an alternative to RC or for those who are medically unfit for surgery. Concurrent chemoradiation (CRT) following TURBT is recognized by several guideline committees as an organ-preservation alternative to radical cystectomy (RC) in selected patients with MIBC (Witjes et al. 2021; Powles et al. 2022; Chang et al. 2017) and should be weighed against RC within a multidisciplinary team including urologists, medical oncologists, and radiation oncologists. There are multiple patient and tumour-related factors that contribute to the selection of trimodal therapy versus RC for MIBC. Trimodal treatment consists of a transurethral resection of the bladder tumor (TURBT), followed by concurrent chemotherapy and radiotherapy of the bladder. The aim is to spare the bladder functionally by aiming for maximum local tumor control while keeping the bladder intact.

The ideal patient for trimodal therapy has a tumor that can undergo a visibly complete resection, has no associated hydronephrosis, does not invade the prostatic urethra, and is not associated with diffuse CIS throughout the bladder. A cystoscopy with bladder biopsy is advised for response evaluation 2–3 months thereafter.

A landmark prospective, randomized trial by James et al. proved that chemoradiotherapy (CRT) using mitomycin C and 5-FU is superior to radiotherapy alone in terms of locoregional survival and disease-free survival (DFS) (67 vs. 54%) (James et al. 2012). The long-term results showed significantly better locoregional disease control in the CRT group than in the RT group, with 5-year recurrence-free rates of 63% (95% CI 54–71%) in the CRT group versus 49% (95% CI 41–57%) in the RT-only group (Hall et al. 2022). The 5-year salvage cystectomy rate was 14% (95% CI 9–21%) with CRT versus 22% (95% CI 16–31%) with RT alone (HR 0.54, [95% CI 0.31–0.95], $p = 0.034$). Improved local control rates were also reported when cisplatin was given with RT (HR 0.50, 90% CI 0.29–0.86) (Coppin et al. 1996). The value of cisplatin-based CRT was confirmed in a retrospective analysis of 475 MIBC patients treated at the Massachusetts General Hospital and enrolled on prospective cisplatin-based protocols. Complete response (CR) rates varied from 66 to 88%, increasing over time, along with improvement of treatment protocols (Giacalone et al. 2017). Weekly gemcitabine can also be combined with RT with comparable high response rates, with CR rates up to 88% (Choudhury et al. 2011). A recent study suggested that mitomycin C combined with daily capecitabine, an oral prodrug of 5-FU, offers a safe and practical chemo-sensitizer alternative to MMC plus continuous 5-FU (Voskuilen et al. 2020). A subsequent retrospective study reporting on patients receiving mitomycin C plus intravenous 5-FU versus mitomycin C plus capecitabine similarly suggested that capecitabine is non-inferior to 5-FU (de Haar-Holleman et al. 2023).

The whole bladder can be treated with radiation, giving an equivalent dose in 2-Gy fractions (EQD2) of 55–60 Gy using intensity modulated radiation therapy (IMRT) or volumetric modulated arc therapy (VMAT) techniques (Foroudi et al. 2012). Depending on availability of daily online adaptive treatment strategies and tumor localization, a simultaneous integrated boost (SIB) can be delivered to the tumor bed, while the rest of the bladder receives a lower dose. MRI-guided irradiation is presently emerging as an even more precise technique (Hijab et al. 2021). Trials of (neoadjuvant) immune therapy combined with trimodality treatment are ongoing and could increase efficacy and potentially broaden the selection of patients who can receive bladder conservation (see Chaps. 22 and 23 for more detailed discussion).

6.4 Perioperative Systemic Therapy

6.4.1 Neoadjuvant Therapy

6.4.1.1 Chemotherapy

Given the efficacy of cisplatin-based chemotherapy in the metastatic setting, various combinations of cisplatin-based chemotherapy have been tested before curative surgery (the neoadjuvant setting) for patients with MIBC. Pathological complete response, or downstaging to non-muscle-invasive bladder cancer, is strongly associated with recurrence-free survival (RFS) and overall survival (OS) (Rosenblatt et al. 2012). However, the benefit in terms of overall survival is more limited. A meta-analysis of 11 randomized trials of 3005 patients receiving neoadjuvant cisplatin-based chemotherapy (NAC) showed a 5% absolute increase in 5-year overall survival (OS) (HR 0.86, 95% CI 0.77–0.95) (Advanced Bladder Cancer Meta-analysis C 2005). Cisplatin/gemcitabine or dose-dense methotrexate, vinblastine, adriamycin, and cisplatin (ddMVAC; chemotherapy cycles are given with shorter interval by administering growth factor support) are the most commonly used regimens (Zargar et al. 2018; Galsky et al. 2015; Pfister et al. 2021). Usually three or (most commonly) four cycles are administered (Grossman et al. 2003). The use of these regimens is extrapolated mostly from data in the metastatic setting, as the largest trials in the meta-analysis were done with three cycles of CMV (cisplatin, methotrexate, vinblastine) or standard MVAC. A recent trial by Pfister et al. compared six cycles of ddMVAC to four cycles of cisplatin/gemcitabine. The primary endpoint was progression-free survival (PFS) in the full perioperative cohort, including adjuvant treatment. This endpoint was borderline significant (HR = 0.77, $p = 0.066$). The majority of patients were treated in the neoadjuvant setting. When only considering the neoadjuvant setting, PFS at 3 years was significantly higher in the ddMVAC arm (66% vs. 56%, HR 0.70) (Pfister et al. 2022). An unanswered question remains whether the additional benefit of six cycles of ddMVAC compared to four cycles of cisplatin/gemcitabine was caused by the treatment regimen or the number of cycles. Of note, only 60% of patients were able to complete all six cycles of ddMVAC.

The benefit of neoadjuvant treatment in patients having histological variants of bladder cancer is unknown (Horwich et al. 2019). Pure squamous cell or adenocarcinoma bladder cancer is generally not treated with neoadjuvant therapy.

Bladder cancers having a significant percentage of small cell neuroendocrine variants are treated with neoadjuvant cisplatin/etoposide and consolidating local therapy, which may consist of RT instead of RC, given the high rate of systemic recurrence (Horwich et al. 2019).

6.4.1.2 Other Neoadjuvant Treatments

Several phase 2 trials have tested immune checkpoint inhibitors as anti-PD-(L)1 monotherapy (Powles et al. 2019; Necchi et al. 2018), in combination with anti-CTLA4 (van Dijk et al. 2020; Gao et al. 2020) or in combination with platinum-based chemotherapy. Whereas promising activity has been observed, phase 3 trials are presently still ongoing.

6.4.2 Adjuvant Therapy

6.4.2.1 Chemotherapy

Given the activity of cisplatin-based chemotherapy in the neoadjuvant setting, a similar efficacy would be expected in the adjuvant setting. As randomized phase 3 studies were negative on the overall survival, this remains a controversial issue in bladder cancer treatment. However, a recent meta-analysis of ten randomized trials with a total of 1183 participants demonstrated a benefit of cisplatin-based adjuvant chemotherapy on overall survival (HR = 0.82, $p = 0.02$). The absolute improvement in overall survival was 6% at 5 year, from 50 to 56% (Advanced Bladder Cancer Meta-analysis Collaborators G 2022). After adjustment for various clinical variables, a 9% absolute benefit was observed. Given these results, which were highly similar to results in the neoadjuvant setting, it is reasonable to consider adjuvant cisplatin-based chemotherapy in patients who have high-risk disease (pT3-4a or N1-3) at cystectomy and are fit to receive this form of chemotherapy. Importantly, a significant subset of patients will not be able to receive adjuvant chemotherapy due to slow recovery from cystectomy or a decline in renal function. Also, some patients who do not receive neoadjuvant chemotherapy will have unresectable disease at surgery, losing the opportunity to undergo curative therapy. Neoadjuvant cisplatin-based chemotherapy is therefore preferred in cisplatin-eligible MIBC patients (Powles et al. 2022).

6.4.2.2 Immunotherapy

In recent years, two randomized phase 3 trials reporting DFS with adjuvant checkpoint inhibition in high-risk urothelial cancer have reported different outcomes (for detailed discussion, see Chap. 23). In the CheckMate 274 trial, investigating adjuvant nivolumab (anti-PD-1) for 1 year versus placebo in 709 high-risk MIBC patients (including upper tract cancers), the median DFS in the intention-to-treat population (ITT) was 20.8 months with nivolumab and 10.8 months with placebo (HR 0.70) (Bajorin et al. 2021). This trial did not yet report OS. Still, the US Food and Drug Administration (FDA) granted registration for the ITT population, whereas the European Medicines Agency (EMA) restricted treatment with nivolumab to the PD-L1+ subpopulation. Within the subgroup analysis, two noteworthy subpopulations stood out. Patients who did not previously receive neoadjuvant chemotherapy seemed to lack benefit in DFS, with a HR of 0.92. Similarly, the HR for patients who had an upper urinary tract cancer were 1.23 (renal pelvis) and 1.56 (ureter).

In the IMVIGOR010 trial, 800 high-risk urothelial cancer patients were randomized to adjuvant atezolizumab (anti-PD-L1) for 1 year, or observation. In contrast to CheckMate 274, this trial did not show a difference in DFS (HR 0.89) or OS (HR 0.85) (Bellmunt et al. 2021). Strikingly, PD-L1 as a biomarker could not select for clinical benefit of adjuvant therapy. A third trial, AMBASSADOR, is investigating adjuvant pembrolizumab (anti-PD1) in the same population. Publication of this trial is pending and could potentially bring more clarity regarding the value of adjuvant checkpoint inhibitors in muscle-invasive urothelial cancer and the role of important subpopulations (PDL-1, prior neoadjuvant chemotherapy, and upper tract cancers).

Given the encouraging HR for DFS in the PD-L1+ subgroup, this represents the most optimal subgroup of patients to consider for adjuvant nivolumab. Given the uncertainties in the robustness of clinical benefit, as a similar trial with atezolizumab reported negative results, some physicians will await OS results before implementing this treatment into clinical practice. The results of the subgroup analyses in CheckMate 274 could provide additional arguments to restrict adjuvant nivolumab to certain subpopulations, for example, by offering adjuvant chemotherapy (instead of immunotherapy) to cisplatin-eligible patients who did not receive neoadjuvant chemotherapy. Additionally, the toxicity of nivolumab should be considered, as treatment-related adverse events of grade 3 or higher occurred in 17.9% (nivolumab), compared to 7.2% in the placebo arm.

6.5 Treatment of Advanced Disease

6.5.1 First-Line Therapy for Advanced UC

For many years, platinum-based combination chemotherapy has been the standard of care for advanced (irresectable, locoregionally advanced, or metastatic) urothelial cancer (UC). Whereas ddMVAC can be used (Sternberg et al. 2006), platinum/gemcitabine combinations are the most widely used regimen, given the easier schedule and lower toxicity (von der Maase et al. 2000; De Santis et al. 2012). Cisplatin is preferred in patients without contraindications, such as decreased glomerular filtration rate (GFR), hearing loss, or neuropathy (Galsky et al. 2011). In patients who are cisplatin-ineligible, carboplatin + gemcitabine can be used. The preference for cisplatin is mainly based on indirect comparisons of prospective trials (mostly single arm for carboplatin).

After having established efficacy in the platinum-refractory setting, immune checkpoint inhibitors have been tested in cisplatin-ineligible first-line patients. Based on the results of phase 2 studies, pembrolizumab and atezolizumab were approved for advanced UC patients not eligible for cisplatin-based chemotherapy. This registration was later restricted to PD-L1-positive patients. Unfortunately, randomized phase 3 trials failed to show a significant improvement in OS compared with standard chemotherapy (Powles et al. 2020a, 2021a; Galsky et al. 2020). The phase 3 trials using pembrolizumab and durvalumab (anti-PD-L1) also failed to show a clear advantage for the PD-L1-positive subpopulation, leading to further uncertainty around this biomarker.

Given the positive results of combinations of chemotherapy with immune checkpoint inhibition in other cancer types, several phase 3 trials compared chemotherapy + anti-PD(L)1 with chemotherapy alone. Two trials combining platinum-based chemotherapy (choice of cisplatin or carboplatin) have failed to show an improvement in OS (Powles et al. 2021a; Galsky et al. 2020). In contrast, maintenance avelumab (anti-PD-L1), initiated within 10 weeks of completion of four to six cycles of first-line platinum-based chemotherapy in patients having disease control (stable disease or partial response), showed a significant OS benefit compared to best supportive care: a HR of 0.69 (95% CI 0.56–0.86) and an improvement in median OS from 14 to 21 months (Powles et al. 2020b). It is unclear why this strategy appeared to be more successful than combined treatment. A better "natural" selection by chemotherapy response of patients who could benefit from immune checkpoint inhibition may have played a role. Biological differences between combined vs. sequential and differential effect of the platinum-combination partner (cisplatin vs. carboplatin) may also play a role. In a recent trial of nivolumab + cisplatin/gemcitabine, a significant OS benefit was demonstrated over cisplatin/gemcitabine alone (van der Heijden et al. 2023). In the landmark phase 3 EV302 trial, the combination of enfortumab vedotin (EV, an antibody-drug conjugate [ADC] targeting nectin-4, with monomethyl auristatin E as the payload drug) with pembrolizumab was shown to have a significant OS (HR 0.47; 95% CI 0.38–0.58; $p < 0.00001$) and PFS (HR 0.45; 95% CI 0.38–0.54; $p < 0.00001$) benefit in comparison to standard chemotherapy (Powles et al. 2024). Pending trials will establish the position of anti-CTLA4 + anti-PD(L)1 combinations in advanced urothelial cancer (Sharma et al. 2019).

6.5.2 Treatment of Advanced UC Following Progression After Platinum-Based Chemotherapy

The first sign that inhibition of PD-L1 could be beneficial in advanced bladder cancer patients came from an expansion cohort of a phase 1 study with atezolizumab (Powles et al. 2014). In this study, durable responses were seen in heavily pre-treated patients. Responses were associated with PD-L1 immunohistochemistry (IHC) positivity on immune cells, though responses were seen in all IHC subgroups. Other checkpoint inhibitors with activity demonstrated in bladder cancer include pembrolizumab, nivolumab, durvalumab, and avelumab. In a phase 3 trial, 542 patients with advanced urothelial cancer that recurred or progressed after platinum-based chemotherapy were randomly assigned to receive pembrolizumab or the investigator's choice of chemotherapy with paclitaxel, docetaxel, or vinflunine. Pembrolizumab was associated with significantly longer OS (by approximately 3 months) and with a lower rate of treatment-related adverse events than chemotherapy as second-line therapy for platinum-refractory advanced urothelial carcinoma (Bellmunt et al. 2017). The IMVigor211 trial tested atezolizumab in PD-L1-positive platinum-refractory advanced UC and (surprisingly) did not show a significant OS advantage (Powles et al. 2018). In the exploratory analysis of the full population, atezolizumab had a HR of 0.85 (95% CI 0.73–0.99) compared to chemotherapy. In an updated analysis, atezolizumab showed a 30-month OS of 18% compared to 10% for chemotherapy (Van der Heijden 2019).

6.5.3 Treatment After Progression Following Chemo- and Immunotherapy

After promising results in single-arm trials, EV was compared to chemotherapy (taxanes or vinflunine) in advanced UC patients who had progressed following platinum-based chemotherapy and immune checkpoint inhibitors. EV showed a significantly improved OS with a HR of 0.70 (95% CI 0.56–0.89) and a median OS benefit of 12.8 versus 9.0 months (Powles et al. 2021b). The response rate was approximately 40%. EV is associated with a specific toxicity spectrum, which can be serious, challenging to treat, and even lethal. Specific toxicities of interest include rash (which may include Stevens-Johnson syndrome), peripheral neuropathy, hyperglycemia, and metabolic acidosis. Based on the results in this study, EV has become the standard of care in patients with progression of disease after first-line chemotherapy and immunotherapy (including maintenance avelumab).

Erdafitinib is a pan-FGFR tyrosine kinase inhibitor and was tested in a phase II trial in 99 patients with advanced UC, progressive after platinum-based chemotherapy, and having *FGFR* genomic alterations (*FGFR2* or *3* gene fusions, or *FGFR3* mutations) (Loriot et al. 2019). The objective response rate in this single-arm trial cohort was 40%. Median PFS and OS were 5.5 months and 13.8 months, respectively. Recently, the phase 3 THOR trial was completed, randomizing advanced UC patients having genomic *FGFR* alterations to erdafitinib investigator's choice chemotherapy after immunotherapy failure (mostly third line, (after chemotherapy and immunotherapy). This trial showed a significant OS benefit for erdafitinib with a HR of 0.64 (95% CI 0.47–0.88) and a median OS benefit of 12.1 versus 7.8 months (Loriot et al. NEJM 2023).

6.6 Conclusion

Major developments, particularly in the use of systemic therapy, have changed the treatment landscape of urothelial cancer. As these novel combination therapies are moving to earlier disease settings, the treatment landscape is likely to evolve in the coming years, particularly in the perioperative setting. Hopefully, these developments will not only lead to improved survival but also to an improved quality of life for patients, for example, by increasing the opportunities for organ-preservation strategies.

References

Advanced Bladder Cancer Meta-analysis C (2005) Neoadjuvant chemotherapy in invasive bladder cancer: update of a systematic review and meta-analysis of individual patient data advanced bladder cancer (ABC) meta-analysis collaboration. Eur Urol 48(2):202–205. discussion 5–6

Advanced Bladder Cancer Meta-analysis Collaborators G (2022) Adjuvant chemotherapy for muscle-invasive bladder cancer: a systematic review and meta-analysis of individual participant data from randomised controlled trials. Eur Urol 81(1):50–61

Alfred Witjes J, Max Bruins H, Carrion A, Cathomas R, Comperat E, Efstathiou JA et al (2024) European Association of Urology Guidelines on muscle-invasive and metastatic bladder cancer: summary of the 2023 guidelines. Eur Urol 85(1):17–31

Bajorin DF, Witjes JA, Gschwend JE, Schenker M, Valderrama BP, Tomita Y et al (2021) Adjuvant Nivolumab versus placebo in muscle-invasive urothelial carcinoma. N Engl J Med 384(22):2102–2114

Bellmunt J, de Wit R, Vaughn DJ, Fradet Y, Lee JL, Fong L et al (2017) Pembrolizumab as second-line therapy for advanced urothelial carcinoma. N Engl J Med 376(11):1015–1026

Bellmunt J, Hussain M, Gschwend JE, Albers P, Oudard S, Castellano D et al (2021) Adjuvant atezolizumab versus observation in muscle-invasive urothelial carcinoma (IMvigor010): a multicentre, open-label, randomised, phase 3 trial. Lancet Oncol 22(4):525–537

Bochner BH, Dalbagni G, Sjoberg DD, Silberstein J, Keren Paz GE, Donat SM et al (2015) Comparing open radical cystectomy and robot-assisted laparoscopic radical cystectomy: a randomized clinical trial. Eur Urol 67(6):1042–1050

Bruins HM, Veskimae E, Hernandez V, Neuzillet Y, Cathomas R, Comperat EM et al (2020) The importance of hospital and surgeon volume as major determinants of morbidity and mortality after radical cystectomy for bladder cancer: a systematic review and recommendations by the European Association of Urology muscle-invasive and metastatic bladder cancer guideline panel. Eur Urol Oncol 3(2):131–144

Catto JWF, Khetrapal P, Ricciardi F, Ambler G, Williams NR, Al-Hammouri T et al (2022) Effect of robot-assisted radical cystectomy with intracorporeal urinary diversion vs open radical cystectomy on 90-day morbidity and mortality among patients with bladder cancer: a randomized clinical trial. JAMA 327(21):2092–2103

Chang SS, Bochner BH, Chou R, Dreicer R, Kamat AM, Lerner SP et al (2017) Treatment of non-metastatic muscle-invasive bladder cancer: AUA/ASCO/ASTRO/SUO guideline. J Urol 198(3):552–559

Choudhury A, Swindell R, Logue JP, Elliott PA, Livsey JE, Wise M et al (2011) Phase II study of conformal hypofractionated radiotherapy with concurrent gemcitabine in muscle-invasive bladder cancer. J Clin Oncol 29(6):733–738

Cicione A, De Nunzio C, Lombardo R, Trucchi A, Manno S, Lima E, Tubaro A (2020) Complications and quality of life of ileal conduit, orthotopic neobladder and ureterocutaneostomy: systematic review of reports using the Clavien-Dindo classification. Minerva Urol Nefrol 72(4):408–419

Coppin CM, Gospodarowicz MK, James K, Tannock IF, Zee B, Carson J et al (1996) Improved local control of invasive bladder cancer by concurrent cisplatin and preoperative or definitive radiation. The National Cancer Institute of Canada clinical trials group. J Clin Oncol 14(11):2901–2907

de Haar-Holleman A, van Hoogstraten LMC, Hulshof M, Tascilar M, Bruck K, Bla ZIBsg et al (2023) Chemoradiation for muscle-invasive bladder cancer using 5-fluorouracil versus capecitabine: a nationwide cohort study. Radiother Oncol 183:109584

De Santis M, Bellmunt J, Mead G, Kerst JM, Leahy M, Maroto P et al (2012) Randomized phase II/III trial assessing gemcitabine/carboplatin and methotrexate/carboplatin/vinblastine in patients with advanced urothelial cancer who are unfit for cisplatin-based chemotherapy: EORTC study 30986. J Clin Oncol 30(2):191–199

Demaegd L, Albersen M, Muilwijk T, Milenkovic U, Moris L, Everaerts W et al (2020) Comparison of postoperative complications of ileal conduits versus orthotopic neobladders. Transl Androl Urol 9(6):2541–2554

Fahmy O, Khairul-Asri MG, Schubert T, Renninger M, Stenzl A, Gakis G (2017) Clinicopathological features and prognostic value of incidental prostatic adenocarcinoma in radical cystoprostatectomy specimens: a systematic review and Meta-analysis of 13,140 patients. J Urol 197(2):385–390

Foroudi F, Wilson L, Bressel M, Haworth A, Hornby C, Pham D et al (2012) A dosimetric comparison of 3D conformal vs intensity modulated vs volumetric arc radiation therapy for muscle invasive bladder cancer. Radiat Oncol 7:111

Galsky MD, Hahn NM, Rosenberg J, Sonpavde G, Hutson T, Oh WK et al (2011) Treatment of patients with metastatic urothelial cancer "unfit" for cisplatin-based chemotherapy. J Clin Oncol 29(17):2432–2438

Galsky MD, Pal SK, Chowdhury S, Harshman LC, Crabb SJ, Wong YN et al (2015) Comparative effectiveness of gemcitabine plus cisplatin versus methotrexate, vinblastine, doxorubicin, plus cisplatin as neoadjuvant therapy for muscle-invasive bladder cancer. Cancer 121(15):2586–2593

Galsky MD, Arija JAA, Bamias A, Davis ID, De Santis M, Kikuchi E et al (2020) Atezolizumab with or without chemotherapy in metastatic urothelial cancer (IMvigor130): a multicentre, randomised, placebo-controlled phase 3 trial. Lancet 395(10236):1547–1557

Gao J, Navai N, Alhalabi O, Siefker-Radtke A, Campbell MT, Tidwell RS et al (2020) Neoadjuvant PD-L1 plus CTLA-4 blockade in patients with cisplatin-ineligible operable high-risk urothelial carcinoma. Nat Med 26(12):1845–1851

Giacalone NJ, Shipley WU, Clayman RH, Niemierko A, Drumm M, Heney NM et al (2017) Long-term outcomes after bladder-preserving tri-modality therapy for patients with muscle-invasive bladder cancer: an updated analysis of the Massachusetts General Hospital experience. Eur Urol 71(6):952–960

Grossman HB, Natale RB, Tangen CM, Speights VO, Vogelzang NJ, Trump DL et al (2003) Neoadjuvant chemotherapy plus cystectomy compared with cystectomy alone for locally advanced bladder cancer. N Engl J Med 349(9):859–866

Hall E, Hussain SA, Porta N, Lewis R, Crundwell M, Jenkins P et al (2022) Chemoradiotherapy in muscle-invasive bladder cancer: 10-yr follow-up of the phase 3 randomised controlled BC2001 trial. Eur Urol 82(3):273–279

Hernandez V, Espinos EL, Dunn J, MacLennan S, Lam T, Yuan Y et al (2017) Oncological and functional outcomes of sexual function-preserving cystectomy compared with standard radical cystectomy in men: a systematic review. Urol Oncol 35(9):539 e17–539 e29

Hijab A, Tocco B, Hanson I, Meijer H, Nyborg CJ, Bertelsen AS et al (2021) MR-guided adaptive radiotherapy for bladder cancer. Front Oncol 11:637591

Horwich A, Babjuk M, Bellmunt J, Bruins HM, De Reijke TM, De Santis M et al (2019) EAU-ESMO consensus statements on the management of advanced and variant bladder cancer-an international collaborative multi-stakeholder effort: under the auspices of the EAU and ESMO guidelines committees. Ann Oncol 30(11):1697–1727

James ND, Hussain SA, Hall E, Jenkins P, Tremlett J, Rawlings C et al (2012) Radiotherapy with or without chemotherapy in muscle-invasive bladder cancer. N Engl J Med 366(16):1477–1488

Jensen JB, Ulhoi BP, Jensen KM (2010) Lymph node mapping in patients with bladder cancer undergoing radical cystectomy and lymph node dissection to the level of the inferior mesenteric artery. BJU Int 106(2):199–205

Khetrapal P, Wong JKL, Tan WP, Rupasinghe T, Tan WS, Williams SB et al (2023) Robot-assisted radical cystectomy versus open radical cystectomy: a systematic review and meta-analysis of perioperative, oncological, and quality of life outcomes using randomized controlled trials. Eur Urol 84(4):393–405

Leissner J, Ghoneim MA, Abol-Enein H, Thuroff JW, Franzaring L, Fisch M et al (2004) Extended radical lymphadenectomy in patients with urothelial bladder cancer: results of a prospective multicenter study. J Urol 171(1):139–144

Loriot Y, Necchi A, Park SH, Garcia-Donas J, Huddart R, Burgess E et al (2019) Erdafitinib in locally advanced or metastatic urothelial carcinoma. N Engl J Med 381(4):338–348

Loriot Y, Matsubara N, Park SH, Huddart RA, Burgess EF, Houede N, Banek S, Guadalupi V, Ku JH, Valderrama BP, Tran B, Triantos S, Kean Y,Akapame S, Deprince K, Mukhopadhyay S, Stone NL, Siefker-Radtke AO; THOR Cohort 1 Investigators.N Engl J Med. 2023 Nov 23;389(21):1961-1971. doi: 10.1056/NEJMoa2308849. Epub 2023 Oct 21.PMID: 37870920

Mossanen M, Krasnow RE, Zlatev DV, Tan WS, Preston MA, Trinh QD et al (2019) Examining the relationship between complications and perioperative mortality following radical cystectomy: a population-based analysis. BJU Int 124(1):40–46

Necchi A, Anichini A, Raggi D, Briganti A, Massa S, Luciano R et al (2018) Pembrolizumab as neoadjuvant therapy before radical cystectomy in patients with muscle-invasive urothelial bladder carcinoma (PURE-01): an open-label, single-arm, Phase II Study. J Clin Oncol 36(34):3353–3360

Pfister C, Gravis G, Flechon A, Soulie M, Guy L, Laguerre B et al (2021) Randomized phase III trial of dose-dense methotrexate, vinblastine, doxorubicin, and cisplatin, or gemcitabine and cisplatin as perioperative chemotherapy for patients with muscle-invasive bladder cancer. Analysis of the GETUG/AFU V05 VESPER trial secondary endpoints: chemotherapy toxicity and pathological responses. Eur Urol 79(2):214–221

Pfister C, Gravis G, Flechon A, Chevreau C, Mahammedi H, Laguerre B et al (2022) Dose-dense methotrexate, vinblastine, doxorubicin, and cisplatin or gemcitabine and cisplatin as perioperative chemotherapy for patients with nonmetastatic muscle-invasive bladder cancer: results of the GETUG-AFU V05 VESPER trial. J Clin Oncol 40(18):2013–2022

Powles T, Eder JP, Fine GD, Braiteh FS, Loriot Y, Cruz C et al (2014) MPDL3280A (anti-PD-L1) treatment leads to clinical activity in metastatic bladder cancer. Nature 515(7528):558–562

Powles T, Duran I, van der Heijden MS, Loriot Y, Vogelzang NJ, De Giorgi U et al (2018) Atezolizumab versus chemotherapy in patients with platinum-treated locally advanced or metastatic urothelial carcinoma (IMvigor211): a multicentre, open-label, phase 3 randomised controlled trial. Lancet 391(10122):748–757

Powles T, Kockx M, Rodriguez-Vida A, Duran I, Crabb SJ, Van Der Heijden MS et al (2019) Clinical efficacy and biomarker analysis of neoadjuvant atezolizumab in operable urothelial carcinoma in the ABACUS trial. Nat Med 25(11):1706–1714

Powles T, van der Heijden MS, Castellano D, Galsky MD, Loriot Y, Petrylak DP et al (2020a) Durvalumab alone and durvalumab plus tremelimumab versus chemotherapy in previously untreated patients with unresectable, locally advanced or metastatic urothelial carcinoma (DANUBE): a randomised, open-label, multicentre, phase 3 trial. Lancet Oncol 21(12):1574–1588

Powles T, Park SH, Voog E, Caserta C, Valderrama BP, Gurney H et al (2020b) Avelumab maintenance therapy for advanced or metastatic urothelial carcinoma. N Engl J Med 383(13):1218–1230

Powles T, Csoszi T, Ozguroglu M, Matsubara N, Geczi L, Cheng SY et al (2021a) Pembrolizumab alone or

combined with chemotherapy versus chemotherapy as first-line therapy for advanced urothelial carcinoma (KEYNOTE-361): a randomised, open-label, phase 3 trial. Lancet Oncol 22(7):931–945
Powles T, Rosenberg JE, Sonpavde GP, Loriot Y, Duran I, Lee JL et al (2021b) Enfortumab Vedotin in previously treated advanced urothelial carcinoma. N Engl J Med 384(12):1125–1135
Powles T, Bellmunt J, Comperat E, De Santis M, Huddart R, Loriot Y et al (2022) Bladder cancer: ESMO clinical practice guideline for diagnosis, treatment and follow-up. Ann Oncol 33(3):244–258
Powles T, Valderrama BP, Gupta S, Bedke J, Kikuchi E, Hoffman-Censits J et al (2024) Enfortumab Vedotin and Pembrolizumab in untreated advanced urothelial cancer. N Engl J Med 390(10):875–888
Richters A, Ripping TM, Kiemeney LA, Leliveld AM, van Rhijn BWG, Oddens JR et al (2021) Hospital volume is associated with postoperative mortality after radical cystectomy for treatment of bladder cancer. BJU Int 128(4):511–518
Rosenblatt R, Sherif A, Rintala E, Wahlqvist R, Ullen A, Nilsson S et al (2012) Pathologic downstaging is a surrogate marker for efficacy and increased survival following neoadjuvant chemotherapy and radical cystectomy for muscle-invasive urothelial bladder cancer. Eur Urol 61(6):1229–1238
Roth B, Furrer MA, Giannakis I, Vartolomei MD, Boxler S, Wuethrich PY et al (2019) Positive pre-cystectomy biopsies of the prostatic urethra or bladder neck do not necessarily preclude Orthotopic bladder substitution. J Urol 201(5):909–915
Sharma P, Siefker-Radtke A, de Braud F, Basso U, Calvo E, Bono P et al (2019) Nivolumab alone and with Ipilimumab in previously treated metastatic urothelial carcinoma: CheckMate 032 Nivolumab 1 mg/kg plus Ipilimumab 3 mg/kg expansion cohort results. J Clin Oncol 37(19):1608–1616
Stein JP, Penson DF, Wu SD, Skinner DG (2007) Pathological guidelines for orthotopic urinary diversion in women with bladder cancer: a review of the literature. J Urol 178(3 Pt 1):756–760
Sternberg CN, de Mulder P, Schornagel JH, Theodore C, Fossa SD, van Oosterom AT et al (2006) Seven year update of an EORTC phase III trial of high-dose intensity M-VAC chemotherapy and G-CSF versus classic M-VAC in advanced urothelial tract tumours. Eur J Cancer 42(1):50–54
Van der Heijden MS (2019) 2600 - Atezolizumab (atezo) vs chemotherapy (chemo) in patients (pts) with platinum-treated locally advanced or metastatic urothelial carcinoma (mUC): a long-term overall survival (OS) and safety update from the phase III IMvigor211 study. Ann Oncol 30:356–402
van der Heijden MS, Sonpavde G, Powles T, Necchi A, Burotto M, Schenker M et al (2023) Nivolumab plus gemcitabine-cisplatin in advanced urothelial carcinoma. N Engl J Med 389(19):1778–1789
van Dijk N, Gil-Jimenez A, Silina K, Hendricksen K, Smit LA, de Feijter JM et al (2020) Preoperative ipilimumab plus nivolumab in locoregionally advanced urothelial cancer: the NABUCCO trial. Nat Med 26(12):1839–1844
Veskimae E, Neuzillet Y, Rouanne M, MacLennan S, Lam TBL, Yuan Y et al (2017) Systematic review of the oncological and functional outcomes of pelvic organ-preserving radical cystectomy (RC) compared with standard RC in women who undergo curative surgery and orthotopic neobladder substitution for bladder cancer. BJU Int 120(1):12–24
von der Maase H, Hansen SW, Roberts JT, Dogliotti L, Oliver T, Moore MJ et al (2000) Gemcitabine and cisplatin versus methotrexate, vinblastine, doxorubicin, and cisplatin in advanced or metastatic bladder cancer: results of a large, randomized, multinational, multicenter, phase III study. J Clin Oncol 18(17):3068–3077
Voskuilen CS, van de Kamp MW, Schuring N, Mertens LS, Noordzij A, Pos F et al (2020) Radiation with concurrent radiosensitizing capecitabine tablets and single-dose mitomycin-C for muscle-invasive bladder cancer: a convenient alternative to 5-fluorouracil. Radiother Oncol 150:275–280
Wijburg CJ, CTJ M, Hannink G, JPC G, Rovers MM, Alfred Witjes J, Group RS (2021) Robot-assisted radical cystectomy versus open radical cystectomy in bladder cancer patients: a multicentre comparative effectiveness study. Eur Urol 79(5):609–618
Witjes JA, Bruins HM, Cathomas R, Comperat EM, Cowan NC, Gakis G et al (2021) European Association of Urology guidelines on muscle-invasive and metastatic bladder cancer: summary of the 2020 guidelines. Eur Urol 79(1):82–104
Zargar H, Shah JB, van Rhijn BW, Daneshmand S, Bivalacqua TJ, Spiess PE et al (2018) Neoadjuvant dose dense MVAC versus gemcitabine and cisplatin in patients with cT3-4aN0M0 bladder cancer treated with radical cystectomy. J Urol 199(6):1452–1458

Part II

Molecular Genetics and Oncogenesis in Bladder Cancer

From Normalcy to Neoplasia: Mutational Events During Bladder Tumor Evolution

7

Khyati Meghani and Joshua J. Meeks

Abstract

Wind back the tape of life, and let it play again. Would the replay ever yield anything like the history that we know—Stephen Jay Gould in a *Wonderful Life*.

The genetic steps resulting in cancer are an evolutionary process that follows Darwinian evolution and natural selection. Normal cells in the human body have limited replicative potential and, in a stepwise fashion, evolve progressively to a neoplastic state that precedes a tumor. Each step allows the cell to gain "hallmark" capabilities, including but not limited to cellular proliferation and immune evasion. During the evolution of a tumor, a shift from "normal" is observed at all scales, from the tiniest of post-translational modifications that can alter how the genome of a tumor cell is packaged in the nucleus, to changes in regulatory networks and metabolic demands. At the molecular level are the mutational events that are unique not just to each patient but also to each tissue type (Haigis et al., Science 363:1150–1151, 2019). Large-scale chromosomal deletions, translocations, and events such as chromothripsis are at the chromosomal scale.

Through transient epigenetic changes or more permanent genetic changes, tumor cells transform the environment within the organ of origin into one suitable for unrestricted growth. By tracing the clonal evolutionary map of mutations, it is possible to understand the needs of a developing tumor, track the events that lead to the genesis of bladder cancer from normal bladder epithelium (urothelium), and understand how these changes help shape the bladder microenvironment into a more hospitable home for the tumor. In this chapter, we explore the ongoing research into mutational events identified in bladder cancer at different disease stages and the role these mutations play in helping the tumor survive and flourish.

Keywords

Cancer evolution · Genomics · Neoplastic progression · Mutations · Evolutionary map

K. Meghani
Department of Urology and Biochemistry and Molecular Genetics, Northwestern University, Feinberg School of Medicine, Chicago, IL, USA

J. J. Meeks (✉)
Department of Urology and Biochemistry and Molecular Genetics, Northwestern University, Feinberg School of Medicine, Chicago, IL, USA

Jesse Brown VA Medical Center, Chicago, IL, USA
e-mail: joshua.meeks@northwestern.edu

M. A. Knowles, L. Dyrskjøt (eds.), *Biology of Bladder Cancer*,
https://doi.org/10.1007/978-3-031-68505-7_7

7.1 Mutations: Cause and Consequence

The human bladder is an epithelial-lined reservoir that temporarily stores liquid waste (urine) produced by the kidneys, containing toxins, and other metabolic waste products. Given its primary role in urinary storage, the bladder is constantly exposed to toxic substances excreted by the body in the hypertonic urine. For instance, concentrated urine could contain large amounts of urea, a byproduct of protein catabolism, chemicals such as carcinogens from tobacco smoking, and industrial pollutants, and compounds such as aristolochic acid found in herbal medicinal plants. Repeated exposure of the urothelium to such endogenous or exogenous carcinogens can lead to inflammation, damage, and, ultimately, DNA mutations.

On average, approximately 70,000 lesions are generated in cells each day (Tubbs and Nussenzweig 2017). Many of these mutations neither confer a competitive advantage to the cells nor disrupt cellular processes sufficiently to trigger stress response pathways. The adult human urothelium, has a low turnover rate (Wang et al. 2017). However, when homeostasis is disrupted, such as through injury or other disturbances, the urothelial cells undergo rapid proliferation (Wang et al. 2017). As a result, cells containing these neutral mutations can undergo clonal expansion, leading to the propagation of mutated cell populations.

Knowing the mutations found in normal non-malignant urothelium is crucial to understanding their role when found in a malignant state and during carcinogenesis. In this chapter, we highlight the genetic alterations that define urothelial tumors at each stage of development. Additionally, we hope to provide insight into the functional role of these pathways and the impact these mutations have on the microenvironment they inhabit.

7.2 Mutations Present in Histologically Normal Urothelium

One of the most widely accepted models of carcinogenesis is based on "evolution", a cancer cell evolving from its non-malignant ancestors through multiple rounds of selection pressure. Recent technological advances in DNA sequencing have provided an endless stream of unbiased genetic information on the driver mutations of cancer. With this progress, attention is now being paid to the mutations present in morphologically normal tissue surrounding benign tissue and tumors, with the aim of understanding early carcinogenic processes.

In malignant tissue, tissue specificity for oncogenes and tumor suppressors is widely acknowledged (Haigis et al. 2019). Different genes are activated or deactivated through genetic and epigenetic alterations, depending on the specific requirements of the tissue of origin. Consequently, a distinct mutation pattern is generated which is characteristic and distinctive to the tissue where the cancer originates. Such specificity also holds for the non-malignant tissue (Kakiuchi and Ogawa 2021).

In specific organ systems such as the hematopoietic lineage, somatic driver mutations have been shown to accumulate with increasing age at a constant rate (Martincorena et al. 2015; Gaisa et al. 2011; Li et al. 2020; Lawson et al. 2020). In other organs such as skin, this process is so extensive that entire tissues can be remodeled by mutated clones, while maintaining their normal non-malignant status (Lawson et al. 2020). Preliminary histopathological analysis supports similar clonal expansion driven by multiple stem cell niches in the aging bladder urothelium (Gaisa et al. 2011).

Using microscale laser capture microdissection, several groups have identified widespread mutation heterogeneity in the urothelium both within and between individuals (Li et al. 2020; Lawson et al. 2020; Majewski et al. 2019; Thomsen et al. 2017). Interestingly, genes determined to be under positive selection in the normal urothelium belong to the chromatin remodeling family of genes that dominate the mutation landscape in the malignant urothelium (Robertson et al. 2017). Exogenous carcinogens, such as aristolochic acid (AA), provide the necessary selective pressure for the accumulation and clonal expansion of somatic mutation-containing cells in the normal urothelium (Li et al. 2020). The mutation burden, quantified as the number of mutations per megabase in normal AA-exposed urothelium, was closer to that in urothelial carcinoma samples than to normal non-AA urothelium (Li et al. 2020).

7.3 Mutations in Bladder Tumors

The unique signaling circuitry present in each cell of the human body, shaped by the demands of its tissue of origin, generally dictates the dysregulated pathways characteristic of cancer originating from that tissue. This will also determine the mutations that a given cancer will harbor to achieve the ideal transcriptional output for optimal survival in its specific tumor microenvironment (Bianchi et al. 2020). Here, we summarize the most commonly mutated genes that contribute to bladder tumor development and progression. Additional information can be found in Chaps. 8–10.

7.3.1 Signaling by Receptor Tyrosine Kinases (RTKs)

7.3.1.1 Alterations in the RAS Family of Proteins

HRAS/KRAS/NRAS mutations are widespread in cancer. In normal cells, RAS protein transitions from an activated to inactivated state are catalyzed by the activity of GTPase activating proteins (GAPs) and guanine nucleotide exchange factors (GEFs). This protein family regulates several pathways crucial to cellular proliferation, programmed cell death, and angiogenesis (Shields et al. 2000).

Mutated RAS proteins are stuck in a constitutively activated form, activating downstream signaling pathways. The downstream effectors activated are protein serine/threonine kinase RAF, phosphatidylinositol 3-kinase (PI3K), and phospholipase C (PLC). RAF activation affects cell cycle progression and activates the MAPK-ERK (mitogen-activated protein kinase-extracellular signal-regulated kinase) signaling pathway, a crucial regulator of proto-oncogene transcription factors cFOS-JUN. PI3K activates several kinases, the most frequent being PDK1 and AKT and RHO family protein RAC, which activates NF-KB. PLC activates PKC, impacting calcium signaling pathways.

Aberrant RAS signaling results from point mutations, most frequently in *KRAS*, and less frequently in *NRAS* and *HRAS* genes. Mutations in the RAS family are rarely detected in normal urothelium, and similar frequencies of mutations in *HRAS* and *KRAS* (10–15%), are found in non-muscle-invasive bladder cancer (NMIBC) and muscle-invasive bladder cancer (MIBC) (Robertson et al. 2017; Pietzak et al. 2017; Dyrskjøt et al. 2023) (Fig. 7.1). This pathway is also activated through the hyperactivity of the EGF family of proteins.

7.3.1.2 FGFR3

FGFR3 belongs to the Fibroblast Growth Factor Receptor family of transmembrane receptor proteins, composed of an extracellular ligand-binding domain, a transmembrane domain, and an intracellular domain. Binding of small signaling molecules, the fibroblast growth factors (FGFs), leads to oligomerization and subsequent autophosphorylation of tyrosine residues in the cytoplasmic domain. This initiates a cascade of intracellular signaling events involved in cell proliferation, differentiation, and survival through the activation of pathways including but not limited to MAPK-ERK, JAK-STAT, and PI3K-AKT. All members of this family play a crucial role in embryonic development and tissue equilibrium.

Point mutations and translocations affecting *FGFR3* are detected in various malignancies and have been shown to activate ligand-independent hyperactive signaling from the receptor (Webster et al. 1996). Translocation t(4;14)(p16.3;q32.3), associated with increased FGFR3 expression, is seen in about 25% of multiple myeloma patients (Chesi et al. 1997) and ectopic expression of FGFR3 has been shown to induce oncogenic transformation in cells of the hematopoietic lineage (Chesi et al. 1997; Li et al. 2001; Chesi et al. 2001). Several autosomal dominant chondrodysplasias are characterized by activating germline mutations in *FGFR3*. Additionally, mutations in *FGFR3* are detected in cervical cancer, a significantly large fraction of low-grade non-muscle-invasive bladder cancer (NMIBC), and upper-tract

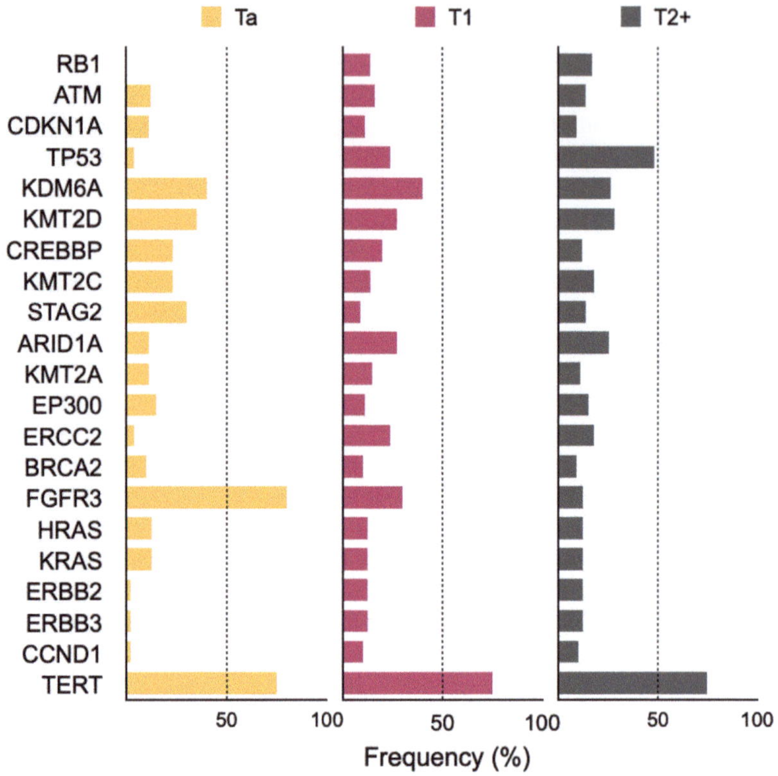

Fig. 7.1 Genomic alterations in bladder cancer by stage. This figure has been adapted from a recent review by Dyrskjøt et al. (2023)

urothelial carcinomas (van Rhijn et al. 2001, 2002; Sibley et al. 2001; van Tilborg et al. 2000; Robinson et al. 2019). While R248C mutations are more prevalent in the germline, S249C is the most common mutation found in 48–71% of NMIBCs. Overexpression of FGFR3 protein is present in 70–80% of Ta stage tumors and 50–60% of stage T1 tumors (Dyrskjøt et al. 2023; Tomlinson et al. 2007). Additionally, an oncogenic *FGFR3-TACC3* fusion event that leads to constitutive *FGFR3* activation has been identified in glioblastoma and bladder cancer (Costa et al. 2016; Frattini et al. 2018). Intriguingly, *FGFR3* mutations are rarely detected in morphologically normal urothelium (Li et al. 2020; Lawson et al. 2020).

Urothelium-restricted overexpression of human FGFR3-IIIb isoform carrying the S249C mutation in genetically engineered mice was sufficient to drive low-grade papillary bladder cancer development, similar in histology and transcriptome to the luminal subtype observed in human FGFR3-driven NMIBC (Lindskrog et al. 2021). In contrast, mice carrying K644E and K644M *Fgfr3* mutations (equivalent to K652E and K652M mutations in human *FGFR3*, which are rare in bladder cancer) could not generate tumors independently; however, upon addition of a heterozygous *Kras* G12D mutation, the mice developed a wide range of urothelial carcinomas (Shi et al. 2023; Ahmad et al. 2011; Foth et al. 2018). MYC has been identified as a critical downstream target in FGFR-addicted bladder cancer cell lines (Liu et al. 2017; Mahe et al. 2018). Interestingly, MYC downregulation in *FGFR* mutant cells was a determinant of response to FGFR inhibition (Liu et al. 2017).

A striking characteristic of *FGFR3*-mutated tumors is the low immune infiltrate observed in these tumors. In particular, *FGFR3*-mutated upper tract urothelial carcinomas with hyperactive FGFR signaling showed a T-cell-depleted immune microenvironment (Robinson et al. 2019). In vitro experiments identified a negative relationship between FGFR3 levels and expression of PD-L1 in bladder cancer cell lines and

FGFR3 inhibition in combination with anti-PD-L1 in a mouse model has shown enhanced anti-tumor immunity (Jing et al. 2022).

7.3.1.3 Human Epidermal Growth Factor (HER) Family

The HER family of four proteins comprising EGFR, ERBB2, ERBB3, and ERBB4 play a significant role in cell growth and division. Signaling through this protein family activates a wide array of intracellular pathways, including but not limited to RAS-ERK, and PI3K-AKT-mTOR, which ultimately controls many cellular processes from cell proliferation and differentiation to migration. Much attention has been paid to this class of proteins in breast cancer, but less is known about their role in bladder cancer.

EGFR is expressed in the normal urothelium and responds to EGF in urine to drive cell proliferation (Chow et al. 1997). Overexpression of EGFR is more commonly noted in MIBC than NMIBC. ERBB2 is an orphan receptor with no identified ligand; however, it is the preferred binding partner for all of the HER family proteins. In particular, ERBB2 promotes wound healing during the urothelial regeneration process (Bindels et al. 2002). ERBB3 lacks intrinsic kinase activity and can only activate intracellular pathways such as PI3K-AKT in a heterodimerized state (Sergina et al. 2007). Levels of ERBB4 correlate with a more differentiated cell state and are known to be downregulated in NMIBC and MIBC tumors (Røtterud et al. 2005).

As with *FGFR3*, mutations in this class of proteins are rare in normal urothelium and stage Ta tumors but much more frequent (10–15%) in T1 and T2+ tumors (Dyrskjøt et al. 2023; Hurst et al. 2021). Relative to other cancers, amplification of *ERBB2* is not common in bladder cancer. A mutual exclusivity pattern is observed between samples with mutations in *ERBB2* and *FGFR3* in bladder tumors, suggesting either a redundant or a potentially divergent path taken by these proteins in bladder carcinogenesis, which warrants further study (Pietzak et al. 2017).

7.3.2 Chromatin Modifiers

Chromatin-modifying proteins are among the most abundantly mutated in normal urothelium and at different stages of bladder cancer (Meghani et al. 2022) (Fig. 7.1). This group of proteins regulates the epigenetic signature of a cell. Higher-order chromatin structure comprises DNA wrapped around a core nucleosome particle. At its core, each subgroup of chromatin modifiers governs the strength of this interaction between DNA and histones. Densely packed chromatin (heterochromatin) is inaccessible to cellular machinery such as transcriptional proteins. In contrast, open chromatin (euchromatin) is more accessible and contains a significant number of actively transcribed genes. The transition between these states is tightly regulated and coordinated for cell-specific gene expression.

Widely grouped into writers, erasers, and remodelers, each working dynamically in coordination with others, these proteins regulate virtually every cellular function. Given the wide range of regulation controlled by these proteins, disruptions to these can have severely detrimental effects. Mutation in at least one chromatin-modifying enzyme is seen in 76% of MIBC (Robertson et al. 2017; Meghani et al. 2022) and in >70% of NMIBC (Morgan and Shilatifard 2015). For brevity, we will focus on histone methyltransferases: *KMT2D*, *KMT2C*, *EZH2*, lysine demethylase *KDM6A*, chromatin remodeler *ARID1A* from the SWI/SNF complex, and acetyltransferase *CREBBP/EP300*. For detailed discussion, see Chap. 10.

7.3.2.1 COMPASS and PRC2

Histone lysine methylation is regulated by the coordinated effort of methyltransferases and demethylases, genes that are mutated in various cancers. In particular, histone methyltransferases belonging to the polycomb (PcG) and trithorax (Trx) group of proteins are evolutionarily conserved from yeast to humans. Polycomb proteins deposit H3K27me3, a marker of gene inactivation, and trithorax proteins deposit H3K4me3, a feature associated with gene activation.

PRC2 is a multiprotein complex containing EZH2, SUZ12, EED, and additional subunits to catalyze mono-, di-, and tri-methylation at lysine 27 on Histone H3. Deposition of this mark marks the underlying DNA for transcriptional silencing. Depending on the context, EZH2 acts as an oncogene or tumor suppressor. In bladder cancer, evidence points to an oncogenic role of EZH2. Increased *EZH2* mRNA levels are measured with increased disease stage. However, mutations in *EZH2* are rare in bladder cancer.

The trithorax group of proteins encompass the MLL family: *MLL1* (*KMT2A*), *MLL2* (*KMT2B*), *MLL3* (*KMT2C*), *MLL4* (*KMT2D*), and histone demethylase *KDM6A* (*UTX*). Members of this family are among the most commonly mutated in normal urothelium and at different stages of bladder cancer (Thomsen et al. 2017; Robertson et al. 2017; Pietzak et al. 2017; Morgan and Shilatifard 2015; Barrows et al. 2020). MLL1/2 drive H3K4me3 at promoters, and MLL3/4 implement H3K4me1 at enhancers. KDM6A, an integral member of the MLL3/4 complex, catalyzes the removal of H3K27 marks deposited by Mll3/4, facilitating the acetylation of that site by CREBBP and EP300 (Morgan and Shilatifard 2015).

KDM6A is a lysine demethylase gene located on the X chromosome. Loss of *KDM6A* was insufficient to drive the growth of mouse bladder organoids in response to PPAR stimulation. However, in combination with *Trp53* loss, a robust growth induction was observed over *Trp53* loss alone (Halstead et al. 2017). Interestingly, loss of *KDM6A* in human bladder tumor cells increased cellular dependence on EZH2 for survival, and genetic/pharmacologic inhibition of EZH2 significantly decreased tumor growth (Ler et al. 2017). Loss-of-function *KDM6A* mutations and activating *FGFR3* mutations have been found to co-occur substantially in MIBC (Barrows et al. 2020). Mutations in *KDM6A* are detected in the normal urothelium (Li et al. 2020; Lawson et al. 2020) and more frequently in bladder tumors (Robertson et al. 2017; Pietzak et al. 2017) (Fig. 7.1). This increase was more prominent when sex was considered as a variable, with increased mutations detected in NMIBC in females relative to males (Hurst et al. 2017). Bladder cancer is three times more prevalent in males relative to females (Fajkovic et al. 2011), and studying the modified epigenome will be crucial to understanding this sex bias in disease incidence.

7.3.2.2 SWI/SNF

ARID1A, a component of the ATP-dependent SWI/SNF family of chromatin remodelers, is mutated in a quarter of bladder tumors and in morphologically normal urothelium (Li et al. 2020; Lawson et al. 2020; Robertson et al. 2017; Pietzak et al. 2017). Loss of *ARID1A* is insufficient to drive bladder cancer in mice despite an increase in pro-oncogenic mRNA due to a concomitant decrease in translation capacity (Jana et al. 2023). *ARID1A*-mutated cells are hyper-dependent on EZH2 and PI3K signaling, making these vulnerable to EZH2 and PI3K inhibitors (Bitler et al. 2015; Wu et al. 2018; Rehman et al. 2022). While limited knowledge exists regarding the function of chromatin modifiers in bladder cancer, it is evident that mutations in this group of proteins alone are not sufficient to initiate bladder cancer. However, when combined with other tumor suppressors or oncogenes, such as *TP53* or *FGFR3*, these genes enhance tumor formation.

To gain deeper insights into the involvement of chromatin modifiers in bladder cancer, future research should concentrate on their role in the normal urothelium to better understand their role in bladder homeostasis. Furthermore, it is crucial to identify the additional genomic or transcriptomic changes required to drive malignant transformation in normal urothelium that has mutations in chromatin modifiers. Such understanding is vital to understand the precise contribution of these proteins to oncogenic transformation of the urothelium and may facilitate the development of improved therapeutic approaches.

7.3.3 DNA Damage Response Genes

7.3.3.1 TP53/RB1

TP53 is a potent tumor suppressor and among the most commonly mutated gene across all cancers. Mutations in *TP53* and *RB1* are detected in about 50% of MIBC, often co-occurring, and in approximately 25% of stage T1 NMIBC (Robertson et al. 2017; Pietzak et al. 2017; Dyrskjøt et al. 2023) (Fig. 7.1). Consistent with this observation, *Trp53* and *Rb1* inactivation by urothelium-restricted expression of SV40T oncogene leads to carcinoma in situ, followed by invasive transitional cell carcinoma in mice (Zhang et al. 1999; Grippo and Sandgren 2000). Inactivation of *TP53*, first identified as a binding partner of SV40 T antigen in transformed cells (Lane and Crawford 1979), is a prerequisite for the genesis of a neoplastic state in most tissue types. Consistent with its function, germline mutations in *TP53*, seen in Li-Fraumeni syndrome, are associated with an increased risk of developing diverse cancers (Li and Fraumeni 1969a, 1969b; Li et al. 1988; Nichols et al. 2001). TP53 responds to many signals falling under the umbrella of acute stress, including but not limited to nutrient deprivation, DNA damage, hypoxia, and chronic stress signals like the activation of oncogenes (Vousden and Lane 2007).

TP53 is the master regulator of multiple cell-autonomous aspects of tumor suppression, maintaining genomic integrity by regulating DNA repair, apoptosis, cell cycle, metabolic homeostasis, and cellular plasticity during processes such as epithelial-mesenchymal transition (Boutelle and Attardi 2021). In addition, TP53 exerts non-cell autonomous effects on cellular processes by inducing the senescence-associated secretory phenotype (SASP) (Xue et al. 2007; Lujambio et al. 2013; Iannello et al. 2013).

RB1, first identified as a prototypical cancer gene in retinoblastoma, stimulated Alfred Knudson's famous two-hit hypothesis for the development of hereditary cancers (Knudson 1971; Friend et al. 1986; Fung et al. 1987; Dunn et al. 1988). Patients with germline *RB1* mutations who survive early childhood retinoblastoma have an increased risk of developing epithelial cancers such as bladder and lung cancers in later life (Fletcher et al. 2004). RB functions as a cell cycle checkpoint protein by binding to transcription factor E2F; this inhibits E2F binding to cyclin, an interaction crucial for cell cycle progression (Weinberg 1995) (see also Chap. 8).

7.3.4 DNA Damage Repair (DDR) Genes

Bladder cancer does not exhibit as high a mutation frequency for DNA damage response and repair genes as breast and ovarian cancers. Nevertheless, the influence of DNA repair genes in bladder cancer is evident from the high tumor mutation burden and mutational patterns seen in MIBC.

ERCC2, encoding a helicase functioning in the nucleotide excision repair (NER) pathway, is among the most commonly mutated DNA damage genes in bladder cancer. NER operates to detect and remove bulk adducts, similar to those formed by platinum-containing drugs such as cisplatin and carboplatin (Wang et al. 2003) and compatible with this, *ERCC2* mutations have been shown to correlate with cisplatin sensitivity in MIBC (Liu et al. 2016; Teo et al. 2017; Van Allen et al. 2014). Mutations in ERCC2 have been detected in 4% of Ta, 24% of T1, and 18% of T2+ tumors (Fig. 7.1). Additionally, the presence of *ERCC2* mutations correlates with the presence of COSMIC signature SBS5 in urothelial tumors (Kim et al. 2016) (see below).

Mutations in other DNA damage repair genes have been associated with a lower risk of metastatic recurrence in a cohort of chemoradiation-treated MIBC (Desai et al. 2016). Mutations in *BRCA2*, a protein involved in homology directed repair, were also associated with improved response in a cohort of MIBC patients treated with cisplatin chemotherapy (Taber et al. 2020). MIBC with other DDR alterations also showed improved clinical outcomes following platinum chemotherapy (Teo et al. 2017). Multiple ongoing clinical trials are exploring the potential of utilizing synthetic lethality in DDR (DNA damage repair) mutated tumors by combining DNA damaging agents such as PARP inhibitors or ATR inhibitors with immunotherapy (Garje et al. 2020) (see also Chap. 9).

7.4 Mutational Signatures

Tumor mutational landscape, or more broadly, the total mutational burden (TMB), serves as a gauge of the distance a normal cell has traversed to evolve into its cancerous state. TMB has been shown to linearly increase with stage (Nassar et al. 2019). In MIBC the TMB is >7 mutations per Mb, surpassed only by lung cancer and melanoma (Alexandrov et al. 2013a).

While knowledge about the total mutation burden of a tumor is important, studying the pattern of individual mutations can provide much information about the addictions and dependencies of a growing tumor. Mutagenic processes that fuel cancer evolution leave traceable "mutational signatures" that can be deconvoluted from somatic mutation profiles. The sources of mutagenesis can be exogenous carcinogens, such as tobacco smoking, or exposure to industrial chemicals. However, they can also be endogenous, such as age-related exposure to reactive oxygen species (ROS) or erroneous DNA editing.

Studies of the genome sequences of large numbers of tumors of multiple types have led to the derivation of so-called "single-base substitution" (SBS) signatures linked to specific mutational processes (available at https://cancer.sanger.ac.uk/cosmic/signatures). In addition to SBS signatures, other mutational patterns such as double base substitution signatures (DBS), small insertions and deletions (ID) signatures, signatures of copy number variations (CN), and structural variations (SV) have also been identified.

For example, carcinogens in tobacco smoke such as benzopyrene, damage DNA, which, when repaired, leaves behind a distinct mutation signature known as COSMIC signature SBS4 that can be identified by analysis of genome sequencing data (Pfeifer et al. 2002; Hainaut and Pfeifer 2001; Alexandrov et al. 2019, 2013b; Nik-Zainal et al. 2012). Similarly, the activity of endogenous mutagenic enzymes APOBEC3A and APOBEC3B is related to signatures SBS2 and SBS13, and aristolochic acid exposure is known to give rise to SBS22 (Alexandrov et al. 2013a; Mertz et al. 2022; Burns et al. 2013; Glaser et al. 2017; Baker et al. 2022). Deconvolution of these signatures from tumor profiles can help decipher the underlying processes leading to tumor development. Analysis of the bladder cancer genome has identified four prominent single-base substitution (SBS) signatures: SBS1, SBS2, SBS5, and SBS13 (Robertson et al. 2017; Lindskrog et al. 2021).

Across all tumors, irrespective of tissue of origin, the presence of SBS1 correlates strongly with age and clock-like mutational processes (Alexandrov et al. 2015). A proposed mechanism for SBS1 is the T:G mismatch arising from the deamination of 5-methylcytosine at CpG dinucleotides. SBS5 is pervasively present in a significant fraction of urothelial tumors and is correlated with *ERCC2* mutation (Kim et al. 2016). In an isogenic human cell line model, loss of *EXO1* and *RNF168* also resulted in a signature similar to SBS5 (Zou et al. 2021), though these genes are not commonly mutated in bladder cancer. Due to numerous factors that can impact the reliability of mutational signatures, such as sample size and the number of mutations per sample, further research is required to unravel the underlying cause of SBS5 in bladder cancer (Alexandrov et al. 2015).

While the SBS signature associated with smoking (SBS4) has only been identified in lung cancer, and not bladder, despite the higher risk of bladder cancer in smokers (Freedman et al. 2011), DBS2 and ID3 signatures also found to be similarly associated with tobacco smoking have been detected in bladder tumors (Alexandrov et al. 2019).

7.5 APOBEC Mutagenesis

MIBC has a very high tumor mutation burden, partly attributable to the hyperactivity of the APOBEC family of enzymes (Robertson et al. 2017; Chalmers et al. 2017). SBS2 and SBS13, signatures of APOBEC activity, are detected in approximately 70% of MIBC. Several different studies have identified APOBEC3 enzymes as the cause of these signatures (Robertson et al. 2017; Burns et al. 2013; Glaser et al. 2017; Petljak et al. 2019). In NMIBC, similar high rates of APOBEC mutagenesis are also found (Hurst et al 2021). APOBEC activity is also implicated in mutations found in normal urothelium (Lawson et al. 2020; Wang et al. 2023). Of the seven APOBEC3 family members, APOBEC3A and APOBEC3B have been implicated in generating the characteristic SBS2 and SBS13 signatures in bladder cancer (Glaser et al. 2017; Petljak et al. 2019, 2022a; Salter et al. 2016; Jarvis et al. 2022).

7.5.1 APOBEC Enzymes

In higher eukaryotes, the cytidine deaminase family consists of eleven proteins: AID (Activation Induced Deaminase) and APOBEC (Apolipoprotein B mRNA editing enzyme catalytic polypeptide-like) proteins. While only a single copy of APOBEC is found in rodents, eleven APOBEC proteins that share a zinc-dependent cytidine deaminase domain are found in primates (Salter et al. 2016). Cytidine deaminases convert cytosine to uracil in RNA and single-stranded DNA (ssDNA). Members of the APOBEC family are highly similar in structure; AID, APOBEC1/2/4, and APOBEC3A/H/C contain one deaminase domain, while APOBEC3B/D/F/G contain two deaminase domains (Salter and Smith 2018).

Each APOBEC enzyme has also been shown to mutate cytosine preferentially within a unique motif and structure. For instance, APOBEC3A preferentially binds cytosine in ssDNA that adopts a U-shaped conformation like those found in hairpin stem-loop structures (Buisson et al. 2019; Shi et al. 2017a). APOBEC3B most frequently mutates cytosines found in a 5'-TCW motif (where W is A or T) with higher efficiency in ssDNA; however, it also mutates cytosines found in hairpin stem-loop structures, albeit at a much lower efficacy. Crystal structure analysis of APOBEC3B catalytic domain constructs has identified the most thermodynamically stable form of the enzyme to be a closed inactive conformation providing evidence for a model where a sequence-specific stable binding induces conformational changes in the enzyme to allow for interaction between ssDNA and the active site pocket in the enzyme (Shi et al. 2015, 2017b).

Both APOBEC3A and APOBEC3B are overexpressed in cancer relative to normal tissue. While APOBEC3B localizes to the nucleus, APOBEC3A has a cell-wide distribution and is translocated to the nucleus in the presence of appropriate signals. To protect genomic DNA from unintended damage, APOBEC3B is excluded from the nucleus during mitosis (Lackey et al. 2013). Correlation analysis indicates a significant but weak association between *APOBEC3A/3B* mRNA levels and APOBEC signature (Robertson et al. 2017). This raises the question of how APOBEC mutagenesis is regulated. Is the presence of APOBEC enzymes sufficient to manifest the APOBEC signature?

Evolutionarily conserved pathways exist in cells to avoid genomic instability. Uracil generated by APOBEC-mediated deamination of cytosine is repaired by base excision repair (BER) or translesion synthesis pathways resulting in a C > T or C > G mutation (Serebrenik et al. 2019; Burns et al. 2015). BER repairs DNA damage caused by spontaneous, chemical, or enzymatic deamination, alkylation, or oxidation. Hyperactivity of APOBEC on ssDNA at replication forks can activate stress response pathways. In cases of acute replication stress, single-strand breaks from abasic sites can cause stalled forks to collapse, converting a single-strand break into a double-strand break. Hence, the consequences of APOBEC activity are not limited to increased base changes but also include deletions and translocations that can arise from the increased frequency of double-strand breaks.

A necessary component of the APOBEC biochemical reaction is single-strand DNA. Several biological processes such as replication, transcription, repair of damaged DNA, sites of actively transcribed genes, newly fired origins, single-strand breaks or stalled replication forks originating from replication-transcription collision events, and uncapped telomeres generate ssDNA as an intermediate (Giglia-Mari et al. 2011). However, ssDNA is thermodynamically less stable than double-stranded DNA (Marceau 2012) and is always bound by proteins, thereby increasing its stability and shielding it from unwarranted nucleolytic activity. RPA, HMCES, RADX, RAD51, and several other ssDNA binding proteins exist in cells to protect it from degradation (Cortez 2019; Bhat and Cortez 2018).

Replication protein A (RPA) is the most abundant, with approximately four million molecules per cell (Bhat and Cortez 2018). RPA is a heterotrimeric complex of three subunits RPA70, RPA32, and RPA14. RPA consists of four microdomains within its structure that bind to ssDNA and facilitate high affinity and low specificity binding to the ssDNA substrate. It binds to ssDNA generated at telomeres, RNA-DNA hybrids, during DNA recombination and damage responses (Bhat and Cortez 2018). Besides shielding ssDNA from nuclease activity, ssDNA binding proteins also promote the recruitment of other proteins, thereby facilitating several DNA metabolic processes in cells, such as replication fork stability, homologous recombination, and several others. Considering the shielded state of ssDNA in cells, the question arises how does APOBEC gain access to ssDNA in a cell?

RPA and APOBEC proteins share a similar ssDNA substrate which posits that at a cellular level, there might be a certain amount of competition between binding sites on ssDNA for these proteins. While RPA can bind to ssDNA with high affinity, it can be displaced to allow binding of other proteins, such as RAD51, which displaces RPA during homologous recombination. ssDNA generated in cells during biological processes such as replication, transcription and DNA repair, and at structures such as stalled forks, RNA-DNA hybrids, and replication templates, is bound by RPA (Bhat and Cortez 2018). While abundant RPA is present in cells under physiologic conditions, coating ssDNA generated during transcription and replication events, brief exhaustion of steady state RPA levels might occur in conditions such as excessive origin firing and increased transcriptional activity, similar to those observed in cells undergoing oncogenic transformation. Under these circumstances, the accessibility of ssDNA to nucleases and other mutagenic proteins, such as APOBEC, might increase.

Recent insights into regulation of global levels of RPA in cells suggest that under conditions of acute replication stress, RPA levels can be exhausted, leaving ssDNA in replication forks exposed and prone to breakage. An increase in free ssDNA accompanied by low levels of RPA leads to a terminal event termed "replication catastrophe" (Toledo et al. 2013; Ercilla et al. 2020). While replication stress is described as a local and reversible event, replication catastrophe is fatal, with a global accumulation of unrepaired double-strand breaks and DNA fragmentation. Haploinsufficiency of RPA is associated with increased genomic instability and cancer incidence. Transient knockdown of RPA2 using siRNA has been shown to destabilize the RPA complex leading to replication defects, excessive amounts of spontaneous DNA damage, and loss of cellular fitness (Jang et al. 2016). Recent work has identified cyclic hypoxic events as a mediator of such a replication catastrophe event capable of inducing APOBEC3B expression and activity (Bader et al. 2021).

In biochemical assays, APOBEC3G shows reduced deaminase activity on ssDNA substrates in the presence of RPA (Lada et al. 2011). In contrast, cooperation between RPA and AID allows for somatic hypermutation and class switch recombination at immunoglobin loci. Phosphorylation by Protein Kinase A (PKA) at Ser 38 activates AID, facilitating its binding to RPA at deamination sites required for AID function in activated B cells (Vuong et al. 2009; Chaudhuri et al. 2004). Using in vitro assays, it has been demonstrated that APOBEC3B forms tetramers. The resulting structure acts as a processive enzyme capable of deaminating substrates found in RNA-DNA hybrids; however, the protein's biochemical properties in this form limit its activity at transcription sites. However, in the presence of RPA, the deamination activity of APOBEC3B on the ssDNA substrate decreased significantly (Adolph et al. 2017). While these findings obtained from biochemical assays point to the role of RPA as an obstructing factor in APOBEC3B accessing ssDNA, these results remain to be demonstrated in a physiologic cellular model. Annotating rate-limiting steps in the

APOBEC mutagenesis process can help identify targets for anti-cancer therapies for bladder cancer.

7.5.2 Cause and Consequence of APOBEC Activity

Cancers are complex ecosystems comprising stroma, immune, and tumor cells. Interactions between these sub-components within the tumor microenvironment have been shown to influence cancer immunoediting and, by extension, disease outcomes. Parallels can be identified between processes during tumor development and anti-viral responses, one of them being the presence of immunostimulatory "foreign" DNA in the cell (Mesri et al. 2014). While the response to viruses depends on cell type, induction of type I interferons is an expected outcome that leads to a robust response, broadly termed as an "anti-viral state" involving upregulation of several interferon-stimulated genes (ISG), members of the APOBEC family, protein kinase R (PKR) and 2′-5″ oligoadenylate synthases (OAS).

Members of the APOBEC3 family, APOBEC3A, APOBEC3B, APOBEC3F, and APOBEC3G, are inducible upon stimulation by interferon-α as a defense mechanism against virus infection (Stetson and Medzhitov 2006). Several virus-driven cancers, such as head and neck, and cervical cancer, exhibit an enrichment of SBS2 and SBS13 mutational signatures (Zapatka et al. 2020). However, viral sequences have not been detected in the majority of bladder tumors (Zapatka et al. 2020). In a pan-cancer analysis, the mutation burden of SBS2 and SBS13 signatures showed no differences between virus-positive non-bladder tumors and virus-negative bladder tumors (Zapatka et al. 2020).

One study has suggested that APOBEC induction in bladder epithelium is due to exposure to polyoma viral particles in the urine (Baker et al. 2022). Latent BK polyomavirus has been detected in renal cells and urine samples (Nickeleit et al. 1999). However, the frequency of this mechanism in bladder cancer is unknown. IFNγ exposure has been shown to upregulate levels of APOBEC3B in bladder cancer cell lines (Glaser et al. 2017). Genotoxic stress from exposure to chemotherapy drugs and viral infection-dependent IFN-mediated signaling have also been shown to upregulate APOBEC3A in cancer cell lines (Oh et al. 2021). Oncogenic viruses and activation of oncogenes stimulate several common pathways. One such pathway is the NF-κB signaling pathway, which can also upregulate APOBEC3B (Maruyama et al. 2016; Leonard et al. 2015). Other conditions commonly encountered during tumorigenesis, such as increased replication stress and hyperactivity of PI3K, and MAPK signaling pathways, have also been associated with increased APOBEC3B levels and activity (Kanu et al. 2016). However, definitive causative endogenous or exogenous agent(s) responsible for the upregulation of these genes in bladder cancer have not been identified.

APOBEC mutagenesis has been proposed to cause higher than normal *FGFR3* S249C mutations and E542K and E545K mutations in *PIK3CA* in bladder cancer (Shi et al. 2019; Henderson et al. 2014). In a longitudinal study of urothelial carcinoma, clonal enrichment of APOBEC mutations was observed in tumors post-chemotherapy relative to chemotherapy naïve tumors (Faltas et al. 2016). In bladder cancer, accumulation of SBS2 mutations has been shown to increase over time, whereas SBS13 mutations seem to accumulate much more during the early stages of tumorigenesis (clonal mutations) and are much less prevalent in the subclonal mutations that arise later during tumorigenesis (McGranahan et al. 2015). Longitudinal studies from lung cancer have demonstrated a similar definitive presence of APOBEC mutational processes in clonal truncal mutations and a higher intratumor heterogeneity in tumors with higher activity of these enzymes (de Bruin et al. 2014).

However, despite extensive research, there is a divided viewpoint regarding the consequence of APOBEC mutagenesis in cancer. Some studies suggest APOBEC-induced mutations can promote clonal heterogeneity and contribute to therapeutic resistance, thus exhibiting a pro-tumorigenic effect (Faltas et al. 2016; Law et al. 2016; Swanton et al. 2015). Conversely, other studies propose an anti-tumorigenic role for APOBEC, wherein these proteins by increasing the overall mutation burden, enhance the tumor's visibility to the immune system, potentially leading to inflammation, immune recognition, and ultimately tumor elimination (Glaser et al. 2017; Driscoll et al. 2020). Indeed, high levels of APOBEC mutational signature are associated with prolonged overall survival in MIBC (Robertson et al. 2017). These differing perspectives highlight the complexity of APOBEC mutagenesis and its impact on cancer development and immune surveillance. While APOBEC mutagenesis is undoubtedly an important feature of bladder cancer, additional work is needed to determine the therapeutic opportunities that can be exploited in APOBEC high or low tumors (Petljak et al. 2022b).

7.6 Macroscale Genetic Events

Genomic instability occurs at different levels, ranging from point mutations to changes at the chromosomal level, such as loss, duplication, and translocations. Over 100 years ago, Theodor Boveri proposed the idea that failure of cell division resulting in tetraploidy could promote oncogenesis (Boveri 2008). Today it is a well-accepted fact that a change in ploidy is a hallmark of cancer. Somatic copy number alterations or aneuploidy can drive tumorigenesis, increase immune evasion, and increase the rate of tumor cell proliferation (Davoli et al. 2017). Alterations in DNA copy number have been associated with increasing stage, grade, recurrence, and outcome in bladder cancer (Blaveri et al. 2005; Koed et al. 2005; Nord et al. 2010; Zieger et al. 2009; Hurst et al. 2012).

One of the earliest studies that monitored tumor ploidy using flow cytometry-based analysis of DNA content, found hypertetraploidy to be associated with aggressive metastatic disease that is resistant to therapeutic interventions (Shackney et al. 1995). Since then, technologies for studying macroscale genetic events have evolved significantly, from traditional cytogenetic methods such as karyotyping to breakthroughs such as fluorescence in situ hybridization (FISH), comparative genomic hybridization (CGH), microarray technology, and next-generation sequencing (NGS). Recent advances include techniques like digital droplet PCR (ddPCR) and single-cell genomics, alongside improvements in bioinformatics and artificial intelligence, all contributing to more precise and comprehensive detection of copy number variations (CNVs).

Common fragile sites, named so for their propensity to exhibit breakage upon replication stress, are common regions of chromosomal rearrangements in early tumorigenesis (Burrell et al. 2013; Le Tallec et al. 2013). Chromosomal instability occurs in part because of inappropriate DNA synthesis during the mitotic phase of the cell cycle (Minocherhomji et al. 2015). Defects in the spindle assembly checkpoint (SAC) can result in chromosome missegregation errors. Chromosomal instability, resulting from SAC defects, has been demonstrated to make these cells hyper-dependent on KIF18A and MPS1, two proteins essential during mitosis; this synthetic lethality can be exploited in the roughly 54% of MIBC tumors that harbor a genome doubling event (Robertson et al. 2017; Quinton et al. 2021; Marquis et al. 2021; Bielski et al. 2018; Jemaà et al. 2015).

One of the most commonly detected events in bladder cancer is the deletion of all or segments of chromosome 9. Several critical genes and regions regulating cell growth and survival are present on this chromosome. *CDKN2A* and *CDKN2B*, two crucial tumor suppressors that regulate the cell cycle, are located at 9p21 (Cairns et al. 1994; Okamoto et al. 1994; Kamb et al. 1994; Serrano 2000; Carnero et al. 2000). These genes regulate the cell cycle by binding to cyclin-dependent kinases CDK4/CDK6 and preventing their association with cyclin D, thereby preventing cell cycle progression. MTAP, an enzyme in the methionine salvage pathway, is coded by the *MTAP* gene located near the *CDKN2A/B* genes and is deleted along with these genes in 33% of MIBC. Loss of MTAP function increases dependency on *PRMT5*, which can be therapeutically exploited by pharmacologic inhibition (Mavrakis et al. 2016; Feustel and Falchook 2022). Another critical tumor suppressor gene on 9q34 is *TSC1* (Tuberous Sclerosis Complex 1) which negatively regulates mTORC1 activity and hence plays an essential role in cell growth (Huang and Manning 2008; van Slegtenhorst et al. 1997).

DNA amplification is rare in Ta stage tumors (Hurst et al. 2012). However, amplifications occur more commonly as tumors progress. Several of the most commonly amplified genes in bladder cancer have crucial roles in regulating cell cycle, cell growth and proliferation. During the G1/S checkpoint, the binding of CCND1 (cyclin D1) to CDK4 forms an active complex that leads to the phosphorylation and deactivation of RB1, causing the release of E2F3 and facilitating cell cycle progression. Each component of this G1-S cell cycle checkpoint is frequently altered in bladder cancer. *CCND1*, present on 11q13, is amplified in 11% of MIBC and 6% of NMIBC tumors (Robertson et al. 2017; Pietzak et al. 2017; Proctor et al. 1991). *E2F3*, located at 6p22, is amplified in 16% MIBC and 3% NMIBC (Robertson et al. 2017; Pietzak et al. 2017; Oeggerli et al. 2004). *CDK4* at 12q14 is amplified in 1.5% of MIBC (Robertson et al. 2017; Pietzak et al. 2017). *RB1* deletions, at 13q14, are detected in 8% of MIBC (Robertson et al. 2017).

Whole genome doubling (WGD) is a macroscale event detected in about 30% of all cancers. It is hypothesized to arise from dysregulation of cell cycle checkpoints and exposure to stressors such as telomere dysfunction, events commonly encountered during tumorigenesis (Artandi et al. 2000; Darp et al. 2022). Tetraploidy has been demonstrated to increase the frequency of chromosomal rearrangements and tumor cell heterogeneity leading to accelerated cancer evolution, and worse prognosis (Bielski et al. 2018; Fujiwara et al. 2005; Dewhurst et al. 2014; Storchova and Pellman 2004). Cells that have undergone WGD exhibit chromosomal instability, providing the selective pressure required for fitter clones to expand (Cahill et al. 1999).

Chromosome shattering or "chromothripsis" is a complex form of genetic instability that causes large-scale genomic rearrangements. It is a relatively common event in several cancer types, including advanced bladder cancer, and can occur at the clonal or sub-clonal level (Cortés-Ciriano et al. 2020; Morrison et al. 2014). While individual mutations allow a gradual accrual of oncogenic features, chromothripsis is a faster way of achieving this goal (Stephens et al. 2011). Chromothriptic DNA is defined by scars made of multiple clustered DNA breaks resulting in unpredictable rearrangement of considerable numbers of genomic fragments, which can activate oncogenes or inactivate tumor suppressors. This can sometimes result in the circularization of the excised segment, which results in small circular DNA molecules (Shoshani et al. 2021). A crucial macro-feature identified from the pan-cancer analysis is "kataegis", clusters of stranded hypermutations at chromothriptic break sites, demonstrated in in vitro models to be a consequence of cytosine deaminase activity on ssDNA (Maciejowski et al. 2015, 2020; Roberts et al. 2012; Bergstrom et al. 2022). In a cell line model, APOBEC3B has been shown to induce kataegis under conditions of telomere crisis, an event believed to occur frequently during the early stages of tumor development (Maciejowski et al. 2020; von Morgen and Maciejowski 2018).

Bladder cancer is characterized by a spectrum of macroscale genetic events, including copy number variations (CNVs), whole genome doubling, and chromothripsis. When considering large scale alterations, it is important to consider the dosage of genes within these segments. Identifying the underlying mechanisms and dependencies for these macroscale genetic events will ultimately be crucial to understanding tumor evolution.

7.7 Conclusion

Cancer is an evolutionary process and each mutational event shapes the tumor, its microenvironment and the response of the tumor to physiologic stressors such as hypoxia, nutrient deprivation and external stressors such as therapeutic agents. Winding back the tape and understanding the early clonal mutations and their contribution to tumor evolution and progression is critical for developing effective cancer therapies. As we continue to unravel the complexity of the mutational landscape in bladder cancer, we will be better equipped to develop personalized treatment strategies that can improve outcomes for patients.

References

Adolph MB, Love RP, Feng Y, Chelico L (2017) Enzyme cycling contributes to efficient induction of genome mutagenesis by the cytidine deaminase APOBEC3B. Nucleic Acids Res 45:11925–11940

Ahmad I et al (2011) K-Ras and β-catenin mutations cooperate with Fgfr3 mutations in mice to promote tumorigenesis in the skin and lung, but not in the bladder. Dis Model Mech 4:548–555

Alexandrov LB et al (2013a) Signatures of mutational processes in human cancer. Nature 500:415–421

Alexandrov LB, Nik-Zainal S, Wedge DC, Campbell PJ, Stratton MR (2013b) Deciphering signatures of mutational processes operative in human cancer. Cell Rep 3:246–259

Alexandrov LB et al (2015) Clock-like mutational processes in human somatic cells. Nat Genet 47:1402–1407

Alexandrov LB et al (2019) The repertoire of mutational signatures in human cancer. Nature 322859. https://doi.org/10.1101/322859

Artandi SE et al (2000) Telomere dysfunction promotes non-reciprocal translocations and epithelial cancers in mice. Nature 406:641–645

Bader SB et al (2021) Replication catastrophe induced by cyclic hypoxia leads to increased APOBEC3B activity. Nucleic Acids Res 49:7492–7506

Baker SC et al (2022) Induction of APOBEC3-mediated genomic damage in urothelium implicates BK polyomavirus (BKPyV) as a hit-and-run driver for bladder cancer. Oncogene 41:2139–2151

Barrows D, Feng L, Carroll TS, Allis CD (2020) Loss of UTX/KDM6A and the activation of FGFR3 converge to regulate differentiation gene-expression programs in bladder cancer. Proc Natl Acad Sci USA 117:25732–25741

Bergstrom EN et al (2022) Mapping clustered mutations in cancer reveals APOBEC3 mutagenesis of ecDNA. Nature 602:510–517

Bhat KP, Cortez D (2018) RPA and RAD51: fork reversal, fork protection, and genome stability. Nat Struct Mol Biol 25:446–453

Bianchi JJ, Zhao X, Mays JC, Davoli T (2020) Not all cancers are created equal: tissue specificity in cancer genes and pathways. Curr Opin Cell Biol 63:135–143

Bielski CM et al (2018) Genome doubling shapes the evolution and prognosis of advanced cancers. Nat Genet 50:1189–1195

Bindels E, van der Kwast T, Izadifar V, Chopin D, de Boer W (2002) Functions of epidermal growth factor-like growth factors during human urothelial reepithelialization in vitro and the role of erbB2. Urol Res 30:240–247

Bitler BG et al (2015) Synthetic lethality by targeting EZH2 methyltransferase activity in ARID1A-mutated cancers. Nat Med 21:231–238

Blaveri E et al (2005) Bladder cancer stage and outcome by array-based comparative genomic hybridization. Clin Cancer Res Off J Am Assoc Cancer Res 11:7012–7022

Boutelle AM, Attardi LD (2021) p53 and tumor suppression: it takes a network. Trends Cell Biol 31:298–310

Boveri, T. (2008). Concerning the origin of malignant tumours by Theodor Boveri. Translated and annotated by Henry Harris. Journal of cell science 121(Supplement_1):1–84

Buisson R et al (2019) Passenger hotspot mutations in cancer driven by APOBEC3A and mesoscale genomic features. Science 364:eaaw2872

Burns MB et al (2013) APOBEC3B is an enzymatic source of mutation in breast cancer. Nature 494:366–370

Burns MB, Leonard B, Harris RS (2015) APOBEC3B: pathological consequences of an innate immune DNA mutator. Biom J 38:102–110

Burrell RA et al (2013) Replication stress links structural and numerical cancer chromosomal instability. Nature 494:492–496

Cahill DP, Kinzler KW, Vogelstein B, Lengauer C (1999) Genetic instability and darwinian selection in tumours. Trends Cell Biol 9:M57–M60

Cairns P et al (1994) Rates of p16 (MTS1) mutations in primary tumors with 9p loss. Science 265:415–417

Carnero A, Hudson JD, Price CM, Beach DH (2000) p16INK4A and p19ARF act in overlapping pathways in cellular immortalization. Nat Cell Biol 2:148–155

Chalmers ZR et al (2017) Analysis of 100,000 human cancer genomes reveals the landscape of tumor mutational burden. Genome Med 9:34

Chaudhuri J, Khuong C, Alt FW (2004) Replication protein A interacts with AID to promote deamination of somatic hypermutation targets. Nature 430:992–998

Chesi M et al (1997) Frequent translocation t(4;14)(p16.3;q32.3) in multiple myeloma is associated with increased expression and activating mutations of fibroblast growth factor receptor 3. Nat Genet 16:260–264

Chesi M et al (2001) Activated fibroblast growth factor receptor 3 is an oncogene that contributes to tumor progression in multiple myeloma. Blood 97:729–736

Chow N-H, Liu H-S, Yang H-B, Chan S-H, Su I-J (1997) Expression patterns of erbB receptor family in normal urothelium and transitional cell carcinoma. Virchows Arch 430:461–466

Cortés-Ciriano I et al (2020) Comprehensive analysis of chromothripsis in 2,658 human cancers using whole-genome sequencing. Nat Genet 52:331–341

Cortez D (2019) Replication-coupled DNA repair. Mol Cell 74:866–876

Costa R et al (2016) FGFR3-TACC3 fusion in solid tumors: mini review. Oncotarget 7:55924–55938
Darp R, Vittoria MA, Ganem NJ, Ceol CJ (2022) Oncogenic BRAF induces whole-genome doubling through suppression of cytokinesis. Nat Commun 13:4109
Davoli T, Uno H, Wooten EC, Elledge SJ (2017) Tumor aneuploidy correlates with markers of immune evasion and with reduced response to immunotherapy. Science 355:eaaf8399
de Bruin EC et al (2014) Spatial and temporal diversity in genomic instability processes defines lung cancer evolution. Science 346:251–256
Desai NB et al (2016) Genomic characterization of response to chemoradiation in urothelial bladder cancer. Cancer 122:3715–3723
Dewhurst SM et al (2014) Tolerance of whole-genome doubling propagates chromosomal instability and accelerates cancer genome evolution. Cancer Discov 4:175–185
Driscoll CB et al (2020) APOBEC3B-mediated corruption of the tumor cell immunopeptidome induces heteroclitic neoepitopes for cancer immunotherapy. Nat Commun 11:790
Dunn JM, Phillips RA, Becker AJ, Gallie BL (1988) Identification of germline and somatic mutations affecting the retinoblastoma gene. Science 241:1797–1800
Dyrskjøt L et al (2023) Bladder cancer. Nat Rev Dis Primer 9:1–21
Ercilla A et al (2020) Physiological tolerance to ssDNA enables strand uncoupling during DNA replication. Cell Rep 30:2416–2429.e7
Fajkovic H et al (2011) Impact of gender on bladder cancer incidence, staging, and prognosis. World J Urol 29:457–463
Faltas BM et al (2016) Clonal evolution of chemotherapy-resistant urothelial carcinoma. Nat Genet 48:1490–1499
Feustel K, Falchook GS (2022) Protein arginine methyltransferase 5 (PRMT5) inhibitors in oncology clinical trials: a review. J Immunother Precis Oncol 5:58–67
Fletcher O et al (2004) Lifetime risks of common cancers among retinoblastoma survivors. J Natl Cancer Inst 96:357–363
Foth M et al (2018) FGFR3 mutation increases bladder tumourigenesis by suppressing acute inflammation. J Pathol 246:331–343
Frattini V et al (2018) A metabolic function of FGFR3-TACC3 gene fusions in cancer. Nature 553:222–227
Freedman ND, Silverman DT, Hollenbeck AR, Schatzkin A, Abnet CC (2011) Association between smoking and risk of bladder cancer among men and women. JAMA J Am Med Assoc 306:737–745
Friend SH et al (1986) A human DNA segment with properties of the gene that predisposes to retinoblastoma and osteosarcoma. Nature 323:643–646
Fujiwara T et al (2005) Cytokinesis failure generating tetraploids promotes tumorigenesis in p53-null cells. Nature 437:1043–1047
Fung Y-KT et al (1987) Structural evidence for the authenticity of the human retinoblastoma gene. Science 236:1657–1661
Gaisa NT et al (2011) The human urothelium consists of multiple clonal units, each maintained by a stem cell. J Pathol 225:163–171
Garje R, Vaddepally RK, Zakharia Y (2020) PARP inhibitors in prostate and urothelial cancers. Front Oncol 10:114
Giglia-Mari G, Zotter A, Vermeulen W (2011) DNA damage response. Cold Spring Harb Perspect Biol 3:a000745
Glaser AP et al (2017) APOBEC-mediated mutagenesis in urothelial carcinoma is associated with improved survival, mutations in DNA damage response genes, and immune response. Oncotarget 9:4537–4548
Grippo PJ, Sandgren EP (2000) Highly invasive transitional cell carcinoma of the bladder in a simian virus 40 T-antigen transgenic mouse model. Am J Pathol 157:805–813
Haigis KM, Cichowski K, Elledge SJ (2019) Tissue-specificity in cancer: the rule, not the exception. Science 363:1150–1151
Hainaut P, Pfeifer GP (2001) Patterns of p53 G→T transversions in lung cancers reflect the primary mutagenic signature of DNA-damage by tobacco smoke. Carcinogenesis 22:367–374
Halstead AM et al (2017) Bladder-cancer-associated mutations in RXRA activate peroxisome proliferator-activated receptors to drive urothelial proliferation. eLife 6:e30862
Henderson S, Chakravarthy A, Su X, Boshoff C, Fenton TR (2014) APOBEC-mediated cytosine deamination links *PIK3CA* helical domain mutations to human papillomavirus-driven tumor development. Cell Rep 7:1833–1841
Huang J, Manning BD (2008) The TSC1–TSC2 complex: a molecular switchboard controlling cell growth. Biochem J 412:179–190
Hurst CD, Platt FM, Taylor CF, Knowles MA (2012) Novel tumor subgroups of urothelial carcinoma of the bladder defined by integrated genomic analysis. Clin Cancer Res Off J Am Assoc Cancer Res 18:5865–5877
Hurst CD et al (2017) Genomic subtypes of non-invasive bladder cancer with distinct metabolic profile and female gender bias in KDM6A mutation frequency. Cancer Cell 32:701–715.e7
Hurst CD et al (2021) Stage-stratified molecular profiling of non-muscle-invasive bladder cancer enhances biological, clinical, and therapeutic insight. Cell Rep Med 2:100472
Iannello A, Thompson TW, Ardolino M, Lowe SW, Raulet DH (2013) p53-dependent chemokine production by senescent tumor cells supports NKG2D-dependent tumor elimination by natural killer cells. J Exp Med 210:2057–2069

Jana S et al (2023) Transcriptional-translational conflict is a barrier to cellular transformation and cancer progression. Cancer Cell S1535-6108(23):00094–00096. https://doi.org/10.1016/j.ccell.2023.03.021

Jang S-W, Jung JK, Kim JM (2016) Replication protein A (RPA) deficiency activates the Fanconi anemia DNA repair pathway. Cell Cycle Georget Tex 15:2336–2345

Jarvis MC et al (2022) Mutational impact of APOBEC3B and APOBEC3A in a human cell line. 2022.04.26.489523 Preprint at https://doi.org/10.1101/2022.04.26.489523

Jemaà M et al (2015) Whole-genome duplication increases tumor cell sensitivity to MPS1 inhibition. Oncotarget 7:885–901

Jing W et al (2022) FGFR3 destabilizes PD-L1 via NEDD4 to control T-cell–mediated bladder cancer immune surveillance. Cancer Res 82:114–129

Kakiuchi N, Ogawa S (2021) Clonal expansion in noncancer tissues. Nat Rev Cancer 21:239–256

Kamb A et al (1994) A cell cycle regulator potentially involved in genesis of many tumor types. Science 264:436–440

Kanu N et al (2016) DNA replication stress mediates APOBEC3 family mutagenesis in breast cancer. Genome Biol 17:185

Kim J et al (2016) Somatic ERCC2 mutations are associated with a distinct genomic signature in urothelial tumors. Nat Genet 48:600–606

Knudson AG (1971) Mutation and cancer: statistical study of retinoblastoma. Proc Natl Acad Sci USA 68:820–823

Koed K et al (2005) High-density single nucleotide polymorphism array defines novel stage and location-dependent allelic imbalances in human bladder tumors. Cancer Res 65:34–45

Lackey L, Law EK, Brown WL, Harris RS (2013) Subcellular localization of the APOBEC3 proteins during mitosis and implications for genomic DNA deamination. Cell Cycle 12:762–772

Lada AG et al (2011) Replication protein A (RPA) hampers the processive action of APOBEC3G cytosine deaminase on single-stranded DNA. PLoS One 6:e24848

Lane DP, Crawford LV (1979) T antigen is bound to a host protein in SV40-transformed cells. Nature 278:261–263

Law EK et al (2016) The DNA cytosine deaminase APOBEC3B promotes tamoxifen resistance in ER-positive breast cancer. Sci Adv 2:e1601737

Lawson ARJ et al (2020) Extensive heterogeneity in somatic mutation and selection in the human bladder. Science 370:75–82

Le Tallec B et al (2013) Common fragile site profiling in epithelial and erythroid cells reveals that most recurrent cancer deletions lie in fragile sites hosting large genes. Cell Rep 4:420–428

Leonard B et al (2015) The PKC/NF-κB signaling pathway induces APOBEC3B expression in multiple human cancers. Cancer Res 75:4538–4547

Ler LD et al (2017) Loss of tumor suppressor KDM6A amplifies PRC2-regulated transcriptional repression in bladder cancer and can be targeted through inhibition of EZH2. Sci Transl Med 9

Li FP, Fraumeni JF (1969a) Soft-tissue sarcomas, breast cancer, and other neoplasms. A familial syndrome? Ann Intern Med 71:747–752

Li FP, Fraumeni JF (1969b) Rhabdomyosarcoma in children: epidemiologic study and identification of a familial cancer syndrome. J Natl Cancer Inst 43:1365–1373

Li FP et al (1988) A cancer family syndrome in twenty-four kindreds. Cancer Res 48:5358–5362

Li Z et al (2001) The myeloma-associated oncogene fibroblast growth factor receptor 3 is transforming in hematopoietic cells. Blood 97:2413–2419

Li R et al (2020) Macroscopic somatic clonal expansion in morphologically normal human urothelium. Science 370:82–89

Lindskrog SV et al (2021) An integrated multi-omics analysis identifies prognostic molecular subtypes of non-muscle-invasive bladder cancer. Nat Commun 12:2301

Liu D et al (2016) Clinical validation of chemotherapy response biomarker ERCC2 in muscle-invasive urothelial bladder carcinoma. JAMA Oncol 2:1094–1096

Liu H et al (2017) C-Myc alteration determines the therapeutic response to FGFR inhibitors. Clin Cancer Res 23:974–984

Lujambio A et al (2013) Non-cell-autonomous tumor suppression by p53. Cell 153:449–460

Maciejowski J, Li Y, Bosco N, Campbell PJ, De Lange T (2015) Chromothripsis and kataegis induced by telomere crisis. Cell 163:1641–1654

Maciejowski J et al (2020) APOBEC3-dependent kataegis and TREX1-driven chromothripsis during telomere crisis. Nat Genet 52:884–890

Mahe M et al (2018) An FGFR3/MYC positive feedback loop provides new opportunities for targeted therapies in bladder cancers. EMBO Mol Med 10:e8163

Majewski T et al (2019) Whole-organ genomic characterization of mucosal field effects initiating bladder carcinogenesis. https://doi.org/10.1016/j.celrep.2019.01.095

Marceau AH (2012) Functions of single-strand DNA-binding proteins in DNA replication, recombination, and repair. Methods Mol Biol Clifton NJ 922:1–21

Marquis C et al (2021) Chromosomally unstable tumor cells specifically require KIF18A for proliferation. Nat Commun 12:1213

Martincorena I et al (2015) Tumor evolution. High burden and pervasive positive selection of somatic mutations in normal human skin. Science 348:880–886

Maruyama W et al (2016) Classical NF-κB pathway is responsible for APOBEC3B expression in cancer cells. Biochem Biophys Res Commun 478:1466–1471

Mavrakis KJ et al (2016) Disordered methionine metabolism in MTAP/CDKN2A-deleted cancers leads to dependence on PRMT5. Science 351:1208–1213

McGranahan N et al (2015) Clonal status of actionable driver events and the timing of mutational processes in cancer evolution. Sci Transl Med 7:283ra54
Meghani K, Folgosa Cooley L, Piunti A, Meeks JJ (2022) Role of chromatin modifying complexes and therapeutic opportunities in bladder cancer. Bladder Cancer Amst Neth 8:101–112
Mertz TM, Collins CD, Dennis M, Coxon M, Roberts SA (2022) APOBEC-induced mutagenesis in cancer. Annu Rev Genet 56:229–252
Mesri EA, Feitelson MA, Munger K (2014) Human viral oncogenesis: a cancer hallmarks analysis. Cell Host Microbe 15:266–282
Minocherhomji S et al (2015) Replication stress activates DNA repair synthesis in mitosis. Nature 528:286–290
Morgan MA, Shilatifard A (2015) Chromatin signatures of cancer. Genes Dev 29:238–249
Morrison CD et al (2014) Whole-genome sequencing identifies genomic heterogeneity at a nucleotide and chromosomal level in bladder cancer. Proc Natl Acad Sci USA 111:E672–E681
Nassar AH et al (2019) Mutational analysis of 472 urothelial carcinoma across grades and anatomic sites. Clin Cancer Res 25:2458–2470 (4AD)
Nichols KE, Malkin D, Garber JE, Fraumeni JF, Li FP (2001) Germ-line p53 mutations predispose to a wide spectrum of early-onset cancers. Cancer Epidemiol Biomark Prev 10:83–87
Nickeleit V et al (1999) Polyomavirus infection of renal allograft recipients: from latent infection to manifest disease. J Am Soc Nephrol JASN 10:1080–1089
Nik-Zainal S et al (2012) Mutational processes molding the genomes of 21 breast cancers. Cell 149:979–993
Nord H et al (2010) Focal amplifications are associated with high grade and recurrences in stage Ta bladder carcinoma. Int J Cancer 126:1390–1402
Oeggerli M et al (2004) E2F3 amplification and overexpression is associated with invasive tumor growth and rapid tumor cell proliferation in urinary bladder cancer. Oncogene 23:5616–5623
Oh S et al (2021) Genotoxic stress and viral infection induce transient expression of APOBEC3A and proinflammatory genes through two distinct pathways. Nat Commun 12:4917
Okamoto A et al (1994) Mutations and altered expression of p16INK4 in human cancer. Proc Natl Acad Sci 91:11045–11049
Petljak M et al (2019) Characterizing mutational signatures in human cancer cell lines reveals episodic APOBEC mutagenesis. Cell 176:1282–1294.e20
Petljak M et al (2022a) Mechanisms of APOBEC3 mutagenesis in human cancer cells. Nature 607:799–807
Petljak M, Green AM, Maciejowski J, Weitzman MD (2022b) Addressing the benefits of inhibiting APOBEC3-dependent mutagenesis in cancer. Nat Genet 54:1599–1608
Pfeifer GP et al (2002) Tobacco smoke carcinogens, DNA damage and p53 mutations in smoking-associated cancers. Oncogene 21:7435–7451
Pietzak EJ et al (2017) Next-generation sequencing of nonmuscle invasive bladder cancer reveals potential biomarkers and rational therapeutic targets. Eur Urol 72:952–959
Proctor AJ, Coombs LM, Cairns JP, Knowles MA (1991) Amplification at chromosome 11q13 in transitional cell tumours of the bladder. Oncogene 6:789–795
Quinton RJ et al (2021) Whole-genome doubling confers unique genetic vulnerabilities on tumour cells. Nature 590:492–497
Rehman H et al (2022) ARID1A-deficient bladder cancer is dependent on PI3K signaling and sensitive to EZH2 and PI3K inhibitors. JCI Insight 7:e155899
Roberts SA et al (2012) Clustered mutations in yeast and in human cancers can arise from damaged long single-strand DNA regions 46:424–435 (5AD)
Robertson AG et al (2017) Comprehensive molecular characterization of muscle-invasive bladder cancer. Cell 171:540–556.e25
Robinson BD et al (2019) Upper tract urothelial carcinoma has a luminal-papillary T-cell depleted contexture and activated FGFR3 signaling. Nat Commun 10:2977
Røtterud R, Nesland JM, Berner A, Fosså SD (2005) Expression of the epidermal growth factor receptor family in normal and malignant urothelium. BJU Int 95:1344–1350
Salter JD, Smith HC (2018) Modeling the embrace of a mutator: APOBEC selection of nucleic acid ligands. Trends Biochem Sci 43:606–622
Salter JD, Bennett RP, Smith HC (2016) The APOBEC protein family: united by structure, divergent in function. Trends Biochem Sci 41:578–594
Serebrenik AA et al (2019) The deaminase APOBEC3B triggers the death of cells lacking uracil DNA glycosylase. Proc Natl Acad Sci USA 116:22158–22163
Sergina NV et al (2007) Escape from HER-family tyrosine kinase inhibitor therapy by the kinase-inactive HER3. Nature 445:437–441
Serrano M (2000) The INK4a/ARF locus in murine tumorigenesis. Carcinogenesis 21:865–869
Shackney SE et al (1995) Origins and clinical implications of aneuploidy in early bladder cancer. Cytometry 22:307–316
Shi K, Carpenter MA, Kurahashi K, Harris RS, Aihara H (2015) Crystal structure of the DNA deaminase APOBEC3B catalytic domain. J Biol Chem 290:28120–28130
Shi K et al (2017a) Structural basis for targeted DNA cytosine deamination and mutagenesis by APOBEC3A and APOBEC3B. Nat Struct Mol Biol 24:131–139
Shi K et al (2017b) Conformational switch regulates the DNA cytosine deaminase activity of human APOBEC3B. Sci Rep 7:17415
Shi M-J et al (2019) APOBEC-mediated mutagenesis as a likely cause of FGFR3 S249C mutation over-representation in bladder cancer. Eur Urol 76:9–13

Shi M-J et al (2023) FGFR3 mutational activation can induce luminal-like papillary bladder tumor formation and favors a male sex bias. Eur Urol 83:70–81
Shields JM, Pruitt K, McFall A, Shaub A, Der CJ (2000) Understanding Ras: 'it ain't over 'til it's over. Trends Cell Biol 10:147–154
Shoshani O et al (2021) Chromothripsis drives the evolution of gene amplification in cancer. Nature 591:137–141
Sibley K, Stern P, Knowles MA (2001) Frequency of fibroblast growth factor receptor 3 mutations in sporadic tumours. Oncogene 20:4416–4418
Stephens PJ et al (2011) Massive genomic rearrangement acquired in a single catastrophic event during cancer development. Cell 144:27–40
Stetson DB, Medzhitov R (2006) Type I interferons in host defense. Immunity 25:373–381
Storchova Z, Pellman D (2004) From polyploidy to aneuploidy, genome instability and cancer. Nat Rev Mol Cell Biol 5:45–54
Swanton C, McGranahan N, Starrett GJ, Harris RS (2015) APOBEC enzymes: mutagenic fuel for cancer evolution and heterogeneity. Cancer Discov 5:704–712
Taber A et al (2020) Molecular correlates of cisplatin-based chemotherapy response in muscle invasive bladder cancer by integrated multi-omics analysis. Nat Commun 11:4858
Teo MY et al (2017) DNA damage response and repair gene alterations are associated with improved survival in patients with platinum-treated advanced urothelial carcinoma. Clin Cancer Res 23:3610–3618
Thomsen MBH et al (2017) Comprehensive multiregional analysis of molecular heterogeneity in bladder cancer. Sci Rep 7:11702
Toledo LI et al (2013) ATR prohibits replication catastrophe by preventing global exhaustion of RPA. Cell 155:1088–1103
Tomlinson D, Baldo O, Harnden P, Knowles M (2007) FGFR3 protein expression and its relationship to mutation status and prognostic variables in bladder cancer. J Pathol 213:91–98
Tubbs A, Nussenzweig A (2017) Endogenous DNA damage as a source of genomic instability in cancer. Cell 168:644–656
Van Allen EM et al (2014) Somatic ERCC2 mutations correlate with cisplatin sensitivity in muscle-invasive urothelial carcinoma. Cancer Discov 4:1140–1153
van Rhijn BW et al (2001) The fibroblast growth factor receptor 3 (FGFR3) mutation is a strong indicator of superficial bladder cancer with low recurrence rate. Cancer Res 61:1265–1268
van Rhijn BWG, Montironi R, Zwarthoff EC, Jöbsis AC, van der Kwast TH (2002) Frequent FGFR3 mutations in urothelial papilloma. J Pathol 198:245–251
van Slegtenhorst M et al (1997) Identification of the tuberous sclerosis gene TSC1 on chromosome 9q34. Science 277:805–808
van Tilborg AAG et al (2000) Molecular evolution of multiple recurrent cancers of the bladder. Hum Mol Genet 9:2973–2980
von Morgen P, Maciejowski J (2018) The ins and outs of telomere crisis in cancer. Genome Med 10:89
Vousden KH, Lane DP (2007) p53 in health and disease. Nat Rev Mol Cell Biol 8:275–283
Vuong BQ et al (2009) Specific recruitment of protein kinase A to the immunoglobulin locus regulates class-switch recombination. Nat Immunol 10:420–426
Wang D, Hara R, Singh G, Sancar A, Lippard SJ (2003) Nucleotide excision repair from site-specifically platinum-modified nucleosomes. Biochemistry 42:6747–6753
Wang C, Ross WT, Mysorekar IU (2017) Urothelial generation and regeneration in development, injury, and cancer. Dev Dyn 246:336–343
Wang Y et al (2023) APOBEC mutagenesis is a common process in normal human small intestine. Nat Genet 55:246–254
Webster MK, d'Avis PY, Robertson SC, Donoghue DJ (1996) Profound ligand-independent kinase activation of fibroblast growth factor receptor 3 by the activation loop mutation responsible for a lethal skeletal dysplasia, Thanatophoric dysplasia type II. Mol Cell Biol 16:4081–4087
Weinberg RA (1995) The retinoblastoma protein and cell cycle control. Cell 81:323–330
Wu S et al (2018) SWI/SNF catalytic subunits' switch drives resistance to EZH2 inhibitors in ARID1A-mutated cells. Nat Commun 9:4116
Xue W et al (2007) Senescence and tumour clearance is triggered by p53 restoration in murine liver carcinomas. Nature 445:656–660
Zapatka M et al (2020) The landscape of viral associations in human cancers. Nat Genet 52:320–330
Zhang Z-T, Pak J, Shapiro E, Sun T-T, Wu X-R (1999) Urothelium-specific expression of an oncogene in transgenic mice induced the formation of carcinoma in situ and invasive transitional cell Carcinoma1. Cancer Res 59:3512–3517
Zieger K, Marcussen N, Borre M, Ørntoft TF, Dyrskjøt L (2009) Consistent genomic alterations in carcinoma in situ of the urinary bladder confirm the presence of two major pathways in bladder cancer development. Int J Cancer 125:2095–2103
Zou X et al (2021) A systematic CRISPR screen defines mutational mechanisms underpinning signatures caused by replication errors and endogenous DNA damage. Nat Cancer 2:643–657

8 Cell Cycle Regulators as Oncogenic Drivers in Bladder Cancer

David J. DeGraff, Xue-Ru Wu, Joshua I. Warrick, Shamara Lawrence, and Moon-Shong Tang

Abstract

The cell cycle serves as a means for the regulation of cellular turnover to maintain normal tissue homeostasis. For this reason, genetic changes resulting in dysregulated cell cycle kinetics are implicated in a wide array of human malignancies. The same is true in bladder cancer, where genes important for normal cell cycle function in urothelium are frequently mutated (see Chap. 7 for discussion of stage-specific genetic alterations). One goal of this chapter is to provide a broad overview of the normal cell cycle, including the molecular machinery required for the maintenance of cell cycle kinetics. Using this as a framework, a separate goal is to provide an overview of identified molecular alterations associated with cell cycle regulation and discuss the physiologic impact of these alterations on bladder cancer pathogenesis.

Keywords

Cell cycle · Cell proliferation · Bladder cancer · TP53 · Oncogene · Recurrence · Progression

8.1 Overview of the Cell Cycle

Within every tissue, homeostasis is maintained by a fine-tuned balance between cell proliferation and turnover. While different tissues (and even different compartments within a tissue) have dif-

D. J. DeGraff (✉)
Department of Pathology and Laboratory Medicine, Pennsylvania State University College of Medicine, Hershey, PA, USA

Department of Urology, Pennsylvania State University College of Medicine, Hershey, PA, USA

Department of Biochemistry and Molecular Biology, Pennsylvania State University College of Medicine, Hershey, PA, USA

X.-R. Wu
Department of Urology, New York University School of Medicine, Veterans Affairs New York Harbor Healthcare System, New York, NY, USA

Department of Pathology, New York University School of Medicine, Veterans Affairs New York Harbor Healthcare System, New York, NY, USA

J. I. Warrick · S. Lawrence
Department of Pathology and Laboratory Medicine, Pennsylvania State University College of Medicine, Hershey, PA, USA

Department of Urology, Pennsylvania State University College of Medicine, Hershey, PA, USA

M.-S. Tang
Department of Pathology and Laboratory Medicine, Pennsylvania State University College of Medicine, Hershey, PA, USA

Department of Medicine, New York University Grossman School of Medicine, New York, NY, USA

M. A. Knowles, L. Dyrskjøt (eds.), *Biology of Bladder Cancer*,
https://doi.org/10.1007/978-3-031-68505-7_8

ferent rates of cell turnover, the foundation for physiologic homeostasis is governed by the replication of genomic material, followed by cell division, controlled by the cell cycle. In 2000, Hanahan and Weinberg provided a cogent summary of the six "hallmarks" of cancer (Hanahan and Weinberg 2000). Dysregulation of the cell cycle is directly related to at least four of the original six hallmarks of cancer (sustained proliferative signaling, resistance to cell death, evading growth suppression, and acquisition of replicative immortality). In 2011, this work was updated to include additional emerging hallmarks and enabling characteristics, with dysregulated cell cycle dynamics directly contributing to genome instability and mutations (Hanahan and Weinberg 2011). As detailed in this chapter, the centrality of alterations in cell cycle control and kinetics to these hallmarks of cancer is clearly demonstrated across the natural history of bladder cancer. While a detailed examination of the research establishing our understanding of cell cycle control is beyond the scope of this chapter, a general knowledge is required to understand the role of dysregulated cell cycle activity in bladder cancer.

8.1.1 Purpose and Phases of the Cell Cycle

Excellent sources are available for a more detailed perspective regarding the cell cycle (Alberts 2002). At its most basic level, the cell cycle is defined as the cellular processes between one cell division and the next in a proliferating cell. The time required for a cell to progress through the cell cycle is cell type-specific, ranging in time from hours to months, or even years. In particular, the urothelium is especially slow cycling, as detailed below. In addition, terminally differentiated cells are often unable to re-enter an active cell cycle phase.

Three essential components of the cell cycle that are separately but coordinately regulated in normal cells include (1) the chromosome cycle (DNA synthesis and mitosis); (2) the cytoplasmic cycle (cell growth and cytokinesis); and (3) the centrosome cycle (duplication and polar movement of the mitotic spindle). To ensure these cell cycle stages progress accurately and in the right order in normal cells, a mechanism enabling control of the cell cycle has evolved. These mechanisms ensure DNA is faithfully replicated, genetic material is equally distributed to daughter cells, and cell growth is sufficient to support cell division. The general principles of these regulatory structures are detailed below.

8.1.2 The Role of Cyclins and Cyclin-Dependent Kinases in Cell Cycle Control

Cyclins are a highly conserved family of proteins, which are characterized by dramatic fluctuations in protein abundance throughout the cell cycle. Cyclins are key regulators of the function of cyclin-dependent kinases (CDKs). During cell cycle progression, individual cyclins form stable pairs with specific CDKs to control cell cycle progression. Specifically, cyclin/CDKs complexes regulate cell cycle progression at three points. These include mitosis (M phase), commitment to cellular division (G1 phase), and DNA synthesis (S phase). Cyclin/CDKs are regulated through three main processes, including phosphorylation, protein-protein interactions, and degradation via the ubiquitin/proteosome pathways. For a visual representation of the cell cycle, as well as associated genetic alterations of cell cycle machinery in bladder cancer, see Fig. 8.1.

8.1.3 Overview of the Normal Cell Cycle

G1 Phase

G1 phase is a period of cell growth when cells commit to cellular division. This period of delayed progression into S phase enables time for cell growth and interpretation of extracellular cues. The G1 checkpoint (also known as restriction point) is a crucial point within the cell cycle, which determines when the cell becomes committed to entering the cell cycle.

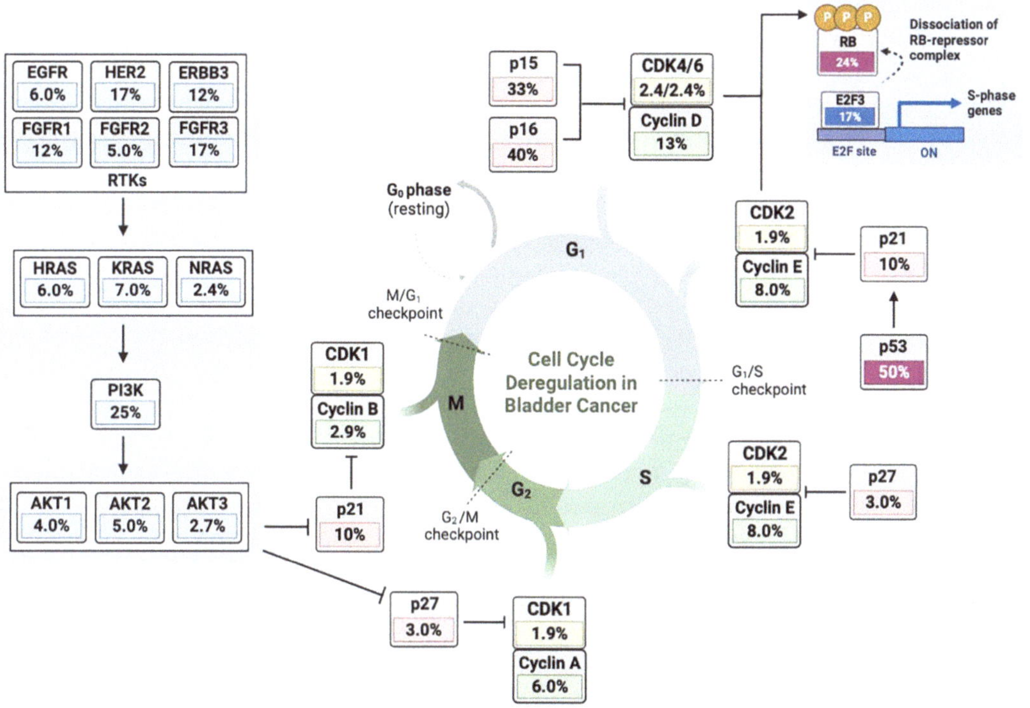

Fig. 8.1 Frequency of genetic alterations in cell cycle regulatory machinery and associated pathways in muscle invasive bladder cancer. Numbers indicate percentage of patients with muscle invasive bladder cancer harboring recurrent genetic alterations (mutations, structural variants, and copy number alterations). Green boxes indicate cyclin genes, yellow boxes indicate CDK genes, red boxes indicate CDK inhibitor genes, dark blue boxes indicate E2F genes, magenta boxes indicate TP53/RB pathway genes, and blue boxes indicate RTK-RAS-PI3K pathway genes. This figure is based on a cbioPortal for Cancer Genomics query of the TCGA MIBC cohort (Robertson et al. 2017). Adapted from "Cell Cycle Checkpoints", by BioRender.com (2023) https://app.biorender.com/biorender-templates

Retinoblastoma protein (RB1) as well as the "pocket proteins" p107 and p130 play an essential role in the G1 checkpoint of the cell cycle. RB1, p107, and p130 function as inhibitors of a subset of E2F transcription factors, which function to transcriptionally activate a plethora of cell cycle control genes. Therefore, RB1, p107, and p130 must be inactivated for a cell to enter S phase. Cell cycle promoting E2Fs are activated following increased Cyclin D expression in response to growth promoting conditions. As Cyclin D levels rise, a complex is formed between Cyclin D and the cyclin-dependent kinases 4 and 6 (CDK4/6). The Cyclin D:CDK4:CDK6 complex monophosphorylates RB1, which in conjunction with phosphorylation of p107 and p130 (also by the Cyclin D:CDK4:CDK6 complex) enables activation of this E2F subset, resulting in increased expression of Cyclin E.

CDK4/6 activity, as well as cell cycle progression is tightly controlled by protein products of the *CDKN2A* gene, which encodes the proteins p16 and p14. p16 serves as an inhibitor of CDK4/6 activity, thus preventing phosphorylation of RB1. p14 inhibits the ubiquitin ligase, MDM2, resulting in p53 stabilization and cell cycle arrest. Therefore, products of the *CDKN2A* gene ensure that RB1 and p53 activity block cell cycle progression to S phase until proper conditions are met. Like the inhibitory role of *CDKN2A*, Cyclin E activity is inhibited by interaction with p27, a product of the *CDKN1B* gene. As Cyclin A levels increase, it additionally forms a complex with CDK2, resulting in the inhibition of p27, and full activation of the CyclinA:CDK2 complex. Active CyclinA:CDK2 serves to phosphorylate activating E2F factors, resulting in their inhibition. In addition, the Cyclin E:CDK2 complex hyperphosphorylates RB1, resulting in complete inactivation of RB1, and increased expression of Cyclin A and Cell Division Cycle 6 (CDC6). At this point, cells are fully committed to enter S phase.

S Phase, G2 and M Phase

The Cyclin A:CDK2 complex functions to initiate DNA replication during S phase, and ensure that this occurs only once in a normal cell cycle. DNA replication origins consist of large protein complexes, which serve as origin recognition complexes for DNA synthesis (Prioleau and MacAlpine 2016). Following binding of the proteins CDC6 and Minichromosome Maintenance (MCM) to DNA, a pre-replication complex is formed, and activation of Cyclin A:CDK2 initiates replication. Activity of the Cyclin A:CDK2 complex remains high during G2 and early mitosis, preventing re-replication.

Following S phase, a secondary growth period ensues (G2), thus preparing the cell for entry and successful completion of cell division during M phase. During G2, levels of Cyclin B rise, and form complexes with CDK1, which is the central regulator of mitosis. Cyclin B serves as the regulatory subunit of CDK1, and for this reason synthesis and degradation of Cyclin B is primarily responsible for entry and exit from the cell cycle. Active CDK1 serves several functions during late G2 in preparation for M phase, as well as during mitosis and subsequent cell division. For example, in late G2, CyclinB:CDK1 activates centrosome separation, golgi organization, nuclear envelope breakdown, and chromosome condensation. Once chromosomes are condensed and aligned at the metaphase plate, CDK1 is inhibited by the serine/threonine G2 checkpoint kinase WEE1, allowing for sister chromatid separation, chromosome de-condensation, reformation of the nuclear envelope, and finally cytokinesis following cleavage furrow formation.

8.2 Cell Cycle of the Normal Urothelium

Normal urothelium, from which all the urothelial carcinoma variants and subtypes originate, is the slowest-cycling epithelium in the body, with a turnover rate ranging from 6 months to a year (Walker 1960; Hicks 1975; Wu et al. 2009; Jost and Potten 1986). Earlier studies using tritium-thymidine incorporation as a surrogate for DNA replication demonstrated that 0.02–0.1% of urothelial cells were undergoing DNA synthesis at any given time point in rats, mice, and ex vivo human bladder tissue (Walker 1960; Jost 1986). The consensus is that under normal circumstances an overwhelming majority of urothelial cells are quiescent, being stationary in the G0/G1 phase (see also Chap. 3).

8.2.1 Normal Urothelial Subpopulations Can Be Polyploid

Several DNA ploidy analyses detected significant proportions of urothelial cells in a tetraploid state (4n), leading to the assumption that these cells were in the G2/M phase and the suggestion that they acted as a reservoir for fast proliferation upon injury (Sharief et al. 1980). It should be emphasized, however, that the superficial (umbrella) cells, and some intermediate cells of the normal urothelium across different species are prone to be bi- or poly-nucleated due to "endoreduplication" and failed cytokinesis (Wang et al. 2018). These polyploid normal urothelial cells should not be confused with active cell division or polyploid urothelial carcinoma cells. Distinguishing low-grade urothelial carcinoma cells from polyploid normal urothelial cells during fluorescence in situ hybridization (FISH)-based ploidy analysis is therefore a challenge (Tapia et al. 2011). The awareness of this issue could help reduce the erroneous interpretation of FISH results. Like normal urothelial cells, normal hepatocytes also tend to exhibit polyploidy.

Hepatocyte polyploidy is age- and injury-dependent, and is regulated by cell cycle regulators, such as p53 and p21 (Wang et al. 2017). Whether these mechanisms underlie urothelial cell polyploidy remains to be seen. The functional importance of normal urothelial polyploidy also needs to be elucidated, although it may play a role at least in part, in innate urothelial defenses against bacterial infections. The presence of multiple nuclei represents a clear advantage over that of single nuclei in mounting sufficient NF-kB-mediated pro-inflammatory signals, without the need for de novo protein synthesis (Liu et al. 2015).

8.2.2 Structural and Cell-Intrinsic Mechanisms Limit Proliferation of Normal Urothelium

Although normal urothelial cells are largely quiescent, they are by no means inert. In fact, when injured by infectious and chemical agents or ionizing radiation, urothelial cells can enter the cell cycle and proliferate rapidly (Erzar et al. 2020). Such rapid responses ensure the restoration of urothelial integrity and function. Experimental evidence, particularly that from lineage-tracing, clearly supports an important role of urothelial basal cells in wound healing (Schäfer et al. 2017). There are studies, however, suggesting that even the intermediate urothelial cells exhibit certain levels of plasticity in repairing urothelial damage (Schäfer et al. 2017; Cheng et al. 2021). Like other epithelia, the proliferative responses to injury by urothelial cells are generally self-contained and subside as soon as the injury is repaired. This is thought to be accomplished not only by the removal of mitogenic signals, but also by negative feedback and growth-inhibiting mechanisms, which overlap, at least partly, with tumor defenses in response to oncogene activation in the urothelium (see below). Urine contains a wide range of toxins and carcinogens, as well as growth factors (Wu 2005). Yet, normal urothelial cells are largely non-proliferating, despite being constantly bathed in this milieu. This is probably because of structural and intrinsic factors which limit access and function of these components of the urine microenvironment. First and foremost, most proliferation-capable urothelial cells reside in the basal layer which is well protected by the highly effective permeability barrier provided by the superficial umbrella cells (Wu et al. 2009; Dalghi et al. 2020). These basal cells express abundant Epidermal Growth Factor Receptor (EGFR) (Messing 1990), but they are precluded from ligand interaction with the extraordinarily high concentrations of Epidermal Growth Factor (EGF) present in urine (Messing et al. 1987). Once the barrier is breached, EGF-EGFR interactions take place that can ignite rapid urothelial proliferation (Messing and Murphy-Brooks 1994). Secondly, while cell cycle machinery including the cyclins and CDKs at the steady state is fully intact and operational, these proteins are kept to a low level, thus ensuring slow cell-cycling. In contrast, negative cell-cycle regulators of G1/S transition, particularly the CDKN1 family (p21, p27, p57), RB, pocket family proteins (RB, p107, and p130), and the CDKN2 family (*CDKN2A*, *CDKN2B*, *CDKN2C*, and *CDKN2D*), are expressed at medium to high levels (Wu 2009). These negative regulators appear to play a redundant role in keeping the urothelial cell cycle in check. The slow rate of cell cycle and renewal of urothelium aligns well with the intended stable and durable functions of the epithelium, which is to maintain a constant permeability barrier and accommodate the dramatic surface area changes during the micturition cycle (Wu et al. 2009; Dalghi et al. 2020). In a macroenvironment full of potent carcinogens, a slow rate of DNA synthesis and replication may be also advantageous to minimizing mutational events from taking place and being propagated.

In addition to its role in the maintenance of homeostasis, the redundancy of negative cell regulators in normal urothelium may also contribute significantly to tumor defense mechanisms during oncogene activation or tumor suppressor gene inactivation. Mounting evidence suggests that the mutational activation of oncogenes found frequently in human bladder cancer, such as

Fibroblast Growth Factor Receptor 3 (*FGFR3*), RAS genes, and Phosphatidylinositol-4,5-bisphosphate 3-kinase Catalytic Subunit Alpha (*PIK3CA*), in urothelia of transgenic mice elicits only minimal urothelial proliferation without full-fledged tumors (Zhou et al. 2016; Ahmad et al. 2011; Zhang et al. 2001; Cheng et al. 2002; Shuman et al. 2023). Analyses of the proliferative lesions often show a marked upregulation of CDK inhibitors normally expressed in urothelium as well as de novo induction of CDKIs not normally expressed (Xia et al. 2021; Mo et al. 2007). Similarly, when a tumor suppressor gene, such as *Rb1*, is inactivated in mouse urothelium, the rest of the family members including *Rbl1* (encoding p107) and *Rbl2* (encoding p130) and the p53 signaling pathway is strongly induced (He et al. 2009, 2015, 2022). Such compensatory induction of a fail-safe mechanism likely acts as a tumor barrier preventing urothelial proliferation from crossing the threshold of tumor formation. These observations from experimental tumorigenesis studies are highly instructive of the insufficiency of single genetic alterations in initiating urothelial tumors and the necessity for combinatorial genetic events to act in concert to drive cell cycle progression and fully transform the urothelial cells (Wu 2005, 2009).

8.3 Clinical Evidence Indicates an Important Role for Cell Cycle Deregulation in Bladder Cancer

8.3.1 Non-muscle Invasive Bladder Cancer

The association between cell cycle activity and clinical outcomes is best exemplified in studies focused on non-muscle invasive bladder cancer (NMIBC). For example, noninvasive papillary urothelial carcinomas (stage Ta) with higher cell cycle activity have higher rates of recurrence and progression to muscle-invasive bladder cancer (MIBC) (Hurst et al. 2021; Zaleski et al. 2019; Lopez-Beltran et al. 2004; Hedegaard et al. 2016; Fristrup et al. 2013). The metrics of cell cycle in these studies have included Ki-67 labelling index, an immunohistochemical test that quantifies the fraction of cells outside of G0 (Lopez-Beltran et al. 2004), and mitotic index, a method that quantifies the number of histologically visible mitotic figures identified per unit area of tissue examined (Zaleski et al. 2019).

Stage Ta NMIBC is classified as either high-grade or low-grade by histology in contemporary clinical practice (Urinary and Male Genital Tumours 2022) (see also Chap. 4). High-grade tumors have higher rates of recurrence and progression (Urinary and Male Genital Tumours 2022). Consistent with this observation, high-grade tumors also tend to have high cell cycle activity (Zaleski et al. 2019; Urinary and Male Genital Tumours 2022). However, the association between tumor grade and cell cycle activity is not perfect. A subset of low-grade cancers demonstrate a high mitotic index, and these tumors have higher rates of recurrence than those with a low mitotic index (Zaleski et al. 2019; Akkalp et al. 2016; Pich et al. 2002). There is also evidence that mitotic index predicts recurrence with greater accuracy than tumor grade. A study demonstrated this using a multivariate model including tumor grade and mitotic index. The model showed that mitotic index significantly associated with recurrence, while tumor grade did not, and conferred a higher hazard of recurrence than tumor grade (Zaleski et al. 2019).

Gene expression-based signatures of cell cycle activity also associate with outcomes in Ta stage disease. These gene expression signatures have been combined with expression signatures indicative of FGFR3 signaling and immune activity to generate a composite signature that reflects these multiple signatures. For example, higher recurrence has been shown in Ta tumors with high cell cycle activity and a low immune signature, as shown with a microarray-based expression signature (Hurst et al. 2021). The study separates these cancers into three expression subtypes (TaE1, TaE2, and TaE3). Signatures of cell cycle and immunity dominated these subtype assignments, with highest rates of recurrence in those with high cell cycle activity and low immune activity. Around 20% of noninvasive papillary urothelial carcinomas harbor biallelic deletion of *CDKN2A* (Rebouissou et al. 2012). As expected, tumors with biallelic deletion of *CDKN2A* exhibit high cell cycle activity (Warrick et al. 2022). Mutations in other cell cycle genes are comparatively less common (Warrick et al. 2022). Stage Ta tumors are enriched in activating *FGFR3* mutations, and the mutations persist as a driver in invasive cancers that evolve from them. Consistent with this observation, MIBC with activating mutations in *FGFR3* are enriched for *CDKN2A* deletion (Rebouissou et al. 2012).

Similar findings are seen with lamina-propria invasive bladder cancer (stage T1). Like Ta tumors, T1 tumors with high cell cycle activity and a low inflammatory signature are more aggressive, demonstrating higher rates of recurrence and stage progression (Lopez-Beltran et al. 2004). These features, among other expression signatures have been used to place these tumors into expression subtypes. For example, Hurst et al. define four subtypes of T1 cancer (designated T1E1 through T1E4) (Hurst et al. 2021). Cell cycle and inflammatory signatures contribute heavily to these subtypes, along with others, including FGFR3 signaling and the "CIS signature," an expression signature seen in both flat urothelial carcinoma in situ and MIBC that present with flat urothelial carcinoma in situ (Dyrskjøt et al. 2004). Those with high cell cycle, high CIS signature, low inflammation, and low FGFR3 signaling had the highest rates of stage progression. Similarly, Robertson et al. describe five expression subtypes of stage T1 carcinoma. These differ in cell cycle and inflammatory signatures, as well as MYC signaling, EZH2 expression, and several others (Robertson et al. 2020). In general, those with high cell cycle activity and low inflammatory signature had the highest rates of rapid recurrence in this study. See Chap. 13 for further description of NMIBC subtypes.

NMIBC with high activity of the cell cycle demonstrate activity of several other signatures, including retinoic acid receptor, sonic hedgehog, and pluripotency, in both noninvasive and lamina propria-invasive cancers (Warrick et al. 2022; Robertson et al. 2020; Lindskrog et al. 2021). There is also evidence that these cancers express signatures of EMT and RHO signaling, even at the noninvasive stage (Warrick et al. 2022). The overall findings suggest cancers with high cell cycle activity likely trigger activity of additional pathways contributing to adverse outcomes.

8.3.2 Muscle Invasive Bladder Cancer

Diversity in cell cycle activity is also seen in muscle-invasive bladder cancer (MIBC). This is readily apparent in studies of molecular subtypes of muscle-invasive disease (Choi et al. 2014; Damrauer et al. 2014; Robertson et al. 2017; Sjödahl et al. 2012, 2017; Marzouka et al. 2018; Kamoun et al. 2020) (see Chap. 14 for details). Several subtyping systems have been developed that highlight different aspects of tumor biology, but in general all have shown that MIBC broadly falls into two subtypes: Luminal and Basal-Squamous. The Basal-squamous subtype expresses markers of squamous differentiation, such as *TP63* and high molecular weight keratins. Luminal cancers express markers of urothelial differentiation, such as *FOXA1* and uroplakins. In addition to playing a role in lineage plasticity, FOXA1 inactivation has been associated with increased proliferation of urothelial cancer cells (Shi et al. 2023) and has a role in G1 to S phase transition in other malignancies (Tsuruta et al. 2006). Neuronal and Basal-Squamous MIBC has high activity of the cell cycle in the vast majority of cases. In contrast, Luminal cancers have diverse activity of the cell cycle, ranging from relatively low to high rates of proliferation.

8.4 Experimental Evidence Indicates that Combinatorial Genetic Events Are Required for Cell Cycle Deregulation in Bladder Cancer

Figure 8.1 illustrates the frequency of common genetic alterations in cell cycle machinery and growth factor signaling in MIBC. Among the cell cycle regulators that are dysregulated in human bladder cancer, those activating the receptor tyrosine kinase-Rat sarcoma virus-phosphoinositide 3-kinase (RTK-RAS-PI3K) mitogenic pathway and those inactivating the p53 tumor suppressor pathway are by far the most common, affecting 71% and 89% of MIBC, respectively (Robertson et al. 2017). The preservation of genetic alterations in advanced tumors is generally considered to be a result of selective advantage, and highly prevalent alterations within a population of a given cancer type are considered driver alterations. Nonetheless, from a biological standpoint, whether a given alteration is tumorigenic and can stand the test of experimental validation is an entirely different matter. As discussed above, single genetic alterations are rarely sufficiently tumorigenic by themselves, regardless of their frequency. For instance, urothelium-specific expression of *Fgfr3* mutants in transgenic mice, whether they be in the extracellular loop or in the cytoplasmic kinase domain, have been mostly reported to result in normal appearing urothelium without overt changes in proliferation (Zhou et al. 2016; Ahmad et al. 2011). However, a recent study shows S249C mutations in *Fgfr3* results in tumor development, particularly at high expression levels of the mutant (Shi et al. 2023). Similarly, activating mutations of *Hras* or *Pik3ca* only elicit mild urothelial hyperplasia but not full-fledged urothelial carcinomas (Zhang et al. 2001). Analagous results have been obtained in knockout mice lacking *Pten* (Tsuruta et al. 2006; Osei-Amponsa et al. 2020), which normally serves as a repressor of PI3K signaling. Deficiency of a single tumor suppressor in the p53 signaling pathway in mice, such as *p53*, *Rb1*, and *Cdkn2a*, also produces no urothelial abnormality (He et al. 2009, 2022; Puzio-Kuter et al. 2009). These data strongly suggest that the urothelial tumorigenicity of single genetic alterations is rather limited, and that combinatorial genetic events are necessary to transform urothelial cells fully. Indeed, while neither mutant *Hras* nor *Tp53* loss is sufficient to independently induce urothelial tumors in mice, together they are highly synergistic in inducing Basal-Squamous MIBC (He et al. 2015). Perhaps unsurprisingly, *Tp53* loss also cooperates with *Pten* loss in triggering the same subtype of MIBC (He et al. 2022; Puzio-Kuter et al. 2009). In the Ta bladder cancer pathway, mutant *Hras* can act synergistically with the loss of *Cdkn2b*, but not *Cdkn2a* in mice, in initiating urothelial tumors (Xia et al. 2021). Loss of both *Tp53* and *Rb1*, however, did not show synergistic effects priming bladder tumor formation (He et al. 2009). It appears therefore that not only the co-occurring events per se, but that functionally relevant co-occurring events are needed to initiate urothelial tumors.

8.5 Growth Promoting Potential: Cell Cycle Regulators Are Not Created Equal

While genetic alterations are often grouped as components of a signaling pathway, experimental evidence suggests that different players within a single signaling pathway frequently exhibit highly variable proliferative potential and tumorigenic potency. For instance, within the RTK-RAS-PI3K pathway, mutated *Ras* exhibits the strongest activity, being able to elicit early-onset and fully penetrant urothelial hyperplasia in mice without mutant overexpression (Zhang et al. 2001; Mo et al. 2007). Bi-allelic loss of *Pten* or mutational activation of *Pik3ca* also leads to urothelial hyperplasia in mice, albeit with much later onset and lower frequency (He et al. 2022; Tsuruta et al. 2006; Yoo et al. 2006). Activating mutations of *Fgfr3* or overexpression of *Egfr* in mice generates normal urothelia or late-onset hyperplasia in some instances (Zhou et al. 2016; Ahmad et al. 2011; Cheng et al. 2002).

Another layer of complexity is that, even with a single gene, different mutation sites may significantly influence the effect on proliferative potential and tumorigenicity (Hobbs et al. 2016). It has been well established in non-urothelial tissues that different *RAS* gene mutations exert different GTPase activities, resulting in different transformation potency (Muñoz-Maldonado et al. 2019). This is also true with *TP53* mutations as, depending on where the mutations are located (e.g., inside or outside the DNA-binding domain), mutant p53 may exert gain-of-function or loss-of-function effects (Vieler and Sanyal 2018). With *FGFR3* mutations, it is suggested that the locations of the mutations in the extracellular, transmembrane or cytoplasmic kinase domains may exert different effects on the kinase activity of the mutant protein (Wu 2005). This is a subject that warrants further investigation in biologically relevant experimental systems. Thus far, the underpinning for the subtypes of MIBC is lacking. It is unclear whether the divergent proliferative and tumorigenic capabilities of the different signaling pathway components may play a role in bladder cancer heterogeneity. Clearly, it would be beneficial if we interpret the genetic alterations in more granular detail by taking into account not only the different components, but also the different mutations' locations and transforming activities.

8.6 p53 and Its Family Gene p63 in Bladder Cancer

TP53 is one of, if not the most mutated gene in MIBC (Fig. 8.1), and experimental evidence confirms a strong role for this "guardian of the genome" in bladder tumorigenesis. It has long been established that TP53, via regulation of p21 and RB1, regulates cell cycle progression. Upon DNA damage, viral infection and various stresses, the expression of TP53 is upregulated, leading to elevated p21, and the release of E2F from RB1-E2F complex via phosphorylation of RB1. In response to TP53 upregulation in G2, cell cycle arrest occurs-enabling DNA repair to take place before entering M phase. Cell cycle arrest at G2 ensures DNA replication fidelity and prevents overlap between DNA repair processes with DNA replication, which may introduce mutations (Engeland 2022). The *TP53* gene encodes a 393 amino acid long peptide; a functional TAp53 that consists of four p53 monomers. It has been found that most of the TAp53 tetramers in cells with a single allele of *TP53* mutation (base substitution and frameshift mutation) will end up containing one or more mutated p53 peptides within the tetramer, and these mutant p53 tetramers no longer have proper transcription activation function (Weinberg 2007). The consequence of cells containing one or two allele *TP53* mutations is loss of cell cycle coordination, including cycle arrest when DNA repair is required. Therefore, *TP53* mutations accelerate DNA damage and cell stress, resulting in enhanced mutagenesis and tumorigenesis (Weinberg 2007). The crucial function of p53 in maintaining genome integrity and avoiding tumorigenesis is illustrated by the finding that 50% of human cancers have *TP53* mutations and 85% of these mutations are base substitutions (Hollstein et al. 1991; Olivier et al. 2010).

Mutant TP53 in MIBC has lost the ability to properly regulate the cell cycle, resulting in uninhibited proliferation. However, NMIBC cells have upregulated wild-type p53, which is supposed to serve as a break on cell proliferation (Wang et al. 2021). The lack of *CDKN1A* and *RB1* mutations (genes regulated by p53) in Ta stage bladder cancer NMIBC raises the intriguing question of how NMIBC escapes cell cycle regulation by wild type and highly expressed p53?

A recent study has shown that while MIBC cells are deficient in nucleotide and base excision repair (NER and BER, respectively) mechanisms and are hypermutable, NMIBC cells are proficient in NER and BER and are normal to hypomutable. This study also reveals that the NER and BER mechanisms in bladder cancer are controlled by the TAp63γ isoform of p63, a *TP53* family gene. MIBC cells have downregulated TAp63γ expression while NMIBC cells have upregulated TAp63γ expression (Wang et al. 2021). TAP63γ regulates the NER gene Xeroderma pigmentosum (*XPC*), and BER genes Human 8-oxoguanine DNA N-glycosylase-1/2 (*HOGG1/2*) and Apurinic/apyrimidinic endodeoxyribonuclease 1 (APEX1/*REF1*) (Wang et al. 2021). These findings raise two intriguing questions on how mutant p53 and lack of TAp63γ in MIBC and the overly expressed TAP63γ and wild-typc p53 in NMIBC deregulate cell cycle control and allow MIBC and NMIBC cells to proliferate. What are the crucial roles of mutant p53 and TAp63γ in bladder carcinogenesis and

MIBC and NMIBC development? Upregulation of TAp63 has been found in lung and cervical cancer (Massion et al. 2003; Wang et al. 2001). One simple possibility is that overwhelmed, wild-type TAp63γ monomers in NMIBC cells form heterotypic associations with p53. This is conceivable due to the high ratio of TAP63γ to p53 within cells. Theoretically, such a TAp63γ-TAp53 association would result in p53 loss of function in a manner similar to *TP53* mutant containing p53 tetramers (Adorno et al. 2009; Natan and Joerger 2012).

It should be noted that besides regulating cell cycle and cell proliferation, p53 and TAp63γ coordinate to regulate the invasion phenotype of BC. It has been found that enforced mutant *TP53* gene expression with knockdown TAp63γ expression can not only reduce NER and BER capacity and mutator phenotype, but also drive invasion. Conversely, suppression of mutant TP53 expression and enforced TAp63γ expression can convert MIBC cells to become NMIBC cells with elevated NER and BER function and normal to hypo-mutator phenotypes (Wang et al. 2021). These results demonstrate the crucial role of mutant P53 and TAp63γ in shaping the invasion, mutator and DNA repair phenotype of MIBC versus NMIBC.

8.7 Summary and Conclusions

For an overview of genetic alterations in cell cycle machinery in MIBC, see Fig. 8.1. As described in this chapter, alterations in cell cycle machinery (and their resulting impacts on cell cycle kinetics) are heavily implicated in disease pathogenesis across the clinical spectrum of bladder cancer. Although significant research has been conducted in this area, more questions remain unexplored, and therefore unanswered. For example, it is unknown if cell cycle kinetics and machinery differ in developing and regenerating urothelium, and if such differences are co-opted during tumorigenesis and/or disease progression. Because of the associations between active cell cycle in risk prediction and disease progression, it is expected that in the future, clinical tests incorporating cell cycle measures will enable patient stratification. Therefore, continued research in this area is warranted and highly significant.

References

Adorno M, Cordenonsi M, Montagner M et al (2009) A mutant-p53/Smad complex opposes p63 to empower TGFbeta-induced metastasis. Cell 137:87–98

Ahmad I, Singh LB, Foth M et al (2011) K-Ras and β-catenin mutations cooperate with Fgfr3 mutations in mice to promote tumorigenesis in the skin and lung, but not in the bladder. Dis Model Mech 4:548–555

Akkalp AK, Onur Ö, Tetikkurt Ü, Tolga D, Özsoy S, Müslümanoğlu AY (2016) Prognostic significance of mitotic activity in noninvasive, low-grade, papillary urothelial carcinoma. Anal Quant Cytopathol Histpathol 38:23–30

Alberts B (2002) Molecular biology of the cell, 4th edn. Garland Science, New York

Cheng J, Huang H, Zhang ZT et al (2002) Overexpression of epidermal growth factor receptor in urothelium elicits urothelial hyperplasia and promotes bladder tumor growth. Cancer Res 62:4157–4163

Cheng X, Lai H, Luo W et al (2021) Single-cell analysis reveals urothelial cell heterogeneity and regenerative cues following cyclophosphamide-induced bladder injury. Cell Death Dis 12:446

Choi W, Porten S, Kim S et al (2014) Identification of distinct basal and luminal subtypes of muscle-invasive bladder cancer with different sensitivities to frontline chemotherapy. Cancer Cell 25:152–165

Dalghi MG, Montalbetti N, Carattino MD, Apodaca G (2020) The Urothelium: life in a liquid environment. Physiol Rev 100:1621–1705

Damrauer JS, Hoadley KA, Chism DD et al (2014) Intrinsic subtypes of high-grade bladder cancer reflect the hallmarks of breast cancer biology. Proc Natl Acad Sci USA 111:3110–3115

Dyrskjøt L, Kruhøffer M, Thykjaer T et al (2004) Gene expression in the urinary bladder: a common carcinoma in situ gene expression signature exists disregarding histopathological classification. Cancer Res 64:4040–4048

Engeland K (2022) Cell cycle regulation: p53-p21-RB signaling. Cell Death Differ 29:946–960

Erzar E, Kerec Kos M, Lakota K, Veranič P, Erman A (2020) Does the Urothelium of old mice regenerate after chitosan injury as quickly as the urothelium of young mice? Int J Mol Sci 21

Fristrup N, Birkenkamp-Demtröder K, Reinert T et al (2013) Multicenter validation of cyclin D1, MCM7, TRIM29, and UBE2C as prognostic protein markers in non-muscle-invasive bladder cancer. Am J Pathol 182:339–349

Hanahan D, Weinberg RA (2000) The hallmarks of cancer. Cell 100:57–70
Hanahan D, Weinberg RA (2011) Hallmarks of cancer: the next generation. Cell 144:646–674
He F, Mo L, Zheng XY et al (2009) Deficiency of pRb family proteins and p53 in invasive urothelial tumorigenesis. Cancer Res 69:9413–9421
He F, Melamed J, Tang MS, Huang C, Wu XR (2015) Oncogenic HRAS activates epithelial-to-mesenchymal transition and confers stemness to p53-deficient urothelial cells to drive muscle invasion of basal subtype carcinomas. Cancer Res 75:2017–2028
He F, Zhang F, Liao Y, Tang MS, Wu XR (2022) Structural or functional defects of PTEN in urothelial cells lacking P53 drive basal/squamous-subtype muscle-invasive bladder cancer. Cancer Lett 550:215924
Hedegaard J, Lamy P, Nordentoft I et al (2016) Comprehensive transcriptional analysis of early-stage urothelial carcinoma. Cancer Cell 30:27–42
Hicks RM (1975) The mammalian urinary bladder: an accommodating organ. Biol Rev Camb Philos Soc 50:215–246
Hobbs GA, Der CJ, Rossman KL (2016) RAS isoforms and mutations in cancer at a glance. J Cell Sci 129:1287–1292
Hollstein M, Sidransky D, Vogelstein B, Harris CC (1991) p53 mutations in human cancers. Science 253:49–53
Hurst CD, Cheng G, Platt FM et al (2021) Stage-stratified molecular profiling of non-muscle-invasive bladder cancer enhances biological, clinical, and therapeutic insight. Cell Rep Med 2:100472
Jost SP (1986) Renewal of normal urothelium in adult mice. Virchows Arch B Cell Pathol Incl Mol Pathol 51:65–70
Jost SP, Potten CS (1986) Urothelial proliferation in growing mice. Cell Tissue Kinet 19:155–160
Kamoun A, de Reyniès A, Allory Y et al (2020) A consensus molecular classification of muscle-invasive bladder cancer. Eur Urol 77:420–433
Lindskrog SV, Prip F, Lamy P et al (2021) An integrated multi-omics analysis identifies prognostic molecular subtypes of non-muscle-invasive bladder cancer. Nat Commun 12:2301
Liu Y, Mémet S, Saban R et al (2015) Dual ligand/receptor interactions activate urothelial defenses against uropathogenic E. coli. Sci Rep 5:16234
Lopez-Beltran A, Luque RJ, Alvarez-Kindelan J et al (2004) Prognostic factors in survival of patients with stage Ta and T1 bladder urothelial tumors: the role of G1-S modulators (p53, p21Waf1, p27Kip1, cyclin D1, and cyclin D3), proliferation index, and clinicopathologic parameters. Am J Clin Pathol 122:444–452
Marzouka NA, Eriksson P, Rovira C, Liedberg F, Sjödahl G, Höglund M (2018) A validation and extended description of the Lund taxonomy for urothelial carcinoma using the TCGA cohort. Sci Rep 8:3737
Massion PP, Taflan PM, Jamshedur Rahman SM et al (2003) Significance of p63 amplification and overexpression in lung cancer development and prognosis. Cancer Res 63:7113–7121
Messing EM (1990) Clinical implications of the expression of epidermal growth factor receptors in human transitional cell carcinoma. Cancer Res 50:2530–2537
Messing EM, Murphy-Brooks N (1994) Recovery of epidermal growth factor in voided urine of patients with bladder cancer. Urology 44:502–506
Messing EM, Hanson P, Ulrich P, Erturk E (1987) Epidermal growth factor--interactions with normal and malignant urothelium: in vivo and in situ studies. J Urol 138:1329–1335
Mo L, Zheng X, Huang HY et al (2007) Hyperactivation of Ha-ras oncogene, but not Ink4a/Arf deficiency, triggers bladder tumorigenesis. J Clin Invest 117:314–325
Muñoz-Maldonado C, Zimmer Y, Medová M (2019) A comparative analysis of individual RAS mutations in cancer biology. Front Oncol 9:1088
Natan E, Joerger AC (2012) Structure and kinetic stability of the p63 tetramerization domain. J Mol Biol 415:503–513
Olivier M, Hollstein M, Hainaut P (2010) TP53 mutations in human cancers: origins, consequences, and clinical use. Cold Spring Harb Perspect Biol 2:a001008
Osei-Amponsa V, Buckwalter JM, Shuman L et al (2020) Hypermethylation of FOXA1 and allelic loss of PTEN drive squamous differentiation and promote heterogeneity in bladder cancer. Oncogene 39:1302–1317
Pich A, Chiusa L, Formiconi A et al (2002) Proliferative activity is the most significant predictor of recurrence in noninvasive papillary urothelial neoplasms of low malignant potential and grade 1 papillary carcinomas of the bladder. Cancer 95:784–790
Prioleau MN, MacAlpine DM (2016) DNA replication origins-where do we begin? Genes Dev 30:1683–1697
Puzio-Kuter AM, Castillo-Martin M, Kinkade CW et al (2009) Inactivation of p53 and Pten promotes invasive bladder cancer. Genes Dev 23:675–680
Rebouissou S, Hérault A, Letouzé E et al (2012) CDKN2A homozygous deletion is associated with muscle invasion in FGFR3-mutated urothelial bladder carcinoma. J Pathol 227:315–324
Robertson AG, Kim J, Al-Ahmadie H et al (2017) Comprehensive molecular characterization of muscle-invasive bladder cancer. Cell 171:540–556.e525
Robertson AG, Groeneveld CS, Jordan B et al (2020) Identification of differential tumor subtypes of T1 bladder cancer. Eur Urol 78:533–537
Schäfer FM, Algarrahi K, Savarino A et al (2017) Mode of surgical injury influences the source of urothelial progenitors during bladder defect repair. Stem Cell Rep 9:2005–2017
Sharief Y, Reich CF, Bonar RA (1980) Polyploidy in mammalian urothelial cells. Urol Res 8:153–161
Shi MJ, Fontugne J, Moreno-Vega A et al (2023) FGFR3 mutational activation can induce luminal-like papillary bladder tumor formation and favors a male sex bias. Eur Urol 83:70–81
Shuman L, Pham J, Wildermuth T et al (2023) Urothelium-specific expression of mutationally activated Pik3ca initiates early lesions of noninvasive bladder cancer. Am J Pathol 193:2133–2143

Sjödahl G, Lauss M, Lövgren K et al (2012) A molecular taxonomy for urothelial carcinoma. Clin Cancer Res 18:3377–3386

Sjödahl G, Eriksson P, Liedberg F, Höglund M (2017) Molecular classification of urothelial carcinoma: global mRNA classification versus tumour-cell phenotype classification. J Pathol 242:113–125

Tapia C, Glatz K, Obermann EC et al (2011) Evaluation of chromosomal aberrations in patients with benign conditions and reactive changes in urinary cytology. Cancer Cytopathol 119:404–410

Tsuruta H, Kishimoto H, Sasaki T et al (2006) Hyperplasia and carcinomas in Pten-deficient mice and reduced PTEN protein in human bladder cancer patients. Cancer Res 66:8389–8396

Urinary and Male Genital Tumours, 5th ed: IARC Publications; 2022; No. 8

Vieler M, Sanyal S (2018) p53 isoforms and their implications in cancer. Cancers (Basel) 10:10

Walker BE (1960) Renewal of cell populations in the female mouse. Am J Anat 107:95–105

Wang TY, Chen BF, Yang YC et al (2001) Histologic and immunophenotypic classification of cervical carcinomas by expression of the p53 homologue p63: a study of 250 cases. Hum Pathol 32:479–486

Wang MJ, Chen F, Lau JTY, Hu YP (2017) Hepatocyte polyploidization and its association with pathophysiological processes. Cell Death Dis 8:e2805

Wang J, Batourina E, Schneider K et al (2018) Polyploid superficial cells that maintain the urothelial barrier are produced via incomplete cytokinesis and Endoreplication. Cell Rep 25:464–477.e464

Wang HT, Lee HW, Weng MW et al (2021) The role of TAp63γ and P53 point mutations in regulating DNA repair, mutational susceptibility and invasion of bladder cancer cells. eLife 10:10

Warrick JI, Knowles MA, Hurst CD et al (2022) A transcriptional network of cell cycle dysregulation in noninvasive papillary urothelial carcinoma. Sci Rep 12:16538

Weinberg RA (2007) The biology of cancer. Garland Science, New York, NY

Wu XR (2005) Urothelial tumorigenesis: a tale of divergent pathways. Nat Rev Cancer 5:713–725

Wu XR (2009) Biology of urothelial tumorigenesis: insights from genetically engineered mice. Cancer Metastasis Rev 28:281–290

Wu XR, Kong XP, Pellicer A, Kreibich G, Sun TT (2009) Uroplakins in urothelial biology, function, and disease. Kidney Int 75:1153–1165

Xia Y, Liu Y, Yang C et al (2021) Dominant role of CDKN2B/p15INK4B of 9p21.3 tumor suppressor hub in inhibition of cell-cycle and glycolysis. Nat Commun 12:2047

Yoo LI, Liu DW, Le Vu S, Bronson RT, Wu H, Yuan J (2006) Pten deficiency activates distinct downstream signaling pathways in a tissue-specific manner. Cancer Res 66:1929–1939

Zaleski M, Gogoj A, Walter V et al (2019) Mitotic activity in noninvasive papillary urothelial carcinoma: its value in predicting tumor recurrence and comparison with the contemporary 2-tier grading system. Hum Pathol 84:275–282

Zhang ZT, Pak J, Huang HY et al (2001) Role of Ha-ras activation in superficial papillary pathway of urothelial tumor formation. Oncogene 20:1973–1980

Zhou H, He F, Mendelsohn CL, Tang MS, Huang C, Wu XR (2016) FGFR3b extracellular loop mutation lacks tumorigenicity in vivo but collaborates with p53/pRB deficiency to induce high-grade papillary urothelial carcinoma. Sci Rep 6:25596

9 DNA Repair Pathway Alterations in Bladder Cancer

Vincent D. D'Andrea and Kent W. Mouw

Abstract

Urothelial cells are under constant exposure to endogenous and exogenous sources of DNA damage. Multiple DNA repair pathways are active in normal urothelial cells and coordinate to repair damage and maintain genomic integrity. However, loss of DNA repair fidelity is common in tumors, and DNA repair genes are among the most frequently mutated genes in bladder cancer. Multiple lines of preclinical and clinical evidence indicate that bladder tumor DNA repair pathway deficiency drives unique biological properties and therapeutic vulnerabilities. This chapter reviews the major sources of DNA damage in urothelial cells and the genomic consequences of mutagen exposure. In addition, we discuss the frequency and biological impact of alterations in critical DNA repair pathways including mismatch repair (MMR), homologous recombination (HR) repair, and nucleotide excision repair (NER). Finally, we highlight several recent and on-going bladder cancer clinical trials designed to test the impact of targeting specific DNA repair-deficient states. DNA repair deficiency is a defining feature of a subset of bladder tumors and efforts to therapeutically exploit DNA repair deficiency hold promise in several bladder cancer clinical settings.

Keywords

Bladder cancer · DNA repair · DNA damage · PARP inhibitor · Biomarker

9.1 DNA Damage and Repair Processes in Urothelium

Urothelial cells play a unique and critical role in acting as a barrier and forming a reservoir for urine. In this role, urothelial cells are constantly exposed to endogenous and exogenous sources of DNA damage (Fig. 9.1) (Crawford 2008). Endogenous damage can arise from errors in DNA replication, reactive oxygen species (ROS), activity of cytidine deaminases (e.g., APOBEC enzymes), and other intracellular sources. Exogenous sources of DNA damage include many known carcinogens and toxic metabolites

V. D. D'Andrea
Department of Surgery, Division of Urology, Brigham and Women's Hospital, Boston, MA, USA

Harvard Medical School, Boston, MA, USA

K. W. Mouw (✉)
Harvard Medical School, Boston, MA, USA

Department of Radiation Oncology, Dana-Farber Cancer Institute, Brigham and Women's Hospital, Boston, MA, USA

Broad Institute of MIT and Harvard, Cambridge, MA, USA
e-mail: kent_mouw@dfci.harvard.edu

M. A. Knowles, L. Dyrskjøt (eds.), *Biology of Bladder Cancer*,
https://doi.org/10.1007/978-3-031-68505-7_9

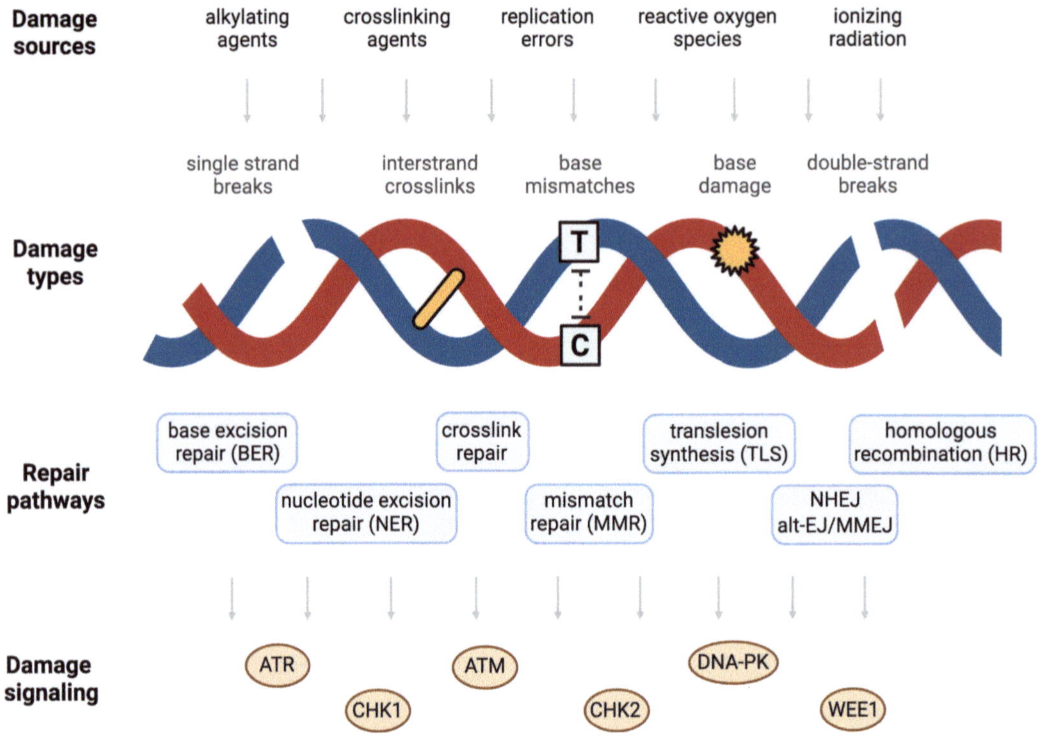

Fig. 9.1 Overview of cellular DNA damage and repair processes

that are filtered by the kidney and excreted in the urine (Cumberbatch et al. 2018).

In order to maintain genomic integrity and ensure cellular homeostasis, urothelial cells rely on DNA repair pathways to detect and repair DNA damage (Mouw 2017). These DNA repair pathways include high-fidelity mechanisms such as homologous recombination (HR), nucleotide excision repair (NER), and mismatch repair (MMR), as well as lower-fidelity pathways including translesion synthesis (TLS) and non-homologous end joining (NHEJ) (Jeggo et al. 2016). Pathway dynamics and repair outcomes depend upon the amount and type of DNA damage as well as on cellular properties including cell cycle state, transcriptional activity, and extracellular signaling cues (Hoeijmakers 2009).

The constant exposure of urothelial cells to genotoxins as well as the frequent loss of DNA repair fidelity conferred by DNA repair gene alterations drive the complexity and heterogeneity of the bladder tumor genome (Robertson et al. 2017; Pelucchi et al. 2006). Bladder tumors have among the highest mutational burden of any solid tumor type, and in addition to frequent single nucleotide variants (SNVs) and short insertions/deletions (indels), bladder tumors also commonly display large-scale copy-number alterations (CNAs) as well as frequent chromosomal translocations (see also Chap. 7) (Robertson et al. 2017). Mutational signature analyses from bladder tumor whole exome and whole genome sequencing (WES/WGS) efforts have identified multiple underlying mutagenic processes that contribute to the complex mutational landscape of bladder tumors (Robertson et al. 2017; Alexandrov et al. 2020; Volkova et al. 2020). Although the total mutational burden as well as the contribution of specific mutagenic processes varies significantly across bladder tumors, the largest contributor in most cohorts is APOBEC-mediated mutagenesis (Glaser et al. 2018). APOBEC enzymes evolved as an anti-viral defense mechanism and primarily deaminate cytosine to uracil within single-stranded DNA and RNA, but APOBEC enzymes can also damage genomic DNA, leading to a characteristic pattern of cytosine to thymine mutations (Liu et al. 2023).

In addition to APOBEC activity, mutational signature analysis has identified several other known mutagenic processes that are active in bladder cancer (Kim et al. 2016). These include signatures that are common across tumors and tumor types, such as an age-related "molecular clock" signature arising from spontaneous deamination of 5-methylcytosine and characterized by cytosine to thymine mutations (Alexandrov et al. 2015). Despite the known association between tobacco exposure and bladder cancer, a tobacco-associated mutational signature identified in smoking-related lung and head and neck cancers is not observed in bladder cancer. However, recent analysis of bladder WGS identified a unique single base substitution signature (SBS92) that was enriched in bladder tumors from patients with a smoking history and is characterized by purine damage with a strong transcriptional strand bias, consistent with DNA damage mediated by known tobacco carcinogens (Islam et al. 2022). Finally, well-characterized mutational signatures due to specific tumor DNA repair pathway defects such as MMR deficiency, HR deficiency, polymerase epsilon (POLE) exonuclease ("proofreading") mutations, or NER deficiency are present in subsets of bladder tumors harboring these specific DNA repair pathway defects and are discussed in detail below.

9.2 DNA Repair Deficiency in Bladder Tumors

DNA repair pathway genes are among the most commonly altered class of genes in numerous cancer types including bladder cancer (Mouw 2017; Robertson et al. 2017). Despite the known prevalence of DNA repair gene alterations in tumors, the biological role of DNA repair dysregulation in tumorigenesis and tumor evolution is poorly understood. It is possible that loss of DNA repair capacity could increase DNA damage tolerance, thereby avoiding damage-induced cell death while also promoting genetic instability and tumor evolution through the upregulation of error-prone back-up DNA repair mechanisms (Jeggo et al. 2016). In addition, DNA repair dysfunction may induce pro-tumorigenic changes in the tumor microenvironment (Kawanishi et al. 2017). Further mechanistic studies are needed to define the role of DNA repair pathway dysregulation during bladder tumor initiation and invasion.

DNA repair genes are commonly organized into DNA repair pathways (Fig. 9.1). Some DNA repair genes have clear and well-defined critical roles in a specific DNA repair pathway (e.g., BRCA1/2 in HR). However, other genes may play a role in several pathways (e.g., RECQL4, SLX4) or are required for DNA damage signaling following activation of multiple pathways (e.g., ATM, ATR). There is no consensus classification scheme for DNA repair genes, and different studies have used different approaches to define DNA repair genes and to organize these genes into pathways. These differences in classification can lead to apparent differences in overall or pathway-specific DNA repair gene mutation frequencies across studies.

Many DNA repair gene alterations arise somatically within tumors as a result of mutagenic processes. However, it is becoming increasingly apparent that a subset of DNA repair gene alterations are inherited (i.e., present in the germline). Several recent studies have included analysis of bladder cancer patients' germline DNA and indicate that 5–15% of bladder cancer patients harbor a potentially deleterious germline DNA repair gene alteration (Carlo et al. 2020). The apparent frequency of germline DNA repair gene alterations depends both upon the DNA sequencing platform and mutation-calling approach as well as on the patient cohort, with rates often higher in younger populations, those without known exposure to bladder cancer risk factors (e.g., tobacco exposure), or those with a significant family history of cancer (Mossanen et al. 2022). These germline DNA repair gene alterations can involve one of several DNA repair pathways including mismatch repair (i.e., Lynch syndrome), homologous recombination (e.g., *BRCA1/2*), or DNA damage signaling (e.g., *ATM*, *CHK2*) and are discussed in detail below.

DNA repair genes typically act as tumor suppressors. Therefore, pathogenic alterations in DNA repair genes are typically those that compromise the normal function of the gene. Some classes of alterations such as frameshift or nonsense mutations result in a truncated protein product that is very unlikely to be able to perform its normal function. The functional impact of other classes of alterations including missense mutations or mutations in non-coding regions such as splice site and 5′ or 3′ untranslated regions (UTRs) are more difficult to predict. Missense mutations in particular present an important challenge because many DNA repair genes are quite large, and given that the overall mutation burden in many bladder tumors is quite high, missense mutations in DNA repair genes are common. Although some missense mutations occur recurrently in critical positions within the protein (i.e., mutational hotspots) leading to loss-of-function, most missense mutations in DNA repair genes arise in non-recurrent positions throughout the protein and thus are less likely to impair protein function or drive a DNA repair-deficient state. Several approaches can be employed to infer the functional impact of specific DNA repair alterations. These include identifying specific amino acid positions that are mutated more frequently than would be expected by chance and/or predicting the biochemical or structural impact of the observed amino acid change (Adzhubei et al. 2010; Vaser et al. 2016; Li and Wang 2017). However, different studies often use markedly different approaches to identify presumed deleterious missense mutations, and these technical differences can lead to dramatic differences in the apparent frequency of DNA repair gene alterations as well as differences in apparent associations between "DNA repair deficiency" (as defined in the specific study) and clinical outcomes.

In addition to germline or somatic mutations detected within tumors, DNA repair gene function can also be impacted via gene loss. Deep (i.e., homozygous) deletion of a DNA repair gene can lead to DNA repair-deficient phenotype. More commonly, loss-of-heterozygosity (LOH), occurs within a tumor harboring a heterozygous pathogenic DNA repair gene alteration, resulting in loss of the second (wild-type) copy of the gene and leading to DNA repair deficiency. Epigenetic silencing of DNA repair genes occurs in some tumor types (e.g., *BRCA1* methylation in breast cancer), but has not been widely observed as a mechanism of DNA repair deficiency in bladder cancer.

Identification of predicted deleterious mutation(s) and/or loss of DNA repair genes through tumor next-generation sequencing (NGS) remains the most common approach used to identify DNA repair deficiency in bladder cancer. However, this approach has several limitations, including a focus on only pre-defined DNA repair genes of interest, thus potentially missing mechanisms of DNA repair deficiency arising via mutations in genes not classically considered to play a role in DNA repair. NGS is also unable to detect non-genetic mechanisms of DNA repair deficiency such as modulation of function at the transcriptional (e.g., epigenetic silencing) or protein (e.g., post-translational modification) levels. Several alternative methods for identifying tumor DNA repair deficiency have been reported and continue to be investigated. Mutational signature analysis also relies on tumor NGS data but attempts to identify mutational patterns reflective of specific DNA repair-deficient settings (Ma et al. 2018). Numerous studies have identified specific mutational signatures driven by mismatch repair (MMR), homologous recombination (HR), and nucleotide excision repair (NER) deficiency and these are discussed in detail below. Immunohistochemical (IHC) approaches detect DNA repair deficiency at the protein level and are commonly employed to detect MMR deficiency. Similar IHC techniques are also being investigated to detect HR deficiency as measured by loss of radiation-induced foci of the central HR protein, Rad51 (Hoppe et al. 2021; Konstantinopoulos et al. 2021). Although these IHC-based approaches are attractive because complete loss of a DNA repair protein is very likely to confer DNA repair deficiency, complete protein loss may not be necessary to confer DNA repair deficiency (as in the case of a deleterious missense mutation).

9.3 Mismatch Repair

The mismatch repair (MRR) pathway is a highly conserved DNA repair pathway that has evolved to repair DNA base mismatches that arise primarily due to nucleotide misincorporation by the replicative DNA polymerases epsilon (POLE) and delta (POLD1) (Pecina-Slaus et al. 2020). Although POLE and POLD1 are high-fidelity polymerases with base misincorporation rates of approximately 1×10^{-5}, which is further improved to ~1×10^{-6} by their exonuclease (proofreading) function, numerous base mismatches occur when replicating a genome of ~3×10^{9} bases. The role of the MMR pathway is to detect and remove misincorporated nucleotides, thereby avoiding the potential for a stable mutation to arise during the following cell division.

The genetics and biochemistry of the MMR pathway have been elucidated over decades of work using bacterial, yeast, and human systems (Li 2008). Mismatched bases lead to loss of the normal helical structure of the DNA duplex and are recognized and bound by the MSH2-MSH6 heterodimer. MSH2-MSH6 recruits the MLH1-PMS2 complex which initiates cleavage of the strand containing the misincorporated base(s). Additional catalytic and regulatory members of the pathway are recruited and ultimately a polymerase (often POLD1) is recruited to fill-in the single-stranded gap, using the remaining (parental) strand as a template. DNA ligation follows to return the duplex to its intact, error-free state.

Mismatch repair deficiency (MMRd) arises when one or more components of the MMR machinery is functionally deficient due to mutation and/or epigenetic silencing. The impact of MMR loss is particularly evident in regions of the genome containing short repeat sequences known as microsatellites. Due to the repetitive nature of these DNA sequences, polymerase slipping can occur, resulting in expansion of the number of microsatellite repeats. In the absence of the MMR pathway to repair these over-replicated regions, the number of microsatellite repeats increases over time, a phenomenon known as microsatellite instability (MSI).

MMRd can arise via germline or somatic events. Lynch syndrome is an autosomal dominant disease caused by inheritance of a mutated copy of one of the MMR genes (e.g., *MLH1, MSH2, MSH6*, or *PMS2*) (Lynch et al. 2015). Lynch syndrome is characterized by increased risk of multiple cancers, including colorectal, endometrial, urothelial, gastric, and ovarian cancer. Although Lynch syndrome patients inherit only one mutated copy of an MMR gene, the second copy is frequently lost or mutated in tissues, leading to complete lack of MMR function and subsequent tumor development. Lynch syndrome-associated tumors can be diagnosed by IHC demonstrating complete loss of one or more of the MMR proteins, by polymerase chain reaction (PCR) showing expansion of known microsatellite regions, or by NGS showing a mutation in an MMR gene and/or a mutational signature characterized by a dramatic increase in characteristic short indels (Stadler et al. 2016).

Lynch syndrome patients are at significantly increased risk of developing urothelial cancer with lifetime risk as high as 25% in some case series (Skeldon et al. 2013; van der Post et al. 2010). For reasons that remain incompletely understood, the increase in risk of upper tract urothelial cancer (UTUC) is significantly higher than bladder cancer in Lynch syndrome patients. Large cohorts of bladder cancer patients with available germline sequencing suggest that the frequency of Lynch syndrome is 1–3% (Carlo et al. 2020). Importantly, Lynch syndrome patients often present at an early age and lack classic risk factors often associated with urothelial cancer.

In addition to MMR loss caused by an inherited MMR gene mutation, somatic loss of MMR function also occurs in a subset of bladder tumors. In The Cancer Genome Atlas (TCGA) cohort of muscle-invasive bladder tumors, approximately 2% of patients harbor loss or mutation of *MLH1, MSH2, MSH6*, or *PMS2* (Robertson et al. 2017). MMR-deficient bladder tumors arising from either germline or somatic events are generally characterized by a high tumor mutational burden (TMB) including frequent short indels. Many MMR-deficient tumors have high levels of

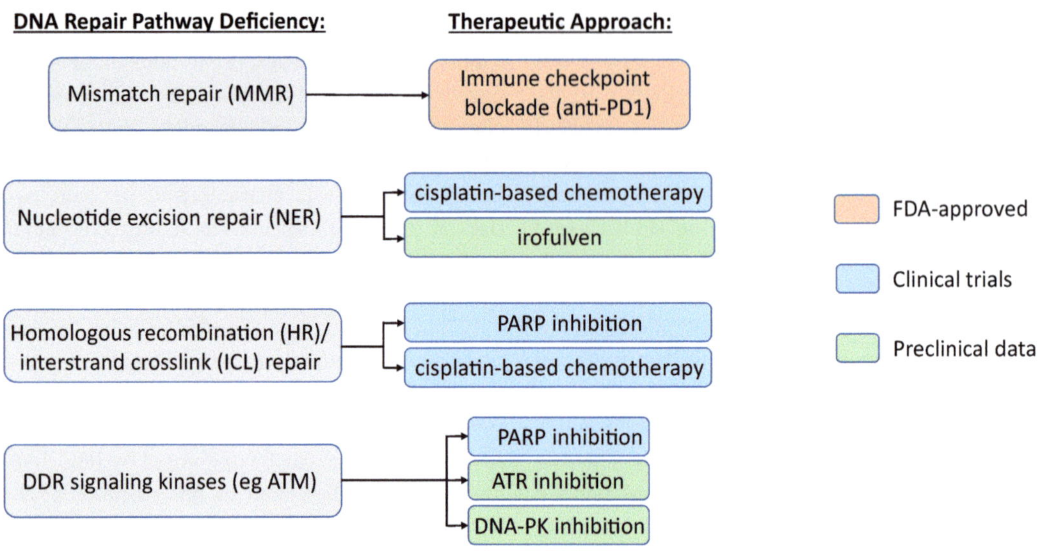

Fig. 9.2 Pathway-specific approaches to target DNA repair deficiency in bladder cancer

immune infiltration due to increased levels of neoantigens and other mechanisms (Le et al. 2015; Kelderman et al. 2015). The rich immune infiltrate present in many MMRd/MSI tumors is the basis for recent exciting therapeutic developments including the tumor-type agnostic FDA approval of the anti-PD1 agent pembrolizumab for treatment of advanced MMRd/MSI tumors, including urothelial cancer (Fig. 9.2). Although MMRd/MSI status is not currently used to inform first-line treatment for muscle-invasive bladder cancer (MIBC), anti-PD1/PD-L1 agents including pembrolizumab have established roles in the metastatic setting (see Chap. 23). Given that molecular testing including tumor DNA sequencing and specialized IHC are increasingly common in clinical practice, bladder cancer patients with MMRd/MSI tumors detected by one of these methods may be prioritized for pembrolizumab or other immune-directed approaches.

9.4 Nucleotide Excision Repair

The NER pathway is a highly conserved DNA repair pathway that primarily repairs bulky intrastrand DNA adducts created by genotoxins such as ultraviolet (UV) irradiation or platinum chemotherapies (Marteijn et al. 2014). There are two distinct sub-pathways through which NER can be activated: the global genome NER pathway (GG-NER or GGR) recognizes lesions throughout the genome whereas the transcription-coupled pathway (TC-NER or TCR) is activated when transcribing RNA polymerase stalls at a lesion. GGR and TCR then converge on a shared pathway that involves DNA duplex unwinding at the lesion site by DNA helicases ERCC2 and ERCC3 followed by removal of a portion of single-stranded DNA that contains the lesion by the DNA nucleases ERCC4/ERCC1 and ERCC5 (Fuss and Tainer 2011). The resulting gap is then filled by a DNA polymerase followed by ligation of the DNA backbone by a DNA ligase to restore an intact DNA duplex with the original (pre-damage) sequence.

The presence of bi-allelic germline inactivating mutations in an NER gene can result in xeroderma pigmentosum (XP), a rare inherited disorder characterized by extreme UV sensitivity and increased cancer predisposition (Kraemer et al. 2007). Although some studies have suggested a higher rate of bladder cancer or other tumor types in heterozygous carriers of an inactivating NER gene alteration (Chang et al. 2012), these reports have not been validated in larger cohorts and there is currently no role for germline testing or increased cancer surveillance in patients with known or suspected heterozygous germline NER gene alterations.

Somatic alterations in NER genes are relatively uncommon in cancer, particularly compared to the frequency in other DNA repair genes such as *BRCA1/2*, *ATM*, and MMR genes across cancer types. However, one notable exception is *ERCC2*. Whereas no other tumor type has an *ERCC2* mutation frequency of greater than ~2–3%, *ERCC2* is recurrently altered in bladder cancer with 8–15% of muscle-invasive bladder cancers (MIBCs) possessing a somatic *ERCC2* missense mutation (Robertson et al. 2017; Van Allen et al. 2014). *ERCC2* mutations are associated with activity of a specific mutational signature in bladder tumors which may in part reflect the unique mutagenic repair events occurring in *ERCC2*-deficient bladder tumors (Kim et al. 2016).

The potential clinical significance of *ERCC2* mutations was first identified in a study which performed whole exome sequencing (WES) of pre-treatment MIBCs in patients treated with neoadjuvant cisplatin-based chemotherapy followed by radical cystectomy (Van Allen et al. 2014). The cohort was comprised of 50 patients, and was selected to include 25 "responders" with no residual invasive disease and 25 "non-responders" with residual MIBC at the time of cystectomy. The only gene with mutations that were significantly enriched in responders compared to non-responders was *ERCC2* (8/25 vs. 0/25, $p < 0.001$). This association between somatic *ERCC2* mutations and improved response to cisplatin-based chemotherapy has been validated in additional clinical cohorts (Liu et al. 2016; Gil-Jimenez et al. 2023); however, other cohorts have failed to identify this association (Christensen et al. 2019; Groenendijk et al. 2016; Taber et al. 2020), perhaps owing to differences in clinical characteristics, sequencing, or mutation-calling approaches. The majority of observed *ERCC2* mutations are missense mutations in one of the two conserved helicase domains of the gene, and functional work has demonstrated that the majority of these clinically observed helicase domain mutations are unable to rescue cellular NER deficiency or cisplatin sensitivity of an ERCC2-deficient cell, suggestive of loss-of-function (Li et al. 2019). Similarly, ERCC2-deficient bladder cancer cells are also sensitive to irofulven, a previously discarded anti-cancer agent that creates DNA adducts that are uniquely recognized and repaired by the TCR pathway (Fig. 9.2) (Borcsok et al. 2021a). A potential role for *ERCC2* mutations to direct therapy decisions in MIBC is currently being tested in several on-going Phase II clinical trials that are discussed below.

In addition to somatic *ERCC2* mutations identified by NGS, other NER genes/proteins have also been associated with clinical outcomes in bladder cancer. Using RT-PCR to investigate the association between mRNA transcript levels of DNA repair genes and clinical outcomes in advanced bladder cancer patients treated with cisplatin-based chemotherapy, an association between low ERCC1 levels and improved clinical outcomes was identified (Bellmunt et al. 2007). This association was more recently validated at the protein level, with lower levels of ERCC1 protein measured by IHC associated with improved outcomes in a separate patient cohort (Mullane et al. 2016). However, other studies in cystectomy- or chemoradiotherapy-treated cohorts have shown the opposite relationship between ERCC1 protein levels and clinical outcomes (Klatte et al. 2015; Sakano et al. 2013). It is unclear at this point if these differences reflect real differences in the biological role of ERCC1 or whether they may be due to issues with technical reproducibility or assay interpretation.

9.5 Homologous Recombination Repair

Double-strand DNA breaks (DSBs) are one of the most toxic DNA lesions and can arise following DNA damage from a variety of sources including ionizing radiation, free radicals, and several types of chemotherapeutics. Given the potential toxicity of DSBs, several DSB repair mechanisms exist within cells and operate in a cell- and context-dependent manner (Scully et al.

2019). The homologous recombination (HR) repair pathway is the primary error-free (non-mutagenic) DSB repair pathway within eukaryotic cells, whereas classic non-homologous end joining (NHEJ) and microhomology-mediated end joining (MMEJ) often generate mutations during the repair process (Ceccaldi et al. 2016). The HR pathway requires an undamaged DNA duplex with homologous sequence to be used as a repair template; therefore, HR can only occur in the S-G2 phases of the cell cycle when two homologous sister chromatids are present. Conversely, NHEJ and MMEJ do not require a homologous DNA sequence and therefore can function during any phase of the cell cycle. For DSBs undergoing HR-mediated repair, the DSB is first processed to generate a 3′ single-strand DNA overhang, which is subsequently coated by Rad51. This Rad51-coated ssDNA invades the undamaged (donor) DNA duplex, searching for and ultimately binding to the homologous sequence. DNA synthesis then occurs to extend the 3′ ssDNA using the homologous sequence as a template. Following extension, the intermediate recombination structures are resolved through strand displacement and re-annealing and/or by structure-specific DNA endonucleases to restore undamaged, intact DNA duplexes (Wright et al. 2018).

HR has been studied extensively in cancer due to the frequency of alterations in the canonical HR genes *BRCA1* and *BRCA2* in several tumor types. *BRCA1/2*-mutant tumors frequently display characteristic features of an HR-deficient phenotype including presence of a mutational signature characterized by high mutation frequency and many short indels which arise when NHEJ and/or MMEJ are upregulated in the absence of HR repair (Nik-Zainal et al. 2016; Polak et al. 2017). Importantly, HR-deficient tumors also display increased sensitivity to some DNA damaging agents including platinum-based chemotherapy, as well as exquisite sensitivity to small molecule inhibitors of poly-(ADP ribose) polymerase (PARP; Fig. 9.2) (Farmer et al. 2005; Bryant et al. 2005). PARP inhibitors disrupt cellular processing of single-strand DNA breaks, thus resulting in a dramatic increase in double-strand breaks which are normally repaired by HR. PARP inhibitors are currently FDA-approved in specific clinical contexts in breast, ovarian, pancreatic, and prostate cancer.

In bladder cancer, large-scale sequencing efforts have identified a small fraction of patients with likely deleterious germline or somatic alterations in HR genes. For example, in TCGA cohort, ~5% of patients harbored a predicted deleterious mutation in an HR gene such as *BRCA1*, *BRCA2, PALB2*, or *RAD51B/C/D* (Robertson et al. 2017; Borcsok et al. 2021b). Similarly, germline studies have also identified that a small percentage of bladder cancer patients harbor inherited mutations in *BRCA1/2* (Carlo et al. 2020; Borcsok et al. 2021b). The apparent frequency of these alterations may depend upon cohort characteristics, with germline alterations in *BRCA1/2* (or other DNA repair genes) more common in younger patients, those without classic bladder cancer risk factors, or those with a family history of bladder cancer or other tumor types.

Although *BRCA1/2* are the HR genes mutated most frequently in bladder cancer (albeit with a low overall frequency), predicted deleterious mutations in other known HR genes (such as *PALB2, RAD51C*, or *BARD1*), or in genes with roles in HR-mediated signaling (such as *ATM* and *CHK2*) also occur in a subset of cases, but the impact of these alterations on HR function is less certain and may depend upon the type of alteration as well as the cell context. In addition, approximately 10–20% of bladder tumors have evidence of HR deficiency identified by the presence of specific HR mutational signatures (Borcsok et al. 2021b). Because only a fraction of these cases harbors a mutation in a known HR gene, it is possible that functional HR deficiency may arise via alternative, as-yet uncharacterized genetic or epigenetic mechanisms in bladder tumors.

Much of the interest in HR deficiency in bladder cancer is appropriately focused on the potential to target HR deficiency with specific therapies such as platinum chemotherapies or PARP inhibitors. Because *BRCA1/2*-mutant cases are relatively rare, the statistical power is limited to identify correlations between HR deficiency mediated by *BRCA1/2* alterations and response to platinum-based chemotherapy. However, a recent study by Taber et al. comprising more than 300 MIBC patients identified an association between *BRCA2* alterations and improved response to platinum-based chemotherapy (Taber et al. 2020). In addition, *BRCA1/2* are included in the DNA repair gene lists being used to enroll patients on several Phase II clinical trials investigating cystectomy avoidance following cisplatin-based neoadjuvant chemotherapy (discussed below). It seems likely that, although rare, deleterious alterations in *BRCA2* (and perhaps *BRCA1*) may confer clinically relevant sensitivity to platinum-based chemotherapy in bladder cancer.

BRCA1/2-mutant bladder tumors are also predicted to show increased sensitivity to PARP inhibition. Several PARP inhibitor clinical trials have now been published in advanced bladder cancer cohorts and are discussed in detail below. In the most recently published trials, there appears to be a clinical benefit of PARP inhibitor treatment in patients with tumors predicted to harbor deleterious DNA repair gene defects. However, data from additional planned and ongoing trials will be required to validate this association and further define the optimal biomarker(s) for PARP inhibitor sensitivity in bladder cancer.

9.6 Other DNA Damage and Repair Genes

MRE11 (encoded by the *MRE11A* gene) is a DNA endonuclease that is part of the MRN complex (MRE11-RAD50-NBS1) that plays a critical role in the sensing and repair of DNA double-strand breaks (Syed and Tainer 2018). MRE11 protein levels measured by IHC were found to be associated with clinical outcomes in a cohort of tumors from MIBC patients treated with curative-intent radiation (Choudhury et al. 2010). Specifically, patients with tumors that had MRE11 expression in the lowest quartile had significantly worse cause-specific survival (CSS) than patients with higher MRE11 expression (3-year CSS, 43% vs. 69%). This association was validated in an independent radiation cohort, and importantly, the association was not observed in a separate cohort of MIBC patients treated with cystectomy. Therefore, the authors concluded that MRE11 expression by IHC was associated with outcomes in MIBC patients treated with radiation, but not in MIBC patients treated with cystectomy. A similar association between low MRE11 expression and worse clinical outcomes with radiation but not cystectomy was subsequently reported by a separate group (Laurberg et al. 2012). However, MRE11 IHC analysis of tumors from BC2001 and BCON, two large randomized trials of radiation-based treatment for MIBC, failed to reproduce this association (Walker et al. 2019). Most recently, a pooled analysis of tumors from six RTOG/NRG radiation-based clinical trials used an immunofluorescence (IF)-based assay to measure the MRE11 nuclear/cytoplasm (N/C) signal ratio (Magliocco et al. 2022). Patients with an MRE11 N/C ratio above the first quartile had significantly lower disease-specific mortality (DSM) than patients with MRE11 N/C ratio below the first quartile (4-year DSM, 21% vs. 41%). However, MRE11 N/C ratio was not associated with overall survival in the study. Additional studies are planned to further characterize the association between MRE11 protein levels and clinical outcomes in MIBC. Functional studies are also needed to define the mechanistic underpinnings of this association since it is somewhat counterintuitive that lower levels of a DNA repair protein such as MRE11 would be associated with worse outcomes. It is possible that lack of MRE11 may fail to trigger appropriate DNA damage signaling, thus leading to continued proliferation despite DNA damage, or that high levels of MRE11 are a futile attempt to upregulate DNA repair within tumor cells that lack sufficient DNA repair capacity due to loss of another required component.

ATM is a kinase that plays a central role in the DNA damage response. ATM is activated following a variety of types of DNA damage and is responsible for coordinating repair events at the damage site as well as regulating downstream effectors including cell cycle, growth, and immune programs. *ATM* mutations are common in a variety of tumor types, and *ATM* is one of the most frequently mutated DNA repair genes in bladder cancer (Robertson et al. 2017). However, the apparent frequency of *ATM* alterations in bladder tumor cohorts depends upon the criteria used to nominate mutations. Because *ATM* is a large gene and because the majority of observed tumor *ATM* alterations are missense mutations, the functional impact of most *ATM* mutations are unknown.

Given its critical role in the DNA damage response, there has been considerable interest in targeting ATM deficiency in bladder cancer and other tumor types (Fig. 9.2) (Brown et al. 2017). Recently, it was reported that MIBC patients with a tumor alteration in *ATM* or one of two other genes (*RB1* or *FANCC*) were more likely to experience complete pathologic response to cisplatin-based neoadjuvant chemotherapy prior to cystectomy (Plimack et al. 2015). *ATM* has also been included in the gene panels for several retrospective studies linking DDR gene alterations with improved outcomes following cisplatin-based chemotherapy in MIBC and metastatic settings (Iyer et al. 2022; Teo et al. 2017). However, the specific contribution of *ATM* alterations (vs. alterations in other panel genes) to these observed associations with clinical response is uncertain. Similarly, *ATM* has also been included in DDR gene panels used to identify bladder cancer patients who may be more likely to respond to a PARP inhibitor. However, reported trial results include only a small number of patients with *ATM*-mutated tumors and additional data will be needed to define the impact of *ATM* mutations on PARP inhibitor response.

9.7 DNA Repair Deficiency and the Immune Response

The clinical development and subsequent regulatory approvals of anti-PD1/PD-L1 agents has transformed the treatment landscape of advanced bladder cancer in recent years (Rhea et al. 2021). However, only a subset of patients benefit from these agents, and despite considerable efforts, there are no validated predictive biomarkers that are routinely used to identify bladder cancer patients who are most likely to benefit (Aggen and Drake 2017).

Tumor DNA repair deficiency can impact the immune microenvironment (Mouw and D'Andrea 2018), and the association between DNA repair deficiency and anti-PD1/PD-L1 response is being studied across DNA repair pathways and tumor types (Mouw et al. 2017). The strongest data linking a specific DNA repair pathway deficiency with anti-PD1/PD-L1 benefit is in the setting of MMRd/MSI. MMRd results in an increased number of short indels which can lead to production of tumor-specific neoantigens that elicit an anti-tumor immune response (Le et al. 2015; Kelderman et al. 2015). Pembrolizumab (anti-PD1) is FDA-approved for treatment of advanced MMRd/MSI tumors independent of histologic subtype, including patients with metastatic MMRd/MSI urothelial cancer arising from the bladder or upper tract.

Although very rare among bladder tumors (~1% of tumors), missense mutations in the exonuclease (proofreading) domain of the replicative DNA polymerases *POLE* or *POLD1* can result in an extremely high number of point (missense) mutations and subsequent production of tumor-specific neoantigens. Accordingly, *POLE/POLD1*-mutant tumors display high response rates to anti-PD1/PD-L1 agents in small case series (Johanns et al. 2016; van Gool et al. 2015). The impact of homologous recombination (HR) deficiency on the immune microenvironment has been studied extensively in tumor types such as breast and ovarian cancer which have high rates of HR deficiency (van Wilpe et al. 2021), but no validated role for HR deficiency as an anti-PD1/PD-L1 response predictor has been defined. The impact of HR deficiency on the immune microenvironment and anti-PD1/PD-L1 response in tumor types with lower rates of HR deficiency such as bladder cancer is less well characterized. NER deficiency is more common in bladder cancer than most other tumor types due to 8–15% of bladder tumors harboring an *ERCC2* mutation; however, the association between NER deficiency and immune dynamics is poorly characterized.

Given that the frequency of alterations for most individual DNA repair genes is relatively low in bladder cancer, several studies have performed pooled analyses by grouping tumors with alterations in one or more DNA repair genes across DNA repair pathways. One such retrospective analysis of metastatic urothelial cancer patients enrolled on several Phase II trials of atezolizumab (anti-PD-L1) or nivolumab (anti-PD1) reported improved response rates (69% vs. 19%) in patients whose tumor had an alteration in at least one gene across a panel of 34 DNA repair genes (Teo et al. 2018). However, analyses of other cohorts have not consistently shown a similar association, although heterogeneity among clinical cohorts and differences in sequencing and mutation-calling approaches limits cross-study comparison.

Tumor mutational burden (TMB) reflects DNA damage and repair events in the tumor, and tumors with DNA repair deficiency conferred by deleterious alterations in specific DNA repair genes (such as *BRCA1/2, ERCC2*, etc.) often have high TMB. However, the relationship between DNA repair gene alterations and TMB is complex: not all tumors with high TMB have obvious DNA repair gene defects, and conversely, alterations (particularly passenger mutations) in DNA repair genes are more likely as TMB increases (Weir et al. 2022). Because tumor mutations can stimulate an anti-tumor immune response through increased neoantigens and other mechanisms, there is significant interest in the correlation between TMB and anti-PD1/PD-L1 response (Queiroz et al. 2021). Multiple studies have demonstrated a positive correlation between TMB and anti-PD1/PD-L1 benefit across tumor types (Samstein et al. 2019; Valero et al. 2021), and pembrolizumab is FDA-approved for patients with advanced solid tumors harboring a TMB equal to or greater than 10 mutations per megabase (Mb) (Subbiah et al. 2020). However, the optimal TMB cut-off in bladder cancer is less clear, and a recent analysis found a TMB of 3 mutations/Mb most strongly separated responders versus non-responders (Sarfaty et al. 2023). However, differences in sequencing platforms and mutation-calling algorithms make standardization of TMB challenging.

9.8 Clinical Trials Investigating Cystectomy Avoidance in MIBC Patients with Tumor DNA Repair Gene Alterations

The impact of DNA repair pathway alterations on sensitivity to DNA damaging agents has been demonstrated in several retrospective analyses (Van Allen et al. 2014; Taber et al. 2020; Plimack et al. 2015; Teo et al. 2017; Iyer et al. 2018). However, these studies have varied significantly in terms of clinical setting (neoadjuvant or metastatic), DNA damaging agents (cisplatin combinations as well as inclusion of carboplatin-based combinations in some studies), and in the DNA repair genes included in the analysis (varying from single genes such as *ERCC2* to panels of dozens of DNA repair genes). Given the inherent limitations of retrospective analyses, several ongoing prospective Phase II clinical trials are now underway. Although the designs vary somewhat, these trials are testing the hypothesis that patients with DNA repair gene alterations are more likely to achieve a clinical complete response (cCR) to neoadjuvant cisplatin-based chemotherapy and therefore may be able to avoid standard-of-care local therapy (radical cystectomy or chemoradiotherapy; Table 9.1).

The first such trial designed to test a risk-adapted approach for select bladder preservation in MIBC was the RETAIN trial (Geynisman et al. 2023). MIBC patients underwent transurethral resection (TURBT) followed by three cycles of accelerated MVAC chemotherapy. Tissue from the diagnostic TURBT was sent for NGS using the Caris platform and mutation-positive patients were defined as those with any alteration in *ATM, RB1, FANCC*, or *ERCC2*. After completing chemotherapy, patients underwent a second TURBT. Mutation-positive patients with no residual tumor on the second TURBT were offered surveillance rather than radical cystectomy. Patients who were mutation-negative or who had residual non-muscle invasive disease on the second TURBT were offered intravesicular therapy, chemoradiotherapy, or radical cystectomy, whereas patients with residual muscle-invasive disease were rec-

Table 9.1 Clinical trials investigating response-guided approaches to MIBC treatment and association with DNA repair gene alterations

Trial	NCT/ISRCTN	DNA repair gene(s)	Regimen	Criteria for cystectomy avoidance	Primary endpoint	Results	Citation
RETAIN	NCT02710734	ERCC2, ATM, FANCC, RB1	Accelerated MVAC	DDR gene alteration + cCR	2-year MFS	2-year MFS 72% (did not meet primary endpoint); 2-year MFS 65% in cystectomy avoidance pop.	Geynisman et al. (2023)
HCRN 16–257	NCT03558087	ERCC2, ATM, FANCC, RB1; TMB	GC + nivolumab	cCR	cCR, ability of cCR to predict 2-year MFS (co-primary)	43% cCR rate; association between cCR and TMB observed	Galsky et al. (2023)
Alliance A031701	NCT03609216	ERCC2, ERCC5, ATM, ATR, FANCC, BRCA1, BRCA2, RECQL4, RAD51C	GC	DDR gene alteration + cCR	3-year EFS	Not reported	Iyer et al. (2018)
RETAIN-2	NCT04506554	ERCC2, ATM, RB1	Accelerated MVAC + nivolumab	DDR gene alteration + cCR	2-year MFS	Not reported	NA

MVAC methotrexate, vinblastine, adriamycin, cisplatin, *DDR* DNA damage repair, *MFS* metastasis-free survival, *GC* gemcitabine plus cisplatin, *cCR* complete clinical response, *EFS* event-free survival ommended to undergo radical cystectomy. The primary endpoint was 2-year metastasis-free survival (MFS) and the risk-adapted approach would be declared non-inferior to the standard of care if the lower bound of an exact one-sided 95% confidence interval (CI) for 2-year MFS was ≥64%. Final results from the trial were recently reported in abstract form (Geynisman et al. 2023). Seventy-one patients were enrolled including 33 (46%) mutation-positive patients. The trial did not meet its primary endpoint: the 2-year MFS for the intention-to-treat population was 72% with a lower bound of 62% for the 95% CI. Among the 33 mutation-positive patients, 26 (79%) had no residual tumor (i.e., clinical stage T0) following MVAC and began active surveillance. However, 18 active surveillance patients had a UC recurrence (69%), including ten (38%) who developed metastatic disease. Nine of the ten patients who developed metastatic disease had a local recurrence prior to development of metastatic disease. These results suggest an unacceptably high rate of disease recurrence in the active surveillance group, and a refined risk-adapted approach is now being tested in RETAIN-2.

Final results from another Phase II clinical trial with a similar design were also reported recently in abstract form (Galsky et al. 2023). The Hoosier Cancer Research Network (HCRN) 16–257 trial treated MIBC patients with four cycles of cisplatin, gemcitabine, and nivolumab followed by clinical re-staging with imaging (CT/MRI), cystoscopy with biopsies, and urine cytology. Patients with a cCR by imaging, biopsy, and cytology were allowed to forego cystectomy and continue with an additional eight cycles of nivolumab whereas patients without a cCR were recommended to undergo cystectomy. All patients had tumor NGS performed from the initial diagnostic TURBT with sequencing of *ERCC2, FANCC, ATM, RB1*, as well as calculation of TMB. The co-primary endpoints were the cCR rate and the association of cCR with 2-year outcomes. A total of 76 patients were enrolled, 33 (43%) of whom achieved a cCR following neoadjuvant chemoimmunotherapy. Among patients who achieved a cCR, 100% were alive and 96.6% were metastasis free at 2 years. Alterations in *ERCC2, FANNC, ATM*, or *RB1* were not associated with likelihood of cCR, but TMB ≥ 10 mut/Mb was associated with higher cCR rate and improved 2-year outcomes.

A third Phase II trial with a similar design is the on-going Alliance A031701 trial (Iyer et al. 2022). Enrolled MIBC patients undergo four cycles of gemcitabine plus cisplatin and sequencing of the diagnostic TURBT. Patients with a predicted deleterious mutation in at least one of nine DNA repair genes (*ERCC2, ERCC5, BRCA1, BRCA2, RAD51C, ATR, RECQL4, ATM, FANCC*) who achieve a cCR or with residual carcinoma in-situ (CIS) are offered surveillance whereas patients with a DNA repair gene mutation with residual ≥T1 disease, as well as all patients without a DNA repair gene mutation, are offered cystectomy or chemoradiotherapy. The study is currently accruing and no results have yet been presented.

When published, the results of these trials will provide critical insights regarding the association of DNA repair gene alterations with cCR following neoadjuvant cisplatin-based chemotherapy as well as the potential to use NAC response to guide local therapy decisions (Fig. 9.3). Several important factors should be considered when interpreting the results of these trials. First, the DNA repair genes assessed as well as the methods used to detect and categorize mutations in the DNA repair genes of interest vary across trials and could strongly influence the apparent mutation frequency of specific genes as well as the association of alterations with clinical outcomes. Second, although each trial included cisplatin, the neoadjuvant regimens varied, and anti-PD1 therapy was used in one of the trials. Finally, the clinical staging tests (imaging, biopsy, etc.) as well as the specific criteria used to define "responders" versus "non-responders" also varied across trials. These subtle but important differences could have important implications for the interpretation of findings when final results are published.

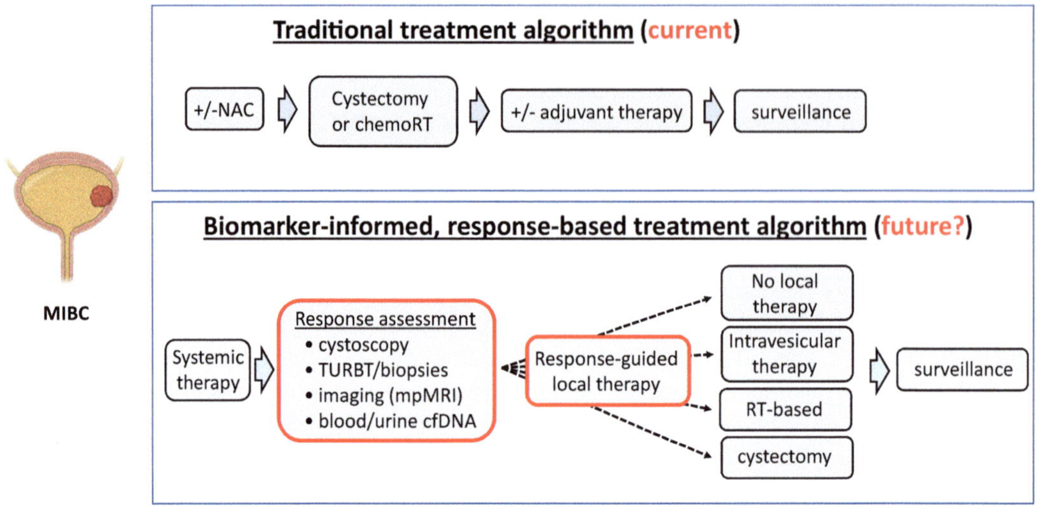

Fig. 9.3 Current and emerging treatment algorithms for muscle-invasive bladder cancer (MIBC)

9.9 Clinical Trials Investigating DNA Repair Gene Alterations and Response to DNA Repair Targeted Agents

Synthetic lethality occurs when tumor-specific loss of a protein or pathway increases dependency on an alternative protein or pathway which can be targeted therapeutically. Synthetic lethality approaches are an attractive strategy to target tumors harboring specific DNA repair defects and this approach has been pioneered by the use of PARP inhibitors to target homologous recombination (HR) deficiency (Bryant et al. 2005; Rose et al. 2020). In the USA, PARP inhibitors are now approved in specific clinical settings for HR-deficient (HRD) breast, ovarian, pancreatic, and prostate cancer. HRD also appears to be present in a subset of bladder tumors (Borcsok et al. 2021b), and several clinical trials have investigated the activity of PARP inhibitors in biomarker-selected and unselected populations (Table 9.2).

One of the first urothelial cancer-specific PARP inhibitor clinical trials to be reported was the ATLAS trial (Grivas et al. 2021). Ninety-seven patients with advanced urothelial cancer previously treated with 1–2 chemotherapy regimens were given rucaparib. Patients with tumors that had genomic loss-of-heterozygosity (LOH) of ≥10% were defined as HRD-positive and the primary endpoint was overall response rate in the intention-to-treat and HRD-positive populations. Among evaluable patients, there were no confirmed responses and the median progression-free survival (PFS) was only 1.8 months. There were no differences in patients with HRD-positive versus negative tumors, and there were also no associations between clinical outcomes and mutations in DNA repair genes for a subset of the trial patients who underwent tumor NGS.

The BISCAY trial was a biomarker-driven basket trial in which metastatic urothelial cancer patients were randomized to durvalumab plus a targeted agent selected based on tumor genomic features (Powles et al. 2021). Durvalumab plus the PARP inhibitor olaparib were given to patients with a predicted deleterious mutation in an HR gene (HRR mutant) as well as in half of the patients who lacked an alteration that would qualify them for any of the other arms of the trial (biomarker-negative). The response rates ranged from 9–36% across arms, which did not meet the pre-defined criteria for further investigation. The response rate to durvalumab plus olaparib was 36% in the HRR-mutant arm and 9% in the biomarker-negative arm, but this difference was not statistically significant and the survival outcomes were similar across arms.

Table 9.2 Clinical trials investigating DNA repair targeted agents in metastatic urothelial cancer

Trial	NCT/ISRCTN	Prior therapies	Trial design	Treatment	Primary endpoint	Biomarker required for enrollment?	DNA repair biomarker(s)	Results	Citation
ATLAS	NCT03397394	1–2 prior chemo regimens	Single arm Phase II	Rucaparib	ORR	No	LOH ≥10%; HR gene alterations	0% ORR; no assoc. between HR deficiency and outcomes	Grivas et al. (2021)
BISCAY	NCT02546661	Previous platinum-based chemo	Adaptive, biomarker-driven phase 1b	Durvalumab + olaparib	Safety	Yes (biomarker determines arm assignment)	HR repair gene mutations	36% response rate in patients with HR gene mutation; 9% response rate in unselected patients	Powles et al. (2021)
BAYOU	NCT03459846	Platinum-ineligible	Randomized Phase II	Durvalumab + olaparib vs. durvalumb + placebo	PFS	No	Alteration in ≥1 of 15 pre-specified HRD genes	No diff. in PFS (trial-wide); PFS higher in HRD-positive subset treated with PARPi (5.8 vs. 1.6 mo)	Rosenberg et al. (2022)
ATLANTIS	ISRCTN25859465	No progression after platinum-based chemo	Randomized Phase II	Maintainence rucaparib vs. placebo	PFS	Yes	≥10% LOH or mutation in ≥1 of 15 DNA repair genes	Increased PFS with PARPi in biomarker-positive patients (35 vs. 15 wks; $p = 0.07$)	Crabb et al. (2022)
ECTCN (Apolo et al)	NCT03375307	At least one prior platinum agent or immune checkpoint inhibitor	Single arm Phase II	Olaparib	ORR	Yes	DNA repair gene alterations as defined by molecular tumor board	Not reported	NA
ECTCN (Pal et al.)	NCT02567409	No prior treatment for metastatic disease	Randomized Phase II	GC +/− berzosertib (ATR inhibitor)	PFS	No	Unselected	No difference in PFS between arms; longer OS in control arm (19.8 vs. 14.4 mo)	Pal et al. (2021)

ORR overall response rate, *LOH* loss-of-heterozygosity, *HR* homologous recombination, *HRD* homologous recombination deficiency, *PFS* progression-free survival, *OS* overall survival, *wks* weeks, *ETCTN* Experimental Therapeutics Clinical Trials Network, *GC* gemcitabine plus cisplatin

Despite the lack of signal for PARP inhibitor activity in the ATLAS and BISCAY trials, two recently reported PARP inhibitor trials do suggest that a subset of HR-deficient urothelial tumors may benefit from PARP inhibition. The BAYOU trial randomized 154 platinum-ineligible metastatic urothelial cancer patients to durvalumab plus olaparib versus durvalumab plus placebo (Rosenberg et al. 2022). Although there was no difference in PFS between the olaparib and placebo arms, there was an improvement in PFS (5.6 vs. 1.8 mo) in the ~20% of patients with HRR-mutant tumors defined by presence of a predicted deleterious mutation in one of 15 HR genes.

The ATLANTIS trial also showed activity of PARP inhibition in a biomarker-selected subset of metastatic urothelial patients, albeit in a somewhat different clinical setting (Crabb et al. 2022). Following platinum-based chemotherapy, 248 metastatic urothelial cancer patients without evidence of progression were screened for presence of DNA repair deficiency (DRD), defined as a predicted deleterious mutation in at least one of 15 DNA repair genes, or genomic LOH of ≥10%. Approximately 30% of screened patients were identified as DRD-positive and were randomized. PFS was 35 weeks in olaparib-treated patients versus 15 weeks in patients treated with placebo ($p = 0.07$). Together, results from the BAYOU and ATLANTIS trial suggest that a subset of bladder cancer patients may benefit from PARP inhibitor therapy, but the optimal clinical setting and the optimal biomarker(s) remain to be defined.

In addition to PARP inhibitors, small molecule inhibitors of other DNA repair enzymes are also being investigated in bladder cancer and other tumor types (Brown et al. 2017). ATR is a DNA damage response kinase that is activated following DNA damage or replication stress, and preclinical data suggests that many tumors have increased dependence on ATR signaling (O'Connor 2015). Pal et al. recently reported findings from a randomized Phase II trial of the ATR inhibitor berzosertib in bladder cancer (Pal et al. 2021). Eighty-seven patients without prior treatment for metastatic urothelial cancer were randomized to cisplatin plus gemcitabine with or without concurrent berzosertib. There was no difference in PFS between arms and OS was numerically higher in the non-berzosertib arm. The cisplatin dose was lower and cisplatin dose reductions were more common in the berzosertib arm than in the control arm, perhaps explaining the trend towards better OS in the control arm. These results suggest that alternative approaches, perhaps including biomarker selection of patients most likely to respond to ATR inhibition (or other DDR-directed therapies), are warranted.

9.10 Conclusion

The unique biological role of urothelial cells results in exposure to multiple DNA damaging agents, and this exposure as well as frequent mutations in DNA repair genes drive the complex and heterogeneous genomic landscape of bladder tumors. Despite the prevalence of DNA repair pathway alterations in bladder tumors, the role of DNA repair dysfunction in tumorigenesis remains poorly understood.

In this chapter, we review the current biological and therapeutic landscape of DNA repair deficiency in bladder cancer. DNA repair genes typically function as tumor suppressors and both somatic and germline alterations occur in bladder tumors. The advent and widespread clinical implementation of NGS has revolutionized the ability to identify DNA repair gene alterations in tumors, yet the biological implications of DNA repair deficiency remain incompletely understood. Therefore, integrated genomic, functional, and clinical studies are needed to elucidate the molecular properties of DNA repair-deficient tumors and inform rational therapeutic approaches.

Several recently reported clinical trials provide important insights regarding the clinical tractability of DNA repair deficiency in bladder cancer. However, important questions remain, including the utility of DNA repair gene mutations to guide bladder preserving approaches for MIBC as well as the optimal biomarker(s) for identifying sensitivity to PARP inhibitors and other DNA repair targeted agents in advanced bladder cancer. On-going preclinical and clinical efforts will continue to shape our understanding of DNA repair biology and refine approaches to personalize therapy in bladder cancer.

References

Adzhubei IA et al (2010) A method and server for predicting damaging missense mutations. Nat Methods 7(4):248–249. PMC2855889

Aggen DH, Drake CG (2017) Biomarkers for immunotherapy in bladder cancer: a moving target. J Immunother Cancer 5(1):94. PMC5697433

Alexandrov LB et al (2015) Clock-like mutational processes in human somatic cells. Nat Genet 47(12):1402–1407. PMC4783858

Alexandrov LB et al (2020) The repertoire of mutational signatures in human cancer. Nature 578(7793):94–101. PMC7054213

Bellmunt J et al (2007) Gene expression of ERCC1 as a novel prognostic marker in advanced bladder cancer patients receiving cisplatin-based chemotherapy. Ann Oncol 18(3):522–528

Borcsok J et al (2021a) Identification of a synthetic lethal relationship between nucleotide excision repair deficiency and irofulven sensitivity in urothelial cancer. Clin Cancer Res 27(7):2011–2022. PMC8026514

Borcsok J et al (2021b) Detection of molecular signatures of homologous recombination deficiency in bladder cancer. Clin Cancer Res 27(13):3734–3743. PMC8896908

Brown JS et al (2017) Targeting DNA repair in cancer: beyond PARP inhibitors. Cancer Discov 7(1):20–37. PMC5300099

Bryant HE et al (2005) Specific killing of BRCA2-deficient tumours with inhibitors of poly(ADP-ribose) polymerase. Nature 434(7035):913–917

Carlo MI et al (2020) Cancer susceptibility mutations in patients with urothelial malignancies. J Clin Oncol 38(5):406–414

Ceccaldi R, Rondinelli B, D'Andrea AD (2016) Repair pathway choices and consequences at the double-Strand break. Trends Cell Biol 26(1):52–64. PMC4862604

Chang DW, Gu J, Wu X (2012) Germline prognostic markers for urinary bladder cancer: obstacles and opportunities. Urol Oncol 30(4):524–532. PMC3824379

Choudhury A et al (2010) MRE11 expression is predictive of cause-specific survival following radical radiotherapy for muscle-invasive bladder cancer. Cancer Res 70(18):7017–7026. PMC2941719

Christensen E et al (2019) Early detection of metastatic relapse and monitoring of therapeutic efficacy by ultra-deep sequencing of plasma cell-free DNA in patients with urothelial bladder carcinoma. J Clin Oncol 37(18):1547–1557

Crabb SJ et al (2022) A randomized, double blind, biomarker selected, phase II clinical trial of maintenance PARP inhibition following chemotherapy for metastatic urothelial carcinoma (mUC): final analysis of the ATLANTIS rucaparib arm. J Clin Oncol 40(6_suppl):436–436

Crawford JM (2008) The origins of bladder cancer. Lab Investig 88(7):686–693

Cumberbatch MGK et al (2018) Epidemiology of bladder cancer: a systematic review and contemporary update of risk factors in 2018. Eur Urol 74(6):784–795

Farmer H et al (2005) Targeting the DNA repair defect in BRCA mutant cells as a therapeutic strategy. Nature 434(7035):917–921

Fuss JO, Tainer JA (2011) XPB and XPD helicases in TFIIH orchestrate DNA duplex opening and damage verification to coordinate repair with transcription and cell cycle via CAK kinase. DNA Repair (Amst) 10(7):697–713. PMC3234290

Galsky MD et al (2023) Co-primary endpoint analysis of HCRN GU 16-257: phase 2 trial of gemcitabine, cisplatin, plus nivolumab with selective bladder sparing in patients with muscle-invasive bladder cancer (MIBC). J Clin Oncol 41(6_suppl):447–447

Geynisman DM et al (2023) A phase II trial of risk-enabled therapy after initiating neoadjuvant chemotherapy for bladder cancer (RETAIN). J Clin Oncol 41(6_suppl):438–438

Gil-Jimenez A et al (2023) Assessment of predictive genomic biomarkers for response to cisplatin-based neoadjuvant chemotherapy in bladder cancer. Eur Urol 83(4):313–317

Glaser AP et al (2018) APOBEC-mediated mutagenesis in urothelial carcinoma is associated with improved survival, mutations in DNA damage response genes, and immune response. Oncotarget 9(4):4537–4548. PMC5796993

Grivas P et al (2021) Efficacy and safety of rucaparib in previously treated, locally advanced or metastatic urothelial carcinoma from a phase 2, open-label trial (ATLAS). BMC Cancer 21(1):593. PMC8147008

Groenendijk FH et al (2016) ERBB2 mutations characterize a subgroup of muscle-invasive bladder cancers with excellent response to neoadjuvant chemotherapy. Eur Urol 69(3):384–388

Hoeijmakers JH (2009) DNA damage, aging, and cancer. N Engl J Med 361(15):1475–1485

Hoppe MM et al (2021) Quantitative imaging of RAD51 expression as a marker of platinum resistance in ovarian cancer. EMBO Mol Med 13(5):e13366. PMC8103098

Islam SMA et al (2022) Uncovering novel mutational signatures by de novo extraction with SigProfilerExtractor. Cell Genom 2(11):PMC9646490

Iyer G et al (2018) Multicenter prospective phase II trial of neoadjuvant dose-dense gemcitabine plus cisplatin in patients with muscle-invasive bladder cancer. J Clin Oncol 36(19):1949–1956

Iyer G et al (2022) A phase II study of gemcitabine plus cisplatin chemotherapy in patients with muscle-invasive bladder cancer with bladder preservation for those patients whose tumors harbor deleterious DNA damage response (DDR) gene alterations (Alliance A031701). J Clin Oncol 40(Suppl 16):TPS4615
Jeggo PA, Pearl LH, Carr AM (2016) DNA repair, genome stability and cancer: a historical perspective. Nat Rev Cancer 16(1):35–42
Johanns TM et al (2016) Immunogenomics of hypermutated glioblastoma: a patient with germline POLE deficiency treated with checkpoint blockade immunotherapy. Cancer Discov 6(11):1230–1236. PMC5140283
Kawanishi S et al (2017) Crosstalk between DNA damage and inflammation in the multiple steps of carcinogenesis. Int J Mol Sci 18(8):PMC5578195
Kelderman S, Schumacher TN, Kvistborg P (2015) Mismatch repair-deficient cancers are targets for anti-PD-1 therapy. Cancer Cell 28(1):11–13
Kim J et al (2016) Somatic ERCC2 mutations are associated with a distinct genomic signature in urothelial tumors. Nat Genet 48(6):600–606. *contributed equally. PMC4936490
Klatte T et al (2015) ERCC1 as a prognostic and predictive biomarker for urothelial carcinoma of the bladder following radical cystectomy. J Urol 194(5):1456–1462
Konstantinopoulos PA et al (2021) A replication stress biomarker is associated with response to gemcitabine versus combined gemcitabine and ATR inhibitor therapy in ovarian cancer. Nat Commun 12(1):5574. PMC8458434
Kraemer KH et al (2007) Xeroderma pigmentosum, trichothiodystrophy and Cockayne syndrome: a complex genotype-phenotype relationship. Neuroscience 145(4):1388–1396. PMC2288663
Laurberg JR et al (2012) Expression of TIP60 (tat-interactive protein) and MRE11 (meiotic recombination 11 homolog) predict treatment-specific outcome of localised invasive bladder cancer. BJU Int 110(11 Pt C):E1228–E1236
Le DT et al (2015) PD-1 blockade in tumors with mismatch-repair deficiency. N Engl J Med 372(26):2509–2520. PMC4481136
Li GM (2008) Mechanisms and functions of DNA mismatch repair. Cell Res 18(1):85–98
Li Q, Wang K (2017) InterVar: clinical interpretation of genetic variants by the 2015 ACMG-AMP guidelines. Am J Hum Genet 100(2):267–280. PMC5294755
Li Q et al (2019) ERCC2 helicase domain mutations confer nucleotide excision repair deficiency and drive cisplatin sensitivity in muscle-invasive bladder cancer. Clin Cancer Res 25(3):977–988. PMC6434536
Liu D et al (2016) Clinical validation of chemotherapy response biomarker ERCC2 in muscle-invasive urothelial bladder carcinoma. JAMA Oncol 2(8):1094–1096. PMC5515075
Liu W et al (2023) The cytidine deaminase APOBEC3G contributes to cancer mutagenesis and clonal evolution in bladder cancer. Cancer Res 83(4):506–520
Lynch HT et al (2015) Milestones of Lynch syndrome: 1895-2015. Nat Rev Cancer 15(3):181–194
Ma J et al (2018) The therapeutic significance of mutational signatures from DNA repair deficiency in cancer. Nat Commun 9(1):3292. PMC6098043
Magliocco AM et al (2022) Analysis of MRE11 and mortality among adults with muscle-invasive bladder cancer managed with trimodality therapy. JAMA Netw Open 5(11):e2242378. PMC9669810
Marteijn JA et al (2014) Understanding nucleotide excision repair and its roles in cancer and ageing. Nat Rev Mol Cell Biol 15(7):465–481
Mossanen M et al (2022) Incidence of germline variants in familial bladder cancer and among patients with cancer predisposition syndromes. Clin Genitourin Cancer 20(6):568–574
Mouw KW (2017) DNA repair pathway alterations in bladder cancer. Cancers (Basel) 9(4):PMC5406703
Mouw KW, D'Andrea AD (2018) DNA repair deficiency and immunotherapy response. J Clin Oncol 36:1710
Mouw KW et al (2017) DNA damage and repair biomarkers of immunotherapy response. Cancer Discov 7(7):675–693. PMC5659200
Mullane SA et al (2016) Expression levels of DNA damage repair proteins are associated with overall survival in platinum-treated advanced urothelial carcinoma. Clin Genitourin Cancer 14(4):352–359
Nik-Zainal S et al (2016) Landscape of somatic mutations in 560 breast cancer whole-genome sequences. Nature 534(7605):47–54. PMC4910866
O'Connor MJ (2015) Targeting the DNA damage response in cancer. Mol Cell 60(4):547–560
Pal SK et al (2021) Effect of cisplatin and gemcitabine with or without berzosertib in patients with advanced urothelial carcinoma: a phase 2 randomized clinical trial. JAMA Oncol 7(10):1536–1543. PMC8391778
Pecina-Slaus N et al (2020) Mismatch repair pathway, genome stability and cancer. Front Mol Biosci 7:122. PMC7332687
Pelucchi C et al (2006) Mechanisms of disease: the epidemiology of bladder cancer. Nat Clin Pract Urol 3(6):327–340
Plimack ER et al (2015) Defects in DNA repair genes predict response to neoadjuvant cisplatin-based chemotherapy in muscle-invasive bladder cancer. Eur Urol 68(6):959–967. PMC4764095
Polak P et al (2017) A mutational signature reveals alterations underlying deficient homologous recombination repair in breast cancer. Nat Genet 49(10):1476–1486
Powles T et al (2021) An adaptive, biomarker-directed platform study of durvalumab in combination with targeted therapies in advanced urothelial cancer. Nat Med 27(5):793–801
Queiroz MM et al (2021) Emerging biomarkers in metastatic urothelial carcinoma: tumour mutational burden, PD-L1 expression and APOBEC polypeptide-like signature in a patient with complete response to anti-programmed cell death protein-1 inhibitor. Ecancermedicalscience 15:1306. PMC8580725

Rhea LP et al (2021) Role of immunotherapy in bladder cancer. Cancer Treat Res Commun 26:100296

Robertson AG et al (2017) Comprehensive molecular characterization of muscle-invasive bladder cancer. Cell 171(3):540–556 e25. PMC5687509

Rose M et al (2020) PARP inhibitors: clinical relevance, mechanisms of action and tumor resistance. Front Cell Dev Biol 8:564601. PMC7509090

Rosenberg JE et al (2022) BAYOU: a phase II, randomized, multicenter, double-blind, study of durvalumab (D) in combination with olaparib (O) for the first-line treatment of platinum-ineligible patients with unresectable, stage IV urothelial carcinoma (UC). J Clin Oncol 40(6_suppl):437–437

Sakano S et al (2013) ERCC1 and XRCC1 expression predicts survival in bladder cancer patients receiving combined trimodality therapy. Mol Clin Oncol 1(3):403–410. PMC3916156

Samstein RM et al (2019) Tumor mutational load predicts survival after immunotherapy across multiple cancer types. Nat Genet 51(2):202–206. PMC6365097

Sarfaty M et al (2023) Novel genetic subtypes of urothelial carcinoma with differential outcomes on immune checkpoint blockade. J Clin Oncol JCO2202144

Scully R et al (2019) DNA double-strand break repair-pathway choice in somatic mammalian cells. Nat Rev Mol Cell Biol 20(11):698–714. PMC7315405

Skeldon SC et al (2013) Patients with Lynch syndrome mismatch repair gene mutations are at higher risk for not only upper tract urothelial cancer but also bladder cancer. Eur Urol 63(2):379–385

Stadler ZK et al (2016) Reliable detection of mismatch repair deficiency in colorectal cancers using mutational load in next-generation sequencing panels. J Clin Oncol 34(18):2141–2147. PMC4962706

Subbiah V et al (2020) The FDA approval of pembrolizumab for adult and pediatric patients with tumor mutational burden (TMB) >/=10: a decision centered on empowering patients and their physicians. Ann Oncol 31(9):1115–1118

Syed A, Tainer JA (2018) The MRE11-RAD50-NBS1 complex conducts the orchestration of damage signaling and outcomes to stress in DNA replication and repair. Annu Rev Biochem 87:263–294. PMC6076887

Taber A et al (2020) Molecular correlates of cisplatin-based chemotherapy response in muscle invasive bladder cancer by integrated multi-omics analysis. Nat Commun 11(1):4858. PMC7519650

Teo MY et al (2017) DNA damage response and repair gene alterations are associated with improved survival in patients with platinum-treated advanced urothelial carcinoma. Clin Cancer Res 23(14):3610–3618

Teo MY et al (2018) Alterations in DNA damage response and repair genes as potential marker of clinical benefit from PD-1/PD-L1 blockade in advanced urothelial cancers. J Clin Oncol 36(17):1685–1694

Valero C et al (2021) The association between tumor mutational burden and prognosis is dependent on treatment context. Nat Genet 53(1):11–15. PMC7796993

Van Allen EM et al (2014) Somatic ERCC2 mutations correlate with cisplatin sensitivity in muscle-invasive urothelial carcinoma. Cancer Discov 4(10):1140–1153. PMC4238969

van der Post RS et al (2010) Risk of urothelial bladder cancer in Lynch syndrome is increased, in particular among MSH2 mutation carriers. J Med Genet 47(7):464–470. PMC2991077

van Gool IC et al (2015) POLE proofreading mutations elicit an antitumor immune response in endometrial cancer. Clin Cancer Res 21(14):3347–3355. PMC4627582

van Wilpe S et al (2021) Homologous recombination repair deficiency and implications for tumor immunogenicity. Cancers (Basel) 13(9):PMC8124836

Vaser R et al (2016) SIFT missense predictions for genomes. Nat Protoc 11(1):1–9

Volkova NV et al (2020) Mutational signatures are jointly shaped by DNA damage and repair. Nat Commun 11(1):2169. PMC7195458

Walker AK et al (2019) MRE11 as a predictive biomarker of outcome after radiation therapy in bladder cancer. Int J Radiat Oncol Biol Phys 104(4):809–818. PMC6588678

Weir WH, Mucha PJ, Kim WY (2022) A bipartite graph-based expected networks approach identifies DDR genes not associated with TMB yet predictive of immune checkpoint blockade response. Cell Rep Med 3(5):100602. PMC9133403

Wright WD, Shah SS, Heyer WD (2018) Homologous recombination and the repair of DNA double-strand breaks. J Biol Chem 293(27):10524–10535. PMC6036207

DNA Methylation and Chromatin Regulators in Bladder Cancer

10

Wolfgang A. Schulz and Michèle J. Hoffmann

Abstract

Pronounced changes in epigenetic regulation contribute crucially to bladder cancer development and progression. DNA methylation patterns are severely disturbed, with—often extensive—hypomethylation across the genome and less pervasive, but significant local hypermethylation. Hypomethylation is thought to contribute to genomic instability, whereas hypermethylation may lead to the transcriptional inactivation of specific genes. Moreover, hypermethylation especially of particular genomic regions known as CpG-islands can be used for diagnostic purposes. Several assays for altered methylation are now approved or in clinical trials for detection and surveillance of bladder cancer. Another characteristic of bladder cancer is a very high prevalence of deleterious mutations in chromatin regulator genes, especially in genes that encode components of the trithorax-like COMPASS and chromatin-remodeling SWI/SNF protein complexes or proteins interacting with these. These complexes establish active enhancers in a cell type-specific fashion and are opposed by polycomb complexes that tend to be overactive in bladder cancer. Collectively, changes in these complexes disturb urothelial differentiation and prevent the downregulation of proliferation during terminal differentiation. The high frequency of epigenetic alterations suggests that bladder cancers may respond well to drugs targeting chromatin regulators (known as epidrugs), especially those with enzymatic activity. A large variety of epidrugs has been explored and some promising results have been obtained in preclinical studies, especially in combination with other established therapies. Clinical trials for some drugs are underway.

Keywords

Cancer epigenetics · DNA methylation · Histone modifications · Chromatin remodeling · Chromatin regulators · Epigenetic drugs · Bladder cancer

10.1 Introduction to Cancer Epigenetics

Genetic changes in cancer, i.e., mutations and chromosomal aberrations, alter the structure of genes, their dosage or their regulation and consequently the function of their protein or RNA products. Genetic changes are complemented

W. A. Schulz (✉) · M. J. Hoffmann
Department of Urology, Medical Faculty, Heinrich Heine University and University Hospital Duesseldorf, Duesseldorf, Germany
e-mail: wolfgang.schulz@hhu.de

M. A. Knowles, L. Dyrskjøt (eds.), *Biology of Bladder Cancer*,
https://doi.org/10.1007/978-3-031-68505-7_10

and aggravated by epigenetic alterations which primarily disturb gene expression and regulation. In bladder cancer, both genetic and epigenetic alterations are abundant and diverse.

According to the currently most prevalent definition, epigenetic mechanisms allow the stable propagation or controlled transitions of cellular states across cell divisions without changes in the amount or sequence of the genomic DNA. In this fashion, epigenetics explains most of all cell differentiation during ontogeny as well as during tissue homeostasis and repair, which proceed as a rule without changes in the sequence or amount of genomic DNA. Since cancer cells assume an aberrantly differentiated state, their epigenetic constitution is—by definition—altered. Like other neoplastic properties, the aberrant differentiation state of cancer cells may be a (secondary) consequence of genetic changes that is implemented via the same epigenetic mechanisms acting in normal cells. Alternatively, it may be directly caused by alterations in epigenetic mechanisms or by incidental mistakes in epigenetic regulation known as "epimutations". These causes contribute to different extents in different cancer types. Bladder cancer in particular is notable for a high prevalence of mutations in epigenetic regulator proteins that likely contribute to the aberrant differentiation and other neoplastic properties of the cancer cells (Hoffmann and Schulz 2021).

Collectively, epigenetic mechanisms regulate the activity of individual genes, but also organize the distribution and activity of the genome in the nucleus at large. For instance, they mediate the fundamental distinction between heterochromatic and euchromatic regions of the genome and support their spatial separation within the nucleus. Within the euchromatic parts of the genome, epigenetic mechanisms ensure the constitutive activity of "house-keeping" genes as well as the cell-type specific expression of developmentally regulated genes. This is achieved by the establishment of specific chromatin states (Table 10.1; ENCODE Project Consortium et al. 2020). As a rule, epigenetic mechanisms do not act in isolation, but in each instance, multiple mechanisms interact. Accordingly, different chromatin states are each characterized by specific histone arrangements and modifications as well as by specific DNA methylation patterns (Table 10.1). Chromatin organization is required for the regulation of transcriptional activity, especially the establishment of cell type-specific expression patterns, but also for appropriate responses to various forms of cellular stress. Importantly, chromatin must also be adapted to allow physiological cellular processes like DNA replication, recombination and mitosis, as well as DNA repair following damage to the genome. Accordingly, some chromatin regulators directly interact with DNA repair factors (Walton et al. 2023).

The basic units of chromatin are nucleosomes formed by approximately 200 bp DNA, of which 147 bp are wound around a histone octamer, consisting of two H2A, H2B, H3, and H4 proteins each. In specific regions of the genome standard histones are substituted by variant forms including H2AX, H2AZ, Macro-H2A, H3.3, and CENP (Ghiraldini et al. 2021). Accessory chromatin proteins binding to nucleosomes or to linker DNA, like histone H1, contribute to variable compaction of the basic nucleosome fiber, which is used for the regulation of gene expression, but is also required for condensation during mitosis.

In the interphase nucleus, chromatin is organized in more than 2000 domains known as topologically associated domains (TADs) each comprising up to several Mbp (Gonzalez-Sandoval and Gasser 2016; Sivakumar et al. 2019). Up to 40% of the genome is present in lamina-associated domains (LAD) close to the nuclear membrane, comprising mainly heterochromatic and transcriptionally inactive sequences. TADs in more active regions of the genome contain one or more enhancers (or in some cases silencers) that regulate the activity of promoters within one TAD, but not across its boundaries. Physically, TADs correspond largely to chromosomal loops (Fig. 10.1; Wang et al. 2021) and serve as units for regulated gene expression and DNA replication. Boundaries between the loops are organized by the CTCF (CCCTC-binding factor) DNA-binding factor in

Table 10.1 Functionally defined regions of the genome[a]

Description	Details	Associated chromatin regulators	DNA methylation
Boundary (CTCF-enriched element)	Few histone modifications, often open chromatin	CTCF, cohesin	Variable
Enhancer	Open chromatin with H3K4me1 and acetylated histones	CBP, p300, KMT2C/D, SWI/SNF	Variable (cell type-specific)
Promoter region including transcription start site (TSS)	Open chromatin with H3K4me3. Enriched for TF known to act close to promoters and polymerases Pol II and Pol III.	HATs, SET1, KMT2A/B	Low or moderate, usually lacking at CpG-islands
Transcribed region	H3K36me3 and H3K4me. Enriched for phosphorylated form of Pol II	SETD2, DNMT3	Higher
Repressed or low activity region	Less open chromatin. Lack of methylation at H3K4 and low histone acetylation, often H3K27me3.	PRC2, PRC1 or other repressive complexes	Moderate to high
Heterochromatic region	Closed chromatin, H3K9me2/3	G9a, SUV39H1, HP1	High

[a] Modified from ENCODE project consortium 2020

conjunction with the cohesin complex. Importantly, the organization of TADs and their distribution within the nucleus change during cell differentiation. Thus, domains may move away from or towards the nuclear membrane, chromatin loops may shrink or expand and enhancers or silencers may become activated or inactivated.

Nucleosomes themselves are often in a dynamic state. During transcription, replication and DNA repair, they may partly or completely dissociate from the associated DNA or may be split into H3-H4 tetramers and H2A-H2B dimers and be newly assembled on DNA. Following DNA replication, old nucleosomes must be distributed and new nucleosomes must be deposited and positioned. Various chaperones load newly synthesized nucleosomes on DNA or exchange standard for variant histones (Martire and Banaszynski 2020). For instance, among its various functions, the ATRX protein organizes the exchange of standard H3 for H3.3 at repeat sequences, (Aguilera and Lopez-Contreras 2023). Activation of genes for transcription requires moving nucleosomes at promoters and enhancers to allow access and binding of activatory transcription factors and the basic transcription machinery. Conversely, gene repression is likewise associated with repositioning of nucleosomes along the DNA helix and compaction of chromatin. These movements are affected or facilitated by one of several chromatin remodeling protein complexes, which usually act in an ATP-dependent manner (Clapier and Cairns 2009). For instance, SWI/SNF remodeling complexes are especially involved in the regulation of cell type-specific gene expression and enhancer functions (Centore et al. 2020).

Posttranslational modifications of histones are instrumental in all aspects of chromatin organization and dynamics. More than 250 different modifications have been described, most but not all taking place at the amino-terminal non-globular domains of the core histones (Zhao et al. 2021). They include acetylation at various lysine residues, methylation at different lysine (abbreviated as K) and arginine (R) residues, phosphorylation at specific serines (S) and threonines (T), but also more exotic modifications like succinylation, crotonylation, lactylation, and ubiquitination (at H2AK119 and H2BK120). Importantly, specific chromatin states are characterized by specific histone modifications (Table 10.1; ENCODE Project Consortium et al. 2020). Histones at active promoters are—often extensively—acetylated, histone H3 is methylated at lysine 4 (H3K4me) and H3s at the transcriptional start site (TSS) are trimethylated at K4 (H3K4me3). Transcribed sequences usually carry H3K36me3,

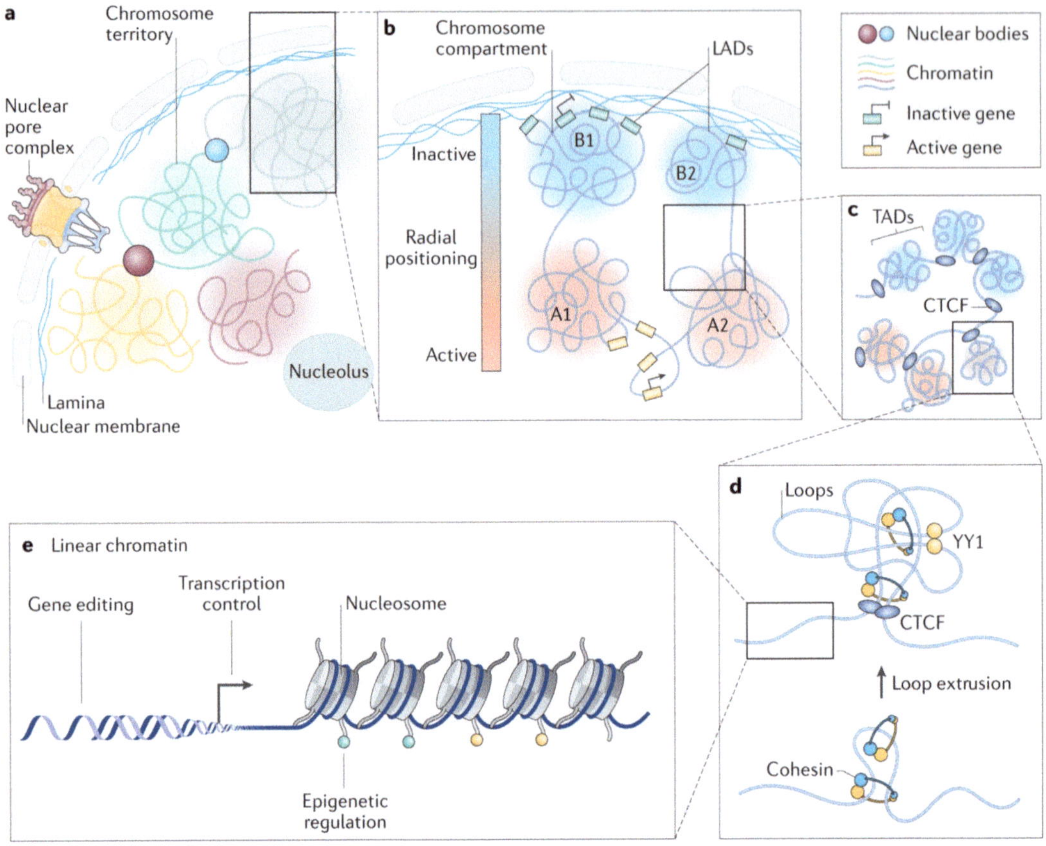

Fig. 10.1 Nuclear structure and chromatin. (**a**) Each interphase chromosome occupies a distinct nuclear region denoted a chromosome territory. Membrane-less nuclear compartments, such as nuclear bodies and the nucleolus, dynamically interact with chromatin. (**b**) The radial positioning of genomic regions in the nucleus is associated with their activity, with inactive regions located close to the nuclear lamina, forming lamina-associated domains. Chromatin compartments are categorized as A with active euchromatin located rather at the nuclear interior, and B with inactive heterochromatin preferentially located at the nuclear periphery. (**c**) Chromatin is organized into self-interacting topologically associating domains, separated by boundaries where CTCF and cohesin are located. (**d**) Loop-extruding factors, especially cohesin, actively extrude loops until they reach the boundary elements. (**e**) Linear chromatin nucleosome fibers are formed by DNA assembling with histones; they carry DNA and histone modifications. Additionally, different DNA motifs can be recognized by structural proteins and transcription factors for genome organization and regulation. From Wang et al. (2021)

whereas intergenic regions contain H3K36me2. Enhancers are distinguished by H3K4me, H3K27 acetylation and binding of the histone acetyltransferases CBP (gene *CREBBP*) or p300 (gene *EP300*). The most characteristic feature of silencers is the H4K20me modification; in transcription activating regions, this lysine is instead acetylated. The most prominent modification in constitutive heterochromatin is tri- or dimethylation of H3K9, in addition to H4K20me3. In contrast, H3K27me3 is rather a mark of facultative heterochromatin and temporarily repressed promoters and enhancers. Bivalent modification, i.e., H3K27me3 with H3K4me or H3K4me3, is a characteristic of "poised" promoters and enhancers. During development and differentiation, but also during cancer development, poised bivalent states may be resolved to active or repressed states. Whereas the above modifications relate to transcriptional regulation, histone phosphorylation is often linked to chromosome condensation for mitosis (e.g., at H3S10, H3S28, and H2AT120) or to DNA repair (e.g., H2AXS139, also known as γH2AX).

Posttranslational modifications are attached by accordingly named enzymes like histone acetyltransferases (HATs), histone methylases (HMTs, or KMTs for lysine methylases), and histone kinases, each enzyme catalyzing modifications at one or a few specific residues (Zhao et al. 2021). For instance, KMT1C (also known as EHMT2 or G9a) catalyzes selectively mono- or dimethylation of H3K9 (Padeken et al. 2022). Such enzymes are collectively considered as "writers". Importantly, many histone methyltransferases also modify non-histone proteins. Many histone modifications can be actively removed by similarly specific enzymes such as histone deacetylases (HDACs), histone demethylases (KDMs for lysine demethylases) or histone phosphatases. For instance, KDM4 demethylases (also known as JMJDs) remove primarily methyl groups at H3K9 and H3K36 (Lee et al. 2020). Such enzymes are considered as "erasers". Some histone modifications, like acetylation, influence the strength of interactions between nucleosomes and DNA, but most influence chromatin states by interacting with specific domains of proteins that bind to nucleosomes. For instance, bromodomains or PHD domains each recognize specific acetylated histone peptides, whereas chromodomains recognize specific methylated histone sequences. Proteins containing such domains are known as (histone modification or chromatin) readers. Readers act as regulators of transcription, but also during DNA replication and repair. For instance, BRD proteins recognize acetylated histones and promote RNA Pol II activity (Donati et al. 2018). Importantly, enzymes modifying chromatin often contain reader domains and furthermore interact with each other. Multiprotein chromatin regulator complexes usually contain reader as well as writer or eraser subunits. Collectively, these interactions result in feed-forward or feedback loops that establish and stabilize particular—active or inactive—chromatin states that can spread from one nucleosome to neighboring ones (Zhao et al. 2021).

The pattern and level of the important regulatory histone modification H3K27me3 is determined by the interplay of two different types of protein complexes that were first identified as developmental regulators in Drosophila and are hence known as polycomb-like vs. trithorax-like or trithorax-related complex (Schuettengruber et al. 2017). In general, polycomb complexes mediate gene repression, whereas trithorax complexes lead to gene activation during development and cell differentiation. Two principal kinds of polycomb complexes exist, PRC1 and PRC2. Core components of PRC2 are the H3K27 methyltransferase EZH2 (or EZH1), SUZ12 (binding to DNA or RNA), EED (binding to H3K27me), and RBBP4 (or RBBP7) recognizing H3K36me3; accessory proteins may comprise among others JARID2 and AEBP2 that recognize ubiquitinated H2A. Ubiquitination of H2A at K119 (H2AK119ub1) is catalyzed by the PRC1 complex, which contains RING1A (or RING1B) and one of the six PCGF RING finger proteins. Additional components may include CBX proteins that bind to H3K27me3 through their chromodomains or the KDM2B demethylase that acts on methylated H3K36. By recognizing each other's histone modification product, the two polycomb complexes can act in either order to initiate and strengthen gene repression. In particular, the H2AK119ub1 mark is used to restore H3K27 trimethylation following replication of repressed gene sequences.

The trithorax complexes are supported by the WRAD (WDR5, RBBP5, ASH2L, and DPY30) core tetramer and contain at least one histone methyltransferase, either SET1, which catalyzes H3K4 trimethylation, or one of the four large KMT2 proteins, which are also known as MLL1–4. Like SET1, KMT2A and KMT2B rather mediate H3K4 methylation at promoters, with the tumor suppressor Menin as another essential subunit (Klonou et al. 2021). In contrast, the H3K4 monomethylases KMT2C and KMT2D associate with the NCOA6, PTIP and PA1 proteins as well as the H3K27me3 demethylase KDM6A (also known as UTX) and primarily activate enhancers. All KMT2-containing complexes are also referred to as COMPASS-like complex (Cenik and Shilatifard 2021; Schulz et al. 2019). They interact with histone acetyltransferases like CBP and p300 that catalyze especially acetylation at H3K27 (Chen et al. 2022) and stimulate chromatin remodeling by the SWI/SNF complex (Centore et al. 2020) to activate enhancers, promoters and ultimately transcription.

In addition to proteins, a number of non-coding RNAs regulate chromatin organization and activity. Whereas miRNAs are indirectly involved by regulating the biogenesis of chromatin proteins in the cytosol, several long non-coding RNAs (lncRNAs) are known or have been postulated to act directly on chromatin in the nucleus (Bhan et al. 2017; Borkiewicz et al. 2021; Mattick et al. 2023). The best-characterized lncRNA of this kind is XIST, a crucial regulator of X-chromosome inactivation in females (Brockdorff et al. 2020). LncRNAs may guide protein chromatin regulators to specific sites, e.g., by forming triplex structures with DNA, they may bring chromatin proteins or protein complexes in close proximity to each other, or they may act as decoys that prevent binding of chromatin regulators to histones or DNA. For instance, the lncRNA HOTAIR, which is aberrantly expressed in some bladder cancers (Heubach et al. 2015), has been reported to bind both PRC2 and the histone demethylase KDM1A (reviewed in Yuan et al. 2020). PRC2 contains RNA-binding subunits; likely via these subunits, nascent RNAs prevent PRC2 binding at many transcribed loci (Song et al. 2023). The functions of lncRNAs in chromatin regulation and especially in cancer are however incompletely understood (Chiu et al. 2018) and are in some cases controversial; in the present chapter, we therefore focus on protein chromatin regulators.

Many chromatin regulators are affected by genomic alterations in many different types of cancer. Alterations may comprise amplification or deletion of their genes, deleterious (truncating, frameshift or missense) mutations or missense mutations that activate chromatin regulators to oncogenes (Table 10.2). In addition, several chromatin regulator genes have been discovered to contribute domains with activator or repressor functions or with enzymatic activity to oncogenic fusion genes. For instance, various KMT2A fusion genes are formed in myeloid leukemias (hence also: MLL1 for KMT2A) and act by gain-of-function to establish a stem cell-like pattern of gene expression (Chan and Chen 2019). Notably, chromatin regulators influence metabolic processes in normal and cancer cells and conversely, their activity is influenced by the levels of normal metabolites such as acetyl-CoA, S-adenosylmethionine, α-ketoglutarate, succinate and many others, but also by oncometabolites like α-hydroxyglutarate (Loras et al. 2021; Miranda-Goncalves et al. 2018).

Epigenetic regulation is furthermore accomplished by modifications of DNA, in particular by DNA methylation (Jones 2012). In mammals, DNA is almost exclusively methylated physiologically at cytosines in the palindromic dinucleotide sequence CG (commonly designated CpG); in specific cell types methylation is found at cytosines in other sequences (denoted as non-CpG methylation). Methylation is introduced by the DNA methyltransferases DNMT1, DNMT3A or DNMT3B; the methyl group is supplied by S-adenosyl methionine (Lyko 2018; Mensah et al. 2021). DNMT1 is the main enzyme restoring symmetrical CpG methylation following DNA replication, interacting directly with components of the replication machinery, whereas the DNMT3 enzymes are mainly responsible for introduction of methylation at previously unmethylated CpGs. DNMT1 is therefore considered a maintenance methylase, whereas the DNMT3s are regarded as de-novo methylases. DNA methylation can be lost over the course of successive replication cycles in a passive manner if DNMTs do not remethylate hemimethylated sites or can be actively removed by TET (ten-eleven translocation) methylcytosine dioxygenases, which generate hydroxymethyl-cytosine. Hydroxymethyl-cytosine may persist, especially in and around active genes, and may influence transcription factor binding, polycomb activity, the transcription process and splicing (Besaratinia et al. 2022). Further oxidation of the cytosine base yields formyl- and carboxy-cytosine that are removed by thymine DNA glycosylase (TDG) whereupon cytosine is substituted by base excision repair. In somatic cells, approximately

Table 10.2 A selection of mutated chromatin regulators in human cancers[a]

Gene	Function	Complex	Examples of cancers with mutations	Effect of most common alterations
DNMT3A	DNA methyltransferase		Acute myeloid leukemia	Oncogenic
KMT2A	H3K4 methyltransferase	Trithorax-like	Leukemia (fusion proteins)	Oncogenic
KMT2B	H3K4 methyltransferase	Trithorax-like	Various	Inactivation
KMT2C	H3K4 methyltransferase	COMPASS	Various, bladder, renal	Inactivation
KMT2D	H3K4 methyltransferase	COMPASS	Various, bladder, renal, lymphomas	Inactivation
KDM6A	H3K4 methyltransferase	COMPASS	Various, bladder, renal, T-ALL	Inactivation
CREBBP	Histone acetyltransferase		Various, bladder	Inactivation
EP300	Histone acetyltransferase		Various, bladder	Inactivation
ARID1A	Chromatin remodeler	SWI/SNF	Various, bladder	Inactivation
ARID2	Chromatin remodeler	SWI/SNF	Various, breast	Inactivation
PBRM1	Chromatin remodeler	SWI/SNF	Renal cell carcinoma	Inactivation
SMARCA4	Chromatin remodeler	SWI/SNF	Various, lung adenocarcinoma	Inactivation
SMARCA2	Chromatin remodeler	SWI/SNF	Rhabdoid tumors, sarcomas	Inactivation
EZH2	H3K27 methyltransferase	PRC2	Various	Oncogenic, in specific tumors inactivation
NSD2	H3K36 methyltransferase		ALL, multiple myeloma	Oncogenic or inactivation
SETD2	H3K36 methyltransferase		Brain, renal	Inactivation
BAP1	H2AK119 deubiquitinase		Renal cell carcinoma, others	Inactivation

[a]Modified from (Schulz 2023)

70–80% of the cytosines in CpG-sites are methylated, depending on the cell type.

Methylated sites are unequally distributed in the genome (Jones 2012). Heterochromatic sequences, especially CpG-rich satellites and endogenous retroelement sequences, are as a rule fully methylated. Conversely, most CpG-islands, CpG-rich sequences straddling the transcriptional start sites of many genes, are unmethylated. In contrast, the actual transcribed regions, known as gene bodies, are typically densely DNA-methylated. Intergenic regions, which typically contain fewer CpGs, are normally also methylated. The sequences bordering CpG-islands, designated CpG-shores (or canyons), carry intermediate levels of methylation. Gene promoters with lower CpG-content (i.e., that do not contain CpG-islands) may be methylated to different extents. Whereas the methylation patterns in all these regions may be quite similar between different cell types, DNA methylation at enhancers and silencers is more variable. These sequences usually contain intermediate proportions of CpG-sites whose methylation reflects the activity state of the respective enhancers (or silencers), with the highest activity associated with the lowest degree of methylation. Methylation at enhancers and to a lower extent at promoters and CpG-shores thus distinguishes individual cell types and tissues. As a rule, methylation patterns are more similar between developmentally related cell types. For instance, DNA methylation at enhancers is more similar between urothelial and prostatic epithelial cells than between either cell type or epithelial cells from the proximal sections of the embryonic endoderm (Loyfer et al. 2023).

DNA methylation acts by modulating protein binding to DNA and—typical of epigenetic mechanisms—is in turn modulated by interactions with DNA-binding proteins, histone modifications and various chromatin regulators. Accordingly, DNMTs contain domains that recognize histone modifications (Hashimoto et al. 2010). For instance, in the establishment of heterochromatin, DNA methyltransferases interact with specific histone methyltransferases that establish H3K9me3 and H4K20me3 (Ren et al. 2021) and the heterochromatin protein HP1. Methylated CpGs are recognized by methyl-binding proteins like MBD1, MBD2, and MeCP2 (Rausch et al. 2019). These proteins can be regarded as subunits of larger repressor protein complexes like SIN3A and NURD which also comprise histone deacetylases (Meier and Brehm 2014). In that manner, DNA methylation promotes histone deacetylation and a repressed chromatin state. DNA methylation may also attract polycomb protein complexes and vice versa. However, DNA methylation and polycomb-mediated histone modifications like H3K27me3 are often successive rather than concomitant modifications, superseding each other.

At CpG-islands, DNMT activity is prevented by H3K4 methylation, which is introduced by histone methyltransferases like SETDB1 (supported by the DNA-binding protein CFP1, which recognizes unmethylated CpGs) or KMT2A/B. In gene bodies, DNMT3 de-novo methylases recognize the H3K36me3 modification (Weinberg et al. 2019) affixed via dimethylation by NSD2 and NSD3 (dimethylation) and SETD2 (trimethylation). The DNA methyltransferases often remain associated with the methylated sequences. In this fashion, gene body methylation prevents spurious transcription initiation (i.e., outside promoters) and allows the recognition of weak splice sites by slowing down RNA Pol II (Wang et al. 2022).

About 30% of all DNA-binding transcription (activating) factors contain CpG-sites in their recognition motifs (Heberle and Bardet 2019). The effect of DNA methylation on the binding of such factors is variable, ranging from strongly inhibitory to insensitive or even strengthening; the effect depends in addition on the precise sequence of the binding site. Thus, CpG-methylation can directly prevent (or in some cases facilitate) the access of transcription factors to gene promoters or enhancers. However, in general, changes in chromatin structure due to interaction of DNA methylation with further chromatin regulators are more decisive. In addition, DNA-binding transcription factors may attract DNA methyltransferases or—like CFP1—repel them. Importantly, binding of CTCF, a protein determining the extension of chromatin loops is inhibited by DNA methylation at some of its potential binding sites, so that DNA methylation affects the size and location of chromatin loops.

Patterns of DNA methylation in cancer cells are often strongly disturbed (Nishiyama and Nakanishi 2021). Two characteristic alterations are known as CpG-island hypermethylation and global hypomethylation (Fig. 10.2). In cancer cells, up to several hundred CpG-islands may aberrantly be densely methylated. CpG-island hypermethylation is associated with inactivation of the affected promoter sequence and decreased expression. Therefore, DNA hypermethylation can lead to the inactivation of tumor suppressor genes by transcriptional repression, such as the *VHL* gene in some renal cell carcinomas (Dizman et al. 2020), the *MLH1* mismatch repair gene in colorectal and other cancers, and a number of secreted WNT antagonist genes in several cancers (Pfeifer 2018) including bladder cancer (see following section). Of note, whereas one promoter in a gene may become hypermethylated and repressed, other promoters in the same gene may remain active, so that expression may be overall decreased or may shift to different transcripts and protein isoforms. Prominent examples are the *CDKN2A* gene, where one or the other or both of its promoters may become hypermethylated or the *TP63* gene, where hypermethylation of its first promoter favors the expression of its ΔN isoform (from a second promoter) over its TA isoform (Pokorna et al. 2022). Importantly, CpG-

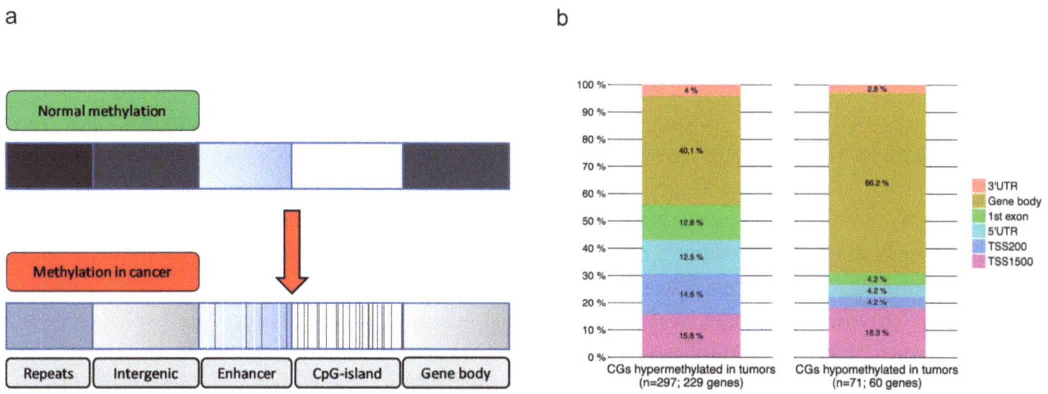

Fig. 10.2 DNA methylation alterations in cancer. (**a**) Schematic representation of DNA methylation distribution in the normal genome and its alterations in cancer. Light to dark shading indicates increasing methylation, from: Schulz (2023). (**b**) Distribution of DNA methylation alterations in and around genes; an example from breast cancer. Note the typical increase in CpG methylation at promoters and 5′-untranslated regions and the likewise typical decrease in gene bodies. From de Almeida et al. (2019)

island hypermethylation commonly results in the methylation of DNA sequences that are not methylated in any other tissue or at any developmental stage. Therefore, assays detecting CpG-island hypermethylation are well-suited for use in cancer diagnostics (Davalos and Esteller 2022; see Sect. 10.3).

The mechanisms underlying CpG-island hypermethylation are not uniform and are in fact incompletely understood in many cancer types, including most cases of bladder cancer. In some cancers, mutations inactivate TET1 or TET2 demethylases or change the specificity of isocitrate dehydrogenases (IDH1 or IDH2) so that they produce α-hydroxyglutarate, an inhibitor of TET and other epigenetic regulator enzymes employing α-ketoglutarate as a substrate. In these cancers, a high number of CpG-islands are aberrantly methylated, because they cannot be actively demethylated. TET mutations occur in a small fraction of bladder cancers, whereas IDH mutations are exceptional. Frequent hypermethylation of CpG-islands is also found in another group of cancers designated as CIMP+ (CpG-island methylation phenotype). CIMP+ cancers were first identified among colorectal carcinomas, but are also observed in other tissues. Their specific methylation phenotype is thought to be elicited by specific repressor proteins acting downstream of oncogenic KRAS and especially BRAF proteins that direct de-novo-methylation to CpG-islands (Serra et al. 2014). Whereas this particular mechanism appears to be rarely responsible in bladder cancers, the general principle may be relevant, namely, that upregulation of transcriptional repressor proteins and DNA methyltransferases leads to aberrant methylation of CpG-island and other gene promoters (Mensah et al. 2021). Finally, a subset of aberrantly hypermethylated genes, with or without CpG-islands, may be susceptible to DNA methylation because they are only weakly expressed in the normal tissue (Schlesinger et al. 2007). Regulatory regions of such genes may carry bivalent histone modifications, i.e., methylation of H3K4 as well as H3K27, and are bound by the PRC2 complex. In cancers, expression of such genes may become completely inactivated with both histone modifications being lost. Consequently, the PRC2 complex dissociates and the gene promoters become DNA-methylated. Increased activity of PRC2, as found in many bladder cancers, may therefore precipitate increased DNA methylation at weakly active promoters and enhancers. As an important corollary, even recurrent hypermethylation of a gene in a cancer type does not necessarily identify it as a tumor suppressor.

Global hypomethylation is a second distinctive cancer-specific alteration. Whereas in normal somatic cells about 3–4% of all cytosines are methylated, the total methylcytosine content of cancer genomes may be dramatically decreased, by 70–80%, despite increased focal hypermethylation. In particular, this decrease affects sequences that are normally densely methylated, such as CpG-rich satellites or endogenous retroelements repressed by DNA methylation. It may therefore destabilize heterochromatin and facilitate reactivation of retroelements like LINE-1 or endogenous retroviral sequences which in turn may contribute to genomic instability (Hoffmann and Schulz 2005). As a consequence, global hypomethylation in cancers may enhance chromosomal instability. Moreover, it contributes to transcriptional deregulation by derepressing certain genes like cancer-testis antigens that are controlled by DNA methylation, by uncovering cryptic promoters within genes or in intergenic regions, by affecting promoter choice, or by altering splicing and transcriptional rates as a consequence of decreased methylation of gene bodies.

The mechanisms eliciting global hypomethylation are not fully understood but are also likely to be manifold. For instance, continuous and rapid replication in cancer cells may interfere especially with the remethylation of late-replicating regions leading to a gradual loss of their methylation (Nishiyama and Nakanishi 2021). As this process has also been observed in senescent cells, global DNA hypomethylation in cancers has been interpreted to represent a failed attempt at undergoing senescence in response to oncogenic stress. A factor likely contributing to global hypomethylation is an insufficient supply of the substrate for cellular methylation reactions, S-adenosylmethionine, resulting from nutritional deficits or from deficiencies in the methyl cycle that regenerates methionine and S-adenosylmethionine from S-adenosylhomocysteine, which are observed in many cancer cells.

CpG-island hypermethylation and global hypomethylation are distinctive and often massive alterations in many cancer types. In addition, more subtle changes take place that alter DNA methylation at specific sites in a more quantitative manner. Especially at promoters and enhancers, they may be linked to transcriptional changes, but they may also affect transcribed, intragenic sequences impinging on splicing and transcription termination. Several techniques are now available to evaluate changes in DNA methylation across the entire genome (Tost 2022). CpG-arrays can quantify methylation at up to 3% of all CpGs across the genome; commonly used arrays cover especially promoter and enhancer sequences, but also a selection of other genomic regions, which are represented by a few CpG each. More comprehensive coverage can be achieved by reduced representation bisulfite sequencing (RRBS) which interrogates mainly CpG-rich regions across the genome and by whole-genome bisulfite sequencing (WGBS), which represents the current gold standard. Capture techniques like methylated-CpG island recovery assay (MIRA) employing proteins binding specifically to methylated or unmethylated DNA represent alternatives to techniques based on bisulfite treatment of DNA. Likewise, third-generation high-throughput techniques allow direct methylation analysis of larger DNA fragments, facilitating analysis of repetitive sequences. Studies on bladder cancer so far have mainly used CpG-arrays (see next section).

An important caveat applying especially to quantitative studies is that DNA methylation is cell type-specific (Loyfer et al. 2023). Methylation patterns of cancer cells are most similar to those of their normal cells of origin, with cancer-specific alterations superimposed. For that reason, quantitative differences between cancer and normal tissues may reflect differences in the cellular composition rather than cancer-specific changes. Global hypomethylation and CpG-island hypermethylation, in comparison, are more distinctive because they are not (or rarely) found in any normal cell type.

10.2 DNA Methylation Changes in Bladder Cancer

The methylation alterations typical of cancers in general, focal CpG-island hypermethylation and global hypomethylation, are also prominent in bladder cancers. Until the first decade of this century, focal DNA hypermethylation was primarily investigated by candidate gene studies or by screening using smaller gene arrays (Kandimalla et al. 2013; Nunes et al. 2020). The methylation events identified in this manner form the basis of several assays that were developed and tested for various applications in bladder cancer diagnostics (see Sect. 10.3). Some hypermethylated genes code for known or presumed tumor suppressors such as APC (a WNT pathway inhibitor), CDH1 (E-Cadherin), DAPK (an apoptotic regulator), FHIT (a potential tumor suppressor located at the fragile site on chromosome 3p), RASSF1A (a Hippo pathway regulator), SFRPs (secreted WNT antagonists), and TIMP3 (a matrix metalloprotease inhibitor). On a note of caution, the correlation of hypermethylation and decreased expression of these genes in bladder cancer was not ascertained in many studies and none of the above genes is recurrently subject to genetic alterations in bladder cancers. A particularly complex case is *CDKN2A*. As in most other cancer types, this tumor suppressor gene is most commonly inactivated in bladder cancer by homozygous deletions, but missense mutations are not infrequent. The effect of DNA hypermethylation depends on the affected sequence within *CDKN2A*; it may inactivate one or both of its promoters, but increased methylation in exon 2 rather reflects increased transcription and expression, which is observed especially in cancers with *RB1* inactivation. In addition, *CDKN2A* is repressed by polycomb factors in conjunction with the lncRNA ANRIL that is expressed from the same genomic region (Aguilo et al. 2011). The large TCGA reference study (Robertson et al. 2017), which used 450 K methylation arrays, noted that DNA hypermethylation was infrequent but mutually exclusive with mutations of *CDKN2A*. In addition, hypermethylation of two additional tumor suppressor genes, *FAT1* (encoding another Hippo regulator) and *CASP8* (encoding another apoptotic regulator), was mutually exclusive with mutations and was associated with their downregulation. More than 150 additional genes were found to be significantly hypermethylated as well as downregulated in that study, but none of them is regarded as a major tumor suppressor.

Global hypomethylation in bladder cancer was initially identified through the highly prevalent and often pronounced decrease of methylation at retroelement sequences like LINE-1 retroelements (reviewed in Hoffmann and Schulz 2005). These observations have been corroborated and extended by more recent investigations applying high-throughput techniques (Li et al. 2022; Olkhov-Mitsel et al. 2017; van der Vos et al. 2020). Notably, the TCGA pan-cancer study of aberrant DNA methylation (Saghafinia et al. 2018) identified bladder cancer as a cancer type with pronounced hypomethylation and relatively low, but significant hypermethylation. Thus, bladder cancer ranked fifth-lowest for hypermethylation, but fourth-highest for hypomethylation among all cancers. Since this conclusion was based on methylation arrays that interrogate DNA methylation prominently at genes and enhancers, global hypomethylation in bladder cancers appears not to be restricted to repeat and heterochromatin sequences. This principal conclusion was corroborated by a study using whole-genome bisulfite sequencing (Li et al. 2022).

A pronounced "hypermethylator" phenotype is rare in bladder cancers. Known mechanisms causing such phenotypes appear to be active in individual cases only. Thus, fewer than 5% of bladder cancers harbor mutations in *TET1*, but only a fraction of these are deletions or otherwise clearly deleterious (Cerami et al. 2012; Gao et al. 2013).[1] Even fewer mutations are found in *TET2*, *IDH1* or *IDH2*; for instance, only a handful of cases have been described to carry the typical oncogenic missense mutations at R112 of *IDH1*. In addition to mutations, oxidative stress and hypoxia can impair the activity of TET enzymes and other dioxygenases (Matuleviciute et al. 2021); these factors might also be relevant in bladder cancer. A CIMP-like phenotype is likewise exceptional in bladder cancers. Instead, the

[1] Statements on the distribution and type of mutations in bladder cancer genomes here and further in the chapter are based on queries using the cBioportal database, www.cbioportal.org, unless stated otherwise.

frequent overexpression of EZH2 and overactivity of PRC2 may underlie repression and DNA hypermethylation of many individual genes in bladder cancers (Schlesinger et al. 2007). This mechanism may particularly target genes encoding developmental regulators and lineage-specific transcription factors that are not or weakly expressed in the normal urothelial lineage.

In the pan-cancer TCGA study (Saghafinia et al. 2018), a high frequency of DNA methylation alterations was statistically associated with mutations affecting IDH1/2 and certain WNT regulator (*CTNNB1*, *RNF43*) genes and alterations in specific chromatin regulator genes, especially the H3K36 methyltransferases *NSD1* and *SETD2*, the SWI/SNF components *ARID2* and *ARID1B*, and the H3K4 methyltransferases *KMT2C* and *KMT2D*; all of which are subject to mutations in bladder cancer (see Sect. 10.4). While those associations may not necessarily reflect causal relationships, in view of the known interactions between chromatin-regulators and DNA methyltransferases (see Sect. 10.1), it seems plausible that some mutations in chromatin regulator genes may contribute to DNA methylation alterations in bladder cancer. In particular, H3K36 methylation directs the activity of DNMT3 enzymes to specific genomic regions, whereas KMT2-containing COMPASS and SWI/SNF complexes antagonize polycomb-mediated gene repression that can precipitate aberrant DNA methylation in cancer cells (see Sect. 10.1).

Aberrant DNA methylation in bladder cancer may also be caused by the impact of chemical carcinogens. As reviewed elsewhere (Schulz and Goering 2016), observational studies and experiments in cell culture models have linked trihalomethane, carcinogens from tobacco smoke and arsenic to DNA methylation alterations in bladder cancer. For instance, DNA methylation alterations detectable in blood were associated with a higher bladder cancer risk in smoking women (Jordahl et al. 2018). This association is likely mediated by elevated levels of methylated metabolites and polycyclic aromatic hydrocarbons that form DNA adducts and cause DNA damage as well as by induction of DNMT1. Accordingly, exposure of bladder cancer cells to the tobacco smoke carcinogens 4-(methyl-nitrosamino)-1-(3-pyridyl)-1-butanone (NNK) or benzopyrene resulted in increased levels of methylated metabolites, DNA adducts, and DNA damage (Jin et al. 2017), which may disturb proper DNA methylation (Goodman et al. 2022). In comparison, epigenetic impacts of arsenic have been thought to be mediated partly through depletion of S-adenosylmethionine, although direct inhibition of DNA methyltransferases and demethylases is now thought to be more relevant (Saintilnord and Fondufe-Mittendorf 2021). Intriguingly, infection by uropathogenic bacteria too may result in altered DNA methylation patterns, although the reported effects appear to be relatively small (Tolg et al. 2011).

Finally, as in most cancers, hydroxymethylcytosine levels are decreased in bladder cancer as well; this may represent an early event during urothelial carcinogenesis (Munari et al. 2016; Peng et al. 2018). In normal cells, up to 0.7% of all cytosine residues are hydroxymethylated. Since hydroxy-methylcytosine and other oxidized forms of methylcytosine are not or are poorly recognized by the maintenance methylase DNMT1, highly proliferative cells including cancer cells lose hydroxy-methylcytosine over successive cell cycles (Besaratinia et al. 2022). In cancers with *TET* or *IDH* mutations, hydroxymethylcytosine is yet more strongly depleted. In bladder cancers, hydroxy-methylcytosine was mostly diminished around active genes, where it is most enriched in normal cells. While the functional consequences of these changes require further elucidation, hydroxymethyl-cytosine content can be determined in DNA from plasma or urine and can be employed for cancer diagnostics (Besaratinia et al. 2022).

10.3 DNA Methylation Diagnostics in Bladder Cancer

Assays detecting alterations in DNA methylation (see Davalos and Esteller (2022) for a general overview) can be applied for a variety of purposes in bladder cancer diagnostics. For initial diagnosis, bladder cancer patients may be identified among persons presenting with hematuria or other suspicious symptoms. DNA methylation-based assays may also be useful for early detection of recurrences during surveillance following transurethral resection of non-muscle-invasive bladder cancers (NMIBC). In addition to assays for detection, assays for prognostication would be valuable in several clinical situations (reviewed by Casadevall et al. 2017; Jeronimo and Henrique 2014; Kandimalla et al. 2013; Yu et al. 2018). Particularly important issues are predicting the likelihood of progression of high-grade NMIBC and choosing appropriate treatments for stage pT1 NMIBC. In the therapy of muscle-invasive bladder cancers, DNA methylation assays—like molecular subtyping—could inform on the optimal application of chemotherapy, conventional or targeted, neo-adjuvant or adjuvant.

DNA from a range of samples can be used for DNA methylation diagnostics of bladder cancer. Cancer tissue samples are suited for prognostic assays, but other samples may be used for this purpose as well. Most assays for detection have been developed for DNA isolated from urine, either from cellular sediments or supernatant (see also Chap. 18). Cell-free DNA from plasma may also be used, especially for detection of invasive cancers. Even DNA from blood cells may be informative since altered DNA methylation patterns in blood cells may reflect the presence of a (bladder) cancer or even an increased risk of developing bladder cancer in the future (Jordahl et al. 2018; Moore et al. 2008).

Several DNA methylation assays for bladder cancer diagnostics have been proposed, developed, and tested, albeit to varying extents. In general, these assays have proved superior to urine cytology or established cytogenetic or biochemical assays and provide higher sensitivity and specificity for initial diagnosis and surveillance. Most methylation assays are based on hypermethylation markers that ought to especially assure high specificity (see Sect. 10.2). A few hypomethylation markers have also been proposed which are usually based on global hypomethylation of repeat sequences such as LINE-1 retrotransposons (Ghanjati et al. 2014), but detection of hypomethylation of one particular LINE-1 sequence located near the *MET* receptor tyrosine kinase gene (*L1-MET*) has also been used as part of an assay panel. Initially, assays were based on hypermethylation of only a few genes (reviewed in Kandimalla et al. 2013; Schulz and Goering 2016), but newer assays use more CpG-sites at larger numbers of genes. Comprehensive DNA methylation analysis techniques may moreover allow classification of bladder cancers into methylation-based molecular subtypes that predict prognosis and responses to specific therapies (Li et al. 2022; Robertson et al. 2017; Tian et al. 2020), especially immunotherapy (Ye et al. 2021).

Several additional methylated gene panels that were proposed more recently (since 2016) for diagnostic purposes are based either on novel assemblies of candidate genes (Hentschel et al. 2022; van der Heijden et al. 2018) or were derived from methylation analyses using high-throughput techniques (Chen et al. 2020a; Kohler et al. 2020; Olkhov-Mitsel et al. 2017). In an interesting approach, several published gene panels for bladder cancer detection have been compared by using RRBS results of a small patient cohort to develop an optimized three-gene methylation panel (Fang et al. 2019). Other panels derived from high-throughput methylation analyses aim at combining detection with tumor grading or risk stratification (Hermanns et al. 2020; Ruan et al. 2021). An analysis of high-grade NMIBC using 450 K CpG arrays confirmed more frequent hypermethylation in these tumors compared to low-grade tumors or normal urothelium and identified several specific hypermethylated genes that might be used for detection of tumors with higher risk for progression (Kitchen et al. 2016). A rare study employing whole-genome bisulfite sequencing in bladder cancer aimed at identifying methylation subtypes that differ in prognosis or in their response to the DNMT inhibitor SGI-110 (Li et al. 2022). While most of these studies employed approaches with separate cohorts for development and validation, the proposed assays still require prospective testing in large cohorts in realistic clinical settings before they can be introduced into clinical practice.

For clinical application, to date, the Bladder EpiCheck assay, which is based on methylation analysis of 15 proprietary CpGs, has been prospectively validated for surveillance of bladder cancer patients (D'Andrea et al. 2019; Witjes et al. 2018; reviewed in Mancini et al. 2020) and is commercially available. A meta-analysis (Laukhtina et al. 2021) confirmed its usefulness to reduce the number of cystoscopies in patients under surveillance following resection of NMIBC. The UroMark assay uses an even larger number (150) of CpG-sites to detect urothelial carcinomas from urine sediment DNA (Feber et al. 2017). Its usefulness in the initial diagnosis of bladder cancer has been tested in a prospective clinical trial (NCT02781428), but the results have not been finally published. A similar trial is ongoing for the AnchorDx UriFind assay, which is based on detection of hypermethylation of the *ONECUT2* and *VIM* genes (Zhang et al. 2019). An MDxHealth assay for bladder cancer is likewise marketed, but no newer publications on its performance in clinical practice are available.

Notably, many published DNA methylation assays achieve values for sensitivity and specificity that would make them useful in their intended clinical applications, but they rarely reach values close to 100% even using increasing numbers of CpG-sites. Low-grade tumors appear to be particularly difficult to detect. This difficulty may be due to the lower degree of methylation disturbances in these tumors as well as to a lower number of tumor cells shed into the urine. The specificity of DNA methylation assays, may also be limited, presumably by methylation changes in normal cells in preneoplastic urothelium. However, if such changes occur, they indicate a higher risk of developing bladder cancer in the future. More generally, limitations of DNA methylation assays may result from the pronounced molecular and clinical heterogeneity of bladder cancer, which is reflected in DNA methylation changes as well (see Sect. 10.2). Some of the above limitations may be ameliorated by adding mutation markers that can be conveniently assayed such as *FGFR3* or *TERT* mutations (van Kessel et al. 2017), which are present in a large fraction of urothelial carcinomas, including low-grade tumors.

10.4 Chromatin Regulator Alterations in Bladder Cancer

A considerable number of chromatin regulator genes have been found to be recurrently mutated in bladder cancer. These include (in increasing order of frequency according to the studies included in the COSMIC cancer database) *JAK2, KDM5A, ASXL2, NSD1, BAP1, NCOR1, ATRX, STAG1, PBRM1, ARID1B, ARID2, SMARCA4, KMT2A, EP300, CREBBP, KMT2C, STAG2, KMT2D, ARID1A*, and *KDM6A*. The relative frequencies of mutations for each gene vary between individual studies, depending on the characteristics of the samples and the study population as well as on the methodology (see below). However, the top ten most frequent mutated genes are essentially the same between the studies. Notably, these genes are more frequently mutated in bladder cancer than on average in all cancers combined (see, e.g., Carrot-Zhang et al. 2020). Overall, therefore, more than 80% of bladder cancers harbor mutations in at least one chromatin regulator gene, meaning that the frequency of alterations in epigenetic regulators is on a par with those deregulating cell cycle control, activating MAPK and PI3K signaling and telomerase.

In addition to the factors encoded by the above genes, RB1 doubles as a chromatin regulator, since the tumor suppressor acts as a repressor that can induce a heterochromatic state at genes promoting cell cycle progression. In a substantial fraction of bladder cancers *RB1* is inactivated by deleterious point mutations, but also quite commonly by partial or complete gene deletions. Deletions may also cause the inactivation of other chromatin regulators. For instance, the *KDM6A* homolog *UTY* is primarily inactivated by loss of the Y-chromosome, where its gene resides, in male patients. Conversely, gene amplification may contribute to overexpression of some chromatin regulators such as EZH2 (Raman et al. 2005). Moreover, as discussed elsewhere in detail (Hoffmann and Schulz 2021), consistent downregulation of their expression may lead to lower activity of certain chromatin regulators.

The most frequently mutated chromatin regulator genes affected by recurrent mutations in bladder cancer encode components of two interacting complexes, namely the trithorax-related COMPASS complex (prominently *KMT2C, KMT2D*, and *KDM6A*) and the SWI/SNF chromatin remodeling complex (*ARID1A, ARID1B, ARID2, SMARCA4*, and *PBRM1*) that cooperate in the activation of enhancers. In comparison, mutations in *KMT2A* and *KMT2B* that encode the H3K4 methyltransferase subunits of trithorax-like complexes acting at promoters (Klonou et al. 2021; Poreba et al. 2020) are less prevalent. In addition, the histone acetyltransferases p300 and CBP encoded by the *EP300* and *CREBBP* genes interact with the KMT2C/D COMPASS complex to establish active enhancers. In bladder cancers, the *EP300* and *CREBBP* genes are affected by truncating mutations or by missense mutations, of which the majority are predicted to inactivate their enzyme activity (Duex et al. 2018). Inactivation of the HATs could constitute an alternative, indirect mechanism of COMPASS inactivation, but notably, in lymphomas, p300 and KMT2C/D inactivation are thought to be synergistic (Zhao et al. 2021). As for the HATs, the overwhelming majority of mutations in all COMPASS-related genes are predicted to be deleterious; nonsense and other truncating mutations abound and missense mutations are distributed throughout the proteins but especially in crucial domains (Fig. 10.3). This pattern is very different from that typically observed in oncogenes—e.g., the majority of mutations in *FGFR3* in bladder cancer are S249C—and rather resembles that observed in canonical tumor suppressor genes. However, different from canonical tumor suppressors, genomic alterations in chromatin regulator genes in bladder cancer do not regularly affect both alleles and are not strictly mutually exclusive with each other. Nevertheless, the great majority of bladder cancers contains inactivating mutations in at least one component of the COMPASS or SWI/SNF complexes or in one of the associated HATs. These observations suggest that the function of COMPASS complexes to establish active enhancers is compromised in almost all bladder cancers, but unlikely to be fully lost (see next section for a detailed discussion).

Conversely, comparatively few genomic alterations are observed in genes encoding components of polycomb complexes which functionally antagonize trithorax complexes (see Sect. 10.1). In particular, the *EZH2* gene is amplified in only a fraction of bladder cancers and is not prone to mutations. EZH2 is however upregulated in a substantial fraction of the cases and particularly in cancers with *RB1* deletions, in keeping with the known negative regulation of EZH2 expression by RB1 (Knudsen et al. 2019). Like EZH2, the methyltransferase G9a that introduces a different repressive histone modification, H3K9me2, is often overexpressed in bladder cancers (Cho et al. 2011).

More than 20% of bladder cancers contain mutations in SWI/SNF components. *ARID1A* (BAF250a), encoding a SWI/SNF subunit, is a commonly mutated gene across human cancers and is mutated in approximately 18–25% of muscle-invasive urothelial carcinomas (MIBC) (Conde and Frew 2022). In other tumor types, inactivation of ARID1A has been linked to deregulation of cell type-specific gene expression, but also to deficiencies in cell cycle regulation, p53 function and checkpoint signaling (Wu and Roberts 2013). ARID1A and ARID1B regulate the target specificities of two different variants of the "canonical" SWI/SNF complex. ARID2 replaces ARID1A/B in a related complex, the polybromo BRG1-associated factor (PBAF) that also contains PBRM1, BRD7, and PHF10 as unique subunits. Since SWI/SNF complexes are essential to maintain accessibility of enhancers in general, their complete inactivation is not compatible with cell growth and survival. Accordingly, *ARID1A* and *ARID1B* inactivating mutations are mutually exclusive with each other; the same holds for the ATPase subunits *SMARCA4* (BRG1) and *SMARCA2* (BRM). In bladder cancers, mutations inactivating *ARID1B* or *ARID2* are also observed at a low frequency, whereas *SMARCA4* mutations are much more common than mutations in *SMARCA2*, as in most other cancer types. Unusually for adult cancers, bladder cancers with *SMARCB1* mutations have also been reported

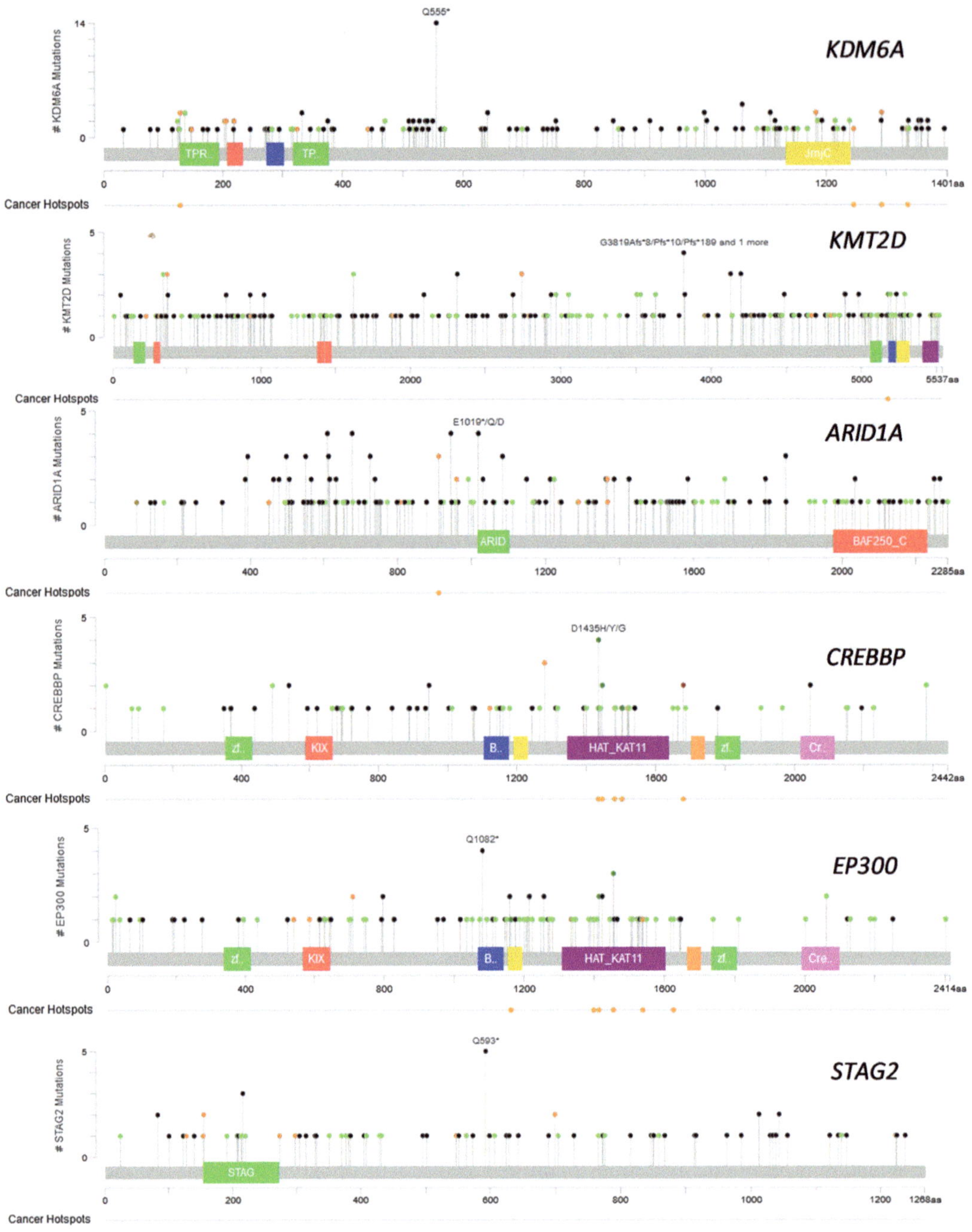

Color code: Missense mutations; truncating mutations (nonsense, nonstop, frameshift deletion or insertion, splice site); **inframe (inframe) mutations** (inframe deletion or insertion); **splice mutations**

Fig. 10.3 Type and distribution of mutations in chromatin regulator genes in muscle-invasive bladder cancer. Top to bottom: Mutations in *KDM6A*, *KMT2C*, *ARID1A*, *CRBBP*, *EP300*, and *STAG2*. At each position, the height of the mark indicates the number of mutations detected and the type of mutations is indicated by the color of the circle as described at the bottom of the figure. At the bottom of each panel, hotspots across all human cancers are indicated in orange. Note hotspots at Q558 of KDM6A (specific to urothelial carcinoma) and in the catalytic domains of the two HATs. The figure is based on the TCGA data on MIBC (Robertson et al. 2017) and the panels were downloaded from the cBioPortal database in April 2023 (Cerami et al. 2012; Gao et al. 2013)

(Gupta et al. 2018). In addition, *PBRM1* mutations are moderately frequent in bladder cancers, if not as frequent as in renal cell carcinoma (Walton et al. 2023). Notably, these mutations underline that all three major variants of the SWI/SNF complex can be affected by deleterious mutations in bladder cancer, albeit not all in the same individual cancer. Given the assumption that the variants serve different functions (Centore et al. 2020), this observation provides a conundrum that needs to be addressed by future research.

Notably, many additional chromatin regulators that are subject to recurrent genomic alterations in bladder cancer (especially MIBC) are functionally related to the COMPASS and polycomb complexes (see next section for details). The *BAP1* gene located at chromosome 3p encodes a H2AK119 deubiquitinase and is affected in about 6% of all cases by deleterious mutations. *ASXL2* encoding a protein interacting and directing BAP1 is subject to inactivating mutations in some cases. The *NSD1* gene, which encodes a lysine methyltransferase specific for H3K36 also known as KMT3B (Tauchmann and Schwaller 2021), is affected in about 7% of all cases by deleterious mutations, as in several other cancer types, in particular squamous carcinomas. KDM5A (also known as JARID1A or RBP2) is a histone demethylase with a jumonji domain that specifically demethylates H3K4me3 and H3K4me2, which are associated with actively transcribed sequences (Yang et al. 2021; Yoo et al. 2022). Depending on the cancer type it can act as an oncogene, e.g., in AML but also in several carcinomas, or in a tumor-suppressive manner. In bladder cancer, genomic alterations are observed in about 5% of the cancers, most are truncating or missense mutations distributed across the gene, fitting rather a tumor suppressor pattern.

The *ATRX* gene is mutated in about 6% of all bladder cancers, but most changes are missense mutations of uncertain significance. It encodes a large multifunctional protein best known for its chaperone function in heterochromatin and telomere maintenance (reviewed in Aguilera and Lopez-Contreras 2023; Valenzuela et al. 2021). Many functions of ATRX require dimerization with its partner protein DAXX which is rarely mutated in bladder cancer. As for other very large genes, it is possible that *ATRX* missense mutations are passenger events resulting from the high mutational rate in bladder cancers (up to 10/Mbp).

The *JAK2* gene is subject to genomic alterations in somewhat more than 5% of all bladder cancers. The large JAK2 kinase activates JAK/STAT signaling at membrane receptors but additionally phosphorylates H3Y41 (Zouein et al. 2011). By preventing binding of HP1, this phosphorylation facilitates especially the activation of STAT target genes. Hotspot mutations in myeloid neoplasms enhance JAK2 protein kinase activity and accordingly JAK/STAT signaling (reviewed by Huang et al. 2022). The alterations in bladder cancers include homozygous deletions of the locus at 9p24 and truncating mutations and rather fit a tumor suppressor pattern. The consequences of JAK2 inactivation in bladder cancer are however unknown to date.

Genomic alterations in *NCOR1* are observed in about 10% of MIBC. Most, but not all of the alterations are clearly inactivating. NCOR1 serves as a corepressor mediating gene repression by nuclear receptors in the absence of their ligands.

STAG2 is a component of the cohesin complex (see next section for details) that alternatively contains STAG1 as well as the SMC1A, SMC3, and RAD21 subunits (Di Nardo et al. 2022). Whereas STAG1 and RAD21 tend to be overexpressed in bladder cancers and their genes are amplified in a few cases, *STAG2* is subject to deletions or truncating mutations in up to 20% of bladder cancers, especially in NMIBC (Balbas-Martinez et al. 2013; Taylor et al. 2014). Missense mutations in *SMC1A* have also been reported.

Importantly, chromatin regulator genes are also regularly affected by inactivating mutations in NMIBC (e.g., in 86% of cases in Hedegaard et al. (2016) and in almost all in Hurst et al. (2017)). Surveying all studies, KDM6A and STAG2 mutations are even more frequent in NMIBC than in MIBC, whereas ARID1A mutations are less common (Hurst and Knowles

2022). For most chromatin regulators, the frequency of genomic alterations does not appear to differ significantly between the molecular subtypes of muscle-invasive bladder cancer. Across many studies, *KDM6A* inactivation was found associated with *FGFR3* mutations and papillary urothelial carcinomas, both non-invasive papillary urothelial carcinoma (Hurst et al. 2017) and the luminal-papillary subtype of MIBC (Kamoun et al. 2020). For *ARID1A* mutations, an association with more aggressive subtypes or higher stage and grades has been reported (Balbas-Martinez et al. 2013; Clinton et al. 2022), but was not confirmed by the comprehensive analysis by Kamoun et al. (2020). However, SWI/SNF inactivation may be pervasive in undifferentiated regions of bladder cancers (Agaimy et al. 2016).

Importantly, like certain DNA methylation alterations, mutations in specific chromatin regulators or specific histone modifications might yield prognostic information. This topic has been discussed by two comprehensive reviews (Casadevall et al. 2017; Martinez et al. 2019) who concluded that the data are not sufficiently mature yet and that prospective studies are required to identify clinically useful biomarkers from any associations observed to date.

10.5 Functional Relevance of Epigenetic Alterations in Bladder Cancer

Mutations in chromatin regulator genes, as detailed in the previous section, are found in the great majority of bladder cancers, including different molecular subtypes, tumor stages and anatomic locations, i.e., they are also detected in urothelial tumors of the upper tract (Karanovic et al. 2022). There are few other cancer types in which chromatin regulator mutations are that prevalent. Evidently, altered functions of chromatin regulators appear to be a prerequisite for the development of bladder cancers. This idea is supported by the detection of mutations in chromatin regulator genes in cell clones expanding in the morphologically normal urothelium of elderly people (Lawson et al. 2020; Li et al. 2020), in a similar fashion as in clonal hematopoiesis. In accord with these observations, knockdown of KDM6A in a normal urothelial cell line and a bladder cancer cell line retaining a urothelial differentiation hierarchy led to the expansion of cells with urothelial stem cell markers (Lang et al. 2020). Similarly, increased epigenetic plasticity allows bladder cancer cells to more easily assume a stem cell state (Xu et al. 2020).

The underlying mechanisms are however far from clarified. Several recent investigations (Barrows et al. 2020; Guo et al. 2022; Lang et al. 2020; Ler et al. 2017; Qiu et al. 2023) suggest that inactivation of specific chromatin regulators disturbs the balance between differentiation and cell proliferation during urothelial differentiation, which are coupled processes in normal cells (Ruijtenberg and van den Heuvel 2016). Notably, these disturbances extend beyond the cancer cells and impinge on their interactions with other cell types, such as stromal cells and cells of the immune system (Chen et al. 2021; Kobatake et al. 2020; Zhu et al. 2020). Moreover, mutations in certain chromatin regulators affect additional processes in the cancer cells, such as DNA repair, contributing to increased mutation rates and chromosomal instability (Rampias et al. 2019; Zhu et al. 2020; reviewed by Walton et al. 2023; Chang et al. 2019), altered cell metabolism (Chang et al. 2019) or cell migration during metastasis (Liu et al. 2021).

The crucial genomic alterations of chromatin regulators in bladder cancer converge on the function of the KMT2C/D COMPASS complex which interacts with CBP and p300 acetyltransferases and SWI/SNF remodeling complexes to establish cell type-specific enhancer activity (Fig. 10.4). Deficiencies in the function of this complex are known to underlie certain inherited syndromes with developmental disturbances like Kabuki syndrome and have been identified as causes of specific cancers (Cenik and Shilatifard 2021; Schulz et al. 2019). For instance, mutations inactivating KDM6A prevent the activation of specific enhancers required for myeloid differentiation in some myeloid leukemias (Gozdecka et al. 2018). In a comparable manner,

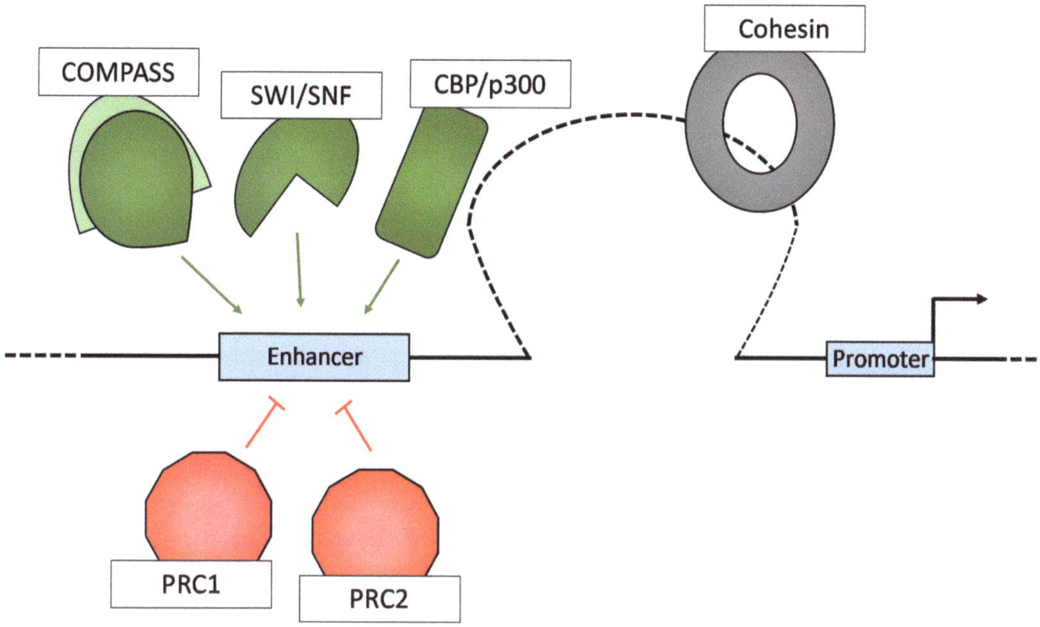

Fig. 10.4 Schematic depiction of regulation of enhancer activity by COMPASS, SWI/SNF, and polycomb complexes

typical chromatin regulator mutations in bladder cancer are likely to lead to deficiencies in establishing proper patterns of cell type-specific enhancer activity during urothelial differentiation. Since chromatin regulator mutations, in particular those in COMPASS and SWI/SNF components, are found across all molecular subtypes of urothelial carcinoma, including luminal subtypes, they do not appear to generally result in a complete lack of differentiation and an arrest of cells at a precursor or stem cell stage. Rather, they may shift the balance between precursor and differentiated cells towards the former (Lang et al. 2020; Richart et al. 2021) or prevent the decrease in proliferation normally associated with terminal differentiation of the urothelium (Qiu et al. 2023).

Notably, as mentioned in the previous section, the less common mutations in several other chromatin regulator genes, such as *BAP1*, *NSD1*, *ATRX*, *KDM5A*, *KDM5B*, and *NCOR1* may influence the same processes. BAP1 directly antagonizes gene repression by PRC1 by deubiquitinating H2AK119, this protein too interacts with KMT2D (Wang et al. 2018). NSD1 catalyzes particularly the dimethylation of H3K36 in intergenic regions (Tauchmann and Schwaller 2021) whereas H3K36 trimethylation in gene bodies is catalyzed by SETD2. NSD1 and polycomb activity oppose each other: NSD1 activity is inhibited by H2A ubiquitination by PRC1, whereas H3K36me2 prevents establishment of the repressive mark H3K27me3 by PRC2. Moreover, H3K36me2 is recognized by de-novo DNA methyltransferases, especially DNMT3A. Accordingly, in several cancers, NSD1 inactivation correlates with stronger DNA hypomethylation (Lee and Wiemels 2016). NSD1 mutations are thus likely to contribute to disturbed deposition of H3K27me3 as well as to DNA hypomethylation in the bladder cancer genome. One of the many interaction partners of ATRX is EZH2, which is recruited to specific chromatin regions by the multifunctional protein. Therefore, ATRX mutations in bladder cancer too may contribute to the deregulation of polycomb function.

The cohesin complex was named for its function during mitosis, where it forms a ring keeping sister chromatids together until it is cleaved at the RAD21 subunit by Separase and the chromatids are distributed into the two daughter cells. A second essential function of cohesin is the epigenetic regulation of chromatin looping, where the complex cooperates with CTCF bound to DNA at the base of the loops. It is thought that cohesin extends chromatin loops until it is blocked by properly bound CTCF with which the complex directly interacts. Cohesin furthermore supports DNA repair, especially homologous recombination repair, and DNA replication. Inherited deficiencies in cohesin function cause defects in DNA repair and gene expression regulation. Because of these multiple functions, it was initially not clear in which way STAG2 inactivation promotes bladder carcinogenesis, but its function in the regulation of tissue-specific gene expression is now considered as most relevant (Richart et al. 2021). In contrast, *STAG2* mutations are not associated with increased chromosomal instability and aneuploidy (Balbas-Martinez et al. 2013) and are in fact more frequent in lower-stage and lower-grade tumors (Taylor et al. 2014).

NCOR1 inactivation by mutations may likewise interfere with proper urothelial differentiation. This corepressor interacts with thyroid hormone, vitamin D and retinoic acid receptors, but also with PPARα and PPARγ. In bladder cancer, *NCOR1* mutations are largely mutually exclusive with mutations in *PPARG*, suggesting that they may act in the same pathway. Although PPARγ is crucially involved in urothelial differentiation, gene amplification, mutations or gene fusions activate the receptor to a lineage-specific oncogene in the luminal non-specified subtype of urothelial carcinoma (Kamoun et al. 2020; Sanchez et al. 2021). Conceivably, NCOR1 inactivation may have similar consequences. Interestingly, *NCOR1* mutations significantly co-occur with *ELF3* mutations, which are found in the same urothelial carcinoma subtype.

Inactivation of KDM5A in cancers may be related to its ability to contribute to repression of genes driving the cell cycle during terminal differentiation or establishment of senescence, partly through cooperation with RB1. The closely related KDM5B demethylase instead supports rather the maintenance of stem and precursor cells by inactivation of genes required for differentiation (Yoo et al. 2022). This may explain why, in bladder cancers, KDM5B inactivation is rare and overexpression has rather been reported (Han et al. 2017).

With respect to individual chromatin regulators, most functional investigations so far have addressed the function of KDM6A in urothelial carcinogenesis (Barrows et al. 2020; Chang et al. 2019; Chen et al. 2021; Kobatake et al. 2020; Koch et al. 2021; Lang et al. 2020; Lang et al. 2019; Ler et al. 2017; Liu et al. 2021) which is reasonable because KDM6A/UTX is the most frequently inactivated chromatin regulator in bladder cancer overall, and particularly so in papillary NMIBC and MIBC. These studies have identified a variety of consequences following KDM6A inactivation in bladder cancer, including effects on proliferation, differentiation, cell migration and interactions with immune cells. In particular, KDM6A inactivation and FGFR3 oncogenic activation were shown to have complementary effects in papillary tumors, explaining their clinical association (Barrows et al. 2020). KDM6A inactivation is nevertheless also frequent in other molecular subtypes. Interestingly, many mutant isoforms of KDM6A, especially those resulting from truncating mutations in its central, structurally disordered domain, disturb the formation of chromatin regulator complex condensates at enhancers (Koch et al. 2021; Shi et al. 2021) in a dominant-negative fashion, potentially causing broad disturbances in gene regulation. As condensates formed by phase separation are considered necessary for the function of chromatin and nuclear subcompartments (Gibson et al. 2019; Strom et al. 2017), such disturbances might represent a more general mechanism by which mutant chromatin regulator proteins act.

In many respects the EZH2 H3K27 methyltransferase is a direct antagonist of KDM6A. Although rarely mutated and not regularly overexpressed in bladder cancer, it has long been considered as a potential oncogene in bladder cancer (reviewed by Hoffmann and Schulz 2021; Martinez-Fernandez et al. 2015). In particular, EZH2 and PRC2 activity may promote cell cycle progression in bladder cancers lacking mutations in direct regulators such as CDKN2A/p16^{INK4A} or RB1 (Warrick et al. 2022). Moreover, inhibitors of EZH2 enzyme activity have been developed as anti-cancer drugs (see Sect. 10.6) and cancers with KDM6A inactivation may respond better to such drugs (Ler et al. 2017).

Unfortunately, beyond KDM6A, very little is known about the biological functions of commonly mutated chromatin regulators in the normal urothelium or the impact of their dysfunction in bladder cancer. In particular, the consequences of mutations in KMT2C and KMT2D have to date only been addressed by single studies (Ding et al. 2019; Rampias et al. 2019). Notably, in bladder cancer cells with *KMT2C/D* mutation, nuclear transfer of KDM6A appears to be impeded and the protein is predominantly or entirely cytosolic (Lang et al. 2019; Zhao et al. 2023). Thus, KDM6A is likely dysfunctional in *KMT2C/D* mutant cancer cells as well. Interestingly, inactivation of STAG2 has been demonstrated to impede the transition from a basal to a luminal transcriptional program via its effects on chromatin looping (Richart et al. 2021). ARID1A has been observed to be essential for normal urothelial development (Guo et al. 2022) and ARID1A deficiencies in bladder cancer are associated with a stronger requirement for PI3K signaling and EZH2 activity, both of which may be addressed by targeted therapies (Rehman et al. 2022). Dedicated experimental studies on the function of other mutated chromatin regulators in bladder cancer are lacking.

An important step towards understanding the consequences of chromatin regulator mutations in bladder cancer should be understanding their global impact on enhancer states and activity in cancer cells. In particular, chromatin regulators are usually recruited to specific genomic regions by DNA-binding transcription factors and interact with transcription factor networks to control and direct cell differentiation; in fact, specific core transcription factor networks are distinctive for each cancer type (Chen et al. 2020b). Accordingly, a recent study found the transcriptional activators FOXA1, GATA3, PPARG as well as a new factor TFAP2 to be essential for luminal subtype-specific gene regulation, whereas TP63, STAT3 and TFAP2A/C characterized basal/squamous cell lines and cancer tissues (Iyyanki et al. 2021), in keeping with their known involvement in the differentiation of the normal urothelium (see Chap. 3). In bladder cancers, binding of these factors at enhancers differed between luminal and basal subtypes along with the overall 3D structure of the nuclear genome. How binding and activity of such factors is influenced by chromatin regulator mutations is still largely unknown, but FOXA1 ability to regulate differentiation and proliferation in urothelial cells has been found to depend on its interaction with KDM6A (Qiu et al. 2023). Large-scale differences in histone modifications, especially in H3K4me1, a mark of active enhancers, have been observed between luminal and basal urothelial carcinoma subtypes (van der Vos et al. 2020). Comprehensive studies on the effect of chromatin regulator mutations on histone modifications and transcription factor binding (compare Nassar et al. 2023 for renal carcinomas) are clearly required.

10.6 Therapeutic Approaches Targeting Epigenetic Alterations in Bladder Cancer

Efficient therapy of UC, particularly of metastatic MIBC, remains an unsolved clinical problem. Beyond surgery, standard of care is cisplatin-based chemotherapy which is now being supplemented with immunotherapies and a still limited arsenal of molecular targeted therapies. Responses to all therapies are often limited by development of resistance. New therapeutic approaches are therefore urgently needed (Bellmunt et al. (2017) and see Chaps. 6, 22, and 23). As detailed above, changes in DNA methylation and chromatin regulators are highly prevalent in UC and contribute crucially to tumor development and progression. Thus, DNA-modifying enzymes and chromatin regulators should be rational therapeutic targets.

A broad range of compounds targeting DNA methyltransferases and chromatin regulators, commonly summarized as epigenetic drugs (or briefly: epidrugs), have been developed and are currently investigated for the treatment of different cancers in preclinical research or in clinical studies or are already approved for clinical use. In general, these compounds are less well investigated for application to solid cancers than for hematological malignancies. Accordingly, very few epidrugs have received FDA approval for treatment of solid cancers (Berdasco and Esteller 2019; Davalos and Esteller 2022) and to our knowledge none for bladder cancer (Table 10.3). Progress in the clinical development of epigenetic drugs into clinical translation has been comprehensively reviewed by several authors (Cheng et al. 2019; Davalos and Esteller 2022; Martinez et al. 2019; Nepali and Liou 2021; Thompson et al. 2023).

Notably, in addition to the cancer cells, epigenetic processes also regulate the phenotype, differentiation or activation status of stromal and immune cells in the tumor microenvironment that crucially affect tumor progression and treatment responses (Liu et al. 2017). For instance, an epigenetic switch mediated by the HAT p300 and DNMTs has been reported to underlie the activation of tumor-promoting cancer-associated fibroblasts (CAFs; Albrengues et al. 2015). Accordingly, epigenetic drugs will also affect the composition of the tumor microenvironment and especially anti-tumor immune responses. For instance, in a mouse model for colorectal cancer, inhibition of EZH2 altered the cellular composition of the tumor microenvironment and in particular enhanced infiltration by anti-tumor CD8+ and CD4+ T cells (Wang et al. 2018). Whether such observations apply to bladder cancer needs to be investigated in the future (Martinez et al. 2019).

Epigenetic drugs may particularly target the catalytic centers of writer or eraser enzymes or binding pockets—like those recognizing specific histone modifications—especially in reader proteins. Below, we discuss epigenetic drugs targeting writers first, followed by compounds targeting erasers and compounds targeting reader domains. Notably, several bifunctional drugs have been developed that bind to more than one target (see examples below). Since many epigenetic regulators act as components of multiprotein or protein-RNA complexes, targeting interactions within such complexes is another option. Targeting the interaction between oncogenic KMT2A fusion proteins and their co-activator Menin is a first successful example of this kind (Krivtsov et al. 2019). Importantly, in bladder cancer, genetic alterations as a rule inactivate epigenetic regulator proteins. Therefore, epidrugs need to target the few epigenetic regulators that are upregulated (like certain HMT and HDACs) or exploit the sensitivities created by deficient chromatin regulators in an approach designated as synthetic lethality (Ryan et al. 2023). In this approach, drugs are directed at proteins that have become essential through the loss of function of another factor (see examples below).

Drugs targeting writers include compounds inhibiting DNA methyltransferases (DNMTi), histone methyltransferases (HMTi), and histone acetyltransferases (HATi). DNMTi are mostly cytidine analogs like decitabine (DAC) or azacytidine (5-Aza; see Table 10.3 for other compounds). These compounds are incorporated into DNA (or RNA in the case of riboside compounds like 5-Aza) instead of cytidine, where they lead to the formation of a covalent bond with a DNMT and irreversible inactivation of the enzyme. DNMT inhibition and depletion results in passive demethylation of the genome in the subsequent replication cycles (Stresemann and Lyko 2008). Additionally, DNMT protein–DNA adducts inhibit DNA replication and transcription, necessitating specialized DNA repair. Since DAC is incorporated only into DNA it may be more specific and less toxic than 5-Aza and may inhibit DNA methylation more efficiently (Jones and Taylor 1980; Lyko and Brown 2005). Both compounds have cytotoxic and myelosuppressive effects (Bender et al. 1998) and were FDA-approved for treatment of myelodysplastic syndrome (MDS) and acute myeloid leukemia (AML) in elderly patients (Dombret et al. 2015; Fenaux et al. 2009; Kantarjian et al. 2012; Lubbert et al. 2011). Interestingly, the treatment response to DAC in AML patients correlates with their p53 mutational status, with leukemias containing p53 mutations responding better (Welch et al.

Table 10.3 Targets of epigenetic drugs for bladder cancer therapy

Target	Clinical trials[a]	Preclinical studies[a]
DNMTs	5-aza-2′deoxycytidine (decitabine), 5-azacytidine (5-Aza) 5-fluoro-2′-deoxycytidine SGI-110 (guadecitabine)	5,6-dihydro-5-azacytidine zebularine
HMT EZH2	CPI-1205 (lirametostat) EPZ6438 (tazemetostat)	GSK126 GSK343 UNC1999 valemetostat
HMT G9a		A-366 BIX-01294 BRD4770 UNC0638
HMT G9a + DNMT		CM-272
HAT EP300/CBP		A-485 B026/ B029-2 C646 CBP30 CCS1477 CCS1477 CCT077791/CCT077792 CPI644 CPI703 FT-7051 GNE-049 GNE-781 I-CBP112 PU141
HDACs	belinostat entinostat mocetinostat romidepsin (FK-228) vorinostat (SAHA)	givinostat panobinostat quisinostat resminostat
KDMs		bomedemstat (IMG-7289) GSK-2879552 iadademstat (ORY-1001) INCB059872 JBI-802 phenelzine pulrodemstat (CC-90011) seclidemstat (SP-2577) tranylcypromine
BETs		iBET762 JQ1 OTX015 (birabresib) PLX51107

[a] For bladder cancer treatment, as of April 2023

2016). Mutations in p53 in urothelial carcinoma may therefore render these tumors more sensitive to DAC. Both compounds have additional effects in cancer cells including induction of DNA damage, cell cycle arrest and apoptosis (Martinez et al. 2019). With regard to bladder cancer DAC was reported to sensitize urothelial carcinoma cell lines to treatment with cisplatin (Xylinas et al. 2016) but also to cytotoxic CAR-T cells (Grunewald et al. 2021). Sensitization of cancer cells to immunotherapies by DNMTi is thought to be caused at least partly by an effect called viral mimicry, because yet more increased DNA hypomethylation in cancer cells induces expression of endogenous retroelements that activate innate immune signaling (Chen et al. 2021). In bladder cancer cells, DAC furthermore synergizes with HDACi with respect to cytotoxicity (Wang et al. 2020).

Since DAC and 5-aza are prone to hydrolysis (Gros et al. 2012), further DNMTi inhibitors have been developed. Zebularine and 5′-fluoro-2′-deoxycytidine are chemically more stable, but not necessarily more efficient. The second-generation DNMTi SGI-110 (guadecitabine) has substantially improved pharmacokinetic properties. This compound too was first investigated in a clinical phase 2 trial with AML patients (Kantarjian et al. 2017) and was also active in MDS patients that did not respond to other FDA-approved DNMTi (Garcia-Manero et al. 2019; Martinez et al. 2019).

Few clinical studies have investigated DNMTi, mainly DAC, for use in the treatment of solid cancers like bladder cancer (see Table 10.3; Davalos and Esteller 2022). A phase 2 study for atezolizumab + guadecitabine in patients with urothelial carcinoma refractory or resistant to immune checkpoint inhibitors is active, and other studies are investigating DNMTi in combination with chemotherapy. Clinical studies on DNMTi in urothelial carcinoma have been comprehensively reviewed (Nunes et al. 2020; Thompson et al. 2023; Cho et al. 2011).

Genomic alterations in bladder cancer inactivate several histone methyltransferases, especially of the KMT2 family. Overexpressed histone methyltransferases like G9a (EHMT2) and EZH2 constitute more promising targets and have been investigated for their functional impact on bladder cancer cells and potential clinical applications. Several inhibitors of the H3K9 methyltransferase G9a (see compounds in Table 10.3), which is overexpressed in bladder cancer (Cho et al. 2011), are available but have not yet proceeded to clinical studies. The new dual inhibitor compound CM-272 targeting G9a and DNMT activity was reported to strongly induce apoptosis and immunogenic cell death in a murine bladder cancer model. It synergized with cisplatin treatment or a PD-L1 immune checkpoint inhibitor (Segovia et al. 2019).

The EZH2 H3K27 methyltransferase is often overexpressed in aggressive bladder cancers (Hinz et al. 2008) and very likely involved in the disturbed balance between proliferation and differentiation that appears to be crucial for the pathogenesis of urothelial carcinomas (see Sect. 10.5; Hoffmann and Schulz 2021). Whereas some inhibitors have only been used in preclinical settings, a clinical trial for CPI-1205 (lirametostat), which inhibits EZH1 as well as EZH2, is ongoing for metastatic bladder cancer. EPZ6438, also known as tazemetostat, has been investigated in more than ten clinical studies, mainly in hematological malignancies, but also in some advanced carcinomas like ovarian and prostate cancer, alone or in combination with, e.g., enzalutamide or abiraterone (clinicaltrials.gov). In advanced urothelial carcinoma, tazemetostat is being clinically investigated in combination with the immune checkpoint inhibitor pembrolizumab. Validation studies will in particular be needed to definitely answer the question whether treatment with EZH2 inhibitors is more efficacious in UC patients with mutated epigenetic enzymes. For example, mutations in *KDM6A*, a direct antagonist of EZH2, have been proposed to sensitize bladder cancers to EZH2 inhibitors (Ler et al. 2017). *ARID1A*-mutated ovarian and gastric cancers were likewise found to be sensitive to EZH2 inhibition (Bitler et al. 2015; Yamada et al. 2021). However, ARID1A expression did not correlate with EZH2 or H3K27me3 levels in urothelial carcinoma tissues and ARID1A depletion in vitro affected neither EZH2 protein expression nor H3K27me levels. Consequently, induced ARID1A-deficiency in urothelial carcinoma cell lines did not result in increased sensitivity to GSK126 (Garczyk et al. 2018). Genomic alterations in other SWI/SNF components may instead provide potential for synthetic lethality (Conde and Frew 2022; Eich et al. 2020).

The histone acetyltransferases CBP and p300 have been studied as potential targets in many different cancer types (Chen et al. 2022). Several targeted compounds have been developed, including CBP/p300 enzyme inhibitors, compounds blocking their bromodomains, CBP/p300 and BET bromodomain dual inhibitors and p300 protein degraders. All diminish H3K27 acetylation, negatively affect transcriptional activity and cell viability of cancer cells in vitro. Some compounds seem to synergize with chemo- or radiotherapy and other epigenetic drugs (Chen et al. 2022). The p300/CBP inhibitor CCS1477 is studied in trials with solid tumors, but no clinical trial for treatment of bladder cancer patients with this or any related compound is registered. In bladder cancers, p300 and CBP are each subject to deleterious mutations in a significant number of cases. The two HATs have overlapping functions, but loss of both is expected to be lethal. Therefore, bladder cancers with *EP300* or *CREBBP* mutations may in fact be oversensitive to inhibition of the respective other histone acetyltransferase, but this presumption has not been formally investigated yet.

Drugs targeting epigenetic erasers may inhibit histone demethylases (KDMi) or histone deacetylases (HDACi). Several HDACi, including vorinostat (SAHA) and panobinostat, have received FDA approval for specific hematological malignancies. HDACs are rarely mutated in bladder cancers, but their expression is frequently deregulated. Some of the overall eleven HDAC isoenzymes are clearly essential for urothelial carcinoma development and progression and present interesting therapeutic targets (Buckwalter et al. 2019; Giannopoulou et al. 2019; Pinkerneil et al. 2017). Initially, especially pan-HDACi like vorinostat and belinostat, which target several different HDAC isoenzymes, were investigated in vitro and in vivo (Castro-Munoz et al. 2023; Cheng et al. 2019). A number of clinical trials for bladder cancer treatment have been performed (summarized by Thompson et al. 2023) using pan-HDAC inhibitors either alone or in combination with cytotoxic chemotherapy or immune checkpoint inhibitors, but revealed significant toxicities (Quinn et al. 2021; Thompson et al. 2023). Publications of three clinical trials for belinostat in UC are still awaited. Half a dozen clinical trials have investigated class I HDACi (romidepsin, entinostat, valproic acid) for the treatment of advanced urothelial carcinoma (Thompson et al. 2023). A phase 1 trial for the HDACi romidepsin (FK-228), which has received FDA approval for use in CTCL, in UC patients demonstrated that it is generally tolerable. Results for valproic acid and entinostat in combination with pembrolizumab in urothelial carcinoma patients are awaited.

Since we had found that pan-HDACi do not efficiently induce cell death in urothelial carcinoma cells, our group delineated which of the HDAC isoenzymes are the best targets for treatment of these cancers and found class I HDAC inhibitors (HDAC1/2/3/8) like romidepsin more efficient than pan-inhibitors (Lehmann et al. 2014; Niegisch et al. 2013; Pinkerneil et al. 2016a, b; Rosik et al. 2014). Moreover, the combination of the HDACi entinostat with DNMTi efficiently killed chemoresistant bladder cancer cells while sparing normal cells (Wang et al. 2020). Other drug combinations may achieve synergistic effects allowing dose reduction to reduce the toxicity observed in clinical trials of HDACi.

The histone demethylase KDM6A—and less commonly KDM5A—is frequently mutated in urothelial carcinoma, but most of the mutations decrease or abolish its function. As discussed in Sect. 10.5, KDM5B should be the better target for cancer treatment. In general, however, while pharmacological inhibitors of histone demethylases are commercially available for research use, they are not highly specific for one particular protein family member. Instead, the histone demethylase LSD1 (encoded by the *KDM1A* gene) has been broadly studied in cancer alone or in combination treatment regimens (Davalos and Esteller 2022); for bladder cancer however little data has been published. We found a dual inhibitor molecule targeting class I HDACs and LSD1 to be quite efficacious on bladder cancer cell lines (Pinkerneil et al. 2016b). To date, nine LSD1 inhibitors are investigated in clinical trials, mainly for hematological, and rarely for solid cancers (see Table 10.3, summarized in Fang et al. 2019; Noce et al. 2023). Since several severe adverse effects have been reported, further studies are needed regarding their precise mode of action, dosing and potential therapeutic windows; likely, more selective compounds may be required (Fang et al. 2019).

The most developed compounds targeting readers aim at proteins recognizing acetylated histone lysine residues, particularly BRD family proteins. In comparison, epigenetic readers recognizing DNA methylation like methyl-CpG binding proteins of the MBD protein family or proteins recognizing histone methylation, e.g., through chromodomains, have rarely been investigated and it is not clear to what extent they are druggable.

Inhibition of BRD family proteins may affect gene transcription globally and additionally impact on DNA repair (Donati et al. 2018), thereby limiting cancer cell survival. First-generation BETi were initially tested as single drugs in clinical studies for hematopoietic and solid cancers (reviewed in Cheng et al. 2019), but dose-limiting hematologic and gastrointestinal toxicities led to the development of second-generation BETi-like PLX51107 with improved pharmaceutical profile. The first developed BET inhibitor (BETi) was JQ1 (Filippakopoulos et al. 2010) which inhibits primarily BRD4 and has been extensively investigated in hematological and solid cancers (reviewed in Martinez et al. 2019). In bladder cancer cells JQ1 is cytostatic, inhibiting proliferation (Wu et al. 2016), but induces significant apoptosis when combined with the HDACi romidepsin, while normal cells are largely spared. The genes affected by BETi treatment appear to be highly cell type-dependent (Holscher et al. 2018). The second-generation BETi PLX51107 with improved pharmaceutical profile displayed anticancer activity in preclinical models of chronic lymphocytic leukemia (Ozer et al. 2018) and melanoma (Tiago et al. 2020). In urothelial carcinoma cells, this compound diminished cell proliferation and induced apoptosis. In line with non-canonical functions of BRD4 in DNA repair (Donati et al. 2018) PLX51107 impaired DNA damage signaling providing a rationale for combination with DNA damaging agents or DNA repair inhibitors (Thy et al. 2021). However, clinical trials have not yet been undertaken.

In summary, given the high prevalence of alterations in chromatin regulators in bladder cancer and the urgent need for additional therapeutic options to treat UC patients, epigenetic drugs represent a novel approach that needs more investigation in preclinical research and clinical studies. Combinations with established treatments like chemotherapy or immunotherapy appear particularly promising to achieve increased efficacy and diminished toxicity. Further improvements may be reached by stratification of patients in order to better select those that may benefit from epidrugs, i.e., by improved prediction of responses and toxicities, based either on specific genomic alterations or on molecular subtyping by transcriptomics.

10.7 Conclusion and Perspectives

Epigenetic alterations contribute to the pathogenesis of many cancers, albeit to various degrees and in different ways. In bladder cancer, DNA methylation alterations had been described for several decades and recent research has confirmed the unusually high prevalence of global hypomethylation and a substantial number of local changes including hypermethylation of specific CpG-islands. While the causes of these changes are still incompletely understood, the exploitation of DNA methylation changes for diagnostic purposes in bladder cancer is advanced. DNA methylation assays may soon become clinical routine especially for the initial diagnosis and the surveillance of patients following transurethral tumor resection (see Sect. 10.3). Furthermore, drugs altering DNA methylation, very likely in combination with chemo- or immunotherapy may provide new options for bladder cancer therapy (see Sect. 10.6).

Although altered activity of polycomb factors like EZH2 had been observed previously, the discovery of frequent (deleterious) mutations in chromatin regulator genes in bladder cancer (Gui et al. 2011) came as a surprise. Following this initial observation, such mutations were found to be present in the vast majority of bladder cancers suggesting that inactivation or impediment of certain chromatin regulators, especially the COMPASS and SWI/SNF complexes, is a crucial requirement for urothelial carcinogenesis. The precise reason why this is so is still not understood, but recent functional studies suggest that chromatin regulator mutations in bladder cancer shift the balance between stem cells and more differentiated progeny, distort urothelial differentiation and prevent the shutdown of cell proliferation associated with terminal differentiation in the normal urothelium. Nevertheless, it remains unclear why inactivation of chromatin regulators is required for urothelial carcinogenesis in addition to the multiple other alterations in cell cycle regulation, proliferation signal transduction, control of genomic stability and the regulation of apoptosis and senescence. Clearly, much more research on these relationships and mechanisms is required. This research may not only provide a better—heuristic—understanding of urothelial carcinogenesis, but also identify optimal points for therapeutic interventions by epigenetic or other drugs. Nevertheless, while precise knowledge on the epigenetic mechanisms of pathogenesis is lacking, preclinical exploration of epigenetic drugs for bladder cancer therapy has begun and for some compounds has already progressed to the stage of clinical trials. Collectively, epigenetic alterations have turned out to be central to bladder cancer pathogenesis and need to be considered in basic, translational and clinical research on this cancer type.

References

Agaimy A, Bertz S, Cheng L, Hes O, Junker K, Keck B, Lopez-Beltran A, Stockle M, Wullich B, Hartmann A (2016) Loss of expression of the SWI/SNF complex is a frequent event in undifferentiated/dedifferentiated urothelial carcinoma of the urinary tract. Virchows Arch 469(3):321–330. https://doi.org/10.1007/s00428-016-1977-y

Aguilera P, Lopez-Contreras AJ (2023) ATRX, a guardian of chromatin. Trends Genet 39:505. https://doi.org/10.1016/j.tig.2023.02.009

Aguilo F, Zhou MM, Walsh MJ (2011) Long noncoding RNA, polycomb, and the ghosts haunting INK4b-ARF-INK4a expression. Cancer Res 71(16):5365–5369. https://doi.org/10.1158/0008-5472.CAN-10-4379

Albrengues J, Bertero T, Grasset E, Bonan S, Maiel M, Bourget I, Philippe C, Herraiz Serrano C, Benamar S, Croce O, Sanz-Moreno V, Meneguzzi G, Feral CC, Cristofari G, Gaggioli C (2015) Epigenetic switch drives the conversion of fibroblasts into proinvasive cancer-associated fibroblasts. Nat Commun 6:10204. https://doi.org/10.1038/ncomms10204

Balbas-Martinez C, Sagrera A, Carrillo-de-Santa-Pau E, Earl J, Marquez M, Vazquez M, Lapi E, Castro-Giner F, Beltran S, Bayes M, Carrato A, Cigudosa JC, Dominguez O, Gut M, Herranz J, Juanpere N, Kogevinas M, Langa X, Lopez-Knowles E, Lorente JA, Lloreta J, Pisano DG, Richart L, Rico D, Salgado RN, Tardon A, Chanock S, Heath S, Valencia A, Losada A, Gut I, Malats N, Real FX (2013) Recurrent inactivation of STAG2 in bladder cancer is not associated with aneuploidy. Nat Genet 45(12):1464–1469. https://doi.org/10.1038/ng.2799

Barrows D, Feng L, Carroll TS, Allis CD (2020) Loss of UTX/KDM6A and the activation of FGFR3 converge to regulate differentiation gene-expression programs in bladder cancer. Proc Natl Acad Sci USA 117(41):25732–25741. https://doi.org/10.1073/pnas.2008017117

Bellmunt J, de Wit R, Vaughn DJ, Fradet Y, Lee JL, Fong L, Vogelzang NJ, Climent MA, Petrylak DP, Choueiri TK, Necchi A, Gerritsen W, Gurney H, Quinn DI, Culine S, Sternberg CN, Mai Y, Poehlein CH, Perini RF, Bajorin DF, Investigators K (2017) Pembrolizumab as second-line therapy for advanced urothelial carcinoma. N Engl J Med 376(11):1015–1026. https://doi.org/10.1056/NEJMoa1613683

Bender CM, Pao MM, Jones PA (1998) Inhibition of DNA methylation by 5-aza-2′-deoxycytidine suppresses the growth of human tumor cell lines. Cancer Res 58(1):95–101

Berdasco M, Esteller M (2019) Clinical epigenetics: seizing opportunities for translation. Nat Rev Genet 20(2):109–127. https://doi.org/10.1038/s41576-018-0074-2

Besaratinia A, Caceres A, Tommasi S (2022) DNA Hydroxymethylation in smoking-associated cancers. Int J Mol Sci 23(5). https://doi.org/10.3390/ijms23052657

Bhan A, Soleimani M, Mandal SS (2017) Long noncoding RNA and cancer: a new paradigm. Cancer Res 77(15):3965–3981. https://doi.org/10.1158/0008-5472.CAN-16-2634

Bitler BG, Aird KM, Garipov A, Li H, Amatangelo M, Kossenkov AV, Schultz DC, Liu Q, Shih Ie M, Conejo-Garcia JR, Speicher DW, Zhang R (2015) Synthetic lethality by targeting EZH2 methyltransferase activity in ARID1A-mutated cancers. Nat Med 21(3):231–238. https://doi.org/10.1038/nm.3799

Borkiewicz L, Kalafut J, Dudziak K, Przybyszewska-Podstawka A, Telejko I (2021) Decoding LncRNAs. Cancers (Basel) 13(11). https://doi.org/10.3390/cancers13112643

Brockdorff N, Bowness JS, Wei G (2020) Progress toward understanding chromosome silencing by Xist RNA. Genes Dev 34(11–12):733–744. https://doi.org/10.1101/gad.337196.120

Buckwalter JM, Chan W, Shuman L, Wildermuth T, Ellis-Mohl J, Walter V, Warrick JI, Wu XR, Kaag M, Raman JD, DeGraff DJ (2019) Characterization of histone deacetylase expression within in vitro and in vivo bladder cancer model systems. Int J Mol Sci 20(10). https://doi.org/10.3390/ijms20102599

Carrot-Zhang J, Chambwe N, Damrauer JS, Knijnenburg TA, Robertson AG, Yau C, Zhou W, Berger AC, Huang KL, Newberg JY, Mashl RJ, Romanel A, Sayaman RW, Demichelis F, Felau I, Frampton GM, Han S, Hoadley KA, Kemal A, Laird PW, Lazar AJ, Le X, Oak N, Shen H, Wong CK, Zenklusen JC, Ziv E, Cancer Genome Atlas Analysis N, Cherniack AD, Beroukhim R (2020) Comprehensive analysis of genetic ancestry and its molecular correlates in cancer. Cancer Cell 37(5):639–654 e636. https://doi.org/10.1016/j.ccell.2020.04.012

Casadevall D, Kilian AY, Bellmunt J (2017) The prognostic role of epigenetic dysregulation in bladder cancer: a systematic review. Cancer Treat Rev 61:82–93. https://doi.org/10.1016/j.ctrv.2017.10.004

Castro-Munoz LJ, Ulloa EV, Sahlgren C, Lizano M, De La Cruz-Hernandez E, Contreras-Paredes A (2023) Modulating epigenetic modifications for cancer therapy (review). Oncol Rep 49:3. https://doi.org/10.3892/or.2023.8496

Cenik BK, Shilatifard A (2021) COMPASS and SWI/SNF complexes in development and disease. Nat Rev Genet 22(1):38–58. https://doi.org/10.1038/s41576-020-0278-0

Centore RC, Sandoval GJ, Soares LMM, Kadoch C, Chan HM (2020) Mammalian SWI/SNF chromatin remodeling complexes: emerging mechanisms and therapeutic strategies. Trends Genet 36(12):936–950. https://doi.org/10.1016/j.tig.2020.07.011

Cerami E, Gao J, Dogrusoz U, Gross BE, Sumer SO, Aksoy BA, Jacobsen A, Byrne CJ, Heuer ML, Larsson E, Antipin Y, Reva B, Goldberg AP, Sander C, Schultz N (2012) The cBio cancer genomics portal: an open platform for exploring multidimensional cancer genomics data. Cancer Discov 2(5):401–404. https://doi.org/10.1158/2159-8290.CD-12-0095

Chan AKN, Chen CW (2019) Rewiring the epigenetic networks in MLL-rearranged leukemias: epigenetic dysregulation and pharmacological interventions. Front Cell Dev Biol 7:81. https://doi.org/10.3389/fcell.2019.00081

Chang S, Yim S, Park H (2019) The cancer driver genes IDH1/2, JARID1C/ KDM5C, and UTX/ KDM6A: crosstalk between histone demethylation and hypoxic reprogramming in cancer metabolism. Exp Mol Med 51(6):1–17. https://doi.org/10.1038/s12276-019-0230-6

Chen X, Zhang J, Ruan W, Huang M, Wang C, Wang H, Jiang Z, Wang S, Liu Z, Liu C, Tan W, Yang J, Chen J, Chen Z, Li X, Zhang X, Xu P, Chen L, Xie R, Zhou Q, Xu S, Irwin DL, Fan JB, Huang J, Lin T (2020a) Urine DNA methylation assay enables early detection and recurrence monitoring for bladder cancer. J Clin Invest 130(12):6278–6289. https://doi.org/10.1172/JCI139597

Chen Y, Xu L, Lin RY, Muschen M, Koeffler HP (2020b) Core transcriptional regulatory circuitries in cancer. Oncogene 39(43):6633–6646. https://doi.org/10.1038/s41388-020-01459-w

Chen X, Lin X, Pang G, Deng J, Xie Q, Zhang Z (2021) Significance of KDM6A mutation in bladder cancer immune escape. BMC Cancer 21(1):635. https://doi.org/10.1186/s12885-021-08372-9

Chen Q, Yang B, Liu X, Zhang XD, Zhang L, Liu T (2022) Histone acetyltransferases CBP/p300 in tumorigenesis and CBP/p300 inhibitors as promising novel anticancer agents. Theranostics 12(11):4935–4948. https://doi.org/10.7150/thno.73223

Cheng Y, He C, Wang M, Ma X, Mo F, Yang S, Han J, Wei X (2019) Targeting epigenetic regulators for cancer therapy: mechanisms and advances in clinical trials. Signal Transduct Target Ther 4:62. https://doi.org/10.1038/s41392-019-0095-0

Chiu HS, Somvanshi S, Patel E, Chen TW, Singh VP, Zorman B, Patil SL, Pan Y, Chatterjee SS, Cancer Genome Atlas Research N, Sood AK, Gunaratne PH, Sumazin P (2018) Pan-cancer analysis of lncRNA regulation supports their targeting of cancer genes in each tumor context. Cell Rep 23 (1):297-312 e212:297. https://doi.org/10.1016/j.celrep.2018.03.064

Cho HS, Kelly JD, Hayami S, Toyokawa G, Takawa M, Yoshimatsu M, Tsunoda T, Field HI, Neal DE, Ponder BA, Nakamura Y, Hamamoto R (2011) Enhanced expression of EHMT2 is involved in the proliferation of cancer cells through negative regulation of SIAH1. Neoplasia 13(8):676–684. https://doi.org/10.1593/neo.11512

Clapier CR, Cairns BR (2009) The biology of chromatin remodeling complexes. Annu Rev Biochem 78:273–304. https://doi.org/10.1146/annurev.biochem.77.062706.153223

Clinton TN, Chen Z, Wise H, Lenis AT, Chavan S, Donoghue MTA, Almassi N, Chu CE, Dason S, Rao P, Rodrigues JA, Vasani NB, Ridouani F, Rosenberg JE, Bajorin DF, Teo MY, Bochner BH, Berger MF, Ostrovnaya I, Pietzak EJ, Iyer G, Gao SP, Hu W, Al-Ahmadie HA, Solit DB (2022) Genomic heterogeneity as a barrier to precision oncology in urothelial cancer. Cell Rep 41(12):111859. https://doi.org/10.1016/j.celrep.2022.111859

Conde M, Frew IJ (2022) Therapeutic significance of ARID1A mutation in bladder cancer. Neoplasia 31:100814. https://doi.org/10.1016/j.neo.2022.100814

D'Andrea D, Soria F, Zehetmayer S, Gust KM, Korn S, Witjes JA, Shariat SF (2019) Diagnostic accuracy, clinical utility and influence on decision-making of a methylation urine biomarker test in the surveillance of non-muscle-invasive bladder cancer. BJU Int 123(6):959–967. https://doi.org/10.1111/bju.14673

Davalos V, Esteller M (2022) Cancer epigenetics in clinical practice. CA Cancer J Clin 73:376. https://doi.org/10.3322/caac.21765

de Almeida BP, Apolonio JD, Binnie A, Castelo-Branco P (2019) Roadmap of DNA methylation in breast cancer identifies novel prognostic biomarkers. BMC Cancer 19(1):219. https://doi.org/10.1186/s12885-019-5403-0

Di Nardo M, Pallotta MM, Musio A (2022) The multifaceted roles of cohesin in cancer. J Exp Clin Cancer Res 41(1):96. https://doi.org/10.1186/s13046-022-02321-5

Ding B, Yan L, Zhang Y, Wang Z, Zhang Y, Xia D, Ye Z, Xu H (2019) Analysis of the role of mutations in the KMT2D histone lysine methyltransferase in bladder cancer. FEBS Open Bio 9(4):693–706. https://doi.org/10.1002/2211-5463.12600

Dizman N, Philip EJ, Pal SK (2020) Genomic profiling in renal cell carcinoma. Nat Rev Nephrol 16(8):435–451. https://doi.org/10.1038/s41581-020-0301-x

Dombret H, Seymour JF, Butrym A, Wierzbowska A, Selleslag D, Jang JH, Kumar R, Cavenagh J, Schuh AC, Candoni A, Recher C, Sandhu I, Bernal del Castillo T, Al-Ali HK, Martinelli G, Falantes J, Noppeney R, Stone RM, Minden MD, McIntyre H, Songer S, Lucy LM, Beach CL, Dohner H (2015) International phase 3 study of azacitidine vs conventional care regimens in older patients with newly diagnosed AML with >30% blasts. Blood 126(3):291–299. https://doi.org/10.1182/blood-2015-01-621664

Donati B, Lorenzini E, Ciarrocchi A (2018) BRD4 and cancer: going beyond transcriptional regulation. Mol Cancer 17(1):164. https://doi.org/10.1186/s12943-018-0915-9

Duex JE, Swain KE, Dancik GM, Paucek RD, Owens C, Churchill MEA, Theodorescu D (2018) Functional impact of chromatin remodeling gene mutations and predictive signature for therapeutic response in bladder cancer. Mol Cancer Res 16(1):69–77. https://doi.org/10.1158/1541-7786.MCR-17-0260

Eich ML, Athar M, Ferguson JE 3rd, Varambally S (2020) EZH2-targeted therapies in cancer: hype or a reality. Cancer Res 80(24):5449–5458. https://doi.org/10.1158/0008-5472.CAN-20-2147

ENCODE Project Consortium; Moore JE, Purcaro MJ, Pratt HE, Epstein CB, Shoresh N, Adrian J, Kawli T, Davis CA, Dobin A, Kaul R, Halow J, Van Nostrand EL, Freese P, Gorkin DU, Shen Y, He Y, Mackiewicz M, Pauli-Behn F, Williams BA, Mortazavi A, Keller CA, Zhang XO, Elhajjajy SI, Huey J, Dickel DE, Snetkova V, Wei X, Wang X, Rivera-Mulia JC, Rozowsky J, Zhang J, Chhetri SB, Zhang J, Victorsen A, White KP, Visel A, Yeo GW, Burge CB, Lecuyer E, Gilbert DM, Dekker J, Rinn J, Mendenhall EM, Ecker JR, Kellis M, Klein RJ, Noble WS, Kundaje A, Guigo R, Farnham PJ, Cherry JM, Myers RM, Ren B, Graveley BR, Gerstein MB, Pennacchio LA, Snyder MP, Bernstein BE, Wold B, Hardison RC, Gingeras TR, Stamatoyannopoulos JA, Weng Z (2020) Expanded encyclopaedias of DNA elements in the human and mouse genomes. Nature 583(7818):699–710. https://doi.org/10.1038/s41586-020-2493-4

Fang Y, Liao G, Yu B (2019) LSD1/KDM1A inhibitors in clinical trials: advances and prospects. J Hematol Oncol 12(1):129. https://doi.org/10.1186/s13045-019-0811-9

Feber A, Dhami P, Dong L, de Winter P, Tan WS, Martinez-Fernandez M, Paul DS, Hynes-Allen A, Rezaee S, Gurung P, Rodney S, Mehmood A, Villacampa F, de la Rosa F, Jameson C, Cheng KK, Zeegers MP, Bryan RT, James ND, Paramio JM, Freeman A, Beck S, Kelly JD (2017) UroMark-a urinary biomarker assay for the detection of bladder cancer. Clin Epigenetics 9:8. https://doi.org/10.1186/s13148-016-0303-5

Fenaux P, Mufti GJ, Hellstrom-Lindberg E, Santini V, Finelli C, Giagounidis A, Schoch R, Gattermann N, Sanz G, List A, Gore SD, Seymour JF, Bennett JM, Byrd J, Backstrom J, Zimmerman L, McKenzie D, Beach C, Silverman LR, International Vidaza High-Risk MDSSSG (2009) Efficacy of azacitidine compared with that of conventional care regimens in the treatment of higher-risk myelodysplastic syndromes: a randomised, open-label, phase III study. Lancet Oncol 10(3):223–232. https://doi.org/10.1016/S1470-2045(09)70003-8

Filippakopoulos P, Qi J, Picaud S, Shen Y, Smith WB, Fedorov O, Morse EM, Keates T, Hickman TT, Felletar I, Philpott M, Munro S, McKeown MR, Wang Y, Christie AL, West N, Cameron MJ, Schwartz B, Heightman TD, La Thangue N, French CA, Wiest O, Kung AL, Knapp S, Bradner JE (2010) Selective inhibition of BET bromodomains. Nature 468(7327):1067–1073. https://doi.org/10.1038/nature09504

Gao J, Aksoy BA, Dogrusoz U, Dresdner G, Gross B, Sumer SO, Sun Y, Jacobsen A, Sinha R, Larsson E, Cerami E, Sander C, Schultz N (2013) Integrative analysis of complex cancer genomics and clinical profiles using the cBioPortal. Sci Signal 6(269):pl1. https://doi.org/10.1126/scisignal.2004088

Garcia-Manero G, Roboz G, Walsh K, Kantarjian H, Ritchie E, Kropf P, O'Connell C, Tibes R, Lunin S, Rosenblat T, Yee K, Stock W, Griffiths E, Mace J, Podoltsev N, Berdeja J, Jabbour E, Issa JJ, Hao Y, Keer HN, Azab M, Savona MR (2019) Guadecitabine (SGI-110) in patients with intermediate or high-risk myelodysplastic syndromes: phase 2 results from a multicentre, open-label, randomised, phase 1/2 trial. Lancet Haematol 6(6):e317–e327. https://doi.org/10.1016/S2352-3026(19)30029-8

Garczyk S, Schneider U, Lurje I, Becker K, Vogeli TA, Gaisa NT, Knuchel R (2018) ARID1A-deficiency in urothelial bladder cancer: no predictive biomarker for EZH2-inhibitor treatment response? PLoS One 13(8):e0202965. https://doi.org/10.1371/journal.pone.0202965

Ghanjati F, Beermann A, Hermanns T, Poyet C, Arauzo-Bravo MJ, Seifert HH, Schmidtpeter M, Goering W, Sorg R, Wernet P, Santourlidis S (2014) Unreserved application of epigenetic methods to define differences of DNA methylation between urinary cellular and cell-free DNA. Cancer Biomark 14(5):295–302. https://doi.org/10.3233/CBM-140407

Ghiraldini FG, Filipescu D, Bernstein E (2021) Solid tumours hijack the histone variant network. Nat Rev Cancer 21(4):257–275. https://doi.org/10.1038/s41568-020-00330-0

Giannopoulou AF, Velentzas AD, Konstantakou EG, Avgeris M, Katarachia SA, Papandreou NC, Kalavros NI, Mpakou VE, Iconomidou V, Anastasiadou E, Kostakis IK, Papassideri IS, Voutsinas GE, Scorilas A, Stravopodis DJ (2019) Revisiting histone deacetylases in human tumorigenesis: the paradigm of urothelial bladder cancer. Int J Mol Sci 20(6). https://doi.org/10.3390/ijms20061291

Gibson BA, Doolittle LK, Schneider MWG, Jensen LE, Gamarra N, Henry L, Gerlich DW, Redding S, Rosen MK (2019) Organization of chromatin by intrinsic and regulated phase separation. Cell 179(2):470–484 e421. https://doi.org/10.1016/j.cell.2019.08.037

Gonzalez-Sandoval A, Gasser SM (2016) On TADs and LADs: spatial control over gene expression. Trends Genet 32(8):485–495. https://doi.org/10.1016/j.tig.2016.05.004

Goodman S, Chappell G, Guyton KZ, Pogribny IP, Rusyn I (2022) Epigenetic alterations induced by genotoxic occupational and environmental human chemical carcinogens: an update of a systematic literature review. Mutat Res Rev Mutat Res 789:108408. https://doi.org/10.1016/j.mrrev.2021.108408

Gozdecka M, Meduri E, Mazan M, Tzelepis K, Dudek M, Knights AJ, Pardo M, Yu L, Choudhary JS, Metzakopian E, Iyer V, Yun H, Park N, Varela I, Bautista R, Collord G, Dovey O, Garyfallos DA, De Braekeleer E, Kondo S, Cooper J, Gottgens B, Bullinger L, Northcott PA, Adams D, Vassiliou GS, Huntly BJP (2018) UTX-mediated enhancer and chromatin remodeling suppresses myeloid leukemogenesis through noncatalytic inverse regulation of ETS and GATA programs. Nat Genet 50(6):883–894. https://doi.org/10.1038/s41588-018-0114-z

Gros C, Fahy J, Halby L, Dufau I, Erdmann A, Gregoire JM, Ausseil F, Vispe S, Arimondo PB (2012) DNA methylation inhibitors in cancer: recent and future approaches. Biochimie 94(11):2280–2296. https://doi.org/10.1016/j.biochi.2012.07.025

Grunewald CM, Haist C, Konig C, Petzsch P, Bister A, Nossner E, Wiek C, Scheckenbach K, Kohrer K, Niegisch G, Hanenberg H, Hoffmann MJ (2021) Epigenetic priming of bladder cancer cells with decitabine increases cytotoxicity of human EGFR and CD44v6 CAR engineered T-cells. Front Immunol 12:782448. https://doi.org/10.3389/fimmu.2021.782448

Gui Y, Guo G, Huang Y, Hu X, Tang A, Gao S, Wu R, Chen C, Li X, Zhou L, He M, Li Z, Sun X, Jia W, Chen J, Yang S, Zhou F, Zhao X, Wan S, Ye R, Liang C, Liu Z, Huang P, Liu C, Jiang H, Wang Y, Zheng H, Sun L, Liu X, Jiang Z, Feng D, Chen J, Wu S, Zou J, Zhang Z, Yang R, Zhao J, Xu C, Yin W, Guan Z, Ye J, Zhang H, Li J, Kristiansen K, Nickerson ML, Theodorescu D, Li Y, Zhang X, Li S, Wang J, Yang H, Wang J, Cai Z (2011) Frequent mutations of chromatin remodeling genes in transitional cell carcinoma of the bladder. Nat Genet 43(9):875–878. https://doi.org/10.1038/ng.907

Guo C, Zhang Y, Tan R, Tang Z, Lam CM, Ye X, Wang Z, Li X (2022) Arid1a regulates bladder urothelium formation and maintenance. Dev Biol 485:61–69. https://doi.org/10.1016/j.ydbio.2022.02.008

Gupta S, Albertson D, Gaston D, Heilbrun ME, Agarwal N, Boucher K, Parnell TJ, Liu T, Morgans A, Madison R, Gowen K, Miller VA, Ross JS, Ali SM, Millis SZ (2018) Comprehensive genomic sequencing of urothelial tumors identifies rare SMARCB1 (INI-1)-deficient carcinomas of the urinary system. Clin Genitourin Cancer 16(2):e373–e382. https://doi.org/10.1016/j.clgc.2017.09.001

Han M, Xu W, Cheng P, Jin H, Wang X (2017) Histone demethylase lysine demethylase 5B in development and cancer. Oncotarget 8(5):8980–8991. https://doi.org/10.18632/oncotarget.13858

Hashimoto H, Vertino PM, Cheng X (2010) Molecular coupling of DNA methylation and histone methylation. Epigenomics 2(5):657–669. https://doi.org/10.2217/epi.10.44

Heberle E, Bardet AF (2019) Sensitivity of transcription factors to DNA methylation. Essays Biochem 63(6):727–741. https://doi.org/10.1042/EBC20190033

Hedegaard J, Lamy P, Nordentoft I, Algaba F, Hoyer S, Ulhoi BP, Vang S, Reinert T, Hermann GG, Mogensen K, Thomsen MBH, Nielsen MM, Marquez M, Segersten U, Aine M, Hoglund M, Birkenkamp-Demtroder K, Fristrup N, Borre M, Hartmann A, Stohr R, Wach S, Keck B, Seitz AK, Nawroth R, Maurer T, Tulic C, Simic T, Junker K, Horstmann M, Harving N, Petersen AC, Calle ML, Steyerberg EW, Beukers W, van Kessel KEM, Jensen JB, Pedersen JS, Malmstrom PU, Malats N, Real FX, Zwarthoff EC, Orntoft TF, Dyrskjot L (2016) Comprehensive transcriptional analysis of early-stage urothelial carcinoma. Cancer Cell 30(1):27–42. https://doi.org/10.1016/j.ccell.2016.05.004

Hentschel AE, Beijert IJ, Bosschieter J, Kauer PC, Vis AN, Lissenberg-Witte BI, van Moorselaar RJA, Steenbergen RDM, Nieuwenhuijzen JA (2022) Bladder cancer detection in urine using DNA methylation markers: a technical and prospective preclinical validation. Clin Epigenetics 14(1):19. https://doi.org/10.1186/s13148-022-01240-8

Hermanns T, Savio AJ, Olkhov-Mitsel E, Mari A, Wettstein MS, Saba K, Bhindi B, Kuk C, Poyet C, Wild PJ, Noon A, Bashir S, Juvet T, Rendon RA, Waltregny D, van der Kwast T, Finelli A, Kulkarni GS, Fleshner NE, Lo K, Bapat B, Zlotta AR (2020) A noninvasive urine-based methylation biomarker panel to detect bladder cancer and discriminate cancer grade. Urol Oncol 38(6):603 e601–603 e607. https://doi.org/10.1016/j.urolonc.2020.01.007

Heubach J, Monsior J, Deenen R, Niegisch G, Szarvas T, Niedworok C, Schulz WA, Hoffmann MJ (2015)

The long noncoding RNA HOTAIR has tissue and cell type-dependent effects on HOX gene expression and phenotype of urothelial cancer cells. Mol Cancer 14:108. https://doi.org/10.1186/s12943-015-0371-8

Hinz S, Kempkensteffen C, Christoph F, Hoffmann M, Krause H, Schrader M, Schostak M, Miller K, Weikert S (2008) Expression of the polycomb group protein EZH2 and its relation to outcome in patients with urothelial carcinoma of the bladder. J Cancer Res Clin Oncol 134(3):331–336. https://doi.org/10.1007/s00432-007-0288-8

Hoffmann MJ, Schulz WA (2005) Causes and consequences of DNA hypomethylation in human cancer. Biochem Cell Biol 83(3):296–321. https://doi.org/10.1139/o05-036

Hoffmann MJ, Schulz WA (2021) Alterations of chromatin regulators in the pathogenesis of urinary bladder urothelial carcinoma. Cancers (Basel) 13(23). https://doi.org/10.3390/cancers13236040

Holscher AS, Schulz WA, Pinkerneil M, Niegisch G, Hoffmann MJ (2018) Combined inhibition of BET proteins and class I HDACs synergistically induces apoptosis in urothelial carcinoma cell lines. Clin Epigenetics 10:1. https://doi.org/10.1186/s13148-017-0434-3

Huang B, Lang X, Li X (2022) The role of IL-6/JAK2/STAT3 signaling pathway in cancers. Front Oncol 12:1023177. https://doi.org/10.3389/fonc.2022.1023177

Hurst CD, Knowles MA (2022) Mutational landscape of non-muscle-invasive bladder cancer. Urol Oncol 40(7):295–303. https://doi.org/10.1016/j.urolonc.2018.10.015

Hurst CD, Alder O, Platt FM, Droop A, Stead LF, Burns JE, Burghel GJ, Jain S, Klimczak LJ, Lindsay H, Roulson JA, Taylor CF, Thygesen H, Cameron AJ, Ridley AJ, Mott HR, Gordenin DA, Knowles MA (2017) Genomic subtypes of non-invasive bladder cancer with distinct metabolic profile and female gender bias in KDM6A mutation frequency. Cancer Cell 32(5):701–715 e707. https://doi.org/10.1016/j.ccell.2017.08.005

Iyyanki T, Zhang B, Wang Q, Hou Y, Jin Q, Xu J, Yang H, Liu T, Wang X, Song F, Luan Y, Yamashita H, Chien R, Lyu H, Zhang L, Wang L, Warrick J, Raman JD, Meeks JJ, DeGraff DJ, Yue F (2021) Subtype-associated epigenomic landscape and 3D genome structure in bladder cancer. Genome Biol 22(1):105. https://doi.org/10.1186/s13059-021-02325-y

Jeronimo C, Henrique R (2014) Epigenetic biomarkers in urological tumors: a systematic review. Cancer Lett 342(2):264–274. https://doi.org/10.1016/j.canlet.2011.12.026

Jin F, Thaiparambil J, Donepudi SR, Vantaku V, Piyarathna DWB, Maity S, Krishnapuram R, Putluri V, Gu F, Purwaha P, Bhowmik SK, Ambati CR, von Rundstedt FC, Roghmann F, Berg S, Noldus J, Rajapakshe K, Godde D, Roth S, Storkel S, Degener S, Michailidis G, Kaipparettu BA, Karanam B, Terris MK, Kavuri SM, Lerner SP, Kheradmand F, Coarfa C, Sreekumar A, Lotan Y, El-Zein R, Putluri N (2017) Tobacco-specific carcinogens induce Hypermethylation, DNA adducts, and DNA damage in bladder cancer. Cancer Prev Res (Phila) 10(10):588–597. https://doi.org/10.1158/1940-6207.CAPR-17-0198

Jones PA (2012) Functions of DNA methylation: islands, start sites, gene bodies and beyond. Nat Rev Genet 13(7):484–492. https://doi.org/10.1038/nrg3230

Jones PA, Taylor SM (1980) Cellular differentiation, cytidine analogs and DNA methylation. Cell 20(1):85–93. https://doi.org/10.1016/0092-8674(80)90237-8

Jordahl KM, Randolph TW, Song X, Sather CL, Tinker LF, Phipps AI, Kelsey KT, White E, Bhatti P (2018) Genome-wide DNA methylation in prediagnostic blood and bladder cancer risk in the Women's Health Initiative. Cancer Epidemiol Biomarkers Prev 27(6):689–695. https://doi.org/10.1158/1055-9965.EPI-17-0951

Kamoun A, de Reynies A, Allory Y, Sjodahl G, Robertson AG, Seiler R, Hoadley KA, Groeneveld CS, Al-Ahmadie H, Choi W, Castro MAA, Fontugne J, Eriksson P, Mo Q, Kardos J, Zlotta A, Hartmann A, Dinney CP, Bellmunt J, Powles T, Malats N, Chan KS, Kim WY, McConkey DJ, Black PC, Dyrskjot L, Hoglund M, Lerner SP, Real FX, Radvanyi F, Bladder Cancer Molecular Taxonomy G (2020) A consensus molecular classification of muscle-invasive bladder cancer. Eur Urol 77(4):420–433. https://doi.org/10.1016/j.eururo.2019.09.006

Kandimalla R, van Tilborg AA, Zwarthoff EC (2013) DNA methylation-based biomarkers in bladder cancer. Nat Rev Urol 10(6):327–335. https://doi.org/10.1038/nrurol.2013.89

Kantarjian HM, Thomas XG, Dmoszynska A, Wierzbowska A, Mazur G, Mayer J, Gau JP, Chou WC, Buckstein R, Cermak J, Kuo CY, Oriol A, Ravandi F, Faderl S, Delaunay J, Lysak D, Minden M, Arthur C (2012) Multicenter, randomized, open-label, phase III trial of decitabine versus patient choice, with physician advice, of either supportive care or low-dose cytarabine for the treatment of older patients with newly diagnosed acute myeloid leukemia. J Clin Oncol 30(21):2670–2677. https://doi.org/10.1200/JCO.2011.38.9429

Kantarjian HM, Roboz GJ, Kropf PL, Yee KWL, O'Connell CL, Tibes R, Walsh KJ, Podoltsev NA, Griffiths EA, Jabbour E, Garcia-Manero G, Rizzieri D, Stock W, Savona MR, Rosenblat TL, Berdeja JG, Ravandi F, Rock EP, Hao Y, Azab M, Issa JJ (2017) Guadecitabine (SGI-110) in treatment-naive patients with acute myeloid leukaemia: phase 2 results from a multicentre, randomised, phase 1/2 trial. Lancet Oncol 18(10):1317–1326. https://doi.org/10.1016/S1470-2045(17)30576-4

Karanovic S, Ardin M, Tang Z, Tomic K, Villar S, Renard C, Venturini E, Lorch AH, Lee DS, Stipancic Z, Slade N, Vukovic Brinar I, Dittrich D, Karlovic K, Borovecki F, Dickman KG, Olivier M, Grollman AP, Jelakovic B, Zavadil J (2022) Molecular profiles and urinary biomarkers of upper tract urothelial carcinomas associated with aristolochic acid exposure. Int J Cancer 150(2):374–386. https://doi.org/10.1002/ijc.33827

Kitchen MO, Bryan RT, Emes RD, Glossop JR, Luscombe C, Cheng KK, Zeegers MP, James ND, Devall AJ, Mein CA, Gommersall L, Fryer AA, Farrell WE (2016) Quantitative genome-wide methylation analysis of high-grade non-muscle invasive bladder cancer. Epigenetics 11(3):237–246. https://doi.org/10.1080/15592294.2016.1154246

Klonou A, Chlamydas S, Piperi C (2021) Structure, activity and function of the MLL2 (KMT2B) protein lysine methyltransferase. Life (Basel) 11(8). https://doi.org/10.3390/life11080823

Knudsen ES, Kumarasamy V, Ruiz A, Sivinski J, Chung S, Grant A, Vail P, Chauhan SS, Jie T, Riall TS, Witkiewicz AK (2019) Cell cycle plasticity driven by MTOR signaling: integral resistance to CDK4/6 inhibition in patient-derived models of pancreatic cancer. Oncogene 38(18):3355–3370. https://doi.org/10.1038/s41388-018-0650-0

Kobatake K, Ikeda KI, Nakata Y, Yamasaki N, Ueda T, Kanai A, Sentani K, Sera Y, Hayashi T, Koizumi M, Miyakawa Y, Inaba T, Sotomaru Y, Kaminuma O, Ichinohe T, Honda ZI, Yasui W, Horie S, Black PC, Matsubara A, Honda H (2020) Kdm6a deficiency activates inflammatory pathways, promotes M2 macrophage polarization, and causes bladder cancer in cooperation with p53 dysfunction. Clin Cancer Res 26(8):2065–2079. https://doi.org/10.1158/1078-0432.CCR-19-2230

Koch J, Lang A, Whongsiri P, Schulz WA, Hoffmann MJ, Greife A (2021) KDM6A mutations promote acute cytoplasmic DNA release, DNA damage response and mitosis defects. BMC Mol Cell Biol 22(1):54. https://doi.org/10.1186/s12860-021-00394-2

Kohler CU, Walter M, Lang K, Plottner S, Roghmann F, Noldus J, Tannapfel A, Tam YC, Kafferlein HU, Bruning T (2020) In-vitro identification and in-vivo confirmation of DNA methylation biomarkers for urothelial cancer. Biomedicines 8(8). https://doi.org/10.3390/biomedicines8080233

Krivtsov AV, Evans K, Gadrey JY, Eschle BK, Hatton C, Uckelmann HJ, Ross KN, Perner F, Olsen SN, Pritchard T, McDermott L, Jones CD, Jing D, Braytee A, Chacon D, Earley E, McKeever BM, Claremon D, Gifford AJ, Lee HJ, Teicher BA, Pimanda JE, Beck D, Perry JA, Smith MA, McGeehan GM, Lock RB, Armstrong SA (2019) A Menin-MLL inhibitor induces specific chromatin changes and eradicates disease in models of MLL-rearranged leukemia. Cancer Cell 36(6):660–673 e611. https://doi.org/10.1016/j.ccell.2019.11.001

Lang A, Yilmaz M, Hader C, Murday S, Kunz X, Wagner N, Wiek C, Petzsch P, Kohrer K, Koch J, Hoffmann MJ, Greife A, Schulz WA (2019) Contingencies of UTX/KDM6A action in urothelial carcinoma. Cancers (Basel) 11(4). https://doi.org/10.3390/cancers11040481

Lang A, Whongsiri P, Yilmaz M, Lautwein T, Petzsch P, Greife A, Gunes C, Kohrer K, Niegisch G, Hoffmann M, Schulz WA (2020) Knockdown of UTX/KDM6A enriches precursor cell populations in urothelial cell cultures and cell lines. Cancers (Basel) 12(4). https://doi.org/10.3390/cancers12041023

Laukhtina E, Shim SR, Mori K, D'Andrea D, Soria F, Rajwa P, Mostafaei H, Comperat E, Cimadamore A, Moschini M, Teoh JY, Enikeev D, Xylinas E, Lotan Y, Palou J, Gontero P, Babjuk M, Witjes JA, Kamat AM, Roupret M, Shariat SF, Pradere B, European Association of Urology-Young Academic Urologists : Urothelial Carcinoma Working G (2021) Diagnostic accuracy of novel urinary biomarker tests in non-muscle-invasive bladder cancer: a systematic review and network meta-analysis. Eur Urol Oncol 4(6):927–942. https://doi.org/10.1016/j.euo.2021.10.003

Lawson ARJ, Abascal F, Coorens THH, Hooks Y, O'Neill L, Latimer C, Raine K, Sanders MA, Warren AY, Mahbubani KTA, Bareham B, Butler TM, Harvey LMR, Cagan A, Menzies A, Moore L, Colquhoun AJ, Turner W, Thomas B, Gnanapragasam V, Williams N, Rassl DM, Vohringer H, Zumalave S, Nangalia J, Tubio JMC, Gerstung M, Saeb-Parsy K, Stratton MR, Campbell PJ, Mitchell TJ, Martincorena I (2020) Extensive heterogeneity in somatic mutation and selection in the human bladder. Science 370(6512):75–82. https://doi.org/10.1126/science.aba8347

Lee ST, Wiemels JL (2016) Genome-wide CpG Island methylation and intergenic demethylation propensities vary among different tumor sites. Nucleic Acids Res 44(3):1105–1117. https://doi.org/10.1093/nar/gkv1038

Lee DH, Kim GW, Jeon YH, Yoo J, Lee SW, Kwon SH (2020) Advances in histone demethylase KDM4 as cancer therapeutic targets. FASEB J 34(3):3461–3484. https://doi.org/10.1096/fj.201902584R

Lehmann M, Hoffmann MJ, Koch A, Ulrich SM, Schulz WA, Niegisch G (2014) Histone deacetylase 8 is deregulated in urothelial cancer but not a target for efficient treatment. J Exp Clin Cancer Res 33(1):59. https://doi.org/10.1186/s13046-014-0059-8

Ler LD, Ghosh S, Chai X, Thike AA, Heng HL, Siew EY, Dey S, Koh LK, Lim JQ, Lim WK, Myint SS, Loh JL, Ong P, Sam XX, Huang D, Lim T, Tan PH, Nagarajan S, Cheng CW, Ho H, Ng LG, Yuen J, Lin PH, Chuang CK, Chang YH, Weng WH, Rozen SG, Tan P, Creasy CL, Pang ST, McCabe MT, Poon SL, Teh BT (2017) Loss of tumor suppressor KDM6A amplifies PRC2-regulated transcriptional repression in bladder cancer and can be targeted through inhibition of EZH2. Sci Transl Med 9(378). https://doi.org/10.1126/scitranslmed.aai8312

Li R, Du Y, Chen Z, Xu D, Lin T, Jin S, Wang G, Liu Z, Lu M, Chen X, Xu T, Bai F (2020) Macroscopic somatic clonal expansion in morphologically normal human urothelium. Science 370(6512):82–89. https://doi.org/10.1126/science.aba7300

Li J, Liang Y, Fan J, Xu C, Guan B, Zhang J, Guo B, Shi Y, Wang P, Tan Y, Zhang Q, Yuan C, Wu Y, Zhou L, Ci W, Li X (2022) DNA methylation subtypes guiding prognostic assessment and linking to responses the DNA methyltransferase inhibitor SGI-110 in urothelial carcinoma. BMC Med 20(1):222. https://doi.org/10.1186/s12916-022-02426-w

Liu M, Zhou J, Chen Z, Cheng AS (2017) Understanding the epigenetic regulation of tumours and their microenvironments: opportunities and problems for epigenetic therapy. J Pathol 241(1):10–24. https://doi.org/10.1002/path.4832

Liu L, Cui J, Zhao Y, Liu X, Chen L, Xia Y, Wang Y, Chen S, Sun S, Shi B, Zou Y (2021) KDM6A-ARHGDIB axis blocks metastasis of bladder cancer by inhibiting Rac1. Mol Cancer 20(1):77. https://doi.org/10.1186/s12943-021-01369-9

Loras A, Segovia C, Ruiz-Cerda JL (2021) Epigenomic and metabolomic integration reveals dynamic metabolic regulation in bladder cancer. Cancers (Basel) 13(11). https://doi.org/10.3390/cancers13112719

Loyfer N, Magenheim J, Peretz A, Cann G, Bredno J, Klochendler A, Fox-Fisher I, Shabi-Porat S, Hecht M, Pelet T, Moss J, Drawshy Z, Amini H, Moradi P, Nagaraju S, Bauman D, Shveiky D, Porat S, Dior U, Rivkin G, Or O, Hirshoren N, Carmon E, Pikarsky A, Khalaileh A, Zamir G, Grinbaum R, Abu Gazala M, Mizrahi I, Shussman N, Korach A, Wald O, Izhar U, Erez E, Yutkin V, Samet Y, Rotnemer Golinkin D, Spalding KL, Druid H, Arner P, Shapiro AMJ, Grompe M, Aravanis A, Venn O, Jamshidi A, Shemer R, Dor Y, Glaser B, Kaplan T (2023) A DNA methylation atlas of normal human cell types. Nature 613(7943):355–364. https://doi.org/10.1038/s41586-022-05580-6

Lubbert M, Suciu S, Baila L, Ruter BH, Platzbecker U, Giagounidis A, Selleslag D, Labar B, Germing U, Salih HR, Beeldens F, Muus P, Pfluger KH, Coens C, Hagemeijer A, Eckart Schaefer H, Ganser A, Aul C, de Witte T, Wijermans PW (2011) Low dose decitabine versus best supportive care in elderly patients with intermediate- or high-risk myelodysplastic syndrome (MDS) ineligible for intensive chemotherapy: final results of the randomized phase III study of the European Organisation for Research and Treatment of Cancer leukemia group and the German MDS study group. J Clin Oncol 29(15):1987–1996. https://doi.org/10.1200/JCO.2010.30.9245

Lyko F (2018) The DNA methyltransferase family: a versatile toolkit for epigenetic regulation. Nat Rev Genet 19(2):81–92. https://doi.org/10.1038/nrg.2017.80

Lyko F, Brown R (2005) DNA methyltransferase inhibitors and the development of epigenetic cancer therapies. J Natl Cancer Inst 97(20):1498–1506. https://doi.org/10.1093/jnci/dji311

Mancini M, Righetto M, Zumerle S, Montopoli M, Zattoni F (2020) The bladder EpiCheck test as a non-invasive tool based on the identification of DNA methylation in bladder cancer cells in the urine: a review of published evidence. Int J Mol Sci 21(18). https://doi.org/10.3390/ijms21186542

Martinez VG, Munera-Maravilla E, Bernardini A, Rubio C, Suarez-Cabrera C, Segovia C, Lodewijk I, Dueñas M, Martinez-Fernandez M, Paramio JM (2019) Epigenetics of bladder cancer: where biomarkers and therapeutic targets meet. Front Genet 10:1125. https://doi.org/10.3389/fgene.2019.01125

Martinez-Fernandez M, Rubio C, Segovia C, Lopez-Calderon FF, Duenas M, Paramio JM (2015) EZH2 in bladder cancer, a promising therapeutic target. Int J Mol Sci 16(11):27107–27132. https://doi.org/10.3390/ijms161126000

Martire S, Banaszynski LA (2020) The roles of histone variants in fine-tuning chromatin organization and function. Nat Rev Mol Cell Biol 21(9):522–541. https://doi.org/10.1038/s41580-020-0262-8

Mattick JS, Amaral PP, Carninci P, Carpenter S, Chang HY, Chen LL, Chen R, Dean C, Dinger ME, Fitzgerald KA, Gingeras TR, Guttman M, Hirose T, Huarte M, Johnson R, Kanduri C, Kapranov P, Lawrence JB, Lee JT, Mendell JT, Mercer TR, Moore KJ, Nakagawa S, Rinn JL, Spector DL, Ulitsky I, Wan Y, Wilusz JE, Wu M (2023) Long non-coding RNAs: definitions, functions, challenges and recommendations. Nat Rev Mol Cell Biol 24:430. https://doi.org/10.1038/s41580-022-00566-8

Matuleviciute R, Cunha PP, Johnson RS, Foskolou IP (2021) Oxygen regulation of TET enzymes. FEBS J 288(24):7143–7161. https://doi.org/10.1111/febs.15695

Meier K, Brehm A (2014) Chromatin regulation: how complex does it get? Epigenetics 9(11):1485–1495. https://doi.org/10.4161/15592294.2014.971580

Mensah IK, Norvil AB, AlAbdi L, McGovern S, Petell CJ, He M, Gowher H (2021) Misregulation of the expression and activity of DNA methyltransferases in cancer. NAR Cancer 3(4):zcab045. https://doi.org/10.1093/narcan/zcab045

Miranda-Goncalves V, Lameirinhas A, Henrique R, Jeronimo C (2018) Metabolism and epigenetic interplay in cancer: regulation and putative therapeutic targets. Front Genet 9:427. https://doi.org/10.3389/fgene.2018.00427

Moore LE, Pfeiffer RM, Poscablo C, Real FX, Kogevinas M, Silverman D, Garcia-Closas R, Chanock S, Tardon A, Serra C, Carrato A, Dosemeci M, Garcia-Closas M, Esteller M, Fraga M, Rothman N, Malats N (2008) Genomic DNA hypomethylation as a biomarker for bladder cancer susceptibility in the Spanish Bladder Cancer Study: a case-control study. Lancet Oncol 9(4):359–366. https://doi.org/10.1016/S1470-2045(08)70038-X

Munari E, Chaux A, Vaghasia AM, Taheri D, Karram S, Bezerra SM, Gonzalez Roibon N, Nelson WG, Yegnasubramanian S, Netto GJ, Haffner MC (2016) Global 5-Hydroxymethylcytosine levels are profoundly reduced in multiple genitourinary malignancies. PLoS One 11(1):e0146302. https://doi.org/10.1371/journal.pone.0146302

Nassar AH, Abou Alaiwi S, Baca SC, Adib E, Corona RI, Seo JH, Fonseca MAS, Spisak S, El Zarif T, Tisza V, Braun DA, Du H, He M, Flaifel A, Alchoueiry M, Denize T, Matar SG, Acosta A, Shukla S, Hou Y,

Steinharter J, Bouchard G, Berchuck JE, O'Connor E, Bell C, Nuzzo PV, Mary Lee GS, Signoretti S, Hirsch MS, Pomerantz M, Henske E, Gusev A, Lawrenson K, Choueiri TK, Kwiatkowski DJ, Freedman ML (2023) Epigenomic charting and functional annotation of risk loci in renal cell carcinoma. Nat Commun 14(1):346. https://doi.org/10.1038/s41467-023-35833-5

Nepali K, Liou JP (2021) Recent developments in epigenetic cancer therapeutics: clinical advancement and emerging trends. J Biomed Sci 28(1):27. https://doi.org/10.1186/s12929-021-00721-x

Niegisch G, Knievel J, Koch A, Hader C, Fischer U, Albers P, Schulz WA (2013) Changes in histone deacetylase (HDAC) expression patterns and activity of HDAC inhibitors in urothelial cancers. Urol Oncol 31(8):1770–1779. https://doi.org/10.1016/j.urolonc.2012.06.015

Nishiyama A, Nakanishi M (2021) Navigating the DNA methylation landscape of cancer. Trends Genet 37(11):1012–1027. https://doi.org/10.1016/j.tig.2021.05.002

Noce B, Di Bello E, Fioravanti R, Mai A (2023) LSD1 inhibitors for cancer treatment: focus on multi-target agents and compounds in clinical trials. Front Pharmacol 14:1120911. https://doi.org/10.3389/fphar.2023.1120911

Nunes SP, Henrique R, Jeronimo C, Paramio JM (2020) DNA methylation as a therapeutic target for bladder cancer. Cells 9(8). https://doi.org/10.3390/cells9081850

Olkhov-Mitsel E, Savio AJ, Kron KJ, Pethe VV, Hermanns T, Fleshner NE, van Rhijn BW, van der Kwast TH, Zlotta AR, Bapat B (2017) Epigenome-wide DNA methylation profiling identifies differential methylation biomarkers in high-grade bladder cancer. Transl Oncol 10(2):168–177. https://doi.org/10.1016/j.tranon.2017.01.001

Ozer HG, El-Gamal D, Powell B, Hing ZA, Blachly JS, Harrington B, Mitchell S, Grieselhuber NR, Williams K, Lai TH, Alinari L, Baiocchi RA, Brinton L, Baskin E, Cannon M, Beaver L, Goettl VM, Lucas DM, Woyach JA, Sampath D, Lehman AM, Yu L, Zhang J, Ma Y, Zhang Y, Spevak W, Shi S, Severson P, Shellooe R, Carias H, Tsang G, Dong K, Ewing T, Marimuthu A, Tantoy C, Walters J, Sanftner L, Rezaei H, Nespi M, Matusow B, Habets G, Ibrahim P, Zhang C, Mathe EA, Bollag G, Byrd JC, Lapalombella R (2018) BRD4 profiling identifies critical chronic lymphocytic leukemia oncogenic circuits and reveals sensitivity to PLX51107, a novel structurally distinct BET inhibitor. Cancer Discov 8(4):458–477. https://doi.org/10.1158/2159-8290.CD-17-0902

Padeken J, Methot SP, Gasser SM (2022) Establishment of H3K9-methylated heterochromatin and its functions in tissue differentiation and maintenance. Nat Rev Mol Cell Biol 23(9):623–640. https://doi.org/10.1038/s41580-022-00483-w

Peng D, Ge G, Gong Y, Zhan Y, He S, Guan B, Li Y, Xu Z, Hao H, He Z, Xiong G, Zhang C, Shi Y, Zhou Y, Ci W, Li X, Zhou L (2018) Vitamin C increases 5-hydroxymethylcytosine level and inhibits the growth of bladder cancer. Clin Epigenetics 10(1):94. https://doi.org/10.1186/s13148-018-0527-7

Pfeifer GP (2018) Defining driver DNA methylation changes in human cancer. Int J Mol Sci 19(4). https://doi.org/10.3390/ijms19041166

Pinkerneil M, Hoffmann MJ, Deenen R, Kohrer K, Arent T, Schulz WA, Niegisch G (2016a) Inhibition of class I histone deacetylases 1 and 2 promotes urothelial carcinoma cell death by various mechanisms. Mol Cancer Ther 15(2):299–312. https://doi.org/10.1158/1535-7163.MCT-15-0618

Pinkerneil M, Hoffmann MJ, Kohlhof H, Schulz WA, Niegisch G (2016b) Evaluation of the therapeutic potential of the novel isotype specific HDAC inhibitor 4SC-202 in urothelial carcinoma cell lines. Target Oncol 11(6):783–798. https://doi.org/10.1007/s11523-016-0444-7

Pinkerneil M, Hoffmann MJ, Schulz WA, Niegisch G (2017) HDACs and HDAC inhibitors in urothelial carcinoma - perspectives for an antineoplastic treatment. Curr Med Chem 24(37):4151–4165. https://doi.org/10.2174/0929867324666170207142740

Pokorna Z, Hrabal V, Tichy V, Vojtesek B, Coates PJ (2022) DNA demethylation switches oncogenic DeltaNp63 to tumor suppressive TAp63 in squamous cell carcinoma. Front Oncol 12:924354. https://doi.org/10.3389/fonc.2022.924354

Poreba E, Lesniewicz K, Durzynska J (2020) Aberrant activity of histone-lysine N-methyltransferase 2 (KMT2) complexes in oncogenesis. Int J Mol Sci 21(24). https://doi.org/10.3390/ijms21249340

Qiu H, Makarov V, Bolzenius JK, Halstead A, Parker Y, Wang A, Iyer GV, Wise H, Kim D, Thayaparan V, Lindner DJ, Haber GP, Ting AH, Ren B, Chan TA, Arora V, Solit DB, Lee BH (2023) KDM6A loss triggers an epigenetic switch that disrupts urothelial differentiation and drives cell proliferation in bladder cancer. Cancer Res 83(6):814–829. https://doi.org/10.1158/0008-5472.CAN-22-1444

Quinn DI, Tsao-Wei DD, Twardowski P, Aparicio AM, Frankel P, Chatta G, Wright JJ, Groshen SG, Khoo S, Lenz HJ, Lara PN, Gandara DR, Newman E (2021) Phase II study of the histone deacetylase inhibitor vorinostat (suberoylanilide hydroxamic acid; SAHA) in recurrent or metastatic transitional cell carcinoma of the urothelium - an NCI-CTEP sponsored: California Cancer Consortium trial, NCI 6879. Investig New Drugs 39(3):812–820. https://doi.org/10.1007/s10637-020-01038-6

Raman JD, Mongan NP, Tickoo SK, Boorjian SA, Scherr DS, Gudas LJ (2005) Increased expression of the polycomb group gene, EZH2, in transitional cell carcinoma of the bladder. Clin Cancer Res 11(24 Pt 1):8570–8576. https://doi.org/10.1158/1078-0432.CCR-05-1047

Rampias T, Karagiannis D, Avgeris M, Polyzos A, Kokkalis A, Kanaki Z, Kousidou E, Tzetis M, Kanavakis E, Stravodimos K, Manola KN, Pantelias

GE, Scorilas A, Klinakis A (2019) The lysine-specific methyltransferase KMT2C/MLL3 regulates DNA repair components in cancer. EMBO Rep 20(3). https://doi.org/10.15252/embr.201846821

Rausch C, Hastert FD, Cardoso MC (2019) DNA modification readers and writers and their interplay. J Mol Biol 432:1731. https://doi.org/10.1016/j.jmb.2019.12.018

Rehman H, Chandrashekar DS, Balabhadrapatruni C, Nepal S, Balasubramanya SAH, Shelton AK, Skinner KR, Ma AH, Rao T, Agarwal S, Eich ML, Robinson AD, Naik G, Manne U, Netto GJ, Miller CR, Pan CX, Sonpavde G, Varambally S, Ferguson JE 3rd (2022) ARID1A-deficient bladder cancer is dependent on PI3K signaling and sensitive to EZH2 and PI3K inhibitors. JCI Insight 7(16). https://doi.org/10.1172/jci.insight.155899

Ren W, Fan H, Grimm SA, Kim JJ, Li L, Guo Y, Petell CJ, Tan XF, Zhang ZM, Coan JP, Yin J, Kim DI, Gao L, Cai L, Khudaverdyan N, Cetin B, Patel DJ, Wang Y, Cui Q, Strahl BD, Gozani O, Miller KM, O'Leary SE, Wade PA, Wang GG, Song J (2021) DNMT1 reads heterochromatic H4K20me3 to reinforce LINE-1 DNA methylation. Nat Commun 12(1):2490. https://doi.org/10.1038/s41467-021-22665-4

Richart L, Lapi E, Pancaldi V, Cuenca-Ardura M, Pau EC, Madrid-Mencia M, Neyret-Kahn H, Radvanyi F, Rodriguez JA, Cuartero Y, Serra F, Le Dily F, Valencia A, Marti-Renom MA, Real FX (2021) STAG2 loss-of-function affects short-range genomic contacts and modulates the basal-luminal transcriptional program of bladder cancer cells. Nucleic Acids Res 49(19):11005–11021. https://doi.org/10.1093/nar/gkab864

Robertson AG, Kim J, Al-Ahmadie H, Bellmunt J, Guo G, Cherniack AD, Hinoue T, Laird PW, Hoadley KA, Akbani R, Castro MAA, Gibb EA, Kanchi RS, Gordenin DA, Shukla SA, Sanchez-Vega F, Hansel DE, Czerniak BA, Reuter VE, Su X, de Sa CB, Chagas VS, Mungall KL, Sadeghi S, Pedamallu CS, Lu Y, Klimczak LJ, Zhang J, Choo C, Ojesina AI, Bullman S, Leraas KM, Lichtenberg TM, Wu CJ, Schultz N, Getz G, Meyerson M, Mills GB, McConkey DJ, Network TR, Weinstein JN, Kwiatkowski DJ, Lerner SP (2017) Comprehensive molecular characterization of muscle-invasive bladder cancer. Cell 171(3):540–556 e525. https://doi.org/10.1016/j.cell.2017.09.007

Rosik L, Niegisch G, Fischer U, Jung M, Schulz WA, Hoffmann MJ (2014) Limited efficacy of specific HDAC6 inhibition in urothelial cancer cells. Cancer Biol Ther 15(6):742–757. https://doi.org/10.4161/cbt.28469

Ruan W, Chen X, Huang M, Wang H, Chen J, Liang Z, Zhang J, Yu Y, Chen S, Xu S, Hu T, Li X, Guo Y, Jiang Z, Chen Z, Huang J, Lin T, Fan JB (2021) A urine-based DNA methylation assay to facilitate early detection and risk stratification of bladder cancer. Clin Epigenetics 13(1):91. https://doi.org/10.1186/s13148-021-01073-x

Ruijtenberg S, van den Heuvel S (2016) Coordinating cell proliferation and differentiation: antagonism between cell cycle regulators and cell type-specific gene expression. Cell Cycle 15(2):196–212. https://doi.org/10.1080/15384101.2015.1120925

Ryan CJ, Mehta I, Kebabci N, Adams DJ (2023) Targeting synthetic lethal paralogs in cancer. Trends Cancer 9(5):397–409. https://doi.org/10.1016/j.trecan.2023.02.002

Saghafinia S, Mina M, Riggi N, Hanahan D, Ciriello G (2018) Pan-cancer landscape of aberrant DNA methylation across human tumors. Cell Rep 25(4):1066–1080. e1068. https://doi.org/10.1016/j.celrep.2018.09.082

Saintilnord WN, Fondufe-Mittendorf Y (2021) Arsenic-induced epigenetic changes in cancer development. Semin Cancer Biol 76:195–205. https://doi.org/10.1016/j.semcancer.2021.03.019

Sanchez DJ, Missiaen R, Skuli N, Steger DJ, Simon MC (2021) Cell-intrinsic tumorigenic functions of PPARgamma in bladder urothelial carcinoma. Mol Cancer Res 19(4):598–611. https://doi.org/10.1158/1541-7786.MCR-20-0189

Schlesinger Y, Straussman R, Keshet I, Farkash S, Hecht M, Zimmerman J, Eden E, Yakhini Z, Ben-Shushan E, Reubinoff BE, Bergman Y, Simon I, Cedar H (2007) Polycomb-mediated methylation on Lys27 of histone H3 pre-marks genes for de novo methylation in cancer. Nat Genet 39(2):232–236. https://doi.org/10.1038/ng1950

Schuettengruber B, Bourbon HM, Di Croce L, Cavalli G (2017) Genome regulation by polycomb and trithorax: 70 years and counting. Cell 171(1):34–57. https://doi.org/10.1016/j.cell.2017.08.002

Schulz WA (2023) Molecular biology of human cancers, 2nd edn. Springer

Schulz WA, Goering W (2016) DNA methylation in uro thelial carcinoma. Epigenomics 8(10):1415–1428. https://doi.org/10.2217/epi-2016-0064

Schulz WA, Lang A, Koch J, Greife A (2019) The histone demethylase UTX/KDM6A in cancer: progress and puzzles. Int J Cancer 145(3):614–620. https://doi.org/10.1002/ijc.32116

Segovia C, San Jose-Eneriz E, Munera-Maravilla E, Martinez-Fernandez M, Garate L, Miranda E, Vilas-Zornoza A, Lodewijk I, Rubio C, Segrelles C, Valcarcel LV, Rabal O, Casares N, Bernardini A, Suarez-Cabrera C, Lopez-Calderon FF, Fortes P, Casado JA, Duenas M, Villacampa F, Lasarte JJ, Guerrero-Ramos F, de Velasco G, Oyarzabal J, Castellano D, Agirre X, Prosper F, Paramio JM (2019) Inhibition of a G9a/DNMT network triggers immune-mediated bladder cancer regression. Nat Med 25(7):1073–1081. https://doi.org/10.1038/s41591-019-0499-y

Serra RW, Fang M, Park SM, Hutchinson L, Green MR (2014) A KRAS-directed transcriptional silencing pathway that mediates the CpG Island methylator phenotype. eLife 3:e02313. https://doi.org/10.7554/eLife.02313

Shi B, Li W, Song Y, Wang Z, Ju R, Ulman A, Hu J, Palomba F, Zhao Y, Le JP, Jarrard W, Dimoff D, Digman MA, Gratton E, Zang C, Jiang H (2021) UTX condensation underlies its tumour-suppressive activity. Nature 597(7878):726–731. https://doi.org/10.1038/s41586-021-03903-7

Sivakumar A, de Las Heras JI, Schirmer EC (2019) Spatial genome organization: from development to disease. Front Cell Dev Biol 7:18. https://doi.org/10.3389/fcell.2019.00018

Song BF, Xu LZ, Jiang K, Cheng F (2023) MiR-124-3p inhibits tumor progression in prostate cancer by targeting EZH2. Funct Integr Genomics 23(2):80. https://doi.org/10.1007/s10142-023-00991-8

Stresemann C, Lyko F (2008) Modes of action of the DNA methyltransferase inhibitors azacytidine and decitabine. Int J Cancer 123(1):8–13. https://doi.org/10.1002/ijc.23607

Strom AR, Emelyanov AV, Mir M, Fyodorov DV, Darzacq X, Karpen GH (2017) Phase separation drives heterochromatin domain formation. Nature 547(7662):241–245. https://doi.org/10.1038/nature22989

Tauchmann S, Schwaller J (2021) NSD1: a lysine methyltransferase between developmental disorders and cancer. Life (Basel) 11(9). https://doi.org/10.3390/life11090877

Taylor CF, Platt FM, Hurst CD, Thygesen HH, Knowles MA (2014) Frequent inactivating mutations of STAG2 in bladder cancer are associated with low tumour grade and stage and inversely related to chromosomal copy number changes. Hum Mol Genet 23(8):1964–1974. https://doi.org/10.1093/hmg/ddt589

Thompson D, Lawrentschuk N, Bolton D (2023) New approaches to targeting epigenetic regulation in bladder cancer. Cancers (Basel) 15(6). https://doi.org/10.3390/cancers15061856

Thy S, Hommel A, Meneceur S, Bartkowiak AL, Schulz WA, Niegisch G, Hoffmann MJ (2021) Epigenetic treatment of urothelial carcinoma cells sensitizes to cisplatin chemotherapy and PARP inhibitor treatment. Cancers (Basel) 13(6). https://doi.org/10.3390/cancers13061376

Tiago M, Capparelli C, Erkes DA, Purwin TJ, Heilman SA, Berger AC, Davies MA, Aplin AE (2020) Targeting BRD/BET proteins inhibits adaptive kinome upregulation and enhances the effects of BRAF/MEK inhibitors in melanoma. Br J Cancer 122(6):789–800. https://doi.org/10.1038/s41416-019-0724-y

Tian Z, Meng L, Long X, Diao T, Hu M, Wang M, Liu M, Wang J (2020) DNA methylation-based classification and identification of bladder cancer prognosis-associated subgroups. Cancer Cell Int 20:255. https://doi.org/10.1186/s12935-020-01345-1

Tolg C, Sabha N, Cortese R, Panchal T, Ahsan A, Soliman A, Aitken KJ, Petronis A, Bagli DJ (2011) Uropathogenic E. coli infection provokes epigenetic downregulation of CDKN2A (p16INK4A) in uroepithelial cells. Lab Investig 91 (6):825-836:825. https://doi.org/10.1038/labinvest.2010.197

Tost J (2022) Current and emerging technologies for the analysis of the genome-wide and locus-specific DNA methylation patterns. Adv Exp Med Biol 1389:395–469. https://doi.org/10.1007/978-3-031-11454-0_16

Valenzuela M, Amato R, Sgura A, Antoccia A, Berardinelli F (2021) The multiple facets of ATRX protein. Cancers (Basel) 13(9). https://doi.org/10.3390/cancers13092211

van der Heijden AG, Mengual L, Ingelmo-Torres M, Lozano JJ, van Rijt-van de Westerlo CCM, Baixauli M, Geavlete B, Moldoveanud C, Ene C, Dinney CP, Czerniak B, Schalken JA, Kiemeney L, Ribal MJ, Witjes JA, Alcaraz A (2018) Urine cell-based DNA methylation classifier for monitoring bladder cancer. Clin Epigenetics 10:71. https://doi.org/10.1186/s13148-018-0496-x

van der Vos KE, Vis DJ, Nevedomskaya E, Kim Y, Choi W, McConkey D, Wessels LFA, van Rhijn BWG, Zwart W, van der Heijden MS (2020) Epigenetic profiling demarcates molecular subtypes of muscle-invasive bladder cancer. Sci Rep 10(1):10952. https://doi.org/10.1038/s41598-020-67850-5

van Kessel KE, Beukers W, Lurkin I, Ziel-van der Made A, van der Keur KA, Boormans JL, Dyrskjot L, Marquez M, Orntoft TF, Real FX, Segersten U, Malats N, Malmstrom PU, Van Criekinge W, Zwarthoff EC (2017) Validation of a DNA methylation-mutation urine assay to select patients with hematuria for cystoscopy. J Urol 197(3 Pt 1):590–595. https://doi.org/10.1016/j.juro.2016.09.118

Walton J, Lawson K, Prinos P, Finelli A, Arrowsmith C, Ailles L (2023) PBRM1, SETD2 and BAP1 - the trinity of 3p in clear cell renal cell carcinoma. Nat Rev Urol 20(2):96–115. https://doi.org/10.1038/s41585-022-00659-1

Wang D, Quiros J, Mahuron K, Pai CC, Ranzani V, Young A, Silveria S, Harwin T, Abnousian A, Pagani M, Rosenblum MD, Van Gool F, Fong L, Bluestone JA, DuPage M (2018) Targeting EZH2 reprograms intratumoral regulatory T cells to enhance cancer immunity. Cell Rep 23(11):3262–3274. https://doi.org/10.1016/j.celrep.2018.05.050

Wang C, Hamacher A, Petzsch P, Kohrer K, Niegisch G, Hoffmann MJ, Schulz WA, Kassack MU (2020) Combination of decitabine and entinostat synergistically inhibits urothelial bladder cancer cells via activation of FoxO1. Cancers (Basel) 12(2). https://doi.org/10.3390/cancers12020337

Wang H, Han M, Qi LS (2021) Engineering 3D genome organization. Nat Rev Genet 22(6):343–360. https://doi.org/10.1038/s41576-020-00325-5

Wang Q, Xiong F, Wu G, Liu W, Chen J, Wang B, Chen Y (2022) Gene body methylation in cancer: molecular mechanisms and clinical applications. Clin Epigenetics 14(1):154. https://doi.org/10.1186/s13148-022-01382-9

Warrick JI, Knowles MA, Hurst CD, Shuman L, Raman JD, Walter V, Putt J, Dyrskjot L, Groeneveld C, Castro MAA, Robertson AG, DeGraff DJ (2022) A transcriptional network of cell cycle dysregulation in noninvasive papillary urothelial carcinoma. Sci Rep 12(1):16538. https://doi.org/10.1038/s41598-022-20927-9

Weinberg DN, Papillon-Cavanagh S, Chen H, Yue Y, Chen X, Rajagopalan KN, Horth C, McGuire JT, Xu X, Nikbakht H, Lemiesz AE, Marchione DM, Marunde MR, Meiners MJ, Cheek MA, Keogh MC, Bareke E, Djedid A, Harutyunyan AS, Jabado N, Garcia BA, Li H, Allis CD, Majewski J, Lu C (2019) The histone mark H3K36me2 recruits DNMT3A and shapes the intergenic DNA methylation landscape. Nature 573(7773):281–286. https://doi.org/10.1038/s41586-019-1534-3

Welch JS, Petti AA, Miller CA, Fronick CC, O'Laughlin M, Fulton RS, Wilson RK, Baty JD, Duncavage EJ, Tandon B, Lee YS, Wartman LD, Uy GL, Ghobadi A, Tomasson MH, Pusic I, Romee R, Fehniger TA, Stockerl-Goldstein KE, Vij R, Oh ST, Abboud CN, Cashen AF, Schroeder MA, Jacoby MA, Heath SE, Luber K, Janke MR, Hantel A, Khan N, Sukhanova MJ, Knoebel RW, Stock W, Graubert TA, Walter MJ, Westervelt P, Link DC, DiPersio JF, Ley TJ (2016) TP53 and decitabine in acute myeloid leukemia and myelodysplastic syndromes. N Engl J Med 375(21):2023–2036. https://doi.org/10.1056/NEJMoa1605949

Witjes JA, Morote J, Cornel EB, Gakis G, van Valenberg FJP, Lozano F, Sternberg IA, Willemsen E, Hegemann ML, Paitan Y, Leibovitch I (2018) Performance of the bladder EpiCheck methylation test for patients under surveillance for non-muscle-invasive bladder cancer: results of a multicenter, prospective. Blinded Clinical Trial Eur Urol Oncol 1(4):307–313. https://doi.org/10.1016/j.euo.2018.06.011

Wu JN, Roberts CW (2013) ARID1A mutations in cancer: another epigenetic tumor suppressor? Cancer Discov 3(1):35–43. https://doi.org/10.1158/2159-8290.CD-12-0361

Wu X, Liu D, Tao D, Xiang W, Xiao X, Wang M, Wang L, Luo G, Li Y, Zeng F, Jiang G (2016) BRD4 regulates EZH2 transcription through upregulation of C-MYC and represents a novel therapeutic target in bladder cancer. Mol Cancer Ther 15(5):1029–1042. https://doi.org/10.1158/1535-7163.MCT-15-0750

Xu T, Li HT, Wei J, Li M, Hsieh TC, Lu YT, Lakshminarasimhan R, Xu R, Hodara E, Morrison G, Gujar H, Rhie SK, Siegmund K, Liang G, Goldkorn A (2020) Epigenetic plasticity potentiates a rapid cyclical shift to and from an aggressive cancer phenotype. Int J Cancer 146(11):3065–3076. https://doi.org/10.1002/ijc.32904

Xylinas E, Hassler MR, Zhuang D, Krzywinski M, Erdem Z, Robinson BD, Elemento O, Clozel T, Shariat SF (2016) An Epigenomic approach to improving response to neoadjuvant cisplatin chemotherapy in bladder cancer. Biomol Ther 6(3). https://doi.org/10.3390/biom6030037

Yamada L, Saito M, Thar Min AK, Saito K, Ashizawa M, Kase K, Nakajima S, Onozawa H, Okayama H, Endo H, Fujita S, Sakamoto W, Saze Z, Momma T, Mimura K, Ohki S, Kono K (2021) Selective sensitivity of EZH2 inhibitors based on synthetic lethality in ARID1A-deficient gastric cancer. Gastric Cancer 24(1):60–71. https://doi.org/10.1007/s10120-020-01094-0

Yang GJ, Zhu MH, Lu XJ, Liu YJ, Lu JF, Leung CH, Ma DL, Chen J (2021) The emerging role of KDM5A in human cancer. J Hematol Oncol 14(1):30. https://doi.org/10.1186/s13045-021-01041-1

Ye F, Liang Y, Hu J, Hu Y, Liu Y, Cheng Z, Ou Y, Xu C, Jiang H (2021) DNA methylation modification map to predict tumor molecular subtypes and efficacy of immunotherapy in bladder cancer. Front Cell Dev Biol 9:760369. https://doi.org/10.3389/fcell.2021.760369

Yoo J, Kim GW, Jeon YH, Kim JY, Lee SW, Kwon SH (2022) Drawing a line between histone demethylase KDM5A and KDM5B: their roles in development and tumorigenesis. Exp Mol Med 54(12):2107–2117. https://doi.org/10.1038/s12276-022-00902-0

Yu Y, Cao H, Zhang M, Shi F, Wang R, Liu X (2018) Prognostic value of DNA methylation for bladder cancer. Clin Chim Acta 484:207–212. https://doi.org/10.1016/j.cca.2018.05.056

Yuan C, Ning Y, Pan Y (2020) Emerging roles of HOTAIR in human cancer. J Cell Biochem 121(5–6):3235–3247. https://doi.org/10.1002/jcb.29591

Zhang N, Chen S, Wu L, Wu Y, Jiang G, Shao J, Chen L, Sun J, Na R, Wang X, Xu J (2019) Identification of cancer-specific methylation of gene combination for the diagnosis of bladder cancer. J Cancer 10(26):6761–6766. https://doi.org/10.7150/jca.28192

Zhao S, Allis CD, Wang GG (2021) The language of chromatin modification in human cancers. Nat Rev Cancer 21(7):413–430. https://doi.org/10.1038/s41568-021-00357-x

Zhao Z, Aoi Y, Philips CN, Meghani KA, Gold SR, Yu Y, John LS, Qian J, Zeidner JM, Meeks JJ, Shilatifard A (2023) Somatic mutations of MLL4/COMPASS induce cytoplasmic localization providing molecular insight into cancer prognosis and treatment. Proc Natl Acad Sci USA 120(52):e2310063120. https://doi.org/10.1073/pnas.2310063120

Zhu G, Pei L, Li Y, Gou X (2020) EP300 mutation is associated with tumor mutation burden and promotes antitumor immunity in bladder cancer patients. Aging (Albany NY) 12(3):2132–2141. https://doi.org/10.18632/aging.102728

Zouein FA, Duhe RJ, Booz GW (2011) JAKs go nuclear: emerging role of nuclear JAK1 and JAK2 in gene expression and cell growth. Growth Factors 29(6):245–252. https://doi.org/10.3109/08977194.2011.614949

Part III

Pathogenesis and Microenvironment Dynamics in Bladder Cancer

11 Molecular Pathogenesis: Field Cancerization and Clonal Evolution in Urothelial Cancer Initiation and Progression

David J. McConkey, Cathy Mendelsohn, Byron Lee, Colin Dinney, and Bogdan Czerniak

Abstract

Early histopathological studies performed on cystectomies from bladder cancer patients demonstrated that large areas of the urothelium display preneoplastic morphological changes. More recent whole-organ mapping studies revealed the presence of widespread genomic changes, including copy-neutral loss of heterozygosity and inactivating mutations in chromatin-modifying enzymes, even in areas that appear normal and in older individuals without cancer. Some of these mutations can be attributed to environmental exposures and apolipoprotein B mRNA editing catalytic polypeptide-like (APOBEC)-mediated mutagenesis, but age-related mutagenic processes predominate in the normal areas and are associated with subclonal expansions that can occupy large areas of the urothelium. Cancer driver mutations and copy number variations then accumulate to produce high-grade dysplasia and carcinoma in situ (CIS) that serve as the immediate precursor lesions for invasive urothelial cancer. The available evidence suggests that basal or luminal molecular subtype commitment occurs very early in bladders with unifocal cancers whereas molecular subtypes can be mixed in bladders with multifocal cancers. More is known about cancer initiation than progression, which is associated with transient inflammation in luminal and chronic inflammation in basal preclinical models. These observations have important implications for cancer prevention and the detection and clinical management of patients with bladder cancer.

Keywords

Field defect · Subclone · Chromatin-modifying enzymes · BBN mouse model

D. J. McConkey (✉)
Johns Hopkins Greenberg Bladder Cancer Institute, Baltimore, MD, USA
e-mail: dmcconk1@jhmi.edu

C. Mendelsohn
Department of Genetics and Development, Columbia University Irving Medical Center, New York, NY, USA

B. Lee · C. Dinney
Department of Urology, U.T. M.D. Anderson Cancer Center, Houston, TX, USA

B. Czerniak
Department of Pathology, U.T. M.D. Anderson Cancer Center, Houston, TX, USA

11.1 Introduction

Environmental exposures, and in particular smoking, are significant risk factors for the development of urothelial bladder cancer (Kamat et al. 2016). The carcinogens in cigarette smoke cause DNA mutations in urothelial

M. A. Knowles, L. Dyrskjøt (eds.), *Biology of Bladder Cancer*,
https://doi.org/10.1007/978-3-031-68505-7_11

cells exposed to them in vitro (Baker et al. 2020) and in rodent models (Fantini et al. 2018), and these and other carcinogens can accumulate in the urine. Therefore, it was long suspected that the whole urothelium in exposed individuals might contain mutations and other genetic and epigenetic changes that set the stage for frank neoplastic transformation. This was termed "field cancerization" or "field effects," and next-generation sequencing analyses of different areas of the urothelium in cystectomy specimens confirmed the presence of field effects in patients with bladder cancer. Mutagenic processes leave genomic "scars" that can be detected by next-generation sequencing (Alexandrov et al. 2013), so we can now estimate their relative contributions to mutagenesis in cancers and normal tissues. Indeed, recent studies revealed somatic mutations characteristic of field effects in many tissues (Martincorena and Campbell 2015), some that are linked to exposure to ultraviolet light, smoking, or aristolochic acid (Martincorena et al. 2015; Alexandrov et al. 2016; Li et al. 2021), and others that appear to be caused by spontaneous replication errors (Tomasetti and Vogelstein 2015a, b; Tomasetti et al. 2017; Lawson et al. 2020; Li et al. 2021). The field effects are characterized by subclonal expansions of cells that contain cancer driver mutations in normal-appearing tissue areas (Martincorena and Campbell 2015; Martincorena et al. 2018; Li et al. 2021). These subclonal expansions accumulate with aging, and they may explain why aging is also the major risk factor for bladder cancer and most other solid and liquid malignancies.

However, even though most of us will acquire cancer driver mutations in many of our tissues if we live long enough, most of us will not develop cancers in these tissues. One explanation for this is that the mutations that accumulate in normal tissues do not provide a strong enough growth advantage unless additional driver mutations are acquired. In addition, many chemicals that are considered carcinogens do not cause mutations (Hill et al. 2023), and early studies of carcinogenesis in the skin and other organs demonstrated that cancer initiation induced by carcinogens that clearly cause DNA mutations (Fujiki et al. 1989) did not produce cancer without exposure to another agent (a "tumor promoter") that increased cell proliferation without necessarily causing DNA damage (Baird and Boutwell 1971). In these early studies phorbol esters were often used, but one common feature of most tumor promoters was that they caused tissue damage and inflammation (Karin 2009). Indeed, non-steroidal anti-inflammatory drugs (NSAIDs) or deletion of one of their targets (cyclooxygenase-2, or COX2) that blocked this inflammation also prevented cancer progression in these preclinical models (Williams et al. 1999; Swamy et al. 2006), and NSAID use was also linked to reduced cancer incidence in humans (Williams et al. 1999). Along with age and smoking, inflammation is probably another major risk factor for bladder cancer. Adaptive immunity appears to counteract cancer by eliminating cells that contain mutations through a process that has been termed "immunoediting" (O'Donnell et al. 2019). Age-related declines also appear to contribute to increased cancer risk.

Here we will review our current understanding of the genetic and epigenetic processes that contribute to cancer initiation and progression in the urothelium. We will focus on the insights gained from histological and genetic mapping studies in cystectomy specimens and mechanistic experiments in a popular carcinogen-induced spontaneous mouse model. Our perspective is shaped by our experience with multi-platform genomic analyses of whole-organ maps and the recognition that urothelial cancers progress along two "tracks" (papillary and non-papillary) that display differences in mutational profiles and gene expression signatures that characterize the luminal and basal/squamous molecular subtypes (Fig. 11.1).

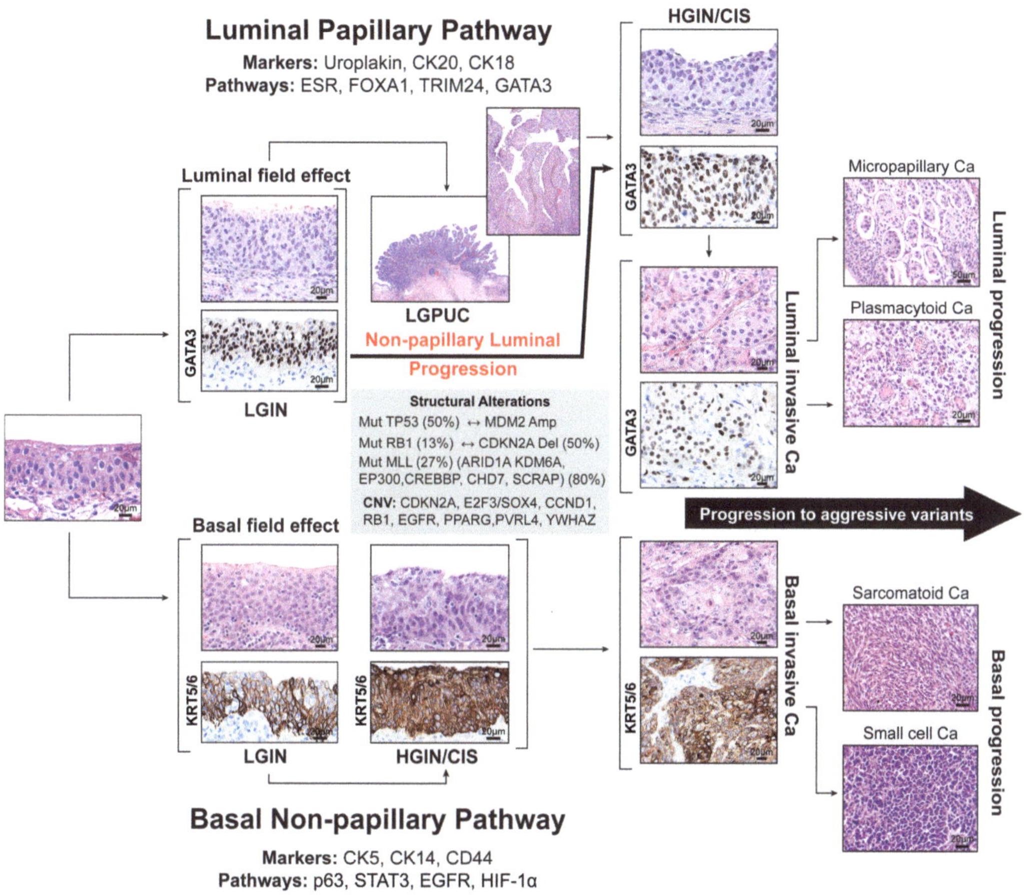

Fig. 11.1 Bladder cancer evolution from mucosal field effects through luminal papillary and basal non-papillary pathways. Dual-track concept of bladder cancer development through luminal papillary and basal non-papillary pathways from their respective luminal and basal field effects. With progression to clinically aggressive subtypes, cancers retain the dual-track dichotomy with micropapillary and plasmacytoid carcinomas evolving via the luminal track, whereas sarcomatoid and small cell develop via the basal track. LGIN, low grade intraepithelial neoplasia; HGIN, high grade intraepithelial neoplasia; CIS, carcinoma in situ. Rearranged and based on figures originally presented in (Majewski et al. 2008; Guo and Czerniak 2019; Guo et al. 2024)

11.2 Histological Whole-Organ Mapping Studies

The basis for the high recurrence rates in patients with urothelial cancer has been an active topic of investigation for decades. Early work by Melicow and colleagues demonstrated that multiple areas of phenotypically abnormal epithelium (including CIS) were often observed distant from areas of cancer in cystectomy specimens (Melicow 1952; Melicow and Hollowell 1952). Subsequently more formal analyses were performed on whole cystectomies preserved by formalin fixation and paraffin-embedding (Koss et al. 1974; Koss 1979). Koss et al. fixed 10 whole mount cystectomies using 10% formalin, cut them into 2 cm × 0.5 cm sections, and made them into blocks (80–120 per cystectomy). Histological maps based on visual inspection of sections from these blocks revealed that in most of the cases, most of the urothelium was affected by hyperplasia, atypia, CIS, and cancer (Koss et al. 1974). Another team produced whole-organ maps of 21 cystectomies from patients with mostly organ-confined bladder cancer and concluded that most regions were affected by atypia and CIS (Farrow et al. 1976). They noted that CIS was always associated with inflammation, which in some cases was severe, and that loss of tight connections between adjacent epithelial cells and between epithelial cells and the basement membrane were also common. Lateral expansion of malignant mucosal cells into areas of benign mucosa was also noted in some cases. Based on the clinical histories of their patients, the authors suggested that progression from CIS to invasive cancer could take many years. Similar observations were made by Skinner et al. (Skinner et al. 1974).

11.3 Urothelial Stem Cells and Clonal Relatedness of Multifocal Tumors

The appreciation that X chromosome inactivation in females results in mosaicism with methylation of maternal or paternal alleles provided investigators with tools to begin to track the clonal relatedness of multifocal urothelial cancers and adjacent normal cells in the urothelium. Sidransky and colleagues examined 13 different tumors from cystectomy specimens from four women (Sidransky et al. 1992). In each of the patients all tumors had inactivation of the same X chromosome, whereas adjacent normal bladder mucosal cells had random patterns of inactivation. In addition, each tumor that could be evaluated had lost the same allele on chromosome 9q, which is an early event in bladder cancer progression (Cairns et al. 1993), whereas losses on 17p and 18q were heterogeneous, probably because they had occurred later in neoplastic progression (Presti Jr. et al. 1991). The authors concluded that "a number of bladder tumors can arise from the uncontrolled spread of a single transformed cell. These tumors can then grow independently with variable subsequent genetic alterations."

A similar approach was used by another group to map the clonal origins of cells in normal areas of the urothelium. They used a highly heterogeneous trinucleotide repeat polymorphism in the androgen receptor gene together with methylation-sensitive restriction enzymes to map maternal and paternal alleles in microdissected strips of urothelium, 0.7–12.2 mm long and 8 mm thick (Tsai et al. 1995). The results revealed monoclonal patches that were estimated to occupy 120 mm^2 in area and contain 2×10^6 daughter cells. The authors estimated that 200–300 progenitor/stem cells would be required to populate the whole urothelium. These early estimates of clonal patch size are consistent with more recent data documenting the locoregional characteristics of the field effect that develops in the ageing urothelium.

11.4 Combined Whole-Organ Histologic and Genomic Mapping in Bladders with Cancer

We first used microsatellite profiling to characterize the relationships between histologic and genomic features in whole cystectomies (Chaturvedi et al. 1997; Czerniak et al. 1999; Lee et al. 2007). Microsatellites are highly polymorphic genomic repeats that allow for the visualization of maternal and paternal alleles and can therefore be used to pinpoint loss of heterozygosity (LOH). A specialized device was created to section the tissues into 1 × 2 cm grids that enabled isolation of DNA and visualization of tissue morphology in adjacent sections. The first study focused on chromosome 17 with embedded analyses of the *TP53* gene (exons 5–9) (Chaturvedi et al. 1997), the second on chromosome 9 (which contains the *CDKN2A*, *CDKN2B*, and *IFNA* loci at 9p21.3 and *TSC1* at 9q34) (Czerniak et al. 1999), and the third on chromosome 13 (which contains the *RB1* locus at 13q14) (Lee et al. 2007). The results revealed that LOH involving all three chromosomes was common and affected large areas of the bladder mucosa in plaques that included regions with normal urothelial histology. The patterns of allele-specific LOH supported the conclusion that these plaques were clonal in origin. Interestingly, although in some cases the deleted regions included canonical tumor suppressors (Chaturvedi et al. 1997) (i.e., *TP53*), in others they did not (Lee et al. 2007). This led us to propose the existence of "forerunner genes" that in some cases are located very near canonical tumor suppressors that play more important roles in the earliest stages of carcinogenesis (reviewed in Czerniak et al. 2016).

The widespread introduction of next-generation sequencing platforms enabled groups to visualize these field changes with greater breadth and depth. One study used multiregional whole exome sequencing (WES, mean read depth = 65x) followed by laser capture microdissection (n = 129 regions) with deep targeted sequencing (mean read depth = 3049x) based on validated mutations that were identified by WES and were predicted to have functional impact to define the extent of intra-tumoral heterogeneity and the characteristics of the urothelial field defect. The authors identified multiple subclones in tumors from two patients with multifocal disease, whereas they observed low clonal heterogeneity in two patients with unifocal disease (Thomsen et al. 2017). Analyses of adjacent urothelium in the patients with multifocal tumors revealed the presence of low-frequency mutations that were enriched with those shared by the tumors, but they only detected few cancer-associated mutations in the histologically normal urothelium in the patients with unifocal tumors (Thomsen et al. 2017). The team also performed RNA expression profiling on the tumor samples to assign the different regions to basal and luminal molecular subtypes (for detailed discussion of the features of these subtypes, see Chaps. 13 and 14). The results revealed subtype heterogeneity in the multifocal tumors whereas the regions in unifocal tumors were more homogeneous. Importantly, all the multifocal tumors were clonal in origin. The results reinforced the conclusion that there is widespread field cancerization in some bladder cancer patients that is characterized by low-frequency driver mutations.

Because their study design limited the characterization of the field defect to the mutations that were identified using WES on primary tumors, the same group explored whether a tumor-uninformed approach would identify additional genomic changes in the visually normal urothelium. To this end, they performed deep sequencing (average target read depth = 634x) using a panel of 509 cancer driver genes on the same four cystectomies they characterized in their original study (Strandgaard et al. 2020). The two patients with multifocal disease had more mutations in their normal urothelial areas than did the two patients with unifocal tumors, and the mutations in the normal samples had lower variant allele frequencies (VAFs), which is a measure of the fraction of sequenced DNA molecules that correspond to a given mutation. In addition, they identified the mutational processes (discussed in Chap. 7) that mediated field cancerization, with age-related processes dominating in normal areas and APOBEC playing a more important role in tumors. In every case the group identified diverse mutations that were only observed in normal urothelial areas. The authors suggested that the mutations that were shared between normal and tumor areas corresponded to the field effect and that the tumor-specific mutations arose through clonal evolution.

In a third study the group characterized field characterization using selected site bladder biopsies (SSBs) and urine from 136 patients with non-muscle invasive bladder cancer (NMIBC) treated with intravesical BCG (Strandgaard et al. 2024). The study leveraged WES data and three tumor-guided sequencing panels developed in a previous study (Strandgaard et al. 2022). The results demonstrated that VAFs were low in the normal-appearing biopsies, were significantly increased in dysplasia and CIS, and were highest in areas that contained tumor. Nevertheless, there was significant heterogeneity in the numbers of mutations detected in the normal samples. Chromatin-modifying enzymes and *TP53* were among the most mutated genes in the normal samples. In the subset of 67 patients with at least three SSBs analyzed with mutations detected in normal biopsies, high-grade recurrence-free survival was shortest in patients with higher field cancerization levels. Not surprisingly, high field levels were associated with higher neoantigen loads and higher tumor mutation burdens (TMBs). Mutations observed in the SSBs were often detected in the urine even when no tumor was visually present. Thus, the mutations present in the urine appear to reflect both field cancerization and shedding of DNA from frank tumors.

Interestingly, smoking history had no significant impact on VAF levels; rather, VAF levels increased with age. One possible explanation for this observation is that smoking plays a more important role in tumor promotion than it does in initiation, potentially by inducing inflammation in the urothelium; additional research is required to address this possibility. If so, the effects of the toxicants in cigarette smoke may be different from those studied in rodent models, where nitrosamine exposure causes clear urothelial mutagenesis (see below). However, another group used cultures of primary differentiated normal urothelium and conditional reprogramming (Baker et al. 2020) to show that the classical smoke procarcinogen, benzo[a]pyrene, can be directly metabolized and activated in the urothelium via a cytochrome P450-mediated mechanism. This process resulted in the accumulation of mutations characterized by mutational signatures (SBS4, DBS2, and ID3) that are also prevalent in lung cancers (Baker et al. 2020).

In an extension of the earlier work with microsatellites (Chaturvedi et al. 1997; Czerniak et al. 1999), we performed multi-platform genomic analyses [WES; average coverage = 37x), copy number analyses (using genome-wide SNP arrays), and DNA methylation analyses] on 37 different tissue areas in a cystectomy from a patient with multifocal high-grade papillary urothelial carcinoma (Majewski et al. 2019). The results revealed the presence of a significant number of non-silent, low-frequency candidate driver mutations (a total of 386) in at least one of the samples. We termed these alterations α mutations. They exhibited very low VAFs that were observed mostly in single or very small clusters of individual samples, suggesting that multiple small subclonal populations were present. Another group of β mutations was identified that exhibited more widespread distributions, but their VAFs did not increase with progression to cancer; the biological significance of these mutations is unclear. Finally, mutations in a third group of γ mutations ($n = 22$) increased with progression, presumably because they served as cancer drivers. A founder mutation was identified in the mRNA splicing regulator, *ACIN1*, that was present in all areas of CIS and cancer but was absent from the field effect. Copy number variations (CNVs) also accumulated in high-grade intraepithelial neoplasia and frank urothelial carcinoma in this map (Majewski et al. 2019), consistent with the conclusion that genome instability increases with stage and grade (Lindgren et al. 2010). Two exceptions were noted—copy number gains in two different regions on 7q and losses in a single region on 8p, which formed large plaques and contained genes implicated in other cancers (Majewski et al. 2019). Large plaques of altered DNA methylation were also observed and included innate inflammatory targets (defensins and the inflammasome component, NALP1), suggesting that downregulation of these targets may have facilitated tumor promotion in response to inflammation. Overall, the results supported the conclusion that the urothelium in patients with multifocal cancers is characterized by clonal field cancerization that gives rise to multiple subclonal tumors. In addition, changes in DNA methylation might alter inflammation in the tumor microenvironment in ways that could promote subclonal expansion.

In a subsequent study we performed whole transcriptome RNAseq, array-based DNA methylation profiling, whole exome sequencing, and SNP-based copy number profiling on multiple 1 × 2 cm regions in two more whole-organ maps, one containing a basal subtype tumor and the other containing a luminal tumor (Bondaruk et al. 2022). Based on the RNA expression profiles, we concluded that commitment to the basal or luminal progression pathway in these bladders with unifocal tumors was already apparent in the areas with normal morphology (Fig. 11.2) and that widespread, plaque-like changes in DNA methylation appeared before the emergence of subclones that ultimately gave rise to CIS and urothelial cancer (Bondaruk et al. 2022). The WES data reinforced the conclusion that small clonal patches containing mostly private α mutations with low VAFs dominated areas of normal urothelium and low-grade dysplasia and that they were associated with a dormant phase that was estimated to last for over a decade (Fig. 11.3) (Bondaruk et al. 2022). The accumulation of γ

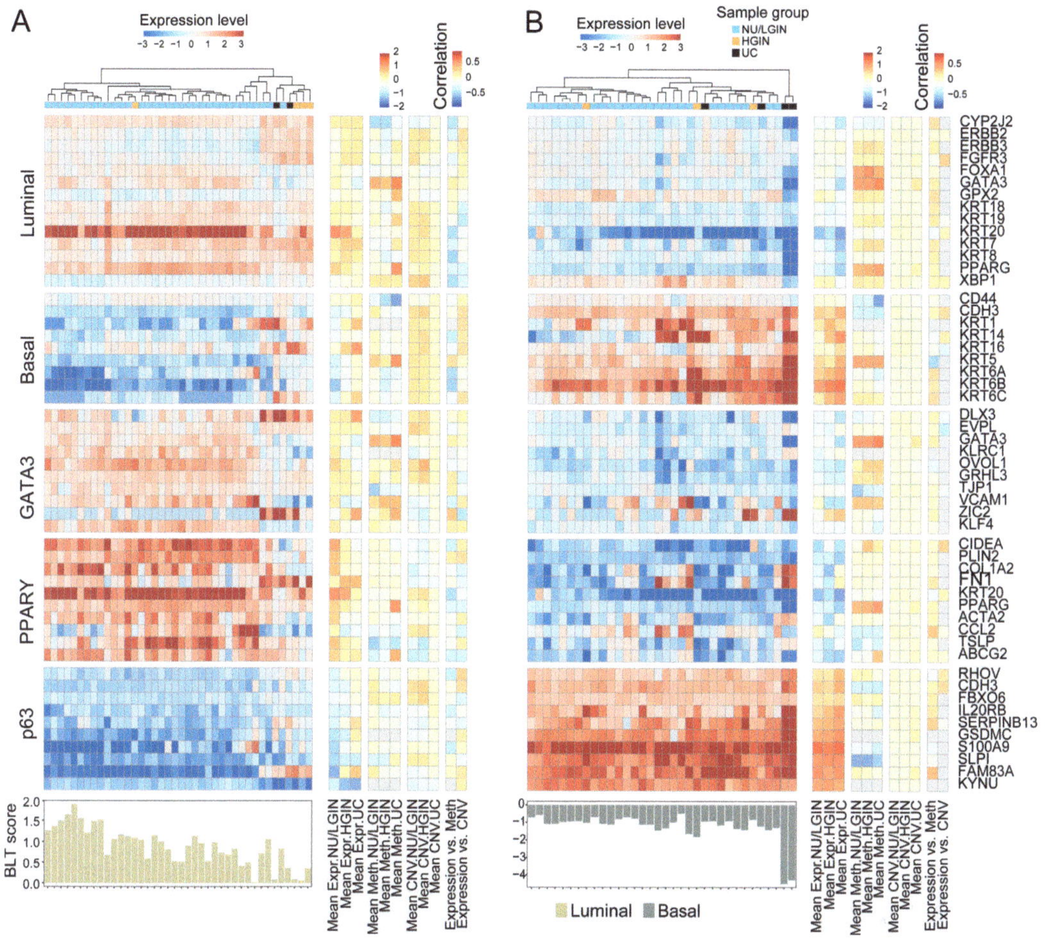

Fig. 11.2 Molecular subtype commitment in whole-organ maps containing unifocal luminal or basal tumors. (**a**) Expression pattern of basal and luminal markers and calculated basal-luminal transition (BLT) scores (positive = luminal, negative = basal) for mucosal and tumor samples on the whole-organ scale from a cystectomy specimen with luminal bladder cancer. (**b**) Expression pattern of basal and luminal markers and BLT scores for mucosal and tumor samples on the whole-organ scale from a cystectomy specimen with basal bladder cancer. Adapted from Bondaruk et al. (2022)

mutations characterized by steady increases in VAFs signaled a progressive phase of disease that was complete within 2 years (Fig. 11.3) (Bondaruk et al. 2022). The biological significance of the dormant phase was not determined, but it seems possible that the genomic changes in the subclones might drive changes in the tumor stroma and provide growth factor support for the tumor cells that subsequently enter the progressive phase.

The conclusions of Thomsen et al. (Thomsen et al. 2017) and Bondaruk et al. (Bondaruk et al. 2022) suggest that the field effects in bladders containing unifocal tumors are more homogeneous than those present in bladders with multifocal tumors. A third study used a combination of Nanostring RNA expression profiling and immunohistochemistry to address the same question in another whole-organ map and samples collected from representative urothelial regions from 22 other patients with muscle-invasive disease (Wullweber et al. 2021). They concluded that subtype commitment was stable in multiple regions in most cystectomies (about 75%) and that it occurred at the CIS stage (Wullweber et al. 2021). Their observation that CIS can display a

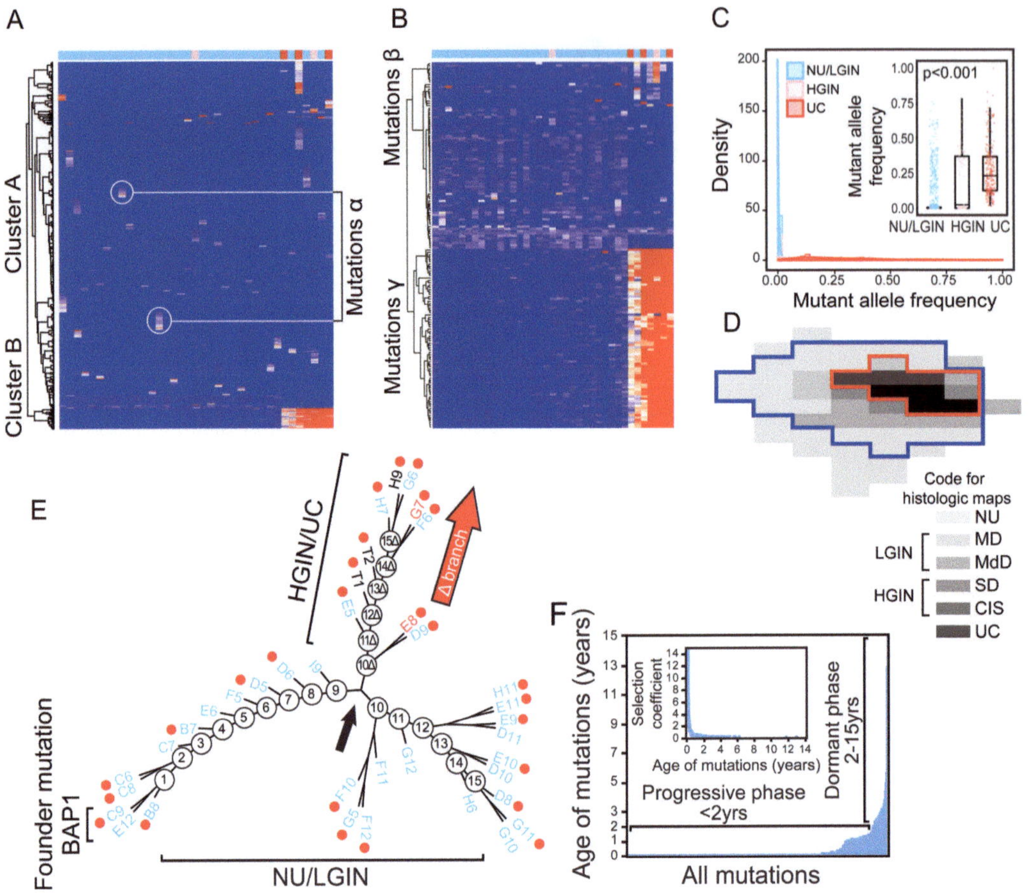

Fig. 11.3 Clonal enrichment of mutations in the evolution of bladder cancer from field effects along the luminal track. (**a**) Heat map of 2811 non-silent mutations showing variant allele frequencies (VAFs) in individual mucosal samples. (**b**) Heat map of VAFs in 157 genes showing variant alleles in at least three samples with VAFs of at least 1%. (**c**) Density plot representing the clonality of non-silent VAFs in cluster γ with a statistically significant increase in clonality with progression to urothelial bladder cancer (UC). Inset: box plot of VAFs in three groups of samples corresponding to NU/LGIN, HGIN, and UC. (**d**) Whole-organ histologic map showing a plaque-like area outlined by the blue line with a founder mutation of BAP1. The red line outlines an area corresponding to widespread CNV alterations. (**e**) Parsimony analysis showing the evolutionary tree with nine nodes of clonal expansion of successive clones in the field effect corresponding to normal urothelium/low-grade intraurothelial neoplasia with major branching at node 9, designated as the Δ branch, which evolved to high-grade intraurothelial neoplasia (HGIN)/carcinoma in situ and urothelial carcinoma. All foci of HGIN and UC evolved from successive waves of clonal expansion in the Δ branch. The main NU/LGIN clone continued to evolve in successive waves of mutational changes (nodes 10–15) with a complex branching pattern that did not progress to HGIN or UC. (**f**) Ages of all synonymous and nonsynonymous mutations predicted by mathematical modeling. Inset: the selection coefficient in relation to the predicted age. Of note is that development of bladder cancer has two distinctive phases: dormant (2–15 years) and progressive (<2 years). Based on data and rearranged figures from (Bondaruk et al. 2022)

basal gene expression profile was striking given that previous work had concluded that CIS was enriched with high level expression of KRT20 (Harnden et al. 1996; McKenney et al. 2001), a canonical luminal marker. Together, the results of the three studies suggest that molecular subtype membership is probably stable in about 75% of cases, and that subtype stability may be more common in bladders containing unifocal tumors. Nevertheless, it is important to emphasize that other studies have demonstrated that molecular subtype membership is subject to significant lineage plasticity and can be different in matched primary tumors and lymph node metastases (Sjodahl et al. 2018), in matched tumors before and after progression (Sjodahl et al. 2020), in human bladder cancer organoids propagated in vitro (Lee et al. 2018; Christin and Shen 2022), in different populations of single tumor cells within the same tumor (Sfakianos et al. 2020), and in different regions of a given tumor (Warrick et al. 2022). The application of single cell and spatial transcriptomics and new methods for measuring chromatin states on whole-organ maps and in preclinical models will reveal the dynamics of basal-luminal lineage plasticity in field cancerization and candidate mechanisms controlling it.

11.5 Multiregional Sequencing in Bladders Without Cancer

The dominance of age-related mutational "scars" in morphologically normal areas of the urothelium in bladders with cancer raises the question of whether subclonal expansions containing mutations in cancer drivers are also present in bladders that do not contain cancer. Recent studies that employed regional sequencing strategies to search for mutations in different epithelial tissues and the blood confirmed that they are widespread and common (Welch et al. 2012; Martincorena and Campbell 2015; Martincorena et al. 2015, 2018). To determine whether cancer-associated mutations are found in normal urothelium, Lawson and coworkers used laser capture microdissection on urothelial microbiopsies from 15 deceased transplant organ donors that had no signs of cancer in their bladders (Lawson et al. 2020). They compared the results to those obtained using the same approach on cystectomies from patients with bladder cancer. They used bioinformatics to identify mutations associated with clonal expansions while correcting for several sequence- and gene-specific factors (Lawson et al. 2020). The results revealed positive selection on 17 genes that included several chromatin-modifying enzymes, *NOTCH2* and *ERCC2* (Lawson et al. 2020). Microbiopsies from different individuals were enriched with different patterns of target gene mutations and different SBS signatures (Lawson et al. 2020), suggesting the involvement of different environmental exposures. One of the signatures (Signature A), characterized by features consistent with transcription-coupled damage or repair, was significantly enriched in smokers in this relatively small cohort, suggesting that it might be caused by a novel carcinogenic process driven by smoking-related metabolites in the urine (Lawson et al. 2020). APOBEC mutagenesis was common in some individuals, where it was associated with an outsized effect on the total mutational burdens (Lawson et al. 2020). In the bladders with cancer, CIS lesions obtained from distant regions were all clonally related and displayed extensive aneuploidy, whereas adjacent normal areas of the urothelium displayed much lower frequencies of chromosome-level abnormalities (Lawson et al. 2020), consistent with the other mapping studies. In addition, driver activating mutations in the *TERT* promoter, *FGFR3*, *PIK3CA*, and the *ERBB* family, and loss-of-function mutations in *TP53* were rare in morphologically normal urothelium (Lawson et al. 2020). This conclusion is consistent with observations made by another group (Li et al. 2020), although others have concluded that *TP53* mutations (Strandgaard et al. 2024) and *TERT* promoter mutations (Hayashi et al. 2020) can be detected in normal biopsies from bladder cancer patients.

In a companion article in the same issue of *Science*, Li et al. used a similar approach to characterize the mutations present in tumors and areas of morphologically normal urothelium in cystectomies and nephroureterectomies from patients with bladder and/or upper tract cancers (Li et al. 2020). Mutation rates in the normal areas displayed a broad range with a median that was higher than is observed in breast cancers or renal cell carcinomas. Focusing on the 19 genes that were significantly mutated in the matched cancers and eight additional significantly mutated genes in The Cancer Genome Atlas (TCGA) study of bladder cancer (Robertson et al. 2017), 37% of the morphologically normal urothelial (MNU) samples contained canonical cancer drivers (Li et al. 2020). De novo deconvolution of the SBSs that were associated with these mutations in the cancers and MNUs revealed three signatures that were like those associated with ageing (SBS1, SBS5), APOBEC (SBS2 and SBS13), and exposure to aristolochic acid (AA, SBS22) (Nik-Zainal et al. 2015), which is found in some Asian herbal supplements and also has a strong impact on mutagenesis in the liver (Li et al. 2021). Overall, AA-associated mutagenesis was a dominant component of field cancerization across the entire study, producing significantly higher mutational burdens and mutant clonal expansion than were associated with age-related processes. Interestingly, mutations in *KMT2D* stood out in being more enriched for ageing-associated mutational signatures (Li et al. 2020), consistent with the idea that mutations in it and other chromatin-modifying enzymes play central roles in the field cancerization that occurs independently of carcinogen exposure. Importantly, while the idea that age-related replication errors in tissue stem cells play a central role in mutagenesis of chromatin-modifying enzymes is gaining acceptance, a role for carcinogen exposure has not been ruled out. Baker et al. combined the SBS signatures that were implicated in *KMT2D* mutagenesis in the Lawson (Lawson et al. 2020) and Li (Li et al. 2020) papers with their benzo[a] pyrene signature (Baker et al. 2020) and derived a novel signature that they showed was enriched in human bladder cancers (Baker et al. 2021).

In summary, the results of the whole-organ mapping studies demonstrated that small clonal expansions containing inactivating mutations in chromatin-modifying genes and others (including *NOTCH2* and *ERCC2*) accumulate in the normal urothelium and in normal-looking areas of the urothelium in patients with cancer. These mutations are linked to both aging and environmental exposures, and APOBEC contributes to mutagenesis in widespread areas of the urothelium in some individuals independently of the other mutagenic processes, which tend to be more spatially restricted (Lawson et al. 2020). The involved areas are equivalent in size to the ones that are thought to be occupied by individual urothelial stem cells, and the mutations produce very modest net increases in clonal expansion. Field cancerization is associated with copy neutral LOH affecting discrete regions of the genome, whereas progression to CIS and cancer is associated with chromosomal instability and aneuploidy. When one of the subclones in the field acquires enough mutations to produce chromosomal instability, it can spread widely throughout the urothelium by direct migration through the tissue or via detachment and reimplantation at distant sites. Non-invasive papillary Ta tumors exhibit two chromosomal subtypes—one with almost no alterations and another characterized by 9q loss and more alterations (Hurst et al. 2017). Papillary lesions progress to become invasive less frequently than do CIS lesions (Czerniak et al. 2016), and when they do, they are also characterized by more chromosomal instability (Hurst et al. 2021).

11.6 Mechanisms of Carcinogenesis in Preclinical Models

Whole-organ mapping studies with cystectomies have revealed some of the temporal changes that occur during urothelial carcinogenesis, but much of what is known has been inferred from genomics data rather than being directly observed. Complementary studies can be performed in preclinical models where the timing of an exposure or introduction of a genomic change can be controlled. Preclinical models are also essential for performing mechanistic studies to identify the molecular mechanisms underlying field cancerization.

N-Butyl-*N*-(4-hydroxybutyl) nitrosamine (BBN) is a carcinogen that is like chemicals found in cigarette smoke (Vasconcelos-Nobrega et al. 2012). It is a potent inducer of bladder cancers in rats (Akagi et al. 1973) and mice (Becci et al. 1978) when it is administered orally via gavage or in drinking water (Vasconcelos-Nobrega et al. 2012). Tumors can also be induced via subcutaneous injection or intravesical instillation (Vasconcelos-Nobrega et al. 2012). Carcinogenesis in the model proceeds over the course of 2–4 months with predictable kinetics and involves histopathological changes that resemble those observed in the human urothelium (Fontugne et al. 2023). Tumors in rats are papillary, whereas tumors in mice progress from CIS (Vasconcelos-Nobrega et al. 2012).

The biological differences in BBN-induced tumors in rats and mice are also illustrated by studies of the anti-diabetic drug and peroxisome proliferator activator receptor (Pparg) agonist rosiglitazone. Pparg is a canonical luminal marker that is downregulated in basal-squamous tumors (Kamoun et al. 2020). Rosiglitazone promoted early disease progression in rats (Tirmenstein et al. 2018) but inhibited progression in mice and eradicated tumors when it was combined with an MEK inhibitor (Tate et al. 2023). Although the molecular subtype(s) of the papillary tumors induced in rats have not been defined, RNA sequencing of murine tumors demonstrated that their gene expression profiles were similar to human basal/squamous tumors, and over time they acquired sarcomatoid histopathological characteristics and signatures associated with epithelial-to-mesenchymal transition (EMT) (Rebouissou et al. 2014; Fantini et al. 2018; Fontugne et al. 2023). WES of murine tumors revealed that they contained genetic alterations that are shared by human muscle-invasive bladder cancers (MIBCs), including mutations in chromatin-modifying enzymes (*Kmt2c*, *Kmt2d*, and *Arid1a*) and in *Tp53* (Fantini et al. 2018). However, they lacked many of the other genomic alterations that are present in humans, including chromosomal copy number alterations or mutations in the *Tert* promoter, *Fgfr3*, *Hras*, *Pik3ca*, *Kdm6a*, or *Ercc2* (Fantini et al. 2018). The SBS mutational signatures in the tumors were most like human SBS5 and SBS22 (Fantini et al. 2018). However, signatures associated with ageing (SBS1) and APOBEC (SBS2 and SBS13) (Fantini et al. 2018), which are ubiquitous in human cancers (Alexandrov et al. 2013), were not observed.

Like its human counterpart, the murine urothelium appears to contain a population of pluripotent progenitors (stem cells) that can repopulate all layers of the urothelium in response to injury. These stem cells were identified by injecting animals with bromodeoxyuridine (BrdU) and harvesting bladders at various time points afterward (up to 1 year) to identify the "label-retaining cells" that correspond to tissue-specific stem cells (Kurzrock et al. 2008). This population was found in the basal layer, made up 9% of total urothelial cells, and expressed Krt14, Tp63, Bcl2, and β4 integrin (Kurzrock et al. 2008). This pattern of biomarker expression was like the one that was subsequently identified in candidate stem cells isolated from human bladder cancers (Chan et al. 2009; He et al. 2009; Ho et al. 2012; Volkmer et al. 2012).

Lineage tracing studies have been performed to precisely visualize clonal expansion and to identify the cancer cells of origin in mice exposed to BBN. One study used it to demonstrate that basal urothelial cells expressing *Sonic hedgehog* (Shh) contained stem cells that could repopulate the urothelium in mice exposed to a uropathogenic strain of *E. coli* (UTI89) or to the damaging chemical protamine sulfate (Shin et al. 2011). Marked basal cells gave rise to patches of geographically restricted columns of intermediate and superficial cells (Shin et al. 2011), consistent with the proposed organization of urothelial stem cells in humans. Other work employing conditional knockout mice demonstrated that the basal genes *Tp63* and *Shh* were required for repopulation of the urothelium in response to injury (Signoretti et al. 2005; Shin et al. 2011; Pignon et al. 2013). However, another study employed a similar strategy to conclude that the Krt5+ basal cell population did not contain the progenitor population that populated the urothelium during embryonic development or injury-induced repopulation in adult animals exposed to intravesical cyclophosphamide (Gandhi et al. 2013).

There is also uncertainty about the populations of cells that serve as stem cells for BBN-induced cancers. One study concluded that Shh + basal cells were solely responsible (Shin et al. 2014), whereas another implicated Krt5+ basal stem cells in the emergence of CIS and muscle-invasive cancers and Upk2+ cells as the progenitor pool for papillary cancers (Van Batavia et al. 2014). A third study employed lineage tracing to demonstrate that inactivation of *Tp53* in Krt5+ cells resulted in more efficient BBN-induced carcinogenesis than did *Tp53* inactivation in Upk2+ cells (Masuda et al. 2020). Considering all the data, they appear to support the conclusion that most of the spontaneous tumors that develop in the BBN mouse model arise from basal stem cells and progress to become basal/squamous tumors. A longitudinal study demonstrated that pTa tumors could be observed at intermediate time points, but they were enriched with basal gene expression profiles and squamous histopathological features (Fontugne et al. 2023), whereas human pTa tumors were exclusively luminal papillary (Hurst et al. 2021). Spatial profiling comparisons of the DNA mutations that are present in BBN-induced papillary and non-papillary tumors could help to resolve the question of whether they arise via distinct molecular mechanisms. It will also be interesting to perform similar studies in rats, where BBN-induced tumors are more clearly papillary in nature.

Lineage tracing is an experimental strategy that employs fluorescent dyes or DNA molecular "barcodes" to permanently mark individual cells so that their fates can be determined unambiguously. One group used a strategy that marked cells with one of four different fluorescent reporters to characterize the clonal expansion that is observed in the urothelium in mice exposed to BBN (Shin et al. 2014). In some animals, widespread areas of CIS were marked by one fluorescent dye, strongly suggesting that they developed via expansion of a single transformed clone. However, in others, areas occupied by CIS were marked by different fluorescent dyes, indicating that transformation of different stem cells was involved. Importantly, the colors in each area were homogeneous, consistent with uniform local expansion of transformed stem cells rather than admixture of multiple stem cells. The results are consistent with human data demonstrating that multiregional CIS can be monoclonal or polyclonal in patients with cancer (Heide et al. 2019).

Pparg and other luminal markers are downregulated in BBN-induced cancers (Rebouissou et al. 2014; Fantini et al. 2018; Saito et al. 2018; Fontugne et al. 2023). To determine what happens when Pparg downregulation is prevented, we generated a mouse model in which a ligand-independent, constitutively active form of Pparg was conditionally expressed in Krt5-positive cells in the urothelium (Tate et al. 2023). Animals were exposed to BBN for 1 month to initiate carcinogenesis before the transgene was activated by intravesical delivery of adenoviral Cre recombinase. Comparison to controls revealed that Pparg activation caused the emergence of luminal papillary tumors as revealed by histopathological assessment and RNA expression profiling. Interestingly, even with enforced Pparg activation, the tumors eventually evolved to become more "basalized" as they progressed, a process that emerged in deeper areas of the urothelium adjacent to the lamina propria and was associated with loss of Pparg signaling, muscle-invasive growth patterns, and a switch in RNA expression profile to one consistent with the basal/squamous molecular subtype (Tate et al. 2023). Therefore, there is strong pressure for "basalization" in the BBN mouse model. Future work is required to identify the specific molecular mechanisms involved.

As discussed above, the clonal expansions that characterize the urothelial field effect in humans are dominated by inactivating mutations in chromatin-modifying enzymes, and in particular *KMT2D* (Lawson et al. 2020; Li et al. 2020). Mutations in *Kmt2d* also dominate the mutational landscapes in murine BBN tumors (Fantini et al. 2018), and in ongoing studies the functional consequences of these mutations are being explored. One hypothesis that has been advanced is that they target Tp63 (Lin-Shiao et al. 2018; Baker et al. 2021), a transcription factor that controls the basal gene expression program (Tran et al. 2013; Choi et al. 2014).

Exposure to BBN or other agents that damage the urothelium (uropathogenic *E. coli* or cyclophosphamide) causes widespread inflammation (Gandhi et al. 2013; Liu et al. 2019; Tate et al. 2021, 2023). This inflammation is associated with downregulation of gene expression signatures activated by Pparg and upregulation of those controlled by nuclear factor kappa-b (Nfκb) (Liu et al. 2019, Tate et al. 2021, 2023). In wild-type animals exposed to these agents transiently, the inflammation ultimately resolves and the urothelium is repaired. However, in animals in which Pparg has been conditionally deleted in the urothelium, chronic inflammation develops which is not resolved, resulting in "basalization" of the urothelium and the development of squamous differentiation (Liu et al. 2019). Thus, inflammation, carcinogenesis, and basalization are tightly interconnected in BBN-exposed murine urothelium, and ongoing studies are investigating the cause-effect relationships among the changes observed.

Other preclinical work has been focused on defining the downstream consequences of *KDM6A* mutations in both human and mouse models. Comparison of *KDM6A* wild-type and mutant human tumors by ATAC-seq revealed that the former were enriched with motifs corresponding to the binding sites for luminal transcription factors that promote urothelial differentiation (FOXA1, GATA3), whereas *KDM6A* mutant tumors were enriched with binding sites for bZIP transcription factors including ATF3 (Qiu et al. 2023), resulting in perturbation of urothelial differentiation. Similarly, another group generated a mouse model in which *Kdm6a* was selectively deleted in the urothelium with or without combined inactivation of one allele of *Tp53*, and they characterized the effects on BBN-induced tumorigenesis and the tumor immune landscape (Kobatake et al. 2020). Loss of *Kdm6a* inhibited cell cycle progression but promoted inflammation. Although the authors did not examine the effects on urothelial differentiation, the results are consistent with the phenotype observed in the *Pparg*-deficient urothelium (Liu et al. 2019). Another group showed that Arid1a expression was enriched in terminally differentiated urothelial cells and that its loss was associated with hyperproliferation and disrupted differentiation (Guo et al. 2022).

11.7 Conclusions

The available evidence supports a model in which mutations in chromatin-modifying enzymes disrupt the transcriptional control of urothelial terminal differentiation, resulting in lineage plasticity that promotes a slightly more basal and stem-like phenotype and is associated with increased inflammation, potentially because of downregulation of Pparg activity. The effects are subtle and result in clonal expansions that set the stage for neoplastic transformation. Tumor progression is mediated by the acquisition of additional driver mutations and chromosomal instability. Environmental contaminants that have been identified as risk factors for bladder cancer may act as tumor promoters rather than initiators, and their effects may also often involve inflammation. Over time, inflammation may cause changes in DNA methylation in the field effect that serves to inhibit innate and adaptive immune surveillance mechanisms that would otherwise act to eliminate mutant cells. Field cancerization is associated with copy neutral LOH and mutations that affect a variety of other genes, but the functional consequences of these effects are unclear and are under active investigation in preclinical models. It seems likely that inactivation of different chromatin-modifying genes would cause different specific downstream effects, potentially by targeting the different transcriptional programs that are controlled by basal (TP63, STAT3, NFkB, AP-1, HIF) versus luminal (PPARG, FOXA1, GATA3) transcription factors. Elucidating these mechanisms requires additional investigation.

References

Akagi G, Akagi A, Kimura M, Otsuka H (1973) Comparison of bladder tumors induced in rats and mice with N-butyl-N-(4-hydroxybutyl)-nitrosoamine. Gan 64(4):331–336

Alexandrov LB, Ju YS, Haase K, Van Loo P, Martincorena I, Nik-Zainal S, Totoki Y, Fujimoto A, Nakagawa H, Shibata T, Campbell PJ, Vineis P, Phillips DH, Stratton MR (2016) Mutational signatures associated with tobacco smoking in human cancer. Science 354(6312):618–622

Alexandrov LB, Nik-Zainal S, Wedge DC, Aparicio SA, Behjati S, Biankin AV, Bignell GR, Bolli N, Borg A, Borresen-Dale AL, Boyault S, Burkhardt B, Butler AP, Caldas C, Davies HR, Desmedt C, Eils R, Eyfjord JE, Foekens JA, Greaves M, Hosoda F, Hutter B, Ilicic T, Imbeaud S, Imielinski M, Jager N, Jones DT, Jones

D, Knappskog S, Kool M, Lakhani SR, Lopez-Otin C, Martin S, Munshi NC, Nakamura H, Northcott PA, Pajic M, Papaemmanuil E, Paradiso A, Pearson JV, Puente XS, Raine K, Ramakrishna M, Richardson AL, Richter J, Rosenstiel P, Schlesner M, Schumacher TN, Span PN, Teague JW, Totoki Y, Tutt AN, Valdes-Mas R, van Buuren MM, van 't Veer L, Vincent-Salomon A, Waddell N, Yates LR, I. Australian Pancreatic Cancer Genome, I. B. C. Consortium, I. M.-S. Consortium, PedBrain I, Zucman-Rossi J, Futreal PA, McDermott U, Lichter P, Meyerson M, Grimmond SM, Siebert R, Campo E, Shibata T, Pfister SM, Campbell PJ, Stratton MR (2013) Signatures of mutational processes in human cancer. Nature 500(7463):415–421

Baird WM, Boutwell RK (1971) Tumor-promoting activity of phorbol and four diesters of phorbol in mouse skin. Cancer Res 31(8):1074–1079

Baker SC, Mason AS, Southgate J (2020) Procarcinogen activation and mutational signatures model the initiation of carcinogenesis in human urothelial tissues in vitro. Eur Urol 78(2):143–147

Baker SC, Mason AS, Southgate J (2021) Does a novel mutagenic process target KMT2D mutation in the Most common first event on the path to bladder cancer? Eur Urol 79(3):435–436

Becci PJ, Thompson HJ, Grubbs CJ, Squire RA, Brown CC, Sporn MB, Moon RC (1978) Inhibitory effect of 13-cis-retinoic acid on urinary bladder carcinogenesis induced in C57BL/6 mice by N-butyl-N-(4-hydroxybutyl)-nitrosamine. Cancer Res 38(12):4463–4466

Bondaruk J, Jaksik R, Wang Z, Cogdell D, Lee S, Chen Y, Dinh KN, Majewski T, Zhang L, Cao S, Tian F, Yao H, Kus P, Chen H, Weinstein JN, Navai N, Dinney C, Gao J, Theodorescu D, Logothetis C, Guo CC, Wang W, McConkey D, Wei P, Kimmel M, Czerniak B (2022) The origin of bladder cancer from mucosal field effects. iScience 25(7):104551

Cairns P, Shaw ME, Knowles MA (1993) Initiation of bladder cancer may involve deletion of a tumour-suppressor gene on chromosome 9. Oncogene 8(4):1083–1085

Chan KS, Espinosa I, Chao M, Wong D, Ailles L, Diehn M, Gill H, Presti J Jr, Chang HY, van de Rijn M, Shortliffe L, Weissman IL (2009) Identification, molecular characterization, clinical prognosis, and therapeutic targeting of human bladder tumor-initiating cells. Proc Natl Acad Sci USA 106(33):14016–14021

Chaturvedi V, Li L, Hodges S, Johnston D, Ro JY, Logothetis C, von Eschenbach AC, Batsakis JG, Czerniak B (1997) Superimposed histologic and genetic mapping of chromosome 17 alterations in human urinary bladder neoplasia. Oncogene 14(17):2059–2070

Choi W, Porten S, Kim S, Willis D, Plimack ER, Hoffman-Censits J, Roth B, Cheng T, Tran M, Lee IL, Melquist J, Bondaruk J, Majewski T, Zhang S, Pretzsch S, Baggerly K, Siefker-Radtke A, Czerniak B, Dinney CP, McConkey DJ (2014) Identification of distinct basal and luminal subtypes of muscle-invasive bladder cancer with different sensitivities to frontline chemotherapy. Cancer Cell 25(2):152–165

Christin JR, Shen MM (2022) Modeling tumor plasticity in organoid models of human cancer. Trends Cancer 8(3):161–163

Czerniak B, Chaturvedi V, Li L, Hodges S, Johnston D, Roy JY, Luthra R, Logothetis C, Von Eschenbach AC, Grossman HB, Benedict WF, Batsakis JG (1999) Superimposed histologic and genetic mapping of chromosome 9 in progression of human urinary bladder neoplasia: implications for a genetic model of multistep urothelial carcinogenesis and early detection of urinary bladder cancer. Oncogene 18(5):1185–1196

Czerniak B, Dinney C, McConkey D (2016) Origins of bladder cancer. Annu Rev Pathol 11:149–174

Fantini D, Glaser AP, Rimar KJ, Wang Y, Schipma M, Varghese N, Rademaker A, Behdad A, Yellapa A, Yu Y, Sze CC, Wang L, Zhao Z, Crawford SE, Hu D, Licht JD, Collings CK, Bartom E, Theodorescu D, Shilatifard A, Meeks JJ (2018) A carcinogen-induced mouse model recapitulates the molecular alterations of human muscle invasive bladder cancer. Oncogene 37(14):1911–1925

Farrow GM, Utz DC, Rife CC (1976) Morphological and clinical observations of patients with early bladder cancer treated with total cystectomy. Cancer Res 36(7 PT 2):2495–2501

Fontugne J, Wong J, Cabel L, Neyret-Kahn H, Karboul N, Maille P, Rapinat A, Gentien D, Nicolas A, Baulande S, Sibony M, Bernard-Pierrot I, Radvanyi F, Allory Y (2023) Progression-associated molecular changes in basal/squamous and sarcomatoid bladder carcinogenesis. J Pathol 259(4):455–467

Fujiki H, Suganuma M, Yoshizawa S, Kanazawa H, Sugimura T, Manam S, Kahn SM, Jiang W, Hoshina S, Weinstein IB (1989) Codon 61 mutations in the c-Harvey-ras gene in mouse skin tumors induced by 7,12-dimethylbenz[a]anthracene plus okadaic acid class tumor promoters. Mol Carcinog 2(4):184–187

Gandhi D, Molotkov A, Batourina E, Schneider K, Dan H, Reiley M, Laufer E, Metzger D, Liang F, Liao Y, Sun TT, Aronow B, Rosen R, Mauney J, Adam R, Rosselot C, Van Batavia J, McMahon A, McMahon J, Guo JJ, Mendelsohn C (2013) Retinoid signaling in progenitors controls specification and regeneration of the urothelium. Dev Cell 26(5):469–482

Guo C, Zhang Y, Tan R, Tang Z, Lam CM, Ye X, Wang Z, Li X (2022) Arid1a regulates bladder urothelium formation and maintenance. Dev Biol 485:61–69

Guo CC, Czerniak B (2019) Bladder cancer in the genomic era. Arch Pathol Lab Med 143(6):695–704

Guo CC, Lee S, Lee JG, Chen H, Zaleski M, Choi W, McConkey DJ, Wei P, Czerniak B (2024) Molecular profile of bladder cancer progression to clinically aggressive subtypes. Nat Rev Urol 21:391

Harnden P, Eardley I, Joyce AD, Southgate J (1996) Cytokeratin 20 as an objective marker of urothelial dysplasia. Br J Urol 78(6):870–875

Hayashi Y, Fujita K, Nojima S, Tomiyama E, Matsushita M, Koh Y, Nakano K, Wang C, Ishizuya Y, Kato

T, Hatano K, Kawashima A, Ujike T, Uemura M, Imamura R, Morii E, Nonomura N (2020) TERT C228T mutation in non-malignant bladder urothelium is associated with intravesical recurrence for patients with non-muscle invasive bladder cancer. Mol Oncol 14(10):2375–2383

He X, Marchionni L, Hansel DE, Yu W, Sood A, Yang J, Parmigiani G, Matsui W, Berman DM (2009) Differentiation of a highly tumorigenic basal cell compartment in urothelial carcinoma. Stem Cells 27(7):1487–1495

Heide T, Maurer A, Eipel M, Knoll K, Geelvink M, Veeck J, Knuechel R, van Essen J, Stoehr R, Hartmann A, Altmueller J, Graham TA, Gaisa NT (2019) Multiregion human bladder cancer sequencing reveals tumour evolution, bladder cancer phenotypes and implications for targeted therapy. J Pathol 248(2):230–242

Hill W, Lim EL, Weeden CE, Lee C, Augustine M, Chen K, Kuan FC, Marongiu F, Evans EJ Jr, Moore DA, Rodrigues FS, Pich O, Bakker B, Cha H, Myers R, van Maldegem F, Boumelha J, Veeriah S, Rowan A, Naceur-Lombardelli C, Karasaki T, Sivakumar M, De S, Caswell DR, Nagano A, Black JRM, Martinez-Ruiz C, Ryu MH, Huff RD, Li S, Fave MJ, Magness A, Suarez-Bonnet A, Priestnall SL, Luchtenborg M, Lavelle K, Pethick J, Hardy S, McRonald FE, Lin MH, Troccoli CI, Ghosh M, Miller YE, Merrick DT, Keith RL, Al Bakir M, Bailey C, Hill MS, Saal LH, Chen Y, George AM, Abbosh C, Kanu N, Lee SH, McGranahan N, Berg CD, Sasieni P, Houlston R, Turnbull C, Lam S, Awadalla P, Gronroos E, Downward J, Jacks T, Carlsten C, Malanchi I, Hackshaw A, Litchfield K, Consortium TR, DeGregori J, Jamal-Hanjani M, Swanton C (2023) Lung adenocarcinoma promotion by air pollutants. Nature 616(7955):159–167

Ho PL, Kurtova A, Chan KS (2012) Normal and neoplastic urothelial stem cells: getting to the root of the problem. Nat Rev Urol 9(10):583–594

Hurst CD, Alder O, Platt FM, Droop A, Stead LF, Burns JE, Burghel GJ, Jain S, Klimczak LJ, Lindsay H, Roulson JA, Taylor CF, Thygesen H, Cameron AJ, Ridley AJ, Mott HR, Gordenin DA, Knowles MA (2017) Genomic subtypes of non-invasive bladder cancer with distinct metabolic profile and female gender bias in KDM6A mutation frequency. Cancer Cell 32(5):701–715 e707

Hurst CD, Cheng G, Platt FM, Castro MAA, Marzouka NS, Eriksson P, Black EVI, Alder O, Lawson ARJ, Lindskrog SV, Burns JE, Jain S, Roulson JA, Brown JC, Koster J, Robertson AG, Martincorena I, Dyrskjot L, Hoglund M, Knowles MA (2021) Stage-stratified molecular profiling of non-muscle-invasive bladder cancer enhances biological, clinical, and therapeutic insight. Cell Rep Med 2(12):100472

Kamat AM, Hahn NM, Efstathiou JA, Lerner SP, Malmstrom PU, Choi W, Guo CC, Lotan Y, Kassouf W (2016) Bladder cancer. Lancet 388(10061):2796–2810

Kamoun A, de Reynies A, Allory Y, Sjodahl G, Robertson AG, Seiler R, Hoadley KA, Groeneveld CS, Al-Ahmadie H, Choi W, Castro MAA, Fontugne J, Eriksson P, Mo Q, Kardos J, Zlotta A, Hartmann A, Dinney CP, Bellmunt J, Powles T, Malats N, Chan KS, Kim WY, McConkey DJ, Black PC, Dyrskjot L, Hoglund M, Lerner SP, Real FX, Radvanyi F, G. Bladder Cancer Molecular Taxonomy (2020) A consensus molecular classification of muscle-invasive bladder cancer. Eur Urol 77(4):420–433

Karin M (2009) NF-kappaB as a critical link between inflammation and cancer. Cold Spring Harb Perspect Biol 1(5):a000141

Kobatake K, Ikeda KI, Nakata Y, Yamasaki N, Ueda T, Kanai A, Sentani K, Sera Y, Hayashi T, Koizumi M, Miyakawa Y, Inaba T, Sotomaru Y, Kaminuma O, Ichinohe T, Honda ZI, Yasui W, Horie S, Black PC, Matsubara A, Honda H (2020) Kdm6a deficiency activates inflammatory pathways, promotes M2 macrophage polarization, and causes bladder cancer in cooperation with p53 dysfunction. Clin Cancer Res 26(8):2065–2079

Koss LG (1979) Mapping of the urinary bladder: its impact on the concepts of bladder cancer. Hum Pathol 10(5):533–548

Koss LG, Tiamson EM, Robbins MA (1974) Mapping cancerous and precancerous bladder changes. A study of the urothelium in ten surgically removed bladders. JAMA 227(3):281–286

Kurzrock EA, Lieu DK, Degraffenried LA, Chan CW, Isseroff RR (2008) Label-retaining cells of the bladder: candidate urothelial stem cells. Am J Physiol Renal Physiol 294(6):F1415–F1421

Lawson ARJ, Abascal F, Coorens THH, Hooks Y, O'Neill L, Latimer C, Raine K, Sanders MA, Warren AY, Mahbubani KTA, Bareham B, Butler TM, Harvey LMR, Cagan A, Menzies A, Moore L, Colquhoun AJ, Turner W, Thomas B, Gnanapragasam V, Williams N, Rassl DM, Vohringer H, Zumalave S, Nangalia J, Tubio JMC, Gerstung M, Saeb-Parsy K, Stratton MR, Campbell PJ, Mitchell TJ, Martincorena I (2020) Extensive heterogeneity in somatic mutation and selection in the human bladder. Science 370(6512):75–82

Lee S, Jeong J, Majewski T, Scherer SE, Kim MS, Tuziak T, Tang KS, Baggerly K, Grossman HB, Zhou JH, Shen L, Bondaruk J, Ahmed SS, Samanta S, Spiess P, Wu X, Filipek S, McConkey D, Bar-Eli M, Issa JP, Benedict WF, Czerniak B (2007) Forerunner genes contiguous to RB1 contribute to the development of in situ neoplasia. Proc Natl Acad Sci USA 104(34):13732–13737

Lee SH, Hu W, Matulay JT, Silva MV, Owczarek TB, Kim K, Chua CW, Barlow LJ, Kandoth C, Williams AB, Bergren SK, Pietzak EJ, Anderson CB, Benson MC, Coleman JA, Taylor BS, Abate-Shen C, McKiernan JM, Al-Ahmadie H, Solit DB, Shen MM (2018) Tumor evolution and drug response in patient-derived organoid models of bladder cancer. Cell 173(2):515–528 e517

Li R, Di L, Li J, Fan W, Liu Y, Guo W, Liu W, Liu L, Li Q, Chen L, Chen Y, Miao C, Liu H, Wang Y, Ma Y, Xu D, Lin D, Huang Y, Wang J, Bai F, Wu C (2021) A body map of somatic mutagenesis in morphologically normal human tissues. Nature 597(7876):398–403

Li R, Du Y, Chen Z, Xu D, Lin T, Jin S, Wang G, Liu Z, Lu M, Chen X, Xu T, Bai F (2020) Macroscopic somatic clonal expansion in morphologically normal human urothelium. Science 370(6512):82–89

Lin-Shiao E, Lan Y, Coradin M, Anderson A, Donahue G, Simpson CL, Sen P, Saffie R, Busino L, Garcia BA, Berger SL, Capell BC (2018) KMT2D regulates p63 target enhancers to coordinate epithelial homeostasis. Genes Dev 32(2):181–193

Lindgren D, Frigyesi A, Gudjonsson S, Sjodahl G, Hallden C, Chebil G, Veerla S, Ryden T, Mansson W, Liedberg F, Hoglund M (2010) Combined gene expression and genomic profiling define two intrinsic molecular subtypes of urothelial carcinoma and gene signatures for molecular grading and outcome. Cancer Res 70(9):3463–3472

Liu C, Tate T, Batourina E, Truschel ST, Potter S, Adam M, Xiang T, Picard M, Reiley M, Schneider K, Tamargo M, Lu C, Chen X, He J, Kim H, Mendelsohn CL (2019) Pparg promotes differentiation and regulates mitochondrial gene expression in bladder epithelial cells. Nat Commun 10(1):4589

Majewski T, Lee S, Jeong J, Yoon DS, Kram A, Kim MS, Tuziak T, Bondaruk J, Lee S, Park WS, Tang KS, Chung W, Shen L, Ahmed SS, Johnston DA, Grossman HB, Dinney CP, Zhou JH, Harris RA, Snyder C, Filipek S, Narod SA, Watson P, Lynch HT, Gazdar A, Bar-Eli M, Wu XF, McConkey DJ, Baggerly K, Issa JP, Benedict WF, Scherer SE, Czerniak B (2008) Understanding the development of human bladder cancer by using a whole-organ genomic mapping strategy. Lab Investig 88(7):694–721

Majewski T, Yao H, Bondaruk J, Chung W, Lee S, Lee JG, Zhang S, Cogdell D, Yang G, Choi W, Dinney C, Grossman HB, Logothetis C, Scherer SE, Guo CC, Zhang L, Wei P, Weinstein JN, Issa JP, Baggerly K, McConkey DJ, Czerniak B (2019) Whole-organ genomic characterization of mucosal field effects initiating bladder carcinogenesis. Cell Rep 26(8):2241–2256 e2244

Martincorena I, Campbell PJ (2015) Somatic mutation in cancer and normal cells. Science 349(6255):1483–1489

Martincorena I, Fowler JC, Wabik A, Lawson ARJ, Abascal F, Hall MWJ, Cagan A, Murai K, Mahbubani K, Stratton MR, Fitzgerald RC, Handford PA, Campbell PJ, Saeb-Parsy K, Jones PH (2018) Somatic mutant clones colonize the human esophagus with age. Science 362(6417):911–917

Martincorena I, Roshan A, Gerstung M, Ellis P, Van Loo P, McLaren S, Wedge DC, Fullam A, Alexandrov LB, Tubio JM, Stebbings L, Menzies A, Widaa S, Stratton MR, Jones PH, Campbell PJ (2015) Tumor evolution. High burden and pervasive positive selection of somatic mutations in normal human skin. Science 348(6237):880–886

Masuda N, Murakami K, Kita Y, Hamada A, Kamada M, Teramoto Y, Sakatani T, Matsumoto K, Sano T, Saito R, Okuno Y, Ogawa O, Kobayashi T (2020) Trp53 mutation in keratin 5 (Krt5)-expressing basal cells facilitates the development of basal squamous-like invasive bladder cancer in the chemical carcinogenesis of mouse bladder. Am J Pathol 190(8):1752–1762

McKenney JK, Desai S, Cohen C, Amin MB (2001) Discriminatory immunohistochemical staining of urothelial carcinoma in situ and non-neoplastic urothelium: an analysis of cytokeratin 20, p53, and CD44 antigens. Am J Surg Pathol 25(8):1074–1078

Melicow MM (1952) Histological study of vesical urothelium intervening between gross neoplasms in total cystectomy. J Urol 68(1):261–279

Melicow MM, Hollowell JW (1952) Intra-urothelial cancer: carcinoma in situ, Bowen's disease of the urinary system: discussion of thirty cases. J Urol 68(4):763–772

Nik-Zainal S, Kucab JE, Morganella S, Glodzik D, Alexandrov LB, Arlt VM, Weninger A, Hollstein M, Stratton MR, Phillips DH (2015) The genome as a record of environmental exposure. Mutagenesis 30(6):763–770

O'Donnell JS, Teng MWL, Smyth MJ (2019) Cancer immunoediting and resistance to T cell-based immunotherapy. Nat Rev Clin Oncol 16(3):151–167

Pignon JC, Grisanzio C, Geng Y, Song J, Shivdasani RA, Signoretti S (2013) p63-expressing cells are the stem cells of developing prostate, bladder, and colorectal epithelia. Proc Natl Acad Sci USA 110(20):8105–8110

Presti JC Jr, Reuter VE, Galan T, Fair WR, Cordon-Cardo C (1991) Molecular genetic alterations in superficial and locally advanced human bladder cancer. Cancer Res 51(19):5405–5409

Qiu H, Makarov V, Bolzenius JK, Halstead A, Parker Y, Wang A, Iyer GV, Wise H, Kim D, Thayaparan V, Lindner DJ, Haber GP, Ting AH, Ren B, Chan TA, Arora V, Solit DB, Lee BH (2023) KDM6A loss triggers an epigenetic switch that disrupts urothelial differentiation and drives cell proliferation in bladder cancer. Cancer Res 83(6):814–829

Rebouissou S, Bernard-Pierrot I, de Reynies A, Lepage ML, Krucker C, Chapeaublanc E, Herault A, Kamoun A, Caillault A, Letouze E, Elarouci N, Neuzillet Y, Denoux Y, Molinie V, Vordos D, Laplanche A, Maille P, Soyeux P, Ofualuka K, Reyal F, Biton A, Sibony M, Paoletti X, Southgate J, Benhamou S, Lebret T, Allory Y, Radvanyi F (2014) EGFR as a potential therapeutic target for a subset of muscle-invasive bladder cancers presenting a basal-like phenotype. Sci Transl Med 6(244):244ra291

Robertson AG, Kim J, Al-Ahmadie H, Bellmunt J, Guo G, Cherniack AD, Hinoue T, Laird PW, Hoadley KA, Akbani R, Castro MAA, Gibb EA, Kanchi RS, Gordenin DA, Shukla SA, Sanchez-Vega F, Hansel DE, Czerniak BA, Reuter VE, Su X, de Sa Carvalho B, Chagas VS, Mungall KL, Sadeghi S, Pedamallu CS, Lu Y, Klimczak LJ, Zhang J, Choo C, Ojesina AI, Bullman S, Leraas KM, Lichtenberg TM, Wu CJ, Schultz N, Getz G, Meyerson M, Mills GB, McConkey DJ, Network TR, Weinstein JN, Kwiatkowski DJ, Lerner SP (2017) Comprehensive molecular characterization of muscle-invasive bladder cancer. Cell 171(3):540–556 e525

Saito R, Smith CC, Utsumi T, Bixby LM, Kardos J, Wobker SE, Stewart KG, Chai S, Manocha U, Byrd KM, Damrauer JS, Williams SE, Vincent BG, Kim WY (2018) Molecular subtype-specific immunocompetent models of high-grade urothelial carcinoma reveal differential Neoantigen expression and response to immunotherapy. Cancer Res 78(14):3954–3968

Sfakianos JP, Daza J, Hu Y, Anastos H, Bryant G, Bareja R, Badani KK, Galsky MD, Elemento O, Faltas BM, Mulholland DJ (2020) Epithelial plasticity can generate multi-lineage phenotypes in human and murine bladder cancers. Nat Commun 11(1):2540

Shin K, Lee J, Guo N, Kim J, Lim A, Qu L, Mysorekar IU, Beachy PA (2011) Hedgehog/Wnt feedback supports regenerative proliferation of epithelial stem cells in bladder. Nature 472(7341):110–114

Shin K, Lim A, Odegaard JI, Honeycutt JD, Kawano S, Hsieh MH, Beachy PA (2014) Cellular origin of bladder neoplasia and tissue dynamics of its progression to invasive carcinoma. Nat Cell Biol 16(5):469–478

Sidransky D, Frost P, Von Eschenbach A, Oyasu R, Preisinger AC, Vogelstein B (1992) Clonal origin of bladder cancer. N Engl J Med 326(11):737–740

Signoretti S, Pires MM, Lindauer M, Horner JW, Grisanzio C, Dhar S, Majumder P, McKeon F, Kantoff PW, Sellers WR, Loda M (2005) p63 regulates commitment to the prostate cell lineage. Proc Natl Acad Sci USA 102(32):11355–11360

Sjodahl G, Eriksson P, Lovgren K, Marzouka NA, Bernardo C, Nordentoft I, Dyrskjot L, Liedberg F, Hoglund M (2018) Discordant molecular subtype classification in the basal-squamous subtype of bladder tumors and matched lymph-node metastases. Mod Pathol 31(12):1869–1881

Sjodahl G, Eriksson P, Patschan O, Marzouka NA, Jakobsson L, Bernardo C, Lovgren K, Chebil G, Zwarthoff E, Liedberg F, Hoglund M (2020) Molecular changes during progression from nonmuscle invasive to advanced urothelial carcinoma. Int J Cancer 146(9):2636–2647

Skinner DG, Richie JP, Cooper PH, Waisman J, Kaufman JJ (1974) The clinical significance of carcinoma in situ of the bladder and its association with overt carcinoma. J Urol 112(1):68–71

Strandgaard T, Lindskrog SV, Nordentoft I, Christensen E, Birkenkamp-Demtroder K, Andreasen TG, Lamy P, Kjaer A, Ranti D, Wang YA, Bieber C, Prip F, Rasmussen J, Steiniche T, Birkbak N, Sfakianos J, Horowitz A, Jensen JB, Dyrskjot L (2022) Elevated T-cell exhaustion and urinary tumor DNA levels are associated with bacillus Calmette-Guerin failure in patients with non-muscle-invasive bladder cancer. Eur Urol 82(6):646–656

Strandgaard T, Nordentoft I, Birkenkamp-Demtroder K, Salminen L, Prip F, Rasmussen J, Andreasen TG, Lindskrog SV, Christensen E, Lamy P, Knudsen M, Steiniche T, Jensen JB, Dyrskjot L (2024) Field cancerization is associated with tumor development, T-cell exhaustion, and clinical outcomes in bladder cancer. Eur Urol 85(1):82–92

Strandgaard T, Nordentoft I, Lamy P, Christensen E, Thomsen MBH, Jensen JB, Dyrskjøt L (2020) Mutational analysis of field cancerization in bladder cancer. Bladder Cancer 6:253–264

Swamy MV, Patlolla JM, Steele VE, Kopelovich L, Reddy BS, Rao CV (2006) Chemoprevention of familial adenomatous polyposis by low doses of atorvastatin and celecoxib given individually and in combination to APCMin mice. Cancer Res 66(14):7370–7377

Tate T, Plumber SA, Al-Ahmadie H, Chen X, Choi W, Lu C, Viny A, Batourina E, Gartensson K, Alija B, Molotkov A, Wiessner G, McKiernan J, McConkey D, Dinney C, Czerniak B, Mendelsohn CL (2023) Combined mek inhibition and pparg activation eradicates muscle invasive bladder cancer in a mouse model of BBN-induced carcinogenesis. bioRxiv

Tate T, Xiang T, Wobker SE, Zhou M, Chen X, Kim H, Batourina E, Lin CS, Kim WY, Lu C, McKiernan JM, Mendelsohn CL (2021) Pparg signaling controls bladder cancer subtype and immune exclusion. Nat Commun 12(1):6160

Thomsen MBH, Nordentoft I, Lamy P, Vang S, Reinert L, Mapendano CK, Hoyer S, Orntoft TF, Jensen JB, Dyrskjot L (2017) Comprehensive multiregional analysis of molecular heterogeneity in bladder cancer. Sci Rep 7(1):11702

Tirmenstein M, Janovitz E, Dorr T, Song Y, Chen SJ, Granaldi K, Chadwick KD, Mangipudy R, Graziano M, Attalla B, Haile S, Czajkowski M, Foster JR, Bergholm AM, Billger M, Soderberg M (2018) Evaluation of uracil, sodium ascorbate, and rosiglitazone as promoters of urinary bladder transitional cell carcinomas in male Sprague-Dawley rats. Toxicol Pathol 46(2):147–157

Tomasetti C, Li L, Vogelstein B (2017) Stem cell divisions, somatic mutations, cancer etiology, and cancer prevention. Science 355(6331):1330–1334

Tomasetti C, Vogelstein B (2015a) Cancer etiology. Variation in cancer risk among tissues can be explained by the number of stem cell divisions. Science 347(6217):78–81

Tomasetti C, Vogelstein B (2015b) Cancer risk: role of environment-response. Science 347(6223):729–731

Tran MN, Choi W, Wszolek MF, Navai N, Lee IL, Nitti G, Wen S, Flores ER, Siefker-Radtke A, Czerniak B, Dinney C, Barton M, McConkey DJ (2013) The p63 protein isoform DeltaNp63alpha inhibits epithelial-mesenchymal transition in human bladder cancer cells: role of MIR-205. J Biol Chem 288(5):3275–3288

Tsai YC, Simoneau AR, Spruck CH 3rd, Nichols PW, Steven K, Buckley JD, Jones PA (1995) Mosaicism in human epithelium: macroscopic monoclonal patches cover the urothelium. J Urol 153(5):1697–1700

Van Batavia J, Yamany T, Molotkov A, Dan H, Mansukhani M, Batourina E, Schneider K, Oyon D, Dunlop M, Wu XR, Cordon-Cardo C, Mendelsohn C (2014) Bladder cancers arise from distinct urothelial sub-populations. Nat Cell Biol 16(10):982-991, 981-985

Vasconcelos-Nobrega C, Colaco A, Lopes C, Oliveira PA (2012) Review: BBN as an urothelial carcinogen. In Vivo 26(4):727–739

Volkmer JP, Sahoo D, Chin RK, Ho PL, Tang C, Kurtova AV, Willingham SB, Pazhanisamy SK, Contreras-Trujillo H, Storm TA, Lotan Y, Beck AH, Chung BI, Alizadeh AA, Godoy G, Lerner SP, van de Rijn M, Shortliffe LD, Weissman IL, Chan KS (2012) Three differentiation states risk-stratify bladder cancer into distinct subtypes. Proc Natl Acad Sci USA 109(6):2078–2083

Warrick JI, Hu W, Yamashita H, Walter V, Shuman L, Craig JM, Gellert LL, Castro MAA, Robertson AG, Kuo F, Ostrovnaya I, Sarungbam J, Chen YB, Gopalan A, Sirintrapun SJ, Fine SW, Tickoo SK, Kim K, Thomas J, Karan N, Gao SP, Clinton TN, Lenis AT, Chan TA, Chen Z, Rao M, Hollman TJ, Li Y, Socci ND, Chavan S, Viale A, Mohibullah N, Bochner BH, Pietzak EJ, Teo MY, Iyer G, Rosenberg JE, Bajorin DF, Kaag M, Merrill SB, Joshi M, Adam R, Taylor JA 3rd, Clark PE, Raman JD, Reuter VE, Chen Y, Funt SA, Solit DB, DeGraff DJ, Al-Ahmadie HA (2022) FOXA1 repression drives lineage plasticity and immune heterogeneity in bladder cancers with squamous differentiation. Nat Commun 13(1):6575

Welch JS, Ley TJ, Link DC, Miller CA, Larson DE, Koboldt DC, Wartman LD, Lamprecht TL, Liu F, Xia J, Kandoth C, Fulton RS, McLellan MD, Dooling DJ, Wallis JW, Chen K, Harris CC, Schmidt HK, Kalicki-Veizer JM, Lu C, Zhang Q, Lin L, O'Laughlin MD, McMichael JF, Delehaunty KD, Fulton LA, Magrini VJ, McGrath SD, Demeter RT, Vickery TL, Hundal J, Cook LL, Swift GW, Reed JP, Alldredge PA, Wylie TN, Walker JR, Watson MA, Heath SE, Shannon WD, Varghese N, Nagarajan R, Payton JE, Baty JD, Kulkarni S, Klco JM, Tomasson MH, Westervelt P, Walter MJ, Graubert TA, DiPersio JF, Ding L, Mardis ER, Wilson RK (2012) The origin and evolution of mutations in acute myeloid leukemia. Cell 150(2):264–278

Williams CS, Mann M, DuBois RN (1999) The role of cyclooxygenases in inflammation, cancer, and development. Oncogene 18(55):7908–7916

Wullweber A, Strick R, Lange F, Sikic D, Taubert H, Wach S, Wullich B, Bertz S, Weyerer V, Stoehr R, Breyer J, Burger M, Hartmann A, Strissel PL, Eckstein M (2021) Bladder tumor subtype commitment occurs in carcinoma in situ driven by key signaling pathways including ECM remodeling. Cancer Res 81(6):1552–1566

The Bladder Tumor Microenvironment

12

Hongbo Gao, Fotis Nikolos, Raj Satkunasivam, and Keith Syson Chan

Abstract

Current bladder cancer studies predominantly investigate tumor cell-intrinsic properties and tumor cell inherent mechanisms driving tumor development. The bladder tumor microenvironment, despite its significance, remains relatively understudied. It serves as a crucial tumor cell extrinsic factor, facilitating the malignant progression of cancer cells during tumor development. This chapter aims to provide an overview of current understanding and recent advances concerning the impact of the stromal cell compartment, associated extracellular matrix components, and the coexisting microbiome within the bladder tumor microenvironment on bladder cancer development.

Keywords

Tumor microenvironment · Bladder stroma · Fibroblast heterogeneity · Collagen · Stromal targeting · Discoidin domain receptor

H. Gao · F. Nikolos · K. S. Chan (✉)
Department of Urology, Houston Methodist Hospital, Houston, TX, USA

Methodist Neal Cancer Center, Houston Methodist Research Institute, Houston, TX, USA
e-mail: kschan@houstonmethodist.org

R. Satkunasivam
Department of Urology, Houston Methodist Hospital, Houston, TX, USA

12.1 The Bladder Tumor Microenvironment

The primary components of the bladder tumor stroma or tumor microenvironment (bTME) consists of both cellular and noncellular elements, which include, among others, (1) stromal cells, (2) the extracellular matrix (ECM), and (3) the coexisting bladder microbiome. The stromal cells comprise various types, such as cancer-associated fibroblasts (CAFs), vascular endothelial cells, pericytes, immune cells, and adipocytes (Hanahan and Coussens 2012). The ECM serves as a supportive structural framework for parenchymal cells, to maintain the normal homeostasis of the bladder. It comprises fibrous proteins (e.g., collagen and fibronectin), glycoproteins (e.g., fibulins, fibrillins, and thrombospondins), elastin, proteoglycans, and hyaluronic acid (HA), a nonprotein glycosaminoglycan polymer (Egeblad et al. 2010).

During tumorigenesis, it was traditionally thought that the stroma and its associated ECM acted as a physical barrier, hindering the dissemination or invasion of cancer cells within the epithelial layer to impede tumor progression. However, recent evidence suggests that activated CAFs and their secreted proteins, including growth factors or ECM components, engage in bidirectional communications with cancer cells and other constituents like immune cells within the TME. These interactions ultimately foster

M. A. Knowles, L. Dyrskjøt (eds.), *Biology of Bladder Cancer*,
https://doi.org/10.1007/978-3-031-68505-7_12

tumor progression, metastasis, and resistance to conventional chemotherapy, radiotherapy, or immunotherapy (Junttila and de Sauvage 2013).

Recent identification of microbiome coexisting within the bTME marks an exciting new finding, although the understanding of its role(s) remains relatively limited. A more in-depth comprehension of the diverse stroma components within this environment holds significant promise for potentially reshaping the TME to impede the uncontrolled proliferation of tumor cells. Elucidating the intricate interplay between the microbiome and various stromal elements could offer insights into modulating the immune response, influencing inflammation, and potentially creating an environment less conducive to tumor growth.

12.1.1 Cancer-Associated Fibroblasts

Cancer-associated fibroblasts (CAFs) constitute a significant portion of the TME and are commonly found near or surrounding cancer cells. A considerable subset of CAFs share remarkable similarities with myofibroblasts that play a critical role during the re-epithelialization stage of wound healing. Myofibroblasts were regarded as the principal contributors to ECM deposition, particularly collagen, which was crucial for wound contraction and tissue repair. It was later believed that as tumorigenesis progressed, these myofibroblasts were co-opted and persistently activated, giving rise to CAFs. Myofibroblasts and their specific gene signatures have gained wide attention among cancer researchers due to their prognostic value and inevitable functional participation in tumorigenesis. It was not until recently that the cellular and functional heterogeneity of CAFs, along with their notorious plasticity, attracted considerable scrutiny. These findings begin to shed light on previous controversial functions of CAFs and call for further biological investigations to reveal new insights.

Prior to the advent of single-cell RNA sequencing (scRNAseq), multiplex immunohistochemistry was the primary technique to identify and evaluate protein markers expressed by stromal cells from normal bladder and bladder carcinomas. Commonly used fibroblast markers include vimentin, tenascin C, alpha smooth muscle actin (αSMA), fibroblast activating protein (FAP), platelet-derived growth factor (PDGFR) α/β, CD34 and CD90, fibroblast-specific protein 1 (FSP1) and others listed in Table 12.1. Unfortunately, none of these markers are uniquely expressed in fibroblasts; they can also be expressed in other stromal cell types, such as endothelial cells and vascular smooth muscle cells. Rapid development and the utilization of the state-of-the-art single cell RNA sequencing (scRNAseq) has reinvigorated the excitement to study fibroblasts and define various subtypes. The increased availability of these published datasets for bioinformatics analyses has further facilitated subclassification and subclustering of CAFs based on their similarity and distinctive gene expression profiles.

12.1.1.1 Relationship of Organ-Specific Fibroblast to CAF Subtypes in Bladder

Tissue Resident Fibroblasts: Potential CAF Precursors

The origins or precursors of CAFs are postulated to arise from diverse cell sources, including tissue-resident fibroblasts (Kojima et al. 2010; Albrengues et al. 2015; Arina et al. 2016), bone marrow-derived mesenchymal stem cells (Quante et al. 2011; Jung et al. 2013), hematopoietic stem cells (McDonald et al. 2015), monocyte-derived fibrocytes (Nimphius et al. 2007; Bellini and Mattoli 2007; Reilkoff et al. 2011), epithelial cells (via EMT) (Iwano et al. 2002; Zeisberg et al. 2007b), and endothelial cells (EndMT) (Zeisberg et al. 2007a). Currently, the relative contributions of these cell types to bladder CAFs are not fully elucidated. In other cancer types, lineage-tracing experiments using hematopoietic cell promoter-driven Cre mice determined that less than 10% of CAFs were the progeny of bone marrow-derived cells. It is generally accepted that a majority of CAFs originate from tissue resident fibroblasts (Sahai et al. 2020), and therefore, these will be our central focus of discussion when comparing different CAF subtypes.

Table 12.1 Markers defining mouse and human fibroblast subtypes

Species	Cell types Nonmalignant bladder		Markers Positive	Low/negative	Ref
Mouse	Urothelium	Car3+	Acta2, Rbp4, Cxcl14, Thy1, Pi16, Fbln1	Cd34, Npy1r, Penk, Dpt, Sult1e1, Dlk1	(Baker et al. 2021)
	Lamina propria	Npy1r+	Pi16, Fbln1, Lum, Cd34, Npy1r	Car3, Acta2, Rbp4, Cxcl14, Thy1, Penk, Dpt	
	Detrusor muscle	Penk+	Pi16, Fbln1, Lum, Cd34, Penk, Dpt, Sult1e1, Dlk1	Car3, Acta2, Rbp4, Cxcl14, Thy1	
Human	Suburothelial layer		SLC14A1	NA	(Benjamin et al. 2023)
	Detrusor muscle layer		DPT+	NA	
	Malignant carcinoma CAFs				
Human	**Subpopulation**		**Positive markers**		
	MyCAFs (RGS5+)		PLA2G2A, RGS5, MYL9, MYL11		(Chen et al. 2020)
	iCAFs (PDGFRA+)		PTGDS, LUM, CFD, FBLN1, APOD, DCN, CXCL14		
	ACTA2hi		DES, ACTG2, SMTN, TAGLN, ACTA2, TGFBR1		(Gouin 3rd et al. 2021)
	PDGFRBhi		MCAM, GJC1, PDE1A, PDGFRB		
	FAPhi		ACTB, COL3A1, COL1A1, POSTN, ANGPT2, GUCY1A2		
	PDPNhi		THBS1, FAP, VCAN, PDGFC, BMP5, ROBO2, PDPN		
	C1_IGFBP6		MFAP5, OGN, CCDC80, PCOLCE2, PI16, EFEMP1		(Ma et al. 2022)
	C2_IL6		APOE, SERPINE2, TNFAIP6, ARID5B, TFP12, PTGS2		
	C3_SLC14A1		STC1, TRPA1, TGFB1, WNT5A,		
	C4_ACTA2		RGS5, GJA4, NDUFA4L2, ANGPT2		
	epiEMT		CTSH, TACSTD2, KRT8, FXYD3, KRT17, KRT19, KRT7		(Qin et al. 2023)
	fibroEMT		COL81, MMP11, TGFBI, SLC14A1, COL12A1, POSTN		
	Myofibroblast		RGS5, NDUFA4L2, PPP1R14A, WFDC1, COL18A1		
	ECM-CAF		CFD, GSN, FBLN1, ITM2A, PLAC9, CCDC80, IGFBP6		

Organ-Site-Specific Fibroblasts: Molecular Similarities and Differences

Comparison of tissue resident fibroblasts across different organs reveals distinct molecular profiles specific to each organ, as demonstrated by both landmark cDNA microarray profiling studies (Chang-HY et al. 2002) and the more recent scRNAseq studies (Zhao et al. 2023). Generally, fibroblasts exhibit greater similarity to those from the same organ rather than from distant tissues, albeit sharing common functions such as contributing to tissue homeostasis by producing extracellular matrix (ECM) and creating a signaling-rich niche (He et al. 2020). In the normal urinary bladder, tissue-resident fibroblasts express specific markers such as the urea transporter *SLC14A1* and the transcription factor *FOXF1*, alongside common fibroblast markers found across various organs like *APOD*, *C7*, *GSN*, and *MMP2*. Conversely, skin-resident fibroblasts are characterized by unique expression of *COCH* and *CXCL14* (Lendahl et al. 2022). These findings suggest that cancer-associated fibroblasts (CAFs) derived from different tissue-resident fibroblasts are likely imprinted with slightly different positional identities.

Urinary Bladder-Specific Fibroblasts and Their Potential Conversion into CAF Subtypes

The derivation of CAFs from normal fibroblasts during bladder tumorigenesis has not been directly demonstrated. Nevertheless, certain markers expressed in normal bladder fibroblasts are retained as markers for CAFs in bladder carcinomas. For instance, *SLC14A1* and dermatopontin (*DPT*) are expressed in both normal bladder resident fibroblasts and as fibroblast markers in bladder carcinomas. In contrast, peptidase inhibitor 16 (*PI16*) and *CXCL14* are detected only in normal bladder fibroblasts and are not found in bladder carcinomas. This suggests that subpopulations of fibroblasts, particularly those expressing *SLC14A1* or *DPT*, may interact with cancer cells and play a role in tumorigenesis (Benjamin et al. 2023).

There is also intriguing relevance in the relative localization patterns of fibroblast subpopulations between normal bladder and tumors. In the normal bladder, *SLC14A1*+ fibroblasts localize to the sub-urothelial layer, while the *DPT*+ fibroblast subset is more diffusely distributed within the detrusor muscle layer. These differential distributions are maintained in bladder cancers, with each subset aligning with discrete microenvironments. *SLC14A1*+ CAFs are more likely associated with vascularization and angiogenesis, whereas a *DPT*+ CAF-rich microenvironment attracts immune-suppressive cells such as M2 macrophages and T regulatory (Treg) cells (Benjamin et al. 2023).

Another investigation utilized cross-species analysis by aligning normal mouse fibroblast markers with human bladder carcinoma RNAseq datasets, which sheds light at the potential relationship between normal fibroblasts (NF) and CAFs, and the possible conversion processes. Spatial transcriptome platforms mapped diverse fibroblast subpopulations distributed across different regions within mouse bladders. For instance, *Car3*+ fibroblasts were found to localize in the sub-urothelial space, *Npy1r* + fibroblasts were found to localize to the lamina propria, and *Penk* + fibroblasts were found within detrusor muscle layers (Baker et al. 2021). To explore whether specific CAFs originated from these normal fibroblast counterparts, gene signatures from scRNAseq of normal mouse bladder were compared with gene profiles from CAFs in clinical cohorts (UROMOL; NMIBC, non-muscle invasive bladder cancer; TCGA: MIBC, muscle invasive bladder cancer). NFs exhibited more similarities with inflammatory CAFs (iCAFs), showing NFs or iCAF-like profiles predominantly in NMIBC without appreciable expression of myofibroblast (myCAFs) genes, such as *ACTA2* (gene name for alpha smooth muscle actin, αSMA). Interestingly, gene signatures for myCAFs were partially or fully represented in MIBC (Kamoun et al. 2020; Caramelo et al. 2023). Refer to the next section for further details.

12.1.1.2 The Current Nomenclature of CAF Subtypes (myCAFs, iCAFs, irCAFs)

The recent subclassification of cancer-associated fibroblasts (CAFs) into distinct subsets primarily relies on scRNAseq data and the unique associated gene signatures, initially described in human and murine pancreatic cancer. Unlike normal fibroblasts that would undergo apoptosis or return to a quiescent state after their activation, CAFs maintain most fibroblast functions but stay in continuous activation processes (Kalluri 2016). The persistent activation of fibroblasts fortifies the pro-tumorigenic TME via matrix remodeling and cytokine secretion (Fig. 12.1).

Myofibroblastic CAFs (myCAFs)

One fundamental shared property of fibroblasts is their ability to synthesize and deposit extracellular matrix (ECM), comprising fiber-forming collagens, proteoglycans, elastin, fibronectin, microfibrillar proteins, and laminins, collectively referred to as the matrisome. In response to injury, αSMA+ myofibroblasts, derived from quiescent fibroblasts, serve as the primary orchestrators of ECM deposition, remodeling and wound healing. myCAFs, the first identified subset of cancer-associated fibroblasts, were initially defined as fibroblasts within tumor beds with positive staining for αSMA, akin to myofibroblasts behavior (Sahai et al. 2020). In addition to collagen deposition, both myofibroblasts and myCAFs modify ECM through the secretion of crosslinking enzymes such as lysyl oxidase and proteases like matrix metalloproteinases (MMPs). Furthermore, myCAFs can dynamically alter the mechanical forces and matrix polarization within the tumor microenvironment through actions resembling "tugging and pulling" on the ECM (Plikus et al. 2021).

The role of αSMA+ CAFs (myCAFs) in inducing cancer fibrosis is well established (Chen et al. 2021). By creating a tumor-favorable niche,

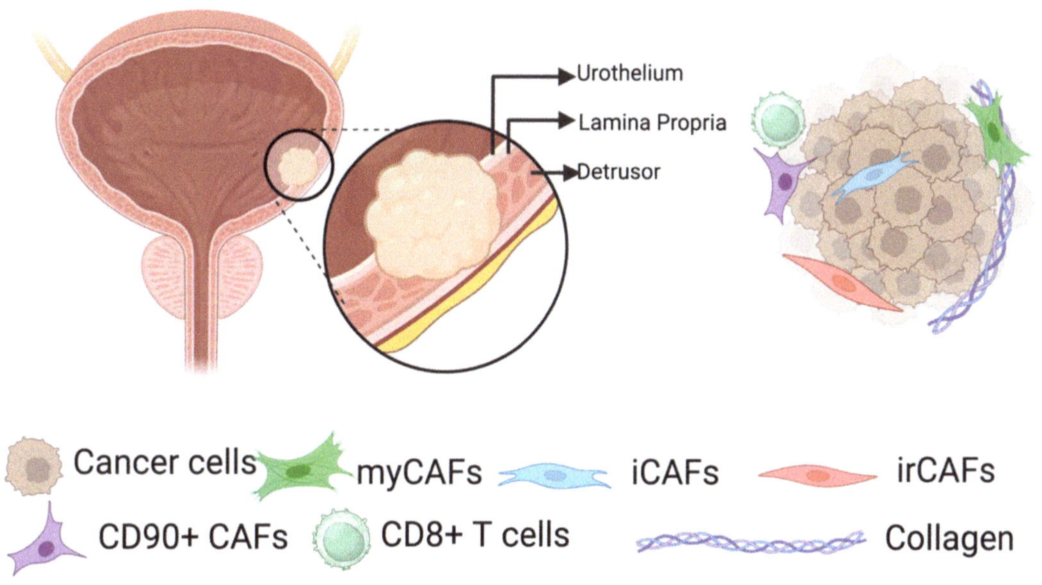

Fig. 12.1 Bladder tissue resident fibroblasts and cancer-associated fibroblasts. Muscle invasive bladder cancer (MIBC) represents an advanced stage bladder cancer, characterized by tumor cell invasion through the basement membrane into the lamina propria and detrusor muscle layers. As the tumor progresses, stromal fibroblasts are converted to cancer-associated fibroblasts (CAFs). At least three subsets of CAFs have been distinguished in human bladder cancers, namely myofibroblast CAFs (myCAFs), inflammatory CAFs (iCAFs) and interferon responding CAFs (irCAFs). Additionally, CD90+ CAFs in bladder carcinomas are associated with CD8+ T cell infiltration with a potential anti-tumor effect. CAFs contribute to the deposition of noncellular components like collagens in the stroma

they serve as a physical barrier that hinders the delivery of chemotherapy and influences tumor cell biology through alterations in matrix stiffness. However, genetic depletion of αSMA+ cells or removal of collagen I from αSMA+ cells in pancreatic cancer models has challenged this assumption (Chen et al. 2021). It was discovered that the absence of αSMA+ collagen-secreting cells resulted in a poor survival rate attributed to an early onset of cancer cell invasion and dissemination associated with deficiency of collagen I deposition (Ozdemir et al. 2014).

The expression of αSMA in the stroma of human bladder carcinomas has also been reported (Mezheyeuski et al. 2020). Based on scRNAseq analysis from eight primary tumors (two low-grade and six high-grade human bladder cancers) and three normal-appearing surrounding tissues adjacent to tumors, a large cluster of the identified CAFs were found to have high expression of *ACTA2* (Chen et al. 2020). Surprisingly, elevated αSMA expression did not correlate with a worse survival rate compared to the αSMA low cluster (Chen et al. 2020). Additionally, an immunohistochemistry (IHC) study indicated that tumors with high αSMA expression were more frequently limited to stage T1 (Mezheyeuski et al. 2020). Integration of scRNAseq with computational analysis identified regulator of G protein signaling 5 + (*RGS5*+) CAFs as myCAFs in bladder cancers, characterized by abundant expression of collagens and enrichment of matrix-related pathways. These findings emphasize the necessity for further investigation into the role of myCAFs in bladder cancers (Chen et al. 2020).

Urothelial transforming growth factor beta (TGFβ) exerts its effect in a paracrine manner on adjacent resident Car3+ NFs, prompting their differentiation into myofibroblastic phenotypes characterized by elevated αSMA expression and increased collagen synthesis. This concept is further supported by findings demonstrating that cancer cell-derived TGFβ promotes the formation of myCAFs in pancreatic cancers through STAT3 activation. Consequently, the thick collagen fibers and contractile stroma resulting from myCAFs enhance tumor tension, leading to a worse prognosis (Biffi et al. 2019).

Inflammatory CAFs (iCAFs)

In addition to producing matrisome, fibroblasts release various cytokines and growth factors, creating signaling niches for tissue-resident stem cells and immune cells. CAFs retain this function, with one subset designated as inflammatory CAFs (iCAFs) distinguished by their high expression of IL6, CXCL12 and other cytokines. iCAFs are functionally different from myCAFs, displaying lower levels of αSMA and matrix expression. The first description of iCAFs was by Tuveson's group in the investigation of pancreatic cancers, which are notorious for their heavy collagen deposition. The matrix-unrelated iCAFs coexist in the distal stroma and are identified by their high IL-6 expression (Öhlund et al. 2017). iCAFs and other newly characterized CAF subtypes have expanded the scope of research in the CAF field through the application of scRNAseq and spatial transcriptome assays. In mouse models, iCAFs are characterized by high expression of Ly6C in pancreatic cancer, breast cancer (Costa et al. 2018), and lung cancers (Louault et al. 2020; Mhaidly and Mechta-Grigoriou 2020). However, it remains unclear whether Ly6C also marks iCAFs in murine bladder cancer models.

To date, scRNAseq studies have pinpointed *PDGFRA+* CAFs as iCAFs in human bladder carcinoma. This categorization is grounded in their distinctive secretome profile, which includes molecules such as *CCL5* (also known as RANTES), connective tissue growth factor (*CTGF*), basic fibroblast growth factor (*FGF2*), colony-stimulating factors (*CSF*s), as well as *CXCL12* and *IL6* (Chen et al. 2020). The functional impacts of iCAFs will be further elaborated in Sect. 2.1.2.

Besides TGFβ, tumor cells release IL1α into the TME, while concurrently, CAFs express high levels of IL1R1 as compared with tumor cells. The paracrine activities of IL1α lead to the activation of the NF-κB pathway in CAFs, promoting p65 translocation into the nucleus. This activation initiates downstream gene expression, culminating in the secretion of leukemia inhibitory factor (LIF), which has been identified as another stimulator of iCAFs. Indeed, neutralizing antibodies against LIF suppressed IL6 expression in IL1α-stimulated CAFs. In murine stellate cells, Lif phosphorylates JAK/STAT (JAK1/2, STAT1/3) in an autocrine manner, consequently promoting *Il6*, *Cxcl1* and *Csf3* expression in iCAFs along with Il1r1 expression. Importantly, the IL1α-initiated positive feedforward loop in iCAF differentiation is blocked upon TGFβ signaling (Biffi et al. 2019). In summary, TGFβ and IL1α direct CAFs towards distinct subsets, namely myCAFs and iCAFs, respectively (Biffi et al. 2019).

Furthermore, the formation of iCAFs can also be facilitated within the TME. iCAFs tend to aggregate particularly in hypoxic regions, where the presence of myCAFs is relatively low, particularly in pancreatic cancers exhibiting high hypoxic gene expression signature. Hypoxia triggers the expression of hypoxia-inducible factor 1 alpha (Hif1α) in CAFs, leading to the suppression of αSMA expression and the upregulation of IL6 protein levels. This phenomenon underscores the contribution of the hypoxic TME to iCAF generation, alongside the influence of cancer-derived IL1α on iCAFs (Schworer et al. 2023).

Interferon Responsive CAFs (irCAFs)

From a human bladder cancer scRNAseq data set, another subset of bladder CAFs was identified, distinguished by high expression of the urea transporter solute carrier family 14-urea transporter-member 1 (*SLC14A1*) (Ma et al. 2022). This subset notably lacks *ACTA2* (myCAFs) or *IL6* (iCAFs) expression. However, *SLC14A1+* CAFs are enriched in expression of genes associated with the type I interferon (*IFNB1*) responsive pathway, leading to their designation as interferon responding CAFs (irCAFs). Furthermore, SLC14A1+ irCAFs are marked by the expression of Wnt family member 5A (WNT5) along with other growth factors such as Neuregulin 1 (*NRG1*), bone morphogenetic protein 5 (*BMP5*) and stanniocalcin-1 (*STC1*). This subset is connected to a poorer prognosis and chemoresistance in bladder cancer, mediated through WNT5-induced cancer stemness (Ma et al. 2022).

Other CAFs

Using scRNAseq to analyze pancreatic cancer models, Tuveson's group has revealed another CAF subset characterized by unique expression of MHC-II and CD74. These CAFs are termed antigen-presenting CAFs (apCAFs) and do not manifest any typical markers associated with myCAFs or iCAFs (Elyada et al. 2019). Despite their presence in pancreatic and lung cancers (approximately 10%), apCAFs have not yet been identified in bladder cancers, possibly due to challenges in dissociation techniques or their presumed extremely low frequency (Tsoumakidou 2023). Pancreatic cancer cells release TGFβ and IL1α, which act on mesothelial cells, prompting their transition into apCAFs. This transition is characterized by the downregulation of mesothelial markers alongside increased expression of major histocompatibility complex class II (MHC-II) and fibroblast markers (Huang et al. 2022). Treatment with anti-mesothelial cell antibodies inhibits the generation of apCAFs, subsequently suppressing regulatory T cell (Treg) populations and inhibiting tumor growth (Kerdidani et al. 2022). However, in lung cancer, apCAFs exhibit similar gene signatures to alveolar type II (AT-II) epithelial cells and also express MHC-II. Intriguingly, lung apCAFs exhibit tumor-suppressive effects in mouse models, contrary to their pro-tumorigenic role in pancreatic and breast cancers (Kerdidani et al. 2022). The function of apCAFs remains a topic of ongoing debate.

12.1.2 Immune Cells

Healthy bladder mucosa is regularly exposed to various elements present in urine, including metabolic waste products, microorganisms such as bacteria and fungi as well as environmental carcinogens (Flores-Mireles et al. 2015). To maintain a balanced and functional environment, the healthy bladder employs homeostatic mechanisms that regulate and promote immune tolerance at the mucosal interface (Ingersoll and Albert 2013). Among the innate immune cells present in a healthy bladder are tissue-resident macrophages, dendritic cells (DCs), mast cells, neutrophils, and natural killer cells (Abraham and Miao 2015). There have been reports of dendritic cells with a phenotype akin to skin-resident Langerhans cells within the lamina propria of human and mouse bladders, contributing to antigen presentation and immune regulation (Seymour et al. 1986; Hart and Fabre 1981).

In mouse models, distinct subsets of tissue-resident macrophages labeled as MacM and MacL, identified based on markers such as CD11c, F4/80, and Cx3cr1 (Schilling et al. 2003; Engel et al. 2008), exhibit different transcriptomic profiles and responses to urinary tract infections (UTIs) (Lacerda Mariano et al. 2020). Understanding these subsets is critical, since a history of recurrent UTIs is associated with an increased risk of bladder cancer.

In the healthy bladder, adaptive immune cells such as helper T cells and cytotoxic T cells along with their innate mucosal counterparts are also present. Moreover, these resident αβ and γδ T cells have been observed within the urothelium and submucosa of healthy human bladders, while they are not found in the detrusor muscle (Christmas 1994).

The bladder TME is heavily infiltrated by various types of innate or myeloid cells, each playing distinct roles that can either promote or inhibit tumor growth. These roles depend on the phenotypes and activation status of these cells. For instance, some myeloid cells exhibit immunosuppressive functions, while others act as antigen-presenting or immunostimulatory cells, thereby inhibiting tumor growth. Interestingly, studies have revealed that dying bladder cancer cells can promote an immunosuppressive tumor microenvironment. They achieve this by releasing prostaglandin E2 (PGE2) as inhibitory damage-associated molecular patterns (iDAMPs). This release skews the resident DCs in the tumor bed toward a tolerogenic phenotype. As a result, these DCs suppress the anti-tumor effect of CD8+ T cells, thereby hindering their ability to kill tumor cells (Fig. 12.2).

The evaluation of stromal cellular components has been used to define MIBC subtypes and differentiation status (Mo et al. 2018). Subtype determination was based on high T cell infiltration with less angiogenesis (inflamed); low T cell and stromal infiltration but high in angiogenesis (termed "immune desert"); or few immune cells and angiogenesis with high stromal distribution in the tumor bed (termed "immune-excluded") (Tiwari et al. 2023). The application of MCPcounter analysis in the 2020 consensus molecular classification of MIBC identified a transcriptionally stroma-rich tumor subtype. This subtype was characterized by high expression of stromal gene signatures (i.e., smooth muscle, endothelial, fibroblast, and myofibroblast gene signatures) alongside an enrichment of T and B cells (Kamoun et al. 2020).

Analysis of MIBC from TCGA data suggested that a high immune gene signature, reflective of immune infiltration within the bTME stroma was associated with a notable improvement in 5-year disease-specific survival (DSS) (80%) (Luo et al. 2019). This contrasts starkly with the less than 25% DSS observed among patients with a low immune gene signature. Moreover, in patients displaying combined low stromal and immune scores, an analysis of commonly downregulated genes revealed enrichment in gene ontology categories such as "ECM" and "collagen-containing ECM" (Luo et al. 2019). Supporting these findings, immunohistochemistry results from an independent study further highlighted the prognostic impact of immune cell presence. Specifically, increased infiltration of CD8+ T cell within a distinct $CD90^+$ stromal microenvironment is associated with a favorable prognosis when compared tumors exhibiting alternative stromal composition in bladder cancer (Mezheyeuski et al. 2020).

These observations strongly suggest that specific stromal components within MIBC play a crucial role in influencing immune cell infiltration, subsequently impacting patient outcomes. Such insights will shed light on the mechanistic interactions during cancer development and therapeutic responses, shaping the direction of clinical management of bladder cancer.

12.1.3 Extracellular Matrix (ECM)

The noncellular components in the bTME primarily comprise the extracellular matrix (ECM), which not only offers structural support but also serves as a niche enriched in signaling molecules that orchestrate cellular behavior and fate. ECM is critical to maintain bladder wall homeostasis and distensibility. In addition to structural support, ECM alone or combined with adhesive molecules exerts other biological effects on inhabited cells through ECM receptors. In the steady state, ECM can direct transformed cells into quiescence and prevent hyperplasia, while the bTME ECM fosters malignancy and facilitates the dissemination of cancer cells. Hence, a better understanding of ECM and its effect on the resident cells holds the potential to restore proper wound healing mechanisms and prevent tumorigenesis.

12.1.3.1 The Basal Lamina (or Basement Membrane)

The basal lamina acts as a structural framework within extracellular matrix (ECM), delineating the basal layer of urothelial cells from the underlying lamina propria and muscularis propria. Comprising primarily of collagen IV, laminin, nidogen, entactin, perlecan, heparan-sulfate proteoglycan, and the anchoring fibril collagen VII, the basal lamina provides essential support and organization to the urothelium (Bryan Brown et al. 2006). Urothelial basal cells adhere to collagen VII and laminins via integrins situated on their basolateral surface, ensuring the maintenance of proper epithelial apical-basal polarity. Disruption in the organization of hemidesmosomal anchoring complexes, attributable to the loss of collagen VII or integrins, is correlated with the onset of invasive bladder cancers (Monica Liebert et al. 1994).

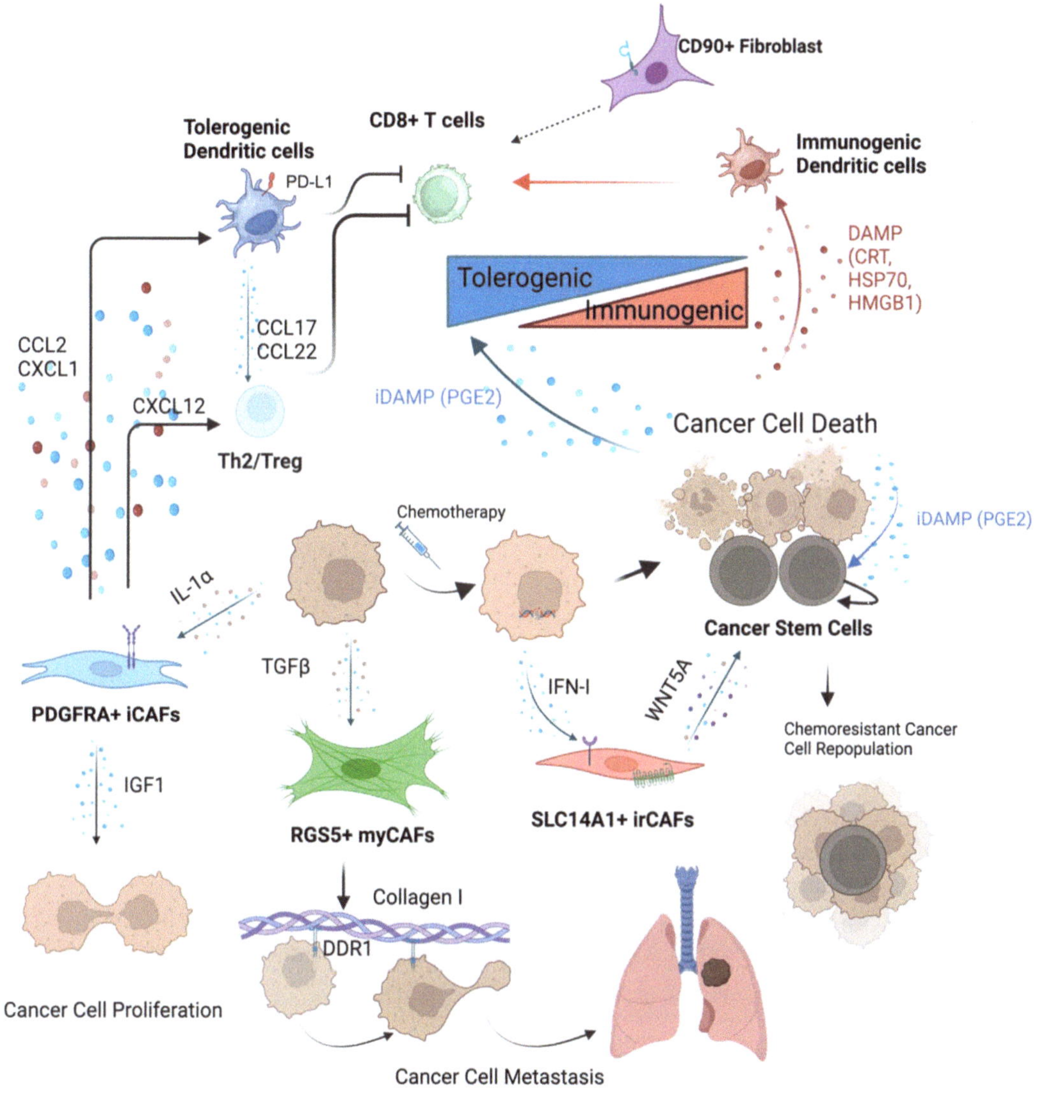

Fig. 12.2 Impact of cancer-associated fibroblasts (CAFs) in the bladder TME and therapy response. The well-defined subsets for bladder CAFs are *PDGFRA*+ iCAFs, *RGS5*+ myCAFs, and *SLC14A1*+ irCAFs. Here, the illustration demonstrates the roles of these three CAF subgroups within the bladder cancer microenvironment. Cancer cells secret IL-1α to promote the emergence of the iCAF subset. scRNAseq assay reveals that *PDGFRA*+ iCAFs express various growth factors, cytokines and chemokines. Among these factors, the released insulin-like growth factor 1 (IGF1) promotes cancer cell proliferation. Additional computational prediction indicates that iCAFs also secret various chemokines, such as chemokine (C-C motif) ligand 2 (CCL2) and C-X-C motif ligand 9 (CXCL9) to promote tolerogenic DCs, and thus, inhibitory effects on CD8+T ceslls. These tolerogenic DCs expressing high CD274 (PD-L1), in turn enhance Th2 and Treg activation via secretion of CCL17 and CCL22. Accompanied with tolerogenic DCs, iCAFs synthesize CXCL12 to further boost Treg activation. The positive association of CD90+ CAFs with CD8+ T cells indicate a better survival rate; however, the mechanism underlying this link is elusive. TGFβ released by cancer cells induces αSMA expression in fibroblasts to promote myCAF formation in a pancreatic cancer model. In bladder cancer, myCAFs are distinguished with exclusively RGS5 expression and display high collagen-containing ECM synthesis. These stroma-derived fibrillar collagens are the ligands for DDR1, which promotes cancer cells to disseminate to collagen III-rich lung airway niches populated by smooth muscle cells. Cancer cells undergo chemotherapy-induced DNA damage-related stress, and release IFN-I to activate SLC14A1+ irCAFs, which subsequently release WNT5A as a mitogen to enhance cancer stem cell proliferation. Chemotherapy-induced dying cancer cells release the multi-function lipid-like PGE_2, functioning as a mitogen to preserve adjacent chemoresistant cancer stem cells (Kurtova et al. 2015). More than that, PGE_2 functions as an iDAMP (Nikolos, Hayashi et al. 2022) that tips the immune response towards a pro-tumor landscape by skewing tolerogenic DCs, regardless of the releasing alarmins or DAMPs that can activate anti-tumor immunogenic DCs (Hayashi et al. 2020)

12.1.3.2 Core Matrisome

The inherent insolubility of the ECM has historically hindered efforts to characterize its protein components. However, an advanced approach has emerged, integrating liquid chromatography and mass spectrometry with in silico definition via bioinformatic prediction. This combined approach has enabled the identification of approximately 300 proteins within the ECM (Naba et al. 2012). Among this list, collagen subunits alone are categorized into over 40 subgroups, while glycoproteins encompass more than 200 proteins, including laminins, fibronectin, tenascins, secreted protein acidic and rich in cysteine (SPARC), and thrombospondin 1, among others. Furthermore, there are over 35 proteoglycans with substantial glycosaminoglycan chains, along with ECM-bound growth factors, cytokines, and ECM-modifying enzymes (Hynes and Naba 2012). Remarkably, comprehensive studies to characterize the non-malignant and tumor bladder matrisome have not been conducted thus far.

12.1.3.3 Collagen

Collagens represent the major ECM within the bTME and can be categorized into the following major subclasses: (i) fibril-forming collagens (COLs) I, II, III, V, XI, XXIV, and XXVII; (ii) fibril-associated COLs IX, XII, XIV, XVI, XIX, XX, XXI, and XXII, which have interrupted triple helices; (iii) network-forming COLs IV, VIII, and X; (iv) membrane-associated COLs XIII, XVII, XXIII, and XXV; (v) COLs XV and XVIII with multiple triple-helix domains and interruptions; (vi) beaded-filament-forming COL VI; (vii) anchoring fibril forming COL VII; and (viii) other COL types XXVI and XXVIII. All collagens consist of repetitions of the proline-rich tripeptide glycine-X-Y, where X and Y typically denote proline and 4-hydroxy-proline, respectively.

Collagens I and III form the bulk of helix fibrils in lamina propria and connective tissue, which are accompanied by smooth muscle cells to keep the tensile strength for maintaining bladder compliance. Collagen III forms thinner fibers with higher distensibility than collagen I, and collagen III is more prevalent in the human bladder than the rodent bladder. Collagen III facilitates collagen I formation of heterotypic microfibres in the bladder. Proper collagen deposition is essential to bladder integrity since high collagen III gene expression is associated with poorer compliance in bladder obstructive disease (Aitken and Bagli 2009). High collagen I deposition is correlated with bladder cancer progression (Ghassemi et al. 2021). Nonetheless, the comprehensive elucidation of collagen components within bTME needs to be investigated further.

12.1.3.4 Other ECM Components

In the bTME, other major non-collagenous ECM proteins include laminin and fibronectin. Laminins are heterotrimeric glycoproteins composed of 15 possible α, β, and γ trimeric combinations (Aitken and Bagli 2009). As the most abundant structural non-collagenous glycoproteins, they play key roles in various biological processes. Laminins are predominant components of the basal lamina and envelop smooth muscle bundles within the detrusor muscle. Structurally, laminins consist of a long arm responsible for integrin binding and a short arm engaged in cell signaling, mediated through laminin–nidogen complex formation and Ca^{2+}-dependent interactions. These properties make laminins essential for maintaining tissue integrity and regulating cellular behavior within the bladder microenvironment (Aitken and Bagli 2009). In bladder cancer, the gene responsible for encoding laminin 5 (*LAMC2*) has been found to be methylated. Interestingly, higher levels of methylation of this gene have been associated with worse patient survival rates (Sathyanarayana et al. 2004).

Fibronectin, another essential ECM glycoprotein present in the urinary bladder, plays a central role in collagen fibrillogenesis in vivo. In nonmalignant bladder tissue, fibronectin is primarily expressed in the lamina propria beneath the basement membrane and surrounding muscle fibers (Wilson et al. 1996). However, in bladder cancer, fibronectin expression shifts to the tumor stroma, with 89% of bladder tumors (in a study of 103 cases) displaying positive expression. Moreover, fibronectin expression correlates positively with tumor stage and proliferative activity (Ioachim et al. 2005). These findings reveal that other non-collagenous ECM proteins also play important roles in bladder tumorigenesis.

12.1.4 Urinary Bladder Microbiome

The term "microbiome" encompasses the collective population of microorganisms residing within and on the human body, along with their genetic components and metabolic byproducts (Berg et al. 2020). These microorganisms establish unique micro-ecosystems in various body regions, including the skin, oral cavity, gastrointestinal tract, and genitourinary system. Now recognized or regarded as the "last organ," the human microbiome holds significant importance in maintaining overall health and exerting influence over a range of physiological processes (Baquero 2012). Extensive research has delved into the microbiome's role in disease states and therapeutic interventions, with particular emphasis on dysbiosis, an imbalance or disruption in the microbiome's composition and function, which has been linked to numerous diseases, including cancer (Scott et al. 2019).

Contrary to earlier beliefs that the urinary bladder is sterile, it is now understood that the urinary bladder hosts its own community of commensal microorganisms (Bučević Popović et al. 2018). Notably, the composition of the urinary microbiome differs not only between the sexes but also between healthy individuals and those with bladder cancer (Andolfi et al. 2020; Pederzoli et al. 2020). The urinary bladder microbiome remains relatively undefined compared to other microbiomes in the body, primarily due to a relatively small number of studies or clinical trials being published. Another limitation is the relatively small sample sizes of these studies, inconsistent urine collection methods, and demographic heterogeneity (Pohl et al. 2020).

Though establishing a universal healthy bladder bacterial profile is challenging, comparative studies have revealed some commonalities as well as intriguing differences. Notably, the urinary microbiome differs between men and women (Andolfi et al. 2020; Pederzoli et al. 2020), much like the gut microbiome (Kim et al. 2020; Fransen et al. 2017). In healthy women the genera, *Streptococcus, Lactobacillus*, and *Prevotella* are more prevalent, whereas men have an abundance of *Lactobacillus, Corynebacterium, Gardnerella, Enterococcus, Proteus*, and *Klebsiella*. It is postulated that the acid-producing *Lactobacillus* species can help maintain a protective acidic environment, guarding against pathogenic bacteria (e.g., Uropathogenic *E. coli*) (Song et al. 2022). Although *Lactobacillus* is associated with a healthy urinary microbiome, specific strains may influence conditions like urinary urge incontinence (Pearce et al. 2014). Nevertheless, defining a single healthy urinary microbiome profile remains very challenging, primarily due to the high variability of the microbiome composition among healthy individuals (Modena et al. 2017; Price et al. 2020).

12.2 Communication Between bTME and Tumor Cells

12.2.1 Stromal-Epithelial Interaction

12.2.1.1 The Inhibitory Effect from Stromal to Epithelial Cells

Stromal cells play a crucial role in the prevention of NMIBC progression into MIBC. In the mouse N-butyl-N-4-hydroxybutyl nitrosamine (BBN)-induced bladder carcinogenesis model, basal urothelial stem cells express Sonic Hedgehog (Shh). This signaling molecule communicates with adjacent stromal cells to secrete bone morphogenetic protein 4 (BMP4) and BMP5. These BMPs act in a paracrine manner, impacting basal stem cells and contributing to the regulation of bladder cancer progression. Indeed, BMPs promote bladder basal cell differentiation and suppress tumor initiation. Loss of Sonic Hedgehog (Shh) expression in malignant tumor cells results in the removal of restraint from stromal cells mediated by BMPs, leading to invasive progression (Baskin et al. 1997; Shin et al. 2014). Studies have shown that the BMP agonist FK506 impedes progression of murine bladder carcinoma induced by BBN. This suggests that restoration of stromal inhibition could potentially retard the early stages of bladder cancer progression.

12.2.1.2 Tumorigenesis Mediated by Various CAF Subtypes

Different subtypes of cancer-associated fibroblasts (CAFs) facilitate diverse interactions with tumor cells, and various types of crosstalk between CAFs and tumor cells have been investigated based on their subtypes. However, the impact of myCAFs on tumor cells remains controversial. One direct effect of myCAFs in their communication with tumor cells is mediated by collagen, given the significant influence of myCAFs on collagen synthesis. In bladder cancer, as well as in many other cancer types, the deposition of collagen I has been demonstrated to enhance tumor cell motility and promote tumor progression (Lee et al. 2019). In contrast, two consecutive studies in pancreatic cancer have revealed that myCAFs could restrain tumor progression, since genetic depletion of myCAFs or collagen I in murine αSMA^+ myofibroblasts was found to promote pancreatic cancer progression (Hanahan and Coussens 2012). Independently, the pro-tumoral effect of iCAFs identified in bladder cancer appears to be conserved in other cancer types, based on their secretory functions. A hallmark feature for iCAFs is IL6 secretion. IL6 released from pancreatic iCAFs distally activates the STAT3 signaling pathway in cancer cells, thereby facilitating cancer growth (Öhlund et al. 2017). Interestingly, scRNAseq has also identified a subset of iCAFs in human bladder carcinoma that specifically express PDGFRA and CXCL12. These iCAFs release insulin-like growth factor 1 (IGF1), which enhances cancer cell proliferation (Chen et al. 2020) (Fig. 12.2). Furthermore, a newly identified subset of type I interferon-responding CAFs (irCAFs) expresses high levels of WNT5A. WNT5A secretion stimulates bladder cancer cell stemness, as demonstrated by a robust 3-dimensional colony formation assay (Ma et al. 2022).

12.2.1.3 Crosstalk Between ECM and Tumor Cells

ECM is not only an inert scaffold in bTME simply for the stabilization of microenvironment structures, but also actively engages with other resident cells via ECM receptors. Although one study demonstrated that the deficiency of collagen I promotes mouse pancreatic cancer metastasis, numerous other studies have shown that the deposition of collagen promotes tumor advancement in various cancer types, correlating with poorer survival rate under chemotherapy/standard-of-care regimens (melanoma, pancreatic, breast, lung cancers). A mouse model revealed that the host CAFs deficient of activating transcription factor 4 (Atf4) lose their ability to deposit collagen I, which in turn delayed pancreatic tumor and melanoma growth, and reduced mortality (DeClerck 2012; Verginadis et al. 2022). In NMIBC, a high collagen I distribution was strongly associated with higher tumor stage and aggressive progression, as well as poor overall survival rate (Brooks et al 2016).

Collagens can exert their function through cognate receptors, such as the discoid domain receptor (DDR) family members, DDR1 and DDR2. DDRs are receptor tyrosine kinases that recognize collagen binding via their extracellular discoidin domain or discoidin-like domain. Upon collagen stimulation, DDR1 undergoes homodimerization or aggregation of multiple dimerized receptors to form larger protein clusters. The dimerized DDR1 initiates autophosphorylation on lateral tyrosine sites and transduces signaling to sequential downstream factors. DDR1 signaling pathway is relatively slower but lasts longer as compared to other tyrosine kinase receptors (Juskaite et al. 2017; Sirvent et al. 2022).

DDR1 is predominantly found in epithelial tumor cells, whereas DDR2 is confined to cells of mesenchymal origin (Alves et al. 1995). Consequently, DDR1 has garnered significant attention in the study of tumorigenesis, particularly in cancer cells responding to cues from the microenvironment. DDRs exhibit a broad collagen-binding specificity and can be activated by various collagen types. Fibrillar collagens serve as ligands for both DDRs (Shrivastava et al.

1997; Vogel et al. 1997). It is important to note that a native, triple-helical conformation is required for DDR activation, as neither DDR binds to heat-denatured collagen (Vogel et al. 1997; Leitinger 2003). DDRs specifically recognize the GVMGFO motif present in the triple helix, which is prevalent in fibrillar collagens, like collagens I, II, and III. Intriguingly, the elevated collagen I and DDR1 expression levels are associated with unfavorable prognosis in bladder cancers that lack E-cadherin (our unpublished data), as well as in other cancers like hepatocellular carcinoma (Lee et al. 2019). Additionally, DDR1 has been reported to respond to collagen IV, a mesh-forming collagen, to regulate oligodendrocyte maturation (Silva et al. 2023).

In bladder cancer, DDR1 plays another crucial role in collagen-induced metastasis by promoting cancer cell migration via the DDR1-mediated non-canonical HSP90-STAT3 pathway (Lee et al. 2019). Furthermore, DDR1 activation has been associated with cancer stem cell (CSC) expansion, leading to increased mortality due to acquired resistance to chemotherapy and/or radiotherapy. Similarly, in hepatocellular carcinoma, DDR1 responds to collagen I stimulation and interacts with CD44 to activate the YAP signaling pathway, thereby promoting hepatocellular cancer stemness, as evidenced by CD133+ CSC expansion (Xiong et al. 2023). Interestingly, in pancreatic cancers, DDR1 signaling dynamics hinge on whether collagen I is cleaved or intact. Matrix metalloprotease (MMP)-mediated collagen I cleavage activates DDR1 and induces mitochondrial biogenesis, which is crucial for tumorigenesis. Conversely, full length or intact collagen I causes DDR1 endocytosis and degradation in pancreatic cancers (Su et al. 2022). Whether cleaved and full-length collagen I exert conserved functions in other cancer types, including bladder cancer, remains unclear and an active area of research.

Interestingly, in a breast cancer xenograft model, dormant breast cancer cells express collagen III, forming a wavy collagen matrix characterized by decreased linear organization of collagen fibers. This collagen III-enriched ECM acts as a paracrine signal to induce neighboring cells into dormancy in a DDR1-dependent manner. Curvy collagen III induces DDR1 activation and leads to the phosphorylation of Stat1, which in turn, promotes collagen III expression in the dormant breast cancer cells to stabilize a pro-dormant ECM niche (Di Martino et al. 2022). Remarkably, genetic depletion of collagen III from dormant cancer cells, causes a highly aligned ECM matrix generated by stromal cells, awakening dormant cells to proliferate (Di Martino et al. 2022). This highlights the profound impact of collagen orientation on cancer cell fate. The low curvature of collagen fibrils seems to promote cancer cell dissemination (Brooks et al 2016; Di Martino et al. 2022). Furthermore, collagen IV maintains breast cancer cells in dormancy. Interestingly, the combination of collagen I with basement membrane extract (BME) restores cell proliferation in dormant cells. The reactivation of dormant cancer cells upon collagen 1 cotreatment relies on activation of autophagy. However, the mechanisms underlying collagen-driven starvation and induction of autophagy are still understudied (Vera-Ramirez et al. 2018).

12.2.2 Cancer Cell Interaction with Stromal Fibroblasts and Immune Cells

12.2.2.1 Microbiome Alters the ECM and Immune Composition of the TME

Mechanistically, urinary microbiota can attach to bladder mucosal surfaces, undergo translocations, and potentially form biofilms, altering the ECM in the bladder (Alfano et al. 2016). Some bacteria release proteases, disrupting ECM renewal and inhibiting immune responses (Alfano et al. 2016). For instance, *Pseudomonas aeruginosa* secretes alkaline proteases in anaerobic conditions within bladder tumors, which degrade ECM components and inhibit lymphocyte proliferation (Alfano ct al. 2016; Vollmer et al. 1996). Proteases can also cleave immune-related molecules like the IL-6 receptor, FAS ligand, TNF and its receptors, influencing urothelial barrier integrity, ECM development, and the bladder's immunological environment (Vollmer et al. 1996; Müllberg et al. 1995; Kayagaki et al. 1995). This altered bladder tissue may facilitate the development of the bladder tumor microenvironment.

12.2.2.2 Cancer-Associated Fibroblast Subtypes and Immune Cell Composition

Stromal cells were originally thought of as immune neutral cells, only playing roles in ECM construction and modification. However, fibroblasts actively serve as immune sentinel partners, for example in the innate immune system by sensing pathological stimuli, and in cancer by infamously fortifying an immunosuppressive TME. CAFs participate in T cell exhaustion and exclusion and induce tumor-favoring phenotypic skew in macrophages and neutrophils (Arpinati and Scherz-Shouval 2023).

CD90+ CAFs are associated with higher numbers of CD8+ cytotoxic T cells in bladder cancers, which correlates with a better survival rate, though the underlying mechanism is still unclear (Mezheyeuski et al. 2020). scRNAseq has been used to identify an association of *PDGFRA*+ iCAFs with Tregs through *CXCL12* secretion and DCs by *CCL17*, *CCL19*, and *CCL21* (Chen et al. 2020) (Fig. 12.2). Careful characterization of these bladder CAF subtypes is still needed. Furthermore, iCAFs from other cancer types were shown to suppress the anti-tumor effects of CD8+ T cells and DCs. In breast cancer, CD73+ CAF-S1 primary fibroblasts promote an increase in Tregs to build up the pro-tumor microenvironment (Magagna et al. 2021). CCL2, released from $IL1r1^{high}$ iCAFs upon IL1β stimulation induces CD8+ T cell exhaustion to facilitate tumorigenesis in colorectal cancer (Koncina et al. 2023).

Furthermore, the application of scRNAseq has advanced our comprehension of the immune landscape involved in mesenchymal cell/fibroblast activation, as well as tissue fibrosis. For instance, in fribrotic liver diseases, scar-associated macrophages (*SPP*+) identified by scRNAseq, distinct from tissue resident macrophages and originating from circulating monocytes, activate hepatic stellate cell and collagen deposition via released factors (Ramachandran et al. 2019). Interaction between macrophages and fibroblasts is communicated by *IL1B-IL-1R1*, *TNFSF12-TNFRSF12A*, *PDGF-PDGFRA*, and *AREG-EGFR*. As a counterpart to scar-associated macrophages (SAmac) from liver, SPP1+ macrophages in lung are also associated with profibrotic activity in idiopathic lung fibrosis via stimulation of myofibroblasts (Bhattacharya and Ramachandran 2023). The above findings revealed an intricate coregulatory network between fibroblasts, immune cells, and ultimate tumor phenotype, yet to be fully elucidated.

12.3 Clinical Relevance

The concept of immunotherapy has long been established in bladder cancer (Pettenati and Ingersoll 2018). Bacillus Calmette-Guérin (BCG), originally an anti-tuberculosis vaccine, has been utilized in managing high-risk NMIBCs since the 1970s (Lobo et al. 2021), greatly predating the successful FDA approval of immune checkpoint inhibitors (ICIs) for bladder cancer treatment in 2017 (Schneider et al. 2019).

12.3.1 Bacillus Calmette-Guerin, the TME and the Microbiome

Bacillus Calmette-Guerin (BCG) immunotherapy is the current standard-of-care therapy for preventing the recurrence and progression of high-risk NMIBC. The impact of various immune cell types in response to BGC has been extensively studied, including those involved in both innate and adaptive immunity (Pettenati and Ingersoll 2018; van Puffelen et al. 2020). In brief, BCG has been shown to induce trained immunity, a process by which innate immune cells, such as monocytes and macrophages, acquire immunologic memory through epigenetic and/or metabolic reprogramming. When challenged by a second stimulus, either related to or unrelated to BCG, these trained innate immune cells can produce higher levels of pro-inflammatory cytokines when compared to non-trained cells, thus promoting an anti-tumoral microenvironment. Furthermore, BCG can be internalized by urothelial cancer cells or antigen-presenting cells, which cross-prime T cells to induce a TH1 response corresponding to an anti-tumoral immunity. Both CD4 + and CD8 + T cells have been shown to be important mediators of this adaptive response, as demonstrated by functional depletion studies using CD4-neutralizing or CD8-neutralizing antibodies, which abolish BCG-induced anti-tumoral activity (Ratliff et al. 1993).

How BCG impacts the stromal bTME is less studied. BCG has been demonstrated to induce fibroblast proliferation and differentiation into αSMA+ myofibroblasts, either directly or indirectly through FGF2 secreted by macrophages (Lodillinsky et al. 2010). A pro-fibrotic stromal bTME phenotype is associated with a favorable response to BCG immunotherapy in patients with NMIBC, whereas a high stroma core signature or stromal bTME is associated with poor response to ICIs in patients with MIBC (Wang et al. 2018). Such varying impacts of the stromal TME on distinct immunotherapies, such as BCG and ICIs, in shaping distinct immune responses leads to speculation that different stromal components could exert either pro-tumoral or anti-tumoral effects (van Puffelen et al. 2020; Lodillinsky et al. 2010; Wang et al. 2018). Thus, future dissection of the stromal TME is crucial to determine which stromal components drive pro-tumoral or anti-tumoral activity. One major technical limitation of studies in NMIBC is the use of mouse NIH3T3 fibroblasts instead of patient-derived CAFs, confounding the assessment of clinically relevant stromal response in the bTME (Lodillinsky et al. 2010). Mechanistically, the connection between the stromal TME and various immune cell types, as well as how their interaction influences BCG-induced response remains to be explored.

Recently, the potential therapeutic applications of the urinary microbiome in the treatment of bladder cancer have begun to be explored. Studies have demonstrated that certain beneficial bacteria, such as *Lactobacillus casei* strain *Shirota* and *Lactobacillus rhamnosus GG* (LGG), exhibit potent anticancer effects, which are comparable to or even surpass those of BCG, in mouse models of NMIBC (Friedrich and Choi 2022). These *Lactobacillus* species have been found to induce bladder cancer cell death through apoptosis and necrosis and enhance the therapeutic efficacy of BCG (Seow et al. 2002). Additionally, LGG promotes tumor regression by recruiting immune cells like T and NK cells and boosting the production of the TNF-α cytokine, which aids in tumor regression. The combination of oral administration of *Lactobacillus* with intravesical chemotherapy has also shown promise in enhancing recurrence-free survival rates in bladder cancer patients compared to chemotherapy alone. Lactobacilli are commonly used as probiotic supplements, making them a safer and potentially effective option for bladder cancer treatment (Naito et al. 2008).

12.3.2 Immune Checkpoint Inhibitor Therapies and Conventional Chemotherapy

Immune checkpoint inhibitors (ICIs), including anti-PD-L1 and anti-PD1 drugs, are becoming a well-tolerated treatment option for patients with advanced bladder cancer (Schneider et al. 2019). The expedited FDA approval of the anti-PD-L1 drug atezolizumab in 2016 and the anti-PD1 drug pembrolizumab in 2017 significantly changed the treatment landscape for advanced MIBC (Balar et al. 2017; Nod for atezolizumab in advanced bladder cancer 2017). However, 70–80% of patients do not respond to ICIs, and the mechanisms behind this resistance are still being intensely studied (see also Chap. 23).

Resistance to ICI treatment in bladder cancer has been linked to the bladder stromal microenvironment and its ECM component receptors. In the CheckMate 275 phase II, single-arm clinical trial, metastatic bladder cancer patients were treated with the anti-PD1 drug nivolumab. Bioinformatic analysis of RNAseq data from this patient cohort identified an eight-gene EMT/stroma signature (including *FLNA*, *EMP3*,

CALD1, *FN1*, *FOXC2*, *LOX*, *FBN1*, and *TNC*) (Wang et al. 2018) that correlated with treatment outcome. Specifically, the study found that patients with high $CD8^+$ T cell infiltration and a low EMT/stromal core signature showed the highest response rates and the longest progression-free and overall survival following nivolumab treatment. Conversely, patients with high $CD8^+$ T cell infiltration and a high EMT/stromal core signature had significantly poorer outcomes (Wang et al. 2018). These findings suggest that the stromal compartment within the bTME may hinder T cell function, thereby contributing to ICI resistance.

In a separate study involving patients with advanced bladder cancer treated with the PD-L1 inhibitor atezolizumab, researchers found that high expression of genes related to the TGFβ1 pathway correlated with non-responsive outcomes—either stable or progressive disease. Notably, an elevated signature indicating heightened TGFβ signaling in fibroblasts significantly predicted poor treatment responses within tumors characterized by immune-exclusion. Conversely, no such correlation was observed in tumors categorized as inflamed or immune-desert (Mariathasan et al. 2018). Preclinical experiments in a mouse mammary carcinoma model showed that blocking the TGFβ pathway with an anti-TGFβ antibody reduced expression of fibroblast genes involved in matrix remodeling. This blockade also synergized with anti-PD-L1 treatment, resulting in a 70% complete response rate compared to 10% with anti-PD-L1-treatment alone. These findings highlight the critical role of stromal TGFβ signaling in restricting T cell movement within the TME. This restriction contributes to an immune-exclusion phenotype observed in advanced MIBCs which is associated with poor response to ICIs (Mariathasan et al. 2018).

In another study utilizing advanced spatial transcriptome analysis (i.e., GeoMX), researchers observed that fibroblast markers (*FAP*, *ACTA2*) were associated with non-responder MIBC patients who underwent treatment with neoadjuvant gemcitabine and cisplatin chemotherapy along with anti-PD1 ICI (Pembrolizumab or Nivolumab). Utilizing machine learning and computational prognostic tools, the study predicted poorer survival outcomes in MIBC characterized by high levels of *ACTA2* and *CD14* (marker for monocytes and macrophages) within the tumor region (detected with Pan-Keratin antibody), and high levels of *FAP* in the tumor margin area. These findings suggest that fibroblasts and macrophages are associated with a diminished response to neoadjuvant chemotherapy and ICI therapy (Beckabir et al. 2023). One potential limitation noted is that FAP expression could also originate from tumor cells with a mesenchymal phenotype.

In a recent study, researchers employed an unbiased in vivo short-hairpin (sh)RNA functional screen to uncover mechanisms of ICI resistance that provided valuable insights into this intruiging area. Using a pooled single guide RNA (sgRNA) library, they identified DDR2, a collagen receptor for fibrillar collagen, as a pivotal modulator of anti-PD1 resistance in murine bladder cancer (Tu et al. 2019). DDR2 ablation either by genetic knockdown or pharmacological inhibition with dasatinib (a receptor tyrosine kinase inhibitor with cross-reactivity towards DDR2) in bladder tumor cells (NA13), sensitized bladder tumors to anti-PD1 therapy. This sensitization was attributed to increased infiltration of $CD8^+$ T cells in both spleen and tumor, validated by CyTOF and multicolor flow cytometry analyses (Tu et al. 2019). DDR2 acts as a collagen receptor, linking it to the finding that lysyl oxidase (LOX), an enzyme involved in collagen cross-linking, was part of the EMT/stroma core signature associated with poor response to ICIs. This suggests a potential connection between collagen modifications, such as crosslinking, and the activation of downstream collagen receptor signaling pathways that promote ICI resistance. Elevated expression of another collagen receptor, DDR1, similarly characterizes immunologically cold or immune-excluded bladder tumors, correlating with diminished responses to immune checkpoint blockade in MIBCs. Together, these results highlight the pivotal role for stromal components within the bTME, particularly collagen

ECM and its receptors, in modulating immune checkpoint responses in MIBCs.

These results clearly indicate that certain stromal components within the bTME play an immunosuppressive role. However, contrasting results from another study suggest a different perspective, implicating ECM components that could foster an immune-stimulatory environment instead. Traditionally, decellularized ECM-based bioscaffolds were believed to be immunologically inert and safe for transplantation. Surprisingly, a bioscaffold derived from porcine urinary bladder created an immune-stimulatory environment that inhibited tumor formation in multiple mouse tumor models (Wolf et al. 2019). This suggested that specific ECM components or ECM-associated growth factors within the scaffold may trigger immune-stimulatory functions. Interestingly, while an elevated ratio of T helper 1 to T helper 2 (T_H1:T_H2) intratumoral T cells is typically associated with ant-tumoral activity, this study found that a skewed ratio towards T_H2 T cells, together with non-classical $CD206^+$ macrophages and eosinophils, contributed to the antitumoral effects that suppressed tumor growth (Wolf et al. 2019). This observation challenges conventional understanding and calls for further validation (Wolf et al. 2019). Nevertheless, given that the bladder bioscaffold contains numerous ECM-related proteins within its core matrisome, identifying the specific ECM components responsible for triggering the immune-stimulatory role remains a complex and unresolved issue. Further investigation is needed to unravel the specific stromal or ECM components within the bTME that drive divergent responses to BCG and ICIs in NMIBC and MIBC contexts.

12.3.3 Microbiome and PD-1/PD-L1 Axis

Immunotherapy, particularly agents targeting the PD-1/PD-L1 axis, has become the gold standard for treating platinum-ineligible urothelial carcinomas. However, chronic inflammation is emerging as an additional risk factor associated with bladder cancer. This chronic inflammation is often attributed to the body's defense mechanisms against microbial infections or cellular damage in response to various stressors. One well-known example is schistosomiasis, a parasitic infection that has been established as a contributor to bladder cancer development (Mostafa et al. 1999). Another factor involved in the pathogenesis of bladder cancer is the urinary microbiome. Commensal microorganisms in the urinary bladder may play a crucial role in maintaining a balanced state and preventing unwanted inflammatory responses. However, disturbances in the urinary microbiome can trigger immune cell infiltration, initiating proinflammatory responses, thereby establishing a chronic inflammatory environment and ultimately contributing to the development of bladder cancer (Alfano et al. 2016).

The significance of the microbiota in bladder cancer extends beyond NMIBC and impacts advanced stage cancer, particularly in the context of immunotherapy. Microbiota has been recognized to play a role in the regulation of PD-L1 expression, suggesting that the composition of the bladder microbiome could influence the response to anti-PD-1/PD-L1 therapy (Chen et al. 2022). While this concept has been explored in other malignancies, such as oral carcinomas and metastatic melanoma, it has not been systematically studied in bladder cancer. Preliminary research comparing the urogenital microbiota between PD-L1-positive and PD-L1-negative groups revealed distinct bacterial taxa associated with PD-L1 expression. For instance, *Leptotrichia*, *Roseomonas*, and *Propionibacterium* were enriched in the PD-L1-positive group, while *Prevotella* and *Massilia* were decreased (Friedrich and Choi 2022). The expanding use of ICIs in neoadjuvant immunotherapy for MIBC presents an intriguing avenue for research into the potential influence of urinary microbiota on treatment outcomes. Recent studies have suggested a connection between antibiotic use and reduced neoadjuvant immunotherapy benefit, raising thc possibility that the diversity and composition of urinary microbiota may play a role in the success of such innovative immunotherapies. Future research is needed to elucidate the complex interaction between urinary microbiota and these evolving immunotherapeutic approaches.

12.4 Future Research Directions

Exciting progress has been made in terms of technologic advances in characterizing and profiling the alterations not only in the bladder tumor cells, but also within the bladder TME at a granular level (e.g., scRNAseq and spatial profiling). These include changes in the fibroblast subtypes and immune landscape that are associated with tumor development and progression, as well as therapy resistance. Functional studies are underway to interrogate whether these alterations and interacting networks within the stroma are driver events, essential co-organizers or contributors in determining the ultimate tumor phenotype and therapy outcome. Integration of profiling studies and mechanistic insights will pave the way to the development of next-generation stromal-oriented therapies that can be exploited as co-targeting approaches in addition to the current standard of care therapies.

References

Abraham SN, Miao Y (2015) The nature of immune responses to urinary tract infections. Nat Rev Immunol 15(10):655–663

Aitken KJ, Bagli DJ (2009) The bladder extracellular matrix. Part I: architecture, development and disease. Nat Rev Urol 6(11):596–611

Albrengues J, Bertero T, Grasset E, Bonan S, Maiel M, Bourget I et al (2015) Epigenetic switch drives the conversion of fibroblasts into proinvasive cancer-associated fibroblasts. Nat Commun 6:10204

Alfano M, Canducci F, Nebuloni M, Clementi M, Montorsi F, Salonia A (2016) The interplay of extracellular matrix and microbiome in urothelial bladder cancer. Nat Rev Urol 13(2):77–90

Alves F, Vogel W, Mossie K, Millauer B, Höfler H, Ullrich A (1995) Distinct structural characteristics of discoidin I subfamily receptor tyrosine kinases and complementary expression in human cancer. Oncogene 10(3):609–618

Andolfi C, Bloodworth JC, Papachristos A, Sweis RF (2020) The urinary microbiome and bladder cancer: susceptibility and immune responsiveness. Bladder Cancer 6(3):225–235

Arina A, Idel C, Hyjek EM, Alegre ML, Wang Y, Bindokas VP et al (2016) Tumor-associated fibroblasts predominantly come from local and not circulating precursors. Proc Natl Acad Sci USA 113(27):7551–7556

Arpinati L, Scherz-Shouval R (2023) From gatekeepers to providers: regulation of immune functions by cancer-associated fibroblasts. Trends Cancer 9(5):421–443

Baker D, Al-Naggar IM, Sivajothi S, Flynn WF, Amiri A, Luo D, Hardy CC, Kuchel GA, Smith PP, Robson P (2021) A cellular reference resource for the mouse urinary bladder. bioRxiv: 2021.2009.2020.461121.

Balar AV, Galsky MD, Rosenberg JE, Powles T, Petrylak DP, Bellmunt J et al (2017) Atezolizumab as first-line treatment in cisplatin-ineligible patients with locally advanced and metastatic urothelial carcinoma: a single-arm, multicentre, phase 2 trial. Lancet 389(10064):67–76

Baquero F (2012) On the shifting balance: the case of Staphylococcus aureus CC398. MBio 3(2)

Baskin LS, Hayward SW, Sutherland RA, DiSandro MS, Thomson AA, Cunha GR (1997) Cellular signaling in the bladder. Front Biosci 2:d592–595

Baskin LS, Hayward SW, Sutherland RA, DiSandro MS, Thomson AA, Cunha GR. Cellular signaling in the bladder. Front Biosci. 1997 Dec 1;2:d592-5. doi: 10.2741/a215. PMID: 9374449.

Beckabir W, Wobker SE, Damrauer JS, Midkiff B, De la Cruz G, Makarov V et al (2023) Spatial relationships in the tumor microenvironment demonstrate association with pathologic response to neoadjuvant Chemoimmunotherapy in muscle-invasive bladder cancer. Eur Urol

Bellini A, Mattoli S (2007) The role of the fibrocyte, a bone marrow-derived mesenchymal progenitor, in reactive and reparative fibroses. Lab Investig 87(9):858–870

Benjamin T, Ristau M, Baker D, Robson P (2023) 'Cancer-associated fibroblasts' are present in normal bladder tissue but differentially located in the bladder tumor microenvironment compared to normal controls. NEAUA 92nd Annual Meeting

Berg G, Rybakova D, Fischer D, Cernava T, Vergès MC, Charles T et al (2020) Microbiome definition revisited: old concepts and new challenges. Microbiome 8(1):103

Bhattacharya M, Ramachandran P (2023) Immunology of human fibrosis. Nat Immunol 24(9):1423–1433

Biffi G, Oni TE, Spielman B, Hao Y, Elyada E, Park Y et al (2019) IL1-induced JAK/STAT signaling is antagonized by TGFbeta to shape CAF heterogeneity in pancreatic ductal adenocarcinoma. Cancer Discov 9(2):282–301

Brooks M, Mo Q, Krasnow R, Ho PL, Yu-Cheng LJX, Kurtova A, Lerner S, Godoy G, Jian W, Castro P, Chen F, Rowley D, Ittmann M, Syson K, Chan (2016) Positive association of collagen type I with non-muscle invasive bladder cancer progression. Oncotarget 7:82609

Brown B, Lindberg K, Reing J, Stolz DB, Badylak SF. The basement membrane component of biologic scaffolds derived from extracellular matrix. Tissue Engineering. 2006;12(3):519-26.

Chang HY, Chi J-T, Dudoit S, Bondre C, van de Rijn M, Botstein D, Brown PO (2002) Diversity, topographic differentiation, and positional memory in human fibroblasts. PNAS 99:8568

Chang HY, Chi JT, Dudoit S, Bondre C, van de Rijn M, Botstein D, et al. Diversity, topographic differentiation, and positional memory in human fibroblasts. Proceedings of the National Academy of Sciences of the United States of America. 2002;99(20):12877-82.

Bučević Popović V, Šitum M, Chow CT, Chan LS, Roje B, Terzić J (2018) The urinary microbiome associated with bladder cancer. Sci Rep 8(1):12157

Caramelo B, Zagorac S, Corral S, Marques M, Real FX (2023) Cancer-associated fibroblasts in bladder cancer: origin, biology, and therapeutic opportunities. Eur Urol Oncol 6(4):366–375

Chen C, Huang Z, Huang P, Li K, Zeng J, Wen Y et al (2022) Urogenital Microbiota:Potentially Important Determinant of PD-L1 Expression in Male Patients with Non-muscle Invasive Bladder Cancer. BMC Microbiol 22(1):7

Chen Y, Kim J, Yang S, Wang H, Wu CJ, Sugimoto H et al (2021) Type I collagen deletion in αSMA(+) myofibroblasts augments immune suppression and accelerates progression of pancreatic cancer. Cancer Cell 39(4):548–65.e6

Chen Z, Zhou L, Liu L, Hou Y, Xiong M, Yang Y et al (2020) Single-cell RNA sequencing highlights the role of inflammatory cancer-associated fibroblasts in bladder urothelial carcinoma. Nat Commun 11(1):5077

Christmas TJ (1994) Lymphocyte sub-populations in the bladder wall in normal bladder, bacterial cystitis and interstitial cystitis. Br J Urol 73(5):508–515

Costa A, Kieffer Y, Scholer-Dahirel A, Pelon F, Bourachot B, Cardon M et al (2018) Fibroblast heterogeneity and immunosuppressive environment in human breast cancer. Cancer Cell 33(3):463–79 e10

DeClerck YA (2012) Desmoplasia: a response or a niche? Cancer Discov 2(9):772–774

Di Martino JS, Nobre AR, Mondal C, Taha I, Farias EF, Fertig EJ et al (2022) A tumor-derived type III collagen-rich ECM niche regulates tumor cell dormancy. Nat Cancer 3(1):90–107

Egeblad M, Nakasone ES, Werb Z (2010) Tumors as organs: complex tissues that interface with the entire organism. Dev Cell 18(6):884–901

Elyada E, Bolisetty M, Laise P, Flynn WF, Courtois ET, Burkhart RA et al (2019) Cross-species single-cell analysis of pancreatic ductal adenocarcinoma reveals antigen-presenting cancer-associated fibroblasts. Cancer Discov 9(8):1102–1123

Engel DR, Maurer J, Tittel AP, Weisheit C, Cavlar T, Schumak B et al (2008) CCR2 mediates homeostatic and inflammatory release of Gr1(high) monocytes from the bone marrow, but is dispensable for bladder infiltration in bacterial urinary tract infection. J Immunol 181(8):5579–5586

Flores-Mireles AL, Walker JN, Caparon M, Hultgren SJ (2015) Urinary tract infections: epidemiology, mechanisms of infection and treatment options. Nat Rev Microbiol 13(5):269–284

Fransen F, van Beek AA, Borghuis T, Aidy SE, Hugenholtz F, van der Gaast-de JC et al (2017) Aged gut microbiota contributes to Systemical Inflammaging after transfer to germ-free mice. Front Immunol 8:1385

Friedrich V, Choi HW (2022) The urinary microbiome: role in bladder cancer and treatment. Diagnostics (Basel) 12(9)

Ghassemi H, Hashemnia M, Mousavibahar SH, Mahmoodzadeh Hosseini H, Mirhosseini SA (2021) Positive Association of Matrix Proteins Alteration with TAZ and the progression of high-grade bladder cancer. Cell J 23(7):742–749

Gouin KH 3rd, Ing N, Plummer JT, Rosser CJ, Ben Cheikh B, Oh C et al (2021) An N-cadherin 2 expressing epithelial cell subpopulation predicts response to surgery, chemotherapy and immunotherapy in bladder cancer. Nat Commun 12(1):4906

Hanahan D, Coussens LM (2012) Accessories to the crime: functions of cells recruited to the tumor microenvironment. Cancer Cell 21(3):309–322

Hart DN, Fabre JW (1981) Demonstration and characterization of Ia-positive dendritic cells in the interstitial connective tissues of rat heart and other tissues, but not brain. J Exp Med 154:154

Hayashi K, Nikolos F, Lee YC, Jain A, Tsouko E, Gao H et al (2020) Tipping the immunostimulatory and inhibitory DAMP balance to harness immunogenic cell death. Nat Commun 11(1)

He S, Wang LH, Liu Y, Li YQ, Chen HT, Xu JH et al (2020) Single-cell transcriptome profiling of an adult human cell atlas of 15 major organs. Genome Biol 21(1):294

Huang H, Wang Z, Zhang Y, Pradhan RN, Ganguly D, Chandra R et al (2022) Mesothelial cell-derived antigen-presenting cancer-associated fibroblasts induce expansion of regulatory T cells in pancreatic cancer. Cancer Cell 40(6):656–73 e7

Hynes RO, Naba A (2012) Overview of the matrisome–an inventory of extracellular matrix constituents and functions. Cold Spring Harb Perspect Biol 4(1):a004903

Ingersoll MA, Albert ML (2013) From infection to immunotherapy: host immune responses to bacteria at the bladder mucosa. Mucosal Immunol 6(6):1041–1053

Ioachim E, Michael M, Stavropoulos NE, Kitsiou E, Salmas M, Malamou-Mitsi V (2005) A clinicopathological study of the expression of extracellular matrix components in urothelial carcinoma. BJU Int 95(4):655–659

Iwano M, Plieth D, Danoff TM, Xue C, Okada H, Neilson EG (2002) Evidence that fibroblasts derive from epithelium during tissue fibrosis. J Clin Invest 110(3):341–350

Jung Y, Kim JK, Shiozawa Y, Wang J, Mishra A, Joseph J et al (2013) Recruitment of mesenchymal stem

cells into prostate tumours promotes metastasis. Nat Commun 4:1795
Junttila MR, de Sauvage FJ (2013) Influence of tumour micro-environment heterogeneity on therapeutic response. Nature 501(7467):346–354
Juskaite V, Corcoran DS, Leitinger B (2017) Collagen induces activation of DDR1 through lateral dimer association and phosphorylation between dimers. eLife 6:6
Kalluri R (2016) The biology and function of fibroblasts in cancer. Nat Rev Cancer 16(9):582–598
Kamoun A, de Reynies A, Allory Y, Sjodahl G, Robertson AG, Seiler R et al (2020) A consensus molecular classification of muscle-invasive bladder cancer. Eur Urol 77(4):420–433
Kayagaki N, Kawasaki A, Ebata T, Ohmoto H, Ikeda S, Inoue S et al (1995) Metalloproteinase-mediated release of human Fas ligand. J Exp Med 182(6):1777–1783
Kerdidani D, Aerakis E, Verrou KM, Angelidis I, Douka K, Maniou MA et al (2022) Lung tumor MHCII immunity depends on in situ antigen presentation by fibroblasts. J Exp Med 219(2)
Kim YS, Unno T, Kim BY, Park MS (2020) Sex differences in gut microbiota. World J Mens Health 38(1):48–60
Kojima Y, Acar A, Eaton EN, Mellody KT, Scheel C, Ben-Porath I et al (2010) Autocrine TGF-beta and stromal cell-derived factor-1 (SDF-1) signaling drives the evolution of tumor-promoting mammary stromal myofibroblasts. Proc Natl Acad Sci USA 107(46):20009–20014
Koncina E, Nurmik M, Pozdeev VI, Gilson C, Tsenkova M, Begaj R et al (2023) IL1R1(+) cancer-associated fibroblasts drive tumor development and immunosuppression in colorectal cancer. Nat Commun 14(1):4251
Kurtova AV, Xiao J, Mo Q, Pazhanisamy S, Krasnow R, Lerner SP, et al (2015) Blocking PGE2-induced tumour repopulation abrogates bladder cancer chemoresistance. Nature. 517(7533):209–13
Lacerda Mariano L, Rousseau M, Varet H, Legendre R, Gentek R, Saenz Coronilla J, Bajenoff M, Gomez Perdiguero E, Ingersoll MA (2020) Functionally distinct resident macrophage subsets differentially shape responses to infection in the bladder. Sci Adv 6(48)
Lee YC, Kurtova AV, Xiao J, Nikolos F, Hayashi K, Tramel Z et al (2019) Collagen-rich airway smooth muscle cells are a metastatic niche for tumor colonization in the lung. Nat Commun 10(1):2131
Leitinger B (2003) Molecular analysis of collagen binding by the human discoidin domain receptors, DDR1 and DDR2. Identification of collagen binding sites in DDR2. J Biol Chem 278(19):16761–16769
Lendahl U, Muhl L, Betsholtz C (2022) Identification, discrimination and heterogeneity of fibroblasts. Nat Commun 13(1):3409
Lobo N, Brooks NA, Zlotta AR, Cirillo JD, Boorjian S, Black PC et al (2021) 100 years of bacillus Calmette-Guérin immunotherapy: from cattle to COVID-19. Nat Rev Urol 18(10):611–622
Lodillinsky C, Langle Y, Guionet A, Góngora A, Baldi A, Sandes EO et al (2010) Bacillus Calmette Guerin induces fibroblast activation both directly and through macrophages in a mouse bladder cancer model. PLoS One 5(10):e13571
Louault K, Li R-R, DeClerck YA (2020) Cancer-associated fibroblasts: understanding their heterogeneity. Cancers 12:11
Luo Y, Zeng G, Wu S (2019) Identification of microenvironment-related prognostic genes in bladder cancer based on gene expression profile. Front Genet 10:1187
Ma Z, Li X, Mao Y, Wei C, Huang Z, Li G et al (2022) Interferon-dependent SLC14A1(+) cancer-associated fibroblasts promote cancer stemness via WNT5A in bladder cancer. Cancer Cell 40(12):1550–65 e7
Magagna I, Gourdin N, Kieffer Y, Licaj M, Mhaidly R, Andre P et al (2021) CD73-mediated immunosuppression is linked to a specific fibroblast population that paves the way for new therapy in breast cancer. Cancers (Basel) 13(23)
Mariathasan S, Turley SJ, Nickles D, Castiglioni A, Yuen K, Wang Y et al (2018) TGFβ attenuates tumour response to PD-L1 blockade by contributing to exclusion of T cells. Nature 554(7693):544–548
McDonald LT, Russell DL, Kelly RR, Xiong Y, Motamarry A, Patel RK et al (2015) Hematopoietic stem cell-derived cancer-associated fibroblasts are novel contributors to the pro-tumorigenic microenvironment. Neoplasia 17(5):434–448
Mezheyeuski A, Segersten U, Leiss LW, Malmstrom PU, Hatina J, Ostman A et al (2020) Fibroblasts in urothelial bladder cancer define stroma phenotypes that are associated with clinical outcome. Sci Rep 10(1):281
Mhaidly R, Mechta-Grigoriou F (2020) Fibroblast heterogeneity in tumor micro-environment: role in immunosuppression and new therapies. Semin Immunol 48:48
Mo Q, Nikolos F, Chen F, Tramel Z, Lee YC, Hayashi K et al (2018) Prognostic power of a tumor differentiation gene signature for bladder urothelial carcinomas. J Natl Cancer Inst 110(5):448–459
Modena BD, Milam R, Harrison F, Cheeseman JA, Abecassis MM, Friedewald JJ et al (2017) Changes in urinary microbiome populations correlate in kidney transplants with interstitial fibrosis and tubular atrophy documented in early surveillance biopsies. Am J Transplant 17(3):712–723
Liebert RW, Wedemeyer G, Carey TE, Grossman HB (1994) Loss of co-localization of a6f34 integrin and collagen VII in bladder cancer. Amnerican journal of'Pathology
Mostafa MH, Sheweita SA, O'Connor PJ (1999) Relationship between schistosomiasis and bladder cancer. Clin Microbiol Rev 12(1):97–111
Müllberg J, Durie FH, Otten-Evans C, Alderson MR, Rose-John S, Cosman D et al (1995) A metalloprotease inhibitor blocks shedding of the IL-6 receptor and the p60 TNF receptor. J Immunol 155(11):5198–5205
Naba A, Clauser KR, Hoersch S, Liu H, Carr SA, Hynes RO (2012) The matrisome: in silico definition and

in vivo characterization by proteomics of normal and tumor extracellular matrices. Mol Cell Proteomics 11(4):M111 014647

Naito S, Koga H, Yamaguchi A, Fujimoto N, Hasui Y, Kuramoto H et al (2008) Prevention of recurrence with epirubicin and lactobacillus casei after transurethral resection of bladder cancer. J Urol 179(2):485–490

Nikolos F, Hayashi K, Hoi XP, Alonzo ME, Mo Q, Kasabyan A et al (2022) Cell death-induced immunogenicity enhances chemoimmunotherapeutic response by converting immune-excluded into T-cell inflamed bladder tumors. Nat Commun 13(1)

Nimphius W, Moll R, Olbert P, Ramaswamy A, Barth PJ (2007) CD34+ fibrocytes in chronic cystitis and noninvasive and invasive urothelial carcinomas of the urinary bladder. Virchows Arch 450(2):179–185

Nod for atezolizumab in advanced bladder cancer (2017) Cancer Discov 7:7

Öhlund D, Handly-Santana A, Biffi G, Elyada E, Almeida AS, Ponz-Sarvise M et al (2017) Distinct populations of inflammatory fibroblasts and myofibroblasts in pancreatic cancer. J Exp Med 214(3):579–596

Ozdemir BC, Pentcheva-Hoang T, Carstens JL, Zheng X, Wu CC, Simpson TR et al (2014) Depletion of carcinoma-associated fibroblasts and fibrosis induces immunosuppression and accelerates pancreas cancer with reduced survival. Cancer Cell 25(6):719–734

Pearce MM, Hilt EE, Rosenfeld AB, Zilliox MJ, Thomas-White K, Fok C et al (2014) The female urinary microbiome: a comparison of women with and without urgency urinary incontinence. MBio 5(4):e01283–e01214

Pederzoli F, Ferrarese R, Amato V, Locatelli I, Alchera E, Lucianò R et al (2020) Sex-specific alterations in the urinary and tissue microbiome in therapy-naïve urothelial bladder cancer patients. Eur Urol Oncol. 3(6):784–788

Pettenati C, Ingersoll MA (2018) Mechanisms of BCG immunotherapy and its outlook for bladder cancer. Nat Rev Urol 15(10):615–625

Plikus MV, Wang X, Sinha S, Forte E, Thompson SM, Herzog EL et al (2021) Fibroblasts: origins, definitions, and functions in health and disease. Cell 184(15):3852–3872

Pohl HG, Groah SL, Pérez-Losada M, Ljungberg I, Sprague BM, Chandal N et al (2020) The urine microbiome of healthy men and women differs by urine collection method. Int Neurourol J 24(1):41–51

Price TK, Wolff B, Halverson T, Limeira R, Brubaker L, Dong Q et al (2020) Temporal dynamics of the adult female lower urinary tract microbiota. MBio 11(2)

Qin Y, Zu X, Li Y, Han Y, Tan J, Cai C et al (2023) A cancer-associated fibroblast subtypes-based signature enables the evaluation of immunotherapy response and prognosis in bladder cancer. iScience 26(9):107722

Quante M, Tu SP, Tomita H, Gonda T, Wang SS, Takashi S et al (2011) Bone marrow-derived myofibroblasts contribute to the mesenchymal stem cell niche and promote tumor growth. Cancer Cell 19(2):257–272

Ramachandran P, Dobie R, Wilson-Kanamori JR, Dora EF, Henderson BEP, Luu NT et al (2019) Resolving the fibrotic niche of human liver cirrhosis at single-cell level. Nature 575(7783):512–518

Ratliff TL, Ritchey JK, Yuan JJ, Andriole GL, Catalona WJ (1993) T-cell subsets required for intravesical BCG immunotherapy for bladder cancer. J Urol 150(3):1018–1023

Reilkoff RA, Bucala R, Herzog EL (2011) Fibrocytes: emerging effector cells in chronic inflammation. Nat Rev Immunol 11(6):427–435

Sahai E, Astsaturov I, Cukierman E, DeNardo DG, Egeblad M, Evans RM et al (2020) A framework for advancing our understanding of cancer-associated fibroblasts. Nat Rev Cancer 20(3):174–186

Sathyanarayana UG, Maruyama R, Padar A, Suzuki M, Bondaruk J, Sagalowsky A et al (2004) Molecular detection of noninvasive and invasive bladder tumor tissues and exfoliated cells by aberrant promoter methylation of laminin-5 encoding genes. Cancer Res 64(4):1425–1430

Schilling JD, Martin SM, Hung CS, Lorenz RG, Hultgren SJ (2003) Tolllike receptor 4 on stromal and hematopoietic cells mediates innate resistance to uropathogenic Escherichia coli. Proc Natl Acad Sci USA 100(7):4203–8

Schneider AK, Chevalier MF, Derré L (2019) The multifaceted immune regulation of bladder cancer. Nat Rev Urol 16(10):613–630

Schworer S, Cimino FV, Ros M, Tsanov KM, Ng C, Lowe SW et al (2023) Hypoxia potentiates the inflammatory fibroblast phenotype promoted by pancreatic cancer cell-derived cytokines. Cancer Res 83(10):1596–1610

Scott AJ, Alexander JL, Merrifield CA, Cunningham D, Jobin C, Brown R et al (2019) International cancer microbiome consortium consensus statement on the role of the human microbiome in carcinogenesis. Gut 68(9):1624–1632

Seow SW, Rahmat JN, Mohamed AA, Mahendran R, Lee YK, Bay BH (2002) Lactobacillus species is more cytotoxic to human bladder cancer cells than mycobacterium Bovis (bacillus Calmette-Guerin). J Urol 168(5):2236–2239

Seymour RAGGJ, Lavin MF, Strutton GM, Gemmell E, Hazan G (1986) Immunohistochemical analysis of the human bladder. Br J Urol 58:19

Shin K, Lim A, Zhao C, Sahoo D, Pan Y, Spiekerkoetter E et al (2014) Hedgehog signaling restrains bladder cancer progression by eliciting stromal production of urothelial differentiation factors. Cancer Cell 26(4):521–533

Shrivastava A, Radziejewski C, Campbell E, Kovac L, McGlynn M, Ryan TE et al (1997) An orphan receptor tyrosine kinase family whose members serve as nonintegrin collagen receptors. Mol Cell 1(1):25–34

Silva ME, Hernandez-Andrade M, Abasolo N, Espinoza-Cruells C, Mansilla JB, Reyes CR et al (2023) DDR1 and its ligand, collagen IV, are involved in in vitro oligodendrocyte maturation. Int J Mol Sci 24(2)

Sirvent A, Espie K, Papadopoulou E, Naim D, Roche S (2022) New functions of DDR1 collagen receptor in tumor dormancy, immune exclusion and therapeutic resistance. Front Oncol 12:956926

Song CH, Kim YH, Naskar M, Hayes BW, Abraham MA, Noh JH et al (2022) Lactobacillus crispatus limits bladder Uropathogenic E. Coli infection by triggering a host type I interferon response. Proc Natl Acad Sci USA 119(33):e2117904119

Su H, Yang F, Fu R, Trinh B, Sun N, Liu J et al (2022) Collagenolysis-dependent DDR1 signalling dictates pancreatic cancer outcome. Nature 610(7931):366–372

Tiwari A, Oravecz T, Dillon LA, Italiano A, Audoly L, Fridman WH et al (2023) Towards a consensus definition of immune exclusion in cancer. Front Immunol 14:1084887

Tsoumakidou M (2023) The advent of immune stimulating CAFs in cancer. Nat Rev Cancer 23:258

Tu MM, Lee FYF, Jones RT, Kimball AK, Saravia E, Graziano RF et al (2019) Targeting DDR2 enhances tumor response to anti-PD-1 immunotherapy. Sci Adv 5(2):eaav2437

van Puffelen JH, Keating ST, Oosterwijk E, van der Heijden AG, Netea MG, Joosten LAB et al (2020) Trained immunity as a molecular mechanism for BCG immunotherapy in bladder cancer. Nat Rev Urol 17(9):513–525

Vera-Ramirez L, Vodnala SK, Nini R, Hunter KW, Green JE (2018) Autophagy promotes the survival of dormant breast cancer cells and metastatic tumour recurrence. Nat Commun 9(1):1944

Verginadis II, Avgousti H, Monslow J, Skoufos G, Chinga F, Kim K et al (2022) A stromal integrated stress response activates perivascular cancer-associated fibroblasts to drive angiogenesis and tumour progression. Nat Cell Biol 24(6):940–953

Vogel W, Gish GD, Alves F, Pawson T (1997) The discoidin domain receptor tyrosine kinases are activated by collagen. Mol Cell 1(1):13–23

Vollmer P, Walev I, Rose-John S, Bhakdi S (1996) Novel pathogenic mechanism of microbial metalloproteinases: liberation of membrane-anchored molecules in biologically active form exemplified by studies with the human interleukin-6 receptor. Infect Immun 64(9):3646–3651

Wang L, Saci A, Szabo PM, Chasalow SD, Castillo-Martin M, Domingo-Domenech J et al (2018) EMT- and stroma-related gene expression and resistance to PD-1 blockade in urothelial cancer. Nat Commun 9(1):3503

Wilson CB, Leopard J, Cheresh DA, Nakamura RM (1996) Extracellular matrix and integrin composition of the normal bladder wall. World J Urol 14(Suppl 1):S30–S37

Wolf MT, Ganguly S, Wang TL, Anderson CW, Sadtler K, Narain R et al (2019) A biologic scaffold-associated type 2 immune microenvironment inhibits tumor formation and synergizes with checkpoint immunotherapy. Sci Transl Med 11(477)

Xiong YX, Zhang XC, Zhu JH, Zhang YX, Pan YL, Wu Y et al (2023) Collagen I-DDR1 signaling promotes hepatocellular carcinoma cell stemness via Hippo signaling repression. Cell Death Differ 30(7):1648–1665

Zeisberg EM, Potenta S, Xie L, Zeisberg M, Kalluri R (2007a) Discovery of endothelial to mesenchymal transition as a source for carcinoma-associated fibroblasts. Cancer Res 67(21):10123–10128

Zeisberg M, Yang C, Martino M, Duncan MB, Rieder F, Tanjore H et al (2007b) Fibroblasts derive from hepatocytes in liver fibrosis via epithelial to mesenchymal transition. J Biol Chem 282(32):23337–23347

Zhao J, Yang C, Liang B, Gao Y, Luo J, Zheng J et al (2023) Single-cell profiling reveals various types of interstitial cells in the bladder. Cell Prolif 56(9):e13431

Part IV

Molecular and Histological Subtypes of Bladder Cancer

13 Molecular Subtypes of Non-Muscle-Invasive Bladder Cancer

Frederik Prip, Sia Viborg Lindskrog, Philippe Lamy, Trine Strandgaard, Iver Nordentoft, Karin Birkenkamp-Demtröder, and Lars Dyrskjøt

Abstract

Non-muscle-invasive bladder cancers (NMIBCs) show large variation in disease aggressiveness and treatment response which is not fully explained by differences in clinical and pathological factors. Researchers have therefore studied different molecular layers of tumors, mainly gene expression profiling, to unravel underlying molecular subtypes that can explain this phenotypic variation. In addition, molecular subtypes can potentially be used for risk stratification of patients and prediction of treatment response based on the biological tumor features. NMIBC subtypes have been investigated in combination with muscle-invasive bladder cancers (MIBCs), using NMIBCs only and separated by tumor stage. Molecularly high-risk tumors across schemes are generally characterized by pronounced cell cycle activity, frequent *TP53* alterations and a high degree of genomic instability. In this chapter, we describe the different NMIBC subtype classification schemes reported. Finally, we discuss the clinical utility of molecular subtypes and what still needs to be answered before clinical implementation.

Keywords

NMIBC · Subtypes · Transcriptomics · Genomics · Proteomics

13.1 Molecular Tumor Subtyping in NMIBC

Generation of high-throughput molecular data and next-generation sequencing have enabled comprehensive molecular subtyping of cancer, i.e., the process of separating tumors into more homogenous groups based on molecular entities and biological differences. Tumor subtyping may constitute a biologically informative division of tumors beyond tumor stage and grade that may translate into improved clinical decision-making and risk stratification of patients. Subtypes of non-muscle-invasive bladder cancer (NMIBC)

F. Prip · S. V. Lindskrog · T. Strandgaard · K. Birkenkamp-Demtröder · L. Dyrskjøt (✉)
Department of Clinical Medicine, Aarhus University, Aarhus, Denmark

Department of Molecular Medicine, Aarhus University Hospital, Aarhus, Denmark
e-mail: frederik.prip@clin.au.dk; svl@clin.au.dk; ts@clin.au.dk; lars@clin.au.dk

P. Lamy · I. Nordentoft
Department of Clinical Medicine, Aarhus University, Aarhus, Denmark
e-mail: philippe.lamy@clin.au.dk; iver.nordentoft@clin.au.dk

M. A. Knowles, L. Dyrskjøt (eds.), *Biology of Bladder Cancer*,
https://doi.org/10.1007/978-3-031-68505-7_13

Table 13.1 Molecular classification systems of NMIBC

	Classification system	Year of publication	Discovery cohort (*n*, NMIBCs/total)	Number of NMIBC subtypes	Subtypes	Reference
Transcriptomic, NMIBC only	UROMOL	2016, 2021	UROMOL2016 (*n* = 460/476), UROMOL2021 (*n* = 535)	4	Class 1, class 2a, class 2b, class 3	(Hedegaard et al. 2016; Lindskrog et al. 2021)
	T1BC	2020	Chicago (*n* = 78)	5	T1-Early, T1-LumGU, T1-Inflam, T1-TLum, T1-Early	(Robertson et al. 2020)
	Leeds	2021	Leeds (*n* = 217)	3 (Ta tumors); 4 (T1 tumors)	TaE1, TaE2, TaE3; T1E1, T1E2, T1E3, T1E4	(Hurst et al. 2021)
	BCPP	2022	Birmingham (*n* = 78)	3	Class A, class B, class C	(Goel et al. 2022)
	BRS	2023	Rotterdam (*n* = 283)	3	BRS1, BRS2, BRS3	(de Jong et al. 2023)
Transcriptomic, pan-bladder cancer	LundTax	2012, 2017	Lund2012 (*n* = 213/308), Lund2017 (*n* = 64/307)	5–7	Urothelial-like A/B/C, Genomically unstable, basal/squamous, mesenchymal-like, small-cell/ neuroendocrine-like	(Sjödahl et al. 2012; Sjödahl et al. 2017)
	BOLD	2018	Meta-dataset (*n* = 653/2411)	6	MC1/NEURAL, MC2/ LUM, MC3/PAP, MC4/ HER2L, MC5/SCC, MC6/MES	(Tan et al. 2019)
	CNUH	2019	CNUH (*n* = 102/165)	4	Class 1, class 2, class 3, class 4	(Song et al. 2019)
Genomic	Leeds	2021	Leeds (*n* = 217)	4	CN1, CN2, CN3, CN4	(Hurst et al. 2021)
Proteomic	NPS	2020	Athens (*n* = 98/117)	3	NSP1, NSP2, NSP3	(Stroggilos et al. 2020)
	UI-III	2022	Shanghai (*n* = 45/116)	3	U-I, U-II, U-III	(Xu et al. 2022)
	uPG	2023	CIT (*n* = 23/63)	5	uPG-A, uPG-B, uPG-C, uPG-D, uPG-E	(Groeneveld et al. 2023)

can be characterized at several levels: from analysis of the full disease spectrum of bladder cancer (pan-bladder cancer studies), NMIBCs only or tumor stages separately (carcinoma in situ [CIS], Ta, T1). Including muscle-invasive bladder cancer (MIBC) in the development of NMIBC subtype schemes might strengthen the ability to identify high-risk NMIBC subtypes, as they will most likely be clustered together with MIBC. However, MIBCs often display more phenotypic variability across tumors compared to NMIBC, and the resulting classification scheme may therefore not fully capture the molecular granularity observed exclusively in NMIBC. Finally, higher granularity and homogeneity of biological subtypes can be obtained when discovering subtypes within Ta or T1 tumors separately.

The following sections will provide an overview of NMIBC subtypes identified using the various groupings of bladder tumors described above with special attention to studies identifying subtypes based on high-throughput profiling of biological entities, including gene expression profiles, copy number alterations, and proteomics (Table 13.1).

13.2 Transcriptomic Subtypes

Subtyping based on transcriptomic profiling of tumors has been widely used to unravel the molecular features of both the tumor and the tumor microenvironment, including infiltrating immune cells. Overall, gene expression

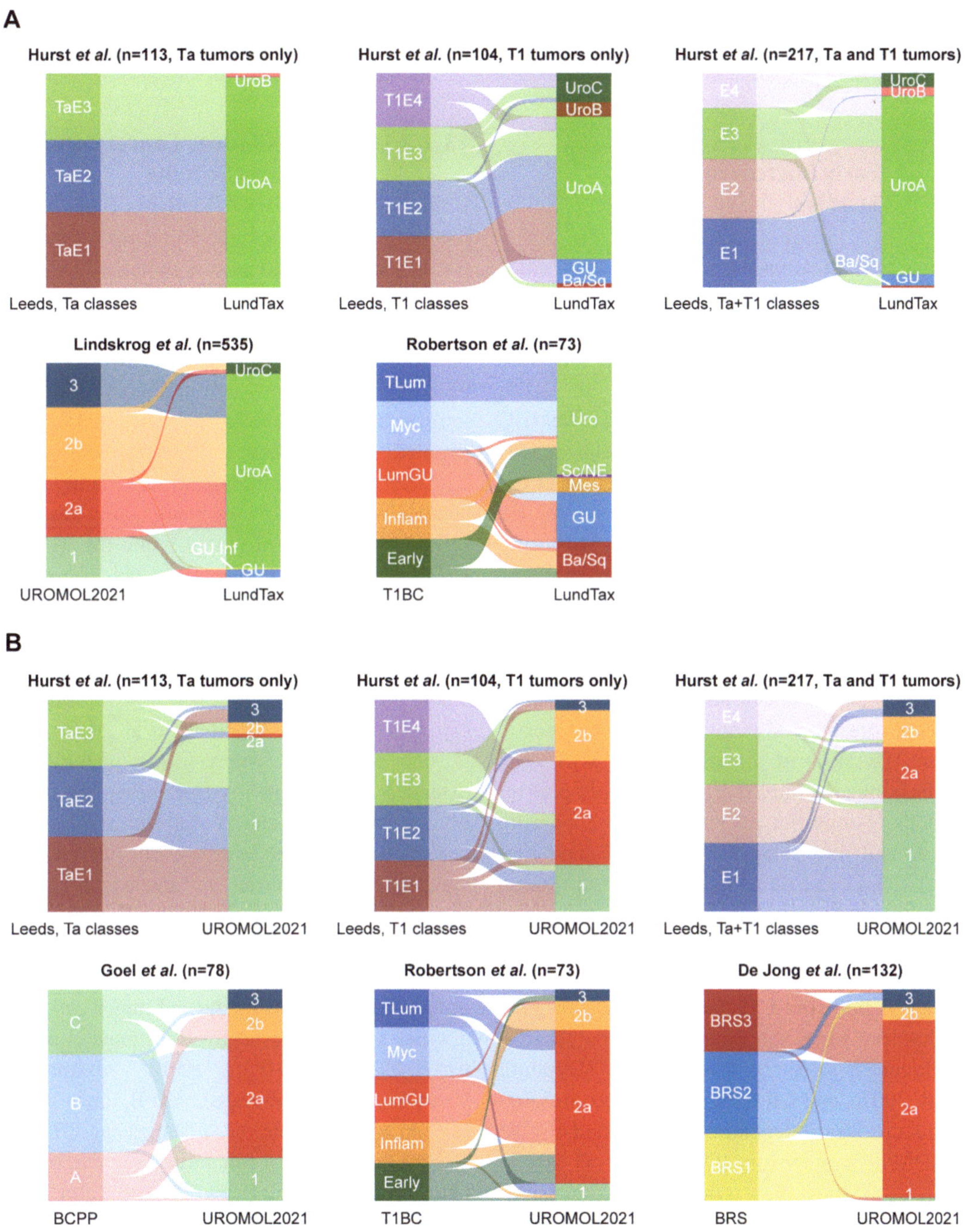

Fig. 13.1 Association between different classification systems and the LundTax (**a**) and UROMOL2021 (**b**) classifiers. Only associations that were reported in the respective publications are included

profiling summarizes the transcriptional landscape of a tumor and reflects cellular composition, biological processes, and intracellular signaling.

To ease the comparison between the different classification systems, the correlation between presented subtype schemes and the pan-bladder cancer Lund taxonomy (Sjödahl et al. 2017; Marzouka et al. 2018) or the NMIBC-specific UROMOL2021 classes (Lindskrog et al. 2021) is shown in Fig. 13.1, when this comparison was included in the respective studies. The Lund taxonomy and UROMOL2021 are the only classification systems that are included consistently as reference across studies.

13.2.1 Early Microarray-Based Studies

Initial hybridization-based microarray studies showed that unsupervised clustering of gene expression profiles can separate NMIBC from MIBC (Dyrskjøt et al. 2003; Mor et al. 2003; Modlich et al. 2004; Blaveri et al. 2005; Sanchez-Carbayo et al. 2006) and that NMIBC can be divided into distinct molecular groups with different clinical risks (Kim et al. 2005; Wild et al. 2005; Lindgren et al. 2006, 2010). Lindgren et al. applied hierarchical clustering of 75 NMIBCs and discovered four subtypes having distinct expression of *FGFR3* and genes related to cell cycle and immune responses (Lindgren et al. 2006). Furthermore, special focus has been on the identification of gene expression signatures with prognostic value. Dyrskjøt et al. identified a CIS gene expression signature that was not only present in CIS lesions but also in normal-appearing tissue and other stages of NMIBC (Dyrskjøt et al. 2004) and developed a gene expression signature of progression using supervised clustering of data from 29 patients with NMIBC (Dyrskjøt et al. 2005). The prognostic value of both the CIS- and progression gene signatures were subsequently validated in a multicenter study of 404 patients (Dyrskjøt et al. 2007), and later, the 12-gene progression signature was independently validated by the UROMOL consortium (Dyrskjøt et al. 2017). Kim et al. have also reported a progression-related gene classifier which was validated in independent cohorts (Kim et al. 2010). These initial microarray-based studies paved the way for subtype discovery in larger patient cohorts using both array-based gene expression profiling and next generation sequencing (NGS) technologies.

13.2.2 NMIBC Subtypes Derived from Pan-Bladder Cancer Studies

13.2.2.1 The Pan-Bladder Cancer Lund Taxonomy Scheme

Building on earlier work (Lindgren et al. 2010), the first version of the Lund molecular taxonomy for urothelial carcinoma was published in 2012 comprising data from 308 tumors, of which 213 were NMIBCs (Sjödahl et al. 2012). Five subtypes, namely urobasal A, genomically unstable, urobasal B, squamous cell carcinoma like and infiltrated, were identified (see Chap. 14 for a detailed description of the subtype characteristics). The NMIBCs were mainly classified as urobasal A (57%), genomically unstable (26%), and infiltrated (11%) while the MIBCs were of any subtype. The Lund taxonomy has subsequently been extended to include both gene expression profiling and immunohistochemistry with the aim of classifying tumors based on carcinoma cells only (see Chap. 14 for details) (Sjödahl et al. 2017; Marzouka et al. 2018). This is one important feature distinguishing the extended Lund taxonomy from other classification systems: non-cancer cell infiltration and cancer cell proliferation are not considered to be class-defining properties of cancer cells in this scheme (Marzouka et al. 2022). The extended LundTax mRNA classifier was established to classify tumors according to the immunohistochemistry-adjusted tumor cell phenotypes and their respective infiltrated counterparts: Urothelial-like (Uro) comprising UroA-Prog, Uro-Infiltrated, UroB, and UroC; genomically unstable (GU) comprising GU and GU-infiltrated; basal/squamous-cell carcinoma like (Ba/Sq) comprising Ba/Sq and Ba/Sq-infiltrated; mesenchymal-like (Mes-like); small-cell/neuroendocrine-like (Sc/NE-like) and Sc/NE-like-infiltrated. Hence, the LundTax scheme comprises five major tumor cell phenotypes (Uro, GU, Ba/Sq, Mes-like, Sc/NE-like) when eliminating the expression signals originating from non-cancer cells in the tumor microenvironment. The LundTax classifier has subsequently been applied to the UROMOL2021 (535 NMIBCs) and Leeds (217 NMIBCs) cohorts to test the translational value of the pan-bladder cancer subtypes in a NMIBC-only setting (Marzouka et al. 2022). For the UROMOL2021 cohort, 507 tumors were classified as Uro (443 UroA, 41 UroB, 23 UroC), 23 as GU, 3 as Ba/Sq, and 2 as Mes-like. For the Leeds cohort, the LundTax classifier identified 183 as UroA, 6 as UroB, 15 as UroC, 12 as GU, and 1 as Ba/Sq. Patients with tumors of the UroA subtype had the best prognosis in both the UROMOL and Leeds cohorts while patients with GU tumors had the highest risk of progression in the UROMOL2021 cohort only. Considering only T1 tumors, patients with GU and UroB tumors had the worst prognosis in the UROMOL2021 cohort while results were not as clear in the Leeds cohort. Exploring intra-subtype variability within the major NMIBC subtype UroA showed varying levels of non-cancer cell infiltration and cancer cell proliferation, overall reflecting some of the characteristics defining the UROMOL2021 subtypes. In conclusion, the study highlights that NMIBCs almost exclusively belong to the luminal subtypes (Uro and GU).

13.2.2.2 Other Pan-Bladder Cancer Subtype Schemes

In 2019, Tan et al. performed a combined reanalysis of previously published microarray-based gene expression data from 2411 tumors encompassing both NMIBC and MIBC (Tan et al. 2019). The authors identified six molecular subtypes, denoted as the BOLD subtypes (MC1/Neural-like, MC2/Luminal-like, MC3/Papillary-like, MC4/HER2-like, MC5/Squamous-cell carcinoma-like, and MC6/Mesenchymal-like). Overall, these subtypes captured the various previously published subtype schemes. Most Ta tumors were of the MC2/Luminal-like subtype whereas most T1 tumors were of the MC3/Papillary-like or MC4/HER2-like subtypes. However, around 20% of all NMIBCs were assigned to one of the MIBC-dominated subtypes: MC1/Neural-like, MC5/Squamous-cell carcinoma-like or MC6/Mesenchymal-like, indicating the presence of MIBC traits in NMIBCs. For the NMIBCs, MC3/Papillary-like tumors showed enrichment of a *FGFR3* gene signature and patients with MC3/Papillary-like tumors had the best outcome compared with the non-papillary subtypes. Furthermore, all the BOLD subtypes were present in the UROMOL2016 cohort (of note, only one tumor was identified as MC1/Neural-like), and patients with tumors classified as MC4/HER2-like and MC5/Squamous-cell carcinoma-like had the worst clinical outcomes (Tan et al. 2019).

A third pan-bladder cancer study by Song et al. performed clustering of microarray-based gene expression profiling of a combined cohort of 102 NMIBCs and 63 MIBCs and identified four subtypes: class 1, 2, 3, and 4 (Song et al. 2019). Overall, these pan-bladder cancer subtypes represented a scheme with a high level of co-clustering of NMIBCs and MIBCs within classes. Class 4 comprised mainly MIBCs with upregulation of immune-related genes and genes involved in epithelial–mesenchymal transition (EMT) and extracellular matrix organization, while the remaining three classes comprised most of the NMIBCs. Class 1 included mainly low-grade NMIBCs and showed low expression of cell cycle-related genes while class 3 comprised both high-grade NMIBCs and MIBCs and was characterized by high cell cycle activity. Class 2, which included both low-grade NMIBCs and some MIBCs, were characterized by high *FGFR3* expression and downregulation of immune-response pathways—a subtype feature observed in other classification schemes as well (e.g., UROMOL2021 class 3 (Lindskrog et al. 2021), T1-TLum (Robertson et al. 2020), BRS2 (de Jong et al. 2023); *introduced in the following sections*). *FGFR3* mutations and overexpression have previously been linked to a non-inflamed tumor microenvironment (Sweis et al. 2016; Damrauer et al. 2021). The subtypes identified by Song et al. were associated with progression-free survival (PFS) in three independent cohorts of patients with NMIBC, with class 3 and 4 patients having the worst outcome.

13.2.3 NMIBC-Specific Subtypes

13.2.3.1 The UROMOL Study

The first comprehensive NGS-based study centered on NMIBC-specific subtypes was published in 2016 by Hedegaard et al. (UROMOL2016) (Hedegaard et al. 2016). Here, the authors performed total RNA-sequencing of 460 NMIBC samples, including both incident and prevalent cases of high- and low-risk tumors. Total RNA-sequencing of 16 MIBCs were additionally included to explore co-clustering between NMIBCs and more advanced tumors. Patients were enrolled prospectively from 2008 to 2012 in the UROMOL consortium, a European multicenter study of NMIBC spanning 10 centers in Denmark, Sweden, the Netherlands, Spain, Germany, and Serbia. In total, fresh frozen tumor tissue was obtained for 1372 patients.

The authors performed unsupervised consensus clustering of gene expression values and identified three classes named class 1, 2, and 3. Class 1 had the highest proportion of Ta and low-grade tumors while class 2 was enriched for T1 and high-grade tumors and contained the majority of the MIBCs (14/16). Even with the large cohort size, the study had a limited number of progression events (31; 6.7%), reflecting the general risk of progression in NMIBC when considering all clinical risk groups (Babjuk et al. 2022). Despite that, the identified subtypes were prognostic of progression to MIBC with class 2 tumors having the highest risk of progression (25 of 31 events).

The classes showed distinct gene expression profiles with class 1 tumors displaying a high expression of early cell cycle genes and class 2 a high expression of late cell cycle genes and genes related to EMT. Both class 1 and 2 tumors showed high expression of uroplakins, which are mainly expressed in luminal cells, compared with class 3 tumors. Class 3 tumors were generally characterized by a repressed gene expression profile but showed high expression of genes related to chromatin remodeling and the basal markers *KRT5* and *KRT15*. In a subsequent analysis, immunohistochemical assessment of the luminal marker GATA3 and the basal cytokeratin marker CK5/6 showed that class 3 tumors expressed both luminal and basal features (Lindskrog et al. 2021). Besides showing differences in expression of protein-coding genes, the classes also showed distinct expression profiles of long non-coding RNAs (lncRNAs) with class 3 showing higher expression of, e.g., *MIR31HG*, *NEAT1* and *MALAT1*. Based on these findings, it was hypothesized that class 1 and 2 tumors are pure luminal, whereas class 3 tumors may represent a more dormant state with basal-like characteristics.

To improve the generalizability of the classification system, a 117-gene classifier was developed. As a validation, the classifier was applied to different datasets. Of note, only few class 3 tumors were observed in datasets based on mRNA-sequencing, indicating that lncRNAs may be essential for identifying class 3 (Hedegaard et al. 2016).

In 2021, Lindskrog et al. published an expansion of the UROMOL2016 study including total RNA-sequencing of tumors from 535 NMIBC patients (UROMOL2021) and updated follow-up for all patients from the UROMOL2016 study (Lindskrog et al. 2021). The additional samples together with the updated follow-up data increased the number of progression events from 31 to 65 (progression rate: 10.3%; median follow-up: 49 months for patients without progression).

Consensus clustering of gene expression values now identified four classes that largely overlapped with the UROMOL2016 classes; class 1 and class 3 were rediscovered, and class 2 was split into two classes named class 2a and 2b. The gene expression signatures, clinicopathological characteristics and risk profiles of class 1 and class 3 aligned with the original paper. Patients with class 2a tumors had the highest risk of progression, followed by patients with class 2b tumors. In addition, class 2a had the highest proportion of T1 and high-grade tumors. Class 2a and 2b showed distinct gene expression profiles with class 2a tumors having a higher expression of genes related to late cell cycle and DNA replication and class 2b tumors showing a higher expression of genes related to EMT, cancer stem cells, and immune infiltration. The high immune infiltration in class 2b tumors was validated by multiplex immunofluorescence for 167 of the tumors; class 2b tumors showed a particularly high infiltration of cytotoxic T-lymphocytes and T helper cells. On the contrary, class 3 tumors were found to have the lowest degree of immune infiltration overall. Using the pan-bladder cancer LundTax scheme (Fig. 13.1a), 91% of the tumors were classified as UroA, while the remaining tumors were classified mainly as GU (4%) or UroC (5%). Tumors classified as GU were almost exclusively class 2a.

The authors also studied differences in the genomic landscape across the UROMOL2021 subtypes. Copy number alterations (CNA) were quantified using single nucleotide polymorphism (SNP)-arrays in a subset of samples and mutations were called from the RNA-sequencing data. Class 2a tumors had the most altered genome and highest mutational load and were enriched for mutations in, e.g., *RB1* and *TP53*, resembling traits of MIBC biology. Class 1 and class 3 tumors had fewer genomic alterations but were enriched for mutations in *FGFR3*.

Finally, a single-sample transcriptomic classifier was constructed to facilitate the use of the UROMOL2021 classification schemes in future research. The UROMOL2021 classifier was applied to 14 independent cohorts comprising 1228 patients with NMIBC, validating the subtype-specific biological traits and the association between class 2a and worse PFS (Lindskrog et al. 2021).

13.2.3.2 Improved Genomic Insights of Transcriptomic Subtypes

In 2022, Goel et al. performed whole exome- and RNA-sequencing of 78 NMIBCs with the majority being T1 high-grade tumors (Goel et al. 2022). This study includes the largest overlap of whole exome and RNA-sequencing data from NMIBC samples to date, which allows for an improved understanding of the underlying genomic landscape of NMIBC subtypes. Consensus clustering of the gene expression data revealed three transcriptomic classes named Bladder Cancer Prognosis Program (BCPP) class A, B, and C. BCPP class A and B were enriched with T1 tumors while class C was enriched with Ta tumors. The BCPP classes highly overlapped with the UROMOL2021 classes (Fig. 13.1b); BCPP class A samples were mainly classified as UROMOL2021 class 2a and 2b, BCPP class B as UROMOL2021 class 2a and BCPP C as UROMOL2021 class 1 and 3. BCPP class A tumors showed high expression of EMT and immune markers, BCPP class B showed high expression of proliferation markers and BCPP class C tumors had a luminal expression profile. However, contrary to the pure luminal profile of class 2a tumors in the UROMOL2021 study, the BCPP class B showed high expression of basal markers. In the UROMOL2021 study, basal-like characteristics were observed mainly for the class 3 tumors (Lindskrog et al. 2021). Genomic profiling of the subtypes revealed that BCPP class B had the highest copy number- and tumor mutational burden. Alterations in *PPARG*, *RAF1*, *GATA3*, *CCND1*, and *MDM2* (all mainly amplifications) were enriched in BCPP class B and/or BCPP class A, and *FGFR3* was preferentially altered in BCPP class C.

13.2.4 Stage-Stratified Subtypes in NMIBC

In addition to pan-bladder cancer and NMIBC-specific subtype schemes, several studies have gained further biological insights on NMIBC and the potential for improved prognostication by focusing on the separate subclassification of Ta and T1 tumors.

Hurst et al. performed a combined and stage-stratified genomic and transcriptomic analysis of 113 Ta tumors and 104 high-grade T1 tumors (Hurst et al. 2021). Most Ta tumors were classified as the LundTax UroA (98%, Fig. 13.1a) and UROMOL2021 class 1 (80%, Fig. 13.1b). Clustering of the gene expression data using non-negative matrix factorization identified three distinct expression subtypes (TaE1-E3) having both distinct expression profiles and genomic alterations. TaE2 tumors had the highest frequency of CNAs, mainly with a loss of chr9q, and high expression of genes associated with cell cycle activity. TaE1 and TaE3 tumors were characterized by a high expression of genes related to urothelial differentiation and had frequent mutations in *STAG2* and *KMT2D*. TaE3 differed from TaE1 by having a higher immune score.

Non-negative matrix factorization analysis of 104 T1 high-grade tumors suggested four classes (T1E1–E4). These subtypes overlapped partially with the UROMOL2021 and LundTax subtypes (Fig. 13.1). T1E1 tumors were mostly classified as UROMOL2021 class 1 and LundTax UroA, T1E2 mostly as UROMOL2021 class 2a and LundTax UroA, T1E3 primarily as UROMOL2021 class 2b and a mix of LundTax UroA-C, and T1E4 mostly as UROMOL2021 class 2a and either LundTax UroA, UroC or GU. This suggests that UROMOL2021 class 2a might contain two distinct subtypes, T1E2 and T1E4. T1E2 and T1E4 shared several common gene expression patterns characteristic of class 2a, but T1E2 tumors had a higher expression of genes related to glucose metabolism and canonical glycolysis whereas T1E4 tumors had a higher expression of genes related to cholesterol, lipid biosynthesis and unfolded protein response. T1E2 and T1E4 also showed different genomic profiles, where T1E4 tumors had more CNAs and more mutations in *ERCC2*, *ATM* and *RB1*. No statistically significant differences in recurrence-free survival (RFS) or PFS across classes were identified, probably due to the limited number of patients in this subanalysis.

In the combined Ta and T1 analysis, four transcriptomic classes (class E1-E4) were identified. Importantly, despite using a different clustering tool than the one used in the UROMOL2021 study (non-negative matrix factorization vs. consensus hierarchical clustering, respectively), the two subtyping schemes showed high alignment (Fig. 13.1b). E1 and E3 aligned with the UROMOL2021 class 1 and 3, E3 aligned with class 2a, and E4 aligned with class 2b. The classes of the two subtyping schemes additionally showed similar gene expression-, copy number-, mutational-, and clinical risk profiles.

Robertson et al. performed transcriptomic analysis focusing on T1 tumors only (T1BC scheme) (Robertson et al. 2020). Five classes (T1-Myc, T1-Luminal genomically unstable [T1-LumGU], T1-Inflamed [T1-Inflam], T1-True Luminals [T1-TLum], T1-Early) were identified using consensus clustering of tumors from 73 Bacillus Calmette-Guérin (BCG)-treated patients. T1-LumGU tumors were associated with high *E2F1* and *EZH2* expression, T1-Inflam tumors showed elevated immune-related signatures and T1-TLum tumors had the highest luminal papillary score and high *FGFR3* expression. Both T1-Myc and T1-Early tumors had a high *MYC* expression; however, T1-Early tumors were distinguishable from T1-Myc tumors by having repressed interferon alpha and interferon gamma hallmarks and a lower estimated inflammation score. The subtypes were not associated with different risk of recurrence, potentially explained by the relatively low number of samples in the different classes (n = 13–16). Furthermore, the low number of progression events in the cohort did not allow for a correlation of the subtypes to progression. All classes but the T1-Inflam subtype were primarily classified as UROMOL2021 class 2a; tumors of the T1-Inflam subtype were mostly classified as UROMOL2021 class 2b (Fig. 13.1b).

A separate subanalysis of Ta low-grade tumors (n = 286) and T1 high-grade tumors (n = 101) was also conducted in the UROMOL2021 study (Lindskrog et al. 2021). Four Ta subtypes, largely corresponding to the four UROMOL classes, and three T1 high-grade subtypes (T1HG-1, T1HG-2, T1HG-3) were identified. The T1HG subtypes were prognostic and T1HG-1 tumors were independently associated with worse PFS and RFS when adjusted for clinical risk scores. Classifying the tumors according to the LundTax (Marzouka et al. 2018) and T1BC (Robertson et al. 2020) schemes showed that the T1HG-1 subtype was enriched for the LundTax GU and UroC and the T1BC T1-LumGU and T1-Myc. Although providing increased granularity, the subtypes did not translate directly into better outcome prediction as more progression events of T1 tumors were "missed" by the T1HG classifier compared to the UROMOL2021 classifier: 89% (32/36) of the progressing T1 tumors were classified as UROMOL2021 class 2a or 2b while 69% (25/36) were classified as T1HG-1 or T1HG-3 (Lindskrog et al. 2021).

13.2.5 Subtypes and BCG Response

As presented above, several subtype schemes have prognostic implications. Another clinical aspect and potential goal of molecular subtyping is to investigate whether subtype-specific molecular hallmarks translate into improved prediction of treatment response. Molecular subtyping may reveal treatment-resistant tumor subtypes, which could potentially serve a purpose in guiding treatment decisions for patients. Patients with high-risk NMIBC are often treated with adjuvant BCG instillations following tumor resection to reduce the risk of recurrence and progression (Babjuk et al. 2022). Unfortunately, up to 30% of patients do not respond to BCG and up to 50% relapse despite an initial response (Sylvester et al. 2005). Studies have sought to identify predictive subtypes to optimize the identification of patients who may benefit from BCG. However, to establish the true predictive value of BCG response subtypes, a control group of BCG-eligible patients not receiving BCG is required, which is not ethically possible. Consequently, studies focusing on BCG-treated patients can therefore per se not differentiate between the prognostic or the predictive value of the identified subtypes (Sjödahl et al. 2023).

The clinical value of the UROMOL2021 subtypes has been explored in a BCG-treated patient cohort including 126 pre-BCG tumors and 44 post-BCG recurrences (Strandgaard et al. 2022). Few patients were treated with BCG maintenance in this study and BCG response was therefore defined as absence of high-grade recurrence within two years after at least five BCG induction instillations and no progression to MIBC at any time during follow-up. The UROMOL2021 classes 2a and 2b were associated with worse high-grade RFS after BCG treatment. Whether this is explained by class 2a/b tumors having a poor response to BCG (predictive value) or because these tumors are generally more aggressive (prognostic value) remains unclear. Additionally, 15% of the pre-BCG tumors were classified as class 2b compared to 43% of post-BCG recurrences, most likely reflecting the increased immune activation following BCG treatment. The five subtypes of T1 tumors presented by Robertson et al. were also evaluated in relation to BCG response as all 73 patients received both induction and maintenance BCG (Robertson et al. 2020). The subtypes T1-Early and T1-Myc included over half of the recurrence events observed in the cohort when combined (14/24, 58%). The T1-Early subtype, characterized by low expression of immune-related gene signatures, had five recurrences within the first 6 months after BCG induction (5/13, 38%) and the T1-Myc subtype comprised the most recurrences after 24 months (12/17, 71%).

De Jong et al. have analyzed total RNA-sequencing data from high-grade NMIBCs from 132 patients treated with BCG (de Jong et al. 2023). BCG response was defined as absence of high-grade recurrence after at least five BCG induction instillations and at least nine maintenance instillations. In line with the LundTax approach, immune-related genes were removed before clustering to prevent potential bias caused by different degrees of immune infiltration. By using unsupervised clustering of the pre-BCG tumors, the study uncovered three molecular BCG response subtypes (BRSs): BRS1, BRS2, and BRS3. Patients with BRS3 tumors had the worst PFS and high-grade RFS after BCG treatment compared to BRS1/2. Furthermore, BRS3 was the dominant subtype when classifying 44 post-BCG recurrences. The BRS stratification of tumors and the association between BRS3 tumors and worse PFS was subsequently validated in a second cohort of 151 BCG-naïve patients with high-grade NMIBC. When classifying tumors according to the UROMOL2021 subtypes, the more aggressive UROMOL class 2a was distributed across all BRSs and class 2b tumors were found to overlap with BRS3 (Fig. 13.1b). BRS3 tumors were characterized by expression of basal and EMT gene markers as well as having higher immune cell infiltration and an immune-suppressive microenvironment, resolved both from bulk RNA-sequencing data and spatial proteomics. This observation is in line with previous findings linking BCG treatment failure to T-cell exhaustion (Kates et al. 2020; Strandgaard et al. 2022). BRS1 and BRS2 tumors shared many luminal features but BRS1 tumors showed an enrichment of pathways involved in cell cycle and mycobacterial processing. BRS2 tumors showed high expression of *FGFR3* and the lowest enrichment of immune-related pathways. Based on these findings, the authors suggest that BRS3 represents a subgroup of patients where the option of early RC may be considered. However, the predictive and clinical value of the BRS classifier remains to be tested in clinical trials.

13.3 Genomic Subtypes

Most classification systems in NMIBC and other cancers are based on transcriptomics data and only few classification systems have been identified from other omics layers such as genomics. Clustering of mutation calls is far less trivial; it contains a high level of noise (passenger mutations) and the number of mutated genes per sample is often low, especially for Ta low-grade tumors. Additionally, it is difficult to account for the binary data structure. Another challenge is that genomic alterations in genes that lead to the same molecular phenotype can be mutually exclusive, but this information would not be accounted for as clustering algorithms cluster samples based on co-occurrence/co-expression. However, CNAs are continuous, making these molecular entities more applicable for clustering and subtype identification.

Initially, Hurst et al. assessed CNAs of 160 tumors (58 Ta, 60 T1, 42 T2–4) using array-based comparative genomic hybridization (CGH). Unsupervised hierarchical clustering identified four and three major genomic subtypes of Ta and T1 high-grade tumors, respectively (Hurst et al. 2012). Subsequently, the cohort of Ta tumors was extended to include 140 tumors and CNAs were assessed using low pass whole genome sequencing or array-CGH (Hurst et al. 2017). Here, two major copy number subtypes of Ta tumors were identified, primarily distinguished by the frequency of chromosome 9 deletions. Furthermore, in the same study where Hurst et al. identified Ta- and T1-specific transcriptomic subtypes, the authors also used unsupervised hierarchical clustering of CNAs derived from low pass whole genome sequencing or array-CGH to identify stage-specific and stage-combined genomic subtypes (Hurst et al. 2017, 2021). In the stage-combined analysis (n = 217), the authors identified four copy number subtypes (CN1–CN4), with increasing genomic instability from CN1 to CN4. CN1 and CN2 contained mainly Ta tumors whereas CN3 and CN4 were dominated by T1 tumors. The classes showed different distribution of mutations in known cancer genes, including *TP53*, which was mostly mutated in CN4 tumors, and *FGFR3*, which was predominantly mutated in CN1 and CN2 tumors. The copy number subtypes were associated with PFS with CN4 tumors, i.e., the tumors with the highest CNA burden, showing the worst prognosis. CNAs were also assessed in the UROMOL2021 study using SNP arrays (Lindskrog et al. 2021). Tumors were stratified into three genomic classes (GC1–3) of equal size based on increasing CNA burden. A higher chromosomal instability was associated with worse PFS, also when restricting the analysis to tumors with high clinical risk scores, highlighting the importance of genomic instability on disease aggressiveness.

13.4 Proteomic Subtypes

In addition to genomic and transcriptomic subtypes, studies identifying subtypes using immunohistochemistry staining or high-throughput proteomics have also been performed. As previously described, the mRNA LundTax classifier classifies tumors according to the immunohistochemistry-adjusted tumor cell phenotypes (Sjödahl et al. 2017; Marzouka et al. 2018). Prior to this, the group defined a histology and immunohistochemistry-based classification scheme to identify the original RNA-based subtypes (Sjödahl et al. 2013) and demonstrated that an independent cohort of 167 T1 tumors could be classified into the major urobasal, genomically unstable and squamous cell carcinoma like subtypes using only nine immunohistochemistry-markers with subtype-specific expression

(Patschan et al. 2015). The application of limited immunohistochemistry markers may ease the implementation of molecular subtyping in routine clinical practice, as it could potentially be added to the standard pathological evaluation of tumors.

Advancing to high-throughput proteomic profiling, Stroggilos et al. performed liquid chromatography-tandem mass spectrometry (LC-MS/MS) analysis of 98 and 19 patients with NMIBC and MIBC, respectively (Stroggilos et al. 2020). Consensus clustering of protein expression from 1309 proteins identified three NMIBC proteomic subtypes (NPS1–3). NPS1 included most T1 and high-grade tumors and the protein expression profiles resembled the 19 MIBC cases, whereas NPS3 was enriched for Ta and low-grade tumors. NPS1 tumors were characterized by enrichment of basal markers, lamina propria components and low levels of proteins that facilitate cell-basal membrane and cell-cell attachment. NPS2 shared basal and cell adhesion expression patterns with NPS1, but NPS2 tumors were distinguished from NPS1 by having a high expression of extracellular matrix/mesenchymal proteins. NPS3 had, amongst others, an enriched expression of proteins denoting high levels of differentiation.

Xu et al. likewise performed a proteomics analysis by LC-MS/MS in NMIBCs ($n = 45$) and MIBCs ($n = 71$) as part of an integrated DNA, RNA, protein, and phosphoproteomic characterization of bladder cancer (Xu et al. 2022). Consensus clustering of 5439 proteins was performed on NMIBC and MIBC samples combined, resulting in three subtypes (U-I, U-II, U-III). The U-I subtype was highly enriched for NMIBCs and was characterized by high protein expression of differentiation markers, FGFR3-related markers and proteins related to different metabolism pathways. The proteomic characteristics of the U-II and U-III subtypes were mainly related to proliferation and EMT, respectively. Overlapping RNA-sequencing data showed that the classes resembled different RNA-based classification systems, including the LundTax with U-I tumors being mainly classified as UroA and GU.

In 2023, Groeneveld et al. conducted an LC-MS/MS proteomic analysis of 40 MIBCs and 23 NMIBCs for which transcriptomic and genomic data was already available (Groeneveld et al. 2023). Unsupervised clustering of the 63 tumors based on filtered proteomic data (3781 proteins) identified five subtypes named uPG-A to uPG-E. The proteomics subtypes were compared with the transcriptomic UROMOL2021 subtypes and the six consensus classes of MIBC (see Chap. 14) and were characterized using the omics data. uPG-A was enriched for MIBC Ba/Sq tumors, uPG-B showed the highest level of genomic instability and higher expression of proteins related to cell cycle and DNA repair and uPG-C was related to the MIBC luminal non-specified subtype. uPG-D was enriched for UROMOL2021 class 2b and MIBC stroma-rich tumors and accordingly showed enrichment of proteins related to smooth muscle and extracellular matrix. Finally, uPG-E consisted mainly of NMIBCs classified as UROMOL2021 class 1 and 3 and showed enrichment of *FGFR3* mutations. Comparing the uPGs to the previously published proteomic subtypes, uPG-D and uPG-E were found to overlap with NPS2 and NPS3 reported by Stroggilos et al. (Stroggilos et al. 2020). For the subtypes reported by Xu et al. (Xu et al. 2022), uPG-E overlapped with a subset of U-I tumors, uPG-B overlapped with U-II tumors and uPG-A and uPG-D showed correspondence to U-III. The added prognostic value of proteomic subtypes is still unclear; however, high-throughput proteomic analysis in bladder cancer may be used to refine other existing classification schemes. Proteogenomic analysis may furthermore be used to identify subtype-specific protein markers that could potentially be targeted in clinical practice as exemplified by Groeneveld et al. (Groeneveld et al. 2023). Besides characterizing the uPG subtypes, the omics data was used to compare *FGFR3*-mutated and wild-type tumors, and TRAIL-induced apoptosis was identified as a potential treatment target for patients with *FGFR3*-mutated tumors.

13.5 Perspectives and Clinical Utility of NMIBC Subtypes

13.5.1 Moving Towards an NMIBC Consensus Classification System?

Transcriptomic subtyping in NMIBC has received increasing attention recently (Table 13.1). Most studies have developed their own classification system focusing on different subgroups of NMIBC, making this field somewhat difficult to navigate. This could be overcome to some extent by developing a consensus classification system, as has been achieved in MIBC (Kamoun et al. 2020). An advantage of reaching a consensus of NMIBC subtypes is that the subtypes could represent a common reference that new cohorts and classification systems should be compared to, to increase comparability across studies. It would have to be decided whether a NMIBC consensus classification should be performed on NMIBCs combined or within tumor stages separately, and whether all tumor biopsy features should be considered in the definition of subtypes (i.e., inclusion or exclusion of signals from stromal/immune infiltration). For reference, the consensus classification of MIBC was developed across all MIBC tumor stages (T2–4) and six previously published classification systems were applied to all available transcriptomic datasets (1750 tumors from 18 cohorts) to construct a graph network of all subtypes across all classification systems and obtain a unified consensus subtyping scheme (see Chap. 14 for further details). The accumulating number of transcriptomic studies of NMIBCs supports the concept that a similar consensus approach could be applied in the context of NMIBC.

13.5.2 Clinical Relevance of NMIBC Subtypes

The ultimate goal of tumor subtyping is to obtain an increased biological understanding of tumors that may aid clinical decision-making, which is currently based solely on clinical and pathological factors. Tumor subtypes may translate into improved risk stratification of patients, explain differences in response to treatment and lead to the identification of potential therapeutic options. Transcriptomic subtypes in NMIBC have been shown to be prognostic of progression independently of clinicopathological factors (Lindskrog et al. 2021); hence, providing prognostic value beyond the conventional clinical risk scores and tumor stage and grade. Molecular risk stratification of tumors can provide a framework for assessing tumor aggressiveness, i.e., if the tumor exhibits a high-risk molecular profile that warrants BCG treatment or early radical cystectomy. In this way, the molecular risk stratification may be used to guide optimal surveillance and additional treatment. However, the prognostic or predictive performance and the added clinical value of the different classification schemes remains to be validated prospectively in clinical trials. In addition, other prognostic biomarkers have been developed and tested, including gene expression signatures (Kim et al. 2010; Dyrskjøt et al. 2017), which might be easier to implement in the clinic with similar prognostic value (Lindskrog et al. 2021). Consequently, if the sole purpose is prognostication, molecular subtypes might not be the biomarker of choice.

Another potential clinical implication of molecular subtypes is that the clinical value of different biomarkers might be subtype dependent. The NMIBC subtypes may provide a framework for future biomarker studies, where novel biomarkers can be identified in the context of the underlying tumor biology. As discussed previously, it is challenging to assess if the different patient outcomes observed across subtypes in BCG-treated patients are due to specific subtypes responding poorly to BCG (predictive value) or due to specific subtypes having a more aggressive tumor biology than others independently of BCG treatment (prognostic value). However, identifying the risk of recurrence and progression in BCG-treated patients is also of high clinical value to, e.g., optimize surveillance programs following treatment or to test subtype-guided BCG administration in clinical trials. In this way, the true predictive value of BCG subtypes can be assessed.

13.5.3 Intra-Tumor Subtype Heterogeneity

All of the above-mentioned classification systems are based on bulk tumor data (i.e., an average measure of all cells in the analyzed tumor biopsy), although gene expression profiling of multiple tumor regions and immunohistochemistry analyses have shown that multiple different subtypes can coexist within a single tumor (Thomsen et al. 2017; Sjödahl et al. 2018). This possibility of intra-tumor heterogeneity, i.e., when different parts of a tumor display distinct molecular traits, represents a challenge for bulk tumor classification systems. Supporting this, single-nucleus RNA-sequencing of 48 human bladder tumors, of which 23 were NMIBCs, has established that some tumors exhibit large intra-tumor subtype heterogeneity, indicating that bulk subtype assignments may lack biological granularity (Lindskrog et al. 2023). Intra-tumor subtype heterogeneity may impact patient clinical outcomes (Lindskrog et al. 2023) and should therefore be considered in subtype-guided clinical trials. Overall, it should be explored whether considering tumors as a continuum of different subtypes instead of assigning a single subtype to each tumor is more appropriate—both to increase our understanding of tumor biology and improve the potential clinical utility of NMIBC subtyping.

13.5.4 Multi-Omics Subtyping

The classification systems discussed in this chapter are all based on a single omics layer. However, multi-omics subtypes may provide improved biological insights and a stronger correlation to clinical outcome compared with single layer studies. Several tools have been developed that integrate different omics layers to identify multi-omics subtypes (Mo et al. 2013; Wu et al. 2015; Subramanian et al. 2020), but none have yet been applied to data on NMIBC. There are only a few studies on NMIBC with overlapping omics layers, including Goel et al. (n = 78) (Goel et al. 2022), Hurst et al. (n = 217) (Hurst et al. 2021), and Lindskrog et al. (n = 303) (Lindskrog et al. 2021), all with overlapping RNA and DNA data. Lindskrog et al. demonstrated that an integrative DNA and RNA approach might provide an improved risk stratification compared to RNA-based subtypes, as a high degree of genomic instability, assessed by DNA analysis, was found to be associated with an increased risk of progression, also within the aggressive UROMOL2021 class 2a/b (Lindskrog et al. 2021).

13.6 Conclusion

Molecular subtyping represents an important tool for understanding and describing divergent tumor biology. So far, several subtyping schemes for NMIBC have been discovered and biologically characterized. Common features across the schemes include the presence of an infiltrated subtype, a low-risk subtype characterized mainly by high *FGFR3* activity and a high-risk subtype with pronounced cell cycle activity, frequent *TP53* alterations and a high degree of genomic instability. Most of the classes in the different schemes show luminal features; however, classes with basal characteristics have also been reported. Whether these classes are pure basal or also show luminal features is not always clear. Before proceeding to subtype-guided clinical trials, the accumulating amount of gene expression data available on NMIBCs warrants establishment of an NMIBC consensus classification system and a common nomenclature, as has been achieved in MIBC. Upcoming studies and trials will hopefully unravel an improved and joint multi-omics characterization of NMIBC subtypes, increase our knowledge of how to handle intra-tumor heterogeneity and establish the clinical utility of NMIBC subtyping.

References

Babjuk M, Burger M, Capoun O et al (2022) European Association of Urology guidelines on non-muscle-invasive bladder cancer (ta, T1, and carcinoma in situ). Eur Urol 81:75–94

Blaveri E, Simko JP, Korkola JE et al (2005) Bladder cancer outcome and subtype classification by gene expression. Clin Cancer Res 11:4044–4055

Damrauer JS, Roell KR, Smith MA et al (2021) Identification of a novel inflamed tumor microenvironment signature as a predictive biomarker of bacillus Calmette-Guérin immunotherapy in non-muscle-invasive bladder cancer. Clin Cancer Res 27:4599–4609

de Jong FC, Laajala TD, Hoedemaeker RF et al (2023) Non–muscle-invasive bladder cancer molecular subtypes predict differential response to intravesical bacillus Calmette-Guérin. Sci Transl Med 15:eabn4118

Dyrskjøt L, Kruhøffer M, Thykjaer T et al (2004) Gene expression in the urinary bladder: a common carcinoma in situ gene expression signature exists disregarding histopathological classification. Cancer Res 64:4040–4048

Dyrskjøt L, Reinert T, Algaba F et al (2017) Prognostic impact of a 12-gene progression score in non-muscle-invasive bladder cancer: a prospective multicentre validation study. Eur Urol 72:461–469

Dyrskjøt L, Thykjaer T, Kruhøffer M et al (2003) Identifying distinct classes of bladder carcinoma using microarrays. Nat Genet 33:90–96

Dyrskjøt L, Zieger K, Kruhøffer M et al (2005) A molecular signature in superficial bladder carcinoma predicts clinical outcome. Clin Cancer Res 11:4029–4036

Dyrskjøt L, Zieger K, Real FX et al (2007) Gene expression signatures predict outcome in non-muscle-invasive bladder carcinoma: a multicenter validation study. Clin Cancer Res 13:3545–3551

Goel A, Ward DG, Noyvert B et al (2022) Combined exome and transcriptome sequencing of non-muscle-invasive bladder cancer: associations between genomic changes, expression subtypes, and clinical outcomes. Genome Med 14:59

Groeneveld CS, Sanchez-Quiles V, Dufour F et al (2023) Proteogenomic characterization of bladder cancer reveals sensitivity to apoptosis induced by tumor necrosis factor-related apoptosis-inducing ligand in FGFR3-mutated tumors. Eur Urol 85:483. https://doi.org/10.1016/j.eururo.2023.05.037

Hedegaard J, Lamy P, Nordentoft I et al (2016) Comprehensive transcriptional analysis of early-stage urothelial carcinoma. Cancer Cell 30:27–42

Hurst CD, Alder O, Platt FM et al (2017) Genomic subtypes of non-invasive bladder cancer with distinct metabolic profile and female gender bias in KDM6A mutation frequency. Cancer Cell 32:701–715.e7

Hurst CD, Cheng G, Platt FM et al (2021) Stage-stratified molecular profiling of non-muscle-invasive bladder cancer enhances biological, clinical, and therapeutic insight. Cell Rep Med 2:100472

Hurst CD, Platt FM, Taylor CF, Knowles MA (2012) Novel tumor subgroups of urothelial carcinoma of the bladder defined by integrated genomic analysis. Clin Cancer Res 18:5865–5877

Kamoun A, de Reyniès A, Allory Y et al (2020) A consensus molecular classification of muscle-invasive bladder cancer. Eur Urol 77:420–433

Kates M, Matoso A, Choi W et al (2020) Adaptive immune resistance to Intravesical BCG in non-muscle invasive bladder cancer: implications for prospective BCG-unresponsive trials. Clin Cancer Res 26:882–891

Kim J-H, Tuziak T, Hu L et al (2005) Alterations in transcription clusters underlie development of bladder cancer along papillary and nonpapillary pathways. Lab Investig 85:532–549

Kim W-J, Kim E-J, Kim S-K et al (2010) Predictive value of progression-related gene classifier in primary non-muscle invasive bladder cancer. Mol Cancer 9:3

Lindgren D, Frigyesi A, Gudjonsson S et al (2010) Combined gene expression and genomic profiling define two intrinsic molecular subtypes of urothelial carcinoma and gene signatures for molecular grading and outcome. Cancer Res 70:3463–3472

Lindgren D, Liedberg F, Andersson A et al (2006) Molecular characterization of early-stage bladder carcinomas by expression profiles, FGFR3 mutation status, and loss of 9q. Oncogene 25:2685–2696

Lindskrog SV, Prip F, Lamy P et al (2021) An integrated multi-omics analysis identifies prognostic molecular subtypes of non-muscle-invasive bladder cancer. Nat Commun 12:2301

Lindskrog SV, Schmøkel SS, Nordentoft I et al (2023) Single-nucleus and spatially resolved Intratumor subtype heterogeneity in bladder cancer. Eur Urol Open Sci 51:78–88

Marzouka N-A-D, Eriksson P, Bernardo C et al (2022) The Lund molecular taxonomy applied to non-muscle-invasive urothelial carcinoma. J Mol Diagn 24:992–1008

Marzouka N-A-D, Eriksson P, Rovira C et al (2018) A validation and extended description of the Lund taxonomy for urothelial carcinoma using the TCGA cohort. Sci Rep 8:3737

Modlich O, Prisack H-B, Pitschke G et al (2004) Identifying superficial, muscle-invasive, and metastasizing transitional cell carcinoma of the bladder: use of cDNA array analysis of gene expression profiles. Clin Cancer Res 10:3410–3421

Mo Q, Wang S, Seshan VE et al (2013) Pattern discovery and cancer gene identification in integrated cancer genomic data. Proc Natl Acad Sci USA 110:4245–4250

Mor O, Nativ O, Stein A et al (2003) Molecular analysis of transitional cell carcinoma using cDNA microarray. Oncogene 22:7702–7710

Patschan O, Sjödahl G, Chebil G et al (2015) A molecular pathologic framework for risk stratification of stage T1 urothelial carcinoma. Eur Urol 68:824–832. discussion 835–6

Robertson AG, Groeneveld CS, Jordan B et al (2020) Identification of differential tumor subtypes of T1 bladder cancer. Eur Urol 78:533–537

Sanchez-Carbayo M, Socci ND, Lozano J et al (2006) Defining molecular profiles of poor outcome in

patients with invasive bladder cancer using oligonucleotide microarrays. J Clin Oncol 24:778–789
Sjödahl G, Bernardo C, Eriksson P et al (2023) Tumor biomarkers for bacillus Calmette-Guérin response: what we get is not what we want. Eur Urol Focus 9:582. https://doi.org/10.1016/j.euf.2023.03.001
Sjödahl G, Eriksson P, Liedberg F, Höglund M (2017) Molecular classification of urothelial carcinoma: global mRNA classification versus tumour-cell phenotype classification. J Pathol 242:113–125
Sjödahl G, Eriksson P, Lövgren K et al (2018) Discordant molecular subtype classification in the basal-squamous subtype of bladder tumors and matched lymph-node metastases. Mod Pathol 31:1869–1881
Sjödahl G, Lauss M, Lövgren K et al (2012) A molecular taxonomy for urothelial carcinoma. Clin Cancer Res 18:3377–3386
Sjödahl G, Lövgren K, Lauss M et al (2013) Toward a molecular pathologic classification of urothelial carcinoma. Am J Pathol 183:681–691
Song B-N, Kim S-K, Mun J-Y et al (2019) Identification of an immunotherapy-responsive molecular subtype of bladder cancer. EBioMedicine 50:238–245
Strandgaard T, Lindskrog SV, Nordentoft I et al (2022) Elevated T-cell exhaustion and urinary tumor DNA levels are associated with bacillus Calmette-Guérin failure in patients with non-muscle-invasive bladder cancer. Eur Urol 82:646. https://doi.org/10.1016/j.eururo.2022.09.008
Stroggilos R, Mokou M, Latosinska A et al (2020) Proteome-based classification of nonmuscle invasive bladder cancer. Int J Cancer 146:281–294
Subramanian I, Verma S, Kumar S et al (2020) Multi-omics data integration, interpretation, and its application. Bioinform Biol Insights 14:1177932219899051
Sweis RF, Spranger S, Bao R et al (2016) Molecular drivers of the non-T-cell-inflamed tumor microenvironment in urothelial bladder cancer. Cancer Immunol Res 4:563–568
Sylvester RJ, van der Meijden APM, Witjes JA, Kurth K (2005) Bacillus calmette-guerin versus chemotherapy for the intravesical treatment of patients with carcinoma in situ of the bladder: a meta-analysis of the published results of randomized clinical trials. J Urol 174:86–91. discussion 91–2
Tan TZ, Rouanne M, Tan KT et al (2019) Molecular subtypes of urothelial bladder cancer: results from a meta-cohort analysis of 2411 tumors. Eur Urol 75:423–432
Thomsen MBH, Nordentoft I, Lamy P et al (2017) Comprehensive multiregional analysis of molecular heterogeneity in bladder cancer. Sci Rep 7:11702
Wild PJ, Herr A, Wissmann C et al (2005) Gene expression profiling of progressive papillary noninvasive carcinomas of the urinary bladder. Clin Cancer Res 11:4415–4429
Wu D, Wang D, Zhang MQ, Gu J (2015) Fast dimension reduction and integrative clustering of multi-omics data using low-rank approximation: application to cancer molecular classification. BMC Genomics 16:1022
Xu N, Yao Z, Shang G et al (2022) Integrated proteogenomic characterization of urothelial carcinoma of the bladder. J Hematol Oncol 15:76

14 Molecular Subtypes of Muscle-Invasive Bladder Cancer

Gottfrid Sjödahl

Abstract

An important tool for understanding the biology of muscle-invasive bladder cancer (MIBC) is molecular subtype classification. Molecular subtypes are qualitatively distinct biological entities that can be identified by molecular analysis of tumor tissue. This chapter describes how such entities have been discovered and described for MIBC and gives an overview of the characteristics that the luminal, basal/squamous, neuroendocrine-like, and other tumor categories possess. Special attention is given to the MIBC Consensus subtypes since they represent a joint effort by all researchers in the field to define a common reference against which all other classification systems can be compared. In addition to outlining the history of MIBC subtype discovery, this chapter also attempts to inform the reader of some understudied aspects of subtype classification. Examples of such aspects include discussion of whether there is a need for further MIBC subtype discovery, to what extent intra-tumor heterogeneity affects classification, and what the advantages of IHC- versus RNA-based classification are.

The chapter comes to the following conclusions: (a) Although there is room for minor modifications, subtype discovery in MIBC is largely completed, (b) Testing the clinical utility of MIBC subtyping is an area of intense ongoing work, (c) The causal origins of the molecular subtypes have not been sufficiently studied and remain largely unknown.

Keywords

MIBC · Molecular subtypes · Tumor classification · Luminal · Basal · Consensus

14.1 Introduction

This chapter will describe the progress that has been achieved in the first decade of research on molecular subtype classification of muscle-invasive bladder cancer (MIBC), from around 2012 to the current day. The purpose is to provide insight into the evolution of this research field over the years and to summarize the current state of knowledge in MIBC subtyping. Thus, each of the early subtype discovery studies will be briefly summarized, followed by an account of how collaboration between many research groups led to the 2019 publication of unified MIBC Consensus subtypes (Kamoun et al. 2020). The chapter will also discuss MIBC subtyping after the Consensus publication and discuss the role of immunohisto-

G. Sjödahl (✉)
Department of Translational Medicine, Lund University, Lund, Sweden
e-mail: gottfrid.sjodahl@med.lu.se

M. A. Knowles, L. Dyrskjøt (eds.), *Biology of Bladder Cancer*,
https://doi.org/10.1007/978-3-031-68505-7_14

chemistry (IHC)-based classification in resolving the influence that stromal content and intra-tumor heterogeneity exert on classification. Only studies aiming for a comprehensive transcriptomic tumor classification are discussed, but these can include both *subtype discovery studies* and *subtype application studies* in which a subtype classifier is applied in order to further characterize subtypes or to achieve clinical translation. There are infinite possibilities of grouping tumors into categories by the expression of any number of specific genes or signatures. What sets molecular subtypes apart from all other ways of grouping tumors is this unbiased and comprehensive approach which differs from a mere grouping of tumors by some chosen molecular signatures, e.g., epithelial to mesenchymal transition (EMT) or cell proliferation. This carries the implication that true molecular subtypes are not weighted toward what is currently considered important in cell biology or medicine. Instead, they should represent the single set of unbiased disease categories that exist objectively, now and in the future, regardless of our current knowledge of the disease and the current treatment of patients. To make it easier to follow, this chapter will use a specific typography when discussing subtype classes of specific classification systems writing the subtype name with capitalized initial letter between single quotation marks. For example, "Luminal" would refer to a category within a specific classification system, whereas luminal refers to the general characteristic without reference to a specific classification system.

14.2 Comprehensive Pre-Consensus Classification Systems

In the first decade of microarray technology (ca. 2000–2010), early transcriptomic cohort studies on bladder cancer performed hierarchical clustering of tumors from bladder cancer patient cohorts (Sanchez-Carbayo et al. 2002; Dyrskjøt et al. 2003; Blaveri et al. 2005; Lindgren et al. 2010). Although in retrospect we can see that these studies identified tumor clusters that we now recognize as different molecular subtypes, too few MIBC tumors were included to robustly identify them as such. Most of these early studies also presented single clustering solutions which are inherently unstable and therefore dependent on arbitrary data pre-processing steps. From 2012 on, starting with work from Lund University, Sweden (Sjödahl et al. 2012), studies included more tumors and subtype identification was becoming based on co-clustering frequencies rather than a single hierarchical clustering solution. This was shown to lead to stable identification of subtypes that could be reproduced in independent datasets and that were robust to preprocessing parameters. The main subtype discovery studies until the MIBC Consensus publication will be described below. Key features of these studies are also summarized in Table 14.1 in the order of granularity, i.e. number of identified subtypes, from the most coarse to the most detailed classification.

The study by Damrauer and colleagues, a group based in the University of North Carolina (UNC), combined four previously available data sets into a meta-dataset which was clustered to identify two main categories termed "Luminal" and "Basal" (Damrauer et al. 2014). Similarities with the intrinsic subtypes of breast cancer were highlighted and a 47-gene nearest-centroid classifier termed BASE47 was devised that could classify an external cohort as "Luminal" and "Basal." The main characteristic of the "Luminal" class was high expression of a set of genes involved in luminal urothelial differentiation, whereas the "Basal" cluster showed low expression of this signature. Furthermore, a subset of the basal cluster was proposed to be claudin-low, another breast cancer phenotype defined as having undergone EMT with low expression of epithelial markers such as tight junction components CLDN3, −4, and − 7. This category corresponds to a double-negative (absence of both luminal and basal urothelial differentiation) phenotype. Thus, the "Basal" class identified by the original UNC BASE47 classifier included both basal and such double-negative cases. In this sense it rather identifies non-luminal cancers, those lacking expression of the luminal urothelial differentia-

Table 14.1 An overview of the pre-consensus molecular classification systems

Classification system	Year of publication	Discovery cohort (n, MIBCs/total)	Number of MIBC subtypes	Subtypes	Reference
UNC	2014	Meta-dataset ($n = 262$)[a]	2	"Luminal," "basal"	(Damrauer et al. 2014)
MDA	2014	MDACC ($n = 73$)	3	"Luminal," "basal," "TP53-like"	(Choi et al. 2014)
GSC	2017	Vancouver-NAC ($n = 223$)	4	"Luminal," "luminal-infiltrated," "basal," "Claudin-low"[b]	(Seiler et al. 2017)
TCGA	2014, 2018	TCGA ($n = 408$)[c]	5	"Luminal-papillary," "luminal-infiltrated," "luminal," "basal-squamous," "neuronal"	(TCGA 2014; Robertson 2018)
LundTax	2012, 2017	Lund2012 ($n = 93/308$), Lund2017 ($n = 243/307$)[d]	5–7[e]	"Urothelial-like A/B/C," "Genomically unstable," "basal/squamous," mesenchymal-like," small-cell/neuroendocrine-like"	(Sjödahl, 2012, Sjödahl 2017)
CIT-curie	2014, 2014	CIT ($n = 92/198$)	7	"MC 1–7," "basal-like," "non-basal-like"	(Rebouissou et al. 2014; Biton et al. 2014)

[a]The UNC Meta-dataset combined data from four public microarray studies
[b]GSC subtypes were defined by a combination of UNC and TCGA systems
[c]A first analysis of 129 tumors was later expanded to the full 408 tumors
[d]LundTax was first defined in both NMIBC and MIBC, then adapted in a mainly MIBC cohort
[e]LundTax has 5 main subtypes of which urothelial-like tumors are subdivided into UroA, UroB, and UroC

tion signature. Since this work was published, several studies have confirmed that luminal versus non-luminal is the first main "split" seen within the hierarchy of bladder cancer molecular classification and that MIBC cohorts are usually divided about evenly between these two categories. The BASE47 classifier captures this first split and, accordingly, several core luminal differentiation markers (e.g., *GATA3*, *PPARG*, *ADIRF*, *UPK1A*, *UPK2*, *SPINK*, and *TBX2*) are included among the genes positively selecting for the UNC "Luminal" subtype. Since the "Basal" subtype includes both basal and double-negative cases, the positive selecting genes for the UNC "Basal" are not canonical basal epithelial genes like *KRT5*, *KRT14*, *CDH3*, or *CD44*. Instead, several genes expressed by stromal cells or by more generally stem-like cancer cells fill the role of being anticorrelated with the luminal differentiation signature in the BASE47 classifier, since these were more uniformly expressed across all non-luminal cases. Thus, the two-tiered "Luminal"–"Basal" dichotomy proposed by the UNC group identifies the most fundamental split in bladder cancer expression data but is insufficient to describe the residual diversity, particularly within the non-luminal half of MIBC. Another very similar division into basal and differentiated tumors was proposed several years later by Mo and colleagues, replicating this main division of MIBC and showing clearly that the luminal, more differentiated cancers are associated with better patient outcomes (Mo et al. 2018).

In the MD Anderson Cancer Center (MDA) classification system, published in 2014 by Choi and colleagues, subtyping is performed on the three-tier level, again identifying clear "Luminal" and "Basal" clusters along with a third cluster termed "TP53-like" (Choi et al. 2014). This third cluster was named based on pathway analysis pointing to a wild-type p53 signature present in these tumors. Upon comparison with other classification systems, it was later clarified that this subtype consists mainly of highly stroma- and immune-cell containing tumor samples. Thus, no specific association with *TP53* alterations or p53 activity in the cancer cells has been documented for this subtype which is thought to be mainly defined by signals from non-cancer cells. The study by Choi and colleagues also identified key transcriptional regulators of their "Luminal" (*PPARG*) and "Basal" (*TP63*) subtypes and suggested therapeutic opportunities in the form of differential sensitivity to chemotherapy. The work by the MDA group resulted in a nearest-centroid classifier which allowed the subtypes to be extensively compared to previous as well as subsequent subtyping efforts.

The first study to split MIBC into four subtypes was the initial 2014 analysis by The Cancer Genome Atlas Research Network (TCGA), based on RNA-seq data from 129 tumors (TCGA 2014). Two of the four identified clusters (Clusters I and II) were of a luminal character of which the first was termed "Papillary," showing an enrichment of *FGFR3* expression and genomic alterations, while the second expressed *ERBB2* but lower levels of *FGFR3*. The third cluster was clearly basal-like, and comparison to other tumor types identified strong similarity to basal-like breast cancer, but also to squamous-cell carcinoma of the head and neck. Thus, the label "Basal-squamous" was used for this cluster. The fourth cluster consisted of non-luminal tumors with lower but variable expression of basal keratins and the basal-expressed oncogenic receptor *EGFR* and less squamous histological features. The TCGA later updated the RNA-based classification to have 5 different classes, as described in detail below, but between 2014 and 2019, several studies referred to this original classification which therefore became influential in the field.

Another four-tier classification of MIBC has been proposed in the GSC (Genomic subtype classifier) system, originally defined by Seiler and colleagues (Seiler et al. 2017). However, the GSC subtypes are different from other pre-consensus classification systems in that they were not defined by performing unsupervised clustering on the discovery cohort. Instead, the cohort studied by Seiler et al. was classified according to other known systems at the time, combining them in order to maximize outcome differences in the chemotherapy treated versus comparator (TCGA) cohort. The four GSC classes were defined by first assigning tumors to a "Luminal" or "Basal" type according to the UNC BASE47 classifier. "Luminal" tumors were then further split according to the initial four TCGA subtypes such that TCGA Class II tumors were termed "luminal-infiltrated" and TCGA class I, III, and IV tumors were termed only "Luminal." Tumors classified as "Basal" by BASE47 were further subdivided by applying a separate "Claudin-low" classifier which had been published a year earlier by the group at UNC as an extension to their "Basal"-subtype (Kardos et al. 2016). In subsequent studies, a neuroendocrine classifier has been used in conjunction with the GSC classifier to also identify NE-like tumors (Grivas et al. 2020). Thus, the GSC classification was identified by sequential application of several UNC and TCGA classifiers for the purpose of stratifying therapeutic responses, and quite different subtypes would probably have been obtained if they had been derived from the discovery cohort in an unsupervised manner.

Four years after the initial TCGA analysis an updated study on 408 tumors was published (Robertson 2018). Part of this major multi-omic MIBC characterization effort was a subtype identification analysis performed by non-negative matrix factorization on RNA-sequencing (RNA-seq) profiles. This represents a technological advance, since before the TCGA projects, studies had been based on microarray technology and not RNA-seq. The result was identification of five clusters which represented a substantial refinement compared to the previous TCGA (I-IV) clusters. The "Luminal-papillary" (previous Class I) and "Luminal-infiltrated" (previous Class II) were complemented on the luminal side by a third, small, cluster termed only "Luminal." This subtype demonstrates an interesting combination of high luminal urothelial expression, along with strong signals of smooth muscle and myofibroblast cells, but low signal of infiltrating B- and T-lymphocytes. The separation of high stromal- but low immune-signals is of particular interest because signals from various non-cancer cell types can otherwise often be artificially positively correlated in cohorts due to variation in sample purity (Wang et al. 2018). The "Luminal"

TCGA subtype had tumor purity scores in between those of "Luminal-papillary" and "Luminal-infiltrated." The updated TCGA analysis also identified the classical "Basal-Squamous" cluster defined by expression of basal keratins *KRT5* and *KRT14*, and a fifth, small, cluster of non-luminal tumors with expression of genes indicative of neuroendocrine biology. Based on the relative upregulation of genes involved in differentiation of neurons this cluster was termed "Neuronal." However, no clear features of nerve cell biology have been validated in these cancer cells and this subtype is now known to overlap with a previously described tumor cluster characterized by distinct neuroendocrine features (Biton et al. 2014; Aine et al. 2015).

As in TCGA, the Lund Taxonomy (LundTax) also classifies MIBC into five main subtypes, of which two are luminal and three are non-luminal (Sjödahl et al. 2017). Being the first molecular subtype classification of urothelial carcinoma (UC), LundTax was originally defined in a mixed non-muscle invasive bladder cancer (NMIBC) and MIBC cohort of 308 tumors (Sjödahl et al. 2012). To ensure that the LundTax classification was appropriate for classification of MIBCs, a follow-up analysis of RNA and matched IHC-profiling data from 307 consecutive tumors treated with radical cystectomy was later performed, and it is this later study that is the basis for the current version of LundTax (Sjödahl et al. 2017). The main difference between LundTax and the other classification systems is its intention to isolate and capture signals from the cancer cells only, minimizing the influence of cells in the tumor environment in classification. This difference is rooted in a viewpoint of the Lund group that the cancer cells are the carriers of the molecular subtype as a property, i.e. that cancer cells can have different molecular subtypes but that adjacent non-cancer cells cannot. In practice, this distinction was achieved by performing both conventional clustering of RNA-profiles and a quite extensive IHC-based profiling of the cancer cells. By having both data types for each tumor, the RNA-profiles with strong stroma signals could still obtain a cancer-cell based subtype label by IHC, which was then used to train an RNA-based classifier. Thus, the earliest version of the LundTax classification that relied only on clustering of RNA-profiles had an "Infiltrated" category of tumors, whereas the current LundTax classifiers can assign subtypes based on the cancer cells' phenotype even for heavily infiltrated/stoma-rich tumors. Compared to the TCGA classification, LundTax identifies two main luminal categories (three in TCGA) and three non-luminal categories (two in TCGA). The two luminal LundTax subtypes are termed "Urothelial-like" (Uro) and "Genomically Unstable" (GU). The "Uro" subtype includes tumors with luminal urothelial differentiation that have a maintained urothelial tissue stratification. For most of these tumors, basal markers like KRT5 are positive in cells adjacent to the basal lamina separating the tumor from adjacent stroma, as would be seen in the normal urothelium. The "Uro" subtype also harbors the *FGFR3*-mutated and overexpressing tumors, and the tumors express *TP63*, in many cases along with anterior *HOXA*/*HOXB* genes (*HOXA2–6* and *HOXB2–8*) indicative of a stratified urothelial cell identity (Eriksson et al. 2015). The "GU" subtype expresses the luminal urothelial differentiation signature equally highly as "Uro" tumors but lacks the cell polarization and tissue stratification into basal and intermediate layers. In the "GU" subtype, basal markers are typically negative in cells adjacent to basal lamina, *FGFR3* is wild-type and not expressed, and *TP63* expression is lost in the majority of cases. The average proliferation rate is higher in "GU" than in "Uro" tumors, and cell divisions are not localized in relation to the tumor-stroma interface but occur randomly throughout the tumor parenchyma. Among the non-luminal tumors, LundTax distinguishes "Basal/squamous" (Ba/Sq) and "Small-cell/Neuroendocrine-like" (Sc/NE) subtypes, very similar to the "Basal-Squamous" and "Neuronal" TCGA subtypes. In addition to these, LundTax also identifies a "Mesenchymal-like" (Mes-like) cancer-cell subtype. In truly "Mes-like" cases, the cancer cells show loss of epithelial markers, e.g. EPCAM and CDH1, and express EMT-markers such as cytoplasmic VIM and nuclear ZEB2. However, any positive identifying marker for "Mes-like" tumors is also expressed in stromal cell types like myofibroblasts present in the tumor environment, making "Mes-like" a very challenging subtype to identify by bulk RNA-profiling. However, by applying IHC, Mes-like cases can be readily identified as a distinct, albeit rare, phenotypic entity.

The MIBC classification work at Institut Curie in Paris on tumors from the French Cartes d'Identité des Tumeurs (CIT-Curie) was heavily focused on identifying and characterizing a "Basal-like" subtype which was shown to be driven by EGFR signaling (Rebouissou et al. 2014). Several non-basal tumor clusters were also identified which were characterized by expression of various independent components in the multi-dimensional expression data reflecting content of non-cancer cells like myofibroblasts, lymphocytes, and early response/inflammatory-cells. Regarding expression in the cancer cells, an identified neuroendocrine signature of 122 genes was associated with a specific "Neuroendocrine" tumor cluster. Furthermore, a clear luminal urothelial differentiation signature was upregulated in non-basal tumors where it was regulated by strong PPARG activity correlating with increased copy number at chromosome 3p25.2 (Biton et al. 2014).

14.3 The Hierarchy of MIBC Subtype Classifiers Evolve to Meet Clinical Needs

Having analyzed all pre-consensus classification systems, the first thing that stands out is that despite being generated in different datasets, they correspond well to each other. In fact, the main difference between any of them is the granularity, i.e. the number of subtypes that they describe. This was also shown to be the case in an analysis of the biological characteristics underlying UNC, MDA, and Lund classification in an early version of the TCGA data set with 234 tumors (Aine et al. 2015). Another feature of all the initial MIBC subtyping systems is that they were generated using similar methodology. In each study, whole transcriptome data from a cohort of MIBC tumors was obtained. The data was then quantile normalized, variance filtered, and subjected to bootstrap- or consensus hierarchical clustering.

Although the MIBC classification systems correspond well to each other and are derived using similar methods, there are still different opinions on what the principles and purpose of classification should be (Höglund 2023). Some researchers focus only on achieving the grouping of the tumors that best captures the variation in measured biological states, arguing that subtypes exist as independent entities regardless of how we treat patients. Other researchers have a more applied, or instrumental, view that subtype classification should be developed to be a useful tool in the current clinical context. An assumption shared by all in the field of MIBC subtyping is that at some point, when it is decided how tumors should be classified, we will stop performing subtype discovery on every new cohort of MIBC tumors, and instead move toward prospective application of classifiers. For clinical use, the applicability of classifiers to individual tumor tissue samples taken during cystoscopy or transurethral resection is a requirement, since a result would need to be available within days after the patient's diagnostic procedure or it would delay treatment. The subtype classifiers that were used in the early subtyping studies used nearest-centroid classifiers which allow subtype classes from one study to be applied to another similar cohort. The centroid-based classifiers can be considered a first-generation of classifiers that had the drawback of needing to be applied to entire cohorts. Currently, centroid-based classifiers are being replaced by single-sample subtype predictors that assign subtype to a sample based on several hundred expression features internal to that sample.

14.4 The Consensus Classification of MIBC

In 2015, an initiative to reach a consensus in MIBC molecular subtype classification was initiated, and the first of three consensus meetings was held in Madrid, Spain. In the resulting consensus publication, all available MIBC subtype classifiers were cross applied to all available transcriptomic datasets (Kamoun et al. 2020). The classification results were constructed as a graph network of all subtypes of all classification systems, which was then analyzed by a Markov clustering algorithm to detect cliques, i.e. sub-structures of the graph network that correspond to subtype clusters. Six consensus subtypes were identified by this method, three luminal-like ("Luminal-papillary," LumP; "Luminal-Non Specified," LumNS; and "Luminal Unstable," LumU), one subtype not defined by the cancer cells ("Stroma-rich"), and two non-luminal types ("Basal-squamous," Ba/Sq; and "Neuroendocrine-like," NE-like). The identification of these consensus subtypes was followed by a full molecular and clinical characterization of the significant features for each subtype. The overlap of each consensus subtype with corresponding subtypes from the contributing classification systems is shown schematically in Fig. 14.1. Below follows a summary of the main features of each subtype.

Consensus "Luminal-papillary" tumors are most clearly characterized by genomic activation of *FGFR3* by mutation and copy number loss of *CDKN2A*. Other genomic alterations that frequently occur in this subtype are mutations in *KDM6A* and *STAG2*, both of which are often found in early-stage cancers. "LumP" tumors have the lowest average levels of both stromal and immune signatures, they often show papillary morphology, and they express *RARG* and *RXRA* regulons, suggesting activity of these retinoid receptors. The tumor stage tends to be T2 rather than T3/T4, and the prognosis of patients with LumP tumors is favorable. Taken together, LumP is a well-defined luminal-like subtype corresponding to TCGA "Luminal-papillary" and LundTax "Urothelial-like A," and it is the MIBC subtype that is most similar to NMIBC.

As indicated by the name, "Luminal Non-Specified" is the least well characterized of the MIBC consensus subtypes. Like "LumP," it shows expression of luminal urothelial differentiation signatures and is enriched for cases with concomitant carcinoma in situ, but this analysis was based on very few LumNS cases. At the genomic level, *ARID1A* and, more significantly, *ELF3* mutations were frequent in this subtype whereas mutational activation of traditional UC oncogenes such as *FGFR3*, *PIK3CA*, and *ERBB2* was rare. Single-copy loss of *CDKN2A* was frequent, but not homozygous deletions as seen in LumP, suggesting that LumP but not LumNS tumors progress through p16^{INK4A}/p14^{ARF} loss of function. Copy number gains of *ERBB2* as well as chromosome 3p25 (*PPARG*, *RAF1*) were also frequent, but high-level amplification of these loci reached higher frequency in the Luminal-unstable subtype. So far, there exist no markers that reliably identify this subtype from the other luminal subtypes by histology, immunostaining, or genomic analysis. The unclear definition of LumNS reflects that it corresponds to three relatively poorly defined subtypes in their original classification systems (TCGA, "Luminal," LundTax "UroC," and CIT-Curie "MC2"). These classes also had lower agreement scores between

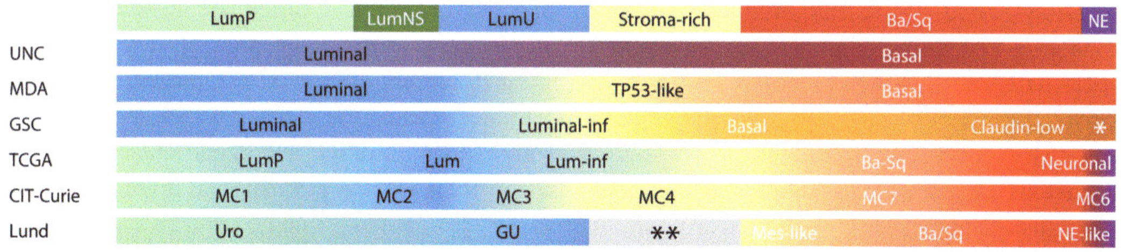

Fig. 14.1 Schematic showing the approximate overlap between the MIBC consensus subtypes (shown in top row; width of each group reflects the subtype proportions in MIBC) and the various disease entities described by the constituent classification systems. * In subsequent studies a neuroendocrine classifier has been applied in conjunction with the GSC classifier. ** The consensus "Stroma-rich" subtype does not have a counterpart in the Lund classification, and "Stroma-rich" tumors could be of any Lund subtype

them than the constituent classes of the other consensus subtypes. It remains to be seen if future studies will be able to consistently root this subtype in biology at different levels or if it will remain as a subtype defined almost entirely by its transcriptomic profile.

"Luminal Unstable" is an interesting category of tumors because it correlates specifically only with two original subtypes (LundTax "Genomically unstable" and CIT-Curie "MC3"). These subtypes form the core of the "LumU" clique in the graph clustering analysis together with the more general luminal/differentiated subtypes of the UNC, Baylor, and MDA classification systems. According to the TCGA classification, however, "LumU" is about evenly split between "Luminal-papillary" versus "Luminal" and "Luminal-infiltrated," meaning that this subtype has no clear counterpart in the TCGA classification. Still, at the molecular level of the cancer cells, "LumU" has a quite distinct profile. In addition to expression of the luminal urothelial differentiation signature, the cancer cells also have a strikingly high proliferation rate, and "LumU" tumors are of the highest histological grade. Thus, the expression of factors like *FOXA1*, *GATA3*, and *PPARG*, or even terminal differentiation markers such as *KRT20* and uroplakins, all associated with differentiation in normal urothelium, does not imply a highly differentiated state in malignancy. "LumU" tumors have a high total burden of both mutations and copy number alterations, indicating that they have undergone genomic instability. This subtype generally has more genomic alterations, and it is also enriched for several specific alterations including *TP53* (loss, mutation), *RB1* (loss, mutation), *ERBB2* (amplification, mutation), 3p25 (*PPARG*, *RAF1*) amplification, 6p22 (*SOX4*, *E2F3*) amplification, and *ERCC2* mutation. Most likely, these specifically enriched alterations are either causally involved in generating this specific cancer-cell state (early tumorigenic events) or they provide a strong fitness advantage in the evolutionary bottleneck that follows an episode of high genomic instability. Due to the high number of genomic alterations found in "LumU" tumors they may be expected to be relatively responsive to various therapeutic approaches. In such a complex genomic background, it will be a challenge to isolate which effects are dependent on the phenotypic state, i.e. general for all "LumU" tumors, and which are a consequence of their complex and frequent genomic alterations. Matching data on phenotypic and genomic levels will therefore be key to further studies aiming to increase the biological understanding of this molecular subtype of UC.

In any bladder cancer cohort subjected to molecular profiling, some tumor samples will be relatively pure, i.e. contain a higher proportion of cancer cells, while others will have less cancer cells and more of other cell types present in the tumor environment. It is therefore expected that any subtype discovery studies that rely on unsupervised clustering will identify clusters associated with signals from non-cancer cells (i.e., "infiltrated" clusters). In the MIBC consensus, such clusters from each classification system collectively formed the "Stroma-rich" consensus subtype, which is thus not defined by any characteristics of the cancer cells. Indeed, "Stroma-rich" tumors show intermediate frequencies of specific genomic alterations, which may be generally slightly underestimated due to the decreased power to detect mutations with low allele frequency in DNA samples of lower purity. However, it is evident from the analysis of RNA signatures that for almost all core "Stroma-rich" tumors, the cancer cells are luminal-like in nature. To understand why this is the case, it is necessary to consider the contrast of stromal- and immune-signals between infiltrated and non-infiltrated clusters. For infiltrated tumors to "break out" and form a specific cluster, the difference in such signals needs to be sufficiently large. If it is not, then these differences would instead remain as residual variance within the other clusters. For luminal tumors (e.g., "LumU" and in particular "LumP"), the average level of stromal- and immune-signals is very low, leading to high contrast compared to "Stroma-rich" tumors. For non-luminal subtypes the average level of stromal- and immune-signals is higher which explains why the "Stroma-rich" subtype does not "pull in" as many tumors of those subtypes. In fact, the "Basal-Squamous" subtype has almost as high average infiltration scores as the "Stroma-rich" subtype has. However, given a sufficiently low-purity sample, even a Basal-Squamous tumor would probably at some point become classified as Stroma-rich. While bulk transcriptomic profiling is not an optimal technique for understanding the complexity of the cell types present in the tumor, some interesting differences were still observed. Signatures of endothelial cells, dendritic cells, and B-cells stand out as particularly high in the "Stroma-rich" subtype. This contrasts with signatures of cytotoxic T cells, NK-cells, and monocytic lineage cells, which are not particularly high. It would be desirable for future work to better characterize the cell type composition of the tumor environment for each of the cancer-cell intrinsic subtypes as well as that of tumors classified as "Stroma-rich." To reach this goal it will be necessary to understand when a tumor's bulk RNA-profile is naturally stroma-rich due to its intrinsic biology, and when it is Stroma rich due to a disproportionate inclusion of non-cancer cells in the tissue piece used for RNA extraction. An answer would therefore likely require carefully matched bulk- and in situ profiling of intact tumors that have not been shredded into unoriented pieces by transurethral resection.

The "Basal-squamous" consensus subtype has probably caused least debate, and researchers in the field agreed early upon a cancer cell-based definition of this subtype (GATA3$^-$FOXA1$^-$KRT5$^+$KRT14$^+$, see (Lerner et al. 2016)). Tumors of this subtype have switched to varying degrees from a urothelial toward a more squamous-like cell identity. This involves heavy upregulation of a keratinization signature that is expressed in squamous epithelia such as the oral mucosa or keratinocytes of the skin. The positive selection markers KRT5 and KRT14 used in the early definition are positive to varying degrees also in the basal cells of the urothelium, but most genes in the keratinization signature that identifies this subtype are restricted to squamous epithelia and not expressed in normal urothelium. Thus, this subtype is not completely described by the term basal-like, but should be seen on a more fundamental level as having adopted a squamous differentiation state. On the other hand, the subtype shares more features with basal urothelial cells than with intermediate- or umbrella cells, including central biologic determinants such as expression of EGFR (Rebouissou et al. 2014). The squamous-like appearance of Ba/Sq tumors under the microscope is often, but not always, apparent and the subtype is heavily enriched for squamous variant histology. Some studies have found a more balanced sex ratio for this subtype compared to the strong male predominance that is generally seen among UC patients. This finding further suggests a role for squamous metaplasia in the origins of this subtype, since this entity is more often found in the bladder of women than in men. The Ba/Sq subtype has high proliferation rate, relatively high mutation burden and genomic complexity, and it is associated with a poor prognosis. However, the poor outcome of patients with this subtype is probably in part due to a more advanced stage at presentation, since the prognostic difference diminishes in more narrowly selected cohorts (Kollberg et al. 2019; Morera et al. 2020). In line with its complex genomic profile, alterations of *TP53* are frequent along with losses of tumor suppressors *RB1* and *CDKN2A* which are about equally prevalent in a mutually exclusive fashion. The frequency of *FGFR3* alterations is intermediate compared to the high frequency and absence in "LumP" and "LumU," respectively. It is unclear if the intermediate frequency of *FGFR3* alterations has any implications for the origin of the Ba/Sq subtype which occurs nearly exclusively in MIBC. It is also not known to what extent the function and/or actionability of *FGFR3* alterations depends on whether it occurs in a "LumP" or in a "Ba/Sq" context.

The second non-luminal molecular subtype of MIBC identified by the Consensus classification was termed "Neuroendocrine-like." Like the "Ba/Sq" subtype, "NE-like" is enriched for the corresponding variant histology (small-cell or neuroendocrine variants) and shares several characteristics of neuroendocrine carcinomas, e.g., very high proliferation index, and frequent alterations in *TP53* and *RB1*, often in conjunction. At the genomic level, the amplification at

6p22 that includes *SOX4* and *E2F3* also stands out as a frequent alteration and, although a joint origin has not been proposed, the NE-like and LumU subtypes share many genomic features. In terms of gene expression, signatures upregulated in this subtype have been published and include regulatory factors *SOX2*, *SOX21* and neuroendocrine markers *CHGA*, *SYP*, and *ENO2* (Aine et al. 2015; Batista da Costa et al. 2019). Among classifiers, the NE-like Consensus subtype clearly overlaps with distinct subtypes of the TCGA, LundTax, and CIT-Curie systems with only minor differences in how inclusive the classification is. The Consensus "NE-like" subtype is therefore in high agreement with all other classifiers for the identification of this molecularly distinct entity which captures nearly all MIBCs with neuroendocrine histology in addition to some tumors with a conventional UC histology.

14.5 Are There More MIBC Molecular Subtypes to Be Discovered?

The largest studies contributing to MIBC subtyping have studied around 300–400 tumors (Robertson 2018; Sjödahl et al. 2017) and the agreement between these and other classification systems is captured well by the Consensus system. The unification in the Consensus makes it very unlikely that either of the underlying classifications is fundamentally wrong, i.e. that they would identify subtypes that don't exist. In this situation, any existing molecular subtype not captured by these systems will either be so rare that it went unrecognized by all previous studies (e.g., estimated below 10 cases among 300–400 which equals below 2–3% prevalence in MIBC) or that it will represent further sub-splits of the already known subtypes. Therefore, a new hypothetical subtype discovery study using a cohort of over a thousand MIBC tumors would likely find an additional small cluster with a yet undescribed expression profile perhaps representing a rare pathologic entity. This would be a discovery of one new molecular subtype but, since it is so rare, the impact of this discovery would be limited. Such a study would also have power to split up existing subtypes into sub-clusters based on the residual variance present within current subtypes. However, new sub-clusters would most likely not be qualitatively distinct but would represent subdivisions based on a cut-point on some signature with a continuous distribution within that subtype. It may, for example, split "LumP"/"Uro" into high and low proliferation subsets or it may split Ba/Sq by the amount of immune infiltration. Such divisions should not be considered new molecular subtypes since they are captured without error by the current classification systems. By applying existing classifiers rather than performing new subtype discovery, transcriptomic data can be efficiently distilled into categories while avoiding the creation of new terminology for every dataset that is analyzed.

By similar reasoning, it also follows that specific clinical subsets of MIBC do not require new subtype discovery. Thus, tumors of stage T2 are clinically, on average, rather different from stage T3–4 tumors, but since they are a sub-category of MIBCs they can be handled by the existing classification systems without need for their own specific subtypes. The same holds true for various patient populations, e.g., MIBC populations that are eligible or ineligible for some therapeutic intervention. A recent example of the latter scenario is a subtyping study for patients treated with neoadjuvant immune checkpoint inhibitors (ICIs) (Robertson et al. 2023). In this study, new subtype discovery was performed based on the idea that subtypes identified in tumors from patients receiving a treatment would better capture response to that treatment. However, the molecular subtype classification of pre-treatment MIBC tissue samples is unaffected by the patients' subsequent treatment. Furthermore, there is nothing that suggests that current MIBC classification was inadequate to apply to the studied cohorts. Importantly, the study did compare its new stratification scheme to several existing systems including the MIBC consensus, making it easier to interpret the results in this context.

Another interesting post-consensus subtype classification study made a case for de novo subtype identification among biopsies of bladder cancer metastases (Nakauma-González et al. 2022). Although disseminated UC disease is directly derived from MIBC, it is conceivable that discrete disease states found only among metastatic lesions could exist. The study identified one cluster that differed from the traditional biology of MIBC subtyping described in this chapter. The novel cluster was negative for all investigated conventional MIBC signatures but was enriched in patients having previously received chemotherapy. While treatment-refractory lesions are both interesting and important to describe, such a phenotype seen only in post-treatment samples falls outside the idea of universal, naturally occurring disease states that MIBC subtypes represent.

A reason why it may be an attractive option to perform subtype discovery rather than applying existing subtype classifiers on a new cohort is that by doing so, gene expression differences between classes may appear more distinct. This occurs because the iterative hierarchical clustering method used for subtype discovery maximizes variance between classes and minimizes variance within classes in that same data set. However, it is important to consider that findings based on subtype classification ought to be valid in the population as a whole. If an existing subtype classifier is applied, it will come with a certain error rate leading to misclassifications. Usually, the error is small if the cohort to which the classifier is applied is not very different, technically or biologically, from the cohort in which it was created. Still, a small error can make the result of an applied classifier seem less distinct than the discovered subtype classes which give the optimal solution for the dataset. Still, if the intent is that the identified molecular subtypes should be applicable also to external tumors, and especially if they are to inform a clinical decision, it will give a more realistic picture to apply an already existing classifier in the translational studies. By this reasoning, the fuzziness that comes with classification error can be avoided in a particular retrospective cohort by performing subtype discovery, but doing so only postpones the error to when the classification is supposed to be applied in the future. Another reason that clustering may look better, but not be better, than applying an existing classifier is in the case of smaller cohorts. With six known consensus subtypes, a cohort smaller than a hundred tumors can easily end up with skewed subtype proportions by chance. It may seem strange if a known subtype is almost completely absent, or if a subtype is too dominating in a cohort, but this is a real statistical possibility. In such cases, clustering often gives more balanced classes, and it will only find the subtypes that are present in the dataset. However, a classifier based on subtypes identified in such a dataset will not perform when confronted with reality where all subtypes exist, including any one(s) that may be absent in a small discovery dataset.

14.6 Intra-Tumor Heterogeneity of Molecular Subtypes

A potential source of error for molecular subtype classification is the existence of intra-tumor heterogeneity (ITH), when different parts of a bladder tumor show distinctly different molecular profiles. Several studies have identified tumors with phenotypic ITH (Thomsen et al. 2017), often in the form of co-existing luminal and Ba/Sq components with a shared clonal origin for both areas (Hovelson et al. 2018; Warrick et al. 2022). Other studies focusing on gene or protein expression have confirmed that subtype ITH exists in MIBC (Sirab et al. 2022; Schallenberg et al. 2023) and heterogeneity of subtypes at the protein levels correlated with components of variant histology (Warrick et al. 2019). However, few of these studies aimed to quantify ITH, which would require defining subtype ITH. One obvious definition is that any area with a different subtype classification would constitute ITH. Adopting such a definition would however greatly overestimate ITH, because it is not unusual that two compared areas which are internally similar can end up being classified differently if they are both close, or "on the border," of being classified as two different subtypes. Up to half of the nominal subtype discrepancies between matched UC samples may show such small absolute phenotypic differences that it is similar to the noise associated with subtype measurement (Sjödahl et al. 2018). Due to such threshold effects, any definition of subtype ITH needs to quantify the absolute difference between areas and not only rely on nominally different classifications. Some efforts to estimate the extent of subtype ITH in larger RNA-based (Cox et al. 2023) or IHC-based (Jakobsson et al. 2018) cohorts have concluded that discordant subtype classification within a patient's disease is relatively uncommon, and that stability rather than heterogeneity is the norm. As spatially resolved profiling techniques become more available, this question will undoubtedly be answered, and defining the minimal areas and differences that constitute subtype ITH will be an important step.

14.7 Subtype Classification by Tissue Immunohistochemistry

In addition to RNA-based methods, several groups have investigated subtype classification based on staining tissue microarrays or sections from tissue blocks of transurethral resection specimens. Thus, by using relatively limited panels of IHC-markers it is possible to identify the same gene expression subtypes that are identified by RNA-seq analyses (Dadhania et al. 2016; Sjödahl et al. 2017). When IHC analyses on TMA cores and transcriptomic classification has been performed on different tissue pieces from the same tumor, they have shown high concordance (91% accuracy reported by Dadhania and colleagues using "Luminal" and "Basal" MDA classification, and around 70–80% for the Lund taxonomy (Hardy et al. 2022)). There are two main factors influencing why such reported numbers are lower than 100%. First, the same subtyping assay may give discordant results on the two different tissue pieces, either due to true subtype ITH or due to subtyping instability because of threshold effects described in the section above on intra-tumor heterogeneity. Second, each of the two classification methods is associated with a certain probability of classification error. For RNA-based classifiers, the probability of misclassification can be estimated by comparing original and predicted class labels for samples in the training dataset that were left-out of classifier training. Optimal RNA-classifier accuracies typically plateau at around 90% depending somewhat on how detailed the classification system is. If either the RNA- or the IHC-classifier gives the wrong subtype due to classifier error, discordance is the most likely outcome for the case.

Given that classifiers are beset with error, the residual discordance due to ITH or instability of subtyping different tissue pieces from the same tumor is relatively small. If used in clinical practice, IHC-subtyping would however not rely on one or two TMA cores but would be performed on full section IHC from tissue blocks. This has recently been shown to be feasible in a clinical pathology lab (Queipo et al. 2022). Once available, this approach opens the possibility of IHC-subtyping in clinical routine, and on archival tissue blocks from decades old clinical trials for which RNA extraction and sequencing may be challenging and lead to dropout of many samples. Finally, the in situ nature of IHC-based subtyping means that it naturally resolves the question of the influence of non-cancer cells. As a full section of a tumor is viewed under the microscope it is clear that only the cancer cells are classified, and that any variation in the type and amount of cancer-associated stroma is a property that tumors have in addition to the molecular subtype of the cancer cells.

14.8 The Biology Behind the Origin of MIBC Molecular Subtypes

This last part of the chapter will focus on some aspects of urothelial cancer biology that are not necessarily subtype-defining (those are described in parts 2 and 4 of this chapter) but that nevertheless vary between molecular subtype in a consistent manner across several studies and classification systems. After all, a major purpose of molecular subtyping is to capture biology very broadly so that the classification serves as a scaffold, or context, in which further biological variation can be better understood.

A central point for UC subtyping is that basal marker protein expression, e.g. KRT5, KRT14, CD44, EGFR, is seen diffusely in the Ba/Sq subtype, but that it is also expressed in the stratified luminal subtypes "LumP" or "Urothelial-like" along the interface between the tumor and the basal membrane (Fig. 14.2). Thus, such stratified expression does not constitute ITH unless the pattern of stratification itself varies radically within a tumor. It is also central to note that the Ba/Sq subtype is not phenotypically equivalent to the basal urothelial cell state in the urothelium or in LumP/Uro tumors. Although basal cells in the normal urothelium are less differentiated than intermediate cells, they still express luminal transcription factors, e.g. GATA3 and are able to differentiate to form urothelium. A typical Basal/Squamous tumor has downregulated these factors completely, taking a much sharper turn in differentiation toward a squamous rather than urothelial state. It has been observed in genetic model systems that tumors with papillary growth pattern (which are enriched among "LumP"/ "Uro") originate in a first transformed intermediate cell, whereas carcinoma in situ and other invasive cancers originate in a basal cell (Van Batavia et al. 2014). It is also worth noting that even completely normal urothelium, when regenerating in response to damage, is capable of transiently upregulating KRT14 in all cell layers (Papafotiou et al. 2016), a phenotype which is reverted when the damage is resolved after which the urothelium once again becomes stratified.

Another interesting aspect of MIBC subtype biology is expression of the sonic hedgehog gene (*SHH*) in "LumP" or "Urothelial-like" subtypes. SHH signaling specifies cell fates in the developing embryo and it is expressed in early-stage bladder cancers and becomes lost as tumors progress. *SHH* and *BMP7*, with which it interacts in urothelial development, has a similar expression in "LumP"/"Uro" that is lost in the "LumU"/"GU" subtype (Aine et al. 2015). In a carcinogen-induced mouse model it has been shown that *Shh* and *Bmp5* and several factors in the same pathway were downregulated as urothelium progressed from carcinoma in situ to basal/squamous and mesenchymal phenotypes. This

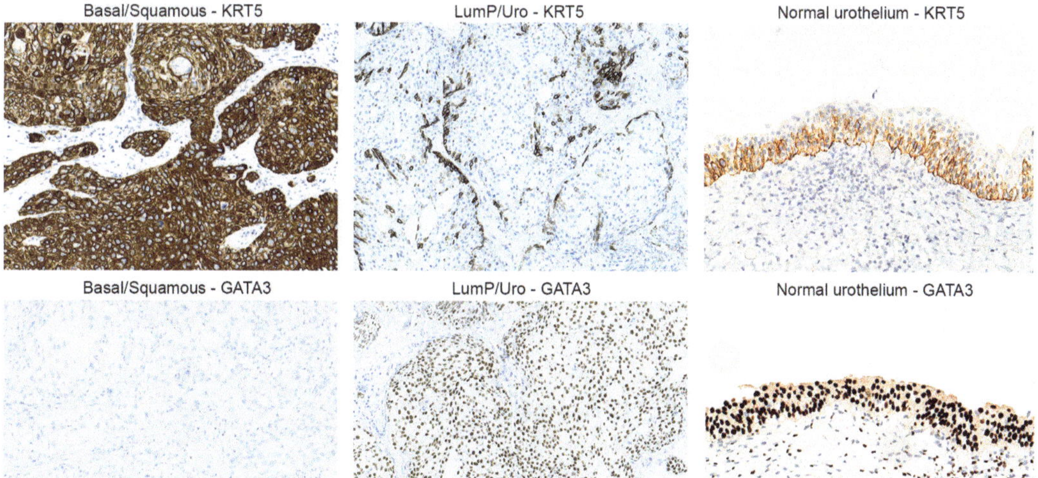

Fig. 14.2 Keratin 5 and GATA3 protein expression in representative cases of a "Basal/Squamous" tumor (left), a "LumP"/"UroA" tumor (middle), and histologically normal, NMIBC adjacent, urothelium (right). Note that basal cells in "LumP"/"UroA" tumor and normal urothelium are KRT5 and GATA3 positive, whereas Ba/Sq tumor cells are GATA3 negative. Images are from tumors in the Lund2017 cohort (Sjödahl et al. 2017). Tumor images are 400 μm and normal urothelium images are 250 μm across

downregulation was accompanied by a metabolic switch from oxidative phosphorylation to glycolysis occurring in both Ba/Sq and mesenchymal-like/sarcomatoid states, whereas a switch from *Egfr* to *Fgfr1* dependency was the main distinguishing biology between these states (Fontugne et al. 2023).

Another important driver of several cancer types including bladder cancer is the Myc family of transcription factors. Although it has eluded therapeutic targeting, its members are differentially expressed in bladder subtypes where *MYC* (coding for c-Myc) shows highest expression in the Ba/Sq subtype, whereas *MYCN* and *MYCL* show low expression in Ba/Sq and higher expression in luminal subtypes with highest expression in Lum-U. It is currently unclear if differential *MYC* expression is due to genomic gain of multiple copies of the gene or if it is a consequence of epigenetic regulation.

Another gene with a unique expression profile is *TP63* which is normally expressed in basal and intermediate cells of the urothelium but negative in umbrella cells. In MIBC, it is expressed at uniformly high levels in the "LumP"/"Uro" subtypes and it is also expressed in Ba/Sq tumors, whereas it drops substantially in "LumU"/"GU," mesenchymal-like and neuroendocrine-like subtypes. In development, *TP63* is a master regulator of stratified epithelia, and its deletion in the developing mouse bladder leads to formation of a simple layer of umbrella-like cells (Pignon et al. 2013). Thus, *TP63* affects how epithelial cells function as a tissue and its absence may be an important cause or consequence of the autonomous dysregulated and invasive character of the *TP63* negative subtypes. Cell–cell adhesion profiles also differ greatly between MIBC subtypes where "LumP"/"Uro" tends to have stratified and polarized expression of integrins, cadherins, junction proteins and claudins, as in the normal urothelium (Sjödahl et al. 2012). In comparison, "LumU"/"GU" seem to overexpress certain tight junction genes (*CLDN3*, *CLDN8*) but show lower expression of *CLDN1*. *CLDN1* is the only tight junction component expressed in the Ba/Sq subtype, which instead has high expression of p-cadherin (*CDH3*), desmosome components, and integrins, which are low in "LumU"/"GU." EpCAM and E-cadherin are expressed in the majority of MIBCs, except for the NE-like subtype which often lack E-cadherin expression and the Mesenchymal-like subtype which lacks both epithelial adhesion proteins. Much more could be included about intrinsic biological differences between the MIBC subtypes. For example, differential immune-cell infiltration, epigenetic profiling, and signatures of stemness and metastatic potential are all topics that were omitted to make this chapter more focused on the subtypes' core biology.

So far, the molecular subtypes of MIBC have been thoroughly described and characterized. Research is also well underway to understand the clinical utility of knowing a patient's molecular subtype—a topic that is not covered in this chapter. When we know precisely which subtypes exist, what are their characteristics, and how they are useful, the final step is to understand their causal origins. At what tumor stage, and in response to which genetic, developmental, or external queues, do the different MIBC subtypes become specified? It should be anticipated that both analysis of large observational omics data, including data from single cells, and experimentation in model systems will be required to fully understand how bladder cancers develop into different molecular subtypes.

References

Aine M, Eriksson P, Liedberg F, Sjödahl G, Höglund M (2015) Biological determinants of bladder cancer gene expression subtypes. Sci Rep 5:10957

Batista da Costa J, Gibb EA, Bivalacqua TJ, Liu Y, Oo HZ, Miyamoto DT, Alshalalfa M, Davicioni E, Wright J, Dall'Era MA, Douglas J, Boormans JL, Van der Heijden MS, Wu CL, van Rhijn BWG, Gupta S, Grivas P, Mouw KW, Murugan P, Fazli L, Ra S, Konety BR, Seiler R, Daneshmand S, Mian OY, Efstathiou JA, Lotan Y, Black PC (2019) Molecular characterization of neuroendocrine-like bladder cancer. Clin Cancer Res 25(13):3908–3920

Biton A, Bernard-Pierrot I, Lou Y, Krucker C, Chapeaublanc E, Rubio-Pérez C, López-Bigas N, Kamoun A, Neuzillet Y, Gestraud P, Grieco L, Rebouissou S, de Reyniès A, Benhamou S, Lebret T, Southgate J, Barillot E, Allory Y, Zinovyev A,

Radvanyi F (2014) Independent component analysis uncovers the landscape of the bladder tumor transcriptome and reveals insights into luminal and basal subtypes. Cell Rep 9(4):1235–1245

Blaveri E, Simko JP, Korkola JE, Brewer JL, Baehner F, Mehta K, Devries S, Koppie T, Pejavar S, Carroll P, Waldman FM (2005) Bladder cancer outcome and subtype classification by gene expression. Clin Cancer Res 11(11):4044–4055

Cancer Genome Atlas Research Network (2014) Comprehensive molecular characterization of urothelial bladder carcinoma. Nature 507(7492):315–322

Choi W, Porten S, Kim S, Willis D, Plimack ER, Hoffman-Censits J, Roth B, Cheng T, Tran M, Lee IL, Melquist J, Bondaruk J, Majewski T, Zhang S, Pretzsch S, Baggerly K, Siefker-Radtke A, Czerniak B, Dinney CP, McConkey DJ (2014) Identification of distinct basal and luminal subtypes of muscle-invasive bladder cancer with different sensitivities to frontline chemotherapy. Cancer Cell 25(2):152–165

Cox A, Klümper N, Stein J, Sikic D, Breyer J, Bolenz C, Roghmann F, Erben P, Wirtz RM, Wullich B, Ritter M, Hölzel M, Schwamborn K, Horn T, Gschwend J, Hartmann A, Weichert W, Erlmeier F, Eckstein M (2023) Molecular urothelial tumor cell subtypes remain stable during metastatic evolution. Eur Urol S0302-2838(23):02698–02692

Dadhania V, Zhang M, Zhang L, Bondaruk J, Majewski T, Siefker-Radtke A, Guo CC, Dinney C, Cogdell DE, Zhang S, Lee S, Lee JG, Weinstein JN, Baggerly K, McConkey D, Czerniak B (2016 Oct) Meta-analysis of the luminal and basal subtypes of bladder cancer and the identification of signature Immunohistochemical markers for clinical use. EBioMedicine 12:105–117

Damrauer JS, Hoadley KA, Chism DD, Fan C, Tiganelli CJ, Wobker SE, Yeh JJ, Milowsky MI, Iyer G, Parker JS, Kim WY (2014) Intrinsic subtypes of high-grade bladder cancer reflect the hallmarks of breast cancer biology. Proc Natl Acad Sci USA 111(8):3110–3115

Dyrskjøt L, Thykjaer T, Kruhøffer M, Jensen JL, Marcussen N, Hamilton-Dutoit S, Wolf H, Orntoft TF (2003) Identifying distinct classes of bladder carcinoma using microarrays. Nat Genet 33(1):90–96

Eriksson P, Aine M, Veerla S, Liedberg F, Sjödahl G, Höglund M (2015) Molecular subtypes of urothelial carcinoma are defined by specific gene regulatory systems. BMC Med Genet 8:25

Fontugne J, Wong J, Cabel L, Neyret-Kahn H, Karboul N, Maillé P, Rapinat A, Gentien D, Nicolas A, Baulande S, Sibony M, Bernard-Pierrot I, Radvanyi F, Allory Y (2023) Progression-associated molecular changes in basal/squamous and sarcomatoid bladder carcinogenesis. J Pathol 259(4):455–467

Grivas P, Bismar TA, Alva AS, Huang HC, Liu Y, Seiler R, Alimohamed N, Cheng L, Hyndman ME, Dabbas B, Black PC, Davicioni E, Wright JL, Ornstein MC, Mian OY, Kaimakliotis HZ, Gibb EA, Lotan Y (2020) Validation of a neuroendocrine-like classifier confirms poor outcomes in patients with bladder cancer treated with cisplatin-based neoadjuvant chemotherapy. Urol Oncol 38(4):262–268

Hardy CSC, Ghaedi H, Slotman A, Sjödahl G, Gooding RJ, Berman DM, Jackson CL (2022) Immunohistochemical assays for bladder cancer molecular subtyping: optimizing parsimony and performance of Lund taxonomy classifiers. J Histochem Cytochem 70(5):357–375

Hovelson DH, Udager AM, McDaniel AS, Grivas P, Palmbos P, Tamura S, Lazo de la Vega L, Palapattu G, Veeneman B, El-Sawy L, Sadis SE, Morgan TM, Montgomery JS, Weizer AZ, Day KC, Neamati N, Liebert M, Keller ET, Day ML, Mehra R, Tomlins SA (2018) Targeted DNA and RNA sequencing of paired urothelial and squamous bladder cancers reveals discordant genomic and transcriptomic events and unique therapeutic implications. Eur Urol 74(6):741–753

Höglund M (2023) What is a bladder cancer molecular subtype? Bladder Cancer 9(4):293–298

Jakobsson L, Chebil G, Marzouka NA, Liedberg F, Sjödahl G (2018) Low frequency of Intratumor heterogeneity in bladder cancer tissue microarrays. Bladder Cancer. 4(3):327–337

Kamoun A, de Reyniès A, Allory Y, Sjödahl G, Robertson AG, Seiler R, Hoadley KA, Groeneveld CS, Al-Ahmadie H, Choi W, Castro MAA, Fontugne J, Eriksson P, Mo Q, Kardos J, Zlotta A, Hartmann A, Dinney CP, Bellmunt J, Powles T, Malats N, Chan KS, Kim WY, McConkey DJ, Black PC, Dyrskjøt L, Höglund M, Lerner SP, Real FX, Radvanyi F (2020) Bladder cancer molecular taxonomy group. A consensus molecular classification of muscle-invasive bladder cancer. Eur Urol 77(4):420–433

Kardos J, Chai S, Mose LE, Selitsky SR, Krishnan B, Saito R, Iglesia MD, Milowsky MI, Parker JS, Kim WY, Vincent BG (2016) Claudin-low bladder tumors are immune infiltrated and actively immune suppressed. JCI Insight 1(3):e85902

Kollberg P, Chebil G, Eriksson P, Sjödahl G, Liedberg F (2019) Molecular subtypes applied to a population-based modern cystectomy series do not predict cancer-specific survival. Urol Oncol 37(10):791–799

Lerner SP, McConkey DJ, Hoadley KA, Chan KS, Kim WY, Radvanyi F, Höglund M, Real FX (2016) Bladder cancer molecular taxonomy: summary from a consensus meeting. Bladder Cancer. 2(1):37–47

Lindgren D, Frigyesi A, Gudjonsson S, Sjödahl G, Hallden C, Chebil G, Veerla S, Ryden T, Månsson W, Liedberg F, Höglund M (2010) Combined gene expression and genomic profiling define two intrinsic molecular subtypes of urothelial carcinoma and gene signatures for molecular grading and outcome. Cancer Res 70(9):3463–3472

Mo Q, Nikolos F, Chen F, Tramel Z, Lee YC, Hayashi K, Xiao J, Shen J, Chan KS (2018) Prognostic power of a tumor differentiation gene signature for bladder urothelial carcinomas. J Natl Cancer Inst 110(5):448–459

Morera DS, Hasanali SL, Belew D, Ghosh S, Klaassen Z, Jordan AR, Wang J, Terris MK, Bollag RJ, Merseburger AS, Stenzl A, Soloway MS, Lokeshwar

VB (2020) Clinical parameters outperform molecular subtypes for predicting outcome in bladder cancer: results from multiple cohorts, Including TCGA. J Urol 203(1):62–72

Nakauma-González JA, Rijnders M, van Riet J, van der Heijden MS, Voortman J, Cuppen E, Mehra N, van Wilpe S, Oosting SF, Rijstenberg LL, Westgeest HM, Zwarthoff EC, de Wit R, van der Veldt AAM, van de Werken HJG, Lolkema MPJ, Boormans JL (2022) Comprehensive molecular characterization reveals genomic and transcriptomic subtypes of metastatic urothelial carcinoma. Eur Urol 81(4):331–336

Papafotiou G, Paraskevopoulou V, Vasilaki E, Kanaki Z, Paschalidis N, Klinakis A (2016) KRT14 marks a subpopulation of bladder basal cells with pivotal role in regeneration and tumorigenesis. Nat Commun 7:11914

Pignon JC, Grisanzio C, Geng Y, Song J, Shivdasani RA, Signoretti S (2013) p63-expressing cells are the stem cells of developing prostate, bladder, and colorectal epithelia. Proc Natl Acad Sci USA 110(20):8105–8110

Queipo FJ, Unamunzaga GM, Negro BF, Fuertes SG, Cortés MÁ, Tejedor EC, Mañas CMB, Ariño AB, Sjödahl G, Beorlegui C (2022) Immunohistochemistry subtyping of urothelial carcinoma is feasible in the daily practice. Virchows Arch 481(2):191–200

Rebouissou S, Bernard-Pierrot I, de Reyniès A, Lepage ML, Krucker C, Chapeaublanc E, Hérault A, Kamoun A, Caillault A, Letouzé E, Elarouci N, Neuzillet Y, Denoux Y, Molinié V, Vordos D, Laplanche A, Maillé P, Soyeux P, Ofualuka K, Reyal F, Biton A, Sibony M, Paoletti X, Southgate J, Benhamou S, Lebret T, Allory Y, Radvanyi F (2014) EGFR as a potential therapeutic target for a subset of muscle-invasive bladder cancers presenting a basal-like phenotype. Sci Transl Med 6(244):244ra91

Robertson AG, Groeneveld CS, Jordan B, Lin X, McLaughlin KA, Das A, Fall LA, Fantini D, Taxter TJ, Mogil LS, Lindskrog SV, Dyrskjøt L, McConkey DJ, Svatek RS, de Reyniès A, Castro MAA, Meeks JJ (2020) Identification of differential tumor subtypes of T1 bladder cancer. Eur Urol 78(4):533–537

Robertson AG, Kim J, Al-Ahmadie H, Bellmunt J, Guo G, Cherniack AD, Hinoue T, Laird PW, Hoadley KA, Akbani R, Castro MAA, Gibb EA, Kanchi RS, Gordenin DA, Shukla SA, Sanchez-Vega F, Hansel DE, Czerniak BA, Reuter VE, Su X, de Sa Carvalho B, Chagas VS, Mungall KL, Sadeghi S, Pedamallu CS, Lu Y, Klimczak LJ, Zhang J, Choo C, Ojesina AI, Bullman S, Leraas KM, Lichtenberg TM, Wu CJ, Schultz N, Getz G, Meyerson M, Mills GB, McConkey DJ, TCGA Research Network, Weinstein JN, Kwiatkowski DJ, Lerner SP (2018) Comprehensive Molecular Characterization of Muscle-Invasive Bladder Cancer. Cell 174(4):1033

Robertson AG, Meghani K, Cooley LF, McLaughlin KA, Fall LA, Yu Y, Castro MAA, Groeneveld CS, de Reyniès A, Nazarov VI, Tsvetkov VO, Choy B, Raggi D, Marandino L, Montorsi F, Powles T, Necchi A, Meeks JJ (2023) Expression-based subtypes define pathologic response to neoadjuvant immune-checkpoint inhibitors in muscle-invasive bladder cancer. Nat Commun. 14(1):2126

Sanchez-Carbayo M, Socci ND, Charytonowicz E, Lu M, Prystowsky M, Childs G, Cordon-Cardo C (2002) Molecular profiling of bladder cancer using cDNA microarrays: defining histogenesis and biological phenotypes. Cancer Res 62(23):6973–6980

Schallenberg S, Dragomir MP, Anders P, Ebner B, Volz Y, Eismann L, Rodler S, Casuscelli J, Buchner A, Klauschen F, Stief C, Horst D, Schulz GB (2023) Intratumoral heterogeneity of molecular subtypes in muscle-invasive bladder cancer-an extensive multiregional Immunohistochemical analysis. Eur Urol Focus S2405-4569(23):00080–00089

Seiler R, Ashab HAD, Erho N, van Rhijn BWG, Winters B, Douglas J, Van Kessel KE, van de Fransen Putte EE, Sommerlad M, Wang NQ, Choeurng V, Gibb EA, Palmer-Aronsten B, Lam LL, Buerki C, Davicioni E, Sjödahl G, Kardos J, Hoadley KA, Lerner SP, McConkey DJ, Choi W, Kim WY, Kiss B, Thalmann GN, Todenhöfer T, Crabb SJ, North S, Zwarthoff EC, Boormans JL, Wright J, Dall'Era M, van der Heijden MS, Black PC (2017) Impact of Molecular Subtypes in Muscle-invasive Bladder Cancer on Predicting Response and Survival after Neoadjuvant Chemotherapy. Eur Urol 72(4):544–554

Sirab N, Drubay D, Maillé P, Popova T, Ngo C, Gentien D, Moktefi A, Soyeux-Porte P, Pelletier R, Reyes C, Henry E, Pouessel D, Vordos D, Lebret T, de Reyniès A, Paoletti X, Radvanyi F, Allory Y (2022) Multilayer spectrum of intratumoral heterogeneity in basal bladder cancer. J Pathol 256(1):108–118

Sjödahl G, Eriksson P, Liedberg F, Höglund M (2017) Molecular classification of urothelial carcinoma: global mRNA classification versus tumour-cell phenotype classification. J Pathol 242(1):113–125

Sjödahl G, Eriksson P, Lövgren K, Marzouka NA, Bernardo C, Nordentoft I, Dyrskjøt L, Liedberg F, Höglund M (2018) Discordant molecular subtype classification in the basal-squamous subtype of bladder tumors and matched lymph-node metastases. Mod Pathol 31(12):1869–1881

Sjödahl G, Lauss M, Lövgren K, Chebil G, Gudjonsson S, Veerla S, Patschan O, Aine M, Fernö M, Ringnér M, Månsson W, Liedberg F, Lindgren D, Höglund M (2012) A molecular taxonomy for urothelial carcinoma. Clin Cancer Res 18(12):3377–3386

Thomsen MBH, Nordentoft I, Lamy P, Vang S, Reinert L, Mapendano CK, Høyer S, Ørntoft TF, Jensen JB, Dyrskjøt L (2017) Comprehensive multiregional analysis of molecular heterogeneity in bladder cancer. Sci Rep 7(1):11702

Van Batavia J, Yamany T, Molotkov A, Dan H, Mansukhani M, Batourina E, Schneider K, Oyon D, Dunlop M, Wu XR, Cordon-Cardo C, Mendelsohn C. Bladder cancers arise from distinct urothelial sub-populations. Nat Cell Biol 2014;16(10):982–91, 1–5

Wang L, Saci A, Szabo PM, Chasalow SD, Castillo-Martin M, Domingo-Domenech J, Siefker-Radtke A, Sharma

P, Sfakianos JP, Gong Y, Dominguez-Andres A, Oh WK, Mulholland D, Azrilevich A, Hu L, Cordon-Cardo C, Salmon H, Bhardwaj N, Zhu J, Galsky MD (2018) EMT- and stroma-related gene expression and resistance to PD-1 blockade in urothelial cancer. Nat Commun 9(1):3503

Warrick JI, Hu W, Yamashita H, Walter V, Shuman L, Craig JM, Gellert LL, Castro MAA, Robertson AG, Kuo F, Ostrovnaya I, Sarungbam J, Chen YB, Gopalan A, Sirintrapun SJ, Fine SW, Tickoo SK, Kim K, Thomas J, Karan N, Gao SP, Clinton TN, Lenis AT, Chan TA, Chen Z, Rao M, Hollman TJ, Li Y, Socci ND, Chavan S, Viale A, Mohibullah N, Bochner BH, Pietzak EJ, Teo MY, Iyer G, Rosenberg JE, Bajorin DF, Kaag M, Merrill SB, Joshi M, Adam R, Taylor JA 3rd, Clark PE, Raman JD, Reuter VE, Chen Y, Funt SA, Solit DB, DeGraff DJ, Al-Ahmadie HA (2022) FOXA1 repression drives lineage plasticity and immune heterogeneity in bladder cancers with squamous differentiation. Nat Commun 13(1):6575

Warrick JI, Sjödahl G, Kaag M, Raman JD, Merrill S, Shuman L, Chen G, Walter V, DeGraff DJ (2019) Intratumoral heterogeneity of bladder cancer by molecular subtypes and histologic variants. Eur Urol 75(1):18–22

Molecular Features of Divergent Differentiation and Histological Subtypes in Bladder Cancer

15

Jacqueline Fontugne and Yves Allory

Abstract

Urothelial carcinoma shows high morphological heterogeneity. Some specific histological features have been defined as divergent differentiation or histological subtypes of invasive urothelial carcinoma. The striking heterogeneity of morphological phenotypes may to some extent reflect an underlying diversity in molecular features. This chapter provides a current overview of the reported associations between histological subtypes of invasive urothelial carcinoma and molecular features, including genomic alterations, transcriptional programs, and molecular subtypes. While some histological subtypes show specific or enriched genomic alterations, others share common genomic profiles with conventional urothelial carcinoma. At the transcriptomic level, some histological subtypes or divergent differentiation is strongly associated with luminal or basal molecular subtypes or shows altered gene expression programs. In rare histological subtypes or divergent differentiation, molecular profiling studies are lacking. More comprehensive analyses of molecular features in the context of histological subtypes require additional studies in larger cohorts.

Keywords

Urothelial carcinoma histological subtypes · Molecular features · Molecular subtyping · Genomics · Transcriptomics

15.1 Introduction

More than 90% of bladder cancers fall into one histological diagnostic category: urothelial carcinoma. However, this common bladder cancer type can display a particularly high heterogeneity of morphological features. In invasive urothelial carcinoma, some morphological features, owing to their high frequency or their uniqueness, have been defined as *histological subtypes* in the 2022 fifth edition of the WHO classification of urinary tumors (IARC 2022). While histological subtypes can be identified in tumors invading only the lamina propria (stage pT1) (Lopez-Beltran et al. 2022), most series comprise tumors invading the bladder muscle or beyond into the perivesical tissue (stages pT2 and above). Of note, in the previous WHO edition, histological subtypes were termed *variants*. As the latter term could

J. Fontugne · Y. Allory (✉)
Department of Pathology, Institut Curie, Saint-Cloud, France

Institut Curie, CNRS, UMR144, Equipe labellisée Ligue Contre le Cancer, Paris, France

Université Paris-Saclay, UVSQ, Saint-Quentin en Yvelines, France
e-mail: jacqueline.fontugne@curie.fr; yves.allory@curie.fr

M. A. Knowles, L. Dyrskjøt (eds.), *Biology of Bladder Cancer*,
https://doi.org/10.1007/978-3-031-68505-7_15

refer to genomic mutations, it has now been excluded to avoid confusion. Histological subtypes follow a morphological definition, based on the visual recognition of specific criteria by pathologists, which are not typically seen in normal tissues. In contrast, invasive urothelial carcinoma may also mirror aspects of normal differentiation of other non-urothelial epithelial tissues. Specifically, invasive urothelial carcinoma may show features of squamous epithelium (such as that of the epidermis), glandular epithelium (such as that of the digestive tract), trophoblastic epithelium (found in the normal placenta), or Müllerian epithelium (found in the normal developing female reproductive tract). Urothelial carcinomas harboring areas resembling other lineages are labeled *urothelial carcinoma with divergent differentiation.*

An area of divergent differentiation and/or a histological subtype—pure or in different combinations of several morphologies—has been identified in 27–47% of invasive urothelial carcinoma in recent series (Warrick et al. 2019; Hajiran et al. 2021). The remaining cases are conventional urothelial carcinoma. The currently described divergent differentiations and histological subtypes of invasive urothelial carcinoma are listed in Table 15.1 (see also Chap. 4).

The striking heterogeneity of morphological phenotypes of muscle-invasive urothelial carcinoma (MIBC) may reflect to some extent an underlying diversity in molecular features. Specifically, genomic alterations or transcriptional programs can modify tumor cell properties, which may translate into changes in cell morphology, or in cell–cell interactions, thus shaping tumor architecture. Several transcriptomic classifications have identified biologically and clinically relevant molecular subtypes of MIBC that could be applied to characterize histological subtypes (Sjödahl et al. 2012; Volkmer et al. 2012; Choi et al. 2014; Damrauer et al. 2014; Rebouissou et al. 2014; Seiler et al. 2017; Marzouka et al. 2018). All classification systems essentially agree that at the lowest level of granularity, MIBC transcriptomic subtypes could be defined in relation to two differentiation states—the basal and luminal phenotypes. Bladder tumors of basal subtype are typically characterized by the overexpression of keratin markers of the basal layer of the normal urothelium, such as *KRT5* and *KRT6,* combined with the under expression of markers of urothelial differentiation, such as *GATA3, FOXA1, KRT20,* and uroplakins. Ba/Sq tumors (see below) also express *KRT14,* a typical basal marker of squamous epithelia and a proposed marker of urothelial stem cells. Luminal tumors essentially display opposite expression patterns, i.e., low expression of basal markers and high expression of luminal markers. Additional genomic alterations or transcriptomic patterns further delineate subgroups of luminal tumors. To facilitate subtype-based studies, leading groups in the field of bladder cancer research recently published a collaborative work on the molecular classification of MIBC defining 6 consensus subtypes, named "luminal papillary" (LumP), "luminal non-specified" (LumNS), "luminal unstable" (LumU), "stroma-rich," "basal/squamous" (Ba/Sq), and "neuroendocrine-like" (NE-like) (Kamoun et al. 2020) (see also Chap. 14). Importantly, luminal and basal marker protein expression patterns can be detected by immunohistochemistry as a surrogate to discriminate, to some extent, between molecular subtypes.

This chapter will provide a current overview of the reported associations between histological

Table 15.1 Divergent differentiation and histological subtypes of invasive urothelial carcinoma

Urothelial carcinoma with divergent differentiation
Urothelial carcinoma with squamous differentiation
Urothelial carcinoma with glandular differentiation
Urothelial carcinoma with trophoblastic differentiation
Urothelial carcinoma with Müllerian differentiation
Micropapillary urothelial carcinoma
Nested urothelial carcinoma
Large nested urothelial carcinoma
Tubular and microcystic urothelial carcinomas
Plasmacytoid urothelial carcinoma
Sarcomatoid urothelial carcinoma
Lipid-rich urothelial carcinoma
Lymphoepithelioma-like urothelial carcinoma
Clear cell (glycogen-rich) urothelial carcinoma
Giant cell urothelial carcinoma
Poorly differentiated urothelial carcinoma

subtypes of MIBC and molecular features, such as genomic alterations and transcriptional programs, particularly in relation to transcriptomic molecular subtypes.

15.2 Molecular Features of Histological Subtypes of Muscle-Invasive Bladder Cancer

Current knowledge regarding the molecular features of histological subtypes of invasive urothelial carcinoma is restricted to frequent and well-studied histological subtypes (Table 15.2), whereas scientific evidence is still lacking for the rarer ones, mostly due to the difficulty in obtaining large cohorts.

15.2.1 Histological Subtypes and Divergent Differentiation with Defined Molecular Features

15.2.1.1 Urothelial Carcinoma with Squamous Differentiation

Urothelial carcinoma with squamous differentiation (UC-SD) is defined by the presence of specific features evocative of squamous epithelia, namely intercellular bridges or keratinization (Fig. 15.1a) (IARC 2022). It is the most frequent histological subtype, found in approximately 20% of MIBC (Warrick et al. 2017).

The most frequent genomic alterations reported in UC-SD are not specific to this histological subtype, involving genes that are commonly mutated in unselected or conventional urothelial carcinoma, such as *TP53, ARID1A,* or *PIK3CA,* with an enrichment in *KMT2D* mutations identified in one study (Hovelson et al. 2018; Tripathi et al. 2022). *TERT* promoter mutations were observed with the same prevalence in UC-SD and conventional urothelial carcinoma (Cheng et al. 2015; Tripathi et al. 2022). Although at a low frequency compared to conventional urothelial carcinoma, targetable *FGFR3* mutations can be identified in UC-SD (Tripathi et al. 2022).

UC-SD is strongly associated with basal subtypes in all transcriptomic classification approaches (Choi et al. 2014; Damrauer et al. 2014; Rebouissou et al. 2014; Robertson et al. 2017; Sjödahl et al. 2017; Kamoun et al. 2020). The gene expression profile of UC-SD is thus characterized by the combined upregulation of basal cell markers and downregulation of luminal markers. Interestingly, tumors including areas of squamous differentiation show the greatest morphological and molecular heterogeneity (Warrick et al. 2019). Specifically, areas with squamous differentiation may be associated with an adjacent non-squamous histological area of luminal subtype within the same tumor (Hovelson et al. 2018; Warrick et al. 2019; Sirab et al. 2022), although both areas partially share genomic profiles (Hovelson et al. 2018; Sirab et al. 2022).

UC-SD also shows *EGFR* upregulation and pathway activation (Rebouissou et al. 2014; Hovelson et al. 2018). EGFR dependence has been demonstrated in basal bladder cancer cell lines, including in those with squamous features (Rebouissou et al. 2014). The basal subtype of UC-SD has also been demonstrated at the protein level, by the immunohistochemical expression of basal cytokeratins, such as CK5/6, and the lack of expression of luminal differentiation markers, such as GATA3 (Fig. 15.1b) (Rebouissou et al. 2014; Paner et al. 2014; Warrick et al. 2017, 2019; Jangir et al. 2019; Font et al. 2020; Bontoux et al. 2021; Ikeda et al. 2021; Labban et al. 2021; Olkhov-Mitsel et al. 2021; Ravanini et al. 2021; Bernardo et al. 2022; Sirab et al. 2022; Jackson et al. 2022). Mouse bladder cancer models further support the relationship between squamous differentiation and basal molecular subtype (Rebouissou et al. 2014; Fantini et al. 2018; Masuda et al. 2020; Fontugne et al. 2023). In vivo studies in mouse models suggest that specific transcription factors, such as FOXA1, are required for the maintenance of urothelial differentiation and that their downregulation induces squamous features (Reddy et al. 2015; Osei-Amponsa et al. 2020).

Table 15.2 Summary of molecular alterations associated with the most common histological subtypes or divergent differentiation of bladder urothelial carcinoma

Histological subtype	Main genomic alterations shared with other UC	Enriched genomic alterations compared to other UC	Transcriptomic subtype	Immunohistochemistry profile
Squamous differentiation	*TERT* promoter *TP53, ARID1A, PIK3CA*	*KMT2D* mutations in one study	Basal	Mostly basal
Glandular differentiation	*TERT* promoter *TP53, RB1, PIK3CA, CDKN1A, CDKN2A, KMT2D, KDM6A*	None reported	Unknown	Mostly luminal
Micropapillary	*TERT* promoter *TP53* *PIK3CA* *FGFR3*	*ERBB2* amplification	Mostly luminal	Mostly luminal
Plasmacytoid	*TERT* promoter *TP53, RB1, CDKN1A, PIK3CA, ERBB2, ARID1*A, and *KDM6A*	Specific *CDH1* inactivation (mostly by mutation)	– (4/4 luminal in TCGA cases)	Mostly luminal
Sarcomatoid	*TERT* promoter	*TP53, RB1* *PIK3CA, MYO1F, CNGB1, FXR1, RBM5, SEMA3D* in one study	Basal	Variable
Nested—tubular and microcystic	*TERT* promoter *TP53, PIK3CA* *FGFR3*	Suggested for *JAK3* and *CTNNB1* in one study	Unknown	Mostly luminal but possible co-expression of basal and luminal markers
Large nested	*TERT* promoter *PIK3CA, CDKN1B, ARID1A, KDM6A*	*FGFR3* mutation	Unknown	Luminal with expression of basal markers at the nest periphery

UC: Urothelial carcinoma

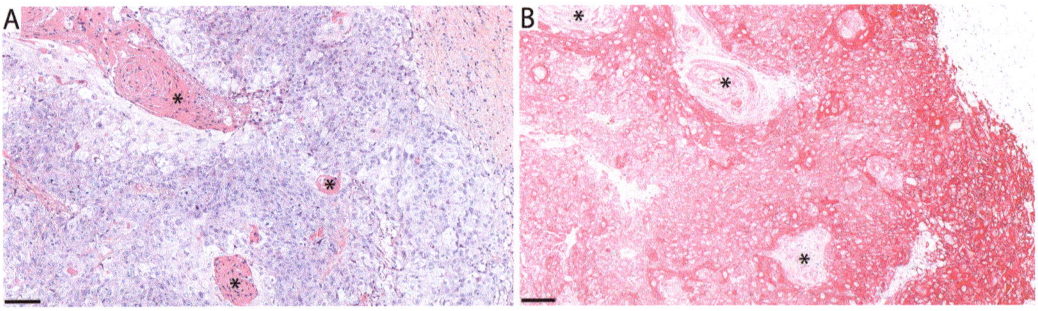

Fig. 15.1 Urothelial carcinoma with squamous differentiation (**a**). Hematoxylin eosin saffron staining of a representative urothelial carcinoma with squamous differentiation defined here by the presence of areas of keratinization (asterisks). (**b**). Dual immunohistochemistry staining using subtype defining markers shows a diffuse expression of the basal cytoplasmic marker CK5/6 (red). No staining with the luminal nuclear marker GATA3 (brown) is seen. Scale bars: 100 µm

15.2.1.2 Urothelial Carcinoma with Glandular Differentiation

Urothelial carcinoma with glandular differentiation (UC-GD) shows structures with gland lumen formation, often resembling that of the digestive tract, with or without extracellular mucin (IARC 2022).

Whole-exome genomic profiling of large series of UC-GD has not currently been performed. In targeted next-generation sequencing studies, UC-GD carried similar genomic alterations to conventional urothelial carcinoma, such as *TP53*, *RB1*, *PIK3CA*, *CDKN1A*, *CDKN2A*, *KMT2D,* or *KDM6A* gene mutations (Maurer et al. 2020; Almassi et al. 2022). *FGFR3* mutations were rare in UC-GD (2/34 cases, 5.9%). Corroborating findings in conventional urothelial carcinoma, the majority of UC-GD exhibited *TERT* promoter mutations (Vail et al. 2015; Maurer et al. 2020; Cheng et al. 2021; Almassi et al. 2022). These studies highlight that although UC-GD seems to lack specific genomic features compared to conventional urothelial carcinoma, genomic profiling may be useful in distinguishing UC-GD from differential diagnoses, such as primary adenocarcinoma or benign glandular lesions.

While the transcriptomic phenotype of UG-GD is unknown, immunohistochemistry analyses in relatively small cohorts revealed high phenotypic variability. Although UC-GD cases most often showed luminal marker expression, some cases could express basal markers or display a double positive or a double negative staining pattern for both luminal and basal markers (Paner et al. 2014; Jangir et al. 2019; Bontoux et al. 2021; Ikeda et al. 2021; Ravanini et al. 2021). This phenotypic variability was further supported in studies using a 13-marker immunohistochemistry panel developed at Lund University (Marzouka et al. 2018) or a simplified 3-marker version, in which UC-GD cases were categorized into the luminal "Urothelial-like" subtype, the luminal "Genomically unstable" subtype or more rarely in the "basal squamous" subtype (Tanaka et al. 2018; Warrick et al. 2019). UC-GD thus might encompass several molecular entities. Comprehensive gene expression profiling studies are needed to elucidate the molecular phenotype of UC-GD.

15.2.1.3 Micropapillary Urothelial Carcinoma

The histological definition of micropapillary urothelial carcinoma (MPUC) includes the presence of micropapillae, formed by a single or multiple small delicate clusters of tumor cells within a lacunar space, which is shaped by peritumoral stromal retraction, mimicking lymphovascular invasion (Fig. 15.2a) (IARC 2022). The outer stroma-facing cell surface of micropapillae is reportedly positive for mucin 1 (MUC1), a glycoprotein typically expressed at the apical surface, suggesting a reversed cell polarity (Sangoi et al. 2009; Yang et al. 2020).

Genomic studies have consistently reported a significant enrichment of *ERBB2* gene alterations in MPUC compared to conventional or unselected invasive urothelial carcinoma. In MPUC cohorts, *ERBB2* amplification has been identified in about 34% of the cases overall, with a wide variability depending on the detection method, the prior selection by immunohistochemistry, the cohort size or composition in terms of tumor stage, or percentage of MPUC component (Table 15.3) (Ching et al. 2011; Schneider et al. 2014; Bertz et al. 2016; Isharwal et al. 2018; Moktefi et al. 2018; Zinnall et al. 2018).

In contrast, conventional or unselected invasive urothelial carcinoma has *ERBB2* amplification in 5–13% of the cases (Hansel et al. 2008; Laé et al. 2009; Fleischmann et al. 2011; Hurst et al. 2012; Schneider et al. 2014; Weinstein et al. 2014; Moktefi et al. 2018). In a reverse approach, analyzing the morphological characteristics of urothelial carcinoma with *ERBB2* amplification, Tschui et al. reported that amplified tumors harbored micropapillary features significantly more frequently than non-amplified tumors (77% vs. 8%) (Tschui et al. 2015). A multisampling study illustrated the intra-tumoral heterogeneity of *ERBB2* amplification in urothelial carcinoma with micropapillary features, showing that the alterations could be found in either the MPUC component alone, in the conventional component

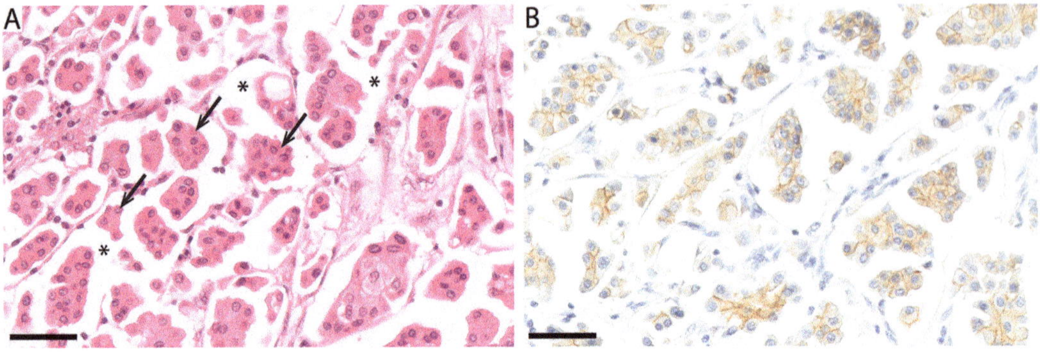

Fig. 15.2 Micropapillary subtype of urothelial carcinoma. (**a**). Hematoxylin eosin staining of a representative micropapillary bladder cancer defined by multiple small delicate clusters of tumor cells (arrows) within lacunar spaces (asterisks). (**b**). Immunohistochemistry staining of micropapillary bladder carcinoma with moderate membranous HER2 overexpression. Scale bars: 50 μm

Table 15.3 Reported prevalence of *ERBB2* amplifications in MPUC series

Study	Number of *ERBB2* amplified MPUCs	Detection method
Ching et al. 2011	8/18 (42%)	CISH
Schneider et al. 2014	8/61 (15%)	FISH
Bertz et al. 2016	3/10 (30%)	CISH
Isharwal et al. 2018	32/43 (74%)	FISH
Moktefi et al. 2018	6/25 (24%) MPUCs with ≥10% moderate/strong membranous HER2 expression by IHC	FISH
Zinnall et al. 2018	21/70 (30%)	CISH
Total	**78/227 (34%)**	

IHC: immunohistochemistry; FISH: fluorescent in situ hybridization; CISH: chromogenic in situ hybridization

alone, or in both (Isharwal et al. 2018). However, *ERBB2* amplification was more commonly found in the MPUC component compared to the conventional one. Overall, these studies provide robust evidence supporting *ERBB2* amplification as a genomic underpinning of micropapillary morphology.

Other studies have suggested an association of MPUC with *ERBB2* gene mutations. In targeted next-generation sequencing studies, *ERBB2* mutations have been identified in 38–40% of MPUC cases and were significantly more frequent than in non-MPUC invasive urothelial carcinoma, in which approximately 5% of *ERBB2* mutated cases were found (Ross et al. 2014, 2016). However, others have reported *ERBB2* mutations in a lower proportion of MPUCs (6.7% of 90 cases), albeit using a less sensitive detection approach, through Sanger sequencing of 2 exons with known hotspot mutations (Zinnall et al. 2018). This proportion was similar to that of *ERBB2* mutations in invasive urothelial carcinoma from the large TCGA cohort, which occurred in 12% of the cases, unselected with regard to histological subtype (Robertson et al. 2017). Thus, additional studies are needed to validate the enrichment of *ERBB2* mutations in MPUC. Regardless of the histological subtype, most *ERBB2* mutations in invasive urothelial carcinoma occur in the region encoding the extracellular domain of ERBB2, S310F/Y being the most frequent alteration (Ross et al. 2014, 2016; Robertson et al. 2017; Zinnall et al. 2018). Of note, MPUC tumors with *ERBB2* amplification, but not mutation, have been reported as associated with high ERBB2 protein expression by immunohistochemistry (Fig. 15.2b) (Hansel et al. 2008; Laé et al. 2009; Ching et al. 2011; Schneider et al. 2014; Tschui et al. 2015) although others have found low concordance (Fleischmann et al. 2011; Isharwal et al. 2018).

Comprehensive genomic profiling studies specifically of MPUC are lacking. However, beyond *ERBB2*, other genomic alterations that are commonly found in conventional urothelial carcinoma have been reported in MPUC in targeted next-generation studies, including *TERT* promoter (Nguyen et al. 2016), *TP53*, *PIK3CA*, or *FGFR3* mutations (Ross et al. 2016).

Regarding transcriptomic molecular subtypes, MPUCs are mostly luminal (Guo et al. 2016; Kamoun et al. 2020). Applying the MDA classification, distinguishing three subtypes (Choi et al. 2014), 98% of 43 MPUCs were "luminal," a subset of which were also "p53-like" (Guo et al. 2016). In the consensus classification study, MPUC cases were categorized into luminal subtypes (Kamoun et al. 2020). Although the strongest association was with the LumNS subcategory of luminal subtypes, pathological review was only available in a cohort subset analysis. Thus, the association of MPUCs with the LumNS group specifically requires validation in larger cohorts combining transcriptomics and pathological data. Using surrogate immunohistochemistry markers of basal and luminal transcriptomic subtypes, most MPUCs consistently displayed high expression of luminal markers and low expression of basal ones (Paner et al. 2014; Guo et al. 2016; Warrick et al. 2017, 2019; Zinnall et al. 2018; Yang et al. 2020; Bontoux et al. 2021; Ikeda et al. 2021). Using the specific immunohistochemistry panel developed at Lund University using 13 markers (Sjödahl et al. 2017; Marzouka et al. 2018), or a simplified 3-marker version, the majority of MPUCs fell into the luminal "genomically unstable" Lund subcategory (Tanaka et al. 2018; Warrick et al. 2019; Olkhov-Mitsel et al. 2021).

Beyond molecular subtypes, Guo et al. explored the transcriptomes of MPUCs in comparison with conventional urothelial carcinoma. MPUCs overexpressed PPARγ and miR-296 target genes and were enriched in pathways related to cell cycle and DNA damage (Guo et al. 2016). The overexpression of miR-296 target genes and cell polarity genes, such as *CLDN3* or *MUC1* (Guo et al. 2016), could contribute to the cell polarity alteration in MPUCs. Transcriptomic analysis of pT1 stage tumors specifically also showed *CLDN3* and *MUC1* overexpression in MPUC compared to conventional urothelial carcinoma (Bowden et al. 2020).

Overall, these data support that the molecular features of MPUC include enrichment in *ERBB2* amplification, and, at the transcriptomic level, an assignment to luminal subtypes with distinct gene expression profiles.

15.2.1.4 Plasmacytoid Urothelial Carcinoma

Plasmacytoid urothelial carcinoma (PUC) is characterized by individual, discohesive, often diffusely infiltrating cells, usually with minimal stromal reaction (Fig. 15.3a) (Lopez-Beltran et al. 2009; IARC 2022). The term "plasmacytoid" refers to the fact that PUC tumor cells may bear resemblance to plasma cells, containing an abundant cytoplasm with an eccentrically placed nucleus, and may even express plasma cell surface markers, such as CD138 (Nigwekar et al. 2009; Keck et al. 2011; Raspollini et al. 2011; Perrino et al. 2019). Others may contain a cytoplasmic vacuole, conferring a signet-ring cell appearance. PUC is characterized by alterations of *CDH1*, a gene encoding a cell–cell adhesion protein, E-cadherin (Al-Ahmadie et al. 2016; Robertson et al. 2017; Sangoi et al. 2020; Teo et al. 2021). The majority of PUCs harbor loss-of-function *CDH1* mutations, most frequently truncating nonsense alterations, often resulting in membranous E-cadherin protein expression loss. In most remaining *CDH1* wild-type PUC tumors, Al-Ahmadie et al. reported another less frequent mechanism of *CDH1* inactivation, through *CDH1* promoter hypermethylation. PUC genomic profiles show co-occurring mutations that are common with those of conventional urothelial carcinoma, the most frequent in *TERT* promoter, *TP53*, *RB1*, *CDKN1A*, *ERBB2*, *PIK3CA*, *ARID1A*, and *KDM6A*. *FGFR3* mutations are very rare in this histological subtype (Al-Ahmadie et al. 2016, Teo et al. 2021). By contrast, *CDH1* mutations are specific to this histological subtype (Al-Ahmadie et al. 2016; Palsgrove et al. 2019; Teo et al. 2021). Importantly, *CDH1* inactivation can be recognized using immunohistochemistry through an aberrant non-membranous CDH1 expression, a decreased expression or more fre-

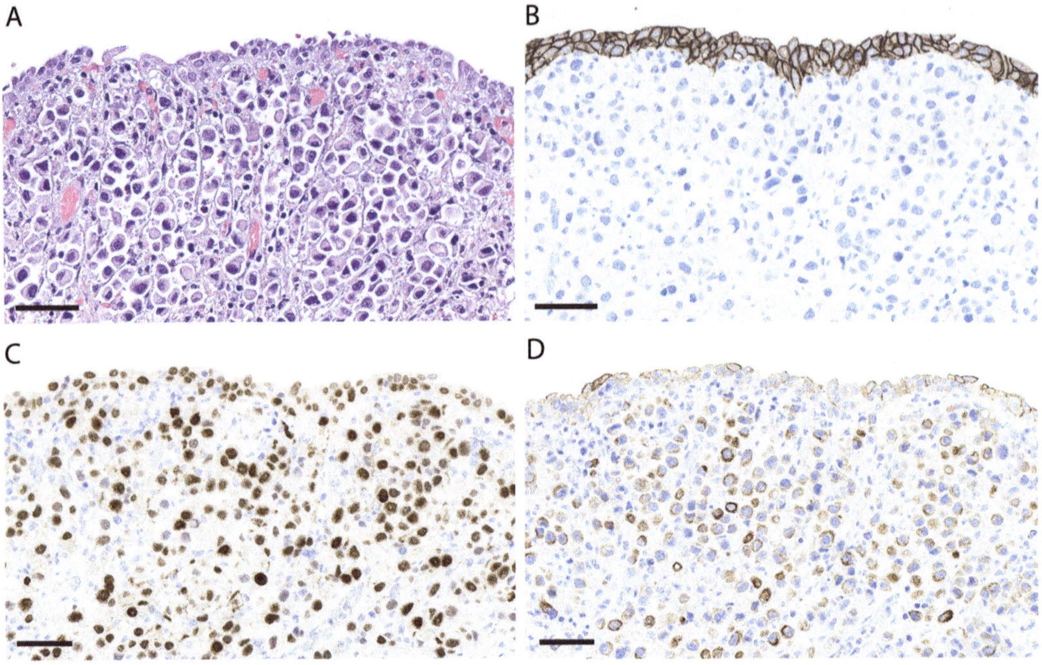

Fig. 15.3 Plasmacytoid subtype of urothelial carcinoma. (**a**). Hematoxylin eosin saffron staining of a representative plasmacytoid bladder cancer displaying sheets of discohesive tumor cells infiltrating the lamina propria. By immunohistochemistry, plasmacytoid urothelial carcinoma classically shows loss of CDH1 expression; Note the retained expression in the overlying urothelium (**b**). Plasmacytoid tumor cells express the nuclear luminal marker GATA3 (**c**) and the cytoplasmic marker CK20 (**d**). Scale bars: 50 μm

quently a complete lack thereof, reported in 65 to 100% of tumors of this subtype, providing a useful tool to confirm the diagnosis (Fig. 15.3b) (Sangoi et al. 2020; Kossaï et al. 2022). Functional in vitro experiments suggest that CDH1 loss increases the migration capacity of bladder cancer cells, providing an underlying mechanism for the discohesive and highly infiltrative nature of PUC (Al-Ahmadie et al. 2016). Finally, in contrast to other cancer types with similar morphology, in particular those of the breast (lobular carcinoma) or the stomach (diffuse type adenocarcinoma), no germline *CDH1* mutations have been identified in patients with PUC (Al-Ahmadie et al. 2016; Massari et al. 2021).

There is currently no transcriptomic profiling study in large PUC cohorts. In the TCGA study, 3 of 4 PUC cases clustered into the "Luminal infiltrated" subtype and the remaining case into the "Luminal papillary" subtype (Robertson et al. 2017). Using immunohistochemistry, most PUCs show expression of luminal markers GATA3, FOXA1, and CK20 and low expression of basal markers (Fig. 15.3c, d) (Lopez-Beltran et al. 2009; Nigwekar et al. 2009; Keck et al. 2011; Raspollini et al. 2011; Paner et al. 2014; Fox et al. 2017; Warrick et al. 2017; Perrino et al. 2019; Bontoux et al. 2021; Ravanini et al. 2021; Ikeda et al. 2021; Kossaï et al. 2022). Using the Lund immunohistochemistry panel or a simplified 3-marker version, PUCs were most frequently luminal "Genomically unstable" followed by "Urothelial-like" subtypes (Sjödahl et al. 2017; Warrick et al. 2019; Olkhov-Mitsel et al. 2021).

Overall, most plasmacytoid urothelial carcinomas are characterized by genomic or epigenetic alterations of *CDH1,* leading to the loss or abnormal expression of the cell–cell adhesion protein E-cadherin, explaining the histological discohesive aspect. At the transcriptomic level, current data suggests that PUCs mostly belong to luminal subtypes, but additional gene expression profiling studies are needed.

15.2.1.5 Sarcomatoid Urothelial Carcinoma

Sarcomatoid urothelial carcinoma (SUC) is an aggressive subtype exhibiting morphological features that are indistinguishable from those of malignant mesenchymal tumors, sarcomas (Cheng et al. 2011; IARC 2022). Most SUCs are composed of elongated pleomorphic cells of spindled appearance (Fig. 15.4a–c).

SUC genomic profiles show recurrent mutations in genes that are commonly altered in conventional urothelial carcinoma but with enrichment in mutations of *TP53*, *RB1,* and *PIK3CA* (Guo et al. 2019). *TERT* promoter mutations have been found in the majority of sarcomatoid urothelial carcinomas (Bertz et al. 2020). Other frequent mutations (>20% of 13 cases) were reported in *MYO1F, CNGB1, FXR1, RBM5,* and *SEMA3D.* No mutation of *FGFR3* has been described in this cohort of sarcomatoid tumors. Genomic comparison between sarcomatoid component and adjacent conventional urothelial carcinoma showed a common ancestor clone supporting phylogenetic association (Sung et al. 2007; Genitsch et al. 2019; Guo et al. 2019; Sirab et al. 2022).

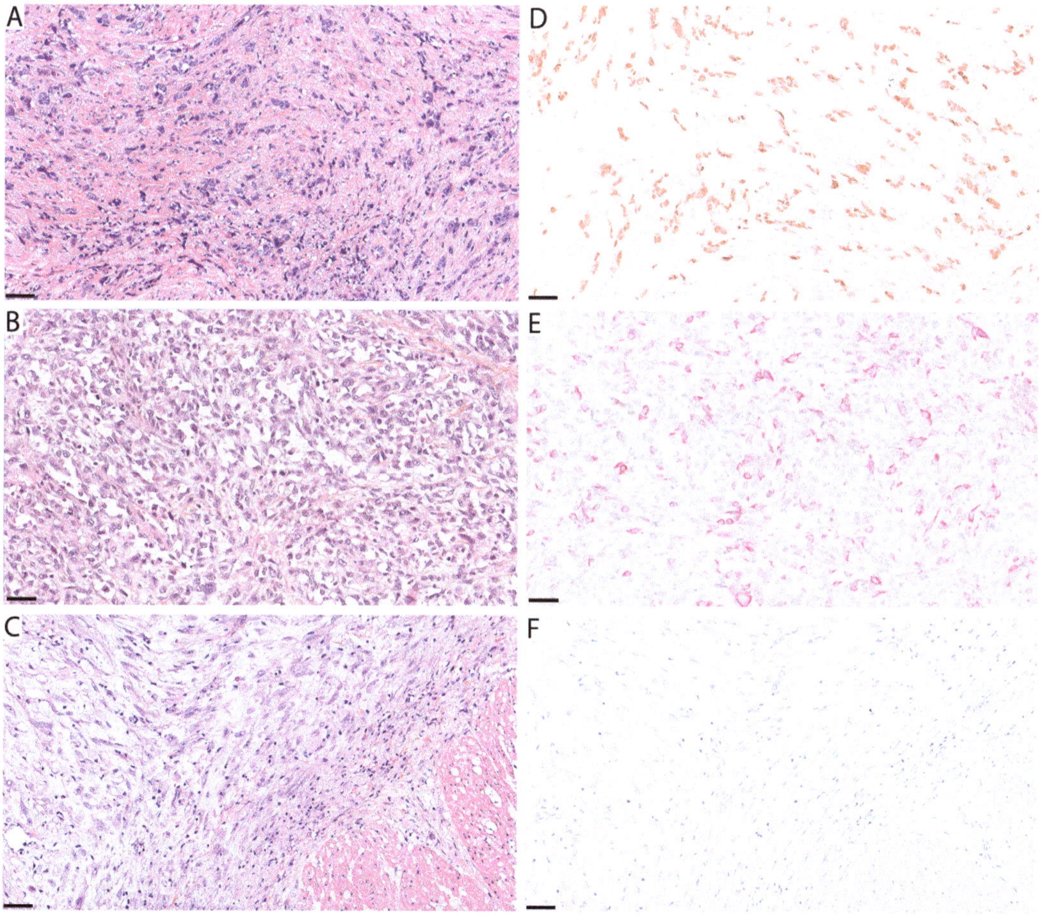

Fig. 15.4 Sarcomatoid urothelial carcinoma. Left panels (**a–c**) represent 3 examples of sarcomatoid urothelial carcinoma with spindle cell morphology (hematoxylin, eosin, and saffron staining). Right panels (**c–f**) illustrate matching dual immunohistochemistry staining of each case combining the nuclear luminal marker GATA3 (brown) and the cytoplasmic basal marker CK5/6 (red). These 3 examples show distinct phenotypes: luminal GATA3 positive/CK5/6 negative (**d**), basal GATA3 negative/CK5/6 positive, (**e**) or double negative (**f**). Scale bars: 50 μm

In transcriptomic classifications, most SUC cases cluster into basal subtypes, i.e., the "Basal" MDA classification subtype (Choi et al. 2014; Guo et al. 2019) or the Ba/Sq consensus class (Genitsch et al. 2019; Kamoun et al. 2020; Fontugne et al. 2023). It has been suggested that most SUC result from the progression through dedifferentiation of basal/squamous non-sarcomatoid urothelial carcinoma (Guo et al. 2019). Consistent with the basal subtype classification, most SUCs are characterized by a downregulation of mRNA expression of luminal markers, combined with an upregulation of basal keratin expression in approximately half of the cases (Guo et al. 2019). In contrast, typical molecular subtype-associated immunostaining, albeit performed in relatively small cohorts, shows disparate results in SUC (Fig. 15.4d–f). In line with the findings of Guo et al., basal marker expression by immunohistochemistry is retained in about half of reported SUC cases (Westfall et al. 2009; Sanfrancesco et al. 2016; Genitsch et al. 2019; Jangir et al. 2019; Ravanini et al. 2021). However, expression of luminal markers, such as GATA3, has been observed in up to 62% of SUCs (Paner et al. 2014; Sanfrancesco et al. 2016; Genitsch et al. 2019; Jangir et al. 2019; Ikeda et al. 2021). In studies using a combined luminal and basal marker analysis as a surrogate to identify molecular subtypes, a subset of SUCs also displayed a non-classified phenotype, most frequently characterized by a double negative pattern for luminal and basal markers (Guo et al. 2019; Bontoux et al. 2021; Ravanini et al. 2021; Sirab et al. 2022). Immunohistochemistry panels related to the Lund classification, although performed in a small number of cases, also demonstrate the heterogeneity of classifications found in SUCs, which can be "Basal/squamous," "Genomically unstable," "Urothelial-like," "Mesenchymal-like," or even "small cell/neuroendocrine" (Sjödahl et al. 2017; Warrick et al. 2019; Olkhov-Mitsel et al. 2021). These results highlight potential discrepancies between SUC immunoprofiles and transcriptomic classification and/or tumor heterogeneity. Thus, additional studies are required to fully unravel the molecular-immunohistochemical correlates in sarcomatoid urothelial carcinoma.

Global analysis of gene expression profiles of SUC also revealed epithelial-mesenchymal transition features, a physiological process by which epithelial cells transiently lose cell polarity and cell–cell adhesion and adopt a mesenchymal phenotype with increased migration capacity. Epithelial-mesenchymal transition features in SUC involved a decreased expression of epithelial adhesion molecules (Guo et al. 2019; Fontugne et al. 2023).

15.2.1.6 Nested, Tubular, and Microcystic Urothelial Carcinoma

Nested urothelial carcinoma (NUC) is recognized by the presence of infiltrating small round or ovoid tumor nests, composed of cells with minimal atypia (Lin et al. 2003; IARC 2022) (Fig. 15.5a). The very rare tubular and microcystic subtypes of urothelial carcinoma (TMUC) have only been studied in case reports or small series (Beltran et al. 2014). TMUC shows similarities with NUC, given their bland cytology, but differs by the presence of tubular structures or cysts of variable sizes (IARC 2022). Tubular and microcystic morphology may be seen adjacent to or admixed with nested features (Dhall et al. 2007; Beltran et al. 2014) and are thus combined in some published cohorts (Mai et al. 2014; Weyerer et al. 2019).

Although comprehensive genomic analyses are lacking, targeted sequencing studies suggest that, similar to conventional urothelial carcinoma, NUC harbors recurrent *TERT* promoter, *TP53* and *PIK3CA* mutations (Zhong et al. 2015; Weyerer et al. 2019; Taylor et al. 2020). In a cohort of 49 NUCs (including cases containing areas of tubular or microcystic morphology), Weyerer et al. also report *JAK3* mutations and *CTNNB1* mutations in 10% and 11.5% of 26 cases, respectively, rates higher than in the TCGA MIBC cohort. *FGFR3* mutation was identified in one case (3.8%) in this cohort (Weyerer et al. 2019).

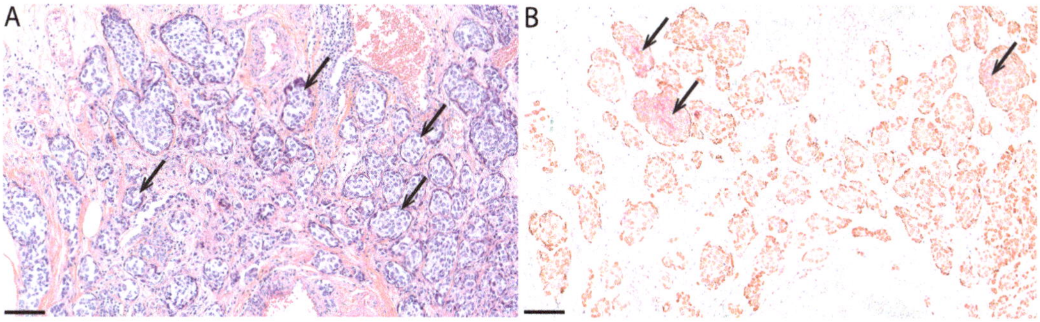

Fig. 15.5 Nested urothelial carcinoma. (**a**). Representative case of nested urothelial carcinoma defined by the presence of infiltrating small round or ovoid tumor nests (arrows), composed of cells with minimal atypia. (**b**). Dual immunohistochemistry staining using subtype defining markers shows a diffuse expression of the luminal marker GATA3 (brown) combined with focal expression of the basal marker CK5/6 (red, arrows). Scale bars: 100 μm

A dedicated gene expression profiling study of NUC or TMUC has not been published so far. Subtype-associated immunohistochemistry studies revealed high expression of luminal markers in most NUC and TMUC (Wasco et al. 2010; Beltran et al. 2014; Paner et al. 2014; Warrick et al. 2017; Weyerer et al. 2019) (Fig. 15.5b). However, conflicting results suggesting high expression of basal markers were reported in a cohort of 14 cases combining NUC and TMUC (Mai et al. 2014). This discrepancy may be partly explained by a specific pattern combining diffuse luminal marker expression, alongside basal marker expression in the outermost layers of tumor nests (Johnson et al. 2021). This expression pattern has previously been described as typical of the "Urothelial-like" Lund subtype (Sjödahl et al. 2017). In studies applying panels related to the Lund approach to a small number of cases, NUCs were in fact mostly classified as "Urothelial-like," or less frequently as "Genomically unstable" (Warrick et al. 2019; Olkhov-Mitsel et al. 2021). In a small series specifically of TMUCs, most cases expressed the luminal marker GATA3 by immunohistochemistry (Beltran et al. 2014). Additional molecular analyses in larger cohorts are needed to precisely define the molecular features of NUC and TMUC.

15.2.1.7 Large Nested Urothelial Carcinoma

In the previous edition of the WHO classification of tumors, large nested urothelial carcinoma (LNUC) was included under the nested variant category, likely due to their similarly bland cytology and nest-forming architecture. However, in contrast to NUC, LNUC is composed of nests that are larger in size, with round contours, or less often, irregularly shaped borders (Cox and Epstein 2011; Hacıhasanoğlu and Behzatoğlu 2019) (Fig. 15.6a). Given these distinct morphological features, as well as distinctive molecular characteristics, LNUC subtype has now been recognized as a specific subtype in the WHO 2022 edition (IARC 2022). This re-classification imposes caution when interpreting previous studies mixing NUC (with small nests) and LNUC without distinction.

There is limited literature regarding the genomic or transcriptomic features of LNUC. In a targeted next-generation study, LNUC cases displayed a higher rate of activating *FGFR3* mutations compared to unselected MIBC, which comprise about 15% of *FGFR3*-mutated cases (Robertson et al. 2017). Specifically, *FGFR3* mutations have been reported in approximately 73% of LNUC, with an even higher proportion in

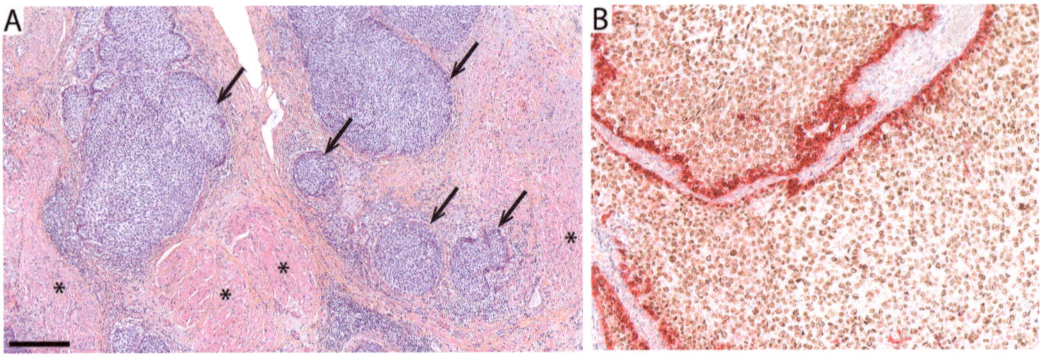

Fig. 15.6 Large nested urothelial carcinoma. (**a**). Representative case of large nested urothelial carcinoma showing large tumor nests with round or irregular borders (arrows), composed of cells with minimal atypia, infiltrating between bladder muscle bundles (asterisks). Scale bar: 250 μm. (**b**). High magnification of a dual immunohistochemistry staining using subtype defining markers shows a typical urothelial-like pattern with diffuse expression of the nuclear luminal marker GATA3 (brown) combined with expression of the basal marker CK5/6 at the periphery of the tumor nests (red)

the subset of tumors with pure large nested morphology (Weyerer et al. 2020). LNUC has also been shown, like conventional urothelial carcinoma, to harbor *TERT* promoter mutation in most cases (Weyerer et al. 2020). In a recent whole-exome sequencing study of 6 metastatic LNUCs, 3 harbored *FGFR3* mutations, followed by mutations in *PIK3CA* and *CDKN1B* in 2 cases each (Gamallat et al. 2023). Other frequently mutated genes in urothelial carcinoma, such as *ARID1A* or *KDM6A,* were each reported in one case. No *TP53* mutation was identified in this small cohort.

Using immunohistochemistry markers as a surrogate for transcriptomic subtyping, most LNUCs exhibit a luminal phenotype. The vast majority of LNUCs express the luminal marker GATA3, and less frequently CK20 (Compérat et al. 2017; Weyerer et al. 2020; Johnson et al. 2021). Basal cell marker expression was often limited to the peripheral cell layer of the nests (Weyerer et al. 2020; Johnson et al. 2021) conferring a typical urothelial-like phenotype, as proposed by the Lund group (Sjödahl et al. 2017) (Fig. 15.6b). These immunohistochemical findings, along with the genomic features described above, suggest that most LNUCs may belong to the *FGFR3* mutation-enriched "Luminal papillary" consensus transcriptomic subtype. Gene expression profiling of LNUCs is needed to confirm this hypothesis.

15.2.2 Histological Subtypes with Unexplored Molecular Features

The literature regarding the very rare remaining subtypes is limited to the description of clinicopathological features in case reports or small series, without molecular data. This is the case for urothelial carcinoma with trophoblastic differentiation, urothelial carcinoma with Müllerian differentiation, lipid-rich urothelial carcinoma, clear cell (glycogen-rich) urothelial carcinoma, giant cell urothelial carcinoma, and poorly differentiated urothelial carcinoma.

Transcriptomic profiling of the rare lymphoepithelioma-like subtype of urothelial carcinoma has been carried out in one study with 14 cases (Manocha et al. 2020). This histological subtype, characterized by sheets of poorly differentiated tumor cells within a dense immune infiltration, was enriched in cases of basal molecular phenotype. In contrast with the molecular profile, using immunohistochemistry most lymphoepithelioma-like tumors expressed the luminal markers FOXA1 or GATA3 to some level, with or without an associated basal marker expression (Manocha et al. 2020). All cases were negative for the luminal marker CK20 in another series of 34 lymphoepithelioma-like cases, with positivity of the basal marker p63 in 53% of cases (Williamson et al. 2011).

15.2.3 Neuroendocrine Carcinoma

Neuroendocrine carcinoma of the urinary bladder (NECUB) is an independent histological type and not a urothelial carcinoma histological subtype in the 2022 fifth edition of the WHO classification of urinary tumors (IARC 2022). Whether with small or large cells expressing immunohistochemical neuroendocrine markers (chromogranin-A, synaptophysin, INSM1) and high Ki-67 proliferation rate, NECUB is not phenotypically different from poorly differentiated neuroendocrine carcinoma developed in other organs (i.e., lung or prostate). However, only one third of the cases are pure and the remaining are admixed with urothelial carcinoma, either conventional, with divergent differentiation or histological subtype, suggesting related oncogenesis. Considering the very poor outcome of NECUB, it is of interest to specify the commonalities and differences between NECUB and urothelial carcinoma at genomic and transcriptomic levels to help the development of new therapeutic approaches.

Similar to neuroendocrine carcinoma from other organs, the combined inactivation of *RB1* and *TP53* was reported as the most recurrent alteration in NECUB (Chang et al. 2018; Shen et al. 2018; Hoffman-Censits et al. 2021). However, the NECUB mutational landscape also included other specific alterations encountered in conventional urothelial carcinoma, including *TERT* promoter mutations and APOBEC-mediated mutagenesis patterns. The specific occurrence of *TERT* promoter mutations in NECUB compared to neuroendocrine carcinoma developed in other organs was confirmed in other studies (Zheng et al. 2014; Priemer et al. 2018). These observations support a common cellular origin between NECUB and UC, and a specific progression pathway compared to other organs. A high tumor mutational burden was also reported in NECUB, raising the potential for immunotherapy approaches in the future.

In transcriptomic classifications, NECUB clusters within the "neuroendocrine-like" molecular subtype in the consensus classification, or in related subtypes of other classifications (Kamoun et al. 2020). The neuroendocrine-like molecular subtype displays high proliferation, low expression of basal and luminal markers, and high expression of neuroendocrine and/or neuronal markers (such as TUBB2B). This profile is mirrored in immunohistochemistry phenotypes: most cases are negative for KRT5, p63, GATA3, KRT20, with a loss of RB1 expression in 80% of cases and frequent over expression of FOXM1 and CCNB1 (Bernardo et al. 2022). As NECUB shares some features with luminal "genomically unstable" tumors, it has been suggested that NECUB might represent a progression from luminal unstable tumors (Bernardo et al. 2022). Of note, several authors noticed that 30 to 50% of tumors molecularly classified as neuroendocrine-like are diagnosed morphologically as UC and not NECUB but shared the same very poor outcome (Da Costa et al. 2019; Kamoun et al. 2020; Bernardo et al. 2022). Further studies are required to determine whether the definition of NECUB should be enlarged to all tumors belonging to the neuroendocrine-like subtype and to determine their oncogenetic relationships.

15.3 Conclusion

Genomic and transcriptomic profiling of urothelial carcinoma in the context of histological subtypes provides important insights into the molecular mechanisms underlying each morphological phenotype (Table 15.2). However, available data is preliminary in most histological subtypes and a comprehensive description of molecular features of each histological subtype will require additional studies in larger cohorts.

References

Al-Ahmadie HA, Iyer G, Lee BH et al (2016) Frequent somatic CDH1 loss-of-function mutations in plasmacytoid variant bladder cancer. Nat Genet 48:356–358. https://doi.org/10.1038/ng.3503

Almassi N, Whiting K, Toubaji A et al (2022) Clinical and genomic characterization of bladder carcinomas with glandular phenotype. JCO Precis Oncol 6:1–10. https://doi.org/10.1200/po.21.00392

Beltran AL, Cheng L, Montironi R et al (2014) Clinicopathological characteristics and outcome of nested carcinoma of the urinary bladder. Virchows Arch 465:199–205. https://doi.org/10.1007/s00428-014-1601-y

Bernardo C, Eriksson P, Marzouka NAD et al (2022) Molecular pathology of the non-luminal Ba/Sq-like and Sc/NE-like classes of urothelial tumours: an integrated immunohistochemical analysis. Hum Pathol 122:11–24. https://doi.org/10.1016/j.humpath.2022.01.006

Bertz S, Wach S, Taubert H et al (2016) Micropapillary morphology is an indicator of poor prognosis in patients with urothelial carcinoma treated with transurethral resection and radiochemotherapy. Virchows Arch 469:339–344. https://doi.org/10.1007/s00428-016-1986-x

Bertz S, Stöhr R, Gaisa NT, Wullich B, Hartmann A, Agaimy A (2020) TERT promoter mutation analysis as a surrogate to morphology and immunohistochemistry in problematic spindle cell lesions of the urinary bladder. Histopathology 77(6):949–962. https://doi.org/10.1111/his.14206. Epub 2020 Sep 22. PMID: 32645760

Bontoux C, Rialland T, Cussenot O, Compérat E (2021) A four-antibody immunohistochemical panel can distinguish clinico-pathological clusters of urothelial carcinoma and reveals high concordance between primary tumor and lymph node metastases. Virchows Arch 478:637–645. https://doi.org/10.1007/s00428-020-02951-0

Bowden M, Nadal R, Zhou CW et al (2020) Transcriptomic analysis of micropapillary high grade T1 urothelial bladder cancer. Sci Rep 10:1–10. https://doi.org/10.1038/s41598-020-76904-7

Chang MT, Penson A, Desai NB et al (2018) Small-cell carcinomas of the bladder and lung are characterized by a convergent but distinct pathogenesis. Clin Cancer Res 24:1965–1973. https://doi.org/10.1158/1078-0432.CCR-17-2655

Cheng L, Zhang S, Alexander R et al (2011) Sarcomatoid carcinoma of the urinary bladder: the final common pathway of urothelial carcinoma dedifferentiation. Am J Surg Pathol 35:34–46. https://doi.org/10.1097/PAS.0b013e3182159dec

Cheng KA, Kurtis B, Babayeva S et al (2015) Heterogeneity of TERT promoter mutations status in squamous cell carcinomas of different anatomical sites. Ann Diagn Pathol 19:146–148. https://doi.org/10.1016/j.anndiagpath.2015.03.005

Cheng L, Lopez-Beltran A, Wang M et al (2021) Telomerase reverse transcriptase (TERT) promoter mutations in primary adenocarcinoma of bladder and urothelial carcinoma with glandular differentiation: pathogenesis and diagnostic implications. Mod Pathol 34:1384–1391. https://doi.org/10.1038/s41379-021-00776-z

Ching CB, Amin MB, Tubbs RR et al (2011) HER2 gene amplification occurs frequently in the micropapillary variant of urothelial carcinoma: analysis by dual-color in situ hybridization. Mod Pathol 24:1111–1119. https://doi.org/10.1038/modpathol.2011.69

Choi W, Porten S, Kim S et al (2014) Identification of distinct basal and luminal subtypes of muscle-invasive bladder cancer with different sensitivities to frontline chemotherapy. Cancer Cell 25:152–165. https://doi.org/10.1016/j.ccr.2014.01.009

Compérat E, McKenney JK, Hartmann A et al (2017) Large nested variant of urothelial carcinoma: a clinicopathological study of 36 cases. Histopathology 71:703–710. https://doi.org/10.1111/his.13280

Cox R, Epstein JI (2011) Large nested variant of urothelial carcinoma: 23 cases mimicking von brunn nests and inverted growth pattern of noninvasive papillary urothelial carcinoma. Am J Surg Pathol 35:1337–1342. https://doi.org/10.1097/PAS.0b013e318222a653

Da Costa JB, Gibb EA, Bivalacqua TJ et al (2019) Molecular characterization of neuroendocrine like bladder cancer. Clin Cancer Res 25:3908–3920. https://doi.org/10.1158/1078-0432.CCR-18-3558

Damrauer JS, Hoadley KA, Chism DD et al (2014) Intrinsic subtypes of high-grade bladder cancer reflect the hallmarks of breast cancer biology. Proc Natl Acad Sci USA 111:3110–3115. https://doi.org/10.1073/pnas.1318376111

Dhall D, Al-Ahmadie H, Olgac S (2007) Nested variant of urothelial carcinoma. Arch Pathol Lab Med 131:1725–1727. https://doi.org/10.5858/2007-131-1725-NVOUC

Fantini D, Glaser AP, Rimar KJ et al (2018) A carcinogen-induced mouse model recapitulates the molecular alterations of human muscle invasive bladder cancer. Oncogene 37:1911–1925. https://doi.org/10.1038/s41388-017-0099-6

Fleischmann A, Rotzer D, Seiler R et al (2011) Her2 amplification is significantly more frequent in lymph node metastases from urothelial bladder cancer than in the primary tumours. Eur Urol 60:350–357. https://doi.org/10.1016/j.eururo.2011.05.035

Font A, Domènech M, Benítez R et al (2020) Immunohistochemistry-based taxonomical classification of bladder cancer predicts response to neoadjuvant chemotherapy. Cancers (Basel) 12:1–13. https://doi.org/10.3390/cancers12071784

Fontugne J, Wong J, Cabel L et al (2023) Progression-associated molecular changes in basal/squamous and sarcomatoid bladder carcinogenesis. J Pathol 259:455–467. https://doi.org/10.1002/path.6060

Fox MD, Xiao L, Zhang M et al (2017) Plasmacytoid urothelial carcinoma of the urinary bladder. Am J Clin

Pathol 147:500–506. https://doi.org/10.1093/ajcp/aqx029

Gamallat Y, Afsharpad M, El Hallani S et al (2023) Large, nested variant of urothelial carcinoma is enriched with activating mutations in fibroblast growth factor Receptor-3 among other targetable mutations. Cancers (Basel) 15:3167. https://doi.org/10.3390/cancers15123167

Genitsch V, Kollár A, Vandekerkhove G et al (2019) Morphologic and genomic characterization of urothelial to sarcomatoid transition in muscle-invasive bladder cancer. Urol Oncol 37:826–836. https://doi.org/10.1016/j.urolonc.2019.09.025

Guo CC, Dadhania V, Zhang L et al (2016) Gene expression profile of the clinically aggressive micropapillary variant of bladder cancer. Eur Urol 70:611–620. https://doi.org/10.1016/j.eururo.2016.02.056

Guo CC, Majewski T, Zhang L et al (2019) Dysregulation of EMT drives the progression to clinically aggressive Sarcomatoid bladder cancer. Cell Rep 27:1781–1793.e4. https://doi.org/10.1016/j.celrep.2019.04.048

Hacıhasanoğlu E, Behzatoğlu K (2019) Large nested urothelial carcinoma: a clinicopathological study of 22 cases on transurethral resection materials. Ann Diagn Pathol 42:7–11. https://doi.org/10.1016/j.anndiagpath.2019.06.005

Hajiran A, Azizi M, Aydin AM et al (2021) Pathological and survival outcomes associated with variant histology bladder cancers managed by cystectomy with or without neoadjuvant chemotherapy. J Urol 205:100–108. https://doi.org/10.1097/JU.0000000000001325

Hansel DE, Swain E, Dreicer R, Tubbs RR (2008) HER2 overexpression and amplification in urothelial carcinoma of the bladder is associated with MYC coamplification in a subset of cases. Am J Clin Pathol 130:274–281. https://doi.org/10.1309/41VLTFX3YPP1HF6F

Hoffman-Censits J, Choi W, Pal S et al (2021) Urothelial cancers with small cell variant histology have confirmed high tumor mutational burden, frequent TP53 and RB mutations, and a unique gene expression profile. Eur Urol Oncol 4:297–300. https://doi.org/10.1016/j.euo.2019.12.002

Hovelson DH, Udager AM, McDaniel AS et al (2018) Targeted DNA and RNA sequencing of paired urothelial and squamous bladder cancers reveals discordant genomic and transcriptomic events and unique therapeutic implications. Eur Urol 74:741–753. https://doi.org/10.1016/j.eururo.2018.06.047

Hurst CD, Platt FM, Taylor CF, Knowles MA (2012) Novel tumor subgroups of urothelial carcinoma of the bladder defined by integrated genomic analysis. Clin Cancer Res 18:5865–5877. https://doi.org/10.1158/1078-0432.CCR-12-1807

IARC (2022) WHO classification of tumours editorial board. Urinary and male genital tumours [internet], WHO classification of tumours series, vol 8, 5th edn. International Agency for Research on Cancer, Lyon (France)

Ikeda J, Ohe C, Yoshida T et al (2021) Comprehensive pathological assessment of histological subtypes, molecular subtypes based on immunohistochemistry, and tumor-associated immune cell status in muscle-invasive bladder cancer. Pathol Int 71:173–182. https://doi.org/10.1111/pin.13060

Isharwal S, Huang H, Nanjangud G et al (2018) Intratumoral heterogeneity of ERBB2 amplification and HER2 expression in micropapillary urothelial carcinoma. Hum Pathol 77:63–69. https://doi.org/10.1016/j.humpath.2018.03.015

Jackson CL, Chen L, Hardy CSC et al (2022) Diagnostic and prognostic implications of a three-antibody molecular subtyping algorithm for non-muscle invasive bladder cancer. J Pathol Clin Res 8:143–154. https://doi.org/10.1002/cjp2.245

Jangir H, Nambirajan A, Seth A et al (2019) Prognostic stratification of muscle invasive urothelial carcinomas using limited immunohistochemical panel of Gata3 and cytokeratins 5/6, 14 and 20. Ann Diagn Pathol 43:151397. https://doi.org/10.1016/j.anndiagpath.2019.08.001

Johnson SM, Khararjian A, Legesse TB et al (2021) Nested variant of urothelial carcinoma is a luminal bladder tumor with distinct coexpression of the basal marker cytokeratin 5/6. Am J Clin Pathol 155:588–596. https://doi.org/10.1093/ajcp/aqaa160

Kamoun A, de Reyniès A, Allory Y et al (2020) A consensus molecular classification of muscle-invasive bladder cancer. Eur Urol 77:420–433. https://doi.org/10.1016/j.eururo.2019.09.006

Keck B, Stoehr R, Wach S et al (2011) The plasmacytoid carcinoma of the bladder-rare variant of aggressive urothelial carcinoma. Int J Cancer 129:346–354. https://doi.org/10.1002/ijc.25700

Kossaï M, Radulescu C, Adam J et al (2022) Plasmacytoid urothelial carcinoma (UC) are luminal tumors with similar CD8+ Tcell density and PD-L1 protein expression on immune cells as compared to conventional UC. Urol Oncol Semin Orig Investig 40:12.e1–12.e11. https://doi.org/10.1016/j.urolonc.2021.07.014

Labban M, Najdi J, Mukherji D et al (2021) Triple-marker immunohistochemical assessment of muscle-invasive bladder cancer: is there prognostic significance? Cancer Rep 4:1–8. https://doi.org/10.1002/cnr2.1313

Laé M, Couturier J, Oudard S et al (2009) Assessing HER2 gene amplification as a potential target for therapy in invasive urothelial bladder cancer with a standardized methodology: results in 1005 patients. Ann Oncol 21:815–819. https://doi.org/10.1093/annonc/mdp488

Lin O, Cardillo M, Dalbagni G et al (2003) Nested variant of urothelial carcinoma: a clinicopathologic and immunohistochemical study of 12 cases. Mod Pathol 16:1289–1298. https://doi.org/10.1097/01.MP.0000094091.04541.FC

Lopez-Beltran A, Requena MJ, Montironi R et al (2009) Plasmacytoid urothelial carcinoma of the bladder. Hum Pathol 40:1023–1028. https://doi.org/10.1016/j.humpath.2009.01.001

Lopez-Beltran A, Blanca A, Cimadamore A et al (2022) T1 bladder carcinoma with variant histology: pathological features and clinical significance. Virchows Arch 480:989–998. https://doi.org/10.1007/s00428-021-03264-6
Mai KT, Hakim SW, Ball CG et al (2014) Nested and microcystic variants of urothelial carcinoma displaying immunohistochemical features of basal-like urothelial cells: an immunohistochemical and histopathogenetic study. Pathol Int 64:375–381. https://doi.org/10.1111/pin.12187
Manocha U, Kardos J, Selitsky S et al (2020) RNA expression profiling of Lymphoepithelioma-like carcinoma of the bladder reveals a basal-like molecular subtype. Am J Pathol 190:134–144. https://doi.org/10.1016/j.ajpath.2019.09.007
Marzouka NAD, Eriksson P, Rovira C et al (2018) A validation and extended description of the Lund taxonomy for urothelial carcinoma using the TCGA cohort. Sci Rep 8:1–12. https://doi.org/10.1038/s41598-018-22126-x
Massari G, Magnoni F, Favia G et al (2021) Frequency of cdh1 germline mutations in non-gastric cancers. Cancers (Basel) 13:4–11. https://doi.org/10.3390/cancers13102321
Masuda N, Murakami K, Kita Y et al (2020) Trp53 mutation in keratin 5 (Krt5)-expressing basal cells facilitates the development of basal squamous-like invasive bladder cancer in the chemical carcinogenesis of mouse bladder. Am J Pathol 190:1752–1762. https://doi.org/10.1016/j.ajpath.2020.04.005
Maurer A, Ortiz-Bruechle N, Guricova K et al (2020) Comparative genomic profiling of glandular bladder tumours. Virchows Arch 477:445–454. https://doi.org/10.1007/s00428-020-02787-8
Moktefi A, Pouessel D, Liu J et al (2018) Reappraisal of HER2 status in the spectrum of advanced urothelial carcinoma: a need of guidelines for treatment eligibility. Mod Pathol 31:1270–1281. https://doi.org/10.1038/s41379-018-0023-9
Nguyen D, Taheri D, Springer S et al (2016) High prevalence of TERT promoter mutations in micropapillary urothelial carcinoma. Virchows Arch 469:427–434. https://doi.org/10.1007/s00428-016-2001-2
Nigwekar P, Tamboli P, Amen MB et al (2009) Plasmacytoid urothelial carcinoma: detailed analysis of morphology with clinicopathologic correlation in 17 cases. Am J Surg Pathol 33:417–424. https://doi.org/10.1097/PAS.0b013e318186c45e
Olkhov-Mitsel E, Hodgson A, Liu SK et al (2021) Three-antibody classifier for muscle invasive urothelial carcinoma and its correlation with p53 expression. J Clin Pathol 75:766–771. https://doi.org/10.1136/jclinpath-2021-207573
Osei-Amponsa V, Buckwalter JM, Shuman L et al (2020) Hypermethylation of FOXA1 and allelic loss of PTEN drive squamous differentiation and promote heterogeneity in bladder cancer. Oncogene 39:1302–1317. https://doi.org/10.1038/s41388-019-1063-4
Palsgrove DN, Taheri D, Springer SU et al (2019) Targeted sequencing of plasmacytoid urothelial carcinoma reveals frequent TERT promoter mutations. Hum Pathol 85:1–9. https://doi.org/10.1016/j.humpath.2018.10.033
Paner GP, Annaiah C, Gulmann C et al (2014) Immunohistochemical evaluation of novel and traditional markers associated with urothelial differentiation in a spectrum of variants of urothelial carcinoma of the urinary bladder. Hum Pathol 45:1473–1482. https://doi.org/10.1016/j.humpath.2014.02.024
Perrino CM, Eble J, Kao CS et al (2019) Plasmacytoid/diffuse urothelial carcinoma: a single-institution immunohistochemical and molecular study of 69 patients. Hum Pathol 90:27–36. https://doi.org/10.1016/j.humpath.2019.04.012
Priemer DS, Wang M, Zhang S et al (2018) Small-cell carcinomas of the urinary bladder and prostate: TERT promoter mutation status differentiates sites of malignancy and provides evidence of common clonality between small-cell carcinoma of the urinary bladder and urothelial carcinoma. Eur Urol Focus 4:880–888. https://doi.org/10.1016/j.euf.2017.03.007
Raspollini MR, Sardi I, Giunti L et al (2011) Plasmacytoid urothelial carcinoma of the urinary bladder: clinicopathologic, immunohistochemical, ultrastructural, and molecular analysis of a case series. Hum Pathol 42:1149–1158. https://doi.org/10.1016/j.humpath.2010.11.011
Ravanini JN, Assato AK, Wakamatsu A, Alves VAF (2021) Combined use of immunohistochemical markers of basal and luminal subtypes in urothelial carcinoma of the bladder: association with clinicopathological features and outcomes. Clinics 76:1–8. https://doi.org/10.6061/CLINICS/2021/E2587
Rebouissou S, Bernard-Pierrot I, De Reyniès A et al (2014) EGFR as a potential therapeutic target for a subset of muscle-invasive bladder cancers presenting a basal-like phenotype. Sci Transl Med 6:244ra91–244ra91. https://doi.org/10.1126/scitranslmed.3008970
Reddy OL, Cates JM, Gellert LL et al (2015) Loss of FOXA1 drives sexually dimorphic changes in urothelial differentiation and is an independent predictor of poor prognosis in bladder cancer. Am J Pathol 185:1385–1395. https://doi.org/10.1016/j.ajpath.2015.01.014
Robertson AG, Kim J, Al-Ahmadie H et al (2017) Comprehensive molecular characterization of muscle-invasive bladder cancer. Cell 171:540–556.e25. https://doi.org/10.1016/j.cell.2017.09.007
Ross JS, Wang K, Gay LM et al (2014) A high frequency of activating extracellular domain ERBB2 (HER2) mutation in micropapillary urothelial carcinoma AC. Clin Cancer Res 20:68–75. https://doi.org/10.1158/1078-0432.CCR-13-1992
Ross JS, Wang K, Khaira D et al (2016) Comprehensive genomic profiling of 295 cases of clinically advanced urothelial carcinoma of the urinary bladder reveals a high frequency of clinically relevant genomic altera-

tions. Cancer 122:702–711. https://doi.org/10.1002/cncr.29826

Sanfrancesco J, McKenney JK, Leivo MZ et al (2016) Sarcomatoid urothelial carcinoma of the bladder: analysis of 28 cases with emphasis on clinicopathologic features and markers of epithelial-to-mesenchymal transition. Arch Pathol Lab Med 140:543–551. https://doi.org/10.5858/arpa.2015-0085-OA

Sangoi AR, Higgins JP, Rouse RV et al (2009) Immunohistochemical comparison of MUC1, CA125, and Her2Neu in invasive micropapillary carcinoma of the urinary tract and typical invasive urothelial carcinoma with retraction artifact. Mod Pathol 22:660–667. https://doi.org/10.1038/modpathol.2009.16

Sangoi AR, Chan E, Stohr BA, Kunju LP (2020) Invasive plasmacytoid urothelial carcinoma: a comparative study of E-cadherin and P120 catenin. Hum Pathol 102:54–59. https://doi.org/10.1016/j.humpath.2020.07.006

Schneider SA, Sukov WR, Frank I et al (2014) Outcome of patients with micropapillary urothelial carcinoma following radical cystectomy: ERBB2 (HER2) amplification identifies patients with poor outcome. Mod Pathol 27:758–764. https://doi.org/10.1038/modpathol.2013.201

Seiler R, Ashab HAD, Erho N et al (2017) Impact of molecular subtypes in muscle-invasive bladder cancer on predicting response and survival after neoadjuvant chemotherapy [figure presented]. Eur Urol 72:544–554. https://doi.org/10.1016/j.eururo.2017.03.030

Shen P, Jing Y, Zhang R et al (2018) Comprehensive genomic profiling of neuroendocrine bladder cancer pinpoints molecular origin and potential therapeutics. Oncogene 37:3039–3044. https://doi.org/10.1038/s41388-018-0192-5

Sirab N, Drubay D, Maillé P et al (2022) Multilayer spectrum of intratumoral heterogeneity in basal bladder cancer. J Pathol 256:108–118. https://doi.org/10.1002/path.5813

Sjödahl G, Lauss M, Lövgren K et al (2012) A molecular taxonomy for urothelial carcinoma. Clin Cancer Res 18:3377–3386. https://doi.org/10.1158/1078-0432.CCR-12-0077-T

Sjödahl G, Eriksson P, Liedberg F, Höglund M (2017) Molecular classification of urothelial carcinoma: global mRNA classification versus tumour-cell phenotype classification. J Pathol 242:113–125. https://doi.org/10.1002/path.4886

Sung M-T, Wang M, MacLennan G et al (2007) Histogenesis of sarcomatoid urothelial carcinoma of the urinary bladder: evidence for a common clonal origin with divergent differentiation. J Pathol 211:420–430. https://doi.org/10.1002/path.2129

Tanaka H, Yoshida S, Koga F et al (2018) Impact of immunohistochemistry-based subtypes in muscle-invasive bladder cancer on response to chemoradiation therapy. Int J Radiat Oncol Biol Phys 102:1408–1416. https://doi.org/10.1016/j.ijrobp.2018.06.030

Taylor AS, McKenney JK, Osunkoya AO et al (2020) PAX8 expression and TERT promoter mutations in the nested variant of urothelial carcinoma: a clinicopathologic study with immunohistochemical and molecular correlates. Mod Pathol 33:1165–1171. https://doi.org/10.1038/s41379-020-0453-z

Teo MY, Al-Ahmadie H, Seier K et al (2021) Natural history, response to systemic therapy, and genomic landscape of plasmacytoid urothelial carcinoma. Br J Cancer 124:1214–1221. https://doi.org/10.1038/s41416-020-01244-2

Tripathi N, Jo Y, Tripathi A et al (2022) Genomic landscape of locally advanced or metastatic urothelial carcinoma with squamous differentiation compared to pure urothelial carcinoma. Urol Oncol Semin Orig Investig 40:493.e1–493.e7. https://doi.org/10.1016/j.urolonc.2022.07.002

Tschui J, Vassella E, Bandi N et al (2015) Morphological and molecular characteristics of HER2 amplified urothelial bladder cancer. Virchows Arch 466:703–710. https://doi.org/10.1007/s00428-015-1729-4

Vail E, Zheng X, Zhou M et al (2015) Telomerase reverse transcriptase promoter mutations in glandular lesions of the urinary bladder. Ann Diagn Pathol 19:301–305. https://doi.org/10.1016/j.anndiagpath.2015.06.007

Volkmer JP, Sahoo D, Chin RK et al (2012) Three differentiation states risk-stratify bladder cancer into distinct subtypes. Proc Natl Acad Sci USA 109:2078–2083. https://doi.org/10.1073/pnas.1120605109

Warrick JI, Kaag M, Raman JD et al (2017) FOXA1 and CK14 as markers of luminal and basal subtypes in histologic variants of bladder cancer and their associated conventional urothelial carcinoma. Virchows Arch 471:337–345. https://doi.org/10.1007/s00428-017-2190-3

Warrick JI, Sjödahl G, Kaag M et al (2019) Intratumoral heterogeneity of bladder cancer by molecular subtypes and histologic variants. Eur Urol 75:18–22. https://doi.org/10.1016/j.eururo.2018.09.003

Wasco MJ, Daignault S, Bradley D, Shah RB (2010) Nested variant of urothelial carcinoma: a clinicopathologic and immunohistochemical study of 30 pure and mixed cases. Hum Pathol 41:163–171. https://doi.org/10.1016/j.humpath.2009.07.015

Weinstein JN, Akbani R, Broom BM et al (2014) Comprehensive molecular characterization of urothelial bladder carcinoma. Nature 507:315–322. https://doi.org/10.1038/nature12965

Westfall DE, Folpe AL, Paner GP et al (2009) Utility of a comprehensive immunohistochemical panel in the differential diagnosis of spindle cell lesions of the urinary bladder. Am J Surg Pathol 33:99–105. https://doi.org/10.1097/PAS.0b013e318180c899

Weyerer V, Weisser R, Moskalev EA et al (2019) Distinct genetic alterations and luminal molecular subtype in nested variant of urothelial carcinoma. Histopathology 75:865–875. https://doi.org/10.1111/his.13958

Weyerer V, Eckstein M, Compérat E et al (2020) Pure large nested variant of urothelial carcinoma (Lnuc)

is the prototype of an fgfr3 mutated aggressive urothelial carcinoma with luminal-papillary phenotype. Cancers (Basel) 12:1–12. https://doi.org/10.3390/cancers12030763

Williamson SR, Zhang S, Lopez-Beltran A et al (2011) Lymphoepithelioma-like carcinoma of the urinary bladder: Clinicopathologic, immunohistochemical, and molecular features. Am J Surg Pathol 35:474–483. https://doi.org/10.1097/PAS.0b013e31820f709e

Yang Y, Kaimakliotis HZ, Williamson SR et al (2020) Micropapillary urothelial carcinoma of urinary bladder displays immunophenotypic features of luminal and p53-like subtypes and is not a variant of adenocarcinoma. Urol Oncol Semin Orig Investig 38:449–458. https://doi.org/10.1016/j.urolonc.2019.10.013

Zheng X, Zhuge J, Bezerra SM et al (2014) High frequency of TERT promoter mutation in small cell carcinoma of bladder, but not in small cell carcinoma of other origins. J Hematol Oncol 7:1–5. https://doi.org/10.1186/s13045-014-0047-7

Zhong M, Tian W, Zhuge J et al (2015) Distinguishing nested variants of urothelial carcinoma from benign mimickers by TERT promoter mutation. Am J Surg Pathol 39:127–131. https://doi.org/10.1097/PAS.0000000000000305

Zinnall U, Weyerer V, Compérat E et al (2018) Micropapillary urothelial carcinoma: evaluation of HER2 status and immunohistochemical characterization of the molecular subtype. Hum Pathol 80:55–64. https://doi.org/10.1016/j.humpath.2018.05.022

Part V

Experimental Models of Bladder Cancer

The Emerging Landscape of Mouse Bladder Cancer Models

16

Tomoko Iwata and Amal Rahil Elgaddafi Yousef

Abstract

Bladder cancer is common and urgently requires new therapies and management strategies. Mouse models are essential platforms that enable interventional studies to address important biological and clinical questions *in vivo* and provide critical evidence complementary to that from human studies. In this chapter, we present an overview of the current mainstream mouse platforms, then outline recent models that present novel insights into the understanding of bladder cancer and proof-of-principle for potential therapies, including the molecular analyses undertaken. Findings from recent models of *Fgfr3* alterations, as well as potential targets to improve response to anti-PD-1/PD-L1 immune checkpoint immunotherapy are discussed. The new generation of mouse models and molecular understanding of them have allowed researchers to address issues that have previously been considered challenging, such as metastasis and sex differences in disease progression and treatment response. Despite technical difficulties and their resource-intensive nature, mouse *in vivo* platforms continue to be an invaluable tool for bladder cancer research.

Keywords

Urothelial carcinoma · Carcinogen · Transgenic mice · Patient-derived xenograft · Organoids · Orthotopic transplantation · Transcriptomics · Immunotherapy · Metastasis · Sex differences

T. Iwata (✉)
School of Medicine, Dentistry and Nursing, College of Medical, Veterinary and Life Sciences, University of Glasgow, Glasgow, UK

Medical Genetics and Pathology, Laboratory Medicine, Queen Elizabeth University Hospital, Glasgow, UK
e-mail: Tomoko.Iwata@glasgow.ac.uk

A. R. E. Yousef
School of Medicine, Dentistry and Nursing, College of Medical, Veterinary and Life Sciences, University of Glasgow, Glasgow, UK
e-mail: 2219759y@student.gla.ac.uk

16.1 Introduction

In vivo models are important platforms that aid understanding of disease mechanisms, identification of new therapeutic targets, and evaluation of drugs prior to clinical trials. Mouse models are by far the most well-established *in vivo* platform in terms of technology, methodology, and their biological characterization. In recent times, disease mechanisms and therapeutic targets can be explored more directly in humans, for example by bioinformatics approaches using publicly available data, such as that from The Cancer Genome Atlas (TCGA) (Robertson et al. 2017).

M. A. Knowles, L. Dyrskjøt (eds.), *Biology of Bladder Cancer*,
https://doi.org/10.1007/978-3-031-68505-7_16

However such evidence provides only correlation rather than direct proof. Bladder cancer is one of the most common cancer types and has major unmet needs in better therapies and management strategies to improve patient survival and quality of life. Research efforts are needed to identify alternatives to Bacillus Calmette-Guerin (BCG) treatment for high-risk non-muscle invasive bladder cancer (NMIBC) and to improve response to chemotherapy and immunotherapy in muscle-invasive bladder cancer (MIBC) and advanced disease. Recent genomic and gene expression profiling of patient samples has led to the identification of molecular subtypes, which has enhanced our understanding of the underlying tumor biology, and has also necessitated the development of models that interrogate potential applications of this new knowledge to clinical management (Ruan et al. 2019; Seyer et al. 2019). Newly developed mouse models can now be used to address questions that have previously been considered challenging, such as the role of immune cells in the tumor microenvironment and metastasis (Hatogai and Sweis 2020; Crispen and Kusmartsev 2020; Seyer et al. 2019; Kobayashi 2016). Importantly, scientific research must also support equality and inclusion in our society. Bladder cancer shows a marked sex-related difference in incidence (see Chap. 1). Variations in biology and therapy response that may arise from sex differences must also be characterized (Koti et al. 2020). Mouse studies are resource intensive, require expert knowledge, and must be ethically justifiable. Thus, before undertaking studies involving mice, researchers should scrutinize the necessity for mouse models and appropriateness of the study design.

16.2 Primer: Basics of Mouse Studies

16.2.1 Overview: Mouse Models and Experimental Design

Mouse models can be categorized as spontaneous (also called "autochthonous") and transplantable ("non-autochthonous") (Wakefield et al. 2023; John and Said 2017) (Fig. 16.1). Spontaneous models are those where tumors arise *in situ* from the bladder, for example, induced by bladder-specific carcinogens (carcinogen-induced models) or by introducing gene deletions or mutations in a mouse chromosome by genetic manipulation (genetically engineered mouse, GEM). In transplantable models, tumor cells are grafted into mice. Modes of transfer could be orthotopic, into the bladder, or heterotopic, to the lower flank, tail vain or footpad of the animal. Tumor cells of human origin can be transplanted to immunocompromised mice as a host (xenograft), or mouse tumor cells to immunocompetent mice of the same strain, i.e., with the same genetic background (allograft, or also called "syngeneic" transplantation). Transplantable tumor materials can be established cell lines ("CellDX" or "CellDA" for human cell-line derived xenografts and mouse syngenetic cell-line derived allografts, respectively), patient-derived tumor xenografts (PDXs), or circulating tumor cells (CTC) (CDXs) (Wakefield et al. 2023).

Like any other experimental platform, mouse models need to be used in the right context. A good bladder cancer model may meet the following basic requirements: (1) tumors are of urothelial origin and reflect molecular and histopathological characteristics; (2) characteristics of tumor progression reflect that of humans; (3) primary tumors grow in the bladder and they can be exposed to drugs by intravesical delivery; (4) primary and metastasized tumors can be monitored real-time and non-invasively; and (5) tumors progress in the immunocompetent tumor microenvironment. It is unlikely that any chosen model would satisfy all criteria, but it should be emphasized that the model needs to be characterized and validated at the outset.

Mouse studies can take a variety of approaches investigating pro- or anti-tumor roles of a gene or obtaining proof-of-principle evidence of a drug's efficacy. Survival of mice is determined by an endpoint, which is normally the timepoint at which animals show clinical signs of morbidity that is ethically acceptable, rather than the actual death of the animal. Tumor progression can be evaluated at set timepoints, either by histopatho-

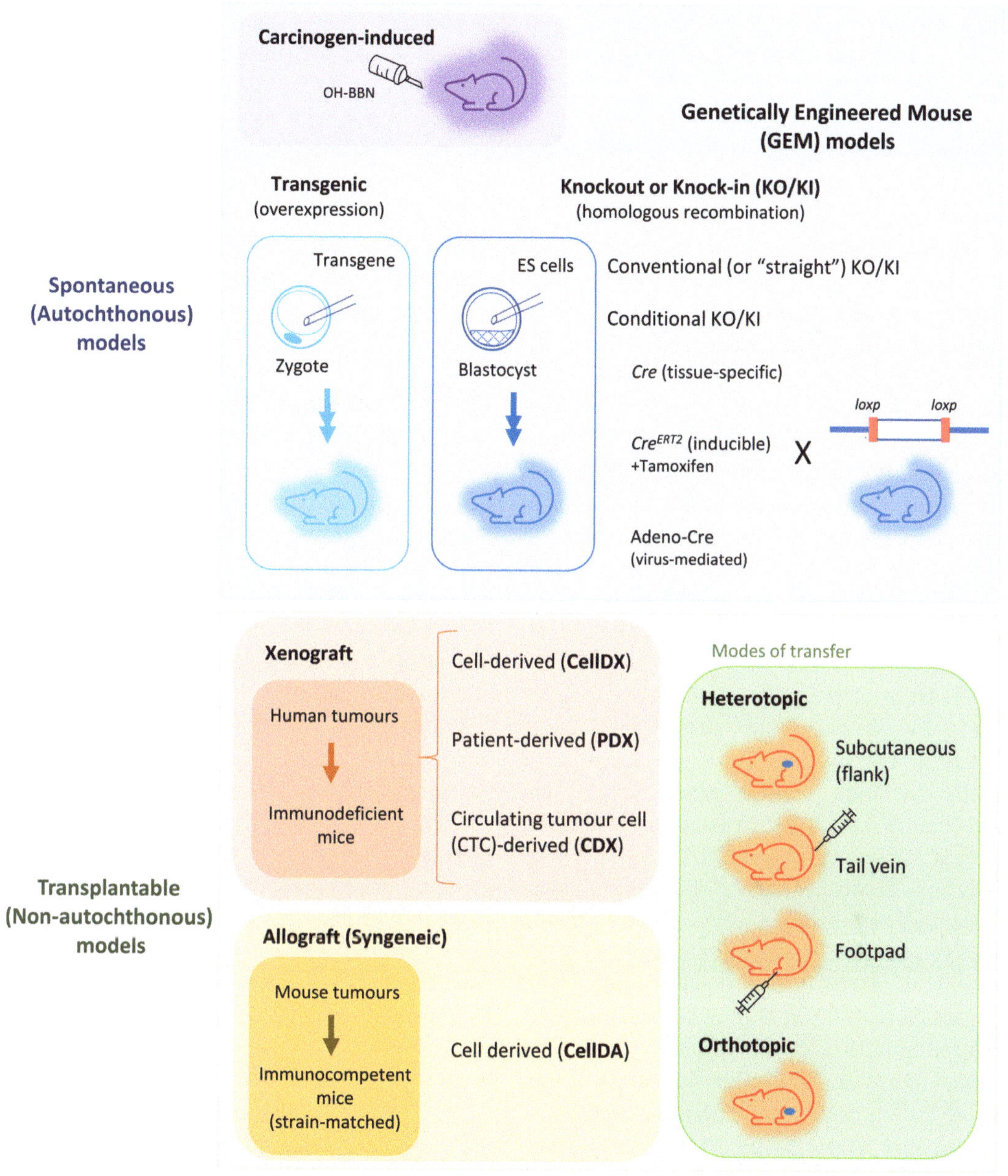

Fig. 16.1 Overview of mouse models

logical evaluation of tumor tissues by killing the mice at each timepoint or by non-invasive imaging of the same mice. Early intervention could be used to evaluate the preventative effects of the drug, while intervention at a later stage would be suitable for evaluating suppression of tumor growth or metastasis. Drugs can be administered short- or long-term to evaluate acute or chronic effects. Evaluation of the drug's toxicity and pharmacokinetics should be incorporated early on in the study.

16.2.2 Models of Bladder Tumors Induced by the Carcinogen OH-BBN

N-butyl-N-(4-hydroxybutyl) nitrosamine (OH-BBN) is widely used as a bladder-specific carcinogen. OH-BBN is metabolized from N-nitroso compounds (NOC) in cigarette smoke, a major risk factor for urothelial cancer (Vasconcelos-Nobrega et al. 2012). OH-BBN covalently binds and causes damage to DNA. By the *in vivo* mutagenicity test with *lacI* (BigBlue™) mice, OH-BBN was shown to induce mutations specifically in the bladder urothelium, but not in the ureter, kidney, liver, or forestomach (He et al. 2012). The tissue specificity of this carcinogen is an important factor, as tumorigenesis in other tissues, such as in the intestine and the lung, would normally kill the mice before bladder tumors form (de la Rosa et al. 2017; Friedrich et al. 2017).

OH-BBN is normally administered to mice aged 6–8 weeks in drinking water for 10–25 weeks at 0.05% v/v, followed by a subsequent time period to allow further tumor progression (Oliveira et al. 2018). Pre-malignant lesions, such as carcinoma *in situ* (CIS), may appear as early as 4–12 weeks from the start of carcinogen induction, and invasive tumors are normally observed in 40–80% of mice at 20–25 weeks (Ismail et al. 2022; Korac-Prlic et al. 2020; Degoricija et al. 2019; Foth et al. 2018). Tumors induced by OH-BBN are clonal and multifocal (Yamamoto et al. 1998). Histopathology of urothelial lesions caused by OH-BBN is well documented and shown to reflect that in humans, including hyperplasia, atypia, dysplasia, CIS, and invasive tumors. However, metastasis is only rarely reported (Degoricija et al. 2019; Foth et al. 2018; Ho et al. 2012; Vasconcelos-Nobrega et al. 2012; Kobayashi 2016). Mouse background may influence susceptibility to carcinogen-induced tumorigenesis (Ohtani et al. 1986).

The main advantages of the OH-BBN-induced model are that it relates to smoking, is relatively simple to generate, and is reliable in terms of tumor generation and histopathological characteristics (John and Said 2017; Kobayashi 2016; Vasconcelos-Nobrega et al. 2012). Disadvantages are that tumor induction takes 4–6 months of continuous carcinogen application, the severity of tumorigenesis can vary from animal to animal, and the model does not represent non-invasive tumors, the most common form of bladder cancer. In addition, mice need to be maintained in filtered-top cages in a facility with appropriate ventilation, under health and safety regulations to protect researchers from carcinogen exposure.

16.2.3 Derivation of Genetically Engineered Mouse Models

GEM models are primarily used to address gene function, by either deleting (knockout mice) or overexpressing a gene (transgenic mice), using germ-line gene transfer (Haruyama et al. 2009; Hall et al. 2009) (Fig. 16.1). Knockout mice are generated by homologous recombination in mouse embryonic stem (ES) cells, delivered by a targeting vector that mediates a deletion of the whole or a part of the gene that is essential to its function. The correctly targeted ES cell clones are isolated by screening and injected to mouse blastocysts, which are then transferred to a foster mother. Offspring are bred for further screening to establish the mouse line. Knock-in mice that carry gene mutations can also be generated in this way. Transgenic mice are traditionally generated by microinjection of an overexpression vector into mouse zygotes.

Models using the *Cre-lox* system can be used to derive tissue-specific, "conditional" recombination. Cre recombinase is a bacterial enzyme that excises a stretch of DNA between two 34 base-pair long "*loxp*" sequences (Kim et al. 2018). Conditional deletion of a gene is achieved by delivery of *Cre*, either by mating or by virus, to mice that carry a "floxed" allele, a cassette of two *loxp* sequences flanking the gene of interest. In reverse, conditional expression can be achieved by *loxp-stop-loxp,* "LSL" cassette inserted upstream of the gene in transgenic vector in mice. Time-dependent, "inducible" gene modification can be achieved by administration of tamoxifen to mice that carry Cre^{ERT2} and *loxp* cassettes.

Cre^{ERT2} encodes Cre recombinase fused with estrogen receptor with a mutated ligand binding domain, which only binds tamoxifen. Binding of tamoxifen by the fusion protein leads to its translocation to the nucleus, where Cre recombination takes place. In order for genetic modification to occur in a bladder-specific context, promoters for uroplakins (*Ukp2, Ukp3*) have often been used to drive Cre expression (John and Said 2017; Saito et al. 2018). Promoters for cytokeratin 5 (*Ck5*), *Ck8, and Ck14* are also used in urothelial cell-type specific recombination in the inducible mode and in adenovirus-mediated *Cre* delivery (Park et al. 2021; Van Batavia et al. 2014). Cre mice could drive recombination incompletely or in unexpected tissues and cells. Therefore, their efficiency should be evaluated at the outset, for example by crossing them with a reporter line that expresses LacZ, GFP, or tdTomato upon recombination.

GEM models develop tumors naturally (or "spontaneously"), originating in the bladder of animals with an intact immune system. This also means that tumors may not develop in all mice and tumor phenotype may be variable, which may make the model unsuitable for drug testing. Furthermore, bladder cancer is one of the most highly mutated cancer types (Alexandrov et al. 2013). Apart from strong tumor inducers, such as *Pten* loss and *p53* mutation, modification of a single gene is normally insufficient to lead to tumor development. In GEM models, the cross-talk of genes can be assessed for no more than 2–3 genes, as mating and genotyping is time-consuming and costly. As an alternative approach, GEM models can be used in conjunction with carcinogen induction. For example, a pro-tumorigenic role of a gene can be identified by evidence of accelerating tumor formation upon carcinogen induction and the converse for an anti-tumor role.

16.2.4 Transplantable Models

In classical xenograft transplantation models, established human tumor cell lines are subcutaneously injected into the lower flank of immunodeficient mice (heterotopic CellDX) (Fig. 16.1). Immunodeficient mouse strains include nude mice that lack thymus and therefore have few or no functional T cells (also called "nude" as they lack fur), severe combined immunodeficiency (SCID) mice that lack T and B cells, and SCID/non-obese diabetic (NOD) mice that lack T, B, and natural killer (NK) cells (Chen et al. 2022). Athymic nude mice have been most typically used in classical xenograft transplantation. Xenografts have been widely used in translational studies as they facilitate drug application and measurement of tumor size. An appropriate model should have a long enough timeframe for drug testing and an efficient "take rate" (rate of successful transplantation). Many cell lines are well characterized molecularly (John and Said 2017; Dancik et al. 2011). The orthotopic mode of transplantation into the bladder has the advantage that tumors develop in the bladder tissue. Tumor grafts are established by intravesical instillation of a cell line, typically of an aggressive type to overcome the lower take rate, by intramural injection via laparotomy, or percutaneous injection guided by ultrasound imaging to facilitate injection precisely to the bladder wall (Jager et al. 2018). However, the tumor microenvironment of xenograft tumors consists of mouse stroma, without immune components.

PDXs are established from surgically removed tumors that are passaged as tissue fragments *in vivo* in highly immunodeficient mice as hosts to ensure reasonable take rates (Wakefield et al. 2023; Bernardo and Santos 2018; Kita et al. 2020). PDXs are more advantageous than CellDX in that the primary tumor's histology and genetic diversity can be retained through passages. The tumor microenvironment is better represented in PDXs, but still lacks immune components. CellDXs and PDXs can be "humanized" by co-transplantation of human lymphocytes (Gong et al. 2015). PDXs are difficult to establish due to a low take rate and the time it takes to establish the first passage. Genetic and phenotypic drift may also occur, so that PDXs are unlikely to be a true "avatar" of the individual patient (Ben-David et al. 2017).

Syngeneic cell lines derived from the same strain of mouse can be transplanted either subcutaneously or orthotopically (CellDA). The two lines used most frequently are MB49, which was established from C57Bl/6 mice treated with the carcinogen 7,12-dimethylbenz[*a*]anthracene (DMBA), and MBT2 from C3H/He mice treated with N-[4-(5-nitro-2-furyl)-2-thiazolyl] formamide (FANFT) (Ruan et al. 2019; John and Said 2017). Syngeneic models are advantageous in having a "natural" tumor microenvironment that consists of both tumor and stromal cells of the mouse of origin, with an intact immune system. However, given the presence of a healthy immune system, tumors may regress spontaneously. Hence, successful syngeneic cell lines tend to be those that are aggressive and grow rapidly, making long-term study challenging. New syngeneic cell lines have been established recently that have shown differential response to therapeutic agents (Kim et al. 2022; Nikolos et al. 2022; Hayashi et al. 2020). These models are one of the promising platforms that are expected to be used more in the coming years.

16.3 Recent Advances in Mouse Models of Spontaneous Urothelial Tumorigenesis

16.3.1 Molecular and Immunological Characterization of Carcinogen-Induced Models

As carcinogens widely induce genomic alterations and perturb gene expression, it is important to characterize their profiles and determine whether they reflect those in human tumors. Early studies showed that OH-BBN models share many differentially regulated genes with those in human bladder tumors (Lu et al. 2011; Williams et al. 2008) (Table 16.1). *p53* mutations are frequently induced, while those in *Hras* and *Kras*, as well as fibroblast growth factor receptor 3 (*Fgfr3),* are infrequent (Yamamoto et al. 1995; Dunois-Larde et al. 2005). A more recent study evaluated the genomic and transcriptional profiles of OH-BBN treated bladders (Fantini et al. 2018). While pre-malignant bladders (4 weeks of carcinogen induction) showed activation of immune-related pathways, tumors (20 weeks of continuous carcinogen application) showed a basal subtype expression signature, with dysregulation of cell cycle and metabolic genes. Tumors contained a high number of mutations in *p53*, and *Kmt2c*, and *Kmt2d* methyltransferases, but not in *Fgfr3* or *Kdm6a.* The study also defined mouse mutational signatures, MOUSIG A and B, corresponding to human COSMIC5 and COSMIC22 signatures, respectively. However, APOBEC signatures were not found in mice, indicating that there is a difference in mutational processes between mouse and human invasive bladder tumors. Tumor size and histopathology were not correlated with mutation load, suggesting that tumor progression is not caused by the overall number of carcinogen-induced mutations, but by key driver mutations.

Earlier studies investigated the effects of nonsteroidal anti-inflammatory drugs (NSAID), indomethacin and celecoxib, in B6D2F1 mice treated with OH-BBN (Lubet et al. 2005; Grubbs et al. 2000). Mice showed a reduction in tumor formation and increased survival, which suggested a pro-tumorigenic role of inflammation. A recent study characterized the immune response and gene expression in the OH-BBN model (Degoricija et al. 2019) (Table 16.1). An inflammatory response was evident at 2 weeks of carcinogen treatment. There was also a notable upregulation of anti-inflammatory interleukin 4 *(Il4)*, which may explain the temporary resolution of inflammation in the following weeks even if carcinogen treatment continued. In tumors, a pro-inflammatory cytokine, *Il18*, and interferon gamma (*Ifnγ*)-responsive genes, as well as immune suppressive genes, cytotoxic T-lymphocyte associated protein 4 (*Ctla4*), programmed death-ligand 1 (*Pd-l1*), and indoleamine 2,3-dioxygenase (*Ido1*), were upregulated. Overall, the model showed similar patterns of gene regulation to those in human MIBC, confirming that they are suitable for pre-clinical studies of immunomodulators.

Table 16.1 Molecular characterization of mouse bladder cancer models

Context of molecular investigation	Mice	Molecular Platform	Main findings	Reference
OH-BBN				
Comparisons of gene expression in humans, rats, and mice	Male C57Bl/6 x DBA/2 F1	Affymetrix MGU74Av2 GeneChips, GSEA	OH-BBN treatment for 12 weeks by gavage. Comparing tumor and normal bladder, 13–34% of total genes were differentially expressed. 20% of them overlapped among mouse, rat, and humans.	(Lu et al. 2011)
Genomic and expression profile of OH-BBN-induced tumors compared to human MIBC	Male C57Bl/6	RNA-seq, pathway enrichment analysis, WES	OH-BBN induced immune-related pathways in pre-tumor samples, while tumors showed basal signatures and were enriched with cell cycle and metabolic pathways.	(Fantini et al. 2018)
Profile of inflammatory response in OH-BBN-induced bladders and tumors	Male C57Bl/6	RNA-seq, RT2 profiler mouse PCR Array, GSEA, Seq- ImmuCC	INFγ-responsive genes were upregulated in the bladders at 2 weeks as a pre-malignant inflammatory response. IL18 was upregulated in tumors at 20 weeks.	(Degoricija et al. 2019)
Comparisons of gene expression and immune profiles of the bladder by age and sex	C57Bl/6, male and female mice	RNA-seq, DESeq2, GSEA, multiplex IF	Differences in gene expression and immune infiltration were identified in age/sex-dependent manner. B-cell-associated pathways were enriched in the bladders of aged females compared to aged males.	(Hamade et al. 2022)
GEM				
Identification of genes expressed in the absence of *Foxa1* comparing males and females	Male and female *UBC-Cre*^{ERT2} *Foxa1*$^{loxp/loxp}$	Affymetrix mouse gene 1.0 ST Array, IPA	*Foxa1* deletion in female mice led to an additional change in the level of cytokeratin gene expression in the bladder, supporting the squamous differentiation observed	(Reddy et al. 2015)
Identification of genes regulated by *Kdm6a* in the urothelium	Female *Upk2Cre Kdm6a* knockout. C57Bl/6 J background	RNA-seq, IPA	p53 tumor suppressor, ERK/MAPK pathways, *Cdkn1* and *perp* genes were among the downregulated pathways and genes in the *Kdm6a* conditional knockout.	(Kaneko and Li 2018)
Identification of the effects of *Pparg* deletion in UTI and pre-malignant bladders	Male and female *Shh*^{Cre};*Pparg*$^{flox/flox}$, *Krt5*^{CreER}; *Pparg*$^{flox/flox}$	RNA-seq, GSEA	*Pparg* in the urothelium regulated genes important for mitochondrial biogenesis and urothelial cell differentiation. UTI model showed that *Pparg* deletion promoted squamous differentiation and upregulation of *Nflb* and its target genes, indicating sustained inflammation.	(Liu et al. 2019)
Gene expression in association with tumor progression caused by urothelial cell-type specific deletion of *p53* and *Pten*	*Ck5-Cre*^{ERT2} *pten*$^{fl/fl}$*p53*$^{fl/fl}$. C57Bl/6 J background	RNA-seq, GSEA	Pre-invasive tumors expressed pro-inflammatory signaling. The mouse 28-gene signature of early tumors predictive of poor prognosis was developed.	(Park et al. 2021)

(continued)

Table 16.1 (continued)

Context of molecular investigation	Mice	Molecular Platform	Main findings	Reference
Identification of genes regulated by FGFR3 S249C overexpression in the urothelium	*UPII-hFGFR3b-S249C.* C57Bl/6 background	Affymetrix mouse exon 1.0 ST Array, GSEA, mMCP counter	While hyperplastic lesions were similar to normal urothelium, tumors showed a distinct transcriptomic profile. FGFR3 S249C tumors showed expression of luminal subtype with lower immune infiltration.	(Shi et al. 2023)
Identification of genes regulated by FGFR3 S249C overexpression in the urothelium	$Upk3a\text{-}Cre^{ERT2};Trp53^{LSL\text{-}R270H/+};LSL\text{-}FGFR3^{S249C/+};Rosa26^{LSL\text{-}luc/+}$ (UFPL)	RNA-seq, GSEA	Tumors resulting from *FGFR3 S249C* and *p53* mutations showed luminal molecular profile and intermediate level of T-cell inflamed immune contexture.	(Okato et al. 2024).
OH-BBN-induced GEM				
Identification of genes regulated by acute and chronic inflammation, and in the absence of Il6	Wild-type and Il6 knockout mice	RNA-seq, RT2 profiler mouse PCR Array	During acute response (2 weeks), the majority of immune response genes were downregulated in the absence of Il6. After chronic inflammation, the majority of innate and adaptive immune cell markers were upregulated at 20 weeks in Il6 knockout bladders.	(Korac-Prlic et al. 2020)
Identification of the effects of *Pparg* overactivation leading to luminal, and immune-cold, invasive tumors	*K5VP16; Pparg*, $VP16;Pparg^{fl/fl}$ and UPPL. C57Bl/6 background	RNA-seq, GSEA	OH-BBN (4 weeks) enhanced expression of basal markers, inflammatory and immune markers, while suppressing luminal markers. OH-BBN-treated *K5VP16;Pparg* tumors showed enhanced luminal marker expression and were immune-cold, in contrast to basal tumor controls, $VP16;Pparg^{fl/fl}$ and UPPL.	(Tate et al. 2021).
Xenograft				
Evaluation of the effects of celecoxib in xenograft tumors treated with gemcitabine and cisplatin (GC)	T24 xenograft	RNA-seq, GSEA	GC induced wound-response gene signature in xenograft tumors, which is suppressed in the presence of COX2 inhibitor, celecoxib.	(Kurtova et al. 2015)
PDX				
Molecular characterization of CoCaB1 PDX and organoids, during early and late passage	CoCaB1 PDX and organoid, early and late passages	RNA-seq, IPA	Molecular subtype signatures and mutational profile were retained through passages in PDX and organoids, CoCaB1, derived from an aggressive, cisplatin-resistant MIBC case.	(Cai et al. 2021)
Syngeneic				
Characterization of UPPL1541 and BBN963 in comparison with MB49	UPPL1541, BBN963, MB49. Cell line and cell-line derived tumors.	RNA-seq, IPA, BASE47 subtype analysis, TCR/BCR repertoire profiling	UPPL1541 and BBN963 cell lines and their tumors showed characteristics of luminal and basal subtypes, respectively, including characteristic immune gene signature profiles. MB49 was more fibroblast-like, showing a signature of epithelial-to-mesenchymal transition.	(Saito et al. 2018)

Abbreviations: GSEA, gene set enrichment analysis; IPA, Ingenuity Pathway Analysis; OH-BBN, N-butyl-N-(4-hydroxybutyl) nitrosamine; WES, whole exome sequencing; UTI, urinary tract infection

16.3.2 New Insights from GEM Models

A previous study has shown that Cre recombinase delivered by adenovirus under the CMV promoter (AdenoCMV-Cre) allows double deletion of *p53* and *Pten* genes in a bladder-specific manner, leading to invasive bladder cancer with poor survival (Puzio-Kuter et al. 2009). In second-generation Adeno-Cre models, highly cell-type specific recombination was achieved under the control of *Ck5* (basal cells) and *Ck8* (intermediate cells) promoters (AdenoCk5-Cre, AdenoCk8-Cre) using surgical delivery, or more efficiently via transurethral injection (Park et al. 2021). In parallel, efficiency of recombination by inducible *Ck5-Cre*^{ERT2} and *Ck8-Cre*^{ERT2} lines was investigated upon intravesical application of tamoxifen, which showed cell-type specific recombination in a highly controllable manner (Park et al. 2021). These approaches are complementary, each with specific advantages and disadvantages, and best used based on the research context. Using both Adeno-Cre and *Cre*^{ERT2} lines, it was shown that *Ck5*-promoter driven deletion of *p53* and *Pten* led to development of invasive urothelial cancer (>T3), while *Ck8*-driven deletion showed a milder, less advanced tumor phenotype, suggesting that basal cells are the populations which contribute to invasive tumors. Comparison of the transcriptomes in *Ck5*- and *Ck8-Cre*^{ERT2} *Pten*$^{fl/fl}$*p53*$^{fl/fl}$ tumors with human data, a 28-gene mouse signature in early-stage tumors was developed that is predictive of poor prognosis (Table 16.1).

Recent GEM models have reported interesting biological findings that are of clinical relevance. Peroxisome proliferator-activated receptor γ (PPARG) is a multifunctional nuclear receptor, which heterodimerizes with retinoid X receptor (RXR) and binds to peroxisome proliferator response elements (Tate et al. 2021; Liu et al. 2019). PPARG is known to be activated by natural ligands, such as eicosanoids and prostaglandins, and it plays a role in control of the inflammatory response, as well as in embryonic development and homeostasis. In MIBC molecular subtypes, PPARG expression is distinctively high in the luminal subtype, while low in the basal subtype, and therefore is considered a key luminal marker (Robertson et al. 2017; Kamoun et al. 2019). The role of Pparg was explored using loss-of-function and overexpression mouse models directed to specific cell populations of the urothelium (Liu et al. 2019; Tate et al. 2021). Deletion of *Pparg* was achieved by crosses with *ShhCre* (all urothelial cells), *Krt5Cre*^{ERT2} (basal cells), and *Upk2Cre*^{ERT2} (Superficial (S) and Intermediate (I) cell in adults) (Liu et al. 2019). Pparg was shown to play a role in differentiation of I and S cells during embryonic development. In contrast, in adults, Pparg was important in all cell types (basal, I, and S cells) and, in particular, in specifying Ck14^{+} basal-cell progenitors by suppressing squamous transformation. In a urinary tract infection (UTI) model, in which the urothelium was infected with uropathogenic E. coli (UPEC), *Pparg* loss induced squamous metaplasia, without tumor development. RNA-seq and pathway enrichment analysis have indicated that Pparg is important for mitochondrial biogenesis and urothelial cell differentiation (Table 16.1). Upregulation of pro-inflammatory nuclear factor-kB *(Nfkb)* is normally transient upon UTI. In the absence of *Pparg*, however, expression of *Nfkb* and its target genes were sustained until long after resolution, with increased F4/80, CD3, and CD45 infiltrations, indicating the overall upregulation of an innate immune response. In the following study, basal-cell specific inducible expression of *Pparg* was achieved by strong HSV *VP16* promoter-driven expression of *Pparg*, induced by *Krt5Cre*^{ERT2} (*K5VP16;Pparg*) (Tate et al. 2021). Contrary to the phenotype of *Pparg* deletion above, Pparg activation induced differentiation of basal cells into superficial cells. OH-BBN applied for 4 weeks was then used to induce mutations in Ck5^{+}Ck14^{+} basal progenitors, which led to the formation of luminal tumors at 4 months after induction. Transcriptomic analysis supported the Pparg activation leading to luminal gene expression in the tumor, immune-cold contexture, and downregulation of *Nfkb* (Tate et al. 2021). Interestingly, a fraction of luminal tumors showed basal phenotype in part of the tumor, indicating a phenotypic drift to basal invasive tumors as they lost *Pparg* expression. This may reflect intratumor heterogeneity in human cases which underlies recurrence or progression (Tate et al. 2021).

Similar to Pparg, the transcription factor, Forkhead box A1 (FOXA1) is a luminal marker in human MIBC, whose mRNA level is high in the luminal subtype, and low in the basal subtype (Robertson et al. 2017; Osei-Amponsa et al. 2020). *FOXA1* expression is associated with methylation of specific CpG islands in human bladder cancer and it is downregulated in human basal-squamous bladder cancer cell lines (Osei-Amponsa et al. 2020). No tumorigenesis was observed in mice when *FoxA1* and *Pten* genes were individually deleted. However, deletion of both genes together (*UpIICre* $Foxa^{loxp/loxp}$ $Pten^{loxp/loxp}$) led to development of tumors with prominent squamous differentiation without OH-BBN induction and accelerated tumorigenesis upon OH-BBN induction. The results suggest that *FOXA1* downregulation in luminal cells plays a role in inducing squamous transformation of invasive tumors.

The transcription factor, STAT3, is upregulated in invasive bladder cancer and its role has been investigated in K5.Stat3C transgenic mice that express dimerized, activated Stat3C under control of the *Ck5* promoter, induced by OH-BBN for 12 weeks and monitored for tumorigenesis (Ho et al. 2012). The results showed that Stat3 activation induced invasive tumors without going through a phase of hyperplasia. Stat3 transgenic tumors harbored more $Ck14^{+}$ progenitors and fewer $Ck16^{+}$ intermediate cells and were more active in sphere formation, indicating that Stat3 tips urothelial populations toward a progenitor state. A recent study further investigated the role of interleukin 6 (Il6)-STAT3 signaling in bladder tumorigenesis and explored the effects of Il6 inhibition in combination with PD-L1 blockade (Korac-Prlic et al. 2020). Inducible $Upk3aCre^{ER}$ $Stat3^{flox/flox}$ mice were treated with tamoxifen to induce *Stat3* deletion. Carcinogen-induced tumorigenesis was reduced in the absence of *Stat3* compared to that in wild-type mice. In contrast, in *Il6* knockout mice in which inflammation was suppressed, tumorigenesis was enhanced (Table 16.1). Combined treatment with Stat3 inhibitor and Il6 blockade showed a cumulative suppression of tumorigenesis. Finally, either Stat3 inhibition or Il6 blockade was able to sensitize bladder tumors to anti-PD-L1 immune checkpoint immunotherapy (ICI) (Table 16.2).

16.4 Recent Advances in Transplantation Models

16.4.1 Improvements in Orthotopic Transplantation

Experimental drugs have been tested in the orthotopic transplantation model, to evaluate a novel theragnostic approach for high-risk NMIBC and in recurrent tumors that progress to MIBC (Huebner et al. 2017; Sun et al. 2020; Naito et al. 2020). An orthotopic xenograft was developed with the human UM-UC-3 urothelial cancer cell line transduced with a luciferase reporter for visualization (UM-UC-3^{Luc}K1) (Huebner et al. 2017). A high rate of engraftment and reproducible period of tumor growth was achieved by transurethral transfer of cells by 24G permanent venous catheters into poly-L-lysine treated bladders of SCID-beige mice. In another study, the UM-UC-3 orthotopic model was evaluated following improved catheter insertion and pretreatment of the bladder wall with trypsin (Naito et al. 2020). Muscle invasion was observed within 21 days, and tumor growth was suppressed upon cisplatin or gemcitabine treatment, indicating that the model is suitable for drug testing. Furthermore, a model with UM-UC-3 with a GFP reporter (UM-UC-3-GFP) was shown to allow real-time monitoring of tumors by noninvasive as well as intra-vital fluorescent imaging (Sun et al. 2020).

One of the limitations of orthotopic models is that the rapidly growing tumors may cause bladder obstruction, making survival time too short for the evaluation of drug efficacy. The MBT-2 syngeneic model develops invasive tumors and metastasis within 2–3 weeks (Seo et al. 2017; Kirschner et al. 2021). To better control mouse

Table 16.2 Strategies to improve response by immune checkpoint inhibitors (ICIs). Recent studies (2018–2023) that addressed strategies to improve the response to ICIs in bladder cancer mouse models are listed

Mouse model	Target to be combined with ICI	Main findings	Reference
OH-BBN			
Male C57BL/6	Anti-PD-1 combined with B7-H4 blocking antibody	Combining anti-PD-1 with anti-B7-H4 antibody reduced tumor size and tumor stage score and also increased $CD8^+$ T cells and decreased Tregs within the tumor.	(Podojil et al. 2020)
Male C57BL/6 J	Anti-PD-L1 combined with STAT3 inhibitor or anti-IL-6 antibody	Stat3 inhibition or Il6 blockade sensitized bladder tumors to anti-PD-L1. Combining Il6 and Stat3 inhibition with anti-PD-L1 resulted in reduced inflammation and downregulation of immune genes including *Il4, Il10, Cd4, Tlr1, Ccr6,* and *Itgam*, and downregulation of B cells (CD19), macrophages (F4/80), and eosinophils (CCR3).	(Korac-Prlic et al. 2020)
GEM			
Adeno-Cre $Pten^{flox/flox}$ $p53^{flox/flox}$	Anti-PD-1 combined with anti-CD40 agonist antibody	Combining anti-PD-1 with anti-CD40 antibody overcame anti-PD-1 resistance by increasing $CD8^+$ T cells in the tumor and shifting from M2 to M1 phenotype through the effect of Ifnγ.	(Leblond et al. 2020)
Syngeneic			
G69, G7, derived from K5.Stat3C transgenic mice, to FVB/N	Anti-PD-1 combined with iDAMP blockers +/− GC	Combining anti-PD-1 with an iDAMP blocker (e.g., COX2 inhibitor, celecoxib) along with chemotherapy (GC) enhanced the response to ICIs. Blocking iDAMPs caused DCs to mature and promoted the recruitment of anti-tumor $CD8^+$ T cells.	(Nikolos et al. 2022)
MB49 to male C57BL/6 J (orthotopic)	Anti-PD-1/PD-L1 combined with CD39i +/− cisplatin	Inhibiting CD39 using POM-1 increased NK cells, cDC1, and $CD8^+$ T cells, while decreasing Treg cells. CD39i showed a synergistic effect with cisplatin, but there was no synergistic effect when combined with anti-PD-1 or anti-PD-L1.	(Liu et al. 2022)
MBT-2 to C3H/HeJ	Anti-PD-1 combined with DC vaccine	Combining anti-PD-1 with activated DCs that were isolated from C3H/HeJ enhanced Ifnγ production and promoted anti-tumor immunity through antigen-specific T cells.	(Lim et al. 2023)
Cisplatin-resistant cell lines MB49R to female C57BL/6	Anti-PD-1 combined with anti-PMN- and Mo-MDSCs antibodies	The combination of anti-Gr1 and anti-Ly6C antibodies to deplete both PMN- and Mo-MDSC significantly suppressed tumor growth and increased $CD8^+$ T cells in the tumor. Combining anti-PD-1 with both anti-MDSC antibodies showed synergistic tumor suppression.	(Takeyama et al. 2020)
MB49 to male C57BL/6 J	Anti-PD-L1 combined with PLAG	Combining anti-PD-L1 with PLAG inhibited the infiltration of neutrophils and increased the cytotoxic activity of $CD8^+$ T cells by regulating cytokines and chemokines.	(Kim et al. 2022)
NA13 (derived by OH-BBN treatment) to female C57BL/6	Anti-PD-1 combined with CCR2 inhibitor	Combination of the CCR2 inhibitor, RS504393, with anti-PD1 increased sensitivity and response compared to anti-PD1 alone. This effect was attributed to the activation and recruitment of $CD8^+$ T cells while reducing $FoxP3^+CD4^+$ T cells.	(Tu et al. 2020)

(continued)

Table 16.2 (continued)

Mouse model	Target to be combined with ICI	Main findings	Reference
MB49 to female C57BL/6 J, MBT-2 to female C3H/HeJ (orthotopic)	Anti-PD-1/PD-L1 combined with IL-2c	Combining anti-PD-1/PD-L1 with IL-2c, that targets Il2 receptor, CD122, improved survival rates by reducing Treg and MDSC cells and promoting CD8^{+} T cells anti-tumor response.	(Reyes et al. 2020)
MB49 to female C57Bl/6 J	Anti-PD1 combined with everolimus	mTOR inhibitor, everolimus, at low dose, in combination with anti-PD1 increased the percentage of CD8^{+} T cells in the spleen and increased the cytotoxic activity of CD8^{+} T cells in the tumor microenvironment that was indicated by elevated GZMB.	(Xia et al. 2022)
BBN963, BBN966 to female C57BL/6	Anti-PD1 combined with entinostat	An inhibitor of HDAC1/3, entinostat, promoted remodeling of the tumor immune microenvironment into anti-tumor, dependent on antigen presentation and increased number of neoantigen-specific T cells. Combining anti-PD-1 with entinostat, complete response was achieved.	(Truong et al. 2021)
MB49 to C57BL6, MBT-2 to C3H	Anti-PD-1/PD-L1 combined with MVAC	Cytotoxic chemotherapy with anti-PD1 or anti-PD-L1 impacted differently depending on the model used. It enhanced anti-tumor effects in the MB49 model, but inhibited ICIs activity in the MBT-2 model.	(Grasselly et al. 2018)
MB49 to male C57BL/6	Anti-PD-L1 combined with radiation therapy	Combining anti-PD-L1 with radiation decreased tumor growth with increased cytotoxic T-cell activity and by downregulating immunosuppressive *Ccl22, Il22*, and *Il13*.	(Rompre-Brodeur et al. 2020)

Abbreviations: cDC1, conventional dendritic cell type 1; DCs, dendritic cells; GC, gemcitabine and cisplatin; GZMB, granzyme B; iDAMP, inhibitory damage-associated molecular pattern; IL-2c, interleukin 2 complex; Mo-MDSC, monocytic myeloid-derived suppressor cell; POM-1, polyoxotungstate-1; PMN-MDSC, polymorphonuclear myeloid-derived suppressor cell; PLAG, 1-palmitoyl-2-linoleoyl-3-acetyl-rac-glycerol; Stat3, signal transducer and activator of transcription 3; Tregs, regulatory T cells

survival and the time window for therapeutic testing, knockdown of *cMYC* by shRNA was used to reduce proliferation of MBT-2 cells, with Luciferase and GFP reporters for monitoring of tumor growth (Seo et al. 2017). The model showed a reduced rate of tumor growth and extended mouse survival. However, the model may not be suitable for testing of drugs that induce p53-dependent apoptosis, as this process is cMYC dependent. Nonetheless the model is useful in evaluating new intravesical treatment approaches, such as immunotherapies, to improve or replace BCG in management of NMIBC. Indeed, the orthotopic MBT-2 model was used to test anti-programmed cell death protein-1 (PD-1) intravesical delivery in comparison with intravesical mitomycin-C or intraperitoneal (systemic) anti-PD-1 treatment (Kirschner et al. 2021). Intravesical anti-PD-1 treatment led to longer overall survival, less toxicity, and increased recruitment of CD8^{+} T cells to the tumor. Both systemic and intravesical treatment with anti-PD-1 led to tumor rejection upon rechallenge after several months, showing long-lasting immunity superior to mitomycin-C treatment.

16.4.2 PDXs as a New Generation of Xenograft Models

Several PDX models have been described (Table 16.3). A recent study reported an establishment of six new PD-L1 expressing PDX models that consist of primary and relapsed cases of NMIBC, with luminal (GATA3^{+}), basal (K5/6^{+}), and *TP53* mutant subtypes (Blinova et al. 2019) (Table 16.3). Following the established method for generation of a humanized immunodeficient model (Gong et al. 2015),

Table 16.3 PDX models used in bladder cancer research

Reference	PDX line	Characteristics of PDX lines developed
(Kurtova et al. 2015)	3 PDXs	PDXs were derived from patients who developed chemoresistance and used in parallel to T24 cell line xenograft to address mechanisms of chemoresistance.
(Blinova et al. 2019)	6 PDXs	PDXs with luminal, basal, and *TP53* mutant subtypes were established from primary and relapsed NMIBC cases. Up to 25% of tumor cells expressed PD-L1, reflecting the original tumors.
(Lee et al. 2019).	1 PDX	A PDX was derived from a metastatic case and evaluated along with T24LungMet cell line to address the role of collagen receptor CD167a in metastasis.
(Blinova et al. 2021)	20 PDXs	PDXs were developed from relapsed NMIBC cases with GATA3$^-$, CK5/6$^-$, PD-L1-high tumors. PDXs were high- and low-grade (10 each).
(Cai et al. 2021)	1 PDX	CoCaB1 was established from an aggressive, cisplatin-resistant MIBC case.
(Jing et al. 2022)	1 PDX	A PDX was established from a high-grade bladder tumor with FGFR3-TACC fusion from a male patient.

Abbreviations: CK, cytokeratin; NMIBC, non-muscle invasive bladder cancer; MIBC, muscle-invasive bladder cancer; PDX, patient-derived xenograft

SCID/NOG mice (severely immunodeficient as SCID/NOD with an additional deletion of interleukin 2 receptor 2γ, $Il\text{-}2r\gamma^{null}$ (Chen et al. 2022)), were X-ray irradiated at 3.5 Gy and simultaneously transplanted with human lymphocytes (intraperitoneal) and with PDX tumor pieces (subcutaneous). Established PDX tumors were metastatic and showed PD-L1 expression in up to 25% of tumor cells, reflective of the original tumors. Durvalumab (anti-PD-L1) suppressed tumor growth and lung metastasis in accordance with levels of PD-L1 expression and CD8$^+$ T-cell infiltration (Blinova et al. 2019). A further 20 PDXs were developed from relapsed cases of NMIBC with GATA$^-$, CK5/6$^-$, and PD-L1^{high} expression (Blinova et al. 2021). CoCaB1 was established as a PDX and a PDX-derived organoid from an aggressive, cisplatin-resistant MIBC case (Cai et al. 2021). Histology and growth properties of the original tumor were maintained through PDX passages. Transcriptomic analysis showed that CoCaB1 PDX retained the signature of basal/squamous subtype at early and late passages, as well as mutational heterogeneity of the original tumor (Table 16.1).

The mechanism underlying acquired resistance to chemotherapy was investigated using a PDX from a patient who developed resistance and the bladder tumor cell line T24 CellDX (Kurtova et al. 2015). Treatment with gemcitabine and cisplatin (GC) was able to suppress tumor growth in both PDX and T24 xenograft models, inducing apoptotic cell death of non-quiescent, dividing cells. However, CK14$^+$ quiescent, label retaining cancer cells (LRCCs) became proliferative and repopulated the remaining tumors. This was accompanied by release of prostaglandin E2 (PGE_2), and expression of cyclooxygenease-2 (COX2) that induces PGE_2 production, in the dying cells adjacent to CK14$^+$ tumors. The COX2 inhibitor, celecoxib, suppressed tumor growth and repopulation of CK14$^+$ cells upon cycles of GC treatment. This finding was further supported by transcriptomic profiling which showed that celecoxib treatment suppressed a wound-response gene signature induced by GC (Table 16.1). Administration of low-dose aspirin could provide protection from blood clots associated with celecoxib treatment, without affecting its anti-tumor effects. The study provides supportive evidence for celecoxib in treating advanced bladder cancer resistant to GC.

A CellDX and a PDX established from a stage T2 bladder tumor were used to investigate the role of the collagen receptor CD167a, Discoidin domain receptor 1 (DDR1), as a factor that promotes lung metastasis of urothelial tumors (Lee et al. 2019). A T24 subline, T24LungMet, that has an increased metastatic capacity, was generated by repeatedly injecting T24 cells via the tail vein. Subcutaneous transplantation of CD167a-overexpressing T24 tumor cells to immunocompromised hosts enhanced distal lung metastasis by increasing lung colonization, but not through intravasation or extravasation. Using the models of spontaneous metastasis from subcutaneous transplantation of the established PDX model and tail vein injection of T24LungMet cells, airway smooth muscle cells (ASMCs) were identified as a novel metastatic niche in the lung. Furthermore, Stat3 was shown to mediate CD167a signaling, and a selective Stat3 inhibitor, napabucasin, inhibited lung metastasis in both T24 and PDX models.

16.4.3 Emerging Syngeneic Models

Recently, several new syngeneic cell lines have been generated and molecularly characterized. A urothelium-specific deletion of *p53* and *Pten* genes (*Upk3a-Cre*^{ERT2};*Trp53*$^{flox/flox}$; *Pten* $^{flox/flox}$; *Rosa26* $^{LSL\text{-}Luc}$, UPPL) was shown to develop invasive urothelial tumors with papillary morphology in the bladder and in the upper tract, with occasional metastasis (Saito et al. 2018). Taking advantage of this GEM model, a cell line, UPPL1541, syngeneic to the C57Bl/6 strain, was derived. BBN963 cell line was also generated from tumors induced by OH-BBN. Transcriptomic analyses showed that both UPPL1541 and BBN963 retained characteristics of urothelial expression reflective of human tumors (Table 16.1). In contrast, the commonly used syngeneic model, MB49, was more mesenchymal and fibroblast-like, indicating that MB49 may have undergone epithelial-to-mesenchymal transition (EMT). UPPL1541 showed higher levels of luminal markers, such as *Pparg* and *Gata3*, than BBN963. In contrast, BBN963 was more basal in phenotype and showed more prominent immune gene signatures than UPPL1541. Immune profiling indicated that UPPL1541 tumors were immune excluded and had lower neoantigen burden than BBN963 tumors. BBN963 tumors were indeed more responsive to anti PD-1 immunotherapy, and within BBN963 tumors, the response was dependent on the balance of CD8/CD4 lymphocytes as well as that of memory and regulatory T cells (Tregs). Limitations of UPPL1541 and BBN963 models are that no driver mutations commonly found in human bladder cancer were identified and that the lack of *Pten* in UPPL1541 may have led to an immune suppressive profile. Nonetheless, the models have excellent utility in future translational studies, with better presentation of luminal and basal characteristics than MB49.

A strategy to reinstall CD8$^+$ T-cell activity from the exhausted state by stimulating dendritic cell (DC) activity by an anti-CD40 agonistic antibody was investigated using UPPL1541 and BBN963 (Garris et al. 2021). CD40 is a membrane protein expressed in conventional dendritic cell type 1 (cDC1) that presents antigens to CD8$^+$ cytotoxic T cells, thereby activating them. High-risk NMIBC requires an alternative to BCG, and in BCG-unresponsive cases, anti-PD-1 checkpoint inhibitors have shown only modest responses (Li et al. 2023). Intravesical treatment with anti-mouse CD40 IgG1 antibody, 1C10, that agonizes CD40 by binding to FcγRs, showed successful reduction of tumor burden in the orthotopic MB49 model. Furthermore, a humanized version of the anti-CD40 antibody, 2141-V11, was tested in mice that express human CD40 and FcγRs (humanized hCD40/hFcγR model). Bilateral subcutaneous implantation was used to test drug efficacy in a tumor on one flank of the animal, while evaluating the drug's systemic effects on a tumor on the other flank. Orthotopic tumors and subcutaneous tumors of MB49, UPPL1541, and BBN963 showed little toxicity in response to 2141-V11. Furthermore, treatment with 2141-V11, as well as with 2141-V11 after BCG, induced a sustained and improved response compared with treatment by BCG alone. Therefore, the intravesical anti-CD40 agonist antibody is a promising new therapy for high-risk NMIBC patients with or without previous treatment with BCG.

Syngeneic cell lines, G69 and G7, were derived from OH-BBN induced tumors from transgenic mice with constitutively active Stat3 (K5.Stat3C) on FVB/N background (Nikolos et al. 2022; Hayashi et al. 2020). These syngeneic lines were used to uncover the role of immunostimulatory and inhibitory damage-associated molecular patterns (DAMPs) in immunogenic cell death (ICD). ICD is one of key mechanisms of tumor rejection by the immune system and influences treatment outcome (Galluzzi et al. 2017; Kroemer et al. 2013). Not all chemotherapeutic agents are able to induce an immunogenic response, including GC (Hayashi et al. 2020). In the *in vivo* vaccination assay, cells pre-treated with chemotherapeutic agents are subcutaneously injected into a host flank. Mice are then challenged with injection of the same cells and monitored for rejection (success of vaccination) or tumor formation (failure of vaccination). While a release of DAMP was confirmed in G69 cells treated with gemcitabine, it was not sufficient for tumor rejection, indicating that ICD may not have occurred. It was revealed that gemcitabine upregulated the expression of COX-2, which induced the release of PGE_2, as an inhibitory DAMP. Indeed, by suppressing PGE_2 release by pre-treatment of G69 with gemcitabine as well as celecoxib, tumor rejection was successfully induced. Furthermore, the status of $CD103^+$ DC maturation was converted from tolerogenic to immunogenic upon COX2/PGE2 inhibition (iDAMP blockade), leading to an appropriate priming of $CD8^+$ T cells and tumor rejection. Footpad vaccination was additionally used to validate the correct priming of $CD8^+$ T cells in the draining lymph node. Application of iDAMP blockade in combination with GC with anti-PD1 ICI was further investigated using G69 and G7 tumors (Nikolos et al. 2022). Cycles of GC treatment increased T cells in the periphery of the tumor, but they were excluded from the tumor core. Accordingly, no tumor regression was observed, despite the fact that $CD8^+$ T cells expressed *granzyme B* and *Ifnγ*, indicating their activation. In line with the earlier study (Hayashi et al. 2020), GC promoted the release of COX2 and PGE2, and their inhibition was effective in restoring DC maturation and promoting antitumor $CD8^+$ T cells (Nikolos et al. 2022). iDAMP blockade in addition to GC and anti-PD1 antibody most effectively suppressed tumor growth in G69 in association with T-cell infiltration in the tumor, while iDAMP blockade and GC was sufficient in G7, without additional suppression by anti-PD-1 antibody, indicating that GC + iDAMP blockade could be sufficient in some cases. Other chemotherapy combinations, such as MVAC and Adriamycin (doxorubicin), should now be evaluated for effectiveness of iDAMP blockade in combination with ICIs.

16.5 Mouse Models for an Oncogenic Role of FGFR3

FGFR3 mutations are associated with papillary, low-grade, low-risk NMIBC with good prognosis (Knowles 2020; Kacew and Sweis 2020). *FGFR3* mutations are also found in 10–15% of MIBC, albeit much less frequently than the ~80% in NMIBC (Knowles 2020; van Rhijn et al. 2020). FGFR3 protein overexpression was found in 40–80% of NMIBC and 30–50% of MIBC (Tomlinson et al. 2007; van Rhijn et al. 2020). *FGFR3* mutated tumors more often overexpress FGFR3 protein (73–85%), in contrast to *FGFR3* wild-type tumors (22–42%) (Tomlinson et al. 2007; van Rhijn et al. 2020). A pan-FGFR inhibitor, erdafitinib, has shown response in 40% of patients with *FGFR2/FGFR3* mutations or gene fusion and was FDA approved for treatment of patients with metastatic bladder cancer (Loriot et al. 2019). Additional pan-FGFR inhibitors, infigratinib and rogaratinib, have also shown promising results and are currently in phase III clinical trials (Pal et al. 2018; Schuler et al. 2019). Identification of predictive biomarkers is key for the success of these trials. Mouse models may assist in their identification and improve understanding of the oncogenic role of FGFR3.

Evidence for an oncogenic role of *FGFR3* activation, either from mutation or overexpression, has been ambiguous *in vivo*. Using a GEM model of *Fgfr3* with K644E mutation that strongly activates FGFR3 tyrosine kinase activity (*UroIICreFgfr3*$^{+/K644E}$), it was shown that *Fgfr3* mutation alone was not sufficient to lead to tumor formation in the bladder urothelium in mice (Ahmad et al. 2011). Two independent studies used transgenic mice that express the epithelial IIIb isoform of human FGFR3 protcin with the most common mutation, S249C, under control of the mouse *UroII* promoter, to investigate the role of *FGFR3* mutations (Foth et al. 2018; Shi et al.

2023). These studies are concordant in showing that few or no spontaneous tumors were formed in the transgenic mice. However, hyperplastic or focal papillary lesions were observed in 10% of aged mice in the transgenic line with four-fold overexpression of *FGFR3 S249C* mutant in the urothelium (Shi et al. 2023), indicating that the severity of phenotype may relate to the level of mutant *FGFR3* overexpression. Results from the ageing cohort (up to 18 months) in this study are valuable, as it is extremely challenging to maintain an aged mouse cohort due to regulations and cost. Inducible urothelial expression of human FGFR3 S249C mutant with an HA tag for visualization provided further mechanistic insight (Zhou et al. 2016). In common with the above studies, no tumors were observed at 12 months, even though MAPK and AKT downstream pathways were activated in the urothelium. p16-pRB and p19-p53-p21 cell cycle inhibitor pathways were upregulated in the urothelium of these mice. A cross with mice that express SV40T, a known functional inhibitor of the above pathways (UPII-SV40T) (Zhang et al. 1999), resulted in non-invasive high-grade (pTaG3) tumors, overcoming cell cycle inhibition. The study explains why only few tumors are formed in mice with *FGFR3* mutations.

Gene expression was explored in the FGFR3 S249C transgenic model without carcinogen induction (Shi et al. 2023) (Table 16.1). Analysis with the BASE47 classifier (Damrauer et al. 2014) showed that FGFR3 S249C mouse tumors were of luminal subtype, in contrast to OH-BBN-induced tumors that were basal (Shi et al. 2023; Rebouissou et al. 2014). An analytical tool, murine Microenvironment Cell Population counter (mMCP counter) (Petitprez et al. 2020) indicated a lower immune infiltration in FGFR3 S249C tumors (Shi et al. 2023).

The lack of tumorigenesis in *FGFR3* mutant mice was also overcome by the additional loss of *Pten* in *UroIICreFgfr3*$^{+/K644E}$*Pten*$^{flox/flox}$ mice, which showed lesions indicative of urothelial tumorigenesis, including hyperplasia and atypia, indicating that *FGFR3* and *Pten* can cooperatively initiate tumor pathogenesis (Foth et al. 2014). The fact that OH-BBN rarely induces *FGFR3* mutations in mice (Fantini et al. 2018; Dunois-Larde et al. 2005) provides an opportunity for carcinogen induction to be used in combination. Accordingly, the role of *FGFR3* mutations in invasive tumors was investigated using *UroIICreFgfr3*$^{+/K644E}$ and *FGFR3 S249C* transgenic lines following OH-BBN induction, which showed conclusive evidence for the pro-tumorigenic role of *FGFR3* mutations (Foth et al. 2018; Shi et al. 2023). *FGFR3* mutations are frequent in non-T cell inflamed MIBC, which shows a lower response to ICI (Kacew and Sweis 2020; Sweis et al. 2016). While clinical studies showed that *FGFR3* mutation status was not directly associated with ICI response or patient survival (Wang et al. 2019; Necchi et al. 2021; Rose et al. 2021), FGFR3 could be involved in the regulation of the tumor immune microenvironment. We showed that the pro-tumorigenic effects of FGFR3 S249C mutation accompanied suppression of an inflammatory response at an early stage of tumorigenesis (Foth et al. 2018). The mechanism of immune suppression by FGFR3 was explored in orthotopic and PDX models (Jing et al. 2022). Effects of erdafitinib and infigratinib in MB49 cells were first compared in immunocompetent and immunodeficient host mice upon orthotopic transplantation. Inhibitors suppressed MB49 tumor growth much more efficiently in the absence of an immune system, indicating that host immunity compromised the effects of FGFR inhibitors. FGFR3 promoted phosphorylation and activation of a ubiquitin ligase NEDD4 (which normally downregulates PD-L1), leading to upregulated PD-L1, thereby inhibiting $CD8^+$ T-cell infiltration and cytotoxic T-cell activity. Erdafitinib and anti-PD-1 dual treatment were shown to enhance suppression of tumor growth and prolonged survival in a PDX tumor with FGFR3-TACC fusion protein.

A recent study has investigated whether FGFR inhibition improves ICI using a model that allows inducible expression of human FGFR3 S249C protein together with *p53* mutation in *Upk3a-Cre*^{ERT2}*;Trp53*$^{LSL\text{-}R270H/+}$*;LSL-FGFR3*$^{S249C/+}$*;Rosa26*$^{LSL\text{-}luc/+}$ (UPFL) mice and UPFL1 and UPFL3 syngeneic lines derived from UPFL tumors (Okato et al. 2024). While co-occurrence of *FGFR3* and *p53* mutations has been known to be rare, that of *FGFR3* mutation and alterations in p53 pathway genes was found in 20–25% of NMIBC and 5–10% in MIBC (Okato et al. 2024). UPFL mice developed high-grade, non-invasive tumors with a papillary morphology in the bladder at a median of 49 weeks, as well as in the upper tract (47% and 22% of the cohort, respectively). UPFL tumors showed luminal gene expression with a medium level of immune infiltration, higher than in UPPL tumors. Effects of erdafitinib and anti-PD-1 treatment were tested *in vivo* using UPFL1 heterotopic transplants. Tumor growth was suppressed by erdafitinib, and most efficiently by the combination of erdafitinib and anti-PD-1 treatment. Erdafitinib was shown to overcome hyperprogression caused by anti-PD-1 treatment, suppressing proliferation of Treg, likely to be via FGFR1 expressed in T cells. Taken together, the study showed that the erdafitinib and ICI combination is effective in suppressing bladder tumors, and the findings above provide mechanistic support for ICI sensitized by FGFR inhibition for the treatment of high-risk NMIBC and MIBC.

16.6 Models of Tumor Immune Suppression in Bladder Cancer

The development of an immunosuppressive tumor microenvironment is a hallmark of cancer progression, as tumors use various strategies to evade the host immune system and suppress antitumor immune responses (Allegrezza and Conejo-Garcia 2017; Schreiber et al. 2011). By controlling both adaptive and innate mechanisms, tumors may evade either by interrupting T-cell trafficking into the tumor microenvironment or by decreasing T-cell activity (Sharma et al. 2017). Antigen detection depends on the presence of antigen-presenting cells (APCs), specifically DCs. Tumors can actively influence the function of infiltrating DCs through a variety of mechanisms, such as the lack of toll-like-receptor ligands and the production of gangliosides, neuropeptides, and mucins, which result in inhibition and death of DCs (Shurin et al. 2013). Tumors may also release immunosuppressive and anti-apoptotic factors, such as transforming growth factor-beta (TGF-β), PGE_2, Il6, and Il10. Furthermore, several types of immune cells with suppressive characteristics, such as myeloid-derived suppressor cells (MDSCs), tolerogenic dendritic cells (tDCs), tumor-associated macrophages (TAMs), and Tregs, contribute to the immunosuppressive tumor microenvironment (Schreiber et al. 2011). Chronic antigen exposure in cancer can lead to T-cell exhaustion, which is characterized by reduced T-cell proliferation, Il2 production, degranulation, and eventual cell death. T-cell exhaustion is consistently associated with expression of PD-1 (Pauken and Wherry 2015; Rotte et al. 2018).

Immune evasion in bladder cancer can also be achieved by a highly immunosuppressive milieu with elevated expression of the inhibitory ligand PD-L1, the increasing presence of MDSCs and TAMs, and enhanced PGE_2 secretion (Hatogai and Sweis 2020; Crispen and Kusmartsev 2020). Bladder cancers have shown good responses to immunotherapy such as intravesical BCG and ICIs (Pettenati and Ingersoll 2018; Roviello et al. 2021), but not all patients respond to treatment (Massari et al. 2018). Factors such as tumor-infiltrating lymphocytes, PD-L1/PD-1 expression, higher tumor mutation burden, and IFNγ gene expression have been associated with response rates to ICIs (Hatogai and Sweis 2020).

Mouse models have recently been increasingly used to investigate the mechanisms of immune suppression in bladder cancer and to explore potential combination therapies (Table 16.2). For example, strategies to improve antigen presentation by activation of DCs have been tested using GEM and syngeneic models (Garris et al. 2021; Nikolos et al. 2022) (Sect. 16.4.3). An anti-CD40 agonistic antibody that targets cDC1 cells increased $CD8^+$ T cells and shifted macrophages from M2 immunosuppressive to M1 inflammatory subtype, increasing response to anti-PD-1 antibody in invasive tumors developed in *Adeno-Cre* $Pten^{fl/fl}p53^{fl/fl}$ mice (Leblond et al. 2020). Similarly, an anti-PD-1 antibody with activated DC vaccines showed synergistic anti-tumor effects, by enhancing *Ifnγ* production and antigen-specific T-cell-mediated immunity in the MBT-2 model (Lim et al. 2023). Inhibiting CD39 (ectonucleoside triphosphate diphosphohydrolase-1) with a novel inhibitor, sodium polyoxotungstate (POM-1) in MB49 orthotopic models increased intratumor NK cells, cDC1, and $CD8^+$ cytotoxic T cells, and decreased Treg, resulting in tumor growth suppression and improved prognosis, though no synergistic effects were observed when combined with anti-PD-1 antibody (Liu et al. 2022). Synergistic effects of ICIs with suppression of MDSCs and tumor-infiltrating neutrophils were also evaluated. Targeting both polymorphonuclear (PMN)- and monocytic (Mo)-MDSCs using α-Gr1 and α-Ly6C antibodies combined with ICIs significantly decreased MB49R cisplatin-resistant syngeneic tumor growth with enhanced infiltration of $CD8^+$ T cells (Takeyama et al. 2020). Combining anti-PD-L1 antibody with 1-palmitoyl-2-linoleoyl-3-acetyl-rac-glycerol (PLAG) compound lowered neutrophil infiltration and increased $CD8^+$ T cells, resulting in enhanced anticancer effects in MB49 tumors (Kim et al. 2022).

The potential of targeting specific signaling pathways to improve the efficacy of ICIs has also been explored. Combining a CCR2 inhibitor with anti-PD-1 antibody increased the sensitivity and response of NA13 syngeneic mouse tumors through increased activation and recruitment of $CD8^+$ T cells and decreased the numbers of inhibitory $FoxP3^+CD4^+$ Treg cells (Tu et al. 2020). A combination of anti-PD-1/PD-L1 and Il2/αIL-complexes (IL-2c) improved survival rates in orthotopic MB49 and MBT-2 models by decreasing Treg and MDSC cell count and stimulating $CD8^+$ T-cell anti-tumor response (Reyes et al. 2020). Application of the mTOR inhibitor, everolimus, at low dose in combination with ICIs improved anti-tumor immunity in the MB49 model, by increasing $CD8^+$ T cells in the spleen and enhancing their cytotoxic activity in the tumor microenvironment (Xia et al. 2022). Finally, combined application of anti-PD-1 antibody with the HDAC1 and HDAC3 inhibitor, entinostat, in BBN963 and BBN966 syngeneic models resulted in complete responses and long-term immunologic memory by promoting immune editing and remodeling of the tumor immune microenvironment (Truong et al. 2021).

The combination of chemotherapy or radiotherapy with ICIs could improve response rates in tumors that lack PD-L1 expression or T-cell infiltration (Peng et al. 2020). Anti-PD-L1 with radiation therapy showed better survival rates in the MB49 model, by boosting the $CD8^+$ T-cell activity and decreasing the expression of immunosuppressive *Ccl22*, *Il22*, and *Il13* (Rompre-Brodeur et al. 2020). In contrast, combination of chemotherapy with anti-PD-1/PD-L1 antibody showed varying effects on anti-tumor activity depending on the model used, whereby tumor suppression was enhanced in MB49 but not in MBT-2 (Grasselly et al. 2018).

OH-BBN models have also been used to evaluate the ICI combination. Blocking of T-cell inhibitory protein, B7-H4, with anti-PD-1 antibody resulted in reduced tumor size, increased $CD8^+$ T-cell infiltration and Ifnγ secretion while Treg numbers were reduced (Podojil et al. 2020). Inhibition of Il6/Stat3 signaling was also shown to sensitize OH-BBN induced bladder tumors to anti-PD-L1 antibody and impaired tumor progression (Korac-Prlic et al. 2020) (Sect. 16.3.2).

16.7 Future Models: Metastasis and Sex Differences

Metastatic bladder cancer has no curative management options, thereby presenting a critical unmet need that requires timely research efforts. The underlying biology of metastasis involves EMT, cancer cell stemness, and the tumor immune microenvironment and is influenced by the cell of origin, and mutational and transcriptional profile of the tumor (Kobayashi 2016). The main metastatic sites are local lymph nodes, bone, lung, liver, and peritoneum in humans. Establishment of mouse models of metastasis has been challenging. Spontaneous metastasis formation in the regional lymph nodes and in the lung can occur in the OH-BBN model (Vasconcelos-Nobrega et al. 2012), but overall this is rare and may not always reflect metastatic sites in humans (DeGraff et al. 2013; John and Said 2017). The Adeno-Cre driven GEM model *Pten*$^{fl/fl}$*p53*$^{fl/fl}$ showed frequent metastases to the local lymph nodes, spleen, liver, and diaphragm (Puzio-Kuter et al. 2009), the UPPL model was metastatic to cervical lymph nodes (Saito et al. 2018) (Sect. 16.4.3) and a combination of GEM with OH-BBN induction can promote metastasis in some models (Overdevest et al. 2012; Said et al. 2013). Orthotopically transplanted xenograft models have also shown metastasis to the lymph nodes (John and Said 2017), kidney and lung (Huebner et al. 2017).

Subcutaneous or orthotopic transplantation of metastatic cells can be used to address spontaneous formation of metastasis, while tail vein injection can be used to measure the ability of cells to colonize at target sites, such as the lung. The tail vein model does not have the long time span normally required in metastatic dissemination and formation of the metastatic niche. Bladder cancer progression takes time and an ageing cohort may be required to model spontaneous progression to metastasis. The lack of an immune system in xenograft hosts is an issue, as the contribution of the immune system in metastasis is now clear.

So far, combinations of transplantation models, either xenograft or syngeneic, and GEM with OH-BBN induction, have been used to examine the molecular mechanisms underlying progression and metastasis, showing a pro-metastatic role of monomeric G protein, RalB (Wang et al. 2010), cancer stem cell marker, CD24 (Overdevest et al. 2011; Overdevest et al. 2012), vasoconstriction factor, endothelin-1 (ET-1) and its receptor ET_AR (Said et al. 2011), loss of RhoGTP dissociation inhibitor 2 (RhoGDL2) (Said and Theodorescu 2012), and loss of SPARC (Said et al. 2013). Some of these studies also indicate the role of inflammation in promoting metastasis (Said et al. 2011; Said and Theodorescu 2012; Said et al. 2013; Kurtova et al. 2015). PDX models with metastatic properties have also been developed recently (Blinova et al. 2019).

The sex-related differences in urothelial cancer are characterized by four-fold higher incidents in males compared to females, with worse prognosis and treatment outcomes in females (Marks et al. 2016). Females have more tumors of basal phenotype and have higher incidence of squamous cell carcinoma of the bladder (Koti et al. 2020). Factors that may influence sex-related differences in bladder cancer may include sex hormones, bladder resident immune cells, differences in genomic profile and gene expression, and the bladder microbiome (Koti et al. 2020).

Several studies have reported sex-related differences in bladder tumorigenesis using carcinogen-treated and GEM mice with C57BL/6 background. Differences in the outcome of carcinogen treatment by sex have been evaluated using the *in vivo* mutagenicity test with *lacI* (Big Blue™) mice (He et al. 2012). The mutant fraction resulting from 2–6 weeks of 0.05% OH-BBN treatment was similar in male and female mice. A more recent study evaluated the age and sex-related differences in gene expression and immune infiltration of normal healthy bladders and tumors developed upon OH-BBN treatment in mice (Hamade et al. 2022) (Table 16.1). In healthy bladders, an enrichment of B-cell function-associated pathways and a higher level of tertiary lymphoid structures (TLSs) were observed in aged females compared to aged males. Invasion to lamina propria was more prominent in males than females when OH-BBN was applied to a 12-month age group. Immune cell infiltrations in the lamina propria were more abundant in young and old female mice.

Sex-related differences in tumor phenotype have been reported in several GEM models. The expression of a cancer stem cell marker, CD24, was shown to be androgen regulated (Overdevest et al. 2012). *Cd24* deletion resulted in fewer tumors in male mice, indicating that males with CD24 overexpression were more susceptible to tumor development and metastasis. Lysine demethylase, *KDM6A* is an X-linked gene and normally expressed at a higher level in females than males (Kaneko and Li 2018). A mouse model of conditional *Kdm6a* deletion in the urothelium was treated with 0.01% OH-BBN for 14 weeks for survival analysis. The result indicated a protective effect of *Kdm6a* in female mice. Whole-body inducible *Foxa1* gene deletion

(*UBC-Cre*^{ERT2} *Foxa1*$^{loxp/loxp}$) resulted in sex-dependent differential phenotype, whereby male mice showed urothelial hyperplasia, while females showed squamous metaplasia with keratinization (Reddy et al. 2015). The pro-tumorigenic effects of *Foxa1* and *Pten* deletion were also compared upon OH-BBN induction in male and female mice (Osei-Amponsa et al. 2020). Female mice showed progression at a slower pace, though overall tumor incidence was similar. Finally, when cell-type specific inducible and Adenovirus-Cre approaches were used, no significant sex-dependent differences were observed in the phenotype of *Pten* and *p53* loss (Park et al. 2021).

16.8 Limitations and Future Perspectives

It is important to be aware of the limitations that mouse models may present when undertaking and evaluating these studies. Firstly, intrinsic biological differences between humans and mice may influence tumorigenesis physiologically, phenotypically, and molecularly. Mice have smaller body size, shorter life span and no menopause (Hamade et al. 2022). Secondly, heterogeneity of human tumors is unlikely to be fully captured in the mouse models. Bladder cancer PDX lines have been shown to preserve heterogeneity of the original tumors well (Sect. 16.4.2). Nonetheless, for conclusive results, studies should examine sufficient numbers of established PDXs, validated statistically and/or taking complementary approaches. Thirdly, there are technical challenges that could influence the characteristics of tumors in the model. For example, the *Cre-lox* system could lead to gene modification in ectopic sites outside the bladder, and this therefore requires careful assessment of the model at the outset. As the tumor immune environment of PDXs is influenced by the mouse host, inclusion of a complementary approach could be considered.

Mouse models are valuable in obtaining mechanistic insights and proof-of-principle for translational approaches. However, mouse models are neither an instant alternative to human studies nor an all-mighty platform that can be used to address all clinical or biological questions with ease. It is imperative to select the right model for the right question, being aware of the intrinsic differences of species and pitfalls that may obscure the interpretation. Animal lives must be used ethically, following the principles of the 3Rs (Reduction, Refinement, Replacement) (Prescott and Lidster 2017) and results must be obtained from otherwise healthy mice that are well taken care of and treated humanely. Finally, most mouse experiments are labor-intensive and time-consuming. Sharing of resources with respect and courtesy is strongly encouraged, including mouse and cell lines derived, tumor tissues, images, and molecular information.

Acknowledgments AREY is sponsored by Ministry of Higher Education of Libya.

References

Ahmad I, Singh LB, Foth M et al (2011) *K-Ras* and *-catenin* mutations cooperate with *Fgfr3* mutations in mice to promote tumorigenesis in the skin and lung, but not in the bladder. Dis Model Mech 4(4):548–555. https://doi.org/10.1242/dmm.006874

Alexandrov LB, Nik-Zainal S, Wedge DC et al (2013) Signatures of mutational processes in human cancer. Nature 500(7463):415–421. https://doi.org/10.1038/nature12477

Allegrezza MJ, Conejo-Garcia JR (2017) Targeted therapy and immunosuppression in the tumor microenvironment. Trends Cancer 3(1):19–27. https://doi.org/10.1016/j.trecan.2016.11.009

Ben-David U, Ha G, Tseng YY et al (2017) Patient-derived xenografts undergo mouse-specific tumor evolution. Nat Genet 49(11):1567–1575. https://doi.org/10.1038/ng.3967

Bernardo C, Santos LL (2018) Patient-derived bladder cancer xenografts. Urothelial Carcinoma 1655:169–175. https://doi.org/10.1007/978-1-4939-7234-0_14

Blinova E, Roshchin D, Kogan E et al (2019) Patient-derived non-muscular invasive bladder cancer xenografts of Main molecular subtypes of the tumor for anti-Pd-l1 treatment assessment. Cells 8(6):526. https://doi.org/10.3390/cells8060526

Blinova E, Samishina E, Deryabina O et al (2021) Expression of p53 protein associates with anti-PD-L1 treatment response on human-derived xenograft model of GATA3/CR5/6-negative recurrent nonmuscular invasive bladder urothelial carcinoma. Int J Mol Sci 22(18):9856. https://doi.org/10.3390/ijms22189856

Cai EY, Garcia J, Liu YZ et al (2021) A bladder cancer patient-derived xenograft displays aggressive growth dynamics *in vivo* and in organoid culture. Sci Rep 11(1):4609. https://doi.org/10.1038/s41598-021-83662-7

Chen J, Liao S, Xiao Z et al (2022) The development and improvement of immunodeficient mice and humanized immune system mouse models. Front Immunol 13:1007579. https://doi.org/10.3389/fimmu.2022.1007579

Crispen PL, Kusmartsev S (2020) Mechanisms of immune evasion in bladder cancer. Cancer Immunol Immunother 69(1):3–14. https://doi.org/10.1007/s00262-019-02443-4

Damrauer JS, Hoadley KA, Chism DD et al (2014) Intrinsic subtypes of high-grade bladder cancer reflect the hallmarks of breast cancer biology. Proc Natl Acad Sci USA 111(8):3110–3115. https://doi.org/10.1073/pnas.1318376111

Dancik GM, Ru Y, Owens CR et al (2011) A framework to select clinically relevant cancer cell lines for investigation by establishing their molecular similarity with primary human cancers. Cancer Res 71(24):7398–7409. https://doi.org/10.1158/0008-5472.CAN-11-2427

de la Rosa J, Weber J, Friedrich MJ et al (2017) A single-copy sleeping beauty transposon mutagenesis screen identifies new PTEN-cooperating tumor suppressor genes. Nat Genet 49(5):730–741. https://doi.org/10.1038/ng.3817

Degoricija M, Korac-Prlic J, Vilovic K et al (2019) The dynamics of the inflammatory response during BBN-induced bladder carcinogenesis in mice. J Transl Med 17(1):394. https://doi.org/10.1186/s12967-019-02146-5

DeGraff DJ, Robinson VL, Shah JB et al (2013) Current preclinical models for the advancement of translational bladder cancer research. Mol Cancer Ther 12(2):121–130. https://doi.org/10.1158/1535-7163.MCT-12-0508

Dunois-Larde C, Levrel O, Brams A et al (2005) Absence of FGFR3 mutations in urinary bladder tumours of rats and mice treated with N-butyl-N-(−4-hydroxybutyl) nitrosamine. Mol Carcinog 42(3):142–149. https://doi.org/10.1002/mc.20075

Fantini D, Glaser AP, Rimar KJ et al (2018) A carcinogen-induced mouse model recapitulates the molecular alterations of human muscle invasive bladder cancer. Oncogene 37(14):1911–1925. https://doi.org/10.1038/s41388-017-0099-6

Foth M, Ahmad I, van Rhijn BW et al (2014) Fibroblast growth factor receptor 3 activation plays a causative role in urothelial cancer pathogenesis in cooperation with *Pten* loss in mice. J Pathol 233(2):148–158. https://doi.org/10.1002/path.4334

Foth M, Ismail NFB, Kung JSC et al (2018) *FGFR3* mutation increases bladder tumourigenesis by suppressing acute inflammation. J Pathol 246(3):331–343. https://doi.org/10.1002/path.5143

Friedrich MJ, Rad L, Bronner IF et al (2017) Genome-wide transposon screening and quantitative insertion site sequencing for cancer gene discovery in mice. Nat Protoc 12(2):289–309. https://doi.org/10.1038/nprot.2016.164

Galluzzi L, Buque A, Kepp O et al (2017) Immunogenic cell death in cancer and infectious disease. Nat Rev Immunol 17(2):97–111. https://doi.org/10.1038/nri.2016.107

Garris CS, Wong JL, Ravetch JV et al (2021) Dendritic cell targeting with fc-enhanced CD40 antibody agonists induces durable antitumor immunity in humanized mouse models of bladder cancer. Sci Transl Med 13(594):eabd1346. https://doi.org/10.1126/scitranslmed.abd1346

Gong Z, Xu H, Su Y et al (2015) Establishment of a novel bladder cancer xenograft model in humanized Immunodeficient mice. Cell Physiol Biochem 37(4):1355–1368. https://doi.org/10.1159/000430401

Grasselly C, Denis M, Bourguignon A et al (2018) The antitumor activity of combinations of cytotoxic chemotherapy and immune checkpoint inhibitors is model-dependent. Fron Immunol 9(9):2100. https://doi.org/10.3389/fimmu.2018.02100

Grubbs CJ, Lubet RA, Koki AT et al (2000) Celecoxib inhibits N-butyl-N-(4-hydroxybutyl)-nitrosamine-induced urinary bladder cancers in male B6D2F1 mice and female Fischer-344 rats. Cancer Res 60(20):5599–5602

Hall B, Limaye A, Kulkarni AB (2009) Overview: generation of gene knockout mice. Curr Protoc Cell Biol, Chapter 19, Unit 19 12 44(1):11–17. https://doi.org/10.1002/0471143030.cb1912s44

Hamade A, Li D, Tyryshkin K et al (2022) Sex differences in the aging murine urinary bladder and influence on the tumor immune microenvironment of a carcinogen-induced model of bladder cancer. Biol Sex Differ 13(1):19. https://doi.org/10.1186/s13293-022-00428-0

Haruyama N, Cho A, Kulkarni AB (2009) Overview: engineering transgenic constructs and mice. Curr Protoc Cell Biol, Chapter 19, Unit 42(1):19–10. https://doi.org/10.1002/0471143030.cb1910s42

Hatogai K, Sweis RF (2020) The tumor microenvironment of bladder cancer. Adv Exp Med Biol 1296:275–290. https://doi.org/10.1007/978-3-030-59038-3_17

Hayashi K, Nikolos F, Lee YC et al (2020) Tipping the immunostimulatory and inhibitory DAMP balance to harness immunogenic cell death. Nat Commun 11(1):6299. https://doi.org/10.1038/s41467-020-19970-9

He Z, Kosinska W, Zhao ZL et al (2012) Tissue-specific mutagenesis by N-butyl-N-(4-hydroxybutyl)nitrosamine as the basis for urothelial carcinogenesis. Mutat Res 742(1–2):92–95. https://doi.org/10.1016/j.mrgentox.2011.11.015

Ho PL, Lay EJ, Jian W et al (2012) Stat3 activation in urothelial stem cells leads to direct progression to invasive bladder cancer. Cancer Res 72(13):3135–3142. https://doi.org/10.1158/0008-5472.CAN-11-3195

Huebner D, Rieger C, Bergmann R et al (2017) An orthotopic xenograft model for high-risk non-muscle invasive bladder cancer in mice: influence of mouse strain, tumor cell count, dwell time and bladder pretreatment. BMC Cancer 17(1):790. https://doi.org/10.1186/s12885-017-3778-3

Ismail NFB, Foth M, Yousef ARE et al (2022) Loss of *Cxcr2* in myeloid cells promotes tumour progression and T cell infiltration in invasive bladder cancer. Bladder Cancer 8(3):277–290. https://doi.org/10.3233/Blc-211645

Jager W, Moskalev I, Raven P et al (2018) Orthotopic mouse models of urothelial cancer. Urothelial Carcinoma 1655:177–197. https://doi.org/10.1007/978-1-4939-7234-0_15

Jing W, Wang G, Cui Z et al (2022) FGFR3 destabilizes PD-L1 via NEDD4 to control T-cell-mediated bladder cancer immune surveillance. Cancer Res 82(1):114–129. https://doi.org/10.1158/0008-5472.CAN-21-2362

John BA, Said N (2017) Insights from animal models of bladder cancer: recent advances, challenges, and opportunities. Oncotarget 8(34):57766–57781. https://doi.org/10.18632/oncotarget.17714

Kacew A, Sweis RF (2020) FGFR3 alterations in the era of immunotherapy for urothelial bladder cancer. Front Immunol 11:575258. https://doi.org/10.3389/fimmu.2020.575258

Kamoun A, de Reynies A, Allory Y et al (2019) A consensus molecular classification of muscle-invasive bladder cancer. Eur Urol 77(4):420–433. https://doi.org/10.1016/j.eururo.2019.09.006

Kaneko S, Li X (2018) X chromosome protects against bladder cancer in females via a KDM6A-dependent epigenetic mechanism. Sci Adv 4(6):eaar5598. https://doi.org/10.1126/sciadv.aar5598

Kim H, Kim M, Im SK et al (2018) Mouse Cre-LoxP system: general principles to determine tissue-specific roles of target genes. Lab Anim Res 34(4):147–159. https://doi.org/10.5625/lar.2018.34.4.147

Kim GT, Kim EY, Shin SH et al (2022) Improving anticancer effect of aPD-L1 through lowering neutrophil infiltration by PLAG in tumor implanted with MB49 mouse urothelial carcinoma. BMC Cancer 22(1):727. https://doi.org/10.1186/s12885-022-09815-7

Kirschner AN, Wang J, Rajkumar-Calkins A et al (2021) Intravesical anti-PD-1 immune checkpoint inhibition treats urothelial bladder cancer in a mouse model. J Urol 205(5):1336–1343. https://doi.org/10.1097/JU.0000000000001576

Kita Y, Saito R, Inoue T et al (2020) Patient-derived urothelial cancer xenograft models: a systematic review and future perspectives. Bladder Cancer 6(2):131–141. https://doi.org/10.3233/Blc-200281

Knowles MA (2020) FGFR3 – a central player in bladder cancer pathogenesis? Bladder Cancer 6(4):403–423. https://doi.org/10.3233/Blc-200373

Kobayashi T (2016) Understanding the biology of urothelial cancer metastasis. Asian J Urol 3(4):211–222. https://doi.org/10.1016/j.ajur.2016.09.005

Korac-Prlic J, Degoricija M, Vilovic K et al (2020) Targeting Stat3 signaling impairs the progression of bladder cancer in a mouse model. Cancer Lett 490:89–99. https://doi.org/10.1016/j.canlet.2020.06.018

Koti M, Ingersoll MA, Gupta S et al (2020) Sex differences in bladder cancer Immunobiology and outcomes: a collaborative review with implications for treatment. Eur Urol Oncol 3(5):622–630. https://doi.org/10.1016/j.euo.2020.08.013

Kroemer G, Galluzzi L, Kepp O et al (2013) Immunogenic cell death in cancer therapy. Annu Rev Immunol 31:51–72. https://doi.org/10.1146/annurev-immunol-032712-100008

Kurtova AV, Xiao J, Mo Q et al (2015) Blocking PGE2-induced tumour repopulation abrogates bladder cancer chemoresistance. Nature 517(7533):209–213. https://doi.org/10.1038/nature14034

Leblond MM, Tille L, Nassiri S et al (2020) CD40 agonist restores the antitumor efficacy of anti-PD1 therapy in muscle-invasive bladder cancer in an IFN I/II-mediated manner. Cancer Immunol Res 8(9):1180–1192. https://doi.org/10.1158/2326-6066.CIR-19-0826

Lee YC, Kurtova AV, Xiao J et al (2019) Collagen-rich airway smooth muscle cells are a metastatic niche for tumor colonization in the lung. Nat Commun 10(1):2131. https://doi.org/10.1038/s41467-019-09878-4

Li R, Sexton WJ, Dhillon J et al (2023) A phase II study of Durvalumab for bacillus Calmette-Guerin (BCG) unresponsive urothelial carcinoma *in situ* of the bladder. Clin Cancer Res 29(19):3875–3881. https://doi.org/10.1158/1078-0432.CCR-23-0354

Lim S, Park JH, Chang H (2023) Enhanced anti-tumor immunity of vaccine combined with anti-PD-1 antibody in a murine bladder cancer model. Investig Clin Urol 64(1):74–81. https://doi.org/10.4111/icu.20220031

Liu C, Tate T, Batourina E et al (2019) Pparg promotes differentiation and regulates mitochondrial gene expression in bladder epithelial cells. Nat Commun 10(1):4589. https://doi.org/10.1038/s41467-019-12332-0

Liu LL, Hou YX, Deng CQ et al (2022) Single cell sequencing reveals that CD39 inhibition mediates changes to the tumor microenvironment. Nat Commun 13(1):6740. https://doi.org/10.1038/s41467-022-34495-z

Loriot Y, Necchi A, Park SH et al (2019) Erdafitinib in locally advanced or metastatic urothelial carcinoma. N Engl J Med 381(4):338–348. https://doi.org/10.1056/NEJMoa1817323

Lu Y, Liu PY, Wen WD et al (2011) Cross-species comparison of orthologous gene expression in human bladder cancer and carcinogen-induced rodent models. Am J Transl Res 3(1):8–27

Lubet RA, Huebner K, Fong LY et al (2005) 4-Hydroxybutyl (butyl)nitrosamine-induced urinary bladder cancers in mice: characterization of FHIT and survivin expression and chemopreventive effects of

indomethacin. Carcinogenesis 26(3):571–578. https://doi.org/10.1093/carcin/bgh352
Marks P, Soave A, Shariat SF et al (2016) Female with bladder cancer: what and why is there a difference? Transl Androl Urol 5(5):668–682. https://doi.org/10.21037/tau.2016.03.22
Massari F, Di Nunno V, Cubelli M et al (2018) Immune checkpoint inhibitors for metastatic bladder cancer. Cancer Treat Rev 64:11–20. https://doi.org/10.1016/j.ctrv.2017.12.007
Naito T, Higuchi T, Shimada Y et al (2020) An improved mouse orthotopic bladder cancer model exhibiting progression and treatment response characteristics of human recurrent bladder cancer. Oncol Lett 19(1):833–839. https://doi.org/10.3892/ol.2019.11172
Necchi A, Raggi D, Giannatempo P et al (2021) Can patients with muscle-invasive bladder cancer and fibroblast growth factor Receptor-3 alterations still be considered for neoadjuvant Pembrolizumab? A comprehensive assessment from the updated results of the PURE-01 study. Eur Urol Oncol 4(6):1001–1005. https://doi.org/10.1016/j.euo.2020.04.005
Nikolos F, Hayashi K, Hoi XP et al (2022) Cell death-induced immunogenicity enhances chemoimmunotherapeutic response by converting immune-excluded into T-cell inflamed bladder tumors. Nat Commun 13(1):1487. https://doi.org/10.1038/s41467-022-29026-9
Ohtani M, Kakizoe T, Sato S et al (1986) Strain differences in mice with invasive bladder carcinomas induced by N-butyl-N-(4-hydroxybutyl)nitrosamine. J Cancer Res Clin Oncol 112(2):107–110. https://doi.org/10.1007/BF00404391
Okato A, Utsumi T, Ranieri M et al (2024) FGFR inhibition augments anti-PD-1 efficacy in murine FGFR3-mutant bladder cancer by abrogating immunosuppression. J Clin Invest 134(2):e169241. https://doi.org/10.1172/JCI169241
Oliveira PA, Vasconcelos-Nobrega C, Gil da Costa RM et al (2018) The N-butyl-N-4-hydroxybutyl nitrosamine mouse urinary bladder cancer model. Methods Mol Biol 1655:155–167. https://doi.org/10.1007/978-1-4939-7234-0_13
Osei-Amponsa V, Buckwalter JM, Shuman L et al (2020) Hypermethylation of FOXA1 and allelic loss of PTEN drive squamous differentiation and promote heterogeneity in bladder cancer. Oncogene 39(6):1302–1317. https://doi.org/10.1038/s41388-019-1063-4
Overdevest JB, Thomas S, Kristiansen G et al (2011) CD24 offers a therapeutic target for control of bladder cancer metastasis based on a requirement for lung colonization. Cancer Res 71(11):3802–3811. https://doi.org/10.1158/0008-5472.CAN-11-0519
Overdevest JB, Knubel KH, Duex JE et al (2012) CD24 expression is important in male urothelial tumorigenesis and metastasis in mice and is androgen regulated. Proc Natl Acad Sci USA 109(51):E3588–E3596. https://doi.org/10.1073/pnas.1113960109
Pal SK, Rosenberg JE, Hoffman-Censits JH et al (2018) Efficacy of BGJ398, a fibroblast growth factor receptor 1-3 inhibitor, in patients with previously treated advanced urothelial carcinoma with FGFR3 alterations. Cancer Discov 8(7):812–821. https://doi.org/10.1158/2159-8290.CD-18-0229
Park S, Rong L, Owczarek TB et al (2021) Novel mouse models of bladder cancer identify a prognostic signature associated with risk of disease progression. Cancer Res 81(20):5161–5175. https://doi.org/10.1158/0008-5472.CAN-21-1254
Pauken KE, Wherry EJ (2015) Overcoming T cell exhaustion in infection and cancer. Trends Immunol 36(4):265–276. https://doi.org/10.1016/j.it.2015.02.008
Peng M, Xiao D, Bu Y et al (2020) Novel combination therapies for the treatment of bladder cancer. Front Oncol 10:539527. https://doi.org/10.3389/fonc.2020.539527
Petitprez F, Levy S, Sun CM et al (2020) The murine microenvironment cell population counter method to estimate abundance of tissue-infiltrating immune and stromal cell populations in murine samples using gene expression. Genome Med 12(1):86. https://doi.org/10.1186/s13073-020-00783-w
Pettenati C, Ingersoll MA (2018) Mechanisms of BCG immunotherapy and its outlook for bladder cancer. Nat Rev Urol 15(10):615–625. https://doi.org/10.1038/s41585-018-0055-4
Podojil JR, Glaser AP, Baker D et al (2020) Antibody targeting of B7-H4 enhances the immune response in urothelial carcinoma. Onco Targets Ther 9(1):1744897. https://doi.org/10.1080/2162402X.2020.1744897
Prescott MJ, Lidster K (2017) Improving quality of science through better animal welfare: the NC3Rs strategy. Lab Anim (NY) 46(4):152–156. https://doi.org/10.1038/laban.1217
Puzio-Kuter AM, Castillo-Martin M, Kinkade CW et al (2009) Inactivation of p53 and Pten promotes invasive bladder cancer. Genes Dev 23(6):675–680. https://doi.org/10.1101/gad.1772909
Rebouissou S, Bernard-Pierrot I, de Reynies A et al (2014) EGFR as a potential therapeutic target for a subset of muscle-invasive bladder cancers presenting a basal-like phenotype. Sci Transl Med 6(244):244ra91–244ra91. https://doi.org/10.1126/scitranslmed.3008970
Reddy OL, Cates JM, Gellert LL et al (2015) Loss of FOXA1 drives sexually dimorphic changes in urothelial differentiation and is an independent predictor of poor prognosis in bladder cancer. Am J Pathol 185(5):1385–1395. https://doi.org/10.1016/j.ajpath.2015.01.014
Reyes R, Deng YL, Zhang DY et al (2020) CD122-directed interleukin-2 complexes and alpha PD-L1 differentially require innate and adaptive immunity to treat local and metastatic bladder cancer. J Immunother Cancer 8:A430–A431. https://doi.org/10.1136/jitc-2020-SITC2020.0719
Robertson AG, Kim J, Al-Ahmadie H et al (2017) Comprehensive molecular characterization of muscle-invasive bladder cancer. Cell 171(3):540–556 e525. https://doi.org/10.1016/j.cell.2017.09.007

Rompre-Brodeur A, Shinde-Jadhav S, Ayoub M et al (2020) PD-1/PD-L1 immune checkpoint inhibition with radiation in bladder cancer: *in situ* and abscopal effects. Mol Cancer Ther 19(1):211–220. https://doi.org/10.1158/1535-7163.MCT-18-0986

Rose TL, Weir WH, Mayhew GM et al (2021) Fibroblast growth factor receptor 3 alterations and response to immune checkpoint inhibition in metastatic urothelial cancer: a real world experience. Br J Cancer 125(9):1251–1260. https://doi.org/10.1038/s41416-021-01488-6

Rotte A, Jin JY, Lemaire V (2018) Mechanistic overview of immune checkpoints to support the rational design of their combinations in cancer immunotherapy. Ann Oncol 29(1):71–83. https://doi.org/10.1093/annonc/mdx686

Roviello G, Catalano M, Santi R et al (2021) Immune checkpoint inhibitors in urothelial bladder cancer: state of the art and future perspectives. Cancers (Basel) 13(17):4411. https://doi.org/10.3390/cancers13174411

Ruan JL, Hsu JW, Browning RJ et al (2019) Mouse models of muscle-invasive bladder cancer: key considerations for clinical translation based on molecular subtypes. Eur Urol Oncol 2(3):239–247. https://doi.org/10.1016/j.euo.2018.08.014

Said N, Theodorescu D (2012) RhoGDI2 suppresses bladder cancer metastasis via reduction of inflammation in the tumor microenvironment. Onco Targets Ther 1(7):1175–1177. https://doi.org/10.4161/onci.20594

Said N, Smith S, Sanchez-Carbayo M et al (2011) Tumor endothelin-1 enhances metastatic colonization of the lung in mouse xenograft models of bladder cancer. J Clin Invest 121(1):132–147. https://doi.org/10.1172/JCI42912

Said N, Frierson HF, Sanchez-Carbayo M et al (2013) Loss of SPARC in bladder cancer enhances carcinogenesis and progression. J Clin Invest 123(2):751–766. https://doi.org/10.1172/JCI64782

Saito R, Smith CC, Utsumi T et al (2018) Molecular subtype-specific immunocompetent models of high-grade urothelial carcinoma reveal differential neoantigen expression and response to immunotherapy. Cancer Res 78(14):3954–3968. https://doi.org/10.1158/0008-5472.CAN-18-0173

Schreiber RD, Old LJ, Smyth MJ (2011) Cancer immunoediting: integrating immunity's roles in cancer suppression and promotion. Science 331(6024):1565–1570. https://doi.org/10.1126/science.1203486

Schuler M, Cho BC, Sayehli CM et al (2019) Rogaratinib in patients with advanced cancers selected by FGFR mRNA expression: a phase 1 dose-escalation and dose-expansion study. Lancet Oncol 20(10):1454–1466. https://doi.org/10.1016/S1470-2045(19)30412-7

Seo HK, Shin SP, Jung NR et al (2017) The establishment of a growth-controllable orthotopic bladder cancer model through the down-regulation of c-myc expression. Oncotarget 8(31):50500–50509. https://doi.org/10.18632/oncotarget.10784

Seyer AK, Lehman HL, DJ DG (2019) Modeling tumor heterogeneity in bladder cancer: the current state of the field and future needs. Bladder Cancer 5(4):251–261. https://doi.org/10.3233/Blc-199009

Sharma P, Hu-Lieskovan S, Wargo JA et al (2017) Primary, adaptive, and acquired resistance to cancer immunotherapy. Cell 168(4):707–723. https://doi.org/10.1016/j.cell.2017.01.017

Shi MJ, Fontugne J, Moreno-Vega A et al (2023) FGFR3 mutational activation can induce luminal-like papillary bladder tumor formation and favors a male sex bias. Eur Urol 83(1):70–81. https://doi.org/10.1016/j.eururo.2022.09.030

Shurin GV, Ma Y, Shurin MR (2013) Immunosuppressive mechanisms of regulatory dendritic cells in cancer. Cancer Microenviron 6(2):159–167. https://doi.org/10.1007/s12307-013-0133-3

Sun YU, Nishino H, Zhao M et al (2020) A non-invasive Imageable GFP-expressing mouse model of Orthotopic human bladder cancer. *In Vivo* 34(6):3225–3231. https://doi.org/10.21873/invivo.12158

Sweis RF, Spranger S, Bao R et al (2016) Molecular drivers of the non-T-cell-inflamed tumor microenvironment in urothelial bladder cancer. Cancer Immunol Res 4(7):563–568. https://doi.org/10.1158/2326-6066.CIR-15-0274

Takeyama Y, Kato M, Tamada S et al (2020) Myeloid-derived suppressor cells are essential partners for immune checkpoint inhibitors in the treatment of cisplatin-resistant bladder cancer. Cancer Lett 479:89–99. https://doi.org/10.1016/j.canlet.2020.03.013

Tate T, Xiang T, Wobker SE et al (2021) Pparg signaling controls bladder cancer subtype and immune exclusion. Nat Commun 12(1):6160. https://doi.org/10.1038/s41467-021-26421-6

Tomlinson DC, Baldo O, Harnden P et al (2007) FGFR3 protein expression and its relationship to mutation status and prognostic variables in bladder cancer. J Pathol 213(1):91–98. https://doi.org/10.1002/path.2207

Truong AS, Zhou M, Krishnan B et al (2021) Entinostat induces antitumor immune responses through immune editing of tumor neoantigens. J Clin Invest 131(16):e138560. https://doi.org/10.1172/JCI138560

Tu MM, Abdel-Hafiz HA, Jones RT et al (2020) Inhibition of the CCL2 receptor, CCR2, enhances tumor response to immune checkpoint therapy. Commun Biol 3(1):720. https://doi.org/10.1038/s42003-020-01441-y

Van Batavia J, Yamany T, Molotkov A et al (2014) Bladder cancers arise from distinct urothelial sub-populations. Nat Cell Biol 16(10):982–991., 981–985. https://doi.org/10.1038/ncb3038

van Rhijn BWG, Mertens LS, Mayr R et al (2020) FGFR3 mutation status and FGFR3 expression in a large bladder cancer cohort treated by radical cystectomy: implications for anti-FGFR3 treatment?(dagger). Eur Urol 78(5):682–687. https://doi.org/10.1016/j.eururo.2020.07.002

Vasconcelos-Nobrega C, Colaco A, Lopes C et al (2012) Review: BBN as an urothelial carcinogen. *In Vivo* 26(4):727–739

Wakefield L, Agarwal S, Tanner K (2023) Preclinical models for drug discovery for metastatic disease. Cell 186(8):1792–1813. https://doi.org/10.1016/j.cell.2023.02.026

Wang H, Owens C, Chandra N et al (2010) Phosphorylation of RalB is important for bladder cancer cell growth and metastasis. Cancer Res 70(21):8760–8769. https://doi.org/10.1158/0008-5472.CAN-10-0952

Wang L, Gong Y, Saci A et al (2019) Fibroblast growth factor receptor 3 alterations and response to PD-1/PD-L1 blockade in patients with metastatic urothelial cancer. Eur Urol 76(5):599–603. https://doi.org/10.1016/j.eururo.2019.06.025

Williams PD, Lee JK, Theodorescu D (2008) Molecular credentialing of rodent bladder carcinogenesis models. Neoplasia 10(8):838–846. https://doi.org/10.1593/neo.08432

Xia W, Zhang S, Duan H et al (2022) The combination therapy of Everolimus and anti-PD-1 improves the antitumor effect by regulating CD8(+) T cells in bladder cancer. Med Oncol 39(3):37. https://doi.org/10.1007/s12032-021-01624-5

Yamamoto S, Masui T, Murai T et al (1995) Frequent mutations of the p53 gene and infrequent H- and K-ras mutations in urinary bladder carcinomas of NON/Shi mice treated with N-butyl-N-(4-hydroxybutyl)nitrosamine. Carcinogenesis 16(10):2363–2368. https://doi.org/10.1093/carcin/16.10.2363

Yamamoto S, Tatematsu M, Yamamoto M et al (1998) Clonal analysis of urothelial carcinomas in C3H/HeN<-->BALB/c chimeric mice treated with N-butyl-N-(4-hydroxybutyl)nitrosamine. Carcinogenesis 19(5):855–860. https://doi.org/10.1093/carcin/19.5.855

Zhang ZT, Pak J, Shapiro E et al (1999) Urothelium-specific expression of an oncogene in transgenic mice induced the formation of carcinoma *in situ* and invasive transitional cell carcinoma. Cancer Res 59(14):3512–3517

Zhou H, He F, Mendelsohn CL et al (2016) FGFR3b extracellular loop mutation lacks Tumorigenicity *in vivo* but collaborates with p53/pRB deficiency to induce high-grade papillary urothelial carcinoma. Sci Rep 6:25596. https://doi.org/10.1038/srep25596

In Vitro Bladder Cancer Models

17

Catalina Berca, Francisco X. Real, and Miriam Marqués

Abstract

Over the past five decades, in vitro models of bladder cancer (BLCA) have been instrumental in understanding tumor biology. These models offer many advantages over animal testing, including bypassing ethical concerns associated with in vivo experiments, cost-effectiveness, and suitability for high-throughput studies like testing small compounds and genetic screens. We review the main in vitro BLCA models, including 2D plastic cultures and more recent three-dimensional (3D) systems such as organoids, tumoroids, and assembloids. Conventional BLCA cell lines are still the primary option for many studies, mainly due to their simple requirements and rapid growth. However, they display shortcomings, favoring the use and optimization of culture techniques designed to tackle these limitations. 3D systems excel regarding efficiency of sustained growth upon primary culture, recapitulating tumor-of-origin features, and usefulness. However, challenges persist, including price, the absence of standardized procedures for establishment and maintenance, and the fact that they generally lack the stroma. Hence, advanced organotypic systems are an important solution to overcome some of these limitations, along with the emergence of nanotechnology and microfluidics advancements that are poised to shape this field in the upcoming decade. Additionally, we discuss the relevance of culturing normal urothelial cells alongside BLCA cells for a better comprehension of cancer-associated biology.

Keywords

Bladder cancer · Cell culture · Two-dimensional · Three-dimensional · Organotypic · Organoids

17.1 Introduction

Over the last five decades, in vitro BLCA models (mainly BLCA cell lines) have played a key role in the study of the biology of this tumor.

C. Berca
Epithelial Carcinogenesis Group, Spanish National Cancer Research Centre-CNIO, Madrid, Spain

F. X. Real (✉)
Epithelial Carcinogenesis Group, Spanish National Cancer Research Centre-CNIO, Madrid, Spain

CIBERONC, Madrid, Spain

Department of Medicine and Life Sciences, Universitat Pompeu Fabra, Barcelona, Spain
e-mail: freal@cnio.es

M. Marqués (✉)
Epithelial Carcinogenesis Group, Spanish National Cancer Research Centre-CNIO, Madrid, Spain

CIBERONC, Madrid, Spain
e-mail: mmarques@cnio.es

M. A. Knowles, L. Dyrskjøt (eds.), *Biology of Bladder Cancer*,
https://doi.org/10.1007/978-3-031-68505-7_17

Such tools present numerous advantages over animal models, the most relevant being that they circumvent the ethical concerns associated with in vivo experimentation. In addition, work with in vitro models is cheaper and amenable to high-throughput studies, such as large-scale testing of small compounds (Agarwal et al. 2022; Merrill et al. 2020; Rinaldetti et al. 2022) and genetic screens (Agarwal et al. 2021; Tortora et al. 2023). However, the BLCA cell lines that have been used most extensively also present important limitations, some of which are overcome by the more recent advent of 3D culture methods. Here, we review the available in vitro models to study BLCA but, while very important, will not discuss in detail the relevance of quality controls of cell line identity, Mycoplasma contamination, absence of stromal components, or endocrine homeostatic effects.

We review the information available on conventional BLCA cells cultured on plastic (2D) and recently reported 3D models, including organoids, tumoroids, and assembloids. In addition, we briefly discuss the state of the art on the culture of normal urothelial cells, since they are critical companions for an improved interpretation of the experimental findings using BLCA cells. Finally, we highlight the use of explants/precision-cut slices as an intermediate step to overcome some of these limitations as well as ongoing technical developments based on nanotechnology and microfluidics that will have an impact over the next decade (Fig. 17.1).

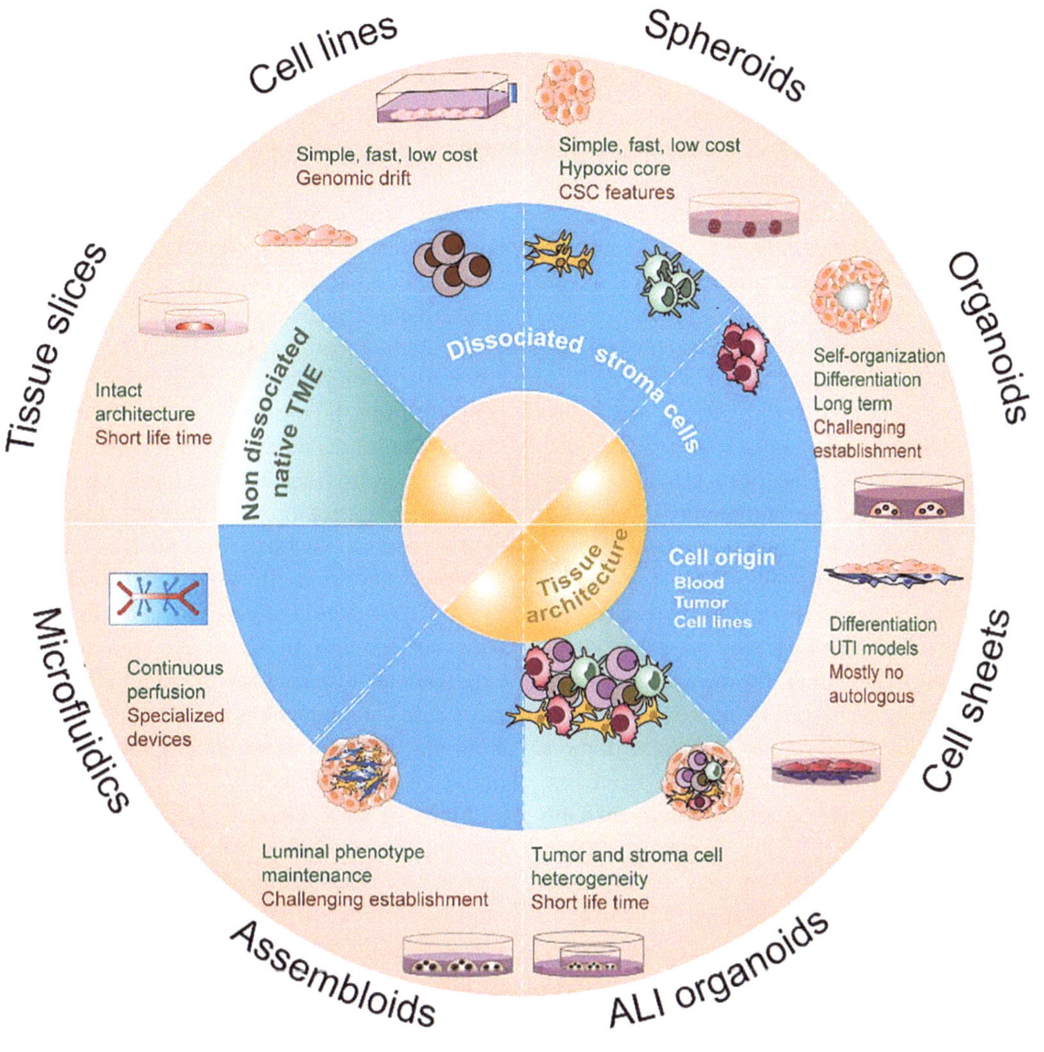

Fig. 17.1 Outline of the in vitro models employed in BLCA research, encompassing both 2D and 3D cultures. In vitro co-cultures of tumor cells with stromal cells can be generated using either **isolated stromal cells** (depicted as blue inserts) or **native stromal cells** (e.g., from minced tumors (depicted as green inserts). ***Isolated Stromal Cells:*** In this approach, stromal cells are either established cell lines or primary cultures isolated from a tissue source (e.g., blood, tumor) that may, or may not, have the same origin as the epithelial cells. Isolating stromal cells from tissues can be technically challenging and generally requires enzymatic digestion, cell sorting, or other purification methods. ***Native Stromal Cells from Minced Tumors:*** Using minced tumors preserves stromal cell heterogeneity and allows for the study of a broader range of stromal cell populations within a culture. The preservation of tissue architecture is highlighted by orange inserts. Green text underscores the system's benefits and red text indicates experimental limitations. ALI: Air-Liquid Interface; CSC: Cancer Stem Cell; UTI:Urinary Tract Infections

17.2 2D Cell Cultures

Monolayer 2D BLCA cultures have been established mainly from human tumors but also from other species, including mouse, rat, and dog (Zuiverloon et al. 2018). In addition, primary 2D cultures from normal urothelium have been reported although their research use has been hampered by their short lifespan (Southgate et al. 1994).

17.2.1 BLCA Cell Lines

Standard methods to establish 2D cell lines from BLCA have met with limited success. Primary growth is often achieved, but less than 10% of cultures give rise to established lines. A recent systematic review compiled information on 127 BLCA cell lines (Zuiverloon et al. 2018) and provides links to the main online BLCA cell line resources.

RT4, the first BLCA cell line established, was derived from a low-grade tumor with superficial invasion of the muscle wall by Rigby and Franks in 1970 (Rigby and Franks 1970). Since then, many BLCA lines have been established and made available to the community, with most notable contributions from the laboratories of H. B. Grossman, C. Reznikoff, M. A. Knowles, and P. Jones, among others. The stage and grade of the tumors from which they were established is not always known but, for the 55 cases where information is available, 19 and 36 lines came from non-muscle- and muscle-invasive tumors, respectively; 20 and 52 lines came from low-grade and high-grade tumors, respectively. Only five of the available lines were established from tumors reported to be G1 grade. Ninety-seven lines came from primary tumors (92 bladder, 2 ureter, and 3 renal pelvis) while 12 were derived from lung, liver, or lymph node metastases. These numbers evidence a selection bias of the samples used to generate BLCA lines, with an over-representation of advanced, high-grade, primary samples. Importantly, histological sections of the original tumors from which the cultures were produced are generally not available either for pathological review or for comparative genomic analyses.

Of all these lines, a handful have been widely used and characterized in terms of their morphology, in vitro behavior, molecular phenotype, genomic alterations, and in vivo performance upon implantation in immunodeficient mice. MGH-U3, RT4, RT112, and SW-780 are the most frequently used lines derived from low-grade tumors, while J82, TCCSUP, T24, and 639V are among the most used lines that were isolated from high-grade tumors (Earl et al. 2015). The biases described above, and the drift associated with long-term culture, imply that these lines do not provide adequate models to assess certain features of bladder tumors. However, they are useful to study urothelial biology and the function of genes involved in BLCA, with due caution in the interpretation of the experimental results. One limitation is that, in most cases, a companion normal cell line/tissue from the subjects from whom the lines was derived is not available.

Many of these lines can be obtained from a few qualified resources which are highly recommended for their quality standards. They are the optimal source to acquire BLCA lines for research given that they place a major effort in quality control (Table 17.1). Of note, the T24 BLCA line is one of the most common sources of cross-contaminations reported in the literature. A few web-based tools are available to compile biological information on selected BLCA lines (Table 17.2).

Table 17.1 Repositories from which to acquire reliable stocks of BLCA lines

Name	Country	Website link
AcceGen Biotechnology	United States	https://www.accegen.com/
American Type Culture Collection (ATCC)	United States	https://www.atcc.org/
Bioresource Collection and Research Center (BCRC)	Taiwan	https://catalog.bcrc.firdi.org.tw/
Cell Lines Service (CLS)	Germany	https://cls.shop/
European Collection of Authenticated Cell Cultures (ECACC)	United Kingdom	https://www.culturecollections.org.uk/
German Collection of Microorganisms and Cell Cultures GMbH (DSMZ)	Germany	https://www.dsmz.de/
Korean Cell Line Bank	Korea	https://cellbank.snu.ac.kr/main/

Table 17.2 Selected web-based tools to mine data related to BLCA lines

Web-based tool	Information available	Website link
Cancer cell line encyclopedia	Human cancer cell lines data: Genotype, gene expression, epigenetic, modifications, proteomics, and drug sensitivity	https://sites.broadinstitute.org/ccle/
Dependency map (DepMap) portal	Public datasets from human cancer cell lines and visualization tools	https://depmap.org/portal/
Cellosaurus	Database of all cell lines used in biomedical research of human, mice, rat, and dog origin	https://www.cellosaurus.org/
Metastasis map (MetMap)	Metastic capacity of human cancer cell lines	https://depmap.org/metmap/
Genomics of drug sensitivity in cancer (GDSC)	Response to drugs (chemotherapy and targeted therapies) and identification of sensitivity-related genomic markers of human cancer cell lines	https://www.cancerrxgene.org/

17.2.1.1 Genomic Studies of BLCA Lines

The DNA alterations of a large number of BLCA cell lines have been summarized by the laboratories of Real and Theodorescu with several collaborators (Earl et al. 2015; Nickerson et al. 2017) (Table 17.3). The most widely used lines harbor many of the prototypical genetic alterations in oncogenes (e.g., *TERT* promoter hotspot mutations, *FGFR3* hotspot mutations and fusions) or tumor suppressor genes (e.g., *STAG2*, *TP53,* and *PTEN* mutations) involved in BLCA. The definite annotation of mutations as somatic is hampered by the lack of normal genomic DNA. However, a series of cell lines with matched Epstein-Barr Virus- (EBV-)immortalized lymphoblasts (lines LUCC1–9) (Ross et al. 2016; Taylor et al. 2014; Williams et al. 2013) has been established recently by the Knowles laboratory and these, together with paired lymphoblasts for the cell lines J82 and DSH1, have been deposited for future distribution by the European Collection of Authenticated Cell Cultures (ECACC).

The available BLCA lines represent useful models to study the biology of urothelial lineage identity. More than 50 lines have been profiled at the transcriptomic level using microarrays or RNA-Seq and their phenotype has been assessed based on the expression of established urothelial markers (e.g., uroplakins and keratins), the transcription factors (TFs) involved in urothelial differentiation (e.g., FOXA1, GATA3, and PPARG) or in loss of lineage commitment (e.g., TP63), and transcriptomic signatures (Earl et al. 2015; Rinaldetti et al. 2022; Warrick et al. 2016). When applied to the cell line transcriptomes, the muscle-invasive bladder cancer (MIBC) BLCA consensus signatures classify the lines as Luminal, Basal/Squamous, and Neuroendocrine-like; the Stromal-rich tumor subtype can, obviously, not be recapitulated (Kamoun et al. 2020) (Table 17.3). These analyses have revealed a bias toward non-luminal phenotypes in vitro, in agreement with their more aggressive features.

RT4, RT112, MGH-U3, and SW-780 represent the best models of luminal/urothelial cell lines (Table 17.3). Interestingly, they all harbor *FGFR3* genetic alterations, thus recapitulating the fact that *FGFR3*-mutant patient tumors generally display luminal phenotypes. SCaBER, VM-CUB-1, and 5637 display basal/squamous transcriptomic features (Earl et al. 2015; Nickerson et al. 2017) (Table 17.3). RT4 and SW-780 cells have been used to assess the genome-wide distribution of FOXA1 and GATA3, two major regulators of the urothelial differentiation program, showing enrichment in gene bodies/intergenic regions, consistent with a reported role at distal enhancers (Iyyanki et al. 2021). Genome-wide chromatin immunoprecipitation of histone marks and urothelial TFs, coupled with RNA sequencing, open chromatin status, and 3D chromatin structure has been used to dissect the gene regulatory networks (GRN) responsible for the phenotype of BLCA cell lines (Iyyanki et al. 2021; Neyret-Kahn et al. 2023). We have recently reviewed the TF landscape involved in the maintenance of urothelial lineage identity, providing detailed information about how BLCA cell lines have contributed to the understanding of these genetic programs (Ramal et al. 2023). These studies suggest that transcrip-

Table 17.3 Summary of the features of the most commonly used BLCA cell lines

Cell line	Source	Origin	Site	Stage	Grade	Sex	Expression data	Consensus class	Consensus class separation	Genome instability group	*TERT*	*FGFR3*	*PIK3CA*	*CDKN2A*	*TP53*	Microsatellite stability	Metastasis potential (MetMap550)	Doubling time (hours)
647V	UCC	Primary	Bladder	T2/3a	G2	M	R	Ba/Sq	Good		c.228C > T Z = unspecified		WT	WT	c.485 T > A c.1006G > T	Stable	Weakly metastatic: Liver, kidney, lung, bone	30
92-1	UCC		Bladder	T4	G3	F	M	Ba/Sq	Good	Intermediate	c.228C > T Z = unspecified	WT	WT	WT	cd 158, 162, 228, 280 & 294/N			
5637	UCC	Primary	Bladder		G2	M	M, R	Ba/Sq	Good	Intermediate	c.228C > T Z = unspecified	WT	WT	WT	c.839G > C Z = homozygous	Stable	Non metastatic	23/24
97-18	UCC		Bladder	T2	G3	Y	M	Ba/Sq	Good	High	MUT	WT	WT	LOH**	cd 220/LOH			
96-1	UCC		Bladder	T3	G2/3	M	M	Ba/Sq	Good	Intermediate	c.228C > T Z = unspecified	WT	WT	HD	cd 175/N			
97-24	UCC		Bladder	T3	G3	M	M	Ba/Sq	Good	High	c.228C > T Z = unspecified	WT	WT	WT	cd 275/N			
SCaBER	SCC	Primary	Bladder	T3		M	M, R	Ba/Sq	Good	Intermediate	c.228C > T Z = unspecified	WT	WT	LOH	c.329G > T/LOH		Metastatic: Lung weakly metastatic: Kidney, brain	
KU-19-19	UCC	Primary	Bladder	T3b	G3	M	R	Ba/Sq	Good		WT	WT	WT	WT	WT		Metastatic: Bone, brain, liver, kidney, lung	48
U-BLC1	UCC	Primary	Bladder	≥T2	G3	F	R	Ba/Sq	Good		c.228C > T Z = unspecified;WT**	WT	WT	WT	c.886C > T; c.991C > T		Non metastatic	
97-7	UCC		Bladder	T1	G2/3	M	M	Ba/Sq	Good	High	c.228C > T Z = unspecified	p.S249C	WT	WT	cd 128/N			
BC-3C	UCC	Primary	Bladder	T3	G4	F	R	Ba/Sq	Good		WT	WT	WT	WT	MUT		Metastatic: Kidney weakly metastatic: Lung	25/30
VM-CUB-1	UCC	Primary	Bladder		G2	M	M, R	Ba/Sq	Good	High	c.228C > T Z = unspecified	WT	WT/p. E542K + p. E674Q**	c.322G > C/ LOH	c.524G > A&c.378C- > G/ LOH		Metastatic: Kidney>bone>brain weakly metastatic: Lung	30–45
UM-UC-18	UCC		Bladder				M	Ba/Sq	Medium	High	MUT	WT	WT	WT	WT/N			
HT1197	UCC		Bladder	T2	G4	M	M, R	Ba/Sq	Medium		c.228C > T Z = unspecified	p.S249C	p.E545K	WT	WT/c.1094A- > G**	Stable		45/60
UM-UC-10	UCC	Primary	Bladder		G3		M, R	Ba/Sq	Medium		MUT	WT	WT		c.853G > A; Z = unspecified			
UM-UC-6	UCC	Primary	Bladder			M	M, R	Ba/Sq	Medium	Low		WT/R248C**	p.E545K	HD	WT/c.592G > T/LOH**			38
HT1376	UCC	Primary	Bladder	T2	G3	F	M, R	Ba/Sq	Medium	Low	c.228C > T Z = unspecified	WT	WT	WT	c.749C > T/LOH	Stable	Metastatic: Lung, kidney weakly metastatic: Bone	30/60
TCCSUP	UCC	Primary	Bladder	T4	G4	F	M, R	Ba/Sq	Medium	Intermediate	c.228C > T Z = unspecified	WT	p.E545K	WT	c.1045G > T/LOH	Stable	Non metastatic	30/49
PSI	UCC		Bladder	T4	G3	M	M	Ba/Sq	Medium		MUT			MUT	WT			
KK47			Bladder		G1	M	M	Ba/Sq	Medium	HIGH	WT	WT/p. S249C**		WT	WT/N			24

UM-UC-15	UCC		Bladder				M	Ba/Sq	Medium		MUT	p.Y375C/p. S249C**	p.E545K					
97-1	UCC		Bladder	T1/2	G1/2	M	M	Ba/Sq	Medium	Low	WT	WT	WT	HD**	WT/LOH**			
BFTC-905	UCC	Primary	Bladder	T4	G3	F	R	Ba/Sq	Medium		WT	WT	WT	WT	c.673-2A > T Z = homozygous	Stable	Metastatic: Kidney weakly metastatic: Brain	
VM-CUB-2	EC		Bladder	T4		M	M	Ba/Sq	Medium	High	c.228C > T Z = unspecified	WT	WT	HD	c.473G- > T&c.488A- > G/LOH			
T24	UCC	Primary	Bladder	Ta	G3	F	M, R	Ba/Sq; NE-like	Medium	Low	c.228C > T Z = unspecified	WT	WT	WT/LOH**	c.378C > G/N Z = homozygous	Stable	Metastatic: Brain weakly metastatic: Lung, bone, kidney	24
SW-1710	UCC	Primary	Bladder		G1	F	M, R	Ba/Sq	Poor	High	c.228C > T Z = unspecified	WT	WT	HD	c.817C > T Z = homozygous	Stable	Non metastatic	25/32
575A	UCC		Bladder		G3	M	M	Ba/Sq	Poor	Intermediate	MUT	WT	WT	WT	WT/LOH**	Stable		50
MGH-U4	Focal severe urothelial atypia		Bladder			M	M	Ba/Sq	Poor	Low	MUT	WT	p.H1047R	HD	WT/N			
BC61	UCC	Primary	Bladder	Ta	G2	M	M	Ba/Sq	Poor	Low		p.G370C	WT	HD**	WT/N			
UM-UC-16	UCC		Bladder				R	Ba/Sq	Poor		MUT	p.S249C			MUT			
CAL-29	UCC	Primary	Bladder	T2	G4	F	R	Ba/Sq	Poor		c.228C > T Z = unspecified	WT	p.H1047R	WT	c.844C > T Z = homozygous	Stable	Non metastatic	30/60
JON	ADC		Bladder			M	M	Ba/Sq	Poor		(c.161A > C)** Z = unspecified		WT		(c.853G > A. Z = homozygous			
SW-780	UCC	Primary	Bladder		G1	F	M, R	LumP	Good	Low	c.228C > T Z = unspecified	WT/p. S773F'FGFR3-BAIAP2L1 fusion**	WT	HD	WT/N	Stable	Metastatic: Lung weakly metastatic: Liver	
KMBC-2		Primary	Bladder				R	LumP	Good		WT	WT	WT	WT	c.839G > C Z = homozygous		Metastatic: Kidney, bone, brain weakly metastatic: Liver, lung	68
UM-UC-14	UCC	Metastasis	Renal pelvis		G4	M	M, R	LumP	Good	Low	c.228C > T Z = unspecified	p.S249C	WT	HD + T45	c.839G > C/LOH			
RT4	UCC	Primary	Bladder	T1/2	G1/2	M	M, R	LumP	Medium	Low	c.228C > T Z = unspecified	WT/ amp'FGFR3-TACC3 fusion**	WT	HD	WT/LOH**	Stable	Non metastatic	60/80
UM-UC-1	UCC	Metastasis	Lymph node	T2-T4	G2	M	M, R	LumP	Medium	Intermediate		WT	WT	HD	c.454C- > T/LOH		Metastatic: Bone	26

Table 17.3 (continued)

Cell line	Source	Origin	Site	Stage	Grade	Sex	Expression data	Consensus class	Consensus class separation	Genome instability group	*TERT*	*FGFR3*	*PIK3CA*	*CDKN2A*	*TP53*	Microsatellite stability	Metastasis potential (MetMap550)	Doubling time (hours)
RT112	UCC	Primary	Bladder	Ta	G2	F	M, R	LumP	Medium	Low	c.228C > T Z = unspecified	WT/amp/ FGFR3- TACC3 fusion**	WT	HD**	c.743G > A&c.548C- > G/ LOH	Stable	Metastatic: Bone>kidney>liver weakly metastatic: Lung	25/35
VM-CUB-3	VM-CUB-1 cells		Bladder		G3	M	M	LumP	Poor	Low	c.228C > T Z = unspecified	WT	p.E545K	HD	c.833C- > T Z = homozygous			26
UM-UC-7	UCC	Primary	Bladder			M	M, R	LumP	Poor	Intermediate	MUT	WT	WT	WT	c.637C > T/LOH			41
UM-UC-17	UCC		Bladder				M	LumP	Poor	Intermediate		p.S249C**	WT	HD	LOH			
UM-UC-5	UCC	Primary	Bladder			F	M, R	LumP	Poor	Intermediate	MUT	WT	p.E545K	HD	c.159G > A/LOH**			19
MGH-U3	UCC		Bladder	Ta/T1	G1	M	M	LumP	Poor	Low	c.228C > T Z = unspecified	p.Y375C/p. Y373C**	WT[4]	HD	WT/N/MUT**			
UM-UC-12	UCC		Bladder			M	M	LumU	Poor	High		WT	WT	WT	WT/N			
UM-UC-4	ADC	Metastasis	Lymph node			F	R	LumU	Poor	High		WT	WT	WT	c.389 T > G/LOH			32
UM-UC-9	UCC	Primary	Bladder		G3	F	M, R	LumU	Poor	Intermediate	MUT	WT	WT	LOH	c.1044delG/LOH			
639V	UCC	Primary	Ureter		G3	M	M, R	NE-like	Medium	High	c.228C > T Z = unspecified	p.R248C	A1066V	LOH	c.743G > A Z = homozygous	Unstable	Weakly metastatic: Kidney>bone>lung	24
UM-UC-3	UCC	Primary	Bladder	T2-T4		M	M, R	NE-like	Medium	High	c.228C > T Z = unspecified	WT	WT	HD/WT**	c.338 T > G/N**	Stable		24
LGWO1-G600	UCC		Bladder				M	NE-like	Medium	Low	WT	WT	WT	HD	LOH			
UM-UC-2	UCC	Primary	Ureter	TIS	*CIS*	F/M**	M	NE-like	Medium		c.228C > T Z = unspecified	WT			c.378C > G/WT**			
UM-UC-11	UCC	Primary	Bladder			M	M, R	NE-like	Medium	High	MUT	WT	WT	HD	WT/N/MUT**			
JMSU-1	UCC	Metastasis	Ascites	T4	G3	M	R	NE-like	Medium		c.228C > T Z = unspecified	WT	WT	WT	(c.839G > C) Z = homozygous		Metastatic: Liver, bone, lung, kidney, brain	30
SW-800	UCC		Bladder		G1	M	M	NE-like	Medium	Low	MUT	WT	WT	HD	WT/N			
253 J-BV	UCC	Metastasis	Lymph node			F	R	NE-like	Poor			WT	p.E545G				Weakly metastatic: Kidney	45/54
UM-UC-13	UCC	Metastasis	Lymph node			M	M, R	NE-like	Poor	High	MUT	WT	WT	LOH	MUT/N			
253J	UCC	Primary	Lymph node	T4	G4	F	M, R	NE-like; Ba/Sq	Poor	Intermediate	WT	WT	p.E545G	HD	WT/N**	Stable	Non metastatic	36
J82	EC	Primary	Bladder	T3	G3	M	M, R	NE-like; Ba/Sq	Poor	Intermediate	c.228C > T Z = unspecified	WT/p. K652E**	p.P124L	WT	c.960G- > C&c.820G- > &c.811G- > A&c.783_919del137/N[1,2,3]	Stable	Weakly metastatic: Kidney, liver	24

Cells are categorized into molecular subclasses using RNAseq (preferred option) or microarray expression data and the consensusMIBC package, accessible on GitHub (https://github.com/cit-bioinfo/consensusMIBC). The "Separation" tab denotes the degree to which a sample accurately represents its assigned consensus class, as determined by the separation level generated in the script. This separation level ranges from 0–1, with 0 indicating that the sample cannot be confidently assigned a specific consensus class label, while a value of 1 means that the sample strongly embodies its assigned consensus class. The labels assigned based on the separation level: "Good" for >0.7, "Medium" for 0.4–0.7, "Poor" < 0.4. Metastatic potential information was extracted from Jin et al. (2020)

(**) indicates data discrepancies between different sources. *UCC* Urothelial Cell Carcinoma, *SCC* Squamous Cell Carcinoma, *ADC* Adenocarcinoma, *EC* Epidermoid Carcinoma, *Ba/Sq* Basal Squamous, *LumP* Luminal Papillary, *NE* Neuroendocrine, *LOH* Loss of Heterozygosity, *HD* Homozygous Deletions, *WT* Wild Type, *MUT* Mutant, *N* Copy number neutral tomic subtypes are driven by specific TFs whose activity is embedded in as yet incompletely characterized GRNs and are associated with distinct epigenetic landscapes.

17.2.1.2 Functional Studies

BLCA cell lines have been used to demonstrate the involvement of urothelial differentiation TFs in the regulation of BLCA transcriptional programs. *FOXA1* knockdown in luminal RT4 cells enhanced cell proliferation (DeGraff et al. 2012) while ectopic GATA3 expression reduced proliferation of T24 and UM-UC-3 cells (Wang et al. 2020). Knockdown of *GRHL3,* another urothelial TF, promoted a more invasive phenotype (DeGraff et al. 2012; Wezel et al. 2021). RT112 have also been widely used as a prototype of luminal BLCA cells: a PPARG-reporter-based genome-wide CRISPR knockout screen using this line identified GATA3, SPT6, and cohesin components as positive regulators of PPARG expression (Tortora et al. 2023). They have also been used to dissect the genomic effect of loss-of-function of *STAG2*, one of the major BLCA tumor suppressor genes (Richart et al. 2021).

In UM-UC-3 mesenchymal-like cells, ELF3 overexpression induced an epithelial phenotype and reduced invasiveness (Gondkar et al. 2019). The combined overexpression of GATA3 and FOXA1 in 5637 basal/squamous-like cells resulted in the activation of a luminal-specific program. T24 cells are undifferentiated and FOXA1 overexpression led to decreased proliferation and invasion and increased E-cadherin expression (DeGraff et al. 2012). Similar effects on invasiveness were observed upon GRHL3 overexpression (Wezel et al. 2021). In non-luminal VM-CUB-1, UM-UC-3, and UM-UC-6 BLCA cells, overexpression of PPARG activated its transcription program and inhibited cell growth, in part, through down-regulation of EGFR expression, while no effect was seen in PPARG high-expressing cells (Coutos-Thévenot et al. 2019).

17.2.1.3 Prediction of Response to Therapy

Many studies have reported the sensitivity of BLCA cells to chemotherapeutic drugs: T24, RT4, J82, and TCCSUP are among the most cisplatin-resistant lines (Shi et al. 2022; Wang et al. 2018). One of the most ambitious projects to leverage the potential of BLCA cell lines to predict response to therapy was COXEN (Coexpression Extrapolation) (Dancik and Theodorescu 2022; Lee et al. 2007). This algorithm identified candidate predictive biomarkers using transcriptomics and in vitro chemosensitivity data to identify patients who might benefit from specific therapies. A clinical trial of neoadjuvant chemotherapy (NCT02177695) analyzed prospectively the predictive value of the COXEN algorithm for response to dose-dense methotrexate-vinblastine-adriamycin-cisplatin vs. gemcitabine-cisplatin. However, the study did not show significant predictive value (Flaig et al. 2021). This work underlines the challenges of using BLCA cell lines for this purpose.

17.2.2 Normal Human Urothelial Cultures

Over the last three decades, the Southgate laboratory has pioneered and led the research to establish methods for the culture of normal human urothelial (NHU) cells (Southgate et al. 1994) (see also Chap. 3). This group has optimized protocols for urothelial digestion and culture; NHU cells proliferate, can be expanded and maintained for a few passages, acquire stratification and, in the presence of PPARG activators and EGFR inhibitors, can undergo urothelial differentiation (Baker et al. 2022; Baker et al. 2020; Baker et al. 2014; Kawakami et al. 2002; Varley and Southgate 2008; Varley et al. 2004). The availability of NHU cultures allows a direct comparison of the features of normal and malignant urothelial cells. This strategy has, for example, allowed the identification of the multiple regional epigenetic silencing phenotype in a subset of human BLCA lines (Vallot et al. 2011). To overcome the short lifespan of NHU, immortalization through hTERT or Human Papillomavirus E6 overexpression has been reported, though this results in compromised differentiation and functional capacity (Chapman et al. 2006;

Georgopoulos et al. 2011). Other researchers have established short-term cultures from exfoliated normal cells in urine (Herz et al. 1985).

Several NHU cell lines are commercially available; for example, HBLAK cells (Cellntec, Bern, Switzerland) are untransformed, can be cultured for longer periods of time, and can be induced to differentiate. These cells contain a few chromosomal aberrations, $p16^{INK4A}$ loss, and harbor the C228T hotspot *TERT* promoter mutation (Hoffmann et al. 2016), two common alterations found in BLCA.

17.2.3 BLCA Cell Lines from Other Species

Tumors from mice, rats, and dogs have been used to generate BLCA lines. A major advantage of rodent lines is that they can be readily implanted in immunocompetent hosts and, therefore, allow questions related to antitumor responses to be addressed (Zhu et al. 2021).

Mouse BLCA lines have been established from tumors induced by chemical carcinogens (Arantes-Rodrigues et al. 2013) or genetically engineered mouse models (GEMM). The most common chemicals used are N-Butyl-N-(−4-hydroxybutyl) nitrosamine (BBN), administered in drinking water for 10–20 weeks; N-Methyl-N-nitrosourea (MNU), administered intravesically for approximately 8 weeks; and N-[4-(5-nitro-2-furyl)-2-thiazolyl] formamide (FANFT), administered in food over longer periods of time (~8 months) (see also Chap. 16). The induced tumors generally resemble human BLCA at the microscopic level, with a wide range of histological variation and considerable inter-species differences (Williams et al. 2008). For example, BBN induces predominantly papillary urothelial tumors in rats whereas it induces basal/squamous muscle-invasive tumors in mice (Vasconcelos-Nobrega et al. 2012). From a genetic standpoint, the tumors resemble, in part, human BLCA (Fantini et al. 2018). Among the available murine BLCA cell lines, MB49 and MBT-2 are the most used (Mickey et al. 1982; Summerhayes and Franks 1979). The rat AY-27 cell line generates high-grade non-muscle-invasive tumors in vivo which rapidly progress to MIBC (Hendricksen et al. 2008).

A relatively small number of BLCA lines have been generated from GEMMs through activation or inactivation of gene function in the bladder (*Pten, Trp53, FGFR3, H-ras*). A novel cell line has been derived from a GEMM where *Pten* and *Trp53* were inactivated in intermediate/umbrella cells (Saito et al. 2018). The resulting line displays a luminal-like phenotype, based on the activity of PPARG and GATA3 transcriptomic signatures.

BLCA cell lines from dog tumors are also frequently used, as BLCA occurs naturally in this species. At the time of diagnosis, most of the tumors are muscle-invasive and some have metastasized. Dog BLCA also display similarities with human BLCA based on both histology and genomic analyses (Knapp et al. 2014; Wong et al. 2023). Several canine urothelial cell lines have been reported and characterized at the genomic level (Shapiro et al. 2015).

An extensive review of non-human BLCA lines has been compiled by Zuiverloon et al. (2018), with information on source and characteristics (e.g., stage/grade, mutations).

17.3 3D Cell Cultures

The concept of culturing cells in 3D was first introduced in the 1970s by radiobiologists who used spheroids to better mimic aspects related to radiation penetration in tissues (Sutherland et al. 1970). However, 3D culture has undergone a dramatic expansion in the last decade, mainly because of the development of "organoids." 3D models recapitulate better the in vivo setting as they mimic the overall tumor architecture and some aspects of the tumor microenvironment (TME), allowing cell–cell and tumor–matrix interactions to be taken into consideration (Kim et al. 2022; Schutgens and Clevers 2020; Yan et al. 2023). Consequently, 3D models are more informative on tumor biology and prediction of response to therapy (Lee et al. 2018; Minoli et al. 2023; Pauli et al. 2017).

When using 3D models, three major elements need to be considered: the matrix, the cells, and the culture medium.

17.3.1 Matrix

Most protocols used to culture cells in 3D involve the use of a matrix, but there are exceptions, particularly in the case of protocols designed for spheroid formation, which are mostly matrix-free. In the latter case, cells are "forced" to grow in 3D by preventing their attachment to the plastic substratum through culture in the absence of fetal bovine serum, using low-adhesion plates, employing the hanging-drop method, or applying specialized devices (e.g., by introducing constant rotation hampering adhesion). All these strategies result in increased cell–cell adhesion (Vakhshiteh et al. 2023).

The matrix-based protocols involve the use of natural components (e.g., Matrigel™, gelatin, type I collagen, laminin), natural matrix mimics (e.g., peptides, alginate), or synthetic hydrogels [e.g., polycaprolactone, polylactic acid (PLA), polyglycolic acid (PGA), and copolymers of PLA-PGA (PLGA)]. Matrigel™ is a complex, non-chemically defined, extracellular matrix derived from Engelbreth-Holm-Swarm (EHS) mouse tumor cells grown in vivo (Kleinman et al. 1982). It contains more than 1800 different components, the main ones being laminin and type IV collagen, two prototypical basement membrane proteins (Kozlowski et al. 2021). The viscoelastic properties of Matrigel depend on the protein concentration, which varies from batch-to-batch, being more elastic at higher concentrations (Borries et al. 2020). In addition, Matrigel biophysical properties change during the culture period, due in part to protease secretion by tumor cells and the associated degradation of the ECM. Matrix stiffness can impact cell proliferation, survival, and migration (Wang et al. 2010).

The Clevers lab used Matrigel at high concentrations and several growth factors to culture intestinal organoids from Lgr5+ stem cells (Sato et al. 2009). Since then, many groups have modified and applied this culture system to grow cells from other tissues (Dekkers et al. 2013; Kim et al. 2020a), including BLCA. Matrigel or similar natural matrices are used in more than 50% of the reports on BLCA 3D cultures (Medle et al. 2022).

Synthetic matrices have a defined chemical structure and are inert, permitting a more refined analysis of experimental variation. The lack of exposure of cells grown on synthetic matrices to animal products facilitates clinical applications. These hydrogels closely mimic the structure and porosity of the natural extracellular matrix (ECM). They generate scaffolds that can be coated with natural molecules (e.g., laminin) and allow growth factor diffusion. Prefabricated scaffolds made of porous natural polymers (e.g., chitosan or collagen) or synthetic polymers (e.g., polycaprolactone) can also provide physical support for spheroids/organoids and compensate for the absence of ECM (Sailer et al. 2023). As they are chemically defined, synthetic polymers can be modified to achieve the desired physical properties (Chaudhuri et al. 2020; Hofer and Lutolf 2021). Presently, Matrigel is superior to the available synthetic matrices and there is a need for their improvement (LeSavage et al. 2022). So far, there is only one report of BLCA cells cultured in 3D using hydrogels (Okuyama et al. 2013).

17.3.2 Cells

A wide variety of cells have been used to study BLCA and normal urothelium in 3D. These include normal urothelial cells, spontaneously immortalized urothelium, oncogene-immortalized cells (e.g., UROtsa, obtained through the overexpression of SV40 large T antigen), BLCA cell lines, primary patient samples, exfoliated urothelial cells, and induced pluripotent stem cells, among others (Cross et al. 2005; Lang et al. 2013; Medle et al. 2022; Rossi et al. 2001; Suzuki et al. 2019).

17.3.2.1 Spheroids

Tumor spheroids can be generated using various approaches which may, or may not, include the use of a matrix (Neuhaus et al. 2023). Spheroids are relatively simple and fast to establish and can offer valuable insights into tumor growth, survival, and differentiation. BLCA cell lines cultured as spheroids have been widely used in studies related to tumor growth and response to therapy (Hortelao et al. 2019; Yoshida et al. 2019). In contrast to cultures in 2D, cells in spheroids face limitations in nutrient and oxygen availability that are reminiscent of conditions found in solid tumors (Leek et al. 2016). As in 2D cultures, BLCA cells grown as spheroids retain their main genetic features but they undergo phenotypic changes (Yoshida et al. 2019). Spheroid size is often difficult to control; this limitation is partially overcome using hanging drops, generated from low cell numbers, to produce BLCA spheroids (Amaral et al. 2017; Miranda et al. 2019). However, this approach does not allow medium replacement.

Spheroids derived from NHU cells and from T24 and J82 BLCA cells have been used to study urothelial biology (e.g., stem cell properties) and the response to anticancer drugs (Namekawa et al. 2020). Spheroid cultures display cancer stem cell properties (Ishiguro et al. 2017): inhibition of the stem cell marker ALDH1A1 in T24 cells grown as spheroids impaired their expansion (Namekawa et al. 2020). Using spheroids derived from UM-UC-3 and 5637 cells, KDM2A inhibition had antiproliferative effects (Lu et al. 2022). Cultures of the same lines have been used to test the combination of BCG immunotherapy with vesicular stomatitis virus-based virotherapy (Rangsitratkul et al. 2022).

17.3.2.2 Organoids

Unlike spheroids, organoids display features that better mimic the organization and function of a given organ or tissue. Three fundamental characteristics of organoids are self-renewal, self-organization capacity, and differentiation potential. These properties emerge from the maintenance of stem cells/progenitors and the establishment of crucial cell–cell and cell–matrix interactions. Consequently, they have proven useful to study morphogenesis, differentiation, and cellular heterogeneity, to establish the foundations for regenerative medicine and gene therapy, and to perform drug and genetic screenings (Lancaster and Knoblich 2014; Lee et al. 2018; Pauli et al. 2017; Shamir and Ewald 2014; Yan et al. 2023).

Compared with other tumor types, relatively few studies have reported the establishment and characterization of BLCA organoids (Medle et al. 2022). Table 17.4 summarizes the main BLCA organoid reports to date. Unlike in the case of intestinal organoids, where a rational design was applied to include growth factors in the medium according to the biological pathways of relevance in homeostasis/regeneration in the corresponding tissue (e.g., Wnt ligands and R-Spondin to activate the WNT pathway) (Sato et al. 2009), a systematic effort to test the growth factors that are required for urothelial homeostasis has not been applied to optimize BLCA organoid establishment.

The lab of M. Shen reported in 2018 a biobank of 22 established BLCA organoids adopting methods previously used to generate prostate cancer organoids (Lee et al. 2018). This work used hepatocyte medium (the composition of which is not known) and charcoal-stripped serum; rho-associated protein kinase (ROCK) inhibitor was used to enhance cell viability upon organoid dissociation. Most of the organoids were derived from tumor samples obtained through transurethral resections (TUR) from patients with non-muscle-invasive bladder cancer (NMIBC) or MIBC and 2 of them were established from patient-derived xenografts. In some cases, organoids grew only for a short period of time but these authors report that, with improved methods, the efficiency to generate established organoid cultures (defined as >6 serial passages) was 70% (12/17). Sixteen of 20 organoids originated from NMIBC and for 3 patients, multiple independent organoid lines were produced. Targeted gene sequencing of 468 genes showed >80% mutational concordance between the organoids and the original tumor for 11 of them, with only 4 showing <60% concordance. Consequently, the biobank includes organoids harboring the more common mutations and gene copy number changes associated with

Table 17.4 BLCA organoids: main reports with associated information

Reference	N° of samples	Paired normal samples	% of success	Passage reached	Success establishment criteria	Base medium	Growth factors	Matrix	Drug sens. Assays	Xenografting	Relevant info
Pauli et al. 2017	8*	No	33	p5-10-15	At least 5 passages	AdvDMEM	A83–01, B27, EGF, FGF2/10, Glutamax, N-acetylcysteine, nicotinamide, noggin, PGE2, ROCK inhibitor, R-spondin, SB202190	Yes, 50%	No	1 line	WES of 4 organoid lines and the paired tumors (3 primary and 1 metastasis from the same patient as 1 primary)
Lee et al. 2018	16	No	70	Up to 26	At least 6 passages	Hepatocyte medium	CS-FBS, EGF, Glutamax, ROCK inhibitor	Yes, 60%	50 compounds (standard-of-care and some tested in clinical trial)	Orthotopic (2 organoid lines established from 2 orthotopic xenografts)	Targeted sequencing of 468 cancer-associated genes, deep sequencing, WES, RNA-seq of organoids and parental tumors
Mullenders et al. 2019	53	Yes (from cystectomy samples)	50	Up to 30	Na	AdvDMEM/F12	A83–01, B27, FGF2/7/10, N-acetylcysteine, nicotinamide	Yes, 100%	Chemotherapy in 3 organoid lines	No	Optimization of culture medium, several lines of organoids from different areas of the same tumor in some cases
Minoli et al. 2023	21	No	Na	Na	Na	AdvDMEM/F12	A83–01, B27, EGF, FBS, FGF10, HGF, N-acetylcysteine, nicotinamide, noggin, ROCK inhibitor, R-spondin, SB202190, Wnt3a	No	21 compounds (standard-of-care, some tested in clinical trial and targeted therapies with tyrosine kinase inhibitors)	No	Successful establishment from fresh and frozen samples, scRNA-seq organoids vs parental tumor, morphological patterns: Solid, hollow, mixed, and correlation with tumor grade/stage, WES

*Bladder and ureter. *AdvDMEM* Advanced Dulbecco's Modified Eagle Medium, *EGF* Epidermal Growth Factor, *FGF* Fibroblast Growth Factor, *PGE2* Prostaglandin E2, *ROCK* Rho Associated Protein Kinase, *WES* Whole Exome Sequencing, *FBS* Fetal Bovine Serum, *CS-FBS* Charcoal-stripped Fetal Bovine Serum, *HGF* Hepatocyte Growth Factor

BLCA. Mutational analysis of multiple organoid samples at different passages showed conservation of the truncal mutations but frequent loss or gain of subclonal mutations. Transcriptomic analysis revealed more variable levels of conservation between the original tumor and the organoids. While several of the cultures retained a luminal phenotype, there was a tendency toward gain of basal marker gene expression in vitro. This phenotypic drift was often reversible upon implantation in immunodeficient mice. An in-depth analysis of the response to 40 drugs, including standard chemotherapy and targeted therapies, using 9 organoid cultures revealed both recurrent and individual responses in the organoids. None of the 3 *FGFR3*-mutant organoids tested showed responses to the FGFR inhibitors studied (which did not include Erdafitinib). Their results also illustrated that the in vitro drug responses largely recapitulated the effects observed in xenografts.

Mullenders et al. cultured tumor and non-neoplastic urothelium from 53 patients undergoing a TUR or a cystectomy (21% and 79%, respectively). They applied a chemically defined medium previously optimized using mouse urothelial cells, containing FGF2, FGF7, FGF10, N-acetylcysteine, Nicotinamide, B27 (optimized serum-free promoter of growth and viability), and A83–01 (inhibitor of activin receptor-like kinase); ROCK inhibitor was also used for cell dissociation. An efficiency of approximately 50% organoid establishment was reported, with some of the lines being in culture for up to 30 passages. As in the study of Lee et al. (Lee et al. 2018), they generated both solid and cystic-type organoids containing cells displaying luminal as well as basal phenotypes. In a more limited drug screen, a range of responses to chemotherapeutic drugs as well as nutlin (inhibitor of the interaction of MDM2 with p53) were reported (Mullenders et al. 2019).

More recently, Minoli et al. have reported 22 organoid lines from TUR and cystectomy samples (59% NMIBC and 41% MIBC), in a matrix-free culture system using ultra-low attachment-plates and following an approach previously used to establish prostate cancer organoids. As in the studies of Lee et al. and Mullenders et al., a similar success rate was noted for NMIBC and MIBC. Histological and molecular analyses also showed a general preservation of the features corresponding to the tumors from which they were derived. Along the same lines, genetic alterations characteristic of BLCA were present in several organoids, allowing the testing of targeted therapies. There was marked heterogeneity in the response to drugs used for BLCA therapy, but they showed higher responses to Erdafitinib in lines harboring *FGFR3* amplification. In a few individual cases, the response of the organoids was compared to that of the patient, suggesting that organoid drug testing can guide therapeutic decisions (Minoli et al. 2023).

The effects of chemotherapy and two novel compounds that interfere with the mitochondrial apoptosis pathway on upper tract urothelial carcinoma and BLCA organoids cultured in 3D and in 2D have been reported recently (Wei et al. 2022).

In summary, despite the fact that there are still few reports on BLCA organoids, the evidence indicates that: (1) the efficiency of establishment of permanent organoid cultures is higher than that of 2D cell lines but lower than for other tumor types, (2) it is possible to establish organoids from low-grade tumors, (3) there is a general conservation of genomic and phenotypic features of the original tumor, (4) organoids recapitulate BLCA heterogeneity better than cell lines, and (5) the wide variation in response to therapy reflects the heterogeneity found in patients.

Despite these advances, several challenges remain: (1) the optimal culture conditions need to be defined, (2) the use of chemically defined matrices and culture medium is needed to facilitate understanding of the biology underlying their establishment, (3) optimized co-cultures with mesenchymal and immune cells should better recapitulate the original TME, and (4) understanding the biology of normal urothelial stem cells may help to design better culture strategies, including the growth selection biases derived from the rich medium in which organoids are cultured. The establishment of methods that consistently support the growth of urothelial stem cells could have a major impact on regenerative medicine applications for diseases of the bladder.

17.3.3 3D Cultures from Other Species

The difficulties in accessing human samples, especially normal human urothelium, have fostered the establishment of urothelial organoids from other species. In addition, the availability of GEMM strains carrying mutations associated with human BLCA facilitates the study of the biology of the corresponding genes.

Our group conducted a comprehensive analysis of the growth factor requirements of normal mouse urothelium grown as organoids and used single cell RNA-Seq to identify urothelial cell states. EGF, Wnt3a, and R-spondin were indispensable for organoid establishment, while Noggin was necessary for their long-term maintenance, beyond 1 year. In the presence of these factors, a population of proliferative cells with basal features was identified. Using growth factor depletion, EGFR inhibition, and PPARG activation we demonstrated the capacity of the organoids to recapitulate normal urothelial differentiation. This included morphological changes, acquisition of barrier function, reduced proliferation, and changes in gene expression. Differentiated organoids exhibited the capacity to revert to a proliferative state when growth factors were reintroduced into the culture medium. Several novel candidate regulators of urothelial proliferation and differentiation were identified, including FOXQ1 and HOPX (Santos et al. 2019). These organoids provide excellent tools to apply knowledge generated through the study of urothelial damage/regeneration in vivo (Shin et al. 2011). Mullenders et al. established organoids from both basal and suprabasal mouse urothelial cells following protocols adopted from other tissues (Mullenders et al. 2019). They reported that EGF was not capable of sustaining long-term culture of organoids, FGF7/FGF10, A83–01 and B27 supplements being required. They also showed the genetic karyotype stability of the organoids up to 60 passages and they used CRISPR-Cas9 editing to introduce mutations in *Stag2* and *Trp53*, two important genes in BLCA. While a distinctive phenotype was not reported, they effectively established genome editing conditions for mouse organoids.

Organoids from GEMMs have also been established to assess the role of important BLCA-related genes, including *Trp53*, *Kdm6a*, *Cdcp1*, and *Stag2* (Halstead et al. 2017; Lapi et al. 2023; Saponaro et al. 2023). Organoids from primary and orthotopic GEMMs of MIBC have been used to study chemoresistance (Wang et al. 2022).

In addition to mice, dogs have been used to establish urothelial organoids. Elbadawy et al. generated canine normal and tumor organoids, the latter derived from urine samples from dogs diagnosed with BLCA. The authors proposed to use them as preclinical models for biomarker and therapeutic discovery for both canine and human BLCA (Elbadawy et al. 2022; Elbadawy et al. 2021; Elbadawy et al. 2019). We have recently used the methods reported by Santos et al. (Santos et al. 2019) to generate pig normal urothelial organoids with high efficiency (unpublished).

This work lays the foundation for the in vitro study of cross-species differences in urothelial biology and neoplastic transformation.

17.4 Co-Cultures, Organotypic Systems, Tissue Engineering, and Tissue Explants

The need to recapitulate the interaction of tumor cells with the TME has been emphasized in recent years, mainly due to the relevance of stromal and immune cells in chemoresistance and response to immune checkpoint blockade (Caramelo et al. 2023; Patwardhan and Mahendran 2023). A range of experimental setups (2D, 2.5D, and 3D) have been employed and are outlined here (Table 17.5). There is some confusion in the literature regarding the nomenclature (e.g., spheroids, tumoroids, organoids).

Table 17.5 Organotypic models: main features. BLCA: Bladder Cancer, CAR-T: Chimeric Antigen Receptor T, PBMCs: Peripheral Blood Mononuclear Cells, ALI: Air Liquid Interphase, HUVEC: Human Umbilical Vein Endothelial Cells, UC: Urothelial Carcinoma, TILs: Tumor-infiltrated Lymphocytes, NK: Natural Killer, CAFs: Cancer Associated Fibroblasts, HULECs: Human Lung Microvascular Endothelial Cells, BMPs: Bone Morphogenetic Proteins, PDMS: poly-di-methyl-siloxane, BCG: Bacille Calmette-Guerin, GelMA: Gelatin methacryloyl, bFGF: Basic Fibroblast Growth Factor, IL-4: Interleukin-4, TGF-b1: Transforming Growth Factor-beta 1

Reference	In vitro model	Epithelial/tumor cells	Stromal cells	Culture conditions	Matrix	Fabrication technique
Booth et al. 2002	3D co-cultures	RT4, RT112, EJ	De-epithelialized human urinary tract basement membrane	bFGF, IL-4, TGF-b1		
Camargo et al. 2021	3D co-cultures	Primary normal and human bladder carcinoma cells	De-epithelialized human urinary tract basement membrane	Primary BLCA-secreted factors		
Palmer et al. 2016	3D co-cultures	5637	Porcine bladder scaffold			
Gelbrich et al. 2023	3D co-cultures	RT4, RT112, SCaBER, T24	Hen's egg test of the chorioallantoic membrane (HET-CAM) in chicken embryos	Gas plasma	Matrigel	
Burgués et al. 2007	Tumoroids	Tumor cells from fragmented tumor biopsies	Native stromal cells	Intravesical therapies	None	Medium submerged spheroids
Yu et al. 2021	Organoid co-cultures	Patient-derived organoids from minced + collagenase/ TrypLE digested tumor tissues	CAR-T cells derived from PBMCs of healthy donors	CAR-T cells	Matrigel	Medium submerged organoids
Mou et al. 2023	Organoid co-cultures	Patient-derived organoids from minced + collagenase/ trypsin digested tumor tissues	Autologous T cells isolated from PBMCs collected before and after cryoablation	Cryoablation-induced microenvironment	Matrigel	Medium submerged organoids
Ringuette Goulet et al. 2017	ALI cell sheets	Urothelial cells isolated from trypsin digested human bladder biopsies. Cell lines: RT4 and T24 spheroids	HUVEC and fibroblasts isolated from human bladder biopsies	Mitomycin C	Collagen: Rat tail type I	Superimposed cell types + ALI cultures to induce UC differentiation

Neal et al. 2018	ALI organoids	Patient-derived organoids from minced tumor tissues	Tumor native TILs, macrophages, dendritic, NK	Anti-PD-1 blocking antibody	Collagen: Cell matrix type I-A / rat tail type I	ALI cultures
Shin et al. 2011	Assembloids	Patient-derived organoids	Human- derived CAFs and HULECs	BMPs	Matrigel	Cultures in spinning bioreactor and 3D bioprinting
van de Merbel et al. 2018	Tumor slices	Tumor slices	Tumor slices	Chemotherapy drugs		Tissue slices on nitrocellulose filter inserts
van der Host et al. 2020	Tumor slices	Tumor slices	Tumor slices	Penfluridol		Tissue slices on nitrocellulose filter inserts
Relph et al. 2020	Precision-cut slices	Tumor slices	Tumor slices	Oncolytic immunotherapy and mitomycin C		Vibratome-sliced tumor tissue
Donelan et al. 2023	Precision-cut slices	Tumor slices	Tumor slices			Compresstome sliced tumor tissue
Liu et al. 2015	Microfluidics	T24	Macrophages (raw 264.7), fibroblasts (BJ-5Ta) and HUVECs	Chemotherapy drugs	Matrigel	Photolithography, PDMS
Choi et al. 2023	Microfluidics	T24, 253 J	THP-1 monocytes	Recombinant BCG	GelMA prepolymer solution	Milling and soft lithography, PDMS

17.4.1 2D co-Cultures

In 2D, co-cultures of primary normal fibroblasts or cancer-associated fibroblasts (CAF) and BLCA cell lines (mainly T24 cells) in transwells have been used to evaluate the ability of CAFs to promote BLCA cell proliferation, invasive properties, epithelial-mesenchymal transition (EMT), and chemotherapy resistance (Chen et al. 2022; Long et al. 2019; Ping et al. 2023; Rastegar-Pouyani et al. 2023). These studies have also underscored the importance of secreted signaling molecules, such as IGF-1 and TGF-β1, in the communication between tumor and stromal cells. In this context, the ability of CAF-derived extracellular vesicles, in co-culture with T24 and CD8+ T cells, to enhance tumor invasiveness and increase T cell immunosuppression was highlighted (Feng et al. 2023). In addition to CAFs, other cell types have been employed, including human adipose-derived stem cells, primary monocytes, and the monocyte THP-1 cell line (Huang et al. 2020; Maj et al. 2022; Miyake et al. 2016; Zhang and Chen 2018). Primary patient-derived BLCA cells have been co-cultured in 2D with autologous tumor-infiltrating CD4+ T cells to evaluate their cytotoxic potential (Oh et al. 2020).

17.4.2 3D co-Cultures

In the early 2000s, the Southgate laboratory reported 3D cultures whereby cells from BLCA lines were seeded onto de-epithelialized human urinary tract basement membrane (Booth et al. 2002; Booth et al. 1997), allowing the testing of paracrine signaling to BLCA cells (Camargo et al. 2021). Subsequently, the human scaffold was replaced by a porcine source (Palmer et al. 2016). The chicken chorioallantoic membrane has also been used as a vascularized scaffold for in vitro tumor growth (Gelbrich et al. 2023).

More recently, organoids have been co-cultured with CAFs in a variety of tumor types but little work has been done in BLCA. Organoid co-cultures with immune cells are useful to evaluate both innate and adaptive immune responses, as tumor cells partially recapitulate the antigen expression profiles of the original tumors. Co-cultures with chimeric antigen receptor (CAR)-T cells derived from peripheral blood mononuclear cells (PBMCs) of healthy donors have been used to determine the cytotoxic activity of the latter (Yu et al. 2021). Recently, co-cultures with autologous PBMCs isolated before and after treatment were used to assess cryoablation-induced antitumor immunity (Mou et al. 2023).

17.4.3 Cell Sheets

Cell sheets are produced by sequentially plating epithelial and stromal cells. Most of these layer-reconstituted models use immortalized cells or cell lines and do not rely on autologous tumor cells. Following this approach, vesical equivalents have been generated with dermal fibroblasts, primary bladder smooth muscle cells, and human umbilical vein endothelial cells (HUVEC)-based stroma. The superficial epithelial layers can be exposed to air to induce urothelial differentiation (Bouhout et al. 2010; Orabi et al. 2017; Ringuette Goulet et al. 2017). Bladder equivalents have been used to model BLCA invasion or urinary tract infections (Jafari and Rohn 2023).

17.4.4 Air–Liquid Interface (ALI) Cultures

Cells/organoids are embedded in a collagen gel in a chamber separated from the culture medium (liquid phase) by a permeable membrane (air phase). In these systems, medium components and oxygen diffuse through the membrane and the collagen gel. These cultures can be used to reproduce the immune contexture and are useful for short-term studies, for example to recapitulate the tumor T-cell TCR repertoire. However, tumor-infiltrating lymphocytes progressively decrease from day 7 of culture (Neal et al. 2018).

17.4.5 Microfluidic-Based Cultures

Microfluidic-based cultures (i.e., organ chips) can use cells from BLCA lines, from organoids, or from tumor digests, placed in a 3D matrix in the central zone of a device where the medium flows through microchannels adjacent to the matrix. Among the common microfluidic chip fabrication methods are soft lithography, laser ablation, micro-milling, injection molding, and 3D printing (Hou et al. 2023). Microfluidic devices constitute flexible systems that allow real-time monitoring of physical and chemical changes in the tme. As with ALI cultures, microfluidic systems allow the interaction of inflammatory cells with tumor cells and can also introduce endothelial cells. One of the first reported microfluidic systems simulating the BLCA TME used T24 tumor cells, macrophages (Raw 264.7), fibroblasts (BJ-5Ta), and human umbilical vein endothelial cells (HUVECs) (Liu et al. 2015) to assess the effect of six different chemotherapy combinations on tumor cell viability. A high-throughput 3D bio-printed BLCA-on-a-chip incorporating tumor cells and THP-1 monocytes was recently used to evaluate the efficacy of a recombinant Bacillus Calmette-Guérin (Choi et al. 2023).

17.4.6 Assembloids

Kim et al. applied a highly sophisticated approach to establish organotypic cultures/assembloids with either normal or malignant urothelial cells (Kim et al. 2020b). Using a spinning bioreactor and 3D bioprinting to produce BLCA assembloids from organoids, matched patient-derived CAFs, and human endothelial cells, they showed that the luminal-basal phenotypic switch that often occurs in vitro can be inhibited. The assembloids recapitulate the invasive properties of the original tumor, highlighting the role of stromal BMP signaling on FOXA1-driven luminal tumor cell differentiation.

17.4.7 Tissue Explants

A major concern when using dissociated cells/tissues are the effects of digestion on cell physiology, potential loss of heterogeneity, and the loss of cell–cell interactions. These limitations are partially bypassed when using organotypic tumor explants and tissue slices cultured in vitro. Biopsy material or surgically resected tissues are carefully collected, kept in cold medium, and processed. Tissue explants cut into small pieces have long been used as preclinical drug screening tools and they have attracted a great deal of interest in recent years. Undissociated "tumoroid-like" fragments from cold-cup biopsies of non-muscle-invasive BLCA maintaining the native stroma have been reported, consisting of a superficial layer of urothelial cells covering the inner stromal cell layer (Burgues et al. 2007).

17.4.8 Tissue Slices

Thick sections of 30–500 microns, precision-cut slices, can be obtained using a vibratome or similar devices and maintained in culture (He and Deng 2022). An advantage of tissue explants and slices, in comparison with other 3D culture systems, lies in their ability to maintain the original 3D architecture with minimal tissue manipulation, thereby preserving essential tumor cell–cell and cell–matrix interactions. Furthermore, they offer a cost-effective approach. Nevertheless, they do come with drawbacks. The main limitations are the restricted tissue availability, short lifespan, and insufficient cell viability (Templeton et al. 2021). Van de Merbel et al. developed a protocol for the ex vivo culture of bladder and prostate cancer cell line xenografts and tumor slices. Tissue integrity was achieved for up to 10 days and these cultures were exploited to assess the antitumor response to chemotherapy, to the antipsychotic drug penfluridol, or to oncolytic immunotherapy (Relph et al. 2020; van de Merbel et al. 2018; van der Horst et al. 2020). A protocol to prepare bladder tissue slice cultures has recently been published (Donelan et al. 2023).

17.5 Concluding Remarks

In summary, the last decade has brought exciting progress in the development of novel in vitro approaches to study BLCA. This will likely continue in the next decade because of increasing knowledge of the cell biology and genomics of BLCA. However, our community is still relatively small and there are areas where research lags behind. The public health relevance of BLCA, the importance of sex-related differences in outcome, the need to better understand resistance to therapy, and to identify biomarkers of disease development and drug response call for an increase in BLCA research. The improved in vitro strategies to study this tumor provide unprecedented opportunities.

Acknowledgments Work in the authors' laboratory is supported, in part, by the Fundación Científica de la Asociación Española Contra el Cáncer (grant PRYGN223005REAL) and US National Institutes of Health (grant R21 CA266660-01A1). C. B. is supported by a grant from the EU (MSCA-ITN-TranSyS). CNIO is supported by Ministerio de Ciencia, Innovación y Universidades as a Centro de Excelencia Severo Ochoa SEV-2015-0510.

References

Agarwal N, Rinaldetti S, Cheikh BB, Zhou Q, Hass EP, Jones RT, Joshi M, LaBarbera DV, Knott SRV, Cech TR, Theodorescu D (2021) TRIM28 is a transcriptional activator of the mutant TERT promoter in human bladder cancer. Proc Natl Acad Sci USA 118(38):e2102423118. https://doi.org/10.1073/pnas.2102423118

Agarwal N, Zhou Q, Arya D, Rinaldetti S, Duex J, LaBarbera DV, Theodorescu D (2022) AST-487 inhibits RET kinase driven TERT expression in bladder cancer. Int J Mol Sci 23(18):10819. https://doi.org/10.3390/ijms231810819

Amaral RLF, Miranda M, Marcato PD, Swiech K (2017) Comparative analysis of 3D bladder tumor spheroids obtained by forced floating and hanging drop methods for drug screening. Front Physiol 8:605. https://doi.org/10.3389/fphys.2017.00605

Arantes-Rodrigues R, Colaco A, Pinto-Leite R, Oliveira PA (2013) In vitro and in vivo experimental models as tools to investigate the efficacy of antineoplastic drugs on urinary bladder cancer. Anticancer Res 33(4):1273–1296. https://www.ncbi.nlm.nih.gov/pubmed/23564765

Baker SC, Shabir S, Southgate J (2014) Biomimetic urothelial tissue models for the in vitro evaluation of barrier physiology and bladder drug efficacy. Mol Pharm 11(7):1964–1970. https://doi.org/10.1021/mp500065m

Baker SC, Mason AS, Southgate J (2020) Procarcinogen activation and mutational signatures model the initiation of carcinogenesis in human urothelial tissues in vitro. Eur Urol 78(2):143–147. https://doi.org/10.1016/j.eururo.2020.03.049

Baker SC, Mason AS, Slip RG, Eriksson P, Sjodahl G, Trejdosiewicz LK, Southgate J (2022) The urothelial transcriptomic response to interferon gamma: implications for bladder cancer prognosis and immunotherapy. Cancers (Basel) 14(21):5295. https://doi.org/10.3390/cancers14215295

Booth C, Harnden P, Trejdosiewicz LK, Scriven S, Selby PJ, Southgate J (1997) Stromal and vascular invasion in an human in vitro bladder cancer model. Lab Investig 76(6):843–857. https://www.ncbi.nlm.nih.gov/pubmed/9194860

Booth C, Harnden P, Selby PJ, Southgate J (2002) Towards defining roles and relationships for tenascin-C and TGFbeta-1 in the normal and neoplastic urinary bladder. J Pathol 198(3):359–368. https://doi.org/10.1002/path.1214

Borries M, Barooji YF, Yennek S, Grapin-Botton A, Berg-Sørensen K, Oddershede LB (2020) Quantification of Visco-elastic properties of a Matrigel for organoid development as a function of polymer concentration. Front Phys 8:579168. https://doi.org/10.3389/fphy.2020.579168

Bouhout S, Perron E, Gauvin R, Bernard G, Ouellet G, Cattan V, Bolduc S (2010) In vitro reconstruction of an autologous, watertight, and resistant vesical equivalent. Tissue Eng Part A 16(5):1539–1548. https://doi.org/10.1089/ten.TEA.2009.0473

Burgues JP, Gomez L, Pontones JL, Vera CD, Jimenez-Cruz JF, Ozonas M (2007) A chemosensitivity test for superficial bladder cancer based on three-dimensional culture of tumour spheroids. Eur Urol 51(4):962–969discussion 969–970. https://doi.org/10.1016/j.eururo.2006.10.034

Camargo S, Gofrit ON, Assis A, Mitrani E (2021) Paracrine signaling from a three-dimensional model of bladder carcinoma and from normal bladder switch the phenotype of stromal fibroblasts. Cancers (Basel) 13(12):2972. https://doi.org/10.3390/cancers13122972

Caramelo B, Zagorac S, Corral S, Marques M, Real FX (2023) Cancer-associated fibroblasts in bladder cancer: origin, biology, and therapeutic opportunities. Eur Urol Oncol 6(4):366–375. https://doi.org/10.1016/j.euo.2023.02.011

Chapman EJ, Hurst CD, Pitt E, Chambers P, Aveyard JS, Knowles MA (2006) Expression of hTERT immortalises normal human urothelial cells without inactivation of the p16/Rb pathway. Oncogene 25(36):5037–5045. https://doi.org/10.1038/sj.onc.1209513

Chaudhuri O, Cooper-White J, Janmey PA, Mooney DJ, Shenoy VB (2020) Effects of extracellular matrix viscoelasticity on cellular behaviour. Nature 584(7822):535–546. https://doi.org/10.1038/s41586-020-2612-2

Chen H, Yang W, Xue X, Li Y, Jin Z, Ji Z (2022) Integrated analysis revealed an inflammatory cancer-associated fibroblast-based subtypes with promising implications in predicting the prognosis and immunotherapeutic response of bladder cancer patients. Int J Mol Sci 23(24):15970. https://doi.org/10.3390/ijms232415970

Choi J, Jung TY, Kim JH, Maeng S, Kang SJ, Kim M, Choi YW, Choi SY, Kim SH, Chang IH (2023) Efficacy of recombinant bacillus Calmette-Guerin containing dltA in in vivo three-dimensional bio-printed bladder cancer-on-a-chip and ex vivo orthotopic mouse model. Investig Clin Urol 64(3):296–305. https://doi.org/10.4111/icu.20220293

Coutos-Thévenot L, Beji S, Neyret-Kahn H, Pippo Q, Fontugne J, Osz J, Krucker C, Dos C, Groeneveld S, Dufour F, Kamoun A, Ley M, Chapeaublanc E, De Reynies A, Lebret T, Allory Y, Cianférani S, Radvanyi F, Rochel N, Bernard-Pierrot I (2019) PPARγ is a tumor suppressor in basal bladder tumors offering new potential therapeutic opportunities. BioRxiv:868190. https://doi.org/10.1101/868190

Cross WR, Eardley I, Leese HJ, Southgate J (2005) A biomimetic tissue from cultured normal human urothelial cells: analysis of physiological function. Am J Physiol Renal Physiol 289(2):F459–F468. https://doi.org/10.1152/ajprenal.00040.2005

Dancik GM, Theodorescu D (2022) Using cell lines to guide neoadjuvant therapy in bladder cancer: COXEN and SWOG S1314. Eur Urol Focus 8(3):648–650. https://doi.org/10.1016/j.euf.2022.03.013

DeGraff DJ, Clark PE, Cates JM, Yamashita H, Robinson VL, Yu X, Smolkin ME, Chang SS, Cookson MS, Herrick MK, Shariat SF, Steinberg GD, Frierson HF, Wu XR, Theodorescu D, Matusik RJ (2012) Loss of the urothelial differentiation marker FOXA1 is associated with high grade, late stage bladder cancer and increased tumor proliferation. PLoS One 7(5):e36669. https://doi.org/10.1371/journal.pone.0036669

Dekkers JF, Wiegerinck CL, de Jonge HR, Bronsveld I, Janssens HM, de Winter-de Groot KM, Brandsma AM, de Jong NW, Bijvelds MJ, Scholte BJ, Nieuwenhuis EE, van den Brink S, Clevers H, van der Ent CK, Middendorp S, Beekman JM (2013) A functional CFTR assay using primary cystic fibrosis intestinal organoids. Nat Med 19(7):939–945. https://doi.org/10.1038/nm.3201

Donelan W, Crispen PL, Kusmartsev S (2023) Tissue slice culture and analysis of tumor-associated hyaluronan in urothelial carcinoma. Methods Mol Biol 2684:167–175. https://doi.org/10.1007/978-1-0716-3291-8_10

Earl J, Rico D, Carrillo-de-Santa-Pau E, Rodriguez-Santiago B, Mendez-Pertuz M, Auer H, Gomez G, Grossman HB, Pisano DG, Schulz WA, Perez-Jurado LA, Carrato A, Theodorescu D, Chanock S, Valencia A, Real FX (2015) The UBC-40 urothelial bladder cancer cell line index: a genomic resource for functional studies. BMC Genomics 16(1):403. https://doi.org/10.1186/s12864-015-1450-3

Elbadawy M, Usui T, Mori T, Tsunedomi R, Hazama S, Nabeta R, Uchide T, Fukushima R, Yoshida T, Shibutani M, Tanaka T, Masuda S, Okada R, Ichikawa R, Omatsu T, Mizutani T, Katayama Y, Noguchi S, Iwai S et al (2019) Establishment of a novel experimental model for muscle-invasive bladder cancer using a dog bladder cancer organoid culture. Cancer Sci 110(9):2806–2821. https://doi.org/10.1111/cas.14118

Elbadawy M, Sato Y, Mori T, Goto Y, Hayashi K, Yamanaka M, Azakami D, Uchide T, Fukushima R, Yoshida T, Shibutani M, Kobayashi M, Shinohara Y, Abugomaa A, Kaneda M, Yamawaki H, Usui T, Sasaki K (2021) Anti-tumor effect of trametinib in bladder cancer organoid and the underlying mechanism. Cancer Biol Ther 22(5–6):357–371. https://doi.org/10.1080/15384047.2021.1919004

Elbadawy M, Fujisaka K, Yamamoto H, Tsunedomi R, Nagano H, Ayame H, Ishihara Y, Mori T, Azakami D, Uchide T, Fukushima R, Abugomaa A, Kaneda M, Yamawaki H, Shinohara Y, Omatsu T, Mizutani T, Usui T, Sasaki K (2022) Establishment of an experimental model of normal dog bladder organoid using a three-dimensional culture method. Biomed Pharmacother 151:113105. https://doi.org/10.1016/j.biopha.2022.113105

Fantini D, Glaser AP, Rimar KJ, Wang Y, Schipma M, Varghese N, Rademaker A, Behdad A, Yellapa A, Yu Y, Sze CC, Wang L, Zhao Z, Crawford SE, Hu D, Licht JD, Collings CK, Bartom E, Theodorescu D et al (2018) A carcinogen-induced mouse model recapitulates the molecular alterations of human muscle invasive bladder cancer. Oncogene 37(14):1911–1925. https://doi.org/10.1038/s41388-017-0099-6

Feng R, Li Z, Ge G, Wang C, Jia Y, Ouyang J (2023) Cancer-associated fibroblast-derived extracellular vesicles mediate immune escape of bladder cancer via PD-L1/PD-1 expression. Endocr Metab Immune Disord Drug Targets 23(11):1410–1420. https://doi.org/10.2174/1871530323666230228124125

Flaig TW, Tangen CM, Daneshmand S, Alva A, Lerner SP, Lucia MS, McConkey DJ, Theodorescu D, Goldkorn A, Milowsky MI, Bangs R, MacVicar GR, Bastos BR, Fowles JS, Gustafson DL, Plets M, Thompson IM Jr (2021) A randomized phase II study of Coexpression extrapolation (COXEN) with neoadjuvant chemotherapy for bladder cancer (SWOG S1314; NCT02177695). Clin Cancer Res 27(9):2435–2441. https://doi.org/10.1158/1078-0432.CCR-20-2409

Gelbrich N, Miebach L, Berner J, Freund E, Saadati F, Schmidt A, Stope M, Zimmermann U, Burchardt M, Bekeschus S (2023) Medical gas plasma augments bladder cancer cell toxicity in preclinical models and patient-derived tumor tissues. J Adv Res 47:209–223. https://doi.org/10.1016/j.jare.2022.07.012

Georgopoulos NT, Kirkwood LA, Varley CL, MacLaine NJ, Aziz N, Southgate J (2011) Immortalisation of normal human urothelial cells compromises differentiation capacity. Eur Urol 60(1):141–149. https://doi.org/10.1016/j.eururo.2011.02.022

Gondkar K, Patel K, Krishnappa S, Patil A, Nair B, Sundaram GM, Zea TT, Kumar P (2019) E74 like ETS transcription factor 3 (ELF3) is a negative regulator of epithelial- mesenchymal transition in bladder carcinoma. Cancer Biomark 25(2):223–232. https://doi.org/10.3233/CBM-190013

Halstead AM, Kapadia CD, Bolzenius J, Chu CE, Schriefer A, Wartman LD, Bowman GR, Arora VK (2017) Bladder-cancer-associated mutations in RXRA activate peroxisome proliferator-activated receptors to drive urothelial proliferation. elife 6:e30862. https://doi.org/10.7554/eLife.30862

He L, Deng C (2022) Recent advances in organotypic tissue slice cultures for anticancer drug development. Int J Biol Sci 18(15):5885–5896. https://doi.org/10.7150/ijbs.78997

Hendricksen K, Molkenboer-Kuenen J, Oosterwijk E, Hulsbergen-van de Kaa CA, Witjes JA (2008) Evaluation of an orthotopic rat bladder urothelial cell carcinoma model by cystoscopy. BJU Int 101(7):889–893. https://doi.org/10.1111/j.1464-410X.2007.07407.x

Herz F, Gazivoda P, Papenhausen PR, Katsuyama J, Koss LG (1985) Normal human urothelial cells in culture. Subculture procedure, flow cytometric and chromosomal analyses. Lab Investig 53(5):571–574. https://www.ncbi.nlm.nih.gov/pubmed/4057954

Hofer M, Lutolf MP (2021) Engineering organoids. Nat Rev Mater 6(5):402–420. https://doi.org/10.1038/s41578-021-00279-y

Hoffmann MJ, Koutsogiannouli E, Skowron MA, Pinkerneil M, Niegisch G, Brandt A, Stepanow S, Rieder H, Schulz WA (2016) The new immortalized uroepithelial cell line HBLAK contains defined genetic aberrations typical of early stage urothelial tumors. Bladder Cancer 2(4):449–463. https://doi.org/10.3233/BLC-160065

Hortelao AC, Carrascosa R, Murillo-Cremaes N, Patino T, Sanchez S (2019) Targeting 3D bladder cancer spheroids with urease-powered nanomotors. ACS Nano 13(1):429–439. https://doi.org/10.1021/acsnano.8b06610

Hou C, Gu Y, Yuan W, Zhang W, Xiu X, Lin J, Gao Y, Liu P, Chen X, Song L (2023) Application of microfluidic chips in the simulation of the urinary system microenvironment. Mater Today Bio 19:100553. https://doi.org/10.1016/j.mtbio.2023.100553

Huang CP, Liu LX, Shyr CR (2020) Tumor-associated macrophages facilitate bladder cancer progression by increasing cell growth, migration, invasion and cytokine expression. Anticancer Res 40(5):2715–2724. https://doi.org/10.21873/anticanres.14243

Ishiguro T, Ohata H, Sato A, Yamawaki K, Enomoto T, Okamoto K (2017) Tumor-derived spheroids: relevance to cancer stem cells and clinical applications. Cancer Sci 108(3):283–289. https://doi.org/10.1111/cas.13155

Iyyanki T, Zhang B, Wang Q, Hou Y, Jin Q, Xu J, Yang H, Liu T, Wang X, Song F, Luan Y, Yamashita H, Chien R, Lyu H, Zhang L, Wang L, Warrick J, Raman JD, Meeks JJ et al (2021) Subtype-associated epigenomic landscape and 3D genome structure in bladder cancer. Genome Biol 22(1):105. https://doi.org/10.1186/s13059-021-02325-y

Jafari NV, Rohn JL (2023) An immunoresponsive three-dimensional urine-tolerant human urothelial model to study urinary tract infection. Front Cell Infect Microbiol 13:1128132. https://doi.org/10.3389/fcimb.2023.1128132

Jin X, Demere Z, Nair K, Ali A, Ferraro GB, Natoli T, Deik A, Petronio L, Tang AA, Zhu C, Wang L, Rosenberg D, Mangena V, Roth J, Chung K, Jain RK, Clish CB, Vander Heiden MG, Golub TR (2020) A metastasis map of human cancer cell lines. Nature 588(7837):331–336. https://doi.org/10.1038/s41586-020-2969-2

Kamoun A, de Reynies A, Allory Y, Sjodahl G, Robertson AG, Seiler R, Hoadley KA, Groeneveld CS, Al-Ahmadie H, Choi W, Castro MAA, Fontugne J, Eriksson P, Mo Q, Kardos J, Zlotta A, Hartmann A, Dinney CP, Bellmunt J et al (2020) A consensus molecular classification of muscle-invasive bladder cancer. Eur Urol 77(4):420–433. https://doi.org/10.1016/j.eururo.2019.09.006

Kawakami S, Arai G, Hayashi T, Fujii Y, Xia G, Kageyama Y, Kihara K (2002) PPARγ ligands suppress proliferation of human urothelial basal cells in vitro. J Cell Physiol 191(3):310–319. https://doi.org/10.1002/jcp.10099

Kim J, Koo BK, Knoblich JA (2020a) Human organoids: model systems for human biology and medicine. Nat Rev Mol Cell Biol 21(10):571–584. https://doi.org/10.1038/s41580-020-0259-3

Kim E, Choi S, Kang B, Kong J, Kim Y, Yoon WH, Lee HR, Kim S, Kim HM, Lee H, Yang C, Lee YJ, Kang M, Roh TY, Jung S, Kim S, Ku JH, Shin K (2020b) Creation of bladder assembloids mimicking tissue regeneration and cancer. Nature 588(7839):664–669. https://doi.org/10.1038/s41586-020-3034-x

Kim YS, Hsieh AC, Lam HM (2022) Bladder cancer patient-derived organoids and avatars for personalized cancer discovery. Eur Urol Focus 8(3):657–659. https://doi.org/10.1016/j.euf.2022.07.006

Kleinman HK, McGarvey ML, Liotta LA, Robey PG, Tryggvason K, Martin GR (1982) Isolation and characterization of type IV procollagen, laminin, and heparan sulfate proteoglycan from the EHS sarcoma. Biochemistry 21(24):6188–6193. https://doi.org/10.1021/bi00267a025

Knapp DW, Ramos-Vara JA, Moore GE, Dhawan D, Bonney PL, Young KE (2014) Urinary bladder cancer in dogs, a naturally occurring model for cancer biology and drug development. ILAR J 55(1):100–118. https://doi.org/10.1093/ilar/ilu018

Kozlowski MT, Crook CJ, Ku HT (2021) Towards organoid culture without Matrigel. Commun Biol 4(1):1387. https://doi.org/10.1038/s42003-021-02910-8

Lancaster MA, Knoblich JA (2014) Organogenesis in a dish: modeling development and disease using organoid technologies. Science 345(6194):1247125. https://doi.org/10.1126/science.1247125

Lang R, Liu G, Shi Y, Bharadwaj S, Leng X, Zhou X, Liu H, Atala A, Zhang Y (2013) Self-renewal and differentiation capacity of urine-derived stem cells after urine preservation for 24 hours. PLoS One 8(1):e53980. https://doi.org/10.1371/journal.pone.0053980

Lapi E, Ramal M, Martínez de Villareal J, Marques M, Losada A, Real FX (2023) Abstract European Association for Cancer Research: elucidating the tumor suppressor role of STAG2 in bladder cancer. Mol Oncol 17(S1):1–597. https://doi.org/10.1002/1878-0261.13471

Lee JK, Havaleshko DM, Cho H, Weinstein JN, Kaldjian EP, Karpovich J, Grimshaw A, Theodorescu D (2007) A strategy for predicting the chemosensitivity of human cancers and its application to drug discovery. Proc Natl Acad Sci USA 104(32):13086–13091. https://doi.org/10.1073/pnas.0610292104

Lee SH, Hu W, Matulay JT, Silva MV, Owczarek TB, Kim K, Chua CW, Barlow LJ, Kandoth C, Williams AB, Bergren SK, Pietzak EJ, Anderson CB, Benson MC, Coleman JA, Taylor BS, Abate-Shen C, McKiernan JM, Al-Ahmadie H et al (2018) Tumor evolution and drug response in patient-derived organoid models of bladder cancer. Cell 173(2):515–528 e517. https://doi.org/10.1016/j.ccll.2018.03.017

Leek R, Grimes DR, Harris AL, McIntyre A (2016) Methods: using three-dimensional culture (spheroids) as an in vitro model of tumour hypoxia. Adv Exp Med Biol 899:167–196. https://doi.org/10.1007/978-3-319-26666-4_10

LeSavage BL, Suhar RA, Broguiere N, Lutolf MP, Heilshorn SC (2022) Next-generation cancer organoids. Nat Mater 21(2):143–159. https://doi.org/10.1038/s41563-021-01057-5

Liu PF, Cao YW, Zhang SD, Zhao Y, Liu XG, Shi HQ, Hu KY, Zhu GQ, Ma B, Niu HT (2015) A bladder cancer microenvironment simulation system based on a microfluidic co-culture model. Oncotarget 6(35):37695–37705. https://doi.org/10.18632/oncotarget.6070

Long X, Xiong W, Zeng X, Qi L, Cai Y, Mo M, Jiang H, Zhu B, Chen Z, Li Y (2019) Cancer-associated fibroblasts promote cisplatin resistance in bladder cancer cells by increasing IGF-1/ERbeta/Bcl-2 signalling. Cell Death Dis 10(5):375. https://doi.org/10.1038/s41419-019-1581-6

Lu B, Wei J, Zhou H, Chen J, Li Y, Ye L, Zhao W, Wu S (2022) Histone H3K36me2 demethylase KDM2A promotes bladder cancer progression through epigenetically silencing RARRES3. Cell Death Dis 13(6):547. https://doi.org/10.1038/s41419-022-04983-7

Maj M, Kazmierski L, Balik K, Kowalska K, Gackowska L, Bajek A, Drewa T (2022) Bladder cancer cells exert pleiotropic effects on human adipose-derived stem cells. Life (Basel) 12(4):549. https://doi.org/10.3390/life12040549

Medle B, Sjodahl G, Eriksson P, Liedberg F, Hoglund M, Bernardo C (2022) Patient-derived bladder cancer organoid models in tumor biology and drug testing: a systematic review. Cancers (Basel) 14(9):2062. https://doi.org/10.3390/cancers14092062

Merrill NM, Vandecan NM, Day KC, Palmbos PL, Day ML, Udager AM, Merajver SD, Soellner MB (2020) MEK is a promising target in the basal subtype of bladder cancer. Oncotarget 11(44):3921–3932. https://doi.org/10.18632/oncotarget.27767

Mickey DD, Mickey GH, Murphy WM, Niell HB, Soloway MS (1982) In vitro characterization of four N-[4-(5-nitro-2-furyl)-2-thiazolyl] formamide (FANFT) induced mouse bladder tumors. J Urol 127(6):1233–1237. https://doi.org/10.1016/s0022-5347(17)54305-0

Minoli M, Cantore T, Hanhart D, Kiener M, Fedrizzi T, La Manna F, Karkampouna S, Chouvardas P, Genitsch V, Rodriguez-Calero A, Comperat E, Klima I, Gasperini P, Kiss B, Seiler R, Demichelis F, Thalmann GN, Kruithof-de Julio M (2023) Bladder cancer organoids as a functional system to model different disease stages and therapy response. Nat Commun 14(1):2214. https://doi.org/10.1038/s41467-023-37696-2

Miranda MA, Marcato PD, Carvalho IPS, Silva LB, Ribeiro DL, Amaral R, Swiech K, Bastos JK, Paschoal JAR, Dos Reis RB, Bentley M (2019) Assessing the cytotoxic potential of glycoalkaloidic extract in nanoparticles against bladder cancer cells. J Pharm Pharmacol 71(10):1520–1531. https://doi.org/10.1111/jphp.13145

Miyake M, Hori S, Morizawa Y, Tatsumi Y, Nakai Y, Anai S, Torimoto K, Aoki K, Tanaka N, Shimada K, Konishi N, Toritsuka M, Kishimoto T, Rosser CJ, Fujimoto K (2016) CXCL1-mediated interaction of cancer cells with tumor-associated macrophages and cancer-associated fibroblasts promotes tumor progression in human bladder cancer. Neoplasia 18(10):636–646. https://doi.org/10.1016/j.neo.2016.08.002

Mou Z, Chen Y, Zhang Z, Chen X, Hu Y, Zou L, Xu C, Jiang H (2023) Cryoablation inhibits the recurrence and progression of bladder cancer by enhancing tumour-specific immunity. Clin Transl Med 13(5):e1255. https://doi.org/10.1002/ctm2.1255

Mullenders J, de Jongh E, Brousali A, Roosen M, Blom JPA, Begthel H, Korving J, Jonges T, Kranenburg O, Meijer R, Clevers HC (2019) Mouse and human urothelial cancer organoids: a tool for bladder cancer research. Proc Natl Acad Sci USA 116(10):4567–4574. https://doi.org/10.1073/pnas.1803595116

Namekawa T, Ikeda K, Horie-Inoue K, Suzuki T, Okamoto K, Ichikawa T, Yano A, Kawakami S, Inoue

S (2020) ALDH1A1 in patient-derived bladder cancer spheroids activates retinoic acid signaling leading to TUBB3 overexpression and tumor progression. Int J Cancer 146(4):1099–1113. https://doi.org/10.1002/ijc.32505

Neal JT, Li X, Zhu J, Giangarra V, Grzeskowiak CL, Ju J, Liu IH, Chiou SH, Salahudeen AA, Smith AR, Deutsch BC, Liao L, Zemek AJ, Zhao F, Karlsson K, Schultz LM, Metzner TJ, Nadauld LD, Tseng YY et al (2018) Organoid modeling of the tumor immune microenvironment. Cell 175(7):1972–1988.e1916. https://doi.org/10.1016/j.cell.2018.11.021

Neuhaus J, Rabien A, Reinhold A, Koehler L, Berndt-Paetz M (2023) 3D tumor models in urology. Int J Mol Sci 24(7):6232. https://doi.org/10.3390/ijms24076232

Neyret-Kahn H, Fontugne J, Meng XY, Groeneveld CS, Cabel L, Ye T, Guyon E, Krucker C, Dufour F, Chapeaublanc E, Rapinat A, Jeffery D, Tanguy L, Dixon V, Neuzillet Y, Lebret T, Gentien D, Davidson I, Allory Y et al (2023) Epigenomic mapping identifies an enhancer repertoire that regulates cell identity in bladder cancer through distinct transcription factor networks. Oncogene 42(19):1524–1542. https://doi.org/10.1038/s41388-023-02662-1

Nickerson ML, Witte N, Im KM, Turan S, Owens C, Misner K, Tsang SX, Cai Z, Wu S, Dean M, Costello JC, Theodorescu D (2017) Molecular analysis of urothelial cancer cell lines for modeling tumor biology and drug response. Oncogene 36(1):35–46. https://doi.org/10.1038/onc.2016.172

Oh DY, Kwek SS, Raju SS, Li T, McCarthy E, Chow E, Aran D, Ilano A, Pai CS, Rancan C, Allaire K, Burra A, Sun Y, Spitzer MH, Mangul S, Porten S, Meng MV, Friedlander TW, Ye CJ, Fong L (2020) Intratumoral CD4(+) T cells mediate anti-tumor cytotoxicity in human bladder cancer. Cell 181(7):1612–1625e1613. https://doi.org/10.1016/j.cell.2020.05.017

Okuyama H, Yoshida T, Endo H, Nakayama M, Nonomura N, Nishimura K, Inoue M (2013) Involvement of heregulin/HER3 in the primary culture of human urothelial cancer. J Urol 190(1):302–310. https://doi.org/10.1016/j.juro.2012.12.106

Orabi H, Saba I, Rousseau A, Bolduc S (2017) Novel three-dimensional autologous tissue-engineered vaginal tissues using the self-assembly technique. Transl Res 180:22–36. https://doi.org/10.1016/j.trsl.2016.07.019

Palmer S, Litvinova K, Dunaev A, Fleming S, McGloin D, Nabi G (2016) Changes in autofluorescence based organoid model of muscle invasive urinary bladder cancer. Biomed Opt Express 7(4):1193–1200. https://doi.org/10.1364/BOE.7.001193

Patwardhan MV, Mahendran R (2023) The bladder tumor microenvironment components that modulate the tumor and impact therapy. Int J Mol Sci 24(15):12311. https://doi.org/10.3390/ijms241512311

Pauli C, Hopkins BD, Prandi D, Shaw R, Fedrizzi T, Sboner A, Sailer V, Augello M, Puca L, Rosati R, McNary TJ, Churakova Y, Cheung C, Triscott J, Pisapia D, Rao R, Mosquera JM, Robinson B, Faltas BM et al (2017) Personalized in vitro and in vivo cancer models to guide precision medicine. Cancer Discov 7(5):462–477. https://doi.org/10.1158/2159-8290.CD-16-1154

Ping Q, Wang C, Cheng X, Zhong Y, Yan R, Yang M, Shi Y, Li X, Li X, Huang W, Wang L, Bi X, Hu L, Yang Y, Wang Y, Gong R, Tan J, Li R, Li H et al (2023) TGF-beta1 dominates stromal fibroblast-mediated EMT via the FAP/VCAN axis in bladder cancer cells. J Transl Med 21(1):475. https://doi.org/10.1186/s12967-023-04303-3

Ramal M, Corral S, Kalisz M, Lapi E, Real FX (2023) The urothelial gene regulatory network: understanding biology to improve bladder cancer management. Under review

Rangsitratkul C, Lawson C, Bernier-Godon F, Niavarani SR, Boudaud M, Rouleau S, Gladu-Corbin AO, Surendran A, Ekindi-Ndongo N, Koti M, Ilkow CS, Richard PO, Tai LH (2022) Intravesical immunotherapy with a GM-CSF armed oncolytic vesicular stomatitis virus improves outcome in bladder cancer. Mol Ther Oncolytics 24:507–521. https://doi.org/10.1016/j.omto.2022.01.009

Rastegar-Pouyani N, Montazeri V, Marandi N, Aliebrahimi S, Andalib M, Jafarzadeh E, Montazeri H, Ostad SN (2023) The impact of cancer-associated fibroblasts on drug resistance, Stemness, and epithelial-mesenchymal transition in bladder cancer: a comparison between recurrent and non-recurrent patient-derived CAFs. Cancer Investig 41(7):656–671. https://doi.org/10.1080/07357907.2023.2237576

Relph K, Annels N, Smith C, Kostalas M, Pandha H (2020) Oncolytic immunotherapy for bladder cancer using Coxsackie A21 virus: using a bladder tumor precision-cut slice model system to assess viral efficacy. Methods Mol Biol 2058:249–259. https://doi.org/10.1007/978-1-4939-9794-7_16

Richart L, Lapi E, Pancaldi V, Cuenca-Ardura M, Pau EC, Madrid-Mencia M, Neyret-Kahn H, Radvanyi F, Rodriguez JA, Cuartero Y, Serra F, Le Dily F, Valencia A, Marti-Renom MA, Real FX (2021) STAG2 loss-of-function affects short-range genomic contacts and modulates the basal-luminal transcriptional program of bladder cancer cells. Nucleic Acids Res 49(19):11005–11021. https://doi.org/10.1093/nar/gkab864

Rigby CC, Franks LM (1970) A human tissue culture cell line from a transitional cell tumour of the urinary bladder: growth, chromosome pattern and ultrastructure. Br J Cancer 24(4):746–754. https://doi.org/10.1038/bjc.1970.89

Rinaldetti S, Zhou Q, Abbott JM, de Jong FC, Esquer H, Costello JC, Theodorescu D, LaBarbera DV (2022) High-content drug discovery targeting molecular bladder cancer subtypes. Int J Mol Sci 23(18):10605. https://doi.org/10.3390/ijms231810605

Ringuette Goulet C, Bernard G, Chabaud S, Couture A, Langlois A, Neveu B, Pouliot F, Bolduc S (2017) Tissue-engineered human 3D model of bladder cancer for invasion study and drug discovery.

Biomaterials 145:233–241. https://doi.org/10.1016/j.biomaterials.2017.08.041

Ross RL, McPherson HR, Kettlewell L, Shnyder SD, Hurst CD, Alder O, Knowles MA (2016) PIK3CA dependence and sensitivity to therapeutic targeting in urothelial carcinoma. BMC Cancer 16:1–12. https://doi.org/10.1186/s12885-016-2570-0

Rossi MR, Masters JR, Park S, Todd JH, Garrett SH, Sens MA, Somji S, Nath J, Sens DA (2001) The immortalized UROtsa cell line as a potential cell culture model of human urothelium. Environ Health Perspect 109(8):801–808. https://doi.org/10.1289/ehp.01109801

Sailer V, von Amsberg G, Duensing S, Kirfel J, Lieb V, Metzger E, Offermann A, Pantel K, Schuele R, Taubert H, Wach S, Perner S, Werner S, Aigner A (2023) Experimental in vitro, ex vivo and in vivo models in prostate cancer research. Nat Rev Urol 20(3):158–178. https://doi.org/10.1038/s41585-022-00677-z

Saito R, Smith CC, Utsumi T, Bixby LM, Kardos J, Wobker SE, Stewart KG, Chai S, Manocha U, Byrd KM, Damrauer JS, Williams SE, Vincent BG, Kim WY (2018) Molecular subtype-specific immunocompetent models of high-grade urothelial carcinoma reveal differential Neoantigen expression and response to immunotherapy. Cancer Res 78(14):3954–3968. https://doi.org/10.1158/0008-5472.CAN-18-0173

Santos CP, Lapi E, Martinez de Villarreal J, Alvaro-Espinosa L, Fernandez-Barral A, Barbachano A, Dominguez O, Laughney AM, Megias D, Munoz A, Real FX (2019) Urothelial organoids originating from Cd49f(high) mouse stem cells display notch-dependent differentiation capacity. Nat Commun 10(1):4407. https://doi.org/10.1038/s41467-019-12307-1

Saponaro M, Flottmann S, Eckstein M, Hommerding O, Klumper N, Corvino D, Hosni S, Schmidt A, Monig N, Schmidt D, Ellinger J, Toma M, Kristiansen G, Bald T, Alimonti A, Ritter M, Holzel M, Alajati A (2023) CDCP1 expression is frequently increased in aggressive urothelial carcinoma and promotes urothelial tumor progression. Sci Rep 13(1):73. https://doi.org/10.1038/s41598-022-26579-z

Sato T, Vries RG, Snippert HJ, van de Wetering M, Barker N, Stange DE, van Es JH, Abo A, Kujala P, Peters PJ, Clevers H (2009) Single Lgr5 stem cells build crypt-villus structures in vitro without a mesenchymal niche. Nature 459(7244):262–265. https://doi.org/10.1038/nature07935

Schutgens F, Clevers H (2020) Human organoids: tools for understanding biology and treating diseases. Annu Rev Pathol 15:211–234. https://doi.org/10.1146/annurev-pathmechdis-012419-032611

Shamir ER, Ewald AJ (2014) Three-dimensional organotypic culture: experimental models of mammalian biology and disease. Nat Rev Mol Cell Biol 15(10):647–664. https://doi.org/10.1038/nrm3873

Shapiro SG, Knapp DW, Breen M (2015) A cultured approach to canine urothelial carcinoma: molecular characterization of five cell lines. Canine Genet Epidemiol 2:15. https://doi.org/10.1186/s40575-015-0028-3

Shi ZD, Hao L, Han XX, Wu ZX, Pang K, Dong Y, Qin JX, Wang GY, Zhang XM, Xia T, Liang Q, Zhao Y, Li R, Zhang SQ, Zhang JH, Chen JG, Wang GC, Chen ZS, Han CH (2022) Targeting HNRNPU to overcome cisplatin resistance in bladder cancer. Mol Cancer 21(1):37. https://doi.org/10.1186/s12943-022-01517-9

Shin K, Lee J, Guo N, Kim J, Lim A, Qu L, Mysorekar IU, Beachy PA (2011) Hedgehog/Wnt feedback supports regenerative proliferation of epithelial stem cells in bladder. Nature 472(7341):110–114. https://doi.org/10.1038/nature09851

Southgate J, Hutton KA, Thomas DF, Trejdosiewicz LK (1994) Normal human urothelial cells in vitro: proliferation and induction of stratification. Lab Investig 71(4):583–594. https://www.ncbi.nlm.nih.gov/pubmed/7967513

Summerhayes IC, Franks LM (1979) Effects of donor age on neoplastic transformation of adult mouse bladder epithelium in vitro. J Natl Cancer Inst 62(4):1017–1023. https://www.ncbi.nlm.nih.gov/pubmed/107359

Sutherland RM, Inch WR, McCredie JA, Kruuv J (1970) A multi-component radiation survival curve using an in vitro tumour model. Int J Radiat Biol Relat Stud Phys Chem Med 18(5):491–495. https://doi.org/10.1080/09553007014551401

Suzuki K, Koyanagi-Aoi M, Uehara K, Hinata N, Fujisawa M, Aoi T (2019) Directed differentiation of human induced pluripotent stem cells into mature stratified bladder urothelium. Sci Rep 9(1):10506. https://doi.org/10.1038/s41598-019-46848-8

Taylor CF, Platt FM, Hurst CD, Thygesen HH, Knowles MA (2014) Frequent inactivating mutations of STAG2 in bladder cancer are associated with low tumour grade and stage and inversely related to chromosomal copy number changes. Hum Mol Gen 23(8):1964–1974. https://doi.org/10.1093/hmg/ddt589

Templeton AR, Jeffery PL, Thomas PB, Perera MPJ, Ng G, Calabrese AR, Nicholls C, Mackenzie NJ, Wood J, Bray LJ, Vela I, Thompson EW, Williams ED (2021) Patient-derived explants as a precision medicine patient-proximal testing platform informing cancer management. Front Oncol 11:767697. https://doi.org/10.3389/fonc.2021.767697

Tortora D, Roberts ME, Kumar G, Kotapalli SS, Ritch E, Scurll JM, McConeghy B, Sinha S, Wyatt AW, Black PC, Daugaard M (2023) A genome-wide CRISPR screen maps endogenous regulators of PPARG gene expression in bladder cancer. iScience 26(5):106525. https://doi.org/10.1016/j.isci.2023.106525

Vakhshiteh F, Bagheri Z, Soleimani M, Ahvaraki A, Pournemat P, Alavi SE, Madjd Z (2023) Heterotypic tumor spheroids: a platform for nanomedicine evaluation. J Nanobiotechnol 21(1):249. https://doi.org/10.1186/s12951-023-02021-y

Vallot C, Stransky N, Bernard-Pierrot I, Herault A, Zucman-Rossi J, Chapeaublanc E, Vordos D, Laplanche A, Benhamou S, Lebret T, Southgate J, Allory Y, Radvanyi F (2011) A novel epigenetic phenotype associated with the most aggressive pathway of bladder tumor progression. J Natl Cancer Inst 103(1):47–60. https://doi.org/10.1093/jnci/djq470

van de Merbel AF, van der Horst G, van der Mark MH, van Uhm JIM, van Gennep EJ, Kloen P, Beimers L, Pelger RCM, van der Pluijm G (2018) An ex vivo tissue culture model for the assessment of individualized drug responses in prostate and bladder cancer. Front Oncol 8:400. https://doi.org/10.3389/fonc.2018.00400

van der Horst G, van de Merbel AF, Ruigrok E, van der Mark MH, Ploeg E, Appelman L, Tvingsholm S, Jaatela M, van Uhm J, Kruithof-de Julio M, Thalmann GN, Pelger RCM, Bangma CH, Boormans JL, van der Pluijm G, Zwarthoff EC (2020) Cationic amphiphilic drugs as potential anticancer therapy for bladder cancer. Mol Oncol 14(12):3121–3134. https://doi.org/10.1002/1878-0261.12793

Varley CL, Southgate J (2008) Effects of PPAR agonists on proliferation and differentiation in human urothelium. Exp Toxicol Pathol 60(6):435–441. https://doi.org/10.1016/j.etp.2008.04.009

Varley CL, Stahlschmidt J, Lee WC, Holder J, Diggle C, Selby PJ, Trejdosiewicz LK, Southgate J (2004) Role of PPARɣ and EGFR signalling in the urothelial terminal differentiation programme. J Cell Sci 117(Pt 10):2029–2036. https://doi.org/10.1242/jcs.01042

Vasconcelos-Nobrega C, Colaco A, Lopes C, Oliveira PA (2012) Review: BBN as an urothelial carcinogen. In Vivo 26(4):727–739. https://www.ncbi.nlm.nih.gov/pubmed/22773588

Wang LS, Boulaire J, Chan PP, Chung JE, Kurisawa M (2010) The role of stiffness of gelatin-hydroxyphenylpropionic acid hydrogels formed by enzyme-mediated crosslinking on the differentiation of human mesenchymal stem cell. Biomaterials 31(33):8608–8616. https://doi.org/10.1016/j.biomaterials.2010.07.075

Wang F, Zhang H, Ma AH, Yu W, Zimmermann M, Yang J, Hwang SH, Zhu D, Lin TY, Malfatti M, Turteltaub KW, Henderson PT, Airhart S, Hammock BD, Yuan J, de Vere White RW, Pan CX (2018) COX-2/sEH dual inhibitor PTUPB potentiates the antitumor efficacy of cisplatin. Mol Cancer Ther 17(2):474–483. https://doi.org/10.1158/1535-7163.MCT-16-0818

Wang C, Yang S, Jin L, Dai G, Yao Q, Xiang H, Zhang Y, Liu X, Xue B (2020) Biological and clinical significance of GATA3 detected from TCGA database and FFPE sample in bladder cancer patients. Onco Targets Ther 13:945–958. https://doi.org/10.2147/OTT.S237099

Wang M, Chen X, Tan P, Wang Y, Pan X, Lin T, Jiang Y, Wang B, Xu H, Wang Y, Yang Y, Wang J, Zhao L, Zhang J, Zhong A, Peng Y, Du J, Zhang Q, Zheng J et al (2022) Acquired semi-squamatization during chemotherapy suggests differentiation as a therapeutic strategy for bladder cancer. Cancer Cell 40(9):1044–1059.e1048. https://doi.org/10.1016/j.ccell.2022.08.010

Warrick JI, Walter V, Yamashita H, Chung E, Shuman L, Amponsa VO, Zheng Z, Chan W, Whitcomb TL, Yue F, Iyyanki T, Kawasawa YI, Kaag M, Guo W, Raman JD, Park JS, DeGraff DJ (2016) FOXA1, GATA3 and PPARɣ cooperate to drive luminal subtype in bladder cancer: a molecular analysis of established human cell lines. Sci Rep 6(1):38531. https://doi.org/10.1038/srep38531

Wei Y, Amend B, Todenhofer T, Lipke N, Aicher WK, Fend F, Stenzl A, Harland N (2022) Urinary tract tumor organoids reveal eminent differences in drug sensitivities when compared to 2-dimensional culture systems. Int J Mol Sci 23(11):6305. https://doi.org/10.3390/ijms23116305

Wezel F, Lustig J, Azoitei A, Liu J, Meessen S, Najjar G, Zehe V, Faustmann P, Zengerling F, John A, Martini T, Bolenz C, Gunes C (2021) Grainyhead-like 3 influences migration and invasion of urothelial carcinoma cells. Int J Mol Sci 22(6):2959. https://doi.org/10.3390/ijms22062959

Williams PD, Lee JK, Theodorescu D (2008) Molecular credentialing of rodent bladder carcinogenesis models. Neoplasia 10(8):838–846. https://doi.org/10.1593/neo.08432

Williams SV, Hurst CD, Knowles MA (2013) Oncogenic FGFR3 gene fusions in bladder cancer. Hum Mol Gen 22(4):795–803. https://doi.org/10.1093/hmg/dds486

Wong K, Abascal F, Ludwig L, Aupperle-Lellbach H, Grassinger J, Wright CW, Allison SJ, Pinder E, Phillips RM, Romero LP, Gal A, Roady PJ, Pires I, Guscetti F, Munday JS, Peleteiro MC, Pinto CA, Carvalho T, Cota J et al (2023) Cross-species oncogenomics offers insight into human muscle-invasive bladder cancer. Genome Biol 24(1):191. https://doi.org/10.1186/s13059-023-03026-4

Yan HHN, Chan AS, Lai FP, Leung SY (2023) Organoid cultures for cancer modeling. Cell Stem Cell 30(7):917–937. https://doi.org/10.1016/j.stem.2023.05.012

Yoshida T, Sopko NA, Kates M, Liu X, Joice G, McConkey DJ, Bivalacqua TJ (2019) Impact of spheroid culture on molecular and functional characteristics of bladder cancer cell lines. Oncol Lett 18(5):4923–4929. https://doi.org/10.3892/ol.2019.10786

Yu L, Li Z, Mei H, Li W, Chen D, Liu L, Zhang Z, Sun Y, Song F, Chen W, Huang W (2021) Patient-derived organoids of bladder cancer recapitulate antigen expression profiles and serve as a personal evaluation model for CAR-T cells in vitro. Clin Transl Immunol 10(2):e1248. https://doi.org/10.1002/cti2.1248

Zhang Q, Chen Z (2018) Sensitization of cisplatin resistant bladder tumor by combination of cisplatin treatment and co-culture of dendritic cells with apoptotic bladder cancer cells. Cell Mol Biol (Noisy-le-Grand) 64(10):102–107. https://www.ncbi.nlm.nih.gov/pubmed/30084800

Zhu S, Zhu Z, Ma AH, Sonpavde GP, Cheng F, Pan CX (2021) Preclinical models for bladder cancer research. Hematol Oncol Clin North Am 35(3):613–632. https://doi.org/10.1016/j.hoc.2021.02.007

Zuiverloon TCM, de Jong FC, Costello JC, Theodorescu D (2018) Systematic review: characteristics and preclinical uses of bladder cancer cell lines. Bladder Cancer 4(2):169–183. https://doi.org/10.3233/BLC-180167

Part VI

Biomarkers for Diagnosis and Treatment of Bladder Cancer

Urine Biomarkers for Bladder Cancer Diagnosis and Screening

18

Rik Bryan and Doug Ward

Abstract

Flexible cystoscopy is the mainstay of bladder cancer detection but is an imperfect test which is resource-intensive and invasive for patients. A focus of bladder cancer research has been to develop non-invasive tests to reliably detect urothelial cancers without the need for cystoscopy. Bladder cancer is unique in that tumor cells are in prolonged contact with a plentiful and easily-collected liquid biopsy, urine; hence, non-invasive alternatives to cystoscopy have been sought for over 30 years. Despite considerable progress in recent years in identifying and commercializing diagnostic urinary biomarkers (some of which rival the sensitivity and specificity of cystoscopy), none are yet being used routinely at the clinical front line as a replacement for cystoscopy, nor are any recommended for this purpose by international guideline committees. It is recognized that there are challenges to overcome, such as false-negative tests due to low rates of shedding by some tumors, false positives caused by hematuria, urothelial field changes or inflammatory conditions, and clinical study design.

In this chapter, we outline the relevant clinical settings, the molecular changes associated with bladder cancer that can be detected in urine, the mechanisms of release of these biomolecules into urine, and important considerations for their detection, measurement, and validity. Furthermore, we provide an overview of all classes of diagnostic urinary biomarkers, highlighting a new generation of urine tests that have been enabled by the expansion of our understanding of bladder cancer genomics during the course of the last 10 years. Finally, in order to realize the full potential and clinical impact of these biomarkers and to progress beyond simple descriptions of test accuracy, we encourage investigators to conduct randomized interventional studies to assess how such tests can change clinical pathways for the better. Consequently, there is a realistic expectation that the latest nucleic acid-based tests will be in routine clinical use within 5 years.

Keywords

Urine · Biomarker · Non-invasive · Diagnosis · Screening · Liquid biopsy

R. Bryan (✉) · D. Ward
Bladder Cancer Research Centre,
Department of Cancer and Genomic Sciences,
College of Medicine and Health, University of Birmingham, Birmingham, UK
e-mail: r.t.bryan@bham.ac.uk

M. A. Knowles, L. Dyrskjøt (eds.), *Biology of Bladder Cancer*,
https://doi.org/10.1007/978-3-031-68505-7_18

18.1 Introduction

Hematuria is the cardinal symptom of bladder cancer (BC) (Wallace et al. 2002; Babjuk et al. 2022); non-visible hematuria (NVH) has a low positive predictive value (PPV, 1–5%) (Edwards et al. 2006; Mitra and Cote 2010; Larre et al. 2013; Tan et al. 2018; Cumberbatch and Noon 2019), whereas visible hematuria (VH) has a PPV of 10–19% and necessitates urgent investigation (Edwards et al. 2006; Tan et al. 2018; Khadhouri et al. 2021). Such investigations include upper urinary tract imaging and flexible cystoscopy (Babjuk et al. 2022), with millions of individuals worldwide undergoing investigations for hematuria each year.

Currently, initial treatment for all BC patients is by transurethral resection of bladder tumor (TURBT), whereby 75–85% of patients will be pathologically diagnosed with non-muscle-invasive tumors (NMIBC, stages pTa/pT1/pTis), and the remainder as muscle-invasive tumors (MIBC, stages pT2-4) (Bryan et al. 2013; Babjuk et al. 2022) (see Chap. 4).

Subsequent treatment strategies differ markedly: patients with MIBC are likely to undergo radical therapy with combinations of chemotherapy and/or immunotherapy and radiotherapy or cystectomy (Witjes et al. 2021), whereas patients with NMIBC will be treated with intravesical therapy followed by regular cystoscopic surveillance (Babjuk et al. 2022). The nature of intravesical therapy and the schedules of cystoscopic surveillance are determined by the risk category of NMIBC (for example, the European Association of Urology categories of low-, intermediate-, high-, and very high-risk), with immediate radical cystectomy to be considered for patients at very high risk of tumor progression (Babjuk et al. 2022) (see Chaps. 5 and 6).

Disease recurrence is a lifetime risk across all NMIBC categories occurring in up to 80% of patients (van Rhijn et al. 2009), and progression to MIBC is a fundamental consideration for high-risk and very high-risk NMIBC patients, occurring in up to 45% of cases (van Rhijn et al. 2009; Sylvester et al. 2021). Therefore, regular cystoscopic surveillance represents the mainstay of long-term management for all NMIBC patients (Babjuk et al. 2022), as well as MIBC patients treated with bladder-sparing approaches (James et al. 2012). Urine cytology is often used as an adjunct to cystoscopy: the microscopic detection of cancer cells in the urine is a very specific indicator of BC but has poor sensitivity for low-grade BC, resulting in low overall sensitivity (Schmitz-Drager et al. 2015).

For all patients, whether in the setting of primary diagnosis or post-treatment disease surveillance, cystoscopy is inconvenient, invasive, and carries morbidity (Mowatt et al. 2010; Svatek et al. 2014); it is also operator-dependent and fallible, with estimated sensitivity ≤85% and specificity ≤87% (Zheng et al. 2012; Svatek et al. 2014). For healthcare providers, cystoscopy is expensive (Svatek et al. 2014; Leal et al. 2016), such that from diagnosis to death on a per patient basis, BC is one of the most expensive malignancies to manage, if not the most expensive (Sangar et al. 2005; Yeung et al. 2014). Therefore, non-invasive urinary biomarker tests for the accurate and reliable detection of BC have the potential to be transformational for both patients and healthcare providers by reducing dependence on cystoscopy for initial diagnosis and subsequent disease surveillance (D'Costa et al. 2017).

Furthermore, such biomarkers may permit screening or early detection approaches in high-risk populations—a strategy for screening or early detection simply based upon individuals with NVH undergoing flexible cystoscopy is considered impractical (Mitra and Cote 2010; Larre et al. 2013; Cumberbatch and Noon 2019). Instead, it has long been suggested that an accurate "molecular-based" urine test is an essential intermediary between NVH and cystoscopy to enable BC screening (Mitra and Cote 2010, Larre et al. 2013, Cumberbatch and Noon 2019).

BCs are in direct contact with urine for periods of several hours between voids, and so urine is considered to be the most promising biospecimen for developing non-invasive tests to accurately detect bladder tumors (D'Costa et al. 2017). However, BCs are highly heterogeneous with variable mutation and gene expression profiles and copy number changes (Alexandrov et al.

2013; Robertson et al. 2017; Lindskrog et al. 2021; Goel et al. 2022), and so different tumors may release different biomarkers, necessitating multi-marker tests (D'Costa et al. 2017). Early-stage and low-grade tumors may only release very small amounts of such markers, potentially impairing test sensitivity (D'Costa et al. 2017). Markers must also be highly tumor-specific so that hematuria itself and other non-malignant conditions do not generate false positives (D'Costa et al. 2017). In the search for accurate diagnostic urinary biomarkers, genomic, proteomic, and metabolomic approaches have all yielded promising results (D'Costa et al. 2017; Humayun-Zakaria et al. 2021).

Several urine biomarkers have been granted FDA approval, including Nuclear Matrix Protein 22 (NMP22) and Bladder Tumor Antigen (BTA) assays, UroVysion, and ImmunoCyt (Ng et al. 2021); these have been the subject of meta-analyses, comparisons, and reviews over the years (Mowatt et al. 2010; Dong et al. 2021; Ng et al. 2021). However, to date, no urine test for BC diagnosis and screening has been included in guidelines or seen widespread clinical uptake. Although the European Association of Urology acknowledges that recently-developed tests could play a future role in detecting disease recurrence, they conclude that no urinary marker can replace cystoscopy during follow-up or reduce cystoscopy frequency on a routine basis (Laukhtina et al. 2021; Babjuk et al. 2022).

Excitingly, recent technological advances and increased understanding of the molecular biology of bladder cancer mean that we may be on the cusp of clinically useful urine tests for bladder cancer diagnosis and surveillance.

18.2 Identifying the Molecular Changes of Bladder Cancer in Urine

As described elsewhere in this book, BCs are characterized by extensive genomic, epigenomic, transcriptomic, proteomic, and metabolomic changes (Hurst et al. 2012, Sjodahl et al. 2012, 2014; Aine et al. 2015; Robertson et al. 2017; Lindskrog et al. 2021; Goel et al. 2022), all of which can be potentially detected in urine (Cheng et al. 2019; Ward et al. 2023). At the molecular level bladder cancers are extremely diverse: low-grade tumors which are largely diploid with mutations in a few oncogenes, and high-grade tumors with high tumor mutation burden, extensive copy number changes and complex alterations in DNA methylation and gene expression profiles. Although tumors can be categorized into subtypes based on gene expression profiles, heterogeneity still exists within these subtypes (Sirab et al. 2022; Lindskrog et al. 2023). Thus, it seems unlikely that there is a single molecular marker that could be measured in urine to accurately detect all bladder cancers. Recent research efforts have shifted toward panels of biomarkers that are able to detect the whole spectrum of BCs while retaining high specificity. There has also been a historical shift from protein biomarkers toward nucleic acid biomarkers driven by technological advances which enable the detection of trace amounts of tumor DNA or RNA in urine (Humayun-Zakaria et al. 2021).

18.3 Mechanisms of Biomarker Release into the Urine

Urine can be separated into two fractions containing cellular and cell-free material by filtration or, more commonly, by low-speed centrifugation (Togneri et al. 2016). The cellular fraction (urine cell pellet) will contain shed urothelial cells including, in variable proportions, normal and tumor cells, and often in BC cases, red and white blood cells. High-grade cancer cells in the cellular fraction can be identified by microscopy (urine cytology) whereas DNA, RNA, and protein biomarkers can be assayed in both the cell pellet and the cell-free fraction (urine supernatant). Estimates of tumor content from variant allele frequencies (VAFs) obtained by the next generation sequencing (NGS) of urine cell pellet DNA indicate that tumor cell shedding into urine is less in small and low-grade BCs than in larger and high-grade BCs (Fig. 18.1) (Bicocca et al. 2022; Ward et al. 2023). This suggests that, even

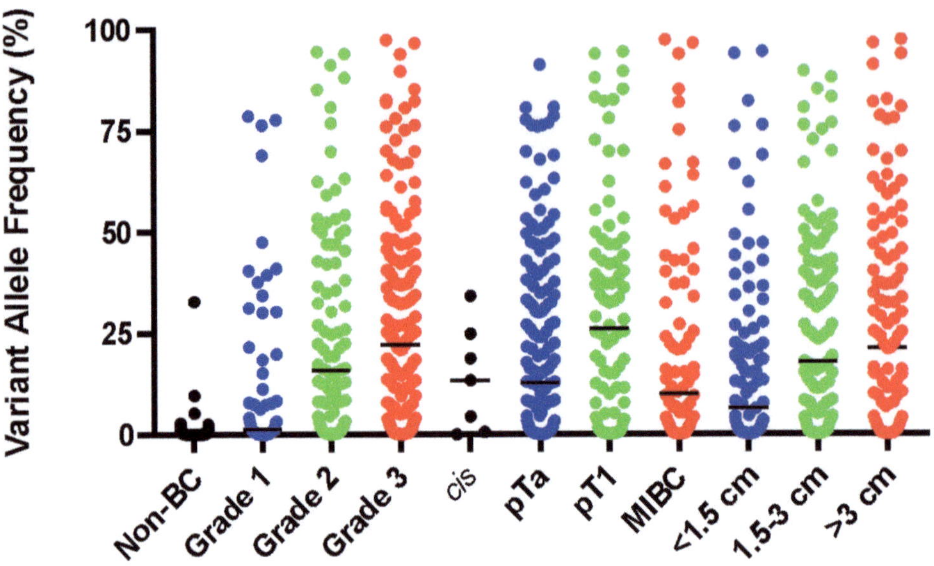

Fig. 18.1 Variant allele frequencies in urine DNA from BC patients with different stages and grades of disease ($n = 343$). Variant allele frequencies were measured using a 23-gene targeted sequencing panel as described in Ward et al. (2023)

with the correct biomarkers, sensitive detection of low-grade BC will require very sensitive analytical techniques.

Cell lysis (due to apoptosis, necrosis, or other mechanisms of cell death) will release cellular contents into the cell-free fraction, as will active biological processes such as secretion, extracellular vesicle (EV) release, proteolytic shedding of the ectodomains of plasma membrane proteins, and proteolysis of extracellular matrix constituents (Fig. 18.2). Increased metalloprotease secretion and activity and shedding of ectodomains appears to be a feature of more aggressive BCs (Arnold Egloff et al. 2017; Snell et al. 2018). EVs can be separated from the remainder of the cell-free fraction by ultracentrifugation or precipitation and have been shown to contain BC biomarkers (Zhan et al. 2018; Tomiyama et al. 2022). EVs protect labile molecules such as RNA from degradation and, particularly if active cancer cells release more EVs than quiescent cells, analyzing EVs may enhance the detection of BC biomarkers, although compelling evidence of high sensitivity and specificity has not been reported to date.

It should also be noted that, subsequent to renal clearance, the cell-free fraction of urine may contain plasma cell-free DNA (cfDNA), including circulating tumor DNA (ctDNA) from non-urothelial malignancies (termed "transrenal ctDNA," TR-ctDNA). This has been reported, for example, with *KRAS*-mutant lung, colorectal, and pancreatic cancers (Su et al. 2004; Wang et al. 2017; Crisafulli et al. 2019; Terasawa et al. 2019; Dermody et al. 2022).

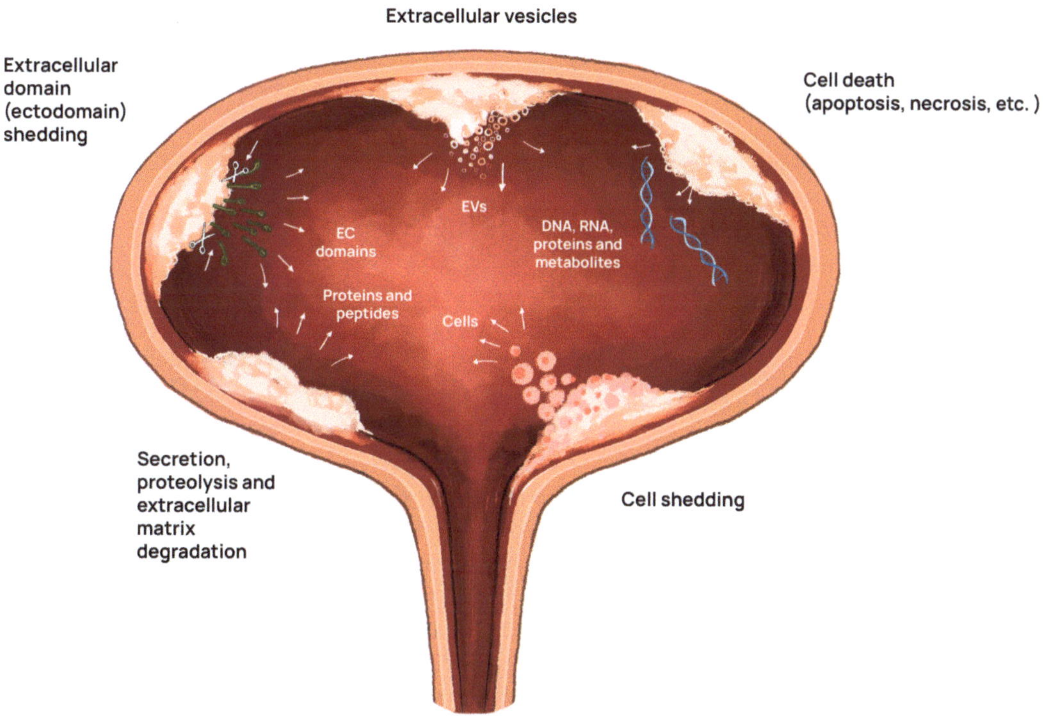

Fig. 18.2 Mechanisms of release and biomarker types found in urine. Biomarkers may be present in tumor cells shed from the urothelium, encapsulated in vesicles, or as free molecules (either actively secreted or released by tumor cell lysis). Tumor-associated proteolysis releases the ectodomains of cell surface proteins and protein fragments arising from extracellular matrix degradation. Non-tumor cells within the tumor microenvironment may also give rise to biomarkers, and some biomarkers may enter the urine via renal clearance

18.4 Confounding Factors and Considerations in the Design of Urine Biomarker Studies

18.4.1 Hematuria

Hematuria is potentially a major confounding factor in urine biomarker discovery and measurement. Although most bladder cancers will cause hematuria, most hematuria is not caused by bladder cancer (Edwards et al. 2006; Tan et al. 2018; Khadhouri et al. 2021). Therefore, any molecules present in blood plasma may appear in urine as seemingly promising BC biomarkers in case–control studies where control subjects are not matched for hematuria (for example, urine samples from cancer patients compared to those from young healthy volunteers) when, in reality, such biomarkers are only surrogates for hematuria. Hence, when evaluated in the real-world setting, those biomarkers will suffer from poor specificity. This is particularly true of proteomic studies which have proposed abundant plasma proteins as urine biomarkers (Bryan et al. 2011; D'Costa et al. 2016).

18.4.2 Other Urological Conditions

Many patients undergoing investigation for possible bladder cancer will instead be diagnosed with other urological conditions including, but not limited to, urinary tract infection and stone disease (Edwards et al. 2006, Tan et al. 2018, Khadhouri ct al. 2021). If these conditions are not included in biomarker evaluation studies, then specificity may be overestimated.

18.4.3 Stage and Grade

Larger and higher grade and stage tumors tend to release higher levels of biomarkers than those of lower stage and grade. Thus, studies with a disproportionately high fraction of high-grade/stage tumors will report inflated sensitivity which will not apply to a real-world bladder cancer patient cohort (D'Costa et al. 2016, 2017).

18.4.4 Field Effect

Genomic and epigenomic changes in apparently normal urothelium precede and accompany urothelial carcinogenesis (Lee et al. 2007; Majewski et al. 2008; di Martino et al. 2015), a phenomenon known as "field change," "field cancerization," or the "field effect" (Murphy 1977; Sidransky et al. 1992; Tsai et al. 1995) (see Chap. 11). As many molecular characteristics are shared between field change urothelium and the cancers themselves (Strandgaard et al. 2024), field change may result in seemingly false-positive urinary biomarker results. Although somatic mutations do genuinely occur in pathologically normal urothelium (Lawson et al. 2020), it should be noted that field change-related "false-positive" urine tests during hematuria investigation or NMIBC surveillance likely indicate an increased risk of bladder cancer and a need for ongoing or more intensive surveillance (Ward et al. 2023)—what is termed "anticipatory" or "pre-emptive" diagnosis (Beukers et al. 2017).

18.4.5 Clinical Context

Urine tests for bladder cancer tend to perform better for initial diagnosis (symptomatic patients with hematuria) than in the surveillance setting (asymptomatic patients). This likely arises from the intent to detect smaller tumors or microscopic residual disease during active surveillance, the field effect, and comparison with an imperfect "gold standard" (flexible cystoscopy).

Furthermore, the requirements for sensitivity and specificity of a urinary marker test depend on the clinical context of the patient: screening asymptomatic individuals will require very high specificity, whereas for triaging hematuria patients, lower specificity may be acceptable.

18.4.6 Sample Collection and Processing

Optimal sample collection and processing is key to test performance. There is little consensus as to what time of day urine should be collected or as to an individual's fluid intake prior to micturition, or whether first void, midstream, or full void specimens are optimal. While many protein biomarker measurements can be made with microliters of urine, yields of nucleic acids benefit from larger volumes, typically 30–50 mL. It is also imperative that urine is either assayed or processed and frozen within a few hours of collection, or preservatives added to prevent bacterial growth and biomarker degradation.

Urine can be centrifuged or filtered to produce supernatant/soluble fractions and a cellular fraction. Some biomarkers are specifically measured in one or other fraction, whereas others (e.g., DNA-based biomarkers) can be measured in either (Ward et al. 2019). Some literature supports supernatant DNA (cell-free DNA, cfDNA) being more representative of the tumor than cell pellet DNA (cpDNA) but this remains to be unequivocally confirmed (Togneri et al. 2016; Ward et al. 2019), albeit cell pellets tend to yield more DNA (Ward et al. 2019).

Urine cell pellets are often too small to be clearly visible and care must be taken to avoid losses when resuspending pellets and transferring between tubes. Occasionally, repeat sampling may be necessary if pellets are too small or samples heavily contaminated with blood.

Furthermore, any systematic difference between sample collection and processing for the cases and controls could introduce bias and generate false biomarker results (particularly for biomarkers related to epiphenomena and not causally linked to BC), e.g. use of different urine preservatives in one or other patient group when collected at different clinics.

18.4.7 Data Analysis

The concentration of urine samples varies enormously due to individuals' fluid uptake. For binary biomarkers (present/absent) this may not be an issue (although it may influence detection), but it may be inappropriate to express quantitative biomarkers as quantity per unit volume of urine. Protein biomarkers may be normalized to the urinary creatinine concentration, whereas RNA biomarkers are often normalized to housekeeping gene expression and DNA biomarkers often presented as variant allele frequencies.

When measuring multiple candidate biomarkers, and in particular, when combining data in complex class prediction models, studies with limited sample size may risk describing overly optimistic biomarker performance due to chance findings. This phenomenon, described as "overfitting" (Han and Jiang 2014; Khan et al. 2019), leads to biomarkers which fail on further validation—in essence, the model learns the training data too well, including its noise and outliers, such that it performs poorly on unseen data. Most studies address this by using independent training and testing cohorts, but when this independence is compromised and biomarkers ("features") are also selected from the test cohort (termed "test data leak into the feature selection step" (Desaire 2022)) overfitting can occur.

18.4.8 Clinical Implementation

A common aim of diagnostic urine tests is to reduce the number of cystoscopies experienced by patients during the course of their disease and to use cystoscopy more selectively. Thus, a line of sight to clinical implementation must be maintained. To be clinically useful, a urine test should be cheaper, faster, easier, or better than existing tests (flexible cystoscopy, urine cytology, and imaging).

No urine tests developed so far have both sufficient performance and validation to be incorporated into routine clinical practice. Recently, guideline committees have acknowledged that some tests could play a future role in detecting high-grade recurrences, with several recently-developed tests appearing to offer high sensitivity and specificity, albeit requiring further validation (Babjuk et al. 2022). However, direct comparisons of different urine tests across different studies are difficult due to different patient cohort compositions. Comparisons within a research study are also difficult for researchers to perform due to limited DNA/RNA and protein yields and the input requirements and financial costs of various tests. A lack of head-to-head comparisons in the same cohort(s) is challenging due to cost and practicalities, and it remains unclear which test(s) could be or should be incorporated into clinical practice.

18.5 Urine Cytology

Urine cytology is a cheap test that is widely used as an adjunct to flexible cystoscopy. The microscopic detection of tumor cells in urine is a very specific way to detect BC (>90% specificity for experienced practitioners), but with poor to modest sensitivity (Hajdinjak 2008; Xie et al. 2016; Nikas et al. 2022). A positive cytology result can indicate the presence of urothelial carcinoma anywhere in the urinary tract, but a negative result cannot be used to rule out the presence of a tumor. Although many publications compare urinary biomarker performance with urine cytology, this is not a particularly useful comparison considering cytology's operator-dependent results and overall poor performance across the spectrum of all grades of BC (Sahai et al. 2020). Due to the high specificity and low cost of urine cytology it could potentially be used in conjunction with novel urine tests. Two FDA approved biomarker tests to improve the performance of cytology based on multiplex FISH or immunofluorescence (UroVysion and ImmunoCyt) have not seen widespread uptake due to increased complexity and cost with minimal benefit (Hajdinjak 2008; Chou et al. 2015). More recently, it has been reported that cytokeratin 17 immunostaining may improve the sensitivity of cytology while retaining high specificity, the URO17™ test (Babu et al. 2021; Vasdev et al. 2021).

18.6 Urine Metabolites as BC Biomarkers

The metabolism of proliferating cancer cells differs from their non-neoplastic counterparts, reflecting transformed cells' greater need for biochemical building blocks and energy (Pavlova and Thompson 2016), which may be reflected in detectable alterations in urinary metabolites. These phenomena were famously exemplified by a 2004 study demonstrating that dogs could be trained to distinguish patients with BC on the basis of urine odor more successfully than would be expected by chance alone, suggesting that tumor-related volatile compounds are present in urine and impart a characteristic odor signature (Willis et al. 2004).

More recently, metabolomic methods such as mass spectrometry, nuclear magnetic resonance spectroscopy, and surface-enhanced Raman spectroscopy have identified distinctly different polar metabolite and lipid profiles in neoplastic and normal urothelium (Putluri et al. 2011; Piyarathna et al. 2018; Loras et al. 2019). It should be noted that these differences comprise changes in the levels of multiple common metabolites rather than production of novel cancer-specific metabolites; thus, dilution in urine (containing metabolites from other sources) and confounding factors (such as hematuria) may mask their detection and, hence, clinical utility. For example, Putluri et al showed that the metabolomic profiles of BC tissue separated perfectly from adjacent benign and normal tissues, but that when 25 of the most discriminatory tissue metabolites were measured in urine samples, only modest discrimination between BC cases and controls could be achieved (Putluri et al. 2011). Many independent studies have directly compared the urine metabolome of BC cases and controls (without attempting to determine the source of the metabolites) and many of these studies report areas under receiver-operator characteristics curves (AUROCs) >0.9 (Lin et al. 2021; Li et al. 2022; Wang et al. 2022), while other studies report more modest performance (Lett et al. 2022; Oto et al. 2022). Potential issues with the high diagnostic accuracies reported include the use of inappropriate controls, limited sample sizes, and the possible over-fitting of class prediction models. There is also a lack of consensus across the studies as to which metabolites discriminate, and large-scale validation is required. If these issues can be overcome, metabolites might ultimately form the basis of a point-of-care (POC) test for BC using portable devices (Hu et al. 2021).

18.7 Protein Biomarkers

Theoretically, overexpression or increased release of proteins from BC cells into the urine should act as a ready source of biomarkers. However, proteins that are normally present in plasma or urine are unlikely to be useful as hematuria will cause false-positive results. Similarly, proteins that are increased in BC but are also increased by infection, inflammation, or calculi will also not offer high specificity. A panel of cancer-specific isoforms of proteins or post-translationally modified versions of proteins (e.g., glycosylation, cleavage, acetylation) could potentially offer a route to an accurate urine test. Candidate cancer-specific isoforms can be inferred from RNA sequencing data (although there is a scarcity of data from normal urothelium) (Humayun-Zakaria et al. 2019), but the in-depth proteomic analyses required to comprehensively identify alterations in post-translational modifications in BC have not been undertaken; the bladder cancer proteome is enormously complex and remains largely unexplored (Shimwell et al. 2013; D'Costa et al. 2016). If suitable protein biomarkers could be identified, this could offer the potential for point-of-care (POC) testing using inexpensive lateral flow devices.

The "first generation" of commercialized protein biomarkers for urine-based detection of bladder cancer (NMP22, BTA, UBC, CYFRA 21-2) were discovered in the 1990s and have been extensively tested, combined, and compared (Glas et al. 2003; van Rhijn et al. 2005; Chou et al. 2015). These biomarkers all show higher overall sensitivity (60–80%) than urine cytology, but poorer specificity (60–80%), and thus have limited clinical utility. More recently, MCM5 (minichromosomal maintenance 5) has been proposed as a biomarker. Again, MCM5 has modest overall diagnostic efficacy, but has high sensitivity for high-grade disease and is marketed as ADXBladder for high-grade NMIBC surveillance (Laukhtina et al. 2021; Sharma et al. 2022). All of these markers have inferior performance to flexible cystoscopy.

Many proteins have been reported as highly promising urine biomarkers for BC but, until validated, must be treated with caution. In 2016 we reviewed the literature and singled out fibronectin, clusterin, CEACAM1, apolipoprotein A4, calprotectin, CD147, coronin-1A, DJ-1, reg-1, stathmin-1, and γ-synuclein as worthy of further investigation (D'Costa et al. 2016). Fibronectin (Dong et al. 2018), clusterin (Duggan et al. 2022), and γ-synuclein (Liu et al. 2016) continue to show promise, most likely as components of multi-marker panels.

As no validated individual proteins appear to have sufficient diagnostic accuracy, multi-marker panels have been explored. For example, the Oncuria multiplex test (comprising angiogenin, apolipoprotein E, alpha-1 antitrypsin, carbonic anhydrase 9, interleukin 8, matrix metallopeptidase 9, matrix metallopeptidase 10, plasminogen activator inhibitor 1, syndecan 1, and vascular endothelial growth factor A) has demonstrated an area under receiver operating characteristic (AUROC) of 0.93 in a single study, with sensitivity and specificity of 93% for diagnosing new cases of BC when combined in an algorithm with age, sex, and race (Hirasawa et al. 2021). However, we note that the individual constituents of this panel do not appear to be particularly promising candidates alone and some are common plasma proteins; further optimization of the assay is ongoing (Murakami et al. 2021).

18.8 RNA Biomarkers

Messenger ribonucleic acids (mRNA) act as the intermediates between genes and their protein products. Measuring mRNA levels is a facile way to quantify gene expression in tumors on a genome-wide scale (by RNA sequencing or microarrays) or for specific genes (e.g., by quantitative reverse transcription PCR, qRT-PCR). As discussed in Chaps. 13 and 14, bladder tumors express many genes at different levels to normal urothelium and these changes in expression could potentially be measured in urine to detect the presence of bladder cancer. Overexpressed genes may be present at very high RNA copy number in each cancer cell, theoretically making them easier to detect than DNA biomarkers (usually one or two copies per cell). Important caveats are that the overexpressed genes should be specific to BC (even modest expression in normal urothelium or benign conditions will compromise specificity) and that mRNA is unstable in solution in urine (although mRNA packaged in sloughed cells or extracellular vesicles may suffice). It should be noted that extraction of usable quantities of mRNA from urine for, for example, RNA sequencing is challenging. Nonetheless, small quantities of RNA are required for qRT-PCR and several urine mRNA biomarkers have been proposed (e.g., *TERT* and survivin *(BIRC5)* (Brems-Eskildsen et al. 2010; Schmidt et al. 2016)), and two tests based on mRNA panels have been commercialized (CxBladder and Xpert Bladder (Chou et al. 2015, Laukhtina et al. 2021)). CxBladder utilizes the expression of *MDK* (angiogenesis), *HOXA13* (differentiation), *CDC2* (proliferation), *IGBP5* (apoptosis), and *CXCR2* to rule out false positives due to inflammation; Xpert Bladder is based on *ABL1*, *UPK1B*, *CRH*, *ANXA10*, and *IGF2*. However, neither test appears to rival flexible cystoscopy with regard to sensitivity and specificity (Laukhtina et al. 2021).

mRNA splicing is often altered in bladder cancer cells. An interesting, but unproven, hypothesis is that rather than quantifying mRNA levels in urine, detection of a panel of cancer-specific isoforms of highly expressed genes could provide sensitive and specific disease detection (Humayun-Zakaria et al. 2019). Another novel type of RNA formed by mRNA back-splicing are circular RNAs (Goel et al. 2020). These are differentially expressed between grades and subtypes of NMIBC and are highly stable compared with linear mRNA (Goel et al. 2020, 2022). To date, there is little concordance as to which circular RNAs are overexpressed or unique in bladder cancer.

In addition to mRNA and housekeeping RNAs (ribosomal and transfer RNAs), there are non-coding RNAs, classified as long non-coding RNA if longer than 200 nucleotides and short non-coding RNA if shorter; the latter group are sub-classified as microRNA, snoRNA, snRNA, siRNA, and piRNA. Several studies have proposed panels of urinary microRNAs as diagnostic for bladder cancer (Suarez-Cabrera et al. 2022; Ye et al. 2022). Individual long non-coding RNAs (lncRNA), including *UCA1* and *MALAT1*, and combinations of lncRNAs have been reported as diagnostic in urine (Yu et al. 2020; Ding et al. 2021; Qiu et al. 2022). However, there are no non-coding RNA-based bladder cancer urine tests that have yet been thoroughly validated or commercialized.

18.9 DNA Biomarkers

As previously discussed, bladder cancer is caused by alterations in the genome of urothelial cells. These changes include single nucleotide variants, insertions, deletions, chromosomal rearrangements, loss of heterozygosity and copy number changes, as well as genome-wide alterations in cytosine methylation. Ideally, to act as biomarkers, these changes should occur early in cancer development, be clonal (i.e., present in all cancer cells) and retained spatially and temporally, and not occur in normal urothelium. The latter criterion may not always be met as cells have to acquire multiple alterations to become cancer cells. Hence, and as discussed above, apparently normal urothelial cells can harbor some alterations (Strandgaard et al. 2024); furthermore, deep-sequencing of microbiopsies has identified that some of these genomic changes can accumulate in entirely normal urothelium (Lawson et al. 2020; Li et al. 2020). However, in the absence of the clonal expansion of carcinogenesis, the levels of these changes in urine DNA are likely to be very low, albeit detectable and measurable. Therefore, establishing thresholds for "positive" and "negative" tests requires careful consideration and the evaluation of urine samples from age- and sex-matched hematuria patients without urothelial cancer (Ward et al. 2023). Nevertheless, detectable genomic changes in urine DNA are theoretically far more specific to cancer cells than changes in levels of RNAs, proteins, or metabolites. DNA is also considered stable relative to RNA, but usually only present at 2 copies per cell (>2 copies in some BC cells but only rarely >10 due to focal amplifications) as opposed to 1000s of copies per BC cell for highly expressed mRNAs, proteins, or metabolites. Therefore, urine samples where BC DNA only comprises a small fraction of the total DNA require very sensitive analytical techniques.

Panels of commonly mutated genes (e.g., *TERT*, *FGFR3*, *ADGRG6*, *TP53*) and/or methylation markers (e.g., *DMRTA2*, *ONECUT*, *OTX1*) have the potential to identify close to 100% of bladder tumors (Kompier et al. 2010; Rachakonda et al. 2013; van Kessel et al. 2017; Garinet et al. 2019; Deng et al. 2022). In reality, when applied to urine, such panels yield high sensitivities and specificities but 100% accuracy is unrealistic. However, it is important to note that there is no "ground truth" of 100% accuracy with any diagnostic investigation for bladder cancer—for example, the use of narrow band imaging (NBI) cystoscopy and photodynamic diagnosis (PDD) has demonstrated that tumors are missed or overlooked by conventional white light (WL) cystoscopy (Bryan et al. 2008; Patel et al. 2011). In a recent systematic review which included a comparison of conventional WL cystoscopy versus imaging, the sensitivity of cystoscopy ranged from 87 to 100% and specificity from 64 to 100% (Devlies et al. 2023). Hence, there will be some BCs that are only detected by a molecular urine test and others that are only detected by cystoscopy; however, with priority currently given to "seeing a tumor" and then "taking a tissue biopsy," it is the reported sensitivity and specificity of the molecular urine test that is more likely to be negatively impacted. As we move into an era of accurate diagnostic urine tests (and ctDNA detection for minimal residual disease (MRD) monitoring), the "seeing a tumor" (by cystoscopy or imaging) and "taking a tissue biopsy" paradigms may need to change. Additionally, some non-bladder cancer cases such as inverted papillomas harbor similar genomic changes to bladder cancer, generating false-positive results.

Nevertheless, the main limitation to such tests is whether the tumor is shedding sufficient DNA to detect and whether in such cases the low levels of tumor DNA can be discriminated from the biological background. This is particularly true in the surveillance setting where field change is highly pertinent. Field changes, combined with recurrent tumors generally being smaller when detected during active surveillance, generally lead to decreased test sensitivity and specificity for surveillance compared with initial diagnosis (albeit, novel tumor clones may be detected by highly sensitive genome-wide testing approaches and result in high sensitivity and specificity). However, the persistence (or reappearance) of DNA biomarkers in NMIBC patients following treatment is predictive of subsequent recurrence ("anticipatory diagnosis") and may signal a requirement for increased surveillance (Ward et al. 2023).

18.9.1 Copy Number Variation (CNV)

With the exception of a few low-grade NMIBCs, copy number changes occur in virtually all BCs (Hurst et al. 2017). The fraction of the genome altered is typically low in low-grade tumors but most have some changes including, commonly, losses of chromosome 9. High-grade tumors have extensive and large-scale losses and gains, and focal deletions and amplifications. Bladder cancer associated copy number changes have been detected in urinary DNA by array-based approaches and shallow whole genome sequencing (WGS); they appear to be better observed in urine supernatant rather than pellet DNA (Togneri et al. 2016). One of the first DNA-based urine tests to be commercialized, BCA-1, was based on CNVs (Larré et al. 2011).

Genome-wide approaches are required as there are few highly recurrent CNVs. Although CNVs are strong candidates as biomarkers (or as an element of a biomarker panel) they are challenging to detect when tumor DNA only represents a small fraction of the total DNA in a urine sample as one is searching for changes in levels rather than the appearance of new mutations/methylation. This requirement for high tumor DNA content in the sample (likely 5–10% tumor DNA required) limits the utility of CNV-based tests.

18.9.2 DNA Methylation

Changes in DNA methylation are considered amongst the earliest events in carcinogenesis (Jones and Baylin 2007). Detection of bladder cancer using DNA methylation was reported as early as 2002 (Chan et al. 2002). Since then, the number of studies that have proposed individual methylation biomarkers or panels of methylation sites as diagnostic tests for bladder cancer is too numerous to list; however, selected publications since 2018–2023 are shown in Table 18.1. Many genes repeatedly appear in these studies, but new methylation markers continue to be reported; it is likely that, in addition to global hypomethylation, there are hundreds or thousands of regions of the genome that are frequently hypermethylated in BC, and that there is an almost infinite number of combinations of these biomarkers that could represent sensitive and specific urinary biomarker panels. Studies using combinations of 2–150 methylation markers to detect BC often report extremely high sensitivity (particularly for high-grade disease) at high specificity (approaching 100%) (Feber et al. 2017; Xiao et al. 2022). However, a widespread consensus on the best combination of these biomarkers has not emerged and few of the tests have progressed from the research phase into thorough validation, commercialization, and clinical uptake. It is unclear whether a small methylation panel (e.g., 2–10 biomarkers measurable by methylation-specific PCR or restriction digest) will be sufficient to capture BC heterogeneity, or if much larger panels (or even genome-wide analysis) involving the cost and complexity of next generation sequencing are required. One methylation test which

Table 18.1 Publications reporting urine DNA methylation for BC diagnosis (2018–2023). Publications based on BC surveillance, or which were inadequately reported have been excluded

Study	Method	Targets	Substrate	No. cases	No. control	Sens (%)	Spec (%)
Wang et al. (2023)	Bisulfite sWGS	Genome-wide	Pellet	109	97[a]	90.8	81.4
Oh et al. (2022)	Bisulfite qMSP	*PENK*	Pellet	55	114[a,b]	76.4	92.5
Pharo et al. (2022)	Bisulfite ddPCR	8 markers	Pellet	93	180[c]	92.1	93.3
Xiao et al. (2022)	Bisulfite amplicon NGS	19 markers	Cell-free	85	72[e]	87.5	100
Deng et al. (2022)	Bisulfite qMSP	*DMRTA2*	Not stated	79	304[b]	78.5	92.1
Fang et al. (2022)	Bisulfite qMSP	*PCDH17, POU4F2, PENK*	Pellet	54	50[e]	87	97
Hentschel et al. (2022)	Bisulfite qMSP	*GHSR, MAL*	Pellet	108	100[d]	80	93
Georgopoulos et al. (2021)	Bisulfite qMSP	*RASSF1, RARB, DAPK, TERT, APC*	Pellet	44	22[d]	61	86
Ruan et al. (2021)	qMSP	*VIM* and *ONECUT2*	Pellet	34	140[c]	91.2	85.7
Piatti et al. (2021)	MSRE-qPCR	*TRNA-Cys, SIM2, NKX1-1*	Not stated	77	136[e]	93.5	92.6
Chen et al. (2020)	MassARRAY	cg21472506 and cg11437784	Pellet	251	237[a]	90.0	83.1
Hermanns et al. (2020)	qMSP	*NID2* and *TWIST1*	Pellet	211	102[a]	76.2	83.3
Wu et al. (2020)	Bisulfite HRM PCR	*HOXA9, PCDH17, POU4F2, ONECUT2*	Pellet	53	58[c]	90.5	73.2
Cheng et al. (2019)	Bisulfite sWGS	Genome-wide	Cell-free	46	39[c]	93.5	95.8

Methods: Bisulfite, bisulfite-modification of DNA; sWGS, shallow whole genome sequencing; qMSP, quantitative methylation-specific real-time polymerase chain reaction (PCR); ddPCR, droplet digital PCR; NGS, next generation sequencing; MSRE, methylation-sensitive restriction enzymes; HRM, high-resolution melting-curve

Nature of controls:

[a]Non-cancer hospital patients

[b]Non-BC urology patients

[c]Non-BC hematuria patients

[d]Age/sex-matched healthy donors

[e]Unknown controls

does appear to be gaining traction in Europe is the Bladder Epicheck test which is based on a proprietary panel of 15 genes and provides 74% sensitivity at 84% specificity in the NMIBC surveillance setting (Laukhtina et al. 2021).

18.9.3 Mutations

High-grade bladder cancers have high tumor mutation burden (TMB), and even low-grade NMIBCs harbor hundreds of exonic somatic mutations (single nucleotide variants; SNVs) (Goel et al. 2022). However, although there may be hundreds to thousands of SNVs in any given bladder tumor, tumor DNA may only comprise a small fraction of urine DNA and, therefore, these mutations are potentially only present at very low variant allele frequencies (VAFs) (Ward et al. 2023). Currently, WGS is too expensive and too error-prone to use for identifying mutations in urine. Decreasing costs, better sequencing accuracy, and using artificial intelligence to search for patterns of mutations in urine WGS data could prove an effective approach for bladder cancer testing in the future; however, for the time-being, most tests focus on the most frequently-mutated genes in bladder cancer. These comprise oncogenes with missense mutation hotspots, genes with non-coding mutation hotspots of unknown significance, and tumor suppressor genes (TSGs) typically with truncating mutations distributed throughout their coding sequence (Table 18.2). By focusing on frequently-mutated genes (in combination with ultra-deep sequencing and unique molecular identifiers, UMIs), the vast majority of tumors can be detected without paired germline sequencing (Ward et al. 2019, 2023), while reducing sequencing costs and false positives due to non-tumor-derived alterations (polymorphisms, clonal hematopoiesis, non-driver mutations in non-tumor urothelium) or sequencing errors.

PCR-based approaches can be used to detect individual SNVs but, with limited multiplexing potential, are only useful for the most frequent hotspots (Table 18.3) or for use in tumor-informed disease monitoring. The most common SNVs in BC are in the *TERT* promoter (approximately 60% of BCs are positive for chr5:1295228 G/A and up to 80% are positive if other nearby SNVs are included). Thus, the *TERT* promoter is a key

Table 18.2 Genes mutated in >15% BCs. Frequency data is taken from analysis of cancer genes in 1313 BC patients, predominantly with high-grade and muscle-invasive BCs (Clinton et al. 2022) and from analysis of non-coding mutation hotpots in a mixed cohort of 302 BCs (Jeeta et al. 2019). One or more of the cancer genes shown are mutated in 95% of BCs and the non-coding mutation hotspots in 74% of BCs. TSG mutation frequencies tend to be much lower and *FGFR3* mutation frequency higher in low-grade disease (van Rhijn et al. 2001)

Gene	%	Ref	Function	Hotspots/distributed
TERT	74	Clinton et al. (2022)	SNVs in promoter region: increased expression	Hotspots
ADGRG6	53	Jeeta et al. (2019)	Non-coding SNVs, unknown function	Hotspots
TP53	50	Clinton et al. (2022)	Missense & truncating mutations	Distributed
PLEKHS1	39	Jeeta et al. (2019)	Non-coding, unknown function	Hotspots
KDM6A	32	Clinton et al. (2022)	Truncating mutations	Distributed
ARID1A	30	Clinton et al. (2022)	Truncating mutations	Distributed
KMT2D	27	Clinton et al. (2022)	Truncating mutations	Distributed
FGFR3	24	Clinton et al. (2022)	Activating missense SNVs increasing activity	Hotspots
LEPROTL1	24	Jeeta et al. (2019)	Non-coding, unknown function	Hotspots
TBC1D12	26	Jeeta et al. (2019)	Non-coding, unknown function	Hotspots
PIK3CA	21	Clinton et al. (2022)	Activating missense SNVs increasing activity	Hotspots
RB1	18	Clinton et al. (2022)	Truncating mutations	Distributed
WDR74	17	Jeeta et al. (2019)	Non-coding, unknown function	Hotspots
ELF3	15	Clinton et al. (2022)	Truncating mutations	Distributed

Table 18.3 Hotspots mutated in >10% of BCs. Frequencies are based on targeted sequencing of BCs all stages and grades (Jeeta et al. 2019; Ward et al. 2019). Many are of unknown consequence but are not detectable in urine in the absence of BC (Baxter et al. 2023). Most of the mutations are due to APOBEC mutagenesis (Jeeta et al. 2019; Shi et al. 2020); the cause of *TERT* promoter mutations is currently unknown

Gene	Frequency (%)	Mutation	APOBEC	Genomic coordinates (Hg37)
TERT	61	Promoter	N	chr5:1295228 G/A
ADGRG6	39	Non-coding	Y	chr6:142706206 G/A
FGFR3	26	Missense (S249C)	Y	chr4:1803568 C/G
ADGRG6	23	Non-coding	Y	chr6:142706209 C/T
PLEKHS1	22	Non-coding	Y	chr10:115511590 G/A
PLEKHS1	19	Non-coding	Y	chr10:115511593 C/T
TBC1D12	14	Non-coding	Y	chr10:96162368 C/T
TBC1D12	14	Non-coding	Y	chr10:96162370 G/A
TERT	13	Promoter	N	chr5:1295250 G/A
WDR54	12	Non-coding	Y	chr11:62609254 G/A
LEPROTL1	12	Non-coding	Y	chr8:29952919 G/A
LEPROTL1	11	Non-coding	Y	chr8:29952921 C/T
PIK3CA	11	Missense (E545K)	Y	chr3:178936091 G/A

constituent of any mutation-based test. Moreover, these mutations are so common that a digital droplet PCR assay for *TERT* promoter mutations has been developed as an inexpensive way to detect bladder cancers (Hosen et al. 2020), although additional biomarkers will be needed to achieve >80% sensitivity. Massively parallel sequencing approaches are better suited to multiplexed mutation detection than PCR (Ward and Bryan 2019). Such approaches use either multiplex PCR-based or capture-based enrichment of the regions of interest in the genome, and then ultra-deep sequencing to detect the mutations. Unique molecular identifiers or complex bioinformatic approaches are used to enable detection of mutations at VAFs well below sequencing error rates. Such targeted sequencing has been shown to reliably detect tumor mutations in paired tumor-urine samples (e.g., Zhang et al. 2021), but sensitivity and specificity for bladder cancer detection has only been presented in a few studies (Dudley et al. 2018; Springer et al. 2018; Ou et al. 2020; Ward et al. 2023). It is likely that a panel of a few tens of genes would provide high sensitivity (Table 18.2) at high specificity, whereas larger panels may provide more in-depth molecular characterization (e.g., TMB) but at additional expense and at the risk of reduced specificity (more sequencing results in a higher risk of false-positive mutation calls).

Increasingly, DNA-based BC detection tests using mutations and/or methylation markers are being commercialized and are available to clinicians and patients; a selection of these is summarized in Table 18.4.

18.10 Conclusion and Outlook

As illustrated in this book, the last 10–15 years have seen a vast expansion in our knowledge of the biology of BC. Among other things, this has produced a raft of nucleic acid biomarkers, many of which are directly mechanistically linked to BC. Alterations in the levels of urine DNA methylation can be used to detect BC very accurately and the presence/absence of mutations can also produce high sensitivity and specificity; such mutation data are intuitive and informative. Using a combination of epigenomic and genomic markers may ultimately be the optimal approach. By detecting these biomarkers using analytically sensitive technologies, such as massively parallel sequencing and digital PCR, potentially in conjunction with the latest imaging methods (Panebianco et al. 2018; Del Giudice et al. 2022), we may, in the very near future, revolutionize the decades-old clinical pathways experienced by BC patients (Bryan et al. 2021).

The current generation of DNA-based biomarkers perform well (Table 18.4) and large-scale trials of how these can be incorporated into clinical practice are required. However, these tests mostly rely on small panels of biomarkers, whereas, in the future, faster, cheaper, and more accurate sequencing in conjunction with advanced data analysis may allow WGS of urine DNA to be the method of choice for accurate BC detection, characterization, and treatment selection. Proteomics and metabolomics also show promise as sensitive and specific diagnostic urinary biomarkers, especially for POC testing, but identification of BC specific molecules has proven challenging thus far.

Artificial intelligence approaches may automate and perpetuate our infatuation with urine cytology and our historical "need" to see cancer in order to diagnose it. Excitingly, incorporation of urine biomarkers for BC detection is almost within reach. While there is still the potential to find better biomarkers (or combinations of biomarkers) and better ways to measure them, the current generation of DNA biomarkers represent the most frequent genomic and epigenomic alterations in BC: we are now at a point where multicenter validation and studying the benefits of their incorporation into clinical practice should be addressed. Moreover, the potential for genuine clinical impact can only be robustly evaluated through interventional randomized studies investigating changes to clinical pathways with outcomes that document clinical benefit (including time to correct treatment) alongside health-related quality of life and economic benefit. As with multiparametric MRI scanning for BC staging (Panebianco et al. 2018; Bryan et al. 2021),

Table 18.4 Examples of commercially available DNA-based multi-marker urine tests for bladder cancer. Overview of marker type and targets, substrates, disease setting, and performance (based on at least one test set of samples not involved in model training)

Test name	Marker type	Targets	Substrate	Setting	No. of cases/ controls	Sens (%)	Spec (%)	Ref
AssureMDx	SNVs + methylation	*TERT, FGFR3, HRAS + OTX1, ONECUT2, TWIST1*	cpDNA	Hematuria	112/726[a]	96	73	van Kessel et al. (2020)
Bladder Care	Methylation	*TRNA-Cys, SIM2, NKX1-1*	Urine DNA	Hematuria	77/136[c]	94	93	Piatti et al. (2021)
Bladder EpiCheck	Methylation	15 proprietary markers	cpDNA	NMIBC surveillance	92/340[b]	64	82	Trenti et al. (2019)
GALEAS Bladder	SNVs	30 genes	cpDNA	Hematuria	165/264[a]	87	85	Ward et al. (2023)
UroAmp	SNVs, CNVs, indels, LOH, aneuploidy	Focus on 60 genes + genome-wide	Total urine DNA	Hematuria	22/96[a]	95	90	Salari et al. (2023)
Uromonitor-V2	SNVs	*TERT, FGFR3, KRAS*	Filtered cellular DNA	NMIBC surveillance	29/68[b]	93	85	Sieverink et al. (2020)

SNVs, single nucleotide variants; CNVs, copy number variants; indels, DNA insertions and deletions; LOH, loss of heterozygosity; sens, sensitivity; spec, specificity; ref, references; cpDNA, urine cell pellet DNA
Nature of controls:
[a]Non-BC hematuria patients
[b]Recurrence-free NMIBC surveillance patients
[c]Unknown controls

the field now needs to venture beyond simply defining sensitivity and specificity for disease detection.

References

Aine M, Sjodahl G, Eriksson P, Veerla S, Lindgren D, Ringner M, Hoglund M (2015) Integrative epigenomic analysis of differential DNA methylation in urothelial carcinoma. Genome Med 7(1):23

Alexandrov LB, Nik-Zainal S, Wedge DC, Aparicio SA, Behjati S, Biankin AV, Bignell GR, Bolli N, Borg A, Borresen-Dale AL, Boyault S, Burkhardt B, Butler AP, Caldas C, Davies HR, Desmedt C, Eils R, Eyfjord JE, Foekens JA, Greaves M, Hosoda F, Hutter B, Ilicic T, Imbeaud S, Imielinski M, Jager N, Jones DT, Jones D, Knappskog S, Kool M, Lakhani SR, Lopez-Otin C, Martin S, Munshi NC, Nakamura H, Northcott PA, Pajic M, Papaemmanuil E, Paradiso A, Pearson JV, Puente XS, Raine K, Ramakrishna M, Richardson AL, Richter J, Rosenstiel P, Schlesner M, Schumacher TN, Span PN, Teague JW, Totoki Y, Tutt AN, Valdes-Mas R, van Buuren MM, van't Veer L, Vincent-Salomon A, Waddell N, Yates LR, Zucman-Rossi J, Futreal PA, McDermott U, Lichter P, Meyerson M, Grimmond SM, Siebert R, Campo E, Shibata T, Pfister SM, Campbell PJ, Stratton MR (2013) Signatures of mutational processes in human cancer. Nature 500(7463):415–421

Arnold Egloff SA, Du L, Loomans HA, Starchenko A, Su PF, Ketova T, Knoll PB, Wang J, Haddad AQ, Fadare O, Cates JM, Lotan Y, Shyr Y, Clark PE, Zijlstra A (2017) Shed urinary ALCAM is an independent prognostic biomarker of three-year overall survival after cystectomy in patients with bladder cancer. Oncotarget 8(1):722–741

Babjuk M, Burger M, Capoun O, Cohen D, Comperat EM, Dominguez Escrig JL, Gontero P, Liedberg F, Masson-Lecomte A, Mostafid AH, Palou J, van Rhijn BWG, Roupret M, Shariat SF, Seisen T, Soukup V, Sylvester RJ (2022) European Association of Urology guidelines on non-muscle-invasive bladder cancer (Ta, T1, and carcinoma in situ). Eur Urol 81(1):75–94

Babu S, Kim NW, Wu M, Chan I, Escobar-Hoyos LF, Shroyer KR (2021) Keratin 17 is a novel cytologic biomarker for urothelial carcinoma diagnosis. Am J Clin Pathol 156(5):926–933

Baxter L, Gordon N, Ott S, Wang J, Patel P, Goel A, Piechocki K, Silcock L, Sale C, Zeegers M, Cheng K, James N, Bryan R, Ward D (2023) Properties of non-coding mutation hotspots as urinary biomarkers for bladder cancer detection. Sci Rep 13(1). https://doi.org/10.1038/s41598-41023-27675-41594

Beukers W, van der Keur KA, Kandimalla R, Vergouwe Y, Steyerberg EW, Boormans JL, Jensen JB, Lorente JA, Real FX, Segersten U, Orntoft TF, Malats N, Malmstrom PU, Dyrskjot L, Zwarthoff EC (2017) FGFR3, TERT and OTX1 as a urinary biomarker combination for surveillance of patients with bladder cancer in a large prospective multicenter study. J Urol 197(6):1410–1418

Bicocca VT, Phillips KG, Fischer DS, Caruso VM, Goudarzi M, Garcia-Ransom M, Lentz PS, MacBride AR, Jensen BW, Mazzarella BC, Koppie T, Korkola JE, Gray JW, Levin TG (2022) Urinary comprehensive genomic profiling correlates urothelial carcinoma mutations with clinical risk and efficacy of intervention. J Clin Med 11(19)

Brems-Eskildsen A, Zieger K, Toldbod H, Holcomb C, Higuchi R, Mansilla F, Munksgaard P, Borre M, Ørntoft T, Dyrskjøt L (2010) Prediction and diagnosis of bladder cancer recurrence based on urinary content of hTERT, SENP1, PPP1CA, and MCM5 transcripts. BMC Cancer 10:646

Bryan RT, Billingham LJ, Wallace DM (2008) Narrow-band imaging flexible cystoscopy in the detection of recurrent urothelial cancer of the bladder. BJU Int 101(6):702–705

Bryan RT, Wei W, Shimwell NJ, Collins SI, Hussain SA, Billingham LJ, Murray PG, Deshmukh N, James ND, Wallace DM, Johnson PJ, Zeegers MP, Cheng KK, Martin A, Ward DG (2011) Assessment of high-throughput high-resolution MALDI-TOF-MS of urinary peptides for the detection of muscle-invasive bladder cancer. Proteomics Clin Appl 5(9–10):493–503

Bryan RT, Zeegers MP, van Roekel EH, Bird D, Grant MR, Dunn JA, Bathers S, Iqbal G, Khan HS, Collins SI, Howman A, Deshmukh NS, James ND, Cheng KK, Wallace DM (2013) A comparison of patient and tumour characteristics in two UK bladder cancer cohorts separated by 20 years. BJU Int 112(2):169–175

Bryan RT, Liu W, Pirrie SJ, Amir R, Gallagher J, Hughes AI, Jefferson KP, Knight A, Nanton V, Mintz HP, Pope AM, Catto JWF, Patel P, James ND (2021) Comparing an imaging-guided pathway with the standard pathway for staging muscle-invasive bladder cancer: preliminary data from the BladderPath Study. Eur Urol 80(1):12–15

Chan M, Chan L, Tang N, Tong J, Lo K, Lee T, Cheung H, Wong W, Chan P, Lai F, K. To (2002) Hypermethylation of multiple genes in tumor tissues and voided urine in urinary bladder cancer patients. Clin Cancer Res 8(2):464–470

Chen X, Zhang J, Ruan W, Huang M, Wang C, Wang H, Jiang Z, Wang S, Liu Z, Liu C, Tan W, Yang J, Chen J, Chen Z, Li X, Zhang X, Xu P, Chen L, Xie R, Zhou Q, Xu S, Irwin D, Fan J, Huang J, Lin T (2020) Urine DNA methylation assay enables early detection and recurrence monitoring for bladder cancer. J Clin Invest 130(12):6278–6289

Cheng THT, Jiang P, Teoh JYC, Heung MMS, Tam JCW, Sun X, Lee WS, Ni M, Chan RCK, Ng CF, Chan KCA, Chiu RWK, Lo YMD (2019) Noninvasive detection of bladder cancer by shallow-depth genome-wide bisulfite sequencing of urinary cell-free DNA for methylation and copy number profiling. Clin Chem 65(7):927–936

Chou R, Gore JL, Buckley D, Fu R, Gustafson K, Griffin JC, Grusing S, Selph S (2015) Urinary biomarkers for diagnosis of bladder cancer: a systematic review and meta-analysis. Ann Intern Med 163(12):922–931

Clinton T, Chen Z, Wise H, Lenis A, Chavan S, Donoghue M, Almassi N, Chu C, Dason S, Rao P, Rodrigues J, Vasani N, Ridouani F, Rosenberg J, Bajorin D, Teo M, Bochner B, Berger M, Ostrovnaya I, Pietzak E, Iyer G, Gao S, Hu W, Al-Ahmadie H, Solit D (2022) Genomic heterogeneity as a barrier to precision oncology in urothelial cancer. Cell Rep 41(12):111859

Crisafulli G, Mussolin B, Cassingena A, Montone M, Bartolini A, Barault L, Martinetti A, Morano F, Pietrantonio F, Sartore-Bianchi A, Siena S, Di Nicolantonio F, Marsoni S, Bardelli A, Siravegna G (2019) Whole exome sequencing analysis of urine trans-renal tumour DNA in metastatic colorectal cancer patients. ESMO Open 4(6)

Cumberbatch MGK, Noon AP (2019) Epidemiology, aetiology and screening of bladder cancer. Transl Androl Urol 8(1):5–11

D'Costa JJ, Goldsmith JC, Wilson JS, Bryan RT, Ward DG (2016) A systematic review of the diagnostic and prognostic value of urinary protein biomarkers in urothelial bladder cancer. Bladder Cancer 2(3):301–317

D'Costa JJ, Ward DG, Bryan RT (2017) Urinary biomarkers for the diagnosis of urothelial bladder cancer. New Horiz Transl Med 3(5):221–223

Del Giudice F, Flammia RS, Pecoraro M, Moschini M, D'Andrea D, Messina E, Pisciotti LM, De Berardinis E, Sciarra A, Panebianco V (2022) The accuracy of Vesical Imaging-Reporting and Data System (VI-RADS): an updated comprehensive multi-institutional, multi-readers systematic review and meta-analysis from diagnostic evidence into future clinical recommendations. World J Urol 40(7):1617–1628

Deng L, Chao H, Deng H, Yu Z, Zhao R, Huang L, Gong Y, Zhu Y, Wang Q, Li F, Liu L, He L, Tang Z, Liao C, Qi Y, Wang X, Zeng T, Zou H (2022) A novel and sensitive DNA methylation marker for the urine-based liquid biopsies to detect bladder cancer. BMC Cancer 22(1):510

Dermody SM, Bhambhani C, Swiecicki PL, Brenner JC, Tewari M (2022) Trans-renal cell-free tumor DNA for urine-based liquid biopsy of cancer. Front Genet 13:879108

Desaire H (2022) How (not) to generate a highly predictive biomarker panel using machine learning. J Proteome Res 21(9):2071–2074

Devlies W, de Jong JJ, Hofmann F, Bruins HM, Zuiverloon TCM, Smith EJ, Yuan Y, van Rhijn BWG, Mostafid H, Santesso N, Violette P, Omar MI (2023) The diagnostic accuracy of cystoscopy for detecting bladder cancer in adults presenting with haematuria: a systematic review from the European Association of Urology Guidelines Office. Eur Urol Focus 10(1):115–122

di Martino E, Kelly G, Roulson JA, Knowles MA (2015) Alteration of cell-cell and cell-matrix adhesion in urothelial cells: an oncogenic mechanism for mutant FGFR3. Mol Cancer Res 13(1):138–148

Ding Z, Ying W, He Y, Chen X, Jiao Y, Wang J, Zhou X (2021) lncRNA-UCA1 in the diagnosis of bladder cancer: A meta-analysis. Medicine (Baltimore) 100(11):e24805

Dong F, Shen Y, Xu T, Wang X, Gao F, Zhong S, Chen S, Shen Z (2018) Effectiveness of urine fibronectin as a non-invasive diagnostic biomarker in bladder cancer patients: a systematic review and meta-analysis. World J Surg Oncol 16(1):61

Dong Y, Zhang T, Li X, Yu F, Yu H, Shao S (2021) Urine biomarkers for the diagnosis of bladder cancer: a network meta-analysis. Urol J 18(6):623–632

Dudley J, Schroers-Martin J, Lazzareschi D, Shi W, Chen S, Esfahani M, Trivedi D, Chabon J, Chaudhuri A, Stehr H, Liu C, Lim H, Costa H, Nabet B, Sin M, Liao J, Alizadeh A, Diehn M (2018) Detection and surveillance of bladder cancer using urine tumor DNA. Cancer Discov. https://doi.org/10.1158/2159-8290.CD-18-0825

Duggan B, O'Rourke D, Anderson N, Reid CN, Watt J, O'Kane H, Boyd R, Curry D, Evans M, Stevenson M, Kurth MJ, Lamont JV, Fitzgerald P, Ruddock MW (2022) Biomarkers to assess the risk of bladder cancer in patients presenting with haematuria are gender-specific. Front Oncol 12:1009014

Edwards TJ, Dickinson AJ, Natale S, Gosling J, McGrath JS (2006) A prospective analysis of the diagnostic yield resulting from the attendance of 4020 patients at a protocol-driven haematuria clinic. BJU Int 97(2):301–305

Fang Q, Zhang X, Nie Q, Hu J, Zhou S, Wang C (2022) Improved urine DNA methylation panel for early bladder cancer detection. BMC Cancer 22(1):237

Feber A, Dhami P, Dong L, de Winter P, Tan W, Martínez-Fernández M, Paul D, Hynes-Allen A, Rezaee S, Gurung P, Rodney S, Mehmood A, Villacampa F, de la Rosa F, Jameson C, Cheng K, Zeegers M, Bryan R, James N, Paramio J, Freeman A, Beck S, Kelly J (2017) UroMark-a urinary biomarker assay for the detection of bladder cancer. Clin Epigenet 9:8

Garinet S, Pignot G, Vacher S, Le Goux C, Schnitzler A, Chemlali W, Sirab N, Barry Delongchamps N, Zerbib M, Sibony M, Allory Y, Damotte D, Bieche I (2019) High prevalence of a hotspot of noncoding somatic mutations in intron 6 of GPR126 in bladder cancer. Mol Cancer Res 17(2):469–475

Georgopoulos P, Papaioannou M, Markopoulou S, Fragou A, Kouvatseas G, Apostolidis A (2021) DNA hypermethylation af a panel of genes as an urinary biomarker for bladder cancer diagnosis. Urol J 19(3):21–220

Glas AS, Roos D, Deutekom M, Zwinderman AH, Bossuyt PM, Kurth KH (2003) Tumor markers in the diagnosis of primary bladder cancer. A systematic review. J Urol 169(6):1975–1982

Goel A, Ward DG, Gordon NS, Abbotts B, Zeegers MP, Cheng KK, James ND, Bryan RT, Arnold R (2020) Back-splicing transcript isoforms (circular RNAs) affect biologically relevant pathways and offer an additional layer of information to stratify NMIBC patients. Front Oncol 10:812

Goel A, Ward DG, Noyvert B, Yu M, Gordon NS, Abbotts B, Colbourne JK, Kissane S, James ND, Zeegers MP, Cheng KK, Cazier JB, Whalley CM, Beggs AD, Palles C, Arnold R, Bryan RT (2022) Combined exome and transcriptome sequencing of non-muscle-invasive bladder cancer: associations between genomic changes, expression subtypes, and clinical outcomes. Genome Med 14(1):59

Hajdinjak T (2008) UroVysion FISH test for detecting urothelial cancers: meta-analysis of diagnostic accuracy and comparison with urinary cytology testing. Urol Oncol 26(6):646–651

Han H, Jiang X (2014) Overcome support vector machine diagnosis overfitting. Cancer Inform 13(Suppl 1):145–158

Hentschel A, Beijert I, Bosschieter J, Kauer P, Vis A, Lissenberg-Witte B, van Moorselaar R, Steenbergen R, Nieuwenhuijzen J (2022) Bladder cancer detection in urine using DNA methylation markers: a technical and prospective preclinical validation. Clin Epigenet 14(1). https://doi.org/10.1186/s13148-13022-01240-13148

Hermanns T, Savio A, Olkhov-Mitsel E, Mari A, Wettstein M, Saba K, Bhindi B, Kuk C, Poyet C, Wild P, Noon A, Bashir S, Juvet T, Rendon R, Waltregny D, van der Kwast T, Finelli A, Kulkarni G, Fleshner N, Lo K, Bapat B, Zlotta A (2020) A noninvasive urine-based methylation biomarker panel to detect bladder cancer and discriminate cancer grade. Urol Oncol 38(6):603.e601–603.e607

Hirasawa Y, Pagano I, Chen R, Sun Y, Dai Y, Gupta A, Tikhonenkov S, Goodison S, Rosser CJ, Furuya H (2021) Diagnostic performance of Oncuria, a urinalysis test for bladder cancer. J Transl Med 19(1):141

Hosen MI, Forey N, Durand G, Voegele C, Bilici S, Avogbe PH, Delhomme TM, Foll M, Manel A, Vian E, Meziani S, De Tilly B, Polo G, Lole O, Francois P, Boureille A, Pisarev E, Salas A, Monteiro-Reis S, Henrique R, Byrnes G, Jeronimo C, Scelo G, McKay JD, Calvez-Kelm FL, Zvereva M (2020) Development of sensitive droplet digital PCR assays for detecting urinary TERT promoter mutations as non-invasive biomarkers for detection of urothelial cancer. Cancers (Basel) 12(12)

Hu D, Xu X, Zhao Z, Li C, Tian Y, Liu Q, Shao B, Chen S, Zhao Y, Li L, Bi H, Chen A, Fu C, Cui X, Zeng Y (2021) Detecting urine metabolites of bladder cancer by surface-enhanced Raman spectroscopy. Spectrochim Acta A Mol Biomol Spectrosc 247:119108

Humayun-Zakaria N, Arnold R, Goel A, Ward D, Savill S, Bryan RT (2019) Tropomyosins: potential biomarkers for urothelial bladder cancer. Int J Mol Sci 20(5)

Humayun-Zakaria N, Ward DG, Arnold R, Bryan RT (2021) Trends in urine biomarker discovery for urothelial bladder cancer: DNA, RNA, or protein? Transl Androl Urol 10(6):2787–2808

Hurst CD, Platt F, Taylor CF, Knowles MA (2012) Novel tumor subgroups of urothelial carcinoma of the bladder defined by integrated genomic analysis. Clin Cancer Res 18(21):5865–5877

Hurst C, Alder O, Platt F, Droop A, Stead L, Burns J, Burghel G, Jain S, Klimczak L, Lindsay H, Roulson J, Taylor C, Thygesen H, Cameron A, Ridley A, Mott H, Gordenin D, Knowles M (2017) Genomic subtypes of non-invasive bladder cancer with distinct metabolic profile and female gender bias in KDM6A mutation frequency. Cancer Cell 32(5):701–715

James ND, Hussain SA, Hall E, Jenkins P, Tremlett J, Rawlings C, Crundwell M, Sizer B, Sreenivasan T, Hendron C, Lewis R, Waters R, Huddart RA (2012) Radiotherapy with or without chemotherapy in muscle-invasive bladder cancer. N Engl J Med 366(16):1477–1488

Jeeta R, Gordon N, Baxter L, Goel A, Noyvert B, Ott S, Boucher R, Humayun-Zakaria N, Arnold R, James N, Zeegers M, Cheng K, Bryan RT, Ward D (2019) Non-coding mutations in urothelial bladder cancer: biological and clinical relevance and potential utility as biomarkers. Bladder Cancer 5(4):263–272

Jones P, Baylin S (2007) The epigenomics of cancer. Cell 128(4):683–692

Khadhouri S, Gallagher KM, MacKenzie KR, Shah TT, Gao C, Moore S, Zimmermann EF, Edison E, Jefferies M, Nambiar A, Mannas MP, Lee T, Marra G, Lillaz B, Gomez Rivas J, Olivier J, Assmus MA, Ucar T, Claps F, Boltri M, Burnhope T, Nkwam N, Tanasescu G, Boxall NE, Downey AP, Lal AA, Anton-Juanilla M, Clarke H, Lau DHW, Gillams K, Crockett M, Nielsen M, Takwoingi Y, Chuchu N, O'Rourke J, MacLennan G, McGrath JS, Kasivisvanathan V, IDENTIFY Study Group (2021) The IDENTIFY study: the investigation and detection of urological neoplasia in patients referred with suspected urinary tract cancer—a multicentre observational study. BJU Int 128(4):440–450

Khan SR, Manialawy Y, Wheeler MB, Cox BJ (2019) Unbiased data analytic strategies to improve biomarker discovery in precision medicine. Drug Discov Today 24(9):1735–1748

Kompier L, Lurkin I, van der Aa M, van Rhijn B, van der Kwast T, Zwarthoff E (2010) FGFR3, HRAS, KRAS, NRAS and PIK3CA mutations in bladder cancer and their potential as biomarkers for surveillance and therapy. PLoS One 5(11):e13821

Larré S, Camparo P, Comperat E, De Medina SGD, Traxer O, Roupret M, Sebe P, Cancel-Tassin G, Sighar K, Lozach F, Cussenot O (2011) Diagnostic, staging, and grading of urothelial carcinomas from urine: performance of BCA-1, a mini-array comparative genomic hybridisation-based test. Eur Urol 59(2):250–257

Larre S, Catto JW, Cookson MS, Messing EM, Shariat SF, Soloway MS, Svatek RS, Lotan Y, Zlotta AR, Grossman HB (2013) Screening for bladder cancer: rationale, limitations, whom to target, and perspectives. Eur Urol 63(6):1049–1058

Laukhtina E, Shim S, Mori K, D'Andrea D, Soria F, Rajwa P, Mostafaei H, Compérat E, Cimadamore A, Moschini M, Teoh J, Enikeev D, Xylinas E, Lotan Y, Palou J, Gontero P, Babjuk M, Witjes J, Kamat A, Roupret M, Shariat S, Pradere B, European Association of Urology–Young Academic Urologists (EAU-YAU): Urothelial Carcinoma Working Group (2021) Diagnostic accuracy of novel urinary biomarker tests in non-muscle-invasive bladder cancer: a systematic review and network meta-analysis. Eur Urol Oncol 4(6):927–942

Lawson ARJ, Abascal F, Coorens THH, Hooks Y, O'Neill L, Latimer C, Raine K, Sanders MA, Warren AY, Mahbubani KTA, Bareham B, Butler TM, Harvey LMR, Cagan A, Menzies A, Moore L, Colquhoun AJ, Turner W, Thomas B, Gnanapragasam V, Williams N, Rassl DM, Vohringer H, Zumalave S, Nangalia J, Tubio JMC, Gerstung M, Saeb-Parsy K, Stratton MR, Campbell PJ, Mitchell TJ, Martincorena I (2020) Extensive heterogeneity in somatic mutation and selection in the human bladder. Science 370(6512):75–82

Leal J, Luengo-Fernandez R, Sullivan R, Witjes JA (2016) Economic burden of bladder cancer across the European Union. Eur Urol 69(3):438–447

Lee S, Jeong J, Majewski T, Scherer SE, Kim MS, Tuziak T, Tang KS, Baggerly K, Grossman HB, Zhou JH, Shen L, Bondaruk J, Ahmed SS, Samanta S, Spiess P, Wu X, Filipek S, McConkey D, Bar-Eli M, Issa JP, Benedict WF, Czerniak B (2007) Forerunner genes contiguous to RB1 contribute to the development of in situ neoplasia. Proc Natl Acad Sci USA 104(34):13732–13737

Lett L, George M, Slater R, De Lacy Costello B, Ratcliffe N, Garcia-Finana M, Lazarowicz H, Probert C (2022) Investigation of urinary volatile organic compounds as novel diagnostic and surveillance biomarkers of bladder cancer. Br J Cancer 127(2):329–336

Li R, Du Y, Chen Z, Xu D, Lin T, Jin S, Wang G, Liu Z, Lu M, Chen X, Xu T, Bai F (2020) Macroscopic somatic clonal expansion in morphologically normal human urothelium. Science 370(6512):82–89

Li J, Cheng B, Xie H, Zhan C, Li S, Bai P (2022) Bladder cancer biomarker screening based on non-targeted urine metabolomics. Int Urol Nephrol 54(1):23–29

Lin JY, Juo BR, Yeh YH, Fu SH, Chen YT, Chen CL, Wu KP (2021) Putative markers for the detection of early-stage bladder cancer selected by urine metabolomics. BMC Bioinformatics 22(1):305

Lindskrog SV, Prip F, Lamy P, Taber A, Groeneveld CS, Birkenkamp-Demtroder K, Jensen JB, Strandgaard T, Nordentoft I, Christensen E, Sokac M, Birkbak NJ,

Maretty L, Hermann GG, Petersen AC, Weyerer V, Grimm MO, Horstmann M, Sjodahl G, Hoglund M, Steiniche T, Mogensen K, de Reynies A, Nawroth R, Jordan B, Lin X, Dragicevic D, Ward DG, Goel A, Hurst CD, Raman JD, Warrick JI, Segersten U, Sikic D, van Kessel KEM, Maurer T, Meeks JJ, DeGraff DJ, Bryan RT, Knowles MA, Simic T, Hartmann A, Zwarthoff EC, Malmstrom PU, Malats N, Real FX, Dyrskjot L (2021) An integrated multi-omics analysis identifies prognostic molecular subtypes of non-muscle-invasive bladder cancer. Nat Commun 12(1):2301

Lindskrog SV, Schmokel SS, Nordentoft I, Lamy P, Knudsen M, Prip F, Strandgaard T, Jensen JB, Dyrskjot L (2023) Single-nucleus and spatially resolved intratumor subtype heterogeneity in bladder cancer. Eur Urol Open Sci 51:78–88

Liu C, Shi B, Hao C, Wang Q, Lv Q, Xing N, Shou J, Qu L, Gao Y, Qin C, Zhao J, Shou C (2016) Urine gamma-synuclein as a biomarker for the diagnosis of bladder cancer. Oncotarget 7(28):43432–43441

Loras A, Suarez-Cabrera C, Martinez-Bisbal MC, Quintas G, Paramio JM, Martinez-Manez R, Gil S, Ruiz-Cerda JL (2019) Integrative metabolomic and transcriptomic analysis for the study of bladder cancer. Cancers (Basel) 11(5)

Majewski T, Lee S, Jeong J, Yoon DS, Kram A, Kim MS, Tuziak T, Bondaruk J, Lee S, Park WS, Tang KS, Chung W, Shen L, Ahmed SS, Johnston DA, Grossman HB, Dinney CP, Zhou JH, Harris RA, Snyder C, Filipek S, Narod SA, Watson P, Lynch HT, Gazdar A, Bar-Eli M, Wu XF, McConkey DJ, Baggerly K, Issa JP, Benedict WF, Scherer SE, Czerniak B (2008) Understanding the development of human bladder cancer by using a whole-organ genomic mapping strategy. Lab Invest 88(7):694–721

Mitra AP, Cote RJ (2010) Molecular screening for bladder cancer: progress and potential. Nat Rev Urol 7(1):11–20

Mowatt G, Zhu S, Kilonzo M, Boachie C, Fraser C, Griffiths TR, N'Dow J, Nabi G, Cook J, Vale L (2010) Systematic review of the clinical effectiveness and cost-effectiveness of photodynamic diagnosis and urine biomarkers (FISH, ImmunoCyt, NMP22) and cytology for the detection and follow-up of bladder cancer. Health Technol Assess 14(4):1–iv

Murakami K, Pagano I, Chen R, Sun Y, Goodison S, Rosser CJ, Furuya H (2021) Influencing factors on the Oncuria urinalysis assay: an experimental model. Diagnostics (Basel) 11(6)

Murphy WM (1977) Falsely positive urinary cytology: pathologist's error or preclinical cancer? J Urol 118(5):811–813

Ng K, Stenzl A, Sharma A, Vasdev N (2021) Urinary biomarkers in bladder cancer: A review of the current landscape and future directions. Urol Oncol 39(1):41–51

Nikas IP, Seide S, Proctor T, Kleinaki Z, Kleinaki M, Reynolds JP (2022) The Paris system for reporting urinary cytology: a meta-analysis. J Pers Med 12(2)

Oh T, Lim E, Bang B, Lee J, Na Y, Shin Y, Lim J, Song K, An S (2022) Identification and validation of methylated PENK gene for early detection of bladder cancer using urine DNA. BMC Cancer 22(1):1195

Oto J, Fernandez-Pardo A, Roca M, Plana E, Cana F, Herranz R, Perez-Ardavin J, Vera-Donoso CD, Martinez-Sarmiento M, Medina P (2022) LC-MS metabolomics of urine reveals distinct profiles for non-muscle-invasive and muscle-invasive bladder cancer. World J Urol 40(10):2387–2398

Ou Z, Li K, Yang T, Dai Y, Chandra M, Ning J, Wang Y, Xu R, Gao T, Xie Y, He Q, Li Y, Lu Q, Wang L, Song Z (2020) Detection of bladder cancer using urinary cell-free DNA and cellular DNA. Clin Transl Med 9(1):4

Panebianco V, Narumi Y, Altun E, Bochner BH, Efstathiou JA, Hafeez S, Huddart R, Kennish S, Lerner S, Montironi R, Muglia VF, Salomon G, Thomas S, Vargas HA, Witjes JA, Takeuchi M, Barentsz J, Catto JWF (2018) Multiparametric magnetic resonance imaging for bladder cancer: development of VI-RADS (vesical imaging-reporting and data system). Eur Urol 74(3):294–306

Patel P, Bryan RT, Wallace DM (2011) Emerging endoscopic and photodynamic techniques for bladder cancer detection and surveillance. ScientificWorldJournal 11:2550–2558

Pavlova NN, Thompson CB (2016) The emerging hallmarks of cancer metabolism. Cell Metab 23(1):27–47

Pharo H, Jeanmougin M, Ager-Wick E, Vedeld H, Sørbø A, Dahl C, Larsen L, Honne H, Brandt-Winge S, Five M, Monteiro-Reis S, Henrique R, Jeronimo C, Steven K, Wahlqvist R, Guldberg P, Lind G (2022) BladMetrix: a novel urine DNA methylation test with high accuracy for detection of bladder cancer in hematuria patients. Clin Epigenet 14(1):115

Piatti P, Chew Y, Suwoto M, Yamada T, Jara B, Jia X, Guo W, Ghodoussipour S, Daneshmand S, Ahmadi H, Rice J, Bhasin J, Holloway F, Tsai Y, Chihara Y, Liang G (2021) Clinical evaluation of Bladder CARE, a new epigenetic test for bladder cancer detection in urine samples. Clin Epigenet 13(1):84

Piyarathna DWB, Rajendiran TM, Putluri V, Vantaku V, Soni T, von Rundstedt FC, Donepudi SR, Jin F, Maity S, Ambati CR, Dong J, Godde D, Roth S, Storkel S, Degener S, Michailidis G, Lerner SP, Pennathur S, Lotan Y, Coarfa C, Sreekumar A, Putluri N (2018) Distinct lipidomic landscapes associated with clinical stages of urothelial cancer of the bladder. Eur Urol Focus 4(6):907–915

Putluri N, Shojaie A, Vasu VT, Vareed SK, Nalluri S, Putluri V, Thangjam GS, Panzitt K, Tallman CT, Butler C, Sana TR, Fischer SM, Sica G, Brat DJ, Shi H, Palapattu GS, Lotan Y, Weizer AZ, Terris MK, Shariat SF, Michailidis G, Sreekumar A (2011) Metabolomic profiling reveals potential markers and bioprocesses altered in bladder cancer progression. Cancer Res 71(24):7376–7386

Qiu T, Xue M, Li X, Li F, Liu S, Yao C, Chen W (2022) Comparative evaluation of long non-coding RNA-based biomarkers in the urinary sediment and urinary exosomes for non-invasive diagnosis of bladder cancer. Mol Omics 18(10):938–947

Rachakonda P, Hosen I, de Verdier P, Fallah M, Heidenreich B, Ryk C, Wiklund N, Steineck G, Schadendorf D, Hemminki K, Kumar R (2013) TERT promoter mutations in bladder cancer affect patient survival and disease recurrence through modification by a common polymorphism. Proc Natl Acad Sci U S A 110(43):17426–17431

Robertson AG, Kim J, Al-Ahmadie H, Bellmunt J, Guo G, Cherniack AD, Hinoue T, Laird PW, Hoadley KA, Akbani R, Castro MAA, Gibb EA, Kanchi RS, Gordenin DA, Shukla SA, Sanchez-Vega F, Hansel DE, Czerniak BA, Reuter VE, Su X, de Sa CB, Chagas VS, Mungall KL, Sadeghi S, Pedamallu CS, Lu Y, Klimczak LJ, Zhang J, Choo C, Ojesina AI, Bullman S, Leraas KM, Lichtenberg TM, Wu CJ, Schultz N, Getz G, Meyerson M, Mills GB, McConkey DJ, Weinstein JN, Kwiatkowski DJ, Lerner SP (2017) Comprehensive molecular characterization of muscle-invasive bladder cancer. Cell 171(3):540–556.e25

Ruan W, Chen X, Huang M, Wang H, Chen J, Liang Z, Zhang J, Yu Y, Chen S, Xu S, Hu T, Li X, Guo Y, Jiang Z, Chen Z, Huang J, Lin T, Fan J (2021) A urine-based DNA methylation assay to facilitate early detection and risk stratification of bladder cancer. Clin Epigenet 13(1):91

Sahai R, Rajkumar B, Joshi P, Singh A, Kumar A, Durgapal P, Gupta A, Kishore S, Chowdhury N (2020) Interobserver reproducibility of The Paris System of Reporting Urine Cytology on cytocentrifuged samples. Diagn Cytopathol 48(11):979–985

Salari K, Sundi D, Lee JJ, Wu S, Wu CL, DiFiore G, Yan QR, Pienkny A, Lee CK, Oberlin D, Barme G, Piser J, Kahn R, Collins E, Phillips KG, Caruso VM, Goudarzi M, Garcia-Ransom M, Lentz PS, Evans-Holm ME, MacBride AR, Fischer DS, Haddadzadeh IJ, Mazzarella BC, Gray JW, Koppie TM, Bicocca VT, Levin TG, Lotan Y, Feldman AS (2023) Development and multicenter case-control validation of urinary comprehensive genomic profiling for urothelial carcinoma diagnosis, surveillance, and risk-prediction. Clin Cancer Res 29(18):3668–3680

Sangar VK, Ragavan N, Matanhelia SS, Watson MW, Blades RA (2005) The economic consequences of prostate and bladder cancer in the UK. BJU Int 95(1):59–63

Schmidt J, Propping C, Siow W, Lohse-Fischer A, Toma M, Baldauf-Twelker A, Hakenberg O, Wirth M, Fuessel S (2016) Diagnostic and prognostic value of bladder cancer-related transcript markers in urine. J Cancer Res Clin Oncol 142(2):401–414

Schmitz-Drager BJ, Droller M, Lokeshwar VB, Lotan Y, Hudson MA, van Rhijn BW, Marberger MJ, Fradet Y, Hemstreet GP, Malmstrom PU, Ogawa O, Karakiewicz PI, Shariat SF (2015) Molecular markers for bladder cancer screening, early diagnosis, and surveillance: the WHO/ICUD Consensus. Urol Int 94(1):1–24

Sharma G, Sharma A, Krishna M, Ahluwalia P, Gautam G (2022) Diagnostic performance of minichromosome maintenance 5 (MCM5) in bladder cancer: A systematic review and meta-analysis. Urol Oncol 40(6):235–242

Shi M-J, Meng X-Y, Fontugne J, Chen C-L, Radvanyi F, Bernard-Pierrot I (2020) Identification of new driver and passenger mutations within APOBEC-induced hotspot mutations in bladder cancer. Genome Med 12(1):85

Shimwell NJ, Bryan RT, Wei W, James ND, Cheng KK, Zeegers MP, Johnson PJ, Martin A, Ward DG (2013) Combined proteome and transcriptome analyses for the discovery of urinary biomarkers for urothelial carcinoma. Br J Cancer 108(9):1854–1861

Sidransky D, Frost P, Von EA, Oyasu R, Preisinger AC, Vogelstein B (1992) Clonal origin bladder cancer. N Engl J Med 326(11):737–740

Sieverink CA, Batista RPM, Prazeres HJM, Vinagre J, Sampaio C, Leao RR, Maximo V, Witjes JA, Soares P (2020) Clinical validation of a urine test (Uromonitor-V2((R))) for the surveillance of non-muscle-invasive bladder cancer patients. Diagnostics (Basel) 10(10)

Sirab N, Drubay D, Maille P, Popova T, Ngo C, Gentien D, Moktefi A, Soyeux-Porte P, Pelletier R, Reyes C, Henry E, Pouessel D, Vordos D, Lebret T, de Reynies A, Paoletti X, Radvanyi F, Allory Y (2022) Multilayer spectrum of intratumoral heterogeneity in basal bladder cancer. J Pathol 256(1):108–118

Sjodahl G, Lauss M, Lovgren K, Chebil G, Gudjonsson S, Veerla S, Patschan O, Aine M, Ferno M, Ringner M, Mansson W, Liedberg F, Lindgren D, Hoglund M (2012) A molecular taxonomy for urothelial carcinoma. Clin Cancer Res 18(12):3377–3386

Snell KIE, Ward DG, Gordon NS, Goldsmith JC, Sutton AJ, Patel P, James ND, Zeegers MP, Cheng KK, Bryan RT (2018) Exploring the roles of urinary HAI-1, EpCAM & EGFR in bladder cancer prognosis & risk stratification. Oncotarget 9(38):25244–25253

Springer S, Chen C, Rodriguez Pena M, Li L, Douville C, Wang Y, Cohen J, Taheri D, Silliman N, Schaefer J, Ptak J, Dobbyn L, Papoli M, Kinde I, Afsari B, Tregnago A, Bezerra S, VandenBussche C, Fujita K, Ertoy D, Cunha I, Yu L, Bivalacqua T, Grollman A, Diaz L, Karchin R, Danilova L, Huang C, Shun C, Turesky R, Yun B, Rosenquist T, Pu Y, Hruban R, Tomasetti C, Papadopoulos N, Kinzler K, Vogelstein B, Dickman K, Netto G (2018) Non-invasive detection of urothelial cancer through the analysis of driver gene mutations and aneuploidy. Elife 7:e32143

Strandgaard T, Nordentoft I, Birkenkamp-Demtroder K, Salminen L, Prip F, Rasmussen J, Andreasen TG, Lindskrog SV, Christensen E, Lamy P, Knudsen M, Steiniche T, Jensen JB, Dyrskjot L (2024) Field cancerization is associated with tumor development, T-cell exhaustion, and clinical outcomes in bladder cancer. Eur Urol 85(1):82–92

Su YH, Wang M, Brenner DE, Ng A, Melkonyan H, Umansky S, Syngal S, Block TM (2004) Human urine contains small, 150 to 250 nucleotide-sized, soluble DNA derived from the circulation and may be useful in the detection of colorectal cancer. J Mol Diagn 6(2):101–107

Suarez-Cabrera C, Estudillo L, Ramon-Gil E, Martinez-Fernandez M, Peral J, Rubio C, Lodewijk I, Martin de Bernardo A, Garcia-Escudero R, Villacampa F, Duarte J, de la Rosa F, Castellano D, Guerrero-Ramos F, Real FX, Malats N, Paramio JM, Duenas M (2022) BlaDimiR: a urine-based miRNA score for accurate bladder cancer diagnosis and follow-up. Eur Urol 82(6):663–667

Svatek RS, Hollenbeck BK, Holmang S, Lee R, Kim SP, Stenzl A, Lotan Y (2014) The economics of bladder cancer: costs and considerations of caring for this disease. Eur Urol 66(2):253–262

Sylvester RJ, Rodriguez O, Hernandez V, Turturica D, Bauerova L, Bruins HM, Brundl J, van der Kwast TH, Brisuda A, Rubio-Briones J, Seles M, Hentschel AE, Kusuma VRM, Huebner N, Cotte J, Mertens LS, Volanis D, Cussenot O, Subiela Henriquez JD, de la Pena E, Pisano F, Pesl M, van der Heijden AG, Herdegen S, Zlotta AR, Hacek J, Calatrava A, Mannweiler S, Bosschieter J, Ashabere D, Haitel A, Cote JF, El Sheikh S, Lunelli L, Algaba F, Alemany I, Soria F, Runneboom W, Breyer J, Nieuwenhuijzen JA, Llorente C, Molinaro L, Hulsbergen-van de Kaa CA, Evert M, Kiemeney L, N'Dow J, Plass K, Capoun O, Soukup V, Dominguez-Escrig JL, Cohen D, Palou J, Gontero P, Burger M, Zigeuner R, Mostafid AH, Shariat SF, Roupret M, Comperat EM, Babjuk M, van Rhijn BWG (2021) European Association of Urology (EAU) Prognostic Factor Risk Groups for Non-muscle-invasive Bladder Cancer (NMIBC) incorporating the WHO 2004/2016 and WHO 1973 classification systems for grade: an update from the EAU NMIBC Guidelines Panel. Eur Urol 79(4):480–488

Tan WS, Feber A, Sarpong R, Khetrapal P, Rodney S, Jalil R, Mostafid H, Cresswell J, Hicks J, Rane A, Henderson A, Watson D, Cherian J, Williams N, Brew-Graves C, Kelly JD, DETECT I trial collaborators (2018) Who should be investigated for haematuria? Results of a contemporary prospective observational study of 3556 patients. Eur Urol 74(1):10–14

Terasawa H, Kinugasa H, Ako S, Hirai M, Matsushita H, Uchida D, Tomoda T, Matsumoto K, Horiguchi S, Kato H, Nouso K, Okada H (2019) Utility of liquid biopsy using urine in patients with pancreatic ductal adenocarcinoma. Cancer Biol Ther 20(10):1348–1353

The Cancer Genome Atlas (2014) Comprehensive molecular characterization of urothelial bladder carcinoma. Nature 507(7492):315–322.

Togneri FS, Ward DG, Foster JM, Devall AJ, Wojtowicz P, Alyas S, Vasques FR, Oumie A, James ND, Cheng KK, Zeegers MP, Deshmukh N, O'Sullivan B, Taniere P, Spink KG, McMullan DJ, Griffiths M, Bryan RT (2016) Genomic complexity of urothelial bladder cancer revealed in urinary cfDNA. Eur J Hum Genet 24(8):1167–1174

Tomiyama E, Fujita K, Matsuzaki K, Narumi R, Yamamoto A, Uemura T, Yamamichi G, Koh Y, Matsushita M, Hayashi Y, Hashimoto M, Banno E, Kato T, Hatano K, Kawashima A, Uemura M, Ukekawa R, Takao T, Takada S, Uemura H, Adachi J, Tomonaga T, Nonomura N (2022) EphA2 on urinary extracellular vesicles as a novel biomarker for bladder cancer diagnosis and its effect on the invasiveness of bladder cancer. Br J Cancer 127(7):1312–1323

Trenti E, D'Elia C, Mian C, Schwienbacher C, Hanspeter E, Pycha A, Kafka M, Degener S, Danuser H, Roth S, Pycha A (2019) Diagnostic predictive value of the Bladder EpiCheck test in the follow-up of patients with non-muscle-invasive bladder cancer. Cancer Cytopathol 127:7

Tsai YC, Simoneau AR, Spruck CH 3rd, Nichols PW, Steven K, Buckley JD, Jones PA (1995) Mosaicism in human epithelium: macroscopic monoclonal patches cover the urothelium. J Urol 153(5):1697–1700

van Kessel K, Beukers W, Lurkin I, Ziel-van der Made A, van der Keur K, Boormans J, Dyrskjøt L, Márquez M, Ørntoft T, Real F, Segersten U, Malats N, Malmström P, Van Criekinge W, Zwarthoff E (2017) Validation of a DNA methylation-mutation urine assay to select patients with hematuria for cystoscopy. J Urol 197:590–595

van Kessel K, de Jong J, Ziel-van der Made A, Roshani H, Haensel S, Wolterbeek J, Boevé E, Oomens E, van Casteren N, Krispin M, Boormans J, Steyerberg E, van Criekinge W, Zwarthoff E (2020) A urine-based genomic assay to triage patients with hematuria for cystoscopy. J Urol 204(1):50–57

van Rhijn B, Lurkin I, Radvanyi F, Kirkels W, van der Kwast T, Zwarthoff E (2001) The fibroblast growth factor receptor 3 (FGFR3) mutation is a strong indicator of superficial bladder cancer with low recurrence rate. Cancer Res 61(4):1265–1268

van Rhijn BW, van der Poel HG, van der Kwast TH (2005) Urine markers for bladder cancer surveillance: a systematic review. Eur Urol 47(6):736–748

van Rhijn BW, Burger M, Lotan Y, Solsona E, Stief CG, Sylvester RJ, Witjes JA, Zlotta AR (2009) Recurrence and progression of disease in non-muscle-invasive bladder cancer: from epidemiology to treatment strategy. Eur Urol 56(3):430–442

Vasdev N, Hampson A, Agarwal S, Swamy R, Chilvers M, Hampson A, Jahanfard S, Kim N (2021) The role of URO17 biomarker to enhance diagnosis of urothelial cancer in new hematuria patients-First European Data. BJUI Compass 2(1):46–52

Wallace DM, Bryan RT, Dunn JA, Begum G, Bathers S (2002) Delay and survival in bladder cancer. BJU Int 89(9):868–878

Wang X, Meng Q, Wang C, Li F, Zhu Z, Liu S, Shi Y, Huang J, Chen S, Li C (2017) Investigation of transrenal KRAS mutation in late stage NSCLC patients correlates to disease progression. Biomarkers 22(7):654–660

Wang R, Kang H, Zhang X, Nie Q, Wang H, Wang C, Zhou S (2022) Urinary metabolomics for discovering metabolic biomarkers of bladder cancer by UPLC-MS. BMC Cancer 22(1):214

Wang P, Shi Y, Zhang J, Shou J, Zhang M, Zou D, Liang Y, Li J, Tan Y, Zhang M, Bi X, Zhou L, Ci W, Li X (2023) UCseek: ultrasensitive early detection and recurrence monitoring of urothelial carcinoma by shallow-depth genome-wide bisulfite sequencing of urinary sediment DNA. EBioMedicine 89:104437

Ward DG, Bryan RT (2019) Massively parallel sequencing of urinary DNA—the dawn of non-invasive bladder cancer detection and surveillance? Transl Cancer Res 8(suppl 2)

Ward D, Gordon N, Boucher R, Pirrie S, Baxter L, Ott S, Silcock L, Whalley C, Stockton J, Beggs A, Griffiths M, Abbotts B, Ijakipour H, Latheef F, Robinson R, White A, James N, Zeegers M, Cheng K, Bryan R (2019) Targeted deep sequencing of urothelial bladder cancers and associated urinary DNA: a 23-gene panel with utility for non-invasive diagnosis and risk stratification. BJU Int. 124(3):532–544

Ward D, Baxter L, Ott S, Gordon N, Wang J, Patel P, Piechocki K, Silcock L, Sale C, Zeegers M, Cheng K, James N, Bryan R, BladderPath Trial Management Group (2023) Highly sensitive and specific detection of bladder cancer via targeted ultra-deep sequencing of urinary DNA. Eur Urol Oncol 6(1):67–75

Willis CM, Church SM, Guest CM, Cook WA, McCarthy N, Bransbury AJ, Church MR, Church JC (2004) Olfactory detection of human bladder cancer by dogs: proof of principle study. BMJ 329(7468):712

Witjes JA, Bruins HM, Cathomas R, Comperat EM, Cowan NC, Gakis G, Hernandez V, Linares Espinos E, Lorch A, Neuzillet Y, Rouanne M, Thalmann GN, Veskimae E, Ribal MJ, van der Heijden AG (2021) European Association of Urology guidelines on muscle-invasive and metastatic bladder cancer: summary of the 2020 guidelines. Eur Urol 79(1):82–104

Wu Y, Jiang G, Zhang N, Liu S, Lin X, Perschon C, Zheng S, Ding Q, Wang X, Na R, Sun J, Xu J (2020) HOXA9, PCDH17, POU4F2, and ONECUT2 as a urinary biomarker combination for the detection of bladder cancer in chinese patients with hematuria. Eur Urol Focus 6(2):284–291

Xiao Y, Ju L, Qian K, Jin W, Wang G, Zhao Y, Jiang W, Nan L, Wu K, Peng M, Cao R, Li S, Shi H, Gong Y, Zheng H, Liu T, Luo Y, Ma H, Chang L, Li G, Cao X, Tian Y, Xu Z, Yang Z, Shan L, Guo Z, Yao D, Zhou X, Chen X, Guo Z, Liu D, Xu S, Ji C, Yu F, Hong X, Luo J, Cao H, Zhang Y, Wang X (2022) Non-invasive diagnosis and surveillance of bladder cancer with driver and passenger DNA methylation in a prospective cohort study. Clin Transl Med 12(8). https://doi.org/10.1002/ctm1002.1008

Xie Q, Huang Z, Zhu Z, Zheng X, Liu J, Zhang M, Zhang Y (2016) Diagnostic value of urine cytology in bladder cancer. A meta-analysis. Anal Quant Cytopathol Histpathol 38(1):38–44

Ye Q, Wang J, Xu D, Liu Y, Zhang D, Ye J, Li H (2022) Diagnostic performance of urine and blood microRNAs for bladder cancer: a meta-analysis. Expert Rev Anticancer Ther 22(12):1357–1369

Yeung C, Dinh T, Lee J (2014) The health economics of bladder cancer: an updated review of the published literature. Pharmacoeconomics 32(11):1093–1104

Yu X, Wang R, Han C, Wang Z, Jin X (2020) A panel of urinary long non-coding RNAs differentiate bladder cancer from urocystitis. J Cancer 11(4):781–787

Zhan Y, Du L, Wang L, Jiang X, Zhang S, Li J, Yan K, Duan W, Zhao Y, Wang L, Wang Y, Wang C (2018) Expression signatures of exosomal long non-coding RNAs in urine serve as novel non-invasive biomarkers for diagnosis and recurrence prediction of bladder cancer. Mol Cancer 17(1):142

Zhang R, Zang J, Xie F, Zhang Y, Wang Y, Jing Y, Zhang Y, Chen Z, Shahatiaili A, Cai M, Zhao Z, Du P, Jia S, Zhuang G, Chen H (2021) Urinary molecular pathology for patients with newly diagnosed urothelial bladder cancer. J Urol 206(4):873–884

Zheng C, Lv Y, Zhong Q, Wang R, Jiang Q (2012) Narrow band imaging diagnosis of bladder cancer: systematic review and meta-analysis. BJU Int 110(11 Pt B):E680–E687

19 Blood-Based Biomarkers for Bladder Cancer Diagnosis and Prognosis

Karin Birkenkamp-Demtröder, Iver Nordentoft, Trine Strandgaard, Sia Viborg Lindskrog, and Lars Dyrskjøt

Abstract

Blood-based biomarkers comprise a number of different analytes including extracellular vesicles, proteins, circulating cells, and circulating nucleic acids. Due to the minimally invasive nature of blood sampling, these biomarkers allow for longitudinal testing, thereby enabling repeated monitoring of the patient's disease over time. This constitutes a unique opportunity for early intervention and monitoring of tumor evolution during the disease course, ultimately providing the possibility to change treatment regimen. Hence, blood-based biomarkers have a great potential in risk stratification, detection of minimal residual disease and relapse as well as for monitoring and guidance of treatment. In this chapter we describe different types of blood-based biomarkers with a special focus on circulating tumor cells and circulating tumor DNA, as these have shown the most promising results for clinical implementation and may prove to be valuable clinical tools following clinical trial validation.

Keywords

Plasma biomarker · cfDNA · ctDNA · CTC · MRD · Treatment monitoring

19.1 Introduction

The most commonly used diagnostic tools for bladder cancer (BC) are cytology, histopathology, and cystoscopy (see Chaps. 4 and 5). Patients with non-muscle invasive BC (NMIBC) often undergo lifelong surveillance with repeated urine cytology and cystoscopy examinations. Patients with muscle invasive BC (MIBC) are followed during neoadjuvant treatment and after cystectomy by radiographic imaging (see Chap. 6). Advanced imaging technologies, e.g. Positron Emission Tomography/Computed Tomography (PET/CT), can detect well-established primary tumors and metastases, whereas 18 F-fluoro-2-deoxy-D-glucose PET/CT (18F-FDG PET/CT) increases the detection rate as metabolic alterations occur before morphological ones (Bacchiani et al. 2023).

K. Birkenkamp-Demtröder · T. Strandgaard · S. V. Lindskrog · L. Dyrskjøt (✉)
Department of Clinical Medicine, Aarhus University, Aarhus, Denmark

Department of Molecular Medicine, Aarhus University Hospital, Aarhus, Denmark
e-mail: ts@clin.au.dk; svl@clin.au.dk; lars@clin.au.dk

I. Nordentoft
Department of Molecular Medicine, Aarhus University Hospital, Aarhus, Denmark
e-mail: iver.nordentoft@clin.au.dk

M. A. Knowles, L. Dyrskjøt (eds.), *Biology of Bladder Cancer*,
https://doi.org/10.1007/978-3-031-68505-7_19

Currently used methods for follow-up and surveillance have limited sensitivity and specificity and/or cannot be repeated frequently, as they might harm the patient and may be associated with high costs to the health care systems. A variety of potential blood-based biomarkers have been suggested as minimally invasive tools for the detection and prognostication of BC. Blood-based analyses have profound advantages compared to tissue-based approaches. They provide rapid, precise, and real-time monitoring of tumor burden in a non-invasive setting with the possibility for frequent testing with less discomfort or disruption to the patient's daily routine and without a risk of inducing DNA damage as is the case for radiographic imaging. Furthermore, they are less costly than tissue biopsies and may be taken at any hospital or by a general practitioner. Tumors are often highly heterogeneous and consist of several different cell types, including carcinoma cells with different genetic backgrounds. Thus, a single tissue biopsy is often not fully representative of the bulk tumor. The challenge of tumor heterogeneity might be overcome by a blood sample, representing the molecular complexity of tumors. Tumor profiling from blood samples is especially valuable in the metastatic disease setting where tissue might not be readily available (Meeks et al. 2020). Furthermore, blood-based analysis offers the potential for longitudinal testing, providing valuable information on disease prognosis and monitoring of tumor evolution, allowing for early intervention and personalized treatment strategies. These advantages make blood-based biomarkers an attractive tool for future clinical decision making.

19.2 Blood-Based Biomarkers

Within the past 10 years, different types of blood-based biomarkers comprising, e.g. RNA, proteins, extracellular vesicles, circulating cells, and DNA have been investigated for potential use in detection and monitoring of cancers (Alix-Panabières and Pantel 2021).

This chapter provides a general overview of blood-based biomarkers analyzed in BC and will especially focus on circulating tumor cells (CTCs), cell-free DNA (cfDNA), and circulating tumor DNA (ctDNA) as multiple studies have shown that these analytes have a high potential for future clinical application.

19.2.1 RNA

Plasma-based RNA molecules can be separated into three categories: total RNA and messenger RNA (mRNA), microRNA (miRNA), and cell-free RNA (cfRNA). An early pilot study analyzed total RNA from blood cells of 16 patients with BC using microarray expression profiling (Osman et al. 2006). Seven transcripts discriminating BC from healthy controls were identified. Serum cell-free mRNA coding for the calcium-binding protein S100A4 was found to be increased in patients with MIBC and sensitivity could be increased by combination with urine cytology (Ismail et al. 2016). miRNAs are small non-coding RNA molecules that regulate gene expression by binding to target mRNAs. A study identified a panel of six miRNAs and showed that higher serum levels of miR-152 and lower levels of miR-3187-3p correlated with advanced tumor stage while lower levels of miR-27a-3p correlated with higher tumor grade (Jiang et al. 2015). A recent study identified higher levels for a subgroup of 379 analyzed circulating microRNAs (miR-1260a, let-7a-3p miR-196b-5p, miR-196a-5p, miR-99a-5p, miR-615-5p, miR-4301, miR-28-3p, miR-4538, miR-1233-3p, miR-4732-5p, miR-1913, miR-1280) in plasma from 34 NMIBC patients compared to 32 control subjects (Kaba et al. 2023). Circulating cell-free mRNA and long non-coding RNA (ncRNA) have been proposed as biomarkers but have had limited success in BC. During cell death, apoptotic bodies shed by Jurkat and HL-60 cancer cell lines were shown to carry ribosomal RNA, miRNA, and mRNA (Stejskal et al. 2023). Thus, apoptosis was suggested as a possible source of circulating tumor RNA with apoptotic bodies being their protective carriers (Battistelli and Falcieri 2020). Moreover, passively released elements of cancer-specific small ncRNAs (termed orphan ncRNAs) have been observed in cancers other than BC (Fish et al. 2018). Thus, miRNAs may serve as potential biomarkers in BC although additional studies are warranted to determine their potential for clinical use.

19.2.2 Proteins

Several studies have sought to identify diagnostic plasma protein biomarkers in BC. Using mass-spectrometry, a pilot study identified three groups of potential plasma protein biomarkers in BC when compared to normal samples. These included plasma transferrin, alpha-2-macroglobulin, and vitamin D-binding protein, which were found to be increased in plasma from patients with urothelial carcinomas (Lemańska-Perek et al. 2019). A total of 13 potential plasma protein biomarkers, including tumor antigens, inflammatory markers, and apolipoproteins (Apo) as well as combinations thereof were assessed by ELISA. Among others, sVCAM-1 levels in particular significantly were higher and ApoA2 significantly lower in 59 BC patients compared to 203 healthy volunteers (Voronova et al. 2019). Potential serum protein markers for NMIBC have been identified using sequential window acquisition of all theoretical mass spectra (SWATH-MS). Three major groups of proteins were found to be deregulated in Ta versus T1 tumors. The most prominent were e.g. AACT or SRTPINA3 found to be upregulated in Ta tumors and APOA2 or APOF which were down-regulated in T1 tumors (Gómez et al. 2021). Inflammation plays a significant role in the development and progression of BC. C-reactive protein (CRP) and interleukin-6 (IL-6) are two inflammatory biomarkers that have been studied in blood samples from BC patients. CRP is an acute-phase protein increasing in response to tissue damage or inflammation (Sproston and Ashworth 2018). A meta-analysis correlated the levels of CRP with the prognosis of urological cancers (Zhou et al. 2015). The study concluded that high baseline serum CRP was a strong prognostic factor of worse cancer-specific survival (CSS). IL-6 is a cytokine that is produced by immune cells in response to inflammation and IL-6 levels have been correlated with advanced stages and poor prognosis (O'Brian et al. 2021). Recently, blood-based proteins have been assessed using 33 cancer-specific aptamers (APTASHAPE) using 1 μL plasma from BC patients. The proteins C4b-binding protein, Complement C3, Fibrinogen, Complement factor H and IgG were found to be differentially expressed between healthy controls and patients with NMIBC or MIBC (Fjelstrup et al. 2022). Additional studies are needed to demonstrate the clinical potential of proteins in blood circulation.

19.2.3 Extracellular Vesicles

Extracellular vesicles (EVs) and tumor-derived extracellular vesicles (TEVs) are membrane-bound vesicles released by cells and cancer cells, respectively, into the circulation. Both are active carriers of cell-derived biological molecules, including nucleic acids, proteins, lipids, and carbohydrates (Rahbarghazi et al. 2019). EVs are classified in three major subtypes according to their size: exosomes (30–120 nm in diameter), microvesicles (0.1–1.0 μm), and apoptotic bodies (0.8–5.0 μm) (Han et al. 2019). The vesicles function as mediators of intercellular communication as they can be taken up by cells in the tumor microenvironment to modulate the molecular and physiological behavior of recipient cells (Liu et al. 2018). Moreover, TEVs carry small DNA fragments on their surface, being amenable to liquid biopsy applications for disease detection and monitoring (Malkin and Bratman 2020). The analysis of exosomal miRNA signatures provides insight into the cellular secreting status (Taylor et al. 2011). Exosomes have been suggested to be used for delivery of therapeutic agents for cancer therapy (Romagnoli et al. 2014). Overall, extracellular vesicles in BC can drive malignant transformation of normal urothelial cells, promote BC progression via stimulation of proliferation, invasion, and migration of recipient neighboring BC cells, and modify the tumor stroma to support tumor growth (Liu et al. 2018). Recently, the involvement of cancer-associated fibroblast-derived EVs in the immune escape of bladder tumors was shown to facilitate the upregulation of PD-L1/PD-1 in mouse models (Feng et al. 2023), providing evidence that EVs may play an important role in BC progression.

19.3 Circulating Tumor Cells

19.3.1 Circulating Tumor Cells: Origin and Characteristics

Circulating tumor cells (CTCs) are cells that have detached from the primary or disseminated tumor and entered the bloodstream. This intravasation can be facilitated by immune cells in the tumor microenvironment (Aceto et al. 2014), e.g. tumor-associated macrophages (TAMs) can promote the dissemination and extravasation of CTCs (Doak et al. 2018). Primary tumor cells acquire stem cell features, such as self-renewal and the ability to differentiate into multiple cell types, by undergoing epithelial-to-mesenchymal transition (EMT). CTCs may extravasate and colonize at distant sites with a favorable host microenvironment, termed the pre-metastatic niche. Formation of a pre-metastatic niche is initiated by local changes involving secretory factors and extracellular vesicles which induce vascular leakage, extracellular matrix, and stroma remodeling as well as immunosuppression (Peinado et al. 2017). CTCs may remain in a dormant state until environmental changes offer the possibility to form distant metastases (Boral et al. 2020). In breast cancer patients, reawakening of dormant cancer cells has been shown to be inducible by gradual increase in bone marrow fat cells, loss of estrogen with aging, inflammation, new blood vessel formation, trauma, surgery, abnormal blood clotting conditions, anxiety, and depression (Wieder 2023). With a mean of 60 ± 693 CTCs per 7.5ml blood in patients with metastatic cancer and lower numbers in non-malignant individuals (Allard et al. 2004), CTCs are a rarity among a high background of blood cells ($50x10^9$ red and $80x10^{67}$ white blood cells per 10 mL, respectively (Au et al. (2017))). The time of blood sampling is an important consideration in capturing a sufficient number of CTCs for downstream analysis, as more CTCs are released during sleep (Diamantopoulou et al. 2022). Leukocytes have a size of 6-20μm in diameter, whereas the size of CTCs varies from <4μm up to >30μm (Allard et al. 2004; Rostami et al. 2019). Patient-derived CTCs from BC and breast cancer patients have been found to be 8.6 μm and 12.4 μm, respectively, indicating size differences between different cancer types (Mendelaar et al. 2021). The smaller size of CTCs from BC patients and the overlap in size with leukocytes may have an impact on CTC enrichment using microfluidic separation methods.

In the bloodstream, single CTCs and CTC clusters have been identified. The origin of the clusters, so-called tumor microemboli, is assumed to be cell jamming or undergo collective migration from a tumor rather than intravascular aggregation of single CTCs as shown in Fig. 19.1 (Amintas et al. 2020). Frequent polyclonal seeding of metastasis has been observed, probably arising from oligoclonal CTC clusters. The clusters have a 20–100 times higher potential for metastasizing compared to single CTCs. CTC clusters are rare and even rarer in early-stage cancers (Amintas et al. 2020). Proliferation is down-regulated within the clusters, allowing cells to potentially escape treatments targeting proliferating cells (Hou et al. 2012). CTC clusters can either be homotypic, containing only cancer cells or heterotypic also containing other cells than cancer cells. For homotypic clusters, intratumor hypoxia may trigger cluster formation with cells overexpressing the cell junction protein plakoglobin (Aceto et al. 2014). In heterotypic CTC clusters, the CTCs ally with white blood cells, including neutrophils, or cancer-associated fibroblasts (CAFs) (Schuster et al. 2021). The crosstalk between CTCs and neutrophils within CTC clusters has been shown to promote CTC extravasation (Szczerba et al. 2019).

Only a small fraction of CTCs survive in circulation and less than 0.01% of cells with high metastatic potential will result in distant

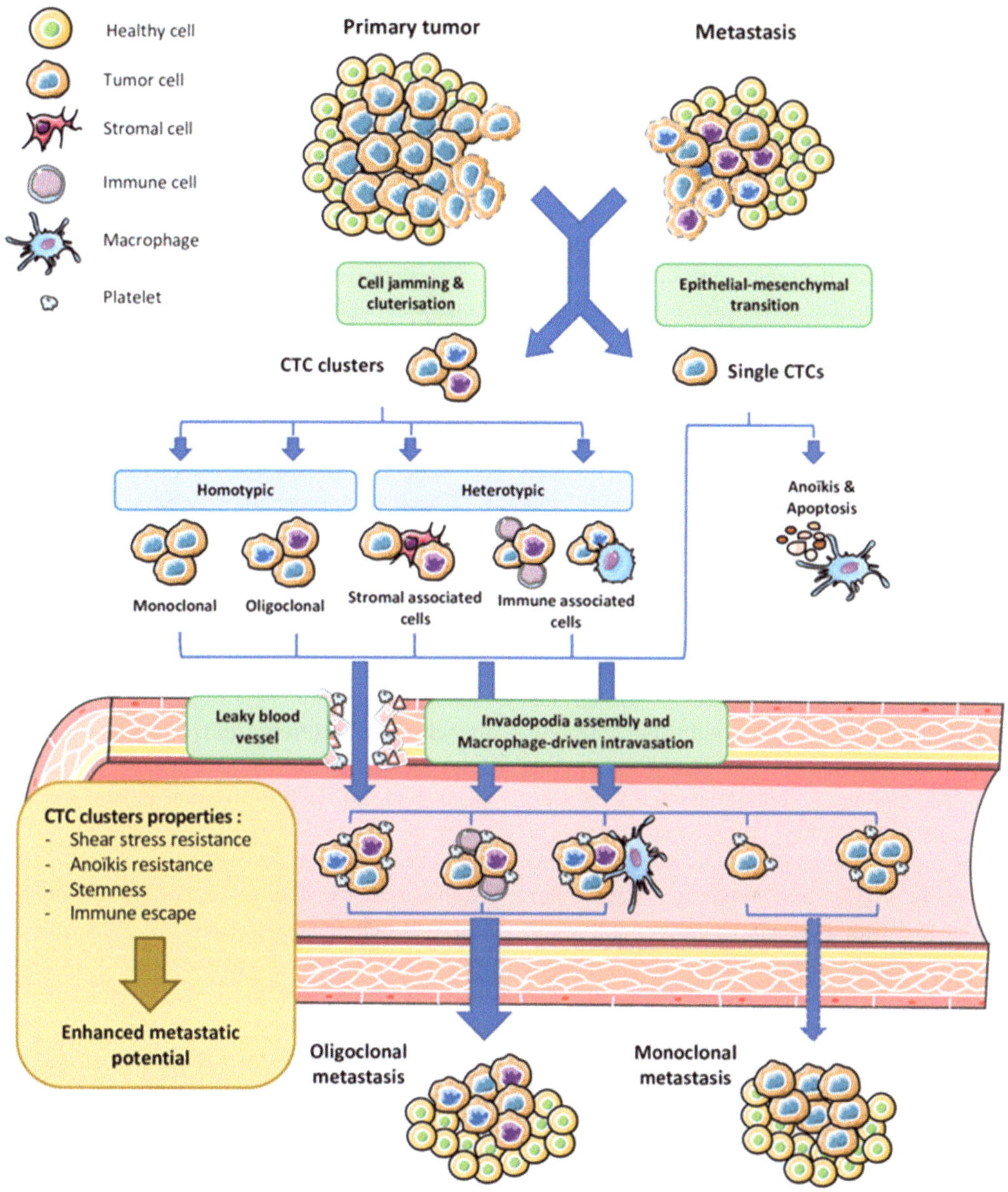

Fig. 19.1 Origin and dissemination of CTCs from Amintas et al. (2020) originally published under CC-BY license

metastasis (Rejniak 2016). Among other factors, survival of CTCs is dependent on their size. While small 6 μm CTCs are still vital, only about 40% of the 3 μm CTCs survive as shear stress induces apoptosis in these cells, which eliminates the potential for seeding and formation of distant metastasis (Mitchell and King 2013). The half-life of CTC clusters is estimated to be 6–10 min, which is significantly shorter than for single-cell CTCs (25–30 min) as those are less likely to be trapped in capillaries (Aceto et al. 2014; Micalizzi ct al. 2017). Small vessels and capillaries establish a distinct blood microenvironment with extensive and narrow branching that can slow, trap, and squeeze CTCs to facilitate their extravasation (Follain et al. 2018). The CTC mechanobiology and interaction with other blood components (e.g., immune cells and platelets inside capillaries) help them to survive the harsh conditions in the circulatory system and to metastasize to distant organs (Kurma and Alix-Panabières 2023).

The isolation of CTCs has been technically challenging and different methods have been developed to isolate CTCs from blood. These include, but are not limited to, immunomagnetic separation using beads coated with antibodies specific for capturing tumor cells or flow cytometry involving labeling cancer cells with fluorescent antibodies and passing them through a laser beam, resulting in sorting tumor cells from other cells in the blood. The "Cell Collector" uses an anti-EpCAM (epithelial cell adhesion molecule) antibody-coated guidewire directly inserted into a cubital vein to capture CTCs in vivo (Saucedo-Zeni et al. 2012). Cellsearch™, which is approved for clinical use, enriches CTCs from blood using antibody-coated ferrofluid particles targeting EpCAM. Captured, immunostained CTCs are subsequently counted using automated cell image capture and analysis (Gorges et al. 2016). However, CTCs may undergo EMT, thus decreasing the expression of epithelial markers (Kalluri and Weinberg 2009). Recently, microfluidic devices for continuous CTC separation, circular microcavity arrays (MCA) to trap CTCs, Pyramidal MCA filter, and The Parsortix™ system, retaining CTCs based on their deformable nature and size have emerged (Descamps et al. 2022), offering novel ways to isolate tumor cells by physical and chemical properties of the cancer cells. For capture of CTC clusters, devices such as "Cluster Chip", "Deterministic Lateral Displacement (DLD) chip," or the "3D scaffold chip" have been applied (Piñeiro et al. 2020). More details, technical advances, and multi-molecular analyses of CTCs are elucidated in Lawrence et al. (2023).

19.3.2 Analyses of CTCs in Bladder Cancer

CTCs in blood samples have been used to study metastatic BC. An early pilot study described the analysis of CTCs from six patients with metastasized, unresectable urothelial carcinomas using a panel covering 50 oncogenes and tumor suppressor genes (Kobayashi et al. 2022). Antibodies against EpCAM, EGFR, Her2, and Trop2 captured an unusually large number of CTCs (median 303 CTCs) from 10 mL of blood of the terminal patients, and 12–17 mutations, including 0–2 hotspot mutations were detected per patient. However, the use of EpCAM-based CTC capture approaches may be limited in BC, as only 32% of patients with BC were EpCAM positive and therefore microfluidics methods are recommended for retrieval of BC CTCs (Went et al. 2004). A study of BC found that preoperative detection of CTCs in patients who underwent radical cystectomy (RC) was associated with a higher risk of recurrence and poor cancer-specific survival compared to CTC-negative patients (Rink et al. 2012). Furthermore, in a prospective study of 102 high-risk NMIBC patients, CTCs were identified in 20% of the patients using "Cellsearch" (median 1 CTC in 7.5 mL blood), and this study demonstrated CTCs to be a strong predictor of disease progression and poor prognosis (Gazzaniga et al. 2014). In addition, the presence of CTCs was associated with poor progression-free survival (PFS), cancer-specific survival (CSS), and overall survival (OS) in patients not receiving adjuvant chemotherapy, indicating a potential role for CTCs in guiding treatment (Soave et al. 2017). A recent study of 48 BC patients using a microfluidic approach identified a higher CTC count in MIBC versus NMIBC as well as in high grade versus low grade BC patients (4.67 vs. 1.88 and 3.69 vs. 1.18 CTCs/3 mL, respectively), offering a complementary tool for risk stratification of BC (Fu et al. 2021). A detailed overview of CTC studies in BC is provided in Li et al. (2023a).

19.3.3 Potential Clinical Applications of CTCs

Several studies and clinical trials aim to implement CTCs for risk and treatment stratification in BC. In the "CirGuidance" trial, CTCs were used for patient stratification for neoadjuvant chemotherapy (NAC) treatment of MIBC patients (T2-T4aN0-N1M0; Netherlands Trial Register NL3954) (Beije et al. 2022). In this multicenter clinical trial, CTC-negative patients (no CTCs detectable using the Cellsearch™ system) underwent RC only, while CTC-positive patients (≥1 detectable CTCs) received NAC followed by RC. The primary endpoint was 2-year OS in the CTC-negative group with a prespecified criterion for trial success of ≥75%. While there was no significant difference with regard to OS, the absence of CTCs was associated with a lower risk of relapse after RC. Moreover, the study showed that CTC-positive patients may benefit from NAC (Beije et al. 2022). A recent pilot study explored the potential of CTCs as predictive biomarkers for NAC response. CTCs were isolated by cell surface markers and enriched by the IsoFlux™ device, using immunofluorescence to confirm the tumor origin of the cells. The number of CTCs decreased significantly after four cycles of NAC and CTC counts in 7.5 mL after four NAC cycles were highly correlated with postoperative pathological T-stage (Jhuo et al. 2023).

Hematogenous dissemination of cancer cells is an early event in patients, often occurring long before primary lesions are clinically detectable. A multi-molecular analysis of the presence, abundance, and biology of CTCs might identify aggressive tumors before metastases are visible, potentially resulting in a unique opportunity to offer personalized, tailored therapy approaches without wasting precious time due to ineffective treatment approaches (Lawrence et al. 2023). In conclusion, the future utility of CTCs for cancer detection provides new perspectives for cancer patients, as high-risk patients can be discriminated from low risk patients. As a consequence, early, personalized treatment might spare patients at low risk from overtreatment.

19.4 Cell-Free DNA

19.4.1 Cell-Free DNA: Origin and Characteristics

cfDNA is released from cells into the bloodstream during cell death (i.e., apoptosis or necrosis), through active secretion into the interstitium or by release from EVs. Apoptosis is the process of programmed cell death that occurs during normal physiological processes, whereas necrosis is a cell death triggered by external factors such as trauma or infection and is characterized by cell swelling, rupture of the plasma membrane, and release of cellular contents into the extracellular environment, including DNA fragments of larger size. Released cfDNA fragments are small-sized double-stranded DNA fragments of nuclear or mitochondrial origin, mainly bound to nucleosomes and thus protected from degradation. About 85% of the DNA fragments in the bloodstream are of hematopoietic origin (Kustanovich et al. 2019). The fragment size corresponds to a nucleosome footprint of 147 bp plus 20 bp protected by histone H1. The length of cfDNA in circulation is between 120 and 220 bp, or multiples thereof with a median size of 167 bp (Alcaide et al. 2020; Cristiano et al. 2019).

The concentration of cfDNA in blood varies significantly both between and within patients and ranges between 0 and 100 ng/mL in healthy subjects to >1000 ng/mL in patients with cancer (Kustanovich et al. 2019). In a study of cfDNA in 114 clinically healthy donors, individuals who developed either a benign neoplasm or cancer were compared to those who did not develop any tumor during 1–10 years of follow-up. High levels of cfDNA were predictive of outcome (Alborelli et al. 2019). The amount of cfDNA in plasma depends on a balance between cfDNA shedding and cfDNA clearance. Three different mechanisms are mainly responsible for cfDNA clearance, namely degradation by DNAses in the circulation, active clearance of nucleosomes and DNA as well as filtration in organs. cfDNA filtration in the liver is mainly achieved by Kupffer cells, stellate macrophages in the hepatic portal vein, responsible for the degradation of 70–85%

of nucleosomes. Additionally, macrophages in the spleen and lymph nodes are also involved in clearance. cfDNA clearance is achieved to a lesser extent by renal clearance where cfDNA is fragmented by DNAse activity in the kidneys, filtered by the glomeruli and excreted in the urine. The clearance rate of cfDNA by the kidneys is lower than that of the liver and cfDNA clearance may be affected by liver diseases such as cirrhosis and hepatitis (Sánchez-Herrero et al. 2022). Other factors may also play a role and the decay kinetics is complex (Sanz-Garcia et al. 2022). The association of cfDNA with molecular or macromolecular complexes, as well as encapsulation in extracellular vesicles, may counterbalance this and prevent rapid degradation of cfDNA (Celec et al. 2018).

Fragmentomics, describing the pattern of fragmentation of cfDNA, aims to understand how DNA in circulation is released and degraded by analyzing the fragment lengths and structure of cfDNA fragments. By examining the size distribution and other structural features of cfDNA fragments, it is possible to gain insight into the underlying biological and biochemical processes that affect their release and stability. The cfDNA fragmentome may be used as a predictor for patient outcome (Keller et al. 2021). Altered fragmentation profiles of cfDNA were initially shown in a study comparing 236 patients with cancer (breast, colorectal, lung, ovarian, pancreatic, gastric, or bile duct cancer) to 245 healthy individuals using a machine learning model (Cristiano et al. 2019). In this approach called "DNA evaluation of fragments for early interception" (DELFI) detection, sensitivities between 57% and 99% were achieved depending on the cancer type and in 75% of cases, it was possible to identify the tissue of origin. Moreover, in the DELFI study, cfDNA was found to carry unique signatures and genome-wide fragmentation profiles across transcription factor binding sites that identified small cell lung cancer with high accuracy. A higher fragmentation score represented an independent prognostic indicator of survival (Mathios et al. 2021). To date, no studies of fragmentomics in BC patients have been described.

19.4.2 Circulating Tumor DNA: Origin and Characteristics

ctDNA is the component of cfDNA originating from carcinoma cells or precancerous lesions where the cells may have acquired genomic alterations. ctDNA usually represents a minor fraction of the total cfDNA and the levels have been reported to constitute <0.1–10% of the total cfDNA detected (Diehl et al. 2008). Patients with disseminated disease may have larger amounts of ctDNA compared to patients with localized disease and the range of ctDNA in plasma may vary between less than 1 copy/mL up to hundreds of copies or even thousands of copies/mL in patients with disseminated disease (Birkenkamp-Demtröder et al. 2016).

The release of ctDNA from cancer cells occurs mainly through apoptosis where ctDNA fragments of about 160 bp are released into the interstitial fluid. DNA fragments longer than 10,000 base pairs (bp) are likely to originate from necrotic cells and are often observed in advanced stages of cancer (Thierry 2023). In addition, secretion of DNA-containing vesicles, such as exosomes and microvesicles, can transport ctDNA to the bloodstream (Hahn et al. 2019) (Fig. 19.2). The short half-life of cfDNA/ctDNA in circulation (15 min to 2.5 h) makes it ideal for monitoring the current state of the disease (disease burden) as well as monitoring disease burden during treatment (García Moreira et al. 2006; Sánchez-Herrero et al. 2022).

An early report on ctDNA in advanced BC described the detection of circulating DNA fragments with point mutations (Bettegowda et al. 2014). Since then, numerous studies have addressed the clinical value of ctDNA and have described several potential clinical applications in BC. ctDNA analysis can provide a non-invasive and sensitive tool for early detection of BC but it may be more challenging for early stages of the disease where levels have been reported to be lower. The genomic variations in ctDNA comprise epigenetic changes in the methylation pattern, single-nucleotide variants (SNV), small insertion or deletion mutations (INDELs), or large chromosomal rearrangements as e.g.

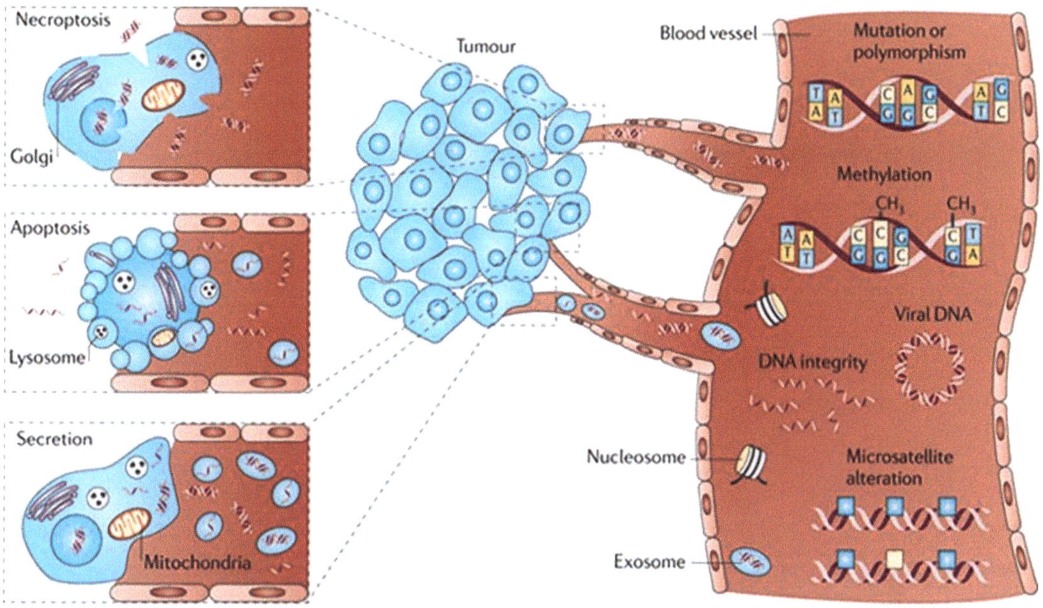

Fig. 19.2 ctDNA in the blood circulation provides information about the tumor such as mutations, DNA methylation, viral DNA, and microsatellite alterations (Schwarzenbach et al. 2011)

inter- or intra-chromosomal translocations (Fig. 19.2). Other analyses of ctDNA include fragmentomics, which comprises ctDNA fragment lengths, tumor-related virus sequence detection, and read depth coverage related to the "footprints" of transcription factors in the tumor (Keller et al. 2021).

These variations in ctDNA can be used for minimally invasive detection throughout all stages of the disease course, e.g. to identify patients at high risk, to monitor treatment response, to detect minimal residual disease (MRD), to guide treatment decisions, to identify actionable targets for treatment approaches, to determine the origin of unknown primary tumors, and many more. Mathematical modeling has demonstrated that molecular ctDNA detection can identify treatment failure much earlier than current imaging technologies (Avanzini et al. 2020) and recent studies have further documented this lead time advantage (Christensen et al. 2019, 2023; Nordentoft et al. 2023b, c).

A combined analysis of CTCs and ctDNA from the same blood sample (Fig. 19.3) offers huge potential to gather specific information about a tumor through minimally invasive sampling and may serve as a diagnostic, prognostic, and treatment-guidance tool without harming the patient.

19.4.3 Technical Challenges of ctDNA Analysis

Somatic mutations in ctDNA can be assessed by a tumor-agnostic or a tumor-informed approach. The tumor-agnostic or tumor-uninformed (tumor-naïve) approach requires only a blood sample without prior knowledge of the genomic profile of the primary tumor of a particular patient (i.e., plasma-only ctDNA analysis). A tumor-agnostic approach is applicable for screening purposes to identify potential cancer patients in a population of healthy individuals but is also valuable when no or very sparse tumor material is available when it is not possible to obtain a biopsy in a metastatic setting (Pascual et al. 2022). The major advantage of tumor-agnostic ctDNA testing is that pre-designed tests targeting, e.g., known cancer genes or hotspot mutations can be directly used for analysis of a blood sample without delay and the turnover time will hence be

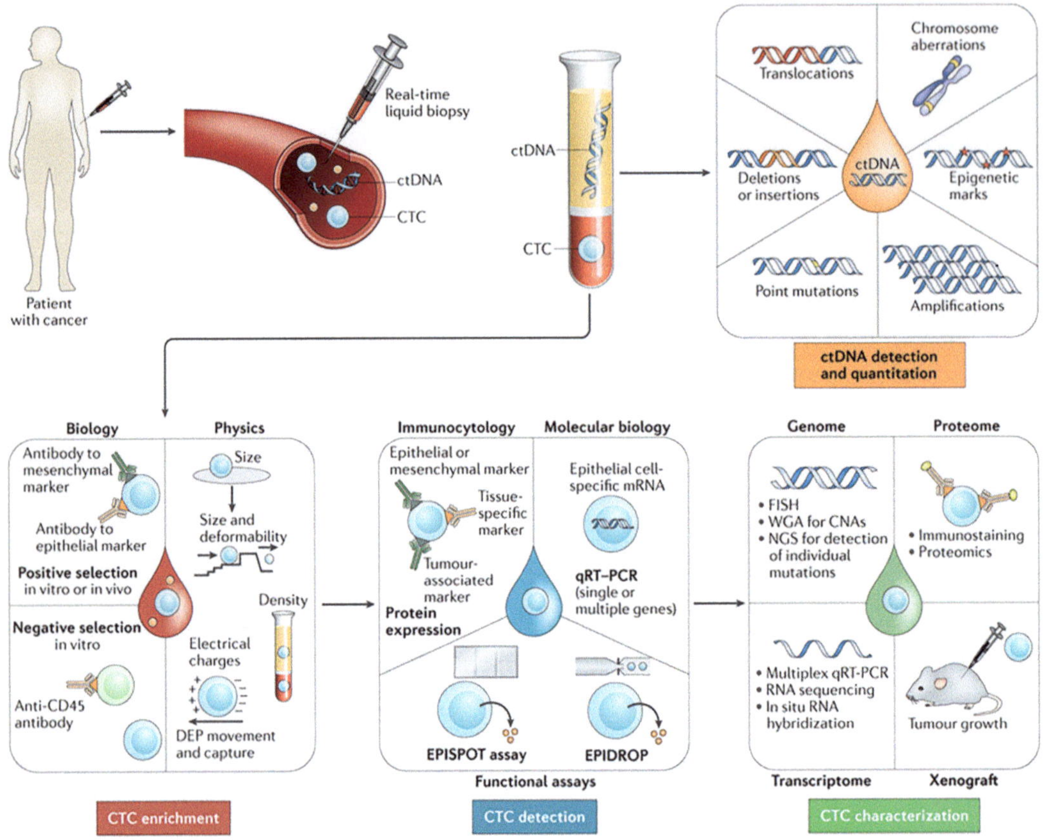

Fig. 19.3 CTCs and ctDNA isolated from the same blood sample may provide additional information (Pantel and Alix-Panabières 2019)

minimized compared to a tumor-informed approach. Despite the identification of tumor-specific mutations, a tumor-agnostic approach might always bear the risk that the mutations identified may have arisen from any tumor process and not necessarily from the cancer of interest, e.g. patients with concomitant lung cancers. For screening approaches it might be recommended to infer the tissue of origin from epigenetic characteristics and combine this with the tumor-agnostic approach (Oberhofer et al. 2022).

The major disadvantage of a tumor-agnostic approach emerges if the specific mutational pattern of a given patient is not sufficiently covered by the applied test or assay. As a consequence, only very few ctDNA molecules might be detected and large test panels combined with deep-sequencing approaches are necessary. As an example, in a tumor-agnostic study on NMIBC, a pre-defined panel of 861 genes was applied to plasma ctDNA and tumor DNA without prior knowledge of the genomic tumor profile. Only a minor fraction of all mutations analyzed were identified in plasma cfDNA (median two mutations per patient, total 165 variants for 54 patients) or in the tumor DNA for comparison (median five mutations per patient, in total 476 variants from 82 NMIBC patients) (Zhang et al. 2021). Furthermore, although some hotspot mutations (same base substitution, same genomic position) are found especially in early-stage BC, the mutational pattern in BC is highly patient-specific and hotspot mutations are uncommon in BC compared to other cancer types such as colon cancer where 50% of the patients harbor hotspot mutations in *KRAS* or *BRAF*. Thus, a tumor-informed approach for assessment of patient-specific mutations in ctDNA is highly recommended for BC. For a tumor-informed approach, mutational profiling by, e.g., whole exome sequencing (WES) or whole genome sequencing (WGS) of tumor DNA and reference germline DNA is necessary to identify and select patient-specific alterations for ctDNA monitoring.

As mentioned above, more than 85% of cfDNA is of hematopoietic cell origin (Moss et al. 2018) and somatic mutations will accumulate in hematopoietic cells as we age. Clonal Hematopoietic mutations of Indeterminate Potential (CHIP) (Steensma et al. 2015) serve as confounding mutations in ctDNA analysis. To distinguish tumor-specific somatic alterations from germline variants, it is highly recommended to sequence DNA derived from peripheral mononuclear blood cells (PBMC) from the buffy coat fraction of the blood sample. Sequencing of a matching germline sample at high coverage is necessary in both the tumor-agnostic and tumor-informed settings to ensure elimination of the confounding effect of CHIP, since CHIP will otherwise be mistaken as true cancer cell mutations.

As the volume of plasma input that can be used for analysis may be limited and the fraction of ctDNA in cfDNA may be extremely small, highly sensitive detection methods are required. A highly sensitive method to assess somatic variants in cfDNA is droplet digital PCR (ddPCR), measuring a few target variants in a sample and next generation sequencing (NGS), detecting few to multiple genomic variants. ddPCR is a highly sensitive and precise method for detecting low levels of mutant DNA, where a limited number of tumor mutations can be analyzed in parallel. It is relatively cheap (compared to NGS) and is particularly useful for the detection of somatic variants at low allele frequencies as a limit of detection down to about 10^{-4} is achievable (Schlenker et al. 2021). Achieving a limit of detection of 10^{-4} using a single ddPCR assay will require a minimum of 1/0.0001 = 10.000 genome equivalents and thus more than 34 ng cfDNA, which may often not be feasible. Applying a multiplex ddPCR assay strategy will increase the probability of variant detection by mitigating the stochasticity of ctDNA presence in plasma sampling.

NGS is more costly per sample but provides a more comprehensive amount of genomic information, as billions of DNA molecules can be interrogated from each sample, thus enabling monitoring of many mutations in a patient's ctDNA profile. Deep sequencing of a limited number of mutations increases the sensitivity and provides the possibility to study the mutational dynamics during a patient's disease course (Nordentoft et al. 2023a). In-silico mathematical probability calculations demonstrate that increasing the sequencing breadth by WGS (thereby increasing the number of detectable mutations) can achieve high detection probability even with a relatively low coverage of, e.g., 20×. For tumors having a tumor mutation burden of >4/Mbp, this approach can detect tumor fractions down to 10^{-5} with high probability (Zviran et al. 2020). The cost of WGS may limit routine clinical utility; however, recent advances in sequencing methods make the $100 genome within reach (Santonja et al. 2023). However, NGS may be affected by sequencing errors or artifacts that need to be eliminated, and bioinformatic procedures may be challenging.

19.4.4 Potential Use of ctDNA for Cancer Screening

High specificity and high sensitivity are a prerequisite for pan-cancer screening tests to mitigate the risk of false-positive findings in a screening approach of a general population (Duffy et al. 2021). The number of multicancer early detection tests (MCED) commercially available or under development is increasing and several tests have been tested on minor cohorts of patients diagnosed with BC, among these cfMeDIP sequencing and fragmentomics (Adela), EVs (Tr(ACE)), LC-MS glycosaminoglycans (MIRAM), multiomics/AI (FMBT), and CpG-cfDNA NGS (Galleri). An overview of MCED tests for several target cancers as well as their performance is provided in Doubeni and Castle (2023) and Hackshaw et al. (2022), respectively.

Four commercially available MCED tests might be potentially appropriate for analysis of ctDNA with regard to BC detection, namely "Guardant360 CDx" (Kim et al. 2017), "CancerSEEK" (Cohen et al. 2018; Lennon et al. 2020), "PanSeer" (Chen et al. 2020), and "Galleri" (Klein et al. 2021). However, none are yet approved as screening tests for BC and larger cohorts are needed to determine sensitivity and specificity for clinical application.

19.4.5 ctDNA in NMIBC

The majority of liquid biopsy biomarkers described in NMIBC are based on urine samples. Many have shown promising implications for recurrence prediction and disease monitoring (see Chap. 18). One of the first studies evaluating ctDNA in patients with NMIBC applied patient-specific ddPCR assays for plasma- and urine-based disease surveillance in 12 patients with either progressive or recurrent NMIBC (Birkenkamp-Demtröder et al. 2016). Patient-specific large chromosomal rearrangements or single-nucleotide variants were identified using WGS and WES of the primary tumors and one to six personalized ddPCR assays were subsequently designed. Longitudinal cfDNA analysis showed a higher ctDNA detection rate among patients with progressive NMIBC and ctDNA was prognostic for disease progression, as it was detected several months to years before clinical evidence of progression to MIBC or metastasis (Birkenkamp-Demtröder et al. 2016). Building on this work, ddPCR assays targeting hotspot mutations in *PIK3CA* and *FGFR3* were designed and used for ctDNA analysis of plasma and urine samples from 25 patients with NMIBC (Christensen et al. 2017). While high urinary tumor DNA (utDNA) levels were associated with increasing tumor size, tumor grade and EORTC risk score, ctDNA analysis did not show significant results for this patient cohort. Advancing to NGS-based approaches for ctDNA detection, Zhang et al. applied targeted sequencing based on an 861-gene panel covering known oncogenes and tumor suppressor genes in BC to detect ctDNA in plasma samples from 82 BCG-treated patients with NMIBC (Zhang et al. 2021). ctDNA was detected in plasma from 43 patients (52.4%) and more frequently in patients with T1 tumors and larger tumor size. While urinary biomarkers have shown promising results in early-stage disease (see Chap. 18), ctDNA analysis in NMIBC may have an important, additional application in staging and prognostication of patients. Additional studies are needed in this setting to investigate the usefulness and clinical relevance of ctDNA in NMIBC.

19.4.6 ctDNA in MIBC

One of the first studies assessing ctDNA in MIBC used tagged amplicon sequencing of a bladder-specific panel in 86 plasma samples from 17 NAC-treated patients (Patel et al. 2017). Detection of ctDNA before NAC was not prognostic in this small cohort, but presence of ctDNA during NAC correlated with disease recurrence. Furthermore, applying targeted sequencing with a 50-gene bladder-specific panel on cfDNA from 51 patients with MIBC revealed a high ctDNA burden in patients with metastatic disease while only 14% of patients with localized disease had detectable ctDNA using this approach (Vandekerkhove et al. 2017). By using a patient-specific approach, Birkenkamp-Demtröder et al. monitored ctDNA in 217 longitudinally collected plasma samples from 24 patients by tumor-informed ddPCR assays (Birkenkamp-Demtröder et al. 2018). The study indicated the prognostic impact of ctDNA and the implications for early detection of metastatic relapse after RC, as ctDNA levels were higher in patients with recurrence compared to disease-free patients and detection of ctDNA had a positive median lead time of 101 days over clinical detection of relapse. Subsequently, ctDNA was assessed in a larger cohort of 68 patients with MIBC who were treated with NAC before RC (Christensen et al. 2019). WES of tumor and matched germline DNA was performed, and ultra-deep sequencing of longitudinal plasma cfDNA using a panel of 16 patient- and tumor-specific mutations

(Signatera™) underlined the biomarker potential and possible clinical relevance of ctDNA. In total, 656 plasma samples collected at diagnosis, during NAC and during surveillance after RC were analyzed. Detection of ctDNA following initial diagnosis and at the completion of NAC was shown to be highly prognostic for disease recurrence (Christensen et al. 2019). Full follow-up results for the cohort were recently published (>5 years follow-up after RC), demonstrating that ctDNA analysis during disease surveillance identified metastatic relapse with a sensitivity of 94% and specificity of 98%, and with a median lead time of 123 days over radiographic imaging (Lindskrog et al. 2023). In addition, total RNA-sequencing of primary tumors was performed to explore the biology underlying ctDNA shedding tumors.

Several studies have subsequently studied ctDNA in larger patient cohorts using pre-designed panels for targeted sequencing. Grivas et al. performed ctDNA analysis of plasma samples from 124 patients using a 73-gene panel (Guardant360) (Grivas et al. 2020). At least one genomic alteration was detected in 112 of the patients (median: 4 genomic alterations) and *BRCA1* and *RAF1* alterations were associated with worse prognosis. Shohdy et al. also utilized the Guardant360 panel for targeted sequencing of 182 serial plasma samples from 53 patients with advanced MIBC (Shohdy et al. 2022). Here, serial ctDNA-derived variant allele fraction values were aggregated (aVAF) and an increase in aVAF of ≥1 predicted disease progression within 6 months in 90% of patients. Furthermore, to explore ctDNA as a tumor tissue surrogate, Vandekerkhove et al. performed ctDNA analysis of 192 cfDNA samples from 104 patients with metastatic UC using targeted sequencing of a custom 50–60 gene panel (Vandekerkhove et al. 2021). Comparison of the mutation profile of ctDNA and tumor tissue from 46 patients revealed a mutation concordance of 83.4%. The ctDNA fraction was >1% in 85% of patients, and 90% of the mutations were identified across serial samples allowing ctDNA to be used as a tumor surrogate. For patients with plasma samples collected prior to first-line platinum-based chemotherapy or immune checkpoint inhibition (n=71), a low ctDNA fraction (<4.9%) was observed in 17 patients and was associated with increased OS compared to the remaining 54 patients with high ctDNA levels.

Using a tumor-informed targeted sequencing approach, a combined analysis of plasma and urine samples was performed for 92 patients with localized MIBC (Christensen et al. 2023). A custom NGS panel capturing approximately 50 mutations per patient was designed and applied to 281 urine-derived DNA and 447 plasma cfDNA samples collected before, during, and after NAC. Presence of ctDNA in plasma before and after NAC was associated with a lower NAC response rate, and a combined measure of plasma ctDNA and urine supernatant tumor DNA dynamics were associated with patient outcomes.

Recently, the feasibility of WGS-based ctDNA detection in patients with MIBC was demonstrated (Nordentoft et al. 2023a, b, c). WGS of the primary tumor from 112 patients was performed to develop patient-specific tumor-informed WGS models of genome-wide somatic alteration patterns. In total, 916 longitudinal plasma samples were collected before NAC, during NAC, before RC, and after RC, and the WGS models were applied to WGS data from plasma cfDNA (20× coverage) to monitor ctDNA status. The tumor-informed WGS of cfDNA proved to be a highly sensitive method for ctDNA detection using very low volumes of 1–2 mL plasma only. The WGS-based analysis of ctDNA additionally facilitates characterization of tumor biology. A platinum therapy-associated mutational signature was discovered in plasma ctDNA after NAC treatment and an evolution of copy number alterations was observed in post-treatment plasma samples compared to the primary tumors (Nordentoft et al. 2023a, b, c).

Results from clinical trials with exploratory ctDNA analysis in MIBC are emerging as well. The phase III IMvigor010 study found no significant benefit of adjuvant atezolizumab when comparing adjuvant treatment with atezolizumab to observation after RC for patients with MIBC (Bellmunt et al. 2021). Retrospective ctDNA analysis using targeted sequencing of 16 tumor- and patient-specific mutations (Signatera™) was subsequently used to investigate the potential of ctDNA-guided adjuvant treatment (Powles et al. 2021, 2023). Before treatment, 37% (214/581) of patients were ctDNA positive and clearance of ctDNA was observed for 18.2% (18/99) of patients treated with adjuvant atezolizumab compared to 3.8% (3/79) of patients undergoing observation. Notably, patients with detectable ctDNA had improved disease-free survival (DFS) and OS after adjuvant atezolizumab compared to patients in the observation arm. On the contrary, no difference in outcome was found between the arms for patients without detectable ctDNA. In 2022, Szabados et al. presented the final results of the phase II ABACUS trial, evaluating two cycles of neoadjuvant atezolizumab prior to RC in patients with MIBC who were ineligible or refused NAC (Szabados et al. 2022). Approximately one third of the patients showed pathological complete response at RC. ctDNA evaluation was performed before neoadjuvant treatment, after treatment and after RC using targeted sequencing of 16 patient- and tumor-specific mutations (Signatera™). Presence of ctDNA was highly prognostic at all timepoints with no detected relapses in patients without detectable ctDNA before and after treatment.

In conclusion, results from the accumulating studies on ctDNA provide substantial evidence of the promising prognostic and predictive value of ctDNA assessment in MIBC with implications for early prognostication, monitoring of treatment response, and early detection of metastatic relapse (Crupi et al. 2023; Rose et al. 2023).

19.4.7 ctDNA in Ongoing Clinical Bladder Cancer Trials

Currently, two ctDNA-guided clinical trials are ongoing to investigate the clinical utility of ctDNA analysis in MIBC, namely the IMvigor011 trial and the TOMBOLA trial.

IMvigor011, ClinicalTrials.gov: https://clinicaltrials.gov/ct2/show/NCT04660344 (2023)

IMvigor011 is a global, phase III, open-label, double-blind randomized trial of atezolizumab versus placebo as adjuvant therapy in patients with high-risk MIBC who are ctDNA positive after RC (Jackson-Spence et al. 2023). The study will provide insight into the clinical benefit of ctDNA-guided adjuvant treatment with atezolizumab and the primary endpoint is DFS within ≤24 weeks after RC (primary analysis population). Key secondary endpoints are OS (primary analysis population) and DFS (randomized population) and ctDNA clearance in patients who are ctDNA positive at baseline and ctDNA negative at cycle three or cycle five. Safety and exploratory predictive, prognostic, and pharmacodynamic biomarkers will also be assessed. The trial is ongoing at 184 sites in 23 different countries and will include a total of 520 patients.

TOMBOLA, ClinicalTrials.gov: https://clinicaltrials.gov/ct2/show/NCT04138628 (2022)

TOMBOLA is an acronym for "Treatment of metastatic BC at the time of biochemical relapse following radical cystectomy" and is a national, non-randomized phase III ctDNA-guided intervention trial for patients with MIBC treated with NAC and RC in Denmark. After surgery, monthly blood samples are analyzed for the presence of ctDNA and ctDNA positive patients will be treated with atezolizumab while ctDNA negative patients will continue the monitoring by monthly blood samples and scheduled CT scans. The aim of the study is to treat patients at a very early time point, where micrometastases are under the limit of detection for radiographic imaging, which may ultimately improve the patient outcomes, and select only high risk patients for oncological treatment. The primary endpoint is response (measured from ctDNA and CT scan results combined) to immunotherapy. Secondary objectives include OS and RFS for patients treated with atezolizumab at the time of biochemical relapse (ctDNA positivity). The trial is ongoing at five centers in Denmark and will include approximately 200 patients.

Several new trials will be initiated in the future, among these, e.g. the "MODERN" trial

(MRD-Based Optimization of ADjuvant ThErapy in URothelial CaNcer) https://classic.clinicaltrials.gov/ct2/show/NCT05987241 (2023). In this phase II/III trial the role of ctDNA in guiding the use of immunotherapy (Nivolumab alone or with Relatlimab) after RC will be investigated.

19.5 Advantages, Limitations, and Future Perspectives of Blood-Based Biomarkers

The major advantages of liquid biopsies in general are that they are minimally invasive and can be drawn repeatedly. A detailed overview of advantages and limitations of different blood-based biomarkers was provided by Li et al. (2023a). The main clinical applications of blood-based biomarkers are for diagnosis and prognosis assessment, while CTCs and ctDNA are also highly appropriate for monitoring of treatment response and for early detection of relapse after RC. In contrast to urine, blood-based analyses are highly reproducible due to the homeostasis of plasma. CTCs or ctDNA measurements may capture tumor heterogeneity, are highly reproducible, and enable achievement of a high test sensitivity and specificity. For implementation of CTCs or ctDNA analysis in a clinical setting, technical variability has to be reduced. This requires detailed standard-operating procedures (SOPs) to avoid differences in sample collection, processing, and storage, as well as in sequencing and bioinformatic analyses.

CTCs offer the possibility to perform a wide range of different analyses, including genomics, epigenomics, transcriptomics, proteomics, metabolomics as well as cancer-related epitope staining approaches. CTC single-cell NGS offers a unique possibility to characterize the tumor biology and the mechanisms of metastasis (Kojima et al. 2023). Moreover, CTCs present a great clinical tool to unravel drug sensitivity (De Renzi et al. 2022). A method for culturing of CTCs from colorectal cancer has recently been described (Nomura et al. 2023). This will be especially valuable for patients with heterogeneous, highly aggressive tumors or patients with multiple metastatic loci. As drugs can be applied to these cultures and drug sensitivity can be tested in vitro, this approach may spare the patient from ineffective treatments. This may facilitate a more personalized and tailored treatment of future patients, which may eradicate micrometastasis before they are detectable by imaging.

Plasma ctDNA analysis is highly dependent on the approach chosen as well as the sensitivity and specificity of the technology used for its detection. Many factors may affect the accuracy of the analysis, including sample quality, tumor heterogeneity, the presence of mutations in non-cancerous cells, and the number of targets analyzed. This can lead to false positives or false negatives, which can compromise the accuracy of the results. The detectability of ctDNA in a blood sample may be regarded as a proxy for the presence of carcinoma cells or micrometastasis and a decrease or increase in ctDNA levels over time is often interpreted as a proxy for treatment response or disease progression, respectively. In contrast, an increase in ctDNA levels during (neo-)adjuvant therapy could also resemble an increase of apoptotic cells and thus treatment response, while a decrease of ctDNA might resemble clonal development and thus progression, escaping detection when tumor-informed approaches are applied and/or few targets are analyzed. At present, ctDNA kinetics are not fully understood. In the future, the establishment of RECIST-ctDNA criteria (Response Evaluation Criteria in Solid Tumors) for ctDNA measurements is necessary to apply ctDNA evaluation of treatment response in the (micro)metastatic setting (Pascual et al. 2022).

A low CTC count in a blood sample or a low ctDNA concentration in a plasma sample represent some of the limitations for CTC and ctDNA analyses. These factors may result in CTCs or ctDNA being undetectable in patients with early-stage disease, where levels are lower. This may limit the usefulness of CTCs or ctDNA in some clinical settings. However, improved sequencing techniques accompanied by decreasing prices for NGS enable analysis with highly sensitive methods, including WGS and ultra-deep panel sequencing. Moreover, methods for cfDNA/

ctDNA extraction and CTC trapping are continuously improving. In the future, therapeutic apheresis or wearable devices may be used for continuous capture of CTCs (Kim et al. 2019). This development is rapidly proceeding, and recently a strategy to implement flexible wearable electronics and injectable nanomaterials to disrupt the hematogenous transport of CTCs was proposed (Li et al. 2023b).

In conclusion, blood-based analysis of CTCs and ctDNA might have large clinical potential. Using the right analyte with the right technique, a combination of the assessment of CTCs, ctDNA, and perhaps urinary tumor DNA may be highly effective for risk stratification, treatment monitoring, MRD detection, and detection of early relapse. However, prospective replication and clinical trial validation is still needed to demonstrate clinical usefulness.

References

Aceto N, Bardia A, Miyamoto DT, Donaldson MC, Wittner BS, Spencer JA, Yu M, Pely A, Engstrom A, Zhu H, Brannigan BW, Kapur R, Stott SL, Shioda T, Ramaswamy S, Ting DT, Lin CP, Toner M, Haber DA, Maheswaran S (2014) Circulating tumor cell clusters are oligoclonal precursors of breast cancer metastasis. Cell 158(5):1110–1122

Alborelli I, Generali D, Jermann P, Cappelletti MR, Ferrero G, Scaggiante B, Bortul M, Zanconati F, Nicolet S, Haegele J, Bubendorf L, Aceto N, Scaltriti M, Mucci G, Quagliata L, Novelli G (2019) Cell-free DNA analysis in healthy individuals by next-generation sequencing: a proof of concept and technical validation study. Cell Death Dis 10(7):534

Alcaide M, Cheung M, Hillman J, Rassekh SR, Deyell RJ, Batist G, Karsan A, Wyatt AW, Johnson N, Scott DW, Morin RD (2020) Evaluating the quantity, quality and size distribution of cell-free DNA by multiplex droplet digital PCR. Sci Rep 10(1):12564

Alix-Panabières C, Pantel K (2021) Liquid biopsy: from discovery to clinical application. Cancer Discov 11(4):858–873

Allard WJ, Matera J, Miller MC, Repollet M, Connelly MC, Rao C, Tibbe AG, Uhr JW, Terstappen LW (2004) Tumor cells circulate in the peripheral blood of all major carcinomas but not in healthy subjects or patients with nonmalignant diseases. Clin Cancer Res 10(20):6897–904. https://doi.org/10.1158/1078-0432.CCR-04-0378

Amintas S, Bedel A, Moreau-Gaudry F, Boutin J, Buscail L, Merlio J-P, Vendrely V, Dabernat S, Buscail E (2020) Circulating tumor cell clusters: united we stand divided we fall. Int J Mol Sci 21(7). https://doi.org/10.3390/ijms21072653

Avanzini S, Kurtz DM, Chabon JJ, Moding EJ, Hori SS, Gambhir SS, Alizadeh AA, Diehn M, Reiter JG (2020) A mathematical model of ctDNA shedding predicts tumor detection size. Sci Adv 6(50). https://doi.org/10.1126/sciadv.abc4308

Au SH, Edd J, Haber DA, Maheswaran S, Stott SL, Toner M (2017) Clusters of circulating tumor cells: a biophysical and technological perspective. Curr Opin Biomed Eng 3:13–19. https://doi.org/10.1016/j.cobme.2017.08.001

Bacchiani M, Salamone V, Massaro E, Sandulli A, Mariottini R, Cadenar A, Di Maida F, Pradere B, Mertens LS, Longoni M, Krajewski W, Del Giudice F, D'Andrea D, Laukhtina E, Shariat SF, Minervini A, Moschini M, Mari A, On Behalf of European Association of Urology-Young Academic Urologists Eau-Yau Urothelial Carcinoma Working Group (2023) Assessing the performance of 18F-FDG PET/CT in bladder cancer: a narrative review of current evidence. Cancers 15(11). https://doi.org/10.3390/cancers15112951

Battistelli M, Falcieri E (2020) Apoptotic bodies: particular extracellular vesicles involved in intercellular communication. Biology 9(1). https://doi.org/10.3390/biology9010021

Beije N, de Kruijff IE, de Jong JJ, Klaver SO, de Vries P, Jacobs RAL, Somford DM, Te Slaa E, van der Heijden AG, Alfred Witjes J, Fossion LMCL, Boevé ER, van der Hoeven J, van Melick HHE, Wijburg CJ, Bickerstaffe H, Martens JWM, de Wit R, Kraan J et al (2022) Circulating tumour cells to drive the use of neoadjuvant chemotherapy in patients with muscle-invasive bladder cancer. ESMO Open 7(2):100416

Bellmunt J, Hussain M, Gschwend JE, Albers P, Oudard S, Castellano D, Daneshmand S, Nishiyama H, Majchrowicz M, Degaonkar V, Shi Y, Mariathasan S, Grivas P, Drakaki A, O'Donnell PH, Rosenberg JE, Geynisman DM, Petrylak DP, Hoffman-Censits J et al (2021) Adjuvant atezolizumab versus observation in muscle-invasive urothelial carcinoma (IMvigor010): a multicentre, open-label, randomised, phase 3 trial. Lancet Oncol 22(4):525–537

Bettegowda C, Sausen M, Leary RJ, Kinde I, Wang Y, Agrawal N, Bartlett BR, Wang H, Luber B, Alani RM, Antonarakis ES, Azad NS, Bardelli A, Brem H, Cameron JL, Lee CC, Fecher LA, Gallia GL, Gibbs P et al (2014) Detection of circulating tumor DNA in early- and late-stage human malignancies. Sci Transl Med 6(224):224ra24

Birkenkamp-Demtröder K, Nordentoft I, Christensen E, Høyer S, Reinert T, Vang S, Borre M, Agerbæk M, Jensen JB, Ørntoft TF, Dyrskjøt L (2016) Genomic alterations in liquid biopsies from patients with bladder cancer. Eur Urol 70(1):75–82

Birkenkamp-Demtröder K, Christensen E, Nordentoft I, Knudsen M, Taber A, Høyer S, Lamy P, Agerbæk M, Jensen JB, Dyrskjøt L (2018) Monitoring treatment response and metastatic relapse in advanced bladder cancer by liquid biopsy analysis. Eur Urol 73(4):535–540

Boral D, Liu HN, Kenney SR, Marchetti D (2020) Molecular interplay between dormant bone marrow-resident cells (BMRCs) and CTCs in breast cancer. Cancers 12(6). https://doi.org/10.3390/cancers12061626

Celec P, Vlková B, Lauková L, Bábíčková J, Boor P (2018) Cell-free DNA: the role in pathophysiology and as a biomarker in kidney diseases. Expert Rev Mol Med 20:e1

Chen X, Gole J, Gore A, He Q, Lu M, Min J, Yuan Z, Yang X, Jiang Y, Zhang T, Suo C, Li X, Cheng L, Zhang Z, Niu H, Li Z, Xie Z, Shi H, Zhang X et al (2020) Non-invasive early detection of cancer four years before conventional diagnosis using a blood test. Nat Commun 11(1):3475

Christensen E, Birkenkamp-Demtröder K, Nordentoft I, Høyer S, van der Keur K, van Kessel K, Zwarthoff E, Agerbæk M, Ørntoft TF, Jensen JB, Dyrskjøt L (2017) Liquid biopsy analysis of FGFR3 and PIK3CA hotspot mutations for disease surveillance in bladder cancer. Eur Urol 71(6):961–969

Christensen E, Birkenkamp-Demtröder K, Sethi H, Shchegrova S, Salari R, Nordentoft I, Wu H-T, Knudsen M, Lamy P, Lindskrog SV, Taber A, Balcioglu M, Vang S, Assaf Z, Sharma S, Tin AS, Srinivasan R, Hafez D, Reinert T et al (2019) Early detection of metastatic relapse and monitoring of therapeutic efficacy by ultra-deep sequencing of plasma cell-free DNA in patients with urothelial bladder carcinoma. J Clin Oncol Off J Am Soc Clin Oncol 37(18):1547–1557

Christensen E, Nordentoft I, Birkenkamp-Demtröder K, Elbæk SK, Lindskrog SV, Taber A, Andreasen TG, Strandgaard T, Knudsen M, Lamy P, Agerbæk M, Jensen JB, Dyrskjøt L (2023) Cell-free urine and plasma DNA mutational analysis predicts neoadjuvant chemotherapy response and outcome in patients with muscle-invasive bladder cancer. Clin Cancer Res 29(8):1582–1591

Cohen JD, Li L, Wang Y, Thoburn C, Afsari B, Danilova L, Douville C, Javed AA, Wong F, Mattox A, Hruban RH, Wolfgang CL, Goggins MG, Dal Molin M, Wang T-L, Roden R, Klein AP, Ptak J, Dobbyn L et al (2018) Detection and localization of surgically resectable cancers with a multi-analyte blood test. Science 359(6378):926–930

Cristiano S, Leal A, Phallen J, Fiksel J, Adleff V, Bruhm DC, Jensen SØ, Medina JE, Hruban C, White JR, Palsgrove DN, Niknafs N, Anagnostou V, Forde P, Naidoo J, Marrone K, Brahmer J, Woodward BD, Husain H et al (2019) Genome-wide cell-free DNA fragmentation in patients with cancer. Nature 570(7761):385–389

Crupi E, de Padua TC, Marandino L, Raggi D, Dyrskjøt L, Spiess PE, Sonpavde GP, Kamat AM, Necchi A (2023) Circulating tumor DNA as a predictive and prognostic biomarker in the perioperative treatment of muscle-invasive bladder cancer: a systematic review. Eur Urol Oncol. https://doi.org/10.1016/j.euo.2023.05.012

De Renzi G, De Marco G, De Meo M, Del Rosso E, Gazzaniga P, Nicolazzo C (2022) In vitro cultures of circulating tumor cells: a potential tool to unravel drug sensitivity. Cancer Drug Resist (Alhambra, Calif.) 5(1):245–260

Descamps L, Le Roy D, Deman A-L (2022) Microfluidic-based technologies for CTC isolation: a review of 10 years of intense efforts towards liquid biopsy. Int J Mol Sci 23(4). https://doi.org/10.3390/ijms23041981

Diamantopoulou Z, Castro-Giner F, Schwab FD, Foerster C, Saini M, Budinjas S, Strittmatter K, Krol I, Seifert B, Heinzelmann-Schwarz V, Kurzeder C, Rochlitz C, Vetter M, Weber WP, Aceto N (2022) The metastatic spread of breast cancer accelerates during sleep. Nature 607(7917):156–162

Diehl F, Schmidt K, Choti MA, Romans K, Goodman S, Li M, Thornton K, Agrawal N, Sokoll L, Szabo SA, Kinzler KW, Vogelstein B, Diaz LA Jr (2008) Circulating mutant DNA to assess tumor dynamics. Nat Med 14(9):985–990

Doak GR, Schwertfeger KL, Wood DK (2018) Distant relations: macrophage functions in the metastatic niche. Trends Cancer Res 4(6):445–459

Doubeni CA, Castle PE (2023) Multicancer early detection: a promise yet to be proven. Am Fam Physician 107(3):224–225A

Duffy MJ, Diamandis EP, Crown J (2021) Circulating tumor DNA (ctDNA) as a pan-cancer screening test: is it finally on the horizon? Clin Chem Lab Med CCLM/FESCC 59(8):1353–1361

Eslami-S Z, Cortés-Hernández LE, Alix-Panabières C (2020) The metastatic cascade as the basis for liquid biopsy development. Front Oncol 10:1055

Feng R, Li Z, Ge G, Wang C, Jia Y, Ouyang J (2023) Cancer-associated fibroblast-derived extracellular vesicles mediate immune escape of bladder cancer via PD-L1/PD-1 expression. Endocr Metab Immune Disord Drug Targets. https://doi.org/10.2174/1871530323666230228124125

Fish L, Zhang S, Yu JX, Culbertson B, Zhou AY, Goga A, Goodarzi H (2018) Cancer cells exploit an orphan RNA to drive metastatic progression. Nat Med 24(11):1743–1751

Fjelstrup S, Dupont DM, Bus C, et al. (2022) Differential RNA aptamer affinity profiling on plasma as a potential diagnostic tool for bladder cancer. NAR Cancer. 4(3):zcac025. Published 2022 Aug 22. https://doi.org/10.1093/narcan/zcac025

Follain G, Osmani N, Azevedo AS, Allio G, Mercier L, Karreman MA, Solecki G, Garcia Leòn MJ, Lefebvre O, Fekonja N, Hille C, Chabannes V, Dollé G, Metivet T, Hovsepian FD, Prudhomme C, Pichot A, Paul N, Carapito R et al (2018) Hemodynamic forces tune the arrest, adhesion, and extravasation of circulating tumor cells. Dev Cell 45(1):33–52.e12

Fu G, Cheng KS, Chen A, Xu Z, Chen X, Tian J, Xu C, Sun Y, Neoh KH, Dai Y, Han RPS, Jin B (2021) Microfluidic assaying of circulating tumor cells and its application in risk stratification of urothelial bladder cancer. Front Oncol 11:701298

García Moreira V, de la Cera Martínez T, Gago González E, Prieto García B, Alvarez Menéndez FV (2006) Increase in and clearance of cell-free plasma DNA in hemodialysis quantified by real-time PCR. Clin Chem Lab Med (CCLM/FESCC) 44(12):1410–1415

Gazzaniga P, de Berardinis E, Raimondi C, Gradilone A, Busetto GM, De Falco E, Nicolazzo C, Giovannone R, Gentile V, Cortesi E, Pantel K (2014) Circulating tumor cells detection has independent prognostic impact in high-risk non-muscle invasive bladder cancer. Int J Cancer 135(8):1978–1982

Gómez BB, López-Cortés R, Casas-Nebra FJ, Vázquez-Estévez S, Pérez-Fentes D, Chantada-Vázquez MDP, Bravo SB, Núñez C (2021) Detection of circulating serum protein biomarkers of non-muscle invasive bladder cancer after protein corona-silver nanoparticles analysis by SWATH-MS. Nanomaterials (Basel, Switzerland) 11(9). https://doi.org/10.3390/nano11092384

Gorges TM, Penkalla N, Schalk T, Joosse SA, Riethdorf S, Tucholski J, Lücke K, Wikman H, Jackson S, Brychta N, Others. (2016) Enumeration and molecular characterization of tumor cells in lung cancer patients using a novel in vivo device for capturing circulating tumor cells detection of CTCs by a novel in vivo approach. Clin Cancer Res 22(9):2197–2206

Grivas P, Lalani A-KA, Pond GR, Nagy RJ, Faltas B, Agarwal N, Gupta SV, Drakaki A, Vaishampayan UN, Wang J, Barata PC, Gopalakrishnan D, Naik G, McGregor BA, Kiedrowski LA, Lanman RB, Sonpavde GP (2020) Circulating tumor DNA alterations in advanced urothelial carcinoma and association with clinical outcomes: a pilot study. Eur Urol Oncol 3(5):695–699

Hackshaw A, Clarke CA, Hartman A-R (2022) New genomic technologies for multi-cancer early detection: Rethinking the scope of cancer screening. Cancer Cell 40(2):109–113

Hahn AW, Nussenzveig RH, Maughan BL, Agarwal N (2019) Cell-free circulating tumor DNA (ctDNA) in metastatic renal cell carcinoma (mRCC): Current knowledge and potential uses. Kidney Cancer 3(1):7–13

Han L, Lam EW-F, Sun Y (2019) Extracellular vesicles in the tumor microenvironment: old stories, but new tales. Mol Cancer 18(1):59

Hou J-M, Krebs MG, Lancashire L, Sloane R, Backen A, Swain RK, Priest LJC, Greystoke A, Zhou C, Morris K, Ward T, Blackhall FH, Dive C (2012) Clinical significance and molecular characteristics of circulating tumor cells and circulating tumor microemboli in patients with small-cell lung cancer. J Clin Oncol Off J Am Soc Clin Oncol 30(5):525–532

Ismail MF, El Boghdady NA, Shabayek MI, Awida HA, Abozeed H (2016) Evaluation and screening of mRNA S100A genes as serological biomarkers in different stages of bladder cancer in Egypt. Tumour Biol 37(4):4621–4631

Jackson-Spence F, Toms C, O'Mahony LF, Choy J, Flanders L, Szabados B, Powles T (2023) IMvigor011: a study of adjuvant atezolizumab in patients with high-risk MIBC who are ctDNA+ post-surgery. Future Oncol 19(7):509–515

Jhuo Y-C, Cha T-L, Kao C-C, Tsai Y-T, Wu S-T, Meng E, Tsao C-W, Chen C-L, Ting H-K, Sun G-H, Yu D-S, Chang S-Y, Yang M-H (2023) Circulating tumor cells predict response of neoadjuvant chemotherapy in patients with bladder cancer: a preliminary study. Diagnostics (Basel, Switzerland) 13(6). https://doi.org/10.3390/diagnostics13061032

Kaba M, Pirinççi N, Demir M, Kaba S, Oztuzcu S, Verep S (2023) The relationship between microRNAs and bladder cancer: are microRNAs useful to predict bladder cancer in suspicious patients? Int Urol Nephrol. https://doi.org/10.1007/s11255-023-03666-2

Kalluri R, Weinberg RA (2009) The basics of epithelial-mesenchymal transition. J Clin Invest 119(6):1420–1428

Keller L, Belloum Y, Wikman H, Pantel K (2021) Clinical relevance of blood-based ctDNA analysis: mutation detection and beyond. Br J Cancer 124(2):345–358

Jiang X, Du L, Wang L, et al. (2015) Serum microRNA expression signatures identified from genome-wide microRNA profiling serve as novel noninvasive biomarkers for diagnosis and recurrence of bladder cancer. Int J Cancer 136(4):854–862. https://doi.org/10.1002/ijc.29041

Kim ST, Banks KC, Lee S-H, Kim K, Park JO, Park SH, Park YS, Lim HY, Kang WK, Lanman RB, Talasaz A, Park K, Lee J (2017) Prospective feasibility study for using cell-free circulating tumor DNA-guided therapy in refractory metastatic solid cancers: an interim analysis. JCO Precis Oncol 1:1–15

Kim TH, Wang Y, Oliver CR, Thamm DH, Cooling L, Paoletti C, Smith KJ, Nagrath S, Hayes DF (2019) A temporary indwelling intravascular aphaeretic system for in vivo enrichment of circulating tumor cells. Nat Commun 10(1):1478

Klein EA, Richards D, Cohn A, Tummala M, Lapham R, Cosgrove D, Chung G, Clement J, Gao J, Hunkapiller N, Jamshidi A, Kurtzman KN, Seiden MV, Swanton C, Liu MC (2021) Clinical validation of a targeted methylation-based multi-cancer early detection test using an independent validation set. Ann Oncol 32(9):1167–1177

Kobayashi M, Abe H, Arai K, Murakami S, Kamai T (2022) Circulating tumor cells and cell-free tumor DNA analyses in urothelial cancer using the LiquidBiopsy platform. Curr Urol Rep 16(2):99–106

Kojima M, Harada T, Fukazawa T, Kurihara S, Touge R, Saeki I, Takahashi S, Hiyama E (2023) Single-cell next-generation sequencing of circulating tumor cells in patients with neuroblastoma. Cancer Sci 114(4):1616–1624

Kurma K, Alix-Panabières C (2023) Mechanobiology and survival strategies of circulating tumor cells: a process towards the invasive and metastatic phenotype. Front Cell Dev Biol 11:1188499

Kustanovich A, Schwartz R, Peretz T, Grinshpun A (2019) Life and death of circulating cell-free DNA. Cancer Biol Ther 20(8):1057–1067

Lawrence R, Watters M, Davies CR, Pantel K, Lu Y-J (2023) Circulating tumour cells for early detection of clinically relevant cancer. Nat Rev Clin Oncol 20(7):487–500

Lemańska-Perek A, Lis-Kuberka J, Lepczyński A, Dratwa-Chałupnik A, Tupikowski K, Kątnik-Prastowska I, Ożgo M (2019) Potential plasma biomarkers of bladder cancer identified by proteomic analysis: A pilot study. Adv Clin Exp Med 28(3):339–346

Lennon AM, Buchanan AH, Kinde I, Warren A, Honushefsky A, Cohain AT, Ledbetter DH, Sanfilippo F, Sheridan K, Rosica D, Adonizio CS, Hwang HJ, Lahouel K, Cohen JD, Douville C, Patel AA, Hagmann LN, Rolston DD, Malani N et al (2020) Feasibility of blood testing combined with PET-CT to screen for cancer and guide intervention. Science 369(6499). https://doi.org/10.1126/science.abb9601

Li S, Xin K, Pan S, Wang Y, Zheng J, Li Z, Liu X, Liu B, Xu Z, Chen X (2023a) Blood-based liquid biopsy: insights into early detection, prediction, and treatment monitoring of bladder cancer. Cell Mol Biol Lett 28(1):28

Li Y, Liu X, Zhang Y, Wu Z, Ling W, Zhang X, Zhou M, Onses MS, Zhou P, Mao S, Huo W, Fan Z, Yang H, Wang H, Huang X (2023b) A flexible wearable device coupled with injectable Fe3O4 nanoparticles for capturing circulating tumor cells and triggering their deaths. Biosens Bioelectron 235:115367

Lindskrog SV, Birkenkamp-Demtroder K, Nordentoft I, Laliotis G, Lamy P, Christensen E, Renner D, Andreasen TG, Lange N, Sharma S, ElNaggar AC, Liu MC, Sethi H, Aleshin A, Agerbæk M, Jensen JB, Dyrskjøt L (2023) Circulating tumor DNA analysis in advanced urothelial carcinoma: insights from biological analysis and extended clinical follow-up. Clin Cancer Res. https://doi.org/10.1158/1078 0432.CCR-23-1860

Liu Y-R, Ortiz-Bonilla CJ, Lee Y-F (2018) Extracellular vesicles in bladder cancer: biomarkers and beyond. Int J Mol Sci 19(9). https://doi.org/10.3390/ijms19092822

Malkin EZ, Bratman SV (2020) Bioactive DNA from extracellular vesicles and particles. Cell Death Dis 11(7):584

Mathios D, Johansen JS, Cristiano S, Medina JE, Phallen J, Larsen KR, Bruhm DC, Niknafs N, Ferreira L, Adleff V, Chiao JY, Leal A, Noe M, White JR, Arun AS, Hruban C, Annapragada AV, Jensen SØ, Ørntoft M-BW et al (2021) Detection and characterization of lung cancer using cell-free DNA fragmentomes. Nat Commun 12(1):5060

Meeks JJ, Al-Ahmadie H, Faltas BM, Taylor JA 3rd, Flaig TW, DeGraff DJ, Christensen E, Woolbright BL, McConkey DJ, Dyrskjøt L (2020) Genomic heterogeneity in bladder cancer: challenges and possible solutions to improve outcomes. Nat Rev Urol 17(5):259–270

Mendelaar PAJ, Kraan J, Van M, Zeune LL, Terstappen LWMM, Oomen-de Hoop E, Martens JWM, Sleijfer S (2021) Defining the dimensions of circulating tumor cells in a large series of breast, prostate, colon, and bladder cancer patients. Mol Oncol 15(1):116–125

Micalizzi DS, Maheswaran S, Haber DA (2017) A conduit to metastasis: circulating tumor cell biology. Genes Dev 31(18):1827–1840

Mitchell MJ, King MR (2013) Fluid shear stress sensitizes cancer cells to receptor-mediated apoptosis via trimeric death receptors. New J Phys 15:015008

Moss J, Magenheim J, Neiman D, Zemmour H, Loyfer N, Korach A, Samet Y, Maoz M, Druid H, Arner P, Fu K-Y, Kiss E, Spalding KL, Landesberg G, Zick A, Grinshpun A, Shapiro AMJ, Grompe M, Wittenberg AD et al (2018) Comprehensive human cell-type methylation atlas reveals origins of circulating cell-free DNA in health and disease. Nat Commun 9(1):5068

Nomura M, Yokoyama Y, Yoshimura D, Minagawa Y, Yamamoto A, Tanaka Y, Sekiguchi N, Marukawa D, Ichihara M, Itakura H, Matsumoto K, Morimoto Y, Tomihara H, Inoue A, Ogino T, Miyoshi N, Takahashi H, Takahashi H, Uemura M et al (2023) Simple detection and culture of circulating tumor cells from colorectal cancer patients using poly(2-methoxyethyl acrylate)-coated plates. Int J Mol Sci 24(4). https://doi.org/10.3390/ijms24043949

Nordentoft I, Birkenkamp-Demtröder K, Dyrskjøt L (2023a) NGS-based tumor-informed analysis of circulating tumor DNA. Methods Mol Biol 2684:179–197

Nordentoft I, Viborg Lindskrog S, Birkenkamp-Demtröder K, Gonzalez S, Kuzman M, Glavas D, Ptashkin RN, Smadbeck J, Afterman D, Lauterman T, Cohen Y, Donenhirsh Z, Tavassoly I, Alon U, Polak P, Oklander B, Agerbaek M, Jensen JB, Zviran A, Dyrskjøt L (2023b) Accuracy of genome-wide mutational analysis for tumor-informed ctDNA-guided MRD monitoring in bladder cancer. J Clin Orthod JCO 41(16_suppl):4589–4589

Nordentoft I, Viborg Lindskrog S, Birkenkamp-Demtroeder K, Gonzalez S, Kuzman M, Levatic J, Glavas D, Ptashkin R, Smadbeck J, Afterman D, Lauterman T, Cohen Y, Donenhirsh Z, Tavassoly I, Alon U, Frydendahl Boll Johansen A, Heilskov Rasmussen M, Lindbjerg Andersen C, Polak P et al (2023c) Whole genome mutational analysis for accurate tumor-informed ctDNA based MRD surveillance, treatment monitoring and biological characterization of urothelial carcinoma. Eur Urol. https://doi.org/10.1101/2023.07.13.23292590

Oberhofer A, Bronkhorst AJ, Uhlig C, Ungerer V, Holdenrieder S (2022) Tracing the origin of cell-free DNA molecules through tissue-specific epigenetic signatures. Diagnostics (Basel, Switzerland) 12(8). https://doi.org/10.3390/diagnostics12081834

O'Brian D, Prunty M, Hill A, Shoag J (2021) The role of C-reactive protein in kidney, bladder, and prostate cancers. Front Immunol 12:721989

Osman I, Bajorin DF, Sun T-T, Zhong H, Douglas D, Scattergood J, Zheng R, Han M, Marshall KW, Liew C-C (2006) Novel blood biomarkers of human urinary bladder cancer. Clin Cancer Res 12(11 Pt 1):3374–3380

Pantel K, Alix-Panabières C (2019) Liquid biopsy and minimal residual disease—latest advances and implications for cure. Nat Rev Clin Oncol 16(7):409–424

Pascual J, Attard G, Bidard F-C, Curigliano G, De Mattos-Arruda L, Diehn M, Italiano A, Lindberg J, Merker JD, Montagut C, Normanno N, Pantel K, Pentheroudakis G, Popat S, Reis-Filho JS, Tie J, Seoane J, Tarazona N, Yoshino T, Turner NC (2022) ESMO recommendations on the use of circulating tumour DNA assays for patients with cancer: a report from the ESMO Precision Medicine Working Group. Ann Oncol 33(8):750–768

Patel KM, van der Vos KE, Smith CG, Mouliere F, Tsui D, Morris J, Chandrananda D, Marass F, van den Broek D, Neal DE, Gnanapragasam VJ, Forshew T, van Rhijn BW, Massie CE, Rosenfeld N, van der Heijden MS (2017) Association of plasma and urinary mutant DNA with clinical outcomes in muscle invasive bladder cancer. Sci Rep 7(1):5554

Peinado H, Zhang H, Matei IR, Costa-Silva B, Hoshino A, Rodrigues G, Psaila B, Kaplan RN, Bromberg JF, Kang Y, Bissell MJ, Cox TR, Giaccia AJ, Erler JT, Hiratsuka S, Ghajar CM, Lyden D (2017) Pre-metastatic niches: organ-specific homes for metastases. Nat Rev Cancer 17(5):302–317

Piñeiro R, Martínez-Pena I, López-López R (2020) Relevance of CTC clusters in breast cancer metastasis. Adv Exp Med Biol 1220:93–115

Powles T, Assaf ZJ, Davarpanah N, Banchereau R, Szabados BE, Yuen KC, Grivas P, Hussain M, Oudard S, Gschwend JE, Albers P, Castellano D, Nishiyama H, Daneshmand S, Sharma S, Zimmermann BG, Sethi H, Aleshin A, Perdicchio M et al (2021) ctDNA guiding adjuvant immunotherapy in urothelial carcinoma. Nature 595(7867):432–437

Powles T, Assaf ZJ, Degaonkar V, Grivas P, Hussain M, Oudard S, Gschwend JE, Albers P, Castellano D, Nishiyama H, Daneshmand S, Sharma S, Sethi H, Aleshin A, Shi Y, Davarpanah N, Carter C, Bellmunt J, Mariathasan S (2023) Updated overall survival by circulating tumor DNA status from the phase 3 IMvigor010 trial: adjuvant atezolizumab versus observation in muscle-invasive urothelial carcinoma. Eur Urol. https://doi.org/10.1016/j.eururo.2023.06.007

Rahbarghazi R, Jabbari N, Sani NA, Asghari R, Salimi L, Kalashani SA, Feghhi M, Etemadi T, Akbariazar E, Mahmoudi M, Rezaie J (2019) Tumor-derived extracellular vesicles: reliable tools for Cancer diagnosis and clinical applications. Cell Commun Signal (CCS) 17(1):73

Rejniak KA (2016) Circulating tumor cells: when a solid tumor meets a fluid microenvironment. Adv Exp Med Biol 936:93–106

Rink M, Chun FK, Dahlem R, Soave A, Minner S, Hansen J, Stoupiec M, Coith C, Kluth LA, Ahyai SA, Friedrich MG, Shariat SF, Fisch M, Pantel K, Riethdorf S (2012) Prognostic role and HER2 expression of circulating tumor cells in peripheral blood of patients prior to radical cystectomy: a prospective study. Eur Urol 61(4):810–817

Romagnoli GG, Zelante BB, Toniolo PA, Migliori IK, Barbuto JAM (2014) Dendritic cell-derived exosomes may be a tool for cancer immunotherapy by converting tumor cells into immunogenic targets. Front Immunol 5:692

Rose KM, Huelster HL, Meeks JJ, Faltas BM, Sonpavde GP, Lerner SP, Ross JS, Spiess PE, Grass GD, Jain RK, Kamat AM, Vosoughi A, Wang L, Wang X, Li R (2023) Circulating and urinary tumour DNA in urothelial carcinoma—upper tract, lower tract and metastatic disease. Nat Rev Urol 20(7):406–419

Rostami P, Kashaninejad N, Moshksayan K, Said Saidi M, Firoozabadi B, Nguyen N-T (2019) Novel approaches in cancer management with circulating tumor cell clusters. J Sci Adv Mater Devices 4(1):1–18. https://doi.org/10.1016/j.jsamd.2019.01.006

Sánchez-Herrero E, Serna-Blasco R, Robado de Lope L, González-Rumayor V, Romero A, Provencio M (2022) Circulating tumor DNA as a cancer biomarker: an overview of biological features and factors that may impact on ctDNA analysis. Front Oncol 12. https://doi.org/10.3389/fonc.2022.943253

Santonja A, Cooper WN, Eldridge MD, Edwards PAW, Morris JA, Edwards AR, Zhao H, Heider K, Couturier D-L, Vijayaraghavan A, Mennea P, Ditter E-J, Smith CG, Boursnell C, Manzano García R, Rueda OM, Beddowes E, Biggs H, Sammut S-J et al (2023) Comparison of tumor-informed and tumor-naïve sequencing assays for ctDNA detection in breast cancer. EMBO Mol Med 15(6):e16505

Sanz-Garcia E, Zhao E, Bratman SV, Siu LL (2022) Monitoring and adapting cancer treatment using circulating tumor DNA kinetics: Current research, opportunities, and challenges. Sci Adv 8(4):eabi8618

Saucedo-Zeni N, Mewes S, Niestroj R, Gasiorowski L, Murawa D, Nowaczyk P, Tomasi T, Weber E, Dworacki G, Morgenthaler NG, Jansen H, Propping C, Sterzynska K, Dyszkiewicz W, Zabel M, Kiechle M, Reuning U, Schmitt M, Lücke K (2012) A novel method for the in vivo isolation of circulating tumor cells from peripheral blood of cancer patients using a functionalized and structured medical wire. Int J Oncol 41(4):1241–1250

Schlenker F, Kipf E, Deuter M, Höffkes I, Lehnert M, Zengerle R, von Stetten F, Scherer F, Wehrle J, von Bubnoff N, Juelg P, Hutzenlaub T, Borst N (2021) Stringent base specific and optimization-free multiplex mediator probe ddPCR for the quantification of point mutations in circulating tumor DNA. Cancers 13(22). https://doi.org/10.3390/cancers13225742

Schuster E, Taftaf R, Reduzzi C, Albert MK, Romero-Calvo I, Liu H (2021) Better together: circulating tumor cell clustering in metastatic cancer. Trends Cancer Res 7(11):1020–1032

Schwarzenbach H, Hoon DSB, Pantel K (2011) Cell-free nucleic acids as biomarkers in cancer patients. Nat Rev Cancer 11(6):426–437

Shohdy KS, Villamar DM, Cao Y, Trieu J, Price KS, Nagy R, Tagawa ST, Molina AM, Sternberg CN, Nanus DM, Mosquera JM, Elemento O, Sonpavde GP, Grivas P, Vogelzang NJ, Faltas BM (2022) Serial ctDNA analysis predicts clinical progression in patients with advanced urothelial carcinoma. Br J Cancer 126(3):430–439

Soave A, Riethdorf S, Dahlem R, von Amsberg G, Minner S, Weisbach L, Engel O, Fisch M, Pantel K, Rink M (2017) A nonrandomized, prospective, clinical study on the impact of circulating tumor cells on outcomes of urothelial carcinoma of the bladder patients treated with radical cystectomy with or without adjuvant chemotherapy. Int J Cancer 140(2):381–389

Sproston NR, Ashworth JJ (2018) Role of C-reactive protein at sites of inflammation and infection. Front Immunol 9:754

Steensma DP, Bejar R, Jaiswal S, Lindsley RC, Sekeres MA, Hasserjian RP, Ebert BL (2015) Clonal hematopoiesis of indeterminate potential and its distinction from myelodysplastic syndromes. Blood 126(1):9–16

Stejskal P, Goodarzi H, Srovnal J, Hajdúch M, van't Veer LJ, Magbanua MJM (2023) Circulating tumor nucleic acids: biology, release mechanisms, and clinical relevance. Mol Cancer 22(1):15

Szabados B, Kockx M, Assaf ZJ, van Dam P-J, Rodriguez-Vida A, Duran I, Crabb SJ, Van Der Heijden MS, Pous AF, Gravis G, Herranz UA, Protheroe A, Ravaud A, Maillet D, Mendez MJ, Suarez C, Linch M, Prendergast A, Tyson C et al (2022) Final results of neoadjuvant atezolizumab in cisplatin-ineligible patients with muscle-invasive urothelial cancer of the bladder. Eur Urol 82(2):212–222

Szczerba BM, Castro-Giner F, Vetter M, Krol I, Gkountela S, Landin J, Scheidmann MC, Donato C, Scherrer R, Singer J, Beisel C, Kurzeder C, Heinzelmann-Schwarz V, Rochlitz C, Weber WP, Beerenwinkel N, Aceto N (2019) Neutrophils escort circulating tumour cells to enable cell cycle progression. Nature 566(7745):553–557

Taylor DD, Zacharias W, Gercel-Taylor C (2011) Exosome isolation for proteomic analyses and RNA profiling. Methods Mol Biol 728:235–246

Thierry AR (2023) Circulating DNA fragmentomics and cancer screening. Cell Genomics 3(1):100242

Vandekerkhove G, Todenhöfer T, Annala M, Struss WJ, Wong A, Beja K, Ritch E, Brahmbhatt S, Volik SV, Hennenlotter J, Nykter M, Chi KN, North S, Stenzl A, Collins CC, Eigl BJ, Black PC, Wyatt AW (2017) Circulating tumor DNA reveals clinically actionable somatic genome of metastatic bladder cancer. Clin Cancer Res 23(21):6487–6497

Vandekerkhove G, Lavoie J-M, Annala M, Murtha AJ, Sundahl N, Walz S, Sano T, Taavitsainen S, Ritch E, Fazli L, Hurtado-Coll A, Wang G, Nykter M, Black PC, Todenhöfer T, Ost P, Gibb EA, Chi KN, Eigl BJ, Wyatt AW (2021) Plasma ctDNA is a tumor tissue surrogate and enables clinical-genomic stratification of metastatic bladder cancer. Nat Commun 12(1):184

Voronova V, Peskov K, Glybochko P, Svistunov A, Fomin V, Kopylov P, Enikeev D, Gitel E, Ragimov A, Poddubskaya E, Sekacheva M (2019) 149P—Evaluation and diagnostic potential of plasma biomarkers in bladder cancer. Ann Oncol 30:v46–v47

Went PT, Lugli A, Meier S, Bundi M, Mirlacher M, Sauter G, Dirnhofer S (2004) Frequent EpCam protein expression in human carcinomas. Hum Pathol 35(1):122–128

Wieder R (2023) Awakening of dormant breast cancer cells in the bone marrow. Cancers 15(11). https://doi.org/10.3390/cancers15113021

Zhang J, Dai D, Tian J, Li L, Bai J, Xu Y, Wang Z, Tang A (2021) Circulating tumor DNA analyses predict disease recurrence in non-muscle-invasive bladder cancer. Front Oncol 11:657483

Zhou L, Cai X, Liu Q, Jian Z-Y, Li H, Wang K-J (2015) Prognostic role of C-reactive protein in urological cancers: a meta-analysis. Sci Rep 5:12733

Zviran A, Schulman RC, Shah M, Hill STK, Deochand S, Khamnei CC, Maloney D, Patel K, Liao W, Widman AJ, Wong P, Callahan MK, Ha G, Reed S, Rotem D, Frederick D, Sharova T, Miao B, Kim T et al (2020) Genome-wide cell-free DNA mutational integration enables ultra-sensitive cancer monitoring. Nat Med 26(7):1114–1124

Mechanisms and Biomarkers of Response to BCG and Chemotherapy in Bladder Cancer

20

Henning Bahlburg and Peter C. Black

Abstract

Almost 50 years after first use, instillation therapy with attenuated strains of *Mycobacterium bovis* (Bacillus Calmette-Guérin, BCG) is still the gold standard in the treatment of high-risk non-muscle invasive bladder cancer (NMIBC). However, up to 26% of patients recur within the first year and 41% within 5 years. Furthermore, progression to muscle-invasive bladder cancer (MIBC) after BCG therapy is observed in about 14% of patients, often resulting in delayed definitive therapy (e.g., radical cystectomy) with worse outcomes. Neoadjuvant platinum-based chemotherapy (NAC) has been shown to improve overall survival for patients with MIBC. However, only 40–50% of patients experience a tumor downstaging and the remaining patients are exposed to potential treatment toxicity and delay in definitive local therapy without apparent benefit.

Several molecular characteristics associated with treatment response have been discovered in both bladder cancer disease states. However, no biomarkers (e.g., extracted from tissue, blood, or urine) have been validated for clinical use that reliably predict response in either NMIBC treated with BCG or MIBC treated with NAC. Therefore, this chapter aims to provide an overview of different known mechanisms of resistance to BCG in high-risk NMIBC and chemotherapy in MIBC, and how this knowledge is informing the development of predictive biomarkers.

Keywords

Non-muscle invasive bladder cancer · Muscle-invasive bladder cancer · Treatment resistance mechanisms · Bacillus Calmette-Guérin · Intravesical therapy · Cisplatin · Neoadjuvant chemotherapy

20.1 Introduction

Optimal treatment for both non-muscle invasive bladder cancer (NMIBC) and muscle-invasive bladder cancer (MIBC) is well-established and driven by appropriate clinical trials evidence (Lamm et al. 2000; Grossman et al. 2003; International Collaboration of Trialists et al. 2011). Across the NMIBC and MIBC disease spectrum, patients are managed primarily with a combination of surgery and medical therapy, as well as radiotherapy in select situations. Intravesical BCG is critical in the management of intermediate and high-risk NMIBC and perioperative chemotherapy is part of the standard of

H. Bahlburg · P. C. Black (✉)
University of British Columbia,
Vancouver, BC, Canada
e-mail: peter.black@ubc.ca

M. A. Knowles, L. Dyrskjøt (eds.), *Biology of Bladder Cancer*,
https://doi.org/10.1007/978-3-031-68505-7_20

care for MIBC. However, both of these long-standing treatments are associated with clinically significant toxicity, and treatment failures are common. Ideally, both BCG and perioperative chemotherapy would be administered only to a subset of patients who are likely to respond, and the remaining patients would proceed to other therapies, thereby avoiding potential toxicity from likely ineffective treatment. Predictive biomarkers are the essential missing link in such a model of precision oncology. Unfortunately, true predictive biomarkers can be difficult to identify and validate because we usually lack the corresponding control cohorts that were treated without the specific treatment being assessed, so that it is impossible to distinguish predictive from prognostic implications of a marker. A putative predictive marker without the adequate control may simply identify an aggressive tumor with a poor prognosis rather than identifying a biological predisposition to the specific treatment. A better understanding of the mechanisms of response to BCG and perioperative chemotherapy will be critical in developing predictive biomarkers. In this chapter, we will review some of what is known about response mechanisms to BCG and chemotherapy, and how this knowledge is informing the discovery of predictive biomarkers.

20.2 Intravesical BCG Therapy for Non-muscle Invasive Bladder Cancer

20.2.1 Natural History of Non-muscle Invasive Bladder Cancer Treated with BCG

The risk of recurrence and progression of NMIBC places a significant burden on patients and the healthcare system (Chamie et al. 2013). Untreated, about 15% of NMIBC progress to MIBC (Fujii 2018). Progression goes hand in hand with an increase in cancer-related death. Superficially invasive T1 tumors, if untreated, progress in >50% of cases and show a mortality of 25% within the first 5 years after initial diagnosis (Herr 1997). Carcinoma in situ (Cis) most commonly presents concomitantly with papillary tumors. Some studies have found a rate of progression to MIBC in >50% of these cases with 20% of patients dying from metastatic bladder cancer when treated conservatively (Aldousari and Kassouf 2010; Jakse et al. 2001). However, several studies have also questioned, whether concomitant Cis contributes to tumor progression (Fujii et al. 1998; Kobayashi et al. 2014; Ali-El-Dein et al. 2013; Yamada et al. 2010).

Progression of high-risk NMIBC to MIBC may be delayed by intravesical instillation with Bacillus Calmette-Guérin (BCG), an attenuated form of *Mycobacterium bovis*. This treatment was established in 1976 by Morales et al. (1976). Instillation therapy with BCG presents a viable alternative to an early radical cystectomy and is superior to intravesical chemotherapy in high-risk NMIBC (Malmstrom et al. 2009; EAU 2022; Chang et al. 2017).

Up to 26% of patients recur within the first year and 41% within 5 years (Cambier et al. 2016). Depending on tumor stage, almost 20% of patients progress to MIBC within 5 years (Cambier et al. 2016). A 20% cancer-related mortality in patients treated with BCG highlights this tumor's aggressiveness and the need for a deeper understanding of tumor biology.

Response seems to decrease with patient age, as patients older than 80 are at particular risk of recurrence (Kamat et al. 2018; Joudi et al. 2006). Although this is often attributed to a waning immune system with aging, the effect is not specific to BCG alone, as similar results have been shown with intravesical epirubicin (Joudi et al. 2006; Fernandez-Gomez et al. 2008; Oddens et al. 2014). Tumors in older patients may have higher risk intrinsic biology (Noon et al. 2013).

Factors such as female sex, tumor multifocality, and the presence of Cis are also predictors of recurrence (Takashi et al. 2002; Davis et al. 2002; Hurle et al. 1999; Saint et al. 2002; Boorjian et al. 2010). High-grade T1 stage (and T1 substage), lymphovascular invasion, histologic subtypes, multifocality, and early recurrence on surveillance are predictors of tumor progression (Cambier et al. 2016; Fernandez-Gomez et al. 2008, 2009; Gontero et al. 2015; Palou et al.

2012; Martin-Doyle et al. 2015). Overall survival in these patients is compromised by delayed definitive therapy (e.g., cystectomy/radiotherapy). Most bladder cancer-related deaths in patients with progressive disease occur within 48 months (van den Bosch and Alfred 2011).

The impact of BCG strain on clinical outcomes remains uncertain (Bandari et al. 2018). A randomized clinical trial showed a significantly improved 5-year recurrence-free survival (RFS) with BCG-Connaught compared to BCG-Tice, although progression-free survival (PFS), overall survival (OS), and disease-specific survival (DSS) were not different. On a molecular basis, BCG-Connaught leads to greater priming of CD8+ T-cells and greater recruitment of T-cells to the bladder and locoregional lymph nodes (Rentsch et al. 2014). In this trial patients received only induction BCG without maintenance therapy. Subsequent large retrospective studies that included patients treated with and without maintenance therapy have refuted the results of this trial. A large randomized clinical trial comparing BCG-Tice with BCG-Tokyo in BCG-naïve high-risk NMIBC has been completed but not yet reported (NCT03091660) and a second trial comparing BCG-Tice with Russian BCG has been launched (NCT05037279).

20.2.2 Molecular Risk Stratification of Non-muscle Invasive Bladder Cancer

The key to advancing a paradigm of precision oncology in patients with NMIBC lies in molecular risk stratification and the development of biomarkers that predict response to BCG and other therapies. Here we will highlight the most promising biomarkers under investigation.

20.2.2.1 RNA Expression Signatures Predicting Response to BCG

Several studies have aimed to stratify risk of disease recurrence and progression in patients with NMIBC based on RNA profiling (Dyrskjot et al. 2004, 2005, 2007) (see also Chap. 13). The Lund group applied to NMIBC the same taxonomy that they described for MIBC. They found that 95% of 752 NMIBC tumors classified to the "luminal" subtypes (UroA, UroB, or UroC) and 5% were "genomically unstable" (GU) (Sjodahl et al. 2012; Patschan et al. 2015; Marzouka et al. 2022). The same authors applied an immunohistochemical classifier to a cohort of 149 high-grade T1 tumors (Patschan et al. 2015). In this subset, 32% were Urobasal, 58% were GU, and 10% were "squamous-cell carcinoma-like" (SCCL). Together the GU and SCCL demonstrated more high-risk features such as lymphovascular invasion and a higher rate of progression. Co-expression of CD3, a global marker of immune cell infiltration, further sub-stratified the risk of progression in the GU/SCCL tumors. However, the poor outcome of high CD3 expressing tumors is discordant with some subsequent reports (see below). Since only 25% of these tumors were treated with BCG, the classification cannot be applied to BCG response.

The UROMOL consortium developed a novel transcriptomic classification in tumors from 834 patients at 10 centers. They initially reported three subtypes that were later expanded to four subtypes, each with different biology and different disease characteristics (Hedegaard et al. 2016; Lindskrog et al. 2021). They layered onto this an analysis of chromosomal instability and spatial proteomics. All but 11 tumors were Ta or T1, and 10.3% progressed to MIBC with a median follow-up of 49 months in those who did not progress.

Class 1 and 3 had the most favorable outcomes, and the high-risk Class 2 was subdivided into Class 2a with the highest risk of progression and Class 2b with intermediate outcomes. Class 1 was characterized by early cell-cycle activation and high uroplakin expression (a marker of urothelial differentiation) while Class 3 was characterized by high FGFR3 and low immune signature (hallmark features of the favorable luminal papillary subtype in the Consensus subtyping (Kamoun et al. 2020)). Class 2a was enriched with T1 and high-grade tumors. These harbored high chromosomal instability, frequent p53-pathway disruption, and a high rate of APOBEC-related mutations. Characteristic features of

Class 2b included immune cell infiltration and high expression of stem cell and mesenchymal markers. Higher immune cell infiltration was associated with a lower recurrence rate in this class.

The prognostic value of the molecular classes using a single sample classifier held up on multivariable analysis controlling for clinical risk parameters in this discovery cohort and in a validation cohort of 1228 patients. The classifier was no longer associated with RFS when the analysis was limited to 83 patients treated with BCG in the UROMOL cohort or 38 patients treated with BCG in an external cohort. The small sample size prevents any definitive conclusions with respect to predicting BCG response, but it is possible that a particularly favorable response to BCG in Class 2 tumors nullifies the differential prognosis observed in the absence of BCG (Damrauer et al. 2021). A bulk RNA expression-based immune signature stratified RFS in patients treated with BCG, with more immune infiltrated tumors having a more favorable outcome.

The Aarhus group also developed a 12-gene quantitative PCR-based classifier to stratify risk of progression in NMIBC that predates these efforts at molecular subtyping (Dyrskjot et al. 2017). This classifier was successfully validated in the same large multicenter NMIBC series as the UROMOL classifier, but it has not been tested in the context of BCG therapy (Dyrskjot et al. 2017).

Other investigators have focused on RNA-based classification specifically in cohorts of patients treated with BCG. Importantly, all of these series have studied exclusively patients treated with BCG so that a potentially predictive marker cannot be distinguished from a prognostic marker that would be equally applicable to patients treated without BCG.

Robertson et al. conducted RNA-sequencing on high-grade T1 tumors from 73 patients treated with repeat transurethral resection of bladder tumors -and induction/maintenance BCG at a single institution (Robertson et al. 2020). They described 5 molecular subtypes: "T1-luminal genomically unstable" (T1-LumGU), "T1-Inflamed" (T1-Inflam), "T1-Myc," "T1-Early" (S5), and "T1-True Luminal" (T1-TLum). These were validated in a second cohort of 26 BCG-naïve patients. T1-LumGU showed a high frequency of Cis and the largest number of copy number gains, but low expression of inflammation genes. T1-Inflam showed a high expression of inflammation-related genes and the highest level of immune cells, while MYC expression was repressed. T1-Myc and T1-Early (S5) were associated with the worst RFS. Both tumor types showed elevated MYC expression, but T1-Early furthermore showed repressed immune response hallmarks for IFN-α and IFN-δ, resulting in an immune-suppressive microenvironment. T1-Lum tumors had the fewest recurrences within 24 months. Although almost all T1 tumors in this series were classified as the highest risk Class 2a according to the UROMOL classification 4 of 13 T1-Lum tumors were Class 1. This subtype showed repressed inflammatory and proliferative hallmarks, but highly expressed markers of luminal differentiation (FGFR3 and RXRA). Regulon analysis identified two major patterns among the subtypes. T1-LumGU and T1-Myc showed activated regulons for transcription factors E2F1 and FOXM1. E2F and its target EZH2 could potentially serve as druggable targets for EZH2 inhibitors. T1-TLum and T1-Early, on the other hand, showed enriched hallmarks for TGF-β signaling, MYC targets, and oxidative phosphorylation. Both patterns of regulon activity were validated in 94 T1-tumors from UROMOL. The classification by Robertson et al. highlights the value of classifying defined patient subsets. A global bladder cancer classifier such as the Lund taxonomy identifies most NMIBC as belonging to the luminal subtypes. A focus on NMIBC alone, as with the UROMOL classifier, defines additional subgroups within this one larger category. The more precise focus on high-grade T1 tumors as conducted by Robertson et al. provides 5 additional subtypes within what is mostly Class 2a tumors from the UROMOL classification. These models therefore resemble a sort of hierarchy of subtyping, although they were not designed in this way. In any case, the discovery of five distinct T1-subtypes could lead to specific therapeutic pathways according to subtype or pattern of regulon activity.

De Jong et al. used RNA-sequencing in a cohort of 144 patients treated with BCG to identify three distinct BCG response subtypes (BRS1, 2, and 3), which were subsequently validated in 151 additional patient tumors (de Jong et al. 2023). BRS3 tumors expressed high epithelial-to-mesenchymal transition, basal, and immunosuppressive markers. Patients with BRS3 tumors had reduced RFS and PFS compared to tumors classified as BRS1 or BRS2, and this effect was retained on multivariable analysis after correction for clinical risk parameters. The BRS3 subtype was also found to be strongly enriched in 34 recurrent tumors that arose after BCG therapy, even in patients with pre-treatment BRS1 and BRS2 tumors. The authors suggested that patients with BRS3 tumors should forgo BCG therapy and move directly to cystectomy or alternative bladder-preserving therapy, pending external validation of their classifier. They also highlight the critical role in BCG-resistant tumors of TGF-β, which has previously been found to induce resistance to immune checkpoint blockade in metastatic urothelial carcinoma (Mariathasan et al. 2018), thus suggesting that targeting of TGF-β could be critical to improve treatment outcomes. Furthermore, they speculate that N803 (an IL-15 heterodimeric agonist) might be effective in overcoming the immunosuppressive tumor microenvironment of BRS3 tumors.

Comparing the BRS classification to the UROMOL classification revealed some overlap, but also clear distinctions. The UROMOL cohort encompasses a broader spectrum of NMIBC, while the BRS cohort included only patients with high-risk NMIBC receiving BCG therapy. Most of these high-risk tumors in the BRS cohort belonged to UROMOL highest risk Class 2a class. However, it is noteworthy that a larger proportion of BRS3 tumors belonged to lower risk groups, especially Class 2b. This was observed in both the BRS3 and UROMOL cohorts. A comparison between the BRS classification and the 5-group classification of Robertson et al. for T1 tumors has not been conducted.

20.2.2.2 Genomic Markers Predicting Response to BCG

Three different groups have drawn similar conclusions after analyzing genomic alteration in tumors that were subsequently treated with BCG. In one of the first efforts of genomic profiling of NMIBC, Pietzak et al. identified *ARID1A* mutations as a single gene alteration that was associated with poor RFS after BCG therapy in 62 patients (Pietzak et al. 2017). A similar association was subsequently reported by Bacon et al. in 90 NMIBC patients and Bellmunt et al. in 62 high-grade T1 patients treated with BCG (Bacon et al. 2022; Bellmunt et al. 2020). Both of these latter groups also identified high total mutational burden as a favorable marker and *CCNE1* amplification as an unfavorable marker of response to BCG. CCNE1 is a cell-cycle protein that has been described as an oncogene in other cancers, especially ovarian cancer. Bastos et al. similarly reported in a series of 35 patients that tumor mutation burden (TMB) and neoantigen load were higher in tumors that responded to BCG compared to those that did not, but they found no association with *ARID1A* mutations (Bastos et al. 2020).

Bellmunt et al. described a favorable response to BCG in high-grade T1 tumors if an *ERCC2* or *BRCA2* mutation was present. Both genes are involved in DNA damage repair (DDR). This finding aligns well with the report of Pietzak et al. that secondary MIBC that arises from prior NMIBC treated with BCG has a reduced rate of alterations in *ERCC2* (0/24 secondary vs. 12/70 primary) and DDR genes, with a resultant poor response to neoadjuvant chemotherapy (Pietzak et al. 2019). The study by Pietzak et al. suggests that tumors with these mutations are less likely to progress because they are more likely to respond to BCG, but the tumors that do progress do not have these chemosensitizing molecular features. Overall, Bellmunt et al. described a high-risk molecular profile with low/intermediate TMB, *TP53* mutations, *ARID1A* mutations, *CCNE1* amplification, or *CDKN2A* deletion and they suggested that these patients should undergo intensive monitoring or proceed directly to cystectomy. They compare these high-risk tumors to low-risk tumors that they postulate may benefit from DNA damaging agents (e.g., cisplatin or PARP inhibitors) and immune checkpoint inhibitors. This is based on the high rate of alterations in DDR genes, especially *BRCA2* and *ERCC2*, and the high TMB in these tumors.

The analysis of Bellmunt et al. identified *CDKN2A* deletion as an adverse prognostic indicator in T1 patients treated with BCG. *CDKN2A* codes for p16, an important cell-cycle control protein. *CDKN2A* deletion has been described previously as a marker of progression in NMIBC (Sherr and McCormick 2002; Warrick et al. 2015; Meeks et al. 2016; Gan et al. 2016). Loss of the short arm of chromosome 9 (9p) is a well-established early event in bladder oncogenesis, and *CDKN2A* is one gene located in this region that is frequently lost (Gan et al. 2016). Interestingly, a cluster of interferon genes including interferon alpha (*IFNA*) is located adjacent to the *CDKN2A* gene on chromosome 9p, and these are often lost together with *CDKN2A*. This is potentially relevant as IFNA-2b has been used clinically as an adjunct with BCG therapy, and nadofaragene firadenovec is a novel intravesical gene therapy that induces *IFNA-2b* expression in the bladder to eradicate cancer cells. *CDKN2A* loss is being explored as a predictive marker of response to this novel agent. Furthermore, loss of the 9p21 locus is associated with a "cold" tumor immune microenvironment (Han et al. 2021). Adib et al. reported that loss-of-function genomic alteration in *CDKN2A* predicted poor outcome after systemic immune checkpoint inhibition but not chemotherapy in metastatic urothelial carcinoma (Adib et al. 2021). The same relationship was not observed in other cancers analyzed. More investigation is needed to delineate the role of *CDKN2A* and *IFN* genes in determining response to BCG.

20.2.2.3 Germline Single Nucleotide Polymorphisms Predicting Response to BCG

Variations in the glutathione pathways may predict disease recurrence after BCG therapy. Glutathione pathways mediate several intracellular processes such as antioxidation and detoxification as well as regulating the function and survival of T-cells and neutrophils. The single nucleotide polymorphism (SNP) rs7265992 in the glutathione synthetase gene is associated with disease recurrence in patients who underwent both BCG induction and maintenance (Ke et al. 2015).

Nitric oxide synthetase (*NOS*)-polymorphisms have been linked to the development and progression of bladder cancer (Ryk et al. 2010, 2011). A Swedish study demonstrated in 88 high-risk NMIBC patients with 15 years of follow-up that polymorphisms in *NOS2* and *3* influenced the outcome of BCG treatment. In particular, these investigators studied the *NOS2* promoter microsatellite (CCTTT)n polymorphism, the *NOS3* promoter polymorphism rs2070744 (-786T>C), and the *NOS3* polymorphism rs1799983 (Glu298Asp), all of which were associated with patient survival outcomes (Ryk et al. 2015). Patients with one or more of these variants showed improved cancer-specific survival (CSS) and significantly lower progression rates. When the analysis was limited to 51 patients who received BCG treatment, the presence of ≥ 1 polymorphisms in the NOS2 promoter, the NOS3 promoter, or the NOS3 exon was also associated with improved CSS and decreased recurrence.

Several functional SNPs in key immune system genes such as *Fas/Fas-ligand (FasL)* and inflammatory response have been discussed as predictors of BCG failure (Alexandroff et al. 2010; Lima et al. 2012, 2014; Gu et al. 2005; Ehrenschwender and Wajant 2009). A large study by Williams et al. investigated polymorphisms in inflammation pathways and their correlation with outcome of BCG treatment. Although several candidate polymorphisms were identified in the discovery cohort of 349 patients treated with BCG, only one *IL2RA* polymorphism (rs7089861) was significantly associated with risk of progression in both the discovery cohort and the validation cohort of another 322 patients (Williams et al. 2017).

A Polish study investigated the role of polymorphisms in cytokine genes on the outcomes of

175 patients with high-risk NMIBC treated with BCG. They identified heterozygosity in the *IL-18* gene (IL-18-137G>C[GC]) to be associated with decreased RFS and PFS, while a homozygous *IL-17A* polymorphism (IL-17A-197G>A[GG]) was associated with the best RFS (Krajewski et al. 2020).

Lima et al. developed a predictive model for BCG responsiveness based on histopathological factors and immune system gene polymorphisms. Several factors were identified as predictors of progressive disease in patients treated with BCG, among them polymorphisms in genes encoding tumor-necrosis factor α (*TNF*), interleukins *IL-2, IL-17, IL-18,* and *FasL* (Lima et al. 2015). Furthermore, a score based on these polymorphisms revealed that patients classified as low-risk have a 90% chance of successful treatment with BCG, whereas patients within the high-risk group have a 75% probability of disease recurrence (Lima et al. 2015).

Buffen et al. reported that a SNP in the autophagy gene *ATG2B* (rs3759601) correlated with progression and recurrence in Dutch patients with high-risk NMIBC treated with BCG (Buffen et al. 2014). However, these results could not be reproduced in a Chinese cohort (Zang et al. 2021). The Dutch study provided experimental evidence in pre-clinical models to demonstrate the effect of autophagy on trained immunity induced by BCG.

A recent study by Pietzak et al. investigated 99 patients with newly diagnosed NMIBC from Memorial Sloan Kettering Cancer Center and an additional cohort of 115 patients with NMIBC initially treated in various centers. Overall, 22 patients (10%) had a gene variant associated with cancer predisposition affecting DDR (*ATM, RECQL4*), nucleotide excision repair (*ERCC2, ERCC3*), and homologous recombination repair (*BRCA1, BRCA2*). While pathogenic or likely pathogenic germline mutations were associated with high-grade disease, an association between RFS, PFS, and germline variants could not be made in patients treated with BCG (Pietzak et al. 2022).

20.2.2.4 Tumor Immune Microenvironment (TIME) Predicting Response to BCG

Generally speaking, BCG therapy is based on two pillars. One pillar is the interaction between BCG and the tumor itself. Sites of urothelial disruption serve as the main points of attack (Bevers et al. 2004; Kuroda et al. 1993). After instillation, BCG is ingested by cells, and bacterial antigens are presented by tumor cells or antigen-presenting cells (Bevers et al. 2004; Ikeda et al. 2002). This induces the production of various cytokines and chemokines, such as IL, interferon-γ, and tumor-necrosis-factor (TNF)-α. Subsequently, the patient's immune system can eliminate residual tumor cells (Alexandroff et al. 2010; Bohle and Brandau 2003; Suttmann et al. 2003).

The second pillar of BCG therapy is the interaction between BCG and the patient's immune system. Macrophages and dendritic cells are the first immunocytes interacting with BCG. After ingestion and processing of BCG, mycobacteria are presented to T-lymphocytes. Simultaneously, co-stimulatory molecules, cytokines, and chemokines such as MHC class II, B7-1 and -2 molecules, IL-1, -6, -8, -10 and -12, TNF, MIP-1a and 1b, MIP-2, and MCP-3 are secreted (Higuchi et al. 2009; Demangel and Britton 2000; Ramoner et al. 1998; Naoe et al. 2007). These cyto- and chemokines then attract regular and γδ T-lymphocytes, natural killer cells, and neutrophils (Higuchi et al. 2009; Naoe et al. 2007; Ratliff et al. 1993; Simons et al. 2008). Dendritic cells and macrophages can exert an additional anti-tumor effect (Higuchi et al. 2009; Pryor et al. 1995; Luo et al. 2006). However, T-lymphocytes remain the key factor to successful BCG therapy. Especially CD4 and CD8 lymphocytes are essential for the elimination of cancer cells and thereby reduction of risk of recurrence (Ratliff et al. 1993). Furthermore, the induction of TH-1 cells (cellular immune response) with concomitant production of IL-2, IL-12, and interferon-γ and suppression of IL-4 and IL-10 leads to a superior anti-tumor effect to the activation of TH2-cells (humoral immune response) (Luo et al. 2006; Jackson et al. 1995; Eto et al. 2005; Saint et al. 2003; Watanabe et al. 2003; Magno et al. 2002;

Sanchez-Carbayo et al. 2001; Kaempfer et al. 1996). The presence of TH1-cytokines in the urine of patients undergoing BCG therapy has been linked to better response and improved cancer-specific survival (Thalmann et al. 2000; Shintani et al. 2007; Pichler et al. 2017). A high level of TH2-lymphocytes arrests the TH1 response and weakens the therapeutic effect of BCG (Luo 2012; Askeland et al. 2012). T-lymphocytes are activated either by lymphokines (IL-2 or interferon-γ) or by BCG-activated killer cells (BAK) (Bohle et al. 1993; Jackson et al. 1992) that both kill through perforin-mediated lysis (Brandau et al. 2000). BAK can distinguish between benign and malignant cells (Durek et al. 1999). Additionally, a longer RFS can be predicted based on baseline CD4 and GATA3+ T-cell abundance. Moreover, tumor-associated macrophages, T-regulatory cells, and T-bet+ cells are associated with shorter RFS (Pichler et al. 2016). Furthermore, increased infiltration of programmed death-ligand 1 (PD-L1) expressing T-regulatory cells (T_{regs}) may predict tumor recurrence (Chevalier et al. 2018). As described above, the aggressive BRS3 subtype of NMIBC displayed immunosuppressive features (higher infiltration with T_{regs}, macrophages, and B cells), further supporting the role of the tumor microenvironment in response to BCG treatment (de Jong et al. 2023). The finding by Damrauer et al. that an inflamed tumor microenvironment is associated with improved RFS after BCG therapy suggests that specific characterization of the immune microenvironment as activating or suppressive is an important distinction (Damrauer et al. 2021).

20.3 Perioperative Chemotherapy in Muscle-Invasive Bladder Cancer

20.3.1 Natural History of Muscle-Invasive Bladder Cancer Treated with Perioperative Chemotherapy

Cisplatin-based neoadjuvant chemotherapy (NAC) before radical cystectomy can significantly increase OS compared to cystectomy alone (Advanced Bladder Cancer Meta-analysis Collaboration 2005; Yin et al. 2016). Adjuvant chemotherapy is also used for patients with high-risk features in the cystectomy pathology specimen if no NAC was administered, although the clinical data is less robust (Advanced Bladder Cancer Meta-analysis Collaborators Group 2022). More recently adjuvant anti-PD1 immunotherapy has also become part of the standard of care in patients with MIBC (see Chap. 23), but we will focus the discussion on chemotherapy.

Response and resistance can be studied particularly well in the context of NAC where tumor is sampled before and after NAC. Response to NAC correlates with subsequent OS, although this relationship has not been demonstrated adequately to be considered a clear surrogate endpoint (Zargar et al. 2016). Response is conventionally defined as either downstaging to at least NMIBC (ypT1/a/Tis) or a complete pathological response (ypT0) in the cystectomy specimen. In real-world experience, a complete response is observed in approximately 25% of patients (Zargar et al. 2015), while in trials this rate can be as high as 38% (Grossman et al. 2003). Downstaging is typically observed in 40–50% of patients. Generally, we believe that only these patients benefit from NAC, while patients with residual MIBC are faced with potential toxicity from NAC and a delay in definite surgical therapy without clear benefit. It is therefore especially critical to understand resistance and response mechanisms and to develop markers to select patients for NAC.

Some clinical factors are associated with response to NAC. The risk of non-response is elevated fourfold in smokers and twofold in former smokers (Boeri et al. 2019). Patients with tumors that include a mix of glandular and/or squamous differentiation with urothelial carcinoma demonstrated improved overall survival in the SWOG 8710 trial (Scosyrev et al. 2011; Kaimakliotis et al. 2016). However, the impact of NAC in patients with histologic subtypes such as micropapillary, plasmacytoid, and sarcomatoid carcinoma is less certain. Although response rates appear to be similar in retrospective analyses, an improvement in OS has not been demonstrated (Abufaraj et al. 2019; Dayyani et al. 2013; Li et al. 2019; Sui et al. 2017).

20.3.2 Resistance Mechanisms to Cisplatin Chemotherapy

Cisplatin causes DNA damage and thereby induces apoptosis (Siddik 2003). Galluzzi et al. highlighted four distinct mechanisms of cisplatin resistance (Table 20.1) (Galluzzi et al. 2012):

1. Mechanism 1, also called "pre-target resistance," involves steps that inhibit cisplatin from binding with DNA, which may result from decreased uptake or increased export of cisplatin. Uptake is mainly dependent on copper transporter 1 (CTR1). If downregulated, cells are two to threefold more resistant to cisplatin (Katano et al. 2002; Holzer et al. 2006; Ishida et al. 2002). Kilari et al. were able to demonstrate a correlation between CTR1 and pathological response in patients undergoing NAC for MIBC (Kilari et al. 2016). On the contrary, upregulated copper-extruding ATPases such as ATP7A and ATP8A can induce chemo-resistance (Safaei et al. 2004; Samimi et al. 2004). Nucleophilic species such as GSH, methionine, and other cysteine-rich proteins may act as cytoplasmic scavengers and thereby reduce cisplatin levels in cancer cells (Kasahara et al. 1991; Sakamoto et al. 2001). Elevated levels of GSH and its catalyzers and mediators have been linked to chemo-resistance (Lewis et al. 1988).
2. "On-target resistance" involves cisplatin-induced DNA damage. Expression of excision repair cross-complementing rodent repair deficiency, complementation group 1 and 2 (*ERCC1, ERCC2*) correlates negatively with survival and cisplatin response (Bellmunt et al. 2007). ERCC genes encode proteins responsible for DNA repair by the nucleotide excision repair (NER) system, which excises damaged nucleotides (Wood et al. 2000; Shuck et al. 2008). Accordingly, NER proficiency and chemo-resistance are linked (Metzger et al. 1998; Li et al. 1998). MSH-2 is an MMR-related protein that transmits a pro-apoptotic signal when cisplatin-induced DNA damage is detected (Vaisman et al. 1998). Altered pathways may lead to chemo-resistance. Further possible "on-target" mechanisms include increased translesional synthesis or replicative bypass, in which DNA synthesis proceeds beyond cisplatin adducts (Bassett et al. 2002).
3. "Post-target resistance" results from alterations in critical signal transduction pathways. Like BCG resistance, cisplatin resistance can occur based on gene mutations, especially the inactivation of the tumor-suppressor gene *TP53*, which occurs in half of all neoplasms (Kirsch and Kastan 1998; Vousden and Lane 2007). In both ovarian and testicular germ-cell tumors, mutations in *TP53* or lack thereof, respectively, have been linked to cisplatin response (Gadducci et al. 2002; Feldman et al. 2008; Peng et al. 1993). In bladder cancer, *TP53* mutations are linked to recurrent disease and shorter overall survival (Esrig et al. 1994). Meanwhile, data concerning the role of *TP53* and chemosensitivity in urothelial cancer are conflicting. A correlation between *TP53* mutations and response to chemotherapy could not be established by Qureshi et al. and Watanabe et al. (Qureshi et al. 1999; Watanabe et al. 2004). On the other hand, studies by Kakehi et al., Sarkis et al., and Cote et al. all linked overexpression of *TP53* (linked to the presence of mutation) to worse overall survival (Kakehi et al. 1998; Sarkis et al. 1994; Cote et al. 1997). BCL-2 as an anti-apoptotic protein may also predict response rates to chemotherapy. A negative BCL-2 status is associated with longer overall survival in patients who underwent neoadjuvant chemotherapy before radiation therapy (Cooke et al. 2000). In addition to breast and prostate cancer, the DNA-mismatch repair genes *BRCA1* and *BRCA2* may also influence sensitivity to platinum-based chemotherapy chemosensitivity in bladder cancer (Quinn et al. 2003). A single study including 57 patients by Font et al. identified *BRCA1* mRNA expression correlated with poor OS

Table 20.1 The four mechanisms of cisplatin resistance

	Mechanism	Altered pathway	Result	References
Pre-target resistance	Inhibition of cisplatin uptake	Down-regulation of CTR1	Decreased intracellular cisplatin concentration	Katano et al. (2002); Holzer et al. (2006); Ishida et al. (2002)
	Upregulation of copper-extruding ATPases	ATP7A, ATP8A		Safaei et al. (2004); Samimi et al. (2004)
	Cytoplasmic scavenging	GSH, methionine		Kasahara et al. (1991); Sakamoto et al. (2001); Lewis et al. (1988)
On-target resistance	Altered nucleotide excision	ERCC1	Deficient protein repair	Bellmunt et al. (2007); Wood et al. (2000); Shuck et al. (2008); Metzger et al. (1998); Li et al. (1998)
	Altered mismatch repair	MSH-2	Induces apoptosis when detecting cisplatin-induced lesions	Vaisman et al. (1998)
	Increased translesional synthesis & replicative bypass		DNA synthesis proceeds beyond cisplatin adducts	Bassett et al. (2002)
Post-target resistance	Gene polymorphisms	p53	Reduced tumor suppression	Qureshi et al. (1999); Watanabe et al. (2004); Kakehi et al. (1998); Sarkis et al. (1994); Cote et al. (1997); Stadler et al. (2011)
		BCL-2	Anti-apoptotic signals	Cooke et al. (2000)
		BRCA1, BRCA2	Differential modulation of apoptosis	Quinn et al. (2003)
Off-target resistance	Autophagy	High-mobility group box 1 (HMGB-1)	Increased autophagy by upregulation	Yin et al. (2017)
	Hypoxia	Hypoxia-induced factor 1 (HIF-1)	Elevated expression of HIF-1 leads to decreased cisplatin-induced apoptosis	Yang et al. (2018)
	Cell-cycle arrest	CDKN1A, CDKN2A (downstream from ERBB2)	Interaction with cell-cycle arrest	Sato et al. (1992); Coombs et al. (1991)
	Proper folding of proteins	Heat-shock proteins	Indirectly down-regulation of tumor suppressors	Ren et al. (2008); Yamamoto et al. (2001)

(Font et al. 2011). Teo et al. demonstrated that the presence of genomic alterations in a panel of 34 DDR genes including *BRCA1/2* is associated with improved outcome after platinum-based chemotherapy in patients with metastatic urothelial carcinoma (Teo et al. 2017). Trials investigating the utility of alterations in DDR genes to predict response to NAC are described below.

4. "Off-target resistance" pertains to pathways and intracellular mechanisms not directly linked to cisplatin that indirectly interfere with cisplatin-induced signals. Autophagy, a process in which molecules from the cytoplasm and organelles are degraded by lysosomal enzymes, is upregulated in chemo-resistant ovarian and lung cancer cells (Ren et al. 2010; Yu et al. 2011). Thus, several

autophagy inhibitors have been investigated as possible targets for tumor therapy. Yin et al. identified high-mobility group box 1 (HMGB1) as a mediator of autophagy which was upregulated in cisplatin-resistant bladder cancer (Yin et al. 2017). Yang et al. demonstrated that gemcitabine-induced apoptosis during hypoxia was significantly reduced and thus identified elevated expression of hypoxia-inducing factor 1 (HIF-1) as triggering chemo-resistance (Yang et al. 2018). *ERBB2*, known for its role in breast and ovarian cancer, encodes the tyrosine-kinase HER2 and is often overexpressed, mutated, or amplified in bladder cancer and thus represents a potential therapeutic target (Sato et al. 1992; Coombs et al. 1991). Downstream connections to CDKN1A and CDKN2A can lead to interference with cell-cycle arrest and cisplatin resistance. Heat-shock proteins (HSP) facilitate the proper folding of proteins. Their role in chemo-resistance has been defined by indirectly influencing markers such as the mammalian sterile 20-like kinase 1 (Mst-1), which functions as a tumor suppressor. Down-regulation of Mst-1 has been linked to chemo-resistance in prostate cancer cells (Ren et al. 2008). Although upregulation of HSP27 in bladder cancer has been linked to taxane resistance (Kamada et al. 2007), the addition of an antisense oligonucleotide targeting HSP27 to chemotherapy has failed to improve patient outcomes compared to chemotherapy alone in the first line (Bellmunt et al. 2017) and the cisplatin-refractory metastatic setting (Rosenberg et al. 2018). Further mechanisms of off-target resistance are still under investigation.

20.3.3 Molecular Risk Stratification of Muscle-Invasive Bladder Cancer

20.3.3.1 RNA Expression Signatures Predicting Response to NAC

Molecular subtyping of MIBC based on RNA expression was described in detail in Chap. 14. Several studies have investigated the association between molecular subtypes and response to NAC. Choi et al. were the first to identify a potential link in their original description of the MD Anderson subtyping model, which classifies MIBC as "basal" (p63 activation, squamous differentiation), "luminal" (active PPARγ and estrogen receptor transcription, enriched with activating *FGFR3* mutations), or "p53-like" (senescence signature, enriched for extracellular matrix gene expression) (Choi et al. 2014). In three different patient cohorts, tumors in the p53-like group had a low rate (<10%) of pathologic response to NAC, while basal and luminal tumors responded similarly (approximately 40-50%). The same group subsequently reported that the basal subtype had the best response rate and survival after NAC in combination with the VEGF inhibitor bevacizumab in a prospective single arm trial (McConkey et al. 2016). In this study it is impossible to subtract the impact of bevacizumab, and other studies have suggested that VEGF pathway inhibition may be most important in basal tumors (van der Heijden et al. 2022).

Multiple studies have demonstrated that "basal" tumors have worse survival compared to other transcriptional subtypes, and luminal tumors generally have more favorable outcomes (Kamoun et al. 2020; Seiler et al. 2017; Robertson et al. 2017; Taber et al. 2020; Sjodahl et al. 2022; Lotan et al. 2022). Luminal tumors are more likely to be organ-confined without NAC and therefore the need for NAC may be less, regardless of the biological implications for response and treatment (Lotan et al. 2019). It is important to note that the impact of subtyping on response and outcome after NAC can only be determined when comparing outcomes in patients who were treated with and without NAC. Otherwise, prognostic effects cannot be separated from predictive effects. Response to NAC is often considered a surrogate for overall survival, so that an impact of subtyping on response rates may be important regardless of a control cohort.

Seiler et al. applied several subtyping models to a large multicenter cohort ($n = 343$) in an attempt to validate whether molecular subtypes predict response to NAC. These authors also analyzed a cohort of 476 patients with MIBC who did not undergo NAC, derived from three publicly available transcriptomic datasets. The investigators developed a single sample classifier that was built on both the University of North Carolina (UNC) and the TCGA classifiers (Damrauer et al. 2014; Cancer Genome Atlas Research Network 2014). The UNC classifier divided tumors into "luminal," "basal," and "claudin-low" (high immune infiltration and strong mesenchymal signature). The TCGA classifier further divided the luminal tumors into "luminal" and "luminal infiltrated," which appeared to be critical to distinguish luminal tumors with an excellent prognosis from "luminal-infiltrated" tumors with a poor prognosis. This genomic subtyping classifier (GSC) was applied to a cohort of 223 patients treated with cisplatin-based NAC. This analysis showed that all subtypes had a poor prognosis except for "luminal" tumors. In comparison, the survival of patients with "basal" tumors was similar to those with "luminal" tumors when treated with NAC. This suggested a differential benefit for "basal" tumors and suggested that molecular subtyping was a predictive marker of outcome after NAC (Seiler et al. 2017). This study did not control for the potential impact of adjuvant chemotherapy.

A subsequent multicenter validation study of the GSC in 601 patients treated with and without NAC at multiple centers generated a somewhat different narrative (Lotan et al. 2022). In this study, "luminal-infiltrated," "claudin-low," and "basal" tumors appeared to benefit from NAC, while "luminal" tumors did not. Rather than prioritizing NAC for patients with "basal" tumors, the conclusion of this validation study was that patients with "luminal" tumors should be spared NAC. Two subsequent studies have demonstrated that patients with "basal" tumors have the worst response and survival after NAC or systemic chemotherapy for metastatic disease (Taber et al. 2020; Sjodahl et al. 2022). While these results are discordant on initial review, the patient cohorts, endpoints, and classifiers are all different between studies. De Jong and Gibb focused in a commentary on the performance of the different classifiers, demonstrating that the classifiers may be identifying the same tumors as having benefit from NAC but attaching different labels to those tumors. For example, "genomically unstable" and "urothelial-like" tumors in the Lund taxonomy were generally "non-luminal" tumors according to the GSC, and both classifiers identified these tumors as having favorable outcomes after NAC (de Jong and Gibb 2022).

Clinical implementation of molecular subtyping to guide neoadjuvant therapy will require prospective validation in clinical trials. Two such trials are being developed, including the GUSTO trial in the UK and the SUBTYP trial in the USA.

20.3.3.2 Genomic Markers Predicting Response to NAC

Groenendijk et al. discovered that presence of an *ERBB2* mutation correlated with response to NAC (Groenendijk et al. 2016), but this has not been validated in other studies (Liu et al. 2016; Gil-Jimenez et al. 2023). All other potential biomarkers for response to NAC discussed below are involved in DDR.

Two pathways, NER and homologous recombination repair (HRR) are responsible for repairing the DNA damage induced by cisplatin. Low *ERCC1* expression affects the NER pathway, which explains an association with longer OS in patients with advanced bladder cancer receiving platinum-based chemotherapy (Bellmunt et al. 2007). However, discordant results were generated in another clinical study that did not show an association between *ERCC1* expression and NAC response (Choueiri et al. 2014).

Loss-of-function mutations in *ERCC2* impair NER function and have been strongly linked to pathologic response and overall survival after treatment of bladder cancer with cisplatin-based NAC in multiple studies, while resistance to chemotherapy was influenced by overexpression (Liu et al. 2016; Gil-Jimenez et al. 2023; Van Allen et al. 2014). These studies showed that most patients with *ERCC2* mutations experience a complete pathologic response to NAC, and the overall survival in the first several years after NAC is nearly 100%. Plimack et al. reported in parallel to the first report on the impact of *ERCC2* that an alteration in one of the three DDR genes (*ATM, RB1, FANCC*) correlated with complete pathologic response and excellent survival in two small single arm phase 2 trials testing different cisplatin-based NAC regimens (dose dense gemcitabine/cisplatin (ddGC) or dose dense methotrexate/vinblastine/Adriamycin/cisplatin (ddMVAC)) (Plimack et al. 2015). The 5-year survival in patients with at least one mutation was 85% compared to 45% in patients lacking a mutation. Such a correlation was not shown by Gil-Jimenez et al. in the NAC setting or a study by Teo et al. in the metastatic setting (Teo et al. 2017; Gil-Jimenez et al. 2023; Miron et al. 2020). While it has not been reported in the literature, our own analysis of TCGA data in patients with MIBC treated without NAC revealed that alterations in *ERCC2, ATM, RB1*, and/or *FANCC* do not impact patient prognosis. This suggests that these markers have no prognostic value but are predictive of response to NAC, although the effects of adjuvant chemotherapy in the TCGA cohort may confound this conclusion.

These potentially predictive genomic markers of outcome after NAC have been tested in three different prospective trials. A031701 is a cooperative group trial (NCT03609216) sponsored by the Alliance for Clinical Trials in Oncology that selects patients for bladder preservation if the tumor harbors a deleterious mutation in one of nine DDR genes (*ERCC2, ERCC5, BRCA1, BRCA2, RAD51C, ATR, RECQL4, ATM, FANCC*) and the patient experiences a complete response to neoadjuvant ddGC. A radical cystectomy is recommended in all other patients. This trial continues to accrue patients and no results have been reported.

The RETAIN trial (NCT02710734) similarly selected patients for bladder conservation if their tumor harbored a mutation in *ERCC2, ATM, RB1*, and/or *FANCC* and they had a complete clinical response to ddMVAC (Geynisman 2023). The trial was designed to be considered positive if the lower bound for the 95% confidence interval for 2-year metastasis-free survival (MFS) was >64%. However, the trial proved to be negative due to a 2-year MFS of 72.8% and a lower bound of the 95% confidence interval of 62.8%. The tumor harbored a DDR mutation in 33 of 70 patients, and 25 of these patients had a complete response to NAC. These 25 and 1 additional patient preserved their bladder and underwent surveillance. A recurrence was observed in 18 (69%) patients, of whom 8 underwent cystectomy and 2 underwent chemoradiation. Ten patients metastasized during follow-up.

In the HCRN GU16-257 trial (NCT03558087) patients were treated with four cycles of neoadjuvant GC plus the immunotherapy drug nivolumab (anti-PD-1) followed by eight cycles of adjuvant nivolumab (Galsky et al. 2023). Bladder preservation was offered to patients who had a complete clinical response after the neoadjuvant phase regardless of the presence of DDR alterations. Thirty-three of 76 (43%) patients had a complete response to neoadjuvant therapy and 32 were monitored, of 10 (30%) recurred and 2 (6%) metastasized. Nine patients (27%) required cystectomy, and 23 (70%) were alive with bladder intact and without metastasis (compared to 46% in the RETAIN trial). Clinical and pathologic response correlated with *ERCC2* mutation status and TMB but not with mutations in *ATM, RB1*, or *FANCC*. The MFS results are more favorable than those of RETAIN, but the reason for the differential outcome is not clear. The assessment of clinical response may have been different between studies, and nivolumab may have affected the results. Regardless, both trials suggest that DDR mutations are not useful for selecting patients for bladder preservation after cisplatin-based NAC. Furthermore, better tools are required to assess clinical response to NAC in an effort to spare the need for cystectomy in more patients.

20.3.3.3 Blood Markers Predicting and Monitoring Response to NAC

An alternative to predicting response to NAC a priori is the strategy of monitoring treatment response at a molecular level during or immediately after NAC and then either intensifying treatment or switching to an alternative regimen or immediate radical cystectomy if the early response is inadequate.

The epithelial tumor markers CA19-9, CA 125, and CEA have been tested as early response markers in patients receiving NAC. Bazargani et al. demonstrate that elevated precystectomy levels of these markers are associated with shorter RFS (HR = 2.81, $p < 0.001$) and OS (HR = 3.97, $p < 0.001$). However, if the markers regressed to normal levels after NAC, the time to recurrence or progression was improved, resulting in significantly prolonged survival compared to those who did not experience a normalization of markers (27.3 months in responders vs. 11.6 months in non-responders, $p = 0.037$) (Bazargani et al. 2019).

As discussed in Chap. 19, circulating tumor DNA offers another tool to predict response to NAC (Christensen et al. 2019, 2023). Clinical implementation of these markers has yet to be tested. The closest clinical application is the use of circulating tumor DNA after radical cystectomy to guide adjuvant immunotherapy (Powles et al. 2021) or early salvage immunotherapy. Three trials are testing this concept prospectively (NCT04660344 "IMvigor011," A032103 "MODERN," NCT04138628 "TOMBOLA").

20.4 Conclusion

We have seen rapid evolution of our understanding of resistance mechanisms to BCG and chemotherapy in bladder cancer over the past several years and an encouraging surge in clinical trial activity testing potentially predictive biomarkers in patients. This activity brings the promise of precision oncology closer to realization. We are seeing a similar surge in the approval of new drug treatments for bladder cancer, which raises the stakes for personalized treatment decisions because individual patients are faced with more treatment choices. Ongoing basic, translational, and clinical investigations into mechanisms of resistance and predictive biomarkers are critical to advance this burgeoning field with the aim of improving survival for patients suffering from NMIBC and MIBC.

References

Abufaraj M, Foerster B, Schernhammer E, Moschini M, Kimura S, Hassler MR et al (2019) Micropapillary urothelial carcinoma of the bladder: a systematic review and meta-analysis of disease characteristics and treatment outcomes. Eur Urol 75:649–658

Adib E, Nassar AH, Akl EW, Abou Alaiwi S, Nuzzo PV, Mouhieddine TH et al (2021) CDKN2A alterations and response to immunotherapy in solid tumors. Clin Cancer Res 27:4025–4035

Advanced Bladder Cancer Meta-analysis Collaboration (2005) Neoadjuvant chemotherapy in invasive bladder cancer: update of a systematic review and meta-analysis of individual patient data advanced bladder cancer (ABC) meta-analysis collaboration. Eur Urol 48:202–205. Discussion 5–6

Advanced Bladder Cancer Meta-analysis Collaborators Group (2022) Adjuvant chemotherapy for muscle-invasive bladder cancer: a systematic review and meta-analysis of individual participant data from randomised controlled trials. Eur Urol 81:50–61

Aldousari S, Kassouf W (2010) Update on the management of non-muscle invasive bladder cancer. Can Urol Assoc J 4:56–64

Alexandroff AB, Nicholson S, Patel PM, Jackson AM (2010) Recent advances in Bacillus Calmette-Guerin immunotherapy in bladder cancer. Immunotherapy 2:551–560

Ali-El-Dein B, Sooriakumaran P, Trinh QD, Barakat TS, Nabeeh A, Ibrahiem el HI. (2013) Construction of predictive models for recurrence and progression in >1000 patients with non-muscle-invasive bladder cancer (NMIBC) from a single centre. BJU Int 111:E331–E341

Askeland EJ, Newton MR, O'Donnell MA, Luo Y (2012) Bladder cancer immunotherapy: BCG and beyond. Adv Urol 2012:181987

Bacon JVW, Muller DC, Ritch E, Annala M, Dugas SG, Herberts C et al (2022) Somatic features of response and relapse in non-muscle-invasive bladder cancer treated with Bacillus Calmette-Guerin immunotherapy. Eur Urol Oncol 5:677–686

Bandari J, Maganty A, MacLeod LC, Davies BJ (2018) Manufacturing and the market: rationalizing the shortage of Bacillus Calmette-Guerin. Eur Urol Focus 4:481–484

Bassett E, Vaisman A, Tropea KA, McCall CM, Masutani C, Hanaoka F et al (2002) Frameshifts and deletions during in vitro translesion synthesis past Pt-DNA adducts by DNA polymerases beta and eta. DNA Repair (Amst) 1:1003–1016

Bastos DA, Mattedi RL, Barreiro R, dos Santos FF, Buzatto V, Masotti C et al (2020) Genomic biomarkers and underlying mechanism of benefit from BCG immunotherapy in non-muscle invasive bladder cancer. Bladder Cancer 171–186

Bazargani ST, Clifford TG, Djaladat H, Schuckman AK, Wayne K, Miranda G et al (2019) Association between precystectomy epithelial tumor marker response to neoadjuvant chemotherapy and oncological outcomes in urothelial bladder cancer. Urol Oncol 37:1–11

Bellmunt J, Paz-Ares L, Cuello M, Cecere FL, Albiol S, Guillem V et al (2007) Gene expression of ERCC1 as a novel prognostic marker in advanced bladder cancer patients receiving cisplatin-based chemotherapy. Ann Oncol 18:522–528

Bellmunt J, Eigl BJ, Senkus E, Loriot Y, Twardowski P, Castellano D et al (2017) Borealis-1: a randomized, first-line, placebo-controlled, phase II study evaluating apatorsen and chemotherapy for patients with advanced urothelial cancer. Ann Oncol 28:2481–2488

Bellmunt J, Kim J, Reardon B, Perera-Bel J, Orsola A, Rodriguez-Vida A et al (2020) Genomic predictors of good outcome, recurrence, or progression in high-grade T1 non-muscle-invasive bladder cancer. Cancer Res 80:4476–4486

Bevers RF, Kurth KH, Schamhart DH (2004) Role of urothelial cells in BCG immunotherapy for superficial bladder cancer. Br J Cancer 91:607–612

Boeri L, Soligo M, Frank I, Boorjian SA, Thompson RH, Tollefson M et al (2019) Cigarette smoking is associated with adverse pathological response and increased disease recurrence amongst patients with muscle-invasive bladder cancer treated with cisplatin-based neoadjuvant chemotherapy and radical cystectomy: a single-centre experience. BJU Int 123:1011–1019

Bohle A, Brandau S (2003) Immune mechanisms in bacillus Calmette-Guerin immunotherapy for superficial bladder cancer. J Urol 170:964–969

Bohle A, Thanhauser A, Ulmer AJ, Ernst M, Flad HD, Jocham D (1993) Dissecting the immunobiological effects of Bacillus Calmette-Guerin (BCG) in vitro: evidence of a distinct BCG-activated killer (BAK) cell phenomenon. J Urol 150:1932–1937

Boorjian SA, Zhu F, Herr HW (2010) The effect of gender on response to Bacillus Calmette-Guerin therapy for patients with non-muscle-invasive urothelial carcinoma of the bladder. BJU Int 106:357–361

Brandau S, Suttmann H, Riemensberger J, Seitzer U, Arnold J, Durek C et al (2000) Perforin-mediated lysis of tumor cells by Mycobacterium bovis Bacillus Calmette-Guerin-activated killer cells. Clin Cancer Res 6:3729–3738

Buffen K, Oosting M, Quintin J, Ng A, Kleinnijenhuis J, Kumar V et al (2014) Autophagy controls BCG-induced trained immunity and the response to intravesical BCG therapy for bladder cancer. PLoS Pathog 10:e1004485

Cambier S, Sylvester RJ, Collette L, Gontero P, Brausi MA, van Andel G et al (2016) EORTC nomograms and risk groups for predicting recurrence, progression, and disease-specific and overall survival in non-muscle-invasive stage Ta-T1 urothelial bladder cancer patients treated with 1-3 years of maintenance Bacillus Calmette-Guerin. Eur Urol 69:60–69

Cancer Genome Atlas Research Network (2014) Comprehensive molecular characterization of urothelial bladder carcinoma. Nature 507:315–322

Chamie K, Litwin MS, Bassett JC, Daskivich TJ, Lai J, Hanley JM et al (2013) Recurrence of high-risk bladder cancer: a population-based analysis. Cancer 119:3219–3227

Chang SS, Bochner BH, Chou R, Dreicer R, Kamat AM, Lerner SP et al (2017) Treatment of non-metastatic muscle-invasive bladder cancer: AUA/ASCO/ASTRO/SUO guideline. J Urol 198:552–559

Chevalier MF, Schneider AK, Cesson V, Dartiguenave F, Lucca I, Jichlinski P et al (2018) Conventional and PD-L1-expressing regulatory T cells are enriched during BCG therapy and may limit its efficacy. Eur Urol 74:540–544

Choi W, Porten S, Kim S, Willis D, Plimack ER, Hoffman-Censits J et al (2014) Identification of distinct basal and luminal subtypes of muscle-invasive bladder cancer with different sensitivities to frontline chemotherapy. Cancer Cell 25:152–165

Choueiri TK, Jacobus S, Bellmunt J, Qu A, Appleman LJ, Tretter C et al (2014) Neoadjuvant dose-dense methotrexate, vinblastine, doxorubicin, and cisplatin with pegfilgrastim support in muscle-invasive urothelial cancer: pathologic, radiologic, and biomarker correlates. J Clin Oncol 32:1889–1894

Christensen E, Birkenkamp-Demtroder K, Sethi H, Shchegrova S, Salari R, Nordentoft I et al (2019) Early detection of metastatic relapse and monitoring of therapeutic efficacy by ultra-deep sequencing of plasma cell-free DNA in patients with urothelial bladder carcinoma. J Clin Oncol 37:1547–1557

Christensen E, Nordentoft I, Birkenkamp-Demtroder K, Elbaek SK, Lindskrog SV, Taber A et al (2023) Cell-free urine and plasma DNA mutational analysis predicts neoadjuvant chemotherapy response and outcome in patients with muscle-invasive bladder cancer. Clin Cancer Res 29:1582–1591

Cooke PW, James ND, Ganesan R, Burton A, Young LS, Wallace DM (2000) Bcl-2 expression identifies patients with advanced bladder cancer treated by radiotherapy who benefit from neoadjuvant chemotherapy. BJU Int 85:829–835

Coombs LM, Pigott DA, Sweeney E, Proctor AJ, Eydmann ME, Parkinson C et al (1991) Amplification and overexpression of c-erbB-2 in transitional cell carcinoma of the urinary bladder. Br J Cancer 63:601–608

Cote RJ, Esrig D, Groshen S, Jones PA, Skinner DG (1997) p53 and treatment of bladder cancer. Nature 385:123–125

Damrauer JS, Hoadley KA, Chism DD, Fan C, Tiganelli CJ, Wobker SE et al (2014) Intrinsic subtypes of high-grade bladder cancer reflect the hallmarks of breast cancer biology. Proc Natl Acad Sci USA 111:3110–3115

Damrauer JS, Roell KR, Smith MA, Sun X, Kirk EL, Hoadley KA et al (2021) Identification of a novel inflamed tumor microenvironment signature as a predictive biomarker of Bacillus Calmette-Guerin immunotherapy in non-muscle-invasive bladder cancer. Clin Cancer Res 27:4599–4609

Davis JW, Sheth SI, Doviak MJ, Schellhammer PF (2002) Superficial bladder carcinoma treated with bacillus Calmette-Guerin: progression-free and disease specific survival with minimum 10-year followup. J Urol 167:494–500. Discussion 1

Dayyani F, Czerniak BA, Sircar K, Munsell MF, Millikan RE, Dinney CP et al (2013) Plasmacytoid urothelial carcinoma, a chemosensitive cancer with poor prognosis, and peritoneal carcinomatosis. J Urol 189:1656–1661

de Jong JJ, Gibb EA (2022) Re: Gottfrid Sjodahl, Johan Abrahamsson, Karin Holmsten, et al. Different responses to neoadjuvant chemotherapy in urothelial carcinoma molecular subtypes. Eur Urol. 2022;81:316–7. Neoadjuvant chemotherapy response in muscle-invasive bladder cancer: Differences in intrinsic biology or subtyping nomenclature? Eur Urol 81:e90–e91

de Jong FC, Laajala TD, Hoedemaeker RF, Jordan KR, van der Made ACJ, Boeve ER et al (2023) Non-muscle-invasive bladder cancer molecular subtypes predict differential response to intravesical Bacillus Calmette-Guerin. Sci Transl Med 15:eabn4118

Demangel C, Britton WJ (2000) Interaction of dendritic cells with mycobacteria: where the action starts. Immunol Cell Biol 78:318–324

Durek C, Brandau S, Ulmer AJ, Flad HD, Jocham D, Bohle A (1999) Bacillus-Calmette-Guerin (BCG) and 3D tumors: an in vitro model for the study of adhesion and invasion. J Urol 162:600–605

Dyrskjot L, Kruhoffer M, Thykjaer T, Marcussen N, Jensen JL, Moller K et al (2004) Gene expression in the urinary bladder: a common carcinoma in situ gene expression signature exists disregarding histopathological classification. Cancer Res 64:4040–4048

Dyrskjot L, Zieger K, Kruhoffer M, Thykjaer T, Jensen JL, Primdahl H et al (2005) A molecular signature in superficial bladder carcinoma predicts clinical outcome. Clin Cancer Res 11:4029–4036

Dyrskjot L, Zieger K, Real FX, Malats N, Carrato A, Hurst C et al (2007) Gene expression signatures predict outcome in non-muscle-invasive bladder carcinoma: a multicenter validation study. Clin Cancer Res 13:3545–3551

Dyrskjot L, Reinert T, Algaba F, Christensen E, Nieboer D, Hermann GG et al (2017) Prognostic impact of a 12-gene progression score in non-muscle-invasive bladder cancer: a prospective multicentre validation study. Eur Urol 72:461–469

EAU guidelines on non-muscle-invasive bladder cancer (TaT1 and CIS) (2022)

Ehrenschwender M, Wajant H (2009) The role of FasL and Fas in health and disease. Adv Exp Med Biol 647:64–93

Esrig D, Elmajian D, Groshen S, Freeman JA, Stein JP, Chen SC et al (1994) Accumulation of nuclear p53 and tumor progression in bladder cancer. N Engl J Med 331:1259–1264

Eto M, Koga H, Noma H, Yamaguchi A, Yoshikai Y, Naito S (2005) Importance of urinary interleukin-18 in intravesical immunotherapy with bacillus Calmette-Guerin for superficial bladder tumors. Urol Int 75:114–118

Feldman DR, Bosl GJ, Sheinfeld J, Motzer RJ (2008) Medical treatment of advanced testicular cancer. JAMA 299:672–684

Fernandez-Gomez J, Solsona E, Unda M, Martinez-Pineiro L, Gonzalez M, Hernandez R et al (2008) Prognostic factors in patients with non-muscle-invasive bladder cancer treated with Bacillus Calmette-Guerin: multivariate analysis of data from four randomized CUETO trials. Eur Urol 53:992–1001

Fernandez-Gomez J, Madero R, Solsona E, Unda M, Martinez-Pineiro L, Gonzalez M et al (2009) Predicting nonmuscle invasive bladder cancer recurrence and progression in patients treated with bacillus Calmette-Guerin: the CUETO scoring model. J Urol 182:2195–2203

Font A, Taron M, Gago JL, Costa C, Sanchez JJ, Carrato C et al (2011) BRCA1 mRNA expression and outcome to neoadjuvant cisplatin-based chemotherapy in bladder cancer. Ann Oncol 22:139–144

Fujii Y (2018) Prediction models for progression of non-muscle-invasive bladder cancer: A review. Int J Urol 25:212–218

Fujii Y, Fukui I, Kihara K, Tsujii T, Ishizaka K, Kageyama Y et al (1998) Significance of bladder neck involvement on progression in superficial bladder cancer. Eur Urol 33:464–468

Gadducci A, Cosio S, Muraca S, Genazzani AR (2002) Molecular mechanisms of apoptosis and chemosensitivity to platinum and paclitaxel in ovarian cancer: biological data and clinical implications. Eur J Gynaecol Oncol 23:390–396

Galluzzi L, Senovilla L, Vitale I, Michels J, Martins I, Kepp O et al (2012) Molecular mechanisms of cisplatin resistance. Oncogene 31:1869–1883

Galsky M et al (2023) Co-primary endpoint analysis of HCRN GU 16-257: phase 2 trial of gemcitabine, cisplatin, plus nivolumab with selective bladder sparing in patients with muscle-invasive bladder cancer (MIBC) ASCO-GU 2023

Gan X, Lin X, He R, Lin X, Wang H, Yan L et al (2016) Prognostic and clinicopathological significance of downregulated p16 expression in patients with bladder cancer: a systematic review and meta-analysis. Dis Markers 2016:5259602

Geynisman DM (2023) A phase II trial of risk-enabled therapy after initiating neoadjuvant chemotherapy for bladder cancer (RETAIN). ASCO-GU 2023

Gil-Jimenez A, van Dorp J, Contreras-Sanz A, van der Vos K, Vis DJ, Braaf L et al (2023) Assessment of predictive genomic biomarkers for response to cisplatin-based neoadjuvant chemotherapy in bladder cancer. Eur Urol 83:313–317

Gontero P, Sylvester R, Pisano F, Joniau S, Vander Eeckt K, Serretta V et al (2015) Prognostic factors and risk groups in T1G3 non-muscle-invasive bladder cancer patients initially treated with Bacillus Calmette-Guerin: results of a retrospective multicenter study of 2451 patients. Eur Urol 67:74–82

Groenendijk FH, de Jong J, Fransen van de Putte EE, Michaut M, Schlicker A, Peters D et al (2016) ERBB2 mutations characterize a subgroup of muscle-invasive bladder cancers with excellent response to neoadjuvant chemotherapy. Eur Urol 69:384–388

Grossman HB, Natale RB, Tangen CM, Speights VO, Vogelzang NJ, Trump DL et al (2003) Neoadjuvant chemotherapy plus cystectomy compared with cystectomy alone for locally advanced bladder cancer. N Engl J Med 349:859–866

Gu J, Grossman HB, Dinney CP, Wu X (2005) The pharmacogenetic impact of inflammatory genes on bladder cancer recurrence. Pharmacogenomics 6:575–584

Han G, Yang G, Hao D, Lu Y, Thein K, Simpson BS et al (2021) 9p21 loss confers a cold tumor immune microenvironment and primary resistance to immune checkpoint therapy. Nat Commun 12:5606

Hedegaard J, Lamy P, Nordentoft I, Algaba F, Hoyer S, Ulhoi BP et al (2016) Comprehensive transcriptional analysis of early-stage urothelial carcinoma. Cancer Cell 30:27–42

Herr HW (1997) Tumour progression and survival in patients with T1G3 bladder tumours: 15-year outcome. Br J Urol 80:762–765

Higuchi T, Shimizu M, Owaki A, Takahashi M, Shinya E, Nishimura T et al (2009) A possible mechanism of intravesical BCG therapy for human bladder carcinoma: involvement of innate effector cells for the inhibition of tumor growth. Cancer Immunol Immunother 58:1245–1255

Holzer AK, Manorek GH, Howell SB (2006) Contribution of the major copper influx transporter CTR1 to the cellular accumulation of cisplatin, carboplatin, and oxaliplatin. Mol Pharmacol 70:1390–1394

Hurle R, Losa A, Manzetti A, Lembo A (1999) Intravesical bacille Calmette-Guerin in Stage T1 grade 3 bladder cancer therapy: a 7 year follow up. Urology 54:258–263

Ikeda N, Toida I, Iwasaki A, Kawai K, Akaza H (2002) Surface antigen expression on bladder tumor cells induced by Bacillus Calmette-Guerin (BCG): A role of BCG internalization into tumor cells. Int J Urol 9:29–35

International Collaboration of Trialists, Medical Research Council Advanced Bladder Cancer Working Party, European Organisation for Research and Treatment of Cancer Genito-Urinary Tract Cancer Group, Australian Bladder Cancer Study Group, National Cancer Institute of Canada Clinical Trials Group et al (2011) International phase III trial assessing neoadjuvant cisplatin, methotrexate, and vinblastine chemotherapy for muscle-invasive bladder cancer: long-term results of the BA06 30894 trial. J Clin Oncol 29:2171–2177

Ishida S, Lee J, Thiele DJ, Herskowitz I (2002) Uptake of the anticancer drug cisplatin mediated by the copper transporter Ctr1 in yeast and mammals. Proc Natl Acad Sci USA 99:14298–14302

Jackson AM, Hawkyard SJ, Prescott S, Ritchie AW, James K, Chisholm GD (1992) An investigation of factors influencing the in vitro induction of LAK activity against a variety of human bladder cancer cell lines. J Urol 147:207–211

Jackson AM, Alexandroff AB, Kelly RW, Skibinska A, Esuvaranathan K, Prescott S et al (1995) Changes in urinary cytokines and soluble intercellular adhesion molecule-1 (ICAM-1) in bladder cancer patients after Bacillus Calmette-Guerin (BCG) immunotherapy. Clin Exp Immunol 99:369–375

Jakse G, Hall R, Bono A, Holtl W, Carpentier P, Spaander JP et al (2001) Intravesical BCG in patients with carcinoma in situ of the urinary bladder: long-term results of EORTC GU Group phase II protocol 30861. Eur Urol 40:144–150

Joudi FN, Smith BJ, O'Donnell MA, Konety BR (2006) The impact of age on the response of patients with superficial bladder cancer to intravesical immunotherapy. J Urol 175:1634–1639. Discussion 9–40

Kaempfer R, Gerez L, Farbstein H, Madar L, Hirschman O, Nussinovich R et al (1996) Prediction of response to treatment in superficial bladder carcinoma through pattern of interleukin-2 gene expression. J Clin Oncol 14:1778–1786

Kaimakliotis HZ, Monn MF, Cho JS, Pedrosa JA, Hahn NM, Albany C et al (2016) Neoadjuvant chemotherapy in urothelial bladder cancer: impact of regimen and variant histology. Future Oncol 12:1795–1804

Kakehi Y, Ozdemir E, Habuchi T, Yamabe H, Hashimura T, Katsura Y et al (1998) Absence of p53 overexpression and favorable response to cisplatin-based neoadjuvant chemotherapy in urothelial carcinomas. Jpn J Cancer Res 89:214–220

Kamada M, So A, Muramaki M, Rocchi P, Beraldi E, Gleave M (2007) Hsp27 knockdown using nucleotide-based therapies inhibit tumor growth and enhance chemotherapy in human bladder cancer cells. Mol Cancer Ther 6:299–308

Kamat AM, Li R, O'Donnell MA, Black PC, Roupret M, Catto JW et al (2018) Predicting response to intravesical Bacillus Calmette-Guerin immunotherapy: are we there yet? A systematic review. Eur Urol 73:738–748

Kamoun A, de Reynies A, Allory Y, Sjodahl G, Robertson AG, Seiler R et al (2020) A consensus molecular classification of muscle-invasive bladder cancer. Eur Urol 77:420–433

Kasahara K, Fujiwara Y, Nishio K, Ohmori T, Sugimoto Y, Komiya K et al (1991) Metallothionein content correlates with the sensitivity of human small cell lung cancer cell lines to cisplatin. Cancer Res 51:3237–3242

Katano K, Kondo A, Safaei R, Holzer A, Samimi G, Mishima M et al (2002) Acquisition of resistance to cisplatin is accompanied by changes in the cellular pharmacology of copper. Cancer Res 62:6559–6565

Ke HL, Lin J, Ye Y, Wu WJ, Lin HH, Wei H et al (2015) Genetic variations in glutathione pathway genes predict cancer recurrence in patients treated with transurethral resection and Bacillus Calmette-Guerin instillation for non-muscle invasive bladder cancer. Ann Surg Oncol 22:4104–4110

Kilari D, Iczkowski KA, Pandya C, Robin AJ, Messing EM, Guancial E et al (2016) Copper transporter-CTR1 expression and pathological outcomes in platinum-treated muscle-invasive bladder cancer patients. Anticancer Res 36:495–501

Kirsch DG, Kastan MB (1998) Tumor-suppressor p53: implications for tumor development and prognosis. J Clin Oncol 16:3158–3168

Kobayashi S, Fujii Y, Koga F, Yokoyama M, Ishioka J, Matsuoka Y et al (2014) Impact of bladder neck involvement on progression in patients with primary non-muscle invasive bladder cancer: a prospective validation study. Urol Oncol 32(38):e29–e36

Krajewski W, Karabon L, Partyka A, Tomkiewicz A, Poletajew S, Tukiendorf A et al (2020) Polymorphisms of genes encoding cytokines predict the risk of high-grade bladder cancer and outcomes of BCG immunotherapy. Cent Eur J Immunol 45:37–47

Kuroda K, Brown EJ, Telle WB, Russell DG, Ratliff TL (1993) Characterization of the internalization of bacillus Calmette-Guerin by human bladder tumor cells. J Clin Invest 91:69–76

Lamm DL, Blumenstein BA, Crissman JD, Montie JE, Gottesman JE, Lowe BA et al (2000) Maintenance Bacillus Calmette-Guerin immunotherapy for recurrent TA, T1 and carcinoma in situ transitional cell carcinoma of the bladder: a randomized Southwest Oncology Group Study. J Urol 163:1124–1129

Lewis AD, Hayes JD, Wolf CR (1988) Glutathione and glutathione-dependent enzymes in ovarian adenocarcinoma cell lines derived from a patient before and after the onset of drug resistance: intrinsic differences and cell cycle effects. Carcinogenesis 9:1283–1287

Li Q, Gardner K, Zhang L, Tsang B, Bostick-Bruton F, Reed E (1998) Cisplatin induction of ERCC-1 mRNA expression in A2780/CP70 human ovarian cancer cells. J Biol Chem 273:23419–23425

Li Q, Assel M, Benfante NE, Pietzak EJ, Herr HW, Donat M et al (2019) The impact of plasmacytoid variant histology on the survival of patients with urothelial carcinoma of bladder after radical cystectomy. Eur Urol Focus 5:104–108

Lima L, Dinis-Ribeiro M, Longatto-Filho A, Santos L (2012) Predictive biomarkers of bacillus Calmette-Guerin immunotherapy response in bladder cancer: where are we now? Adv Urol 2012:232609

Lima L, Ferreira JA, Tavares A, Oliveira D, Morais A, Videira PA et al (2014) FASL polymorphism is associated with response to Bacillus Calmette-Guerin immunotherapy in bladder cancer. Urol Oncol 32(44):e1–e7

Lima L, Oliveira D, Ferreira JA, Tavares A, Cruz R, Medeiros R et al (2015) The role of functional polymorphisms in immune response genes as biomarkers of bacille Calmette-Guerin (BCG) immunotherapy outcome in bladder cancer: establishment of a predictive profile in a Southern Europe population. BJU Int 116:753–763

Lindskrog SV, Prip F, Lamy P, Taber A, Groeneveld CS, Birkenkamp-Demtroder K et al (2021) An integrated multi-omics analysis identifies prognostic molecular subtypes of non-muscle-invasive bladder cancer. Nat Commun 12:2301

Liu D, Plimack ER, Hoffman-Censits J, Garraway LA, Bellmunt J, Van Allen E et al (2016) Clinical validation of chemotherapy response biomarker ERCC2 in muscle-invasive urothelial bladder carcinoma. JAMA Oncol 2:1094–1096

Lotan Y, Boorjian SA, Zhang J, Bivalacqua TJ, Porten SP, Wheeler T et al (2019) Molecular subtyping of clinically localized urothelial carcinoma reveals lower rates of pathological upstaging at radical cystectomy among luminal tumors. Eur Urol 76:200–206

Lotan Y, de Jong JJ, Liu VYT, Bismar TA, Boorjian SA, Huang HC et al (2022) Patients with muscle-invasive bladder cancer with nonluminal subtype derive greatest benefit from platinum based neoadjuvant chemotherapy. J Urol 207:541–550

Luo Y (2012) Blocking IL-10 enhances Bacillus Calmette-Guerin induced T helper Type 1 immune responses and anti-bladder cancer immunity. Onco Targets Ther 1:1183–1185

Luo Y, Yamada H, Evanoff DP, Chen X (2006) Role of Th1-stimulating cytokines in Bacillus Calmette-Guerin (BCG)-induced macrophage cytotoxicity against mouse bladder cancer MBT-2 cells. Clin Exp Immunol 146:181–188

Magno C, Melloni D, Gali A, Mucciardi G, Nicocia G, Morandi B et al (2002) The anti-tumor activity of Bacillus Calmette-Guerin in bladder cancer is associated with an increase in the circulating level of interleukin-2. Immunol Lett 81:235–238

Malmstrom PU, Sylvester RJ, Crawford DE, Friedrich M, Krege S, Rintala E et al (2009) An individual patient data meta-analysis of the long-term outcome of randomised studies comparing intravesical mitomycin C versus Bacillus Calmette-Guerin for non-muscle-invasive bladder cancer. Eur Urol 56:247–256

Mariathasan S, Turley SJ, Nickles D, Castiglioni A, Yuen K, Wang Y et al (2018) TGFbeta attenuates tumour response to PD-L1 blockade by contributing to exclusion of T cells. Nature 554:544–548

Martin-Doyle W, Leow JJ, Orsola A, Chang SL, Bellmunt J (2015) Improving selection criteria for early cystectomy in high-grade t1 bladder cancer: a meta-analysis of 15,215 patients. J Clin Oncol 33:643–650

Marzouka NA, Eriksson P, Bernardo C, Hurst CD, Knowles MA, Sjodahl G et al (2022) The lund molecular taxonomy applied to non-muscle-invasive urothelial carcinoma. J Mol Diagn 24:992–1008

McConkey DJ, Choi W, Shen Y, Lee IL, Porten S, Matin SF et al (2016) A prognostic gene expression signature in the molecular classification of chemotherapy-naive urothelial cancer is predictive of clinical outcomes from neoadjuvant chemotherapy: a phase 2 trial of dose-dense methotrexate, vinblastine, doxorubicin, and cisplatin with bevacizumab in urothelial cancer. Eur Urol 69:855–862

Meeks JJ, Carneiro BA, Pai SG, Oberlin DT, Rademaker A, Fedorchak K et al (2016) Genomic characterization of high-risk non-muscle invasive bladder cancer. Oncotarget 7:75176–75184

Metzger R, Leichman CG, Danenberg KD, Danenberg PV, Lenz HJ, Hayashi K et al (1998) ERCC1 mRNA levels complement thymidylate synthase mRNA levels in predicting response and survival for gastric cancer patients receiving combination cisplatin and fluorouracil chemotherapy. J Clin Oncol 16:309–316

Miron B, Hoffman-Censits JH, Anari F, O'Neill J, Geynisman DM, Zibelman MR et al (2020) Defects in DNA repair genes confer improved long-term survival after cisplatin-based neoadjuvant chemotherapy for muscle-invasive bladder cancer. Eur Urol Oncol 3:544–547

Morales A, Eidinger D, Bruce AW (1976) Intracavitary Bacillus Calmette-Guerin in the treatment of superficial bladder tumors. J Urol 116:180–183

Naoe M, Ogawa Y, Takeshita K, Morita J, Iwamoto S, Miyazaki A et al (2007) Bacillus Calmette-Guerin-pulsed dendritic cells stimulate natural killer T cells and gammadeltaT cells. Int J Urol 14:532–538. Discussion 8.

Noon AP, Albertsen PC, Thomas F, Rosario DJ, Catto JW (2013) Competing mortality in patients diagnosed with bladder cancer: evidence of undertreatment in the elderly and female patients. Br J Cancer 108:1534–1540

Oddens JR, Sylvester RJ, Brausi MA, Kirkels WJ, van de Beek C, van Andel G et al (2014) The effect of age on the efficacy of maintenance Bacillus Calmette-Guerin relative to maintenance epirubicin in patients with stage Ta T1 urothelial bladder cancer: results from EORTC genito-urinary group study 30911. Eur Urol 66:694–701

Palou J, Sylvester RJ, Faba OR, Parada R, Pena JA, Algaba F et al (2012) Female gender and carcinoma in situ in the prostatic urethra are prognostic factors for recurrence, progression, and disease-specific mortality in T1G3 bladder cancer patients treated with bacillus Calmette-Guerin. Eur Urol 62:118–125

Patschan O, Sjodahl G, Chebil G, Lovgren K, Lauss M, Gudjonsson S et al (2015) A molecular pathologic framework for risk stratification of stage T1 urothelial carcinoma. Eur Urol 68:824–832. Discussion 35–6

Peng HQ, Hogg D, Malkin D, Bailey D, Gallie BL, Bulbul M et al (1993) Mutations of the p53 gene do not occur in testis cancer. Cancer Res 53:3574–3578

Pichler R, Fritz J, Zavadil C, Schafer G, Culig Z, Brunner A (2016) Tumor-infiltrating immune cell subpopulations influence the oncologic outcome after intravesical Bacillus Calmette-Guerin therapy in bladder cancer. Oncotarget 7:39916–39930

Pichler R, Gruenbacher G, Culig Z, Brunner A, Fuchs D, Fritz J et al (2017) Intratumoral Th2 predisposition combines with an increased Th1 functional phenotype in clinical response to intravesical BCG in bladder cancer. Cancer Immunol Immunother 66:427–440

Pietzak EJ, Bagrodia A, Cha EK, Drill EN, Iyer G, Isharwal S et al (2017) Next-generation sequencing of nonmuscle invasive bladder cancer reveals potential biomarkers and rational therapeutic targets. Eur Urol 72:952–959

Pietzak EJ, Zabor EC, Bagrodia A, Armenia J, Hu W, Zehir A et al (2019) Genomic differences between "primary" and "secondary" muscle-invasive bladder cancer as a basis for disparate outcomes to cisplatin-based neoadjuvant chemotherapy. Eur Urol 75:231–239

Pietzak EJ, Whiting K, Srinivasan P, Bandlamudi C, Khurram A, Joseph V et al (2022) Inherited germline cancer susceptibility gene variants in individuals with non-muscle-invasive bladder cancer. Clin Cancer Res 28:4267–4277

Plimack ER, Dunbrack RL, Brennan TA, Andrake MD, Zhou Y, Serebriiskii IG et al (2015) Defects in DNA repair genes predict response to neoadjuvant cisplatin-based chemotherapy in muscle-invasive bladder cancer. Eur Urol 68:959–967

Powles T, Assaf ZJ, Davarpanah N, Banchereau R, Szabados BE, Yuen KC et al (2021) ctDNA guiding adjuvant immunotherapy in urothelial carcinoma. Nature 595:432–437

Pryor K, Goddard J, Goldstein D, Stricker P, Russell P, Golovsky D et al (1995) Bacillus Calmette-Guerin (BCG) enhances monocyte- and lymphocyte-mediated bladder tumour cell killing. Br J Cancer 71:801–807

Quinn JE, Kennedy RD, Mullan PB, Gilmore PM, Carty M, Johnston PG et al (2003) BRCA1 functions as a differential modulator of chemotherapy-induced apoptosis. Cancer Res 63:6221–6228

Qureshi KN, Griffiths TR, Robinson MC, Marsh C, Roberts JT, Hall RR et al (1999) TP53 accumulation predicts improved survival in patients resistant to systemic cisplatin-based chemotherapy for muscle-invasive bladder cancer. Clin Cancer Res 5:3500–3507

Ramoner R, Rieser C, Herold M, Klocker H, Bartsch G, Stenzl A et al (1998) Activation of human dendritic cells by bacillus Calmette-Guerin. J Urol 159:1488–1492

Ratliff TL, Ritchey JK, Yuan JJ, Andriole GL, Catalona WJ (1993) T-cell subsets required for intravesical BCG immunotherapy for bladder cancer. J Urol 150:1018–1023

Ren A, Yan G, You B, Sun J (2008) Down-regulation of mammalian sterile 20-like kinase 1 by heat shock protein 70 mediates cisplatin resistance in prostate cancer cells. Cancer Res 68:2266–2274

Ren JH, He WS, Nong L, Zhu QY, Hu K, Zhang RG et al (2010) Acquired cisplatin resistance in human lung adenocarcinoma cells is associated with enhanced autophagy. Cancer Biother Radiopharm 25:75–80

Rentsch CA, Birkhauser FD, Biot C, Gsponer JR, Bisiaux A, Wetterauer C et al (2014) Bacillus Calmette-Guerin strain differences have an impact on clinical outcome in bladder cancer immunotherapy. Eur Urol 66:677–688

Robertson AG, Kim J, Al-Ahmadie H, Bellmunt J, Guo G, Cherniack AD et al (2017) Comprehensive molecular characterization of muscle-invasive bladder cancer. Cell 171(540-56):e25

Robertson AG, Groeneveld CS, Jordan B, Lin X, McLaughlin KA, Das A et al (2020) Identification of differential tumor subtypes of T1 bladder cancer. Eur Urol 78:533–537
Rosenberg JE, Hahn NM, Regan MM, Werner L, Alva A, George S et al (2018) Apatorsen plus docetaxel versus docetaxel alone in platinum-resistant metastatic urothelial carcinoma (Borealis-2). Br J Cancer 118:1434–1441
Ryk C, Steineck G, Wiklund NP, Nyberg T, de Verdier PJ (2010) The (CCTTT)n microsatellite polymorphism in the nitric oxide synthase 2 gene may influence bladder cancer pathogenesis. J Urol 184:2150–2157
Ryk C, Wiklund NP, Nyberg T, de Verdier PJ (2011) Polymorphisms in nitric-oxide synthase 3 may influence the risk of urinary-bladder cancer. Nitric Oxide 25:338–343
Ryk C, Koskela LR, Thiel T, Wiklund NP, Steineck G, Schumacher MC et al (2015) Outcome after BCG treatment for urinary bladder cancer may be influenced by polymorphisms in the NOS2 and NOS3 genes. Redox Biol 6:272–277
Safaei R, Holzer AK, Katano K, Samimi G, Howell SB (2004) The role of copper transporters in the development of resistance to Pt drugs. J Inorg Biochem 98:1607–1613
Saint F, Patard JJ, Maille P, Soyeux P, Hoznek A, Salomon L et al (2002) Prognostic value of a T helper 1 urinary cytokine response after intravesical Bacillus Calmette-Guerin treatment for superficial bladder cancer. J Urol 167:364–367
Saint F, Kurth N, Maille P, Vordos D, Hoznek A, Soyeux P et al (2003) Urinary IL-2 assay for monitoring intravesical Bacillus Calmette-Guerin response of superficial bladder cancer during induction course and maintenance therapy. Int J Cancer 107:434–440
Sakamoto M, Kondo A, Kawasaki K, Goto T, Sakamoto H, Miyake K et al (2001) Analysis of gene expression profiles associated with cisplatin resistance in human ovarian cancer cell lines and tissues using cDNA microarray. Hum Cell 14:305–315
Samimi G, Safaei R, Katano K, Holzer AK, Rochdi M, Tomioka M et al (2004) Increased expression of the copper efflux transporter ATP7A mediates resistance to cisplatin, carboplatin, and oxaliplatin in ovarian cancer cells. Clin Cancer Res 10:4661–4669
Sanchez-Carbayo M, Urrutia M, Romani R, Herrero M, Gonzalez de Buitrago JM, Navajo JA (2001) Serial urinary IL-2, IL-6, IL-8, TNFalpha, UBC, CYFRA 21-1 and NMP22 during follow-up of patients with bladder cancer receiving intravesical BCG. Anticancer Res 21:3041–3047
Sarkis AS, Dalbagni G, Cordon-Cardo C, Melamed J, Zhang ZF, Sheinfeld J et al (1994) Association of P53 nuclear overexpression and tumor progression in carcinoma in situ of the bladder. J Urol 152:388–392
Sato K, Moriyama M, Mori S, Saito M, Watanuki T, Terada K et al (1992) An immunohistologic evaluation of C-erbB-2 gene product in patients with urinary bladder carcinoma. Cancer 70:2493–2498
Scosyrev E, Ely BW, Messing EM, Speights VO, Grossman HB, Wood DP et al (2011) Do mixed histological features affect survival benefit from neoadjuvant platinum-based combination chemotherapy in patients with locally advanced bladder cancer? A secondary analysis of Southwest Oncology Group-Directed Intergroup Study (S8710). BJU Int 108:693–699
Seiler R, Ashab HAD, Erho N, van Rhijn BWG, Winters B, Douglas J et al (2017) Impact of molecular subtypes in muscle-invasive bladder cancer on predicting response and survival after neoadjuvant chemotherapy. Eur Urol 72:544–554
Sherr CJ, McCormick F (2002) The RB and p53 pathways in cancer. Cancer Cell 2:103–112
Shintani Y, Sawada Y, Inagaki T, Kohjimoto Y, Uekado Y, Shinka T (2007) Intravesical instillation therapy with Bacillus Calmette-Guerin for superficial bladder cancer: study of the mechanism of Bacillus Calmette-Guerin immunotherapy. Int J Urol 14:140–146
Shuck SC, Short EA, Turchi JJ (2008) Eukaryotic nucleotide excision repair: from understanding mechanisms to influencing biology. Cell Res 18:64–72
Siddik ZH (2003) Cisplatin: mode of cytotoxic action and molecular basis of resistance. Oncogene 22:7265–7279
Simons MP, O'Donnell MA, Griffith TS (2008) Role of neutrophils in BCG immunotherapy for bladder cancer. Urol Oncol 26:341–345
Sjodahl G, Lauss M, Lovgren K, Chebil G, Gudjonsson S, Veerla S et al (2012) A molecular taxonomy for urothelial carcinoma. Clin Cancer Res 18:3377–3386
Sjodahl G, Abrahamsson J, Holmsten K, Bernardo C, Chebil G, Eriksson P et al (2022) Different responses to neoadjuvant chemotherapy in urothelial carcinoma molecular subtypes. Eur Urol 81:523–532
Stadler WM, Lerner SP, Groshen S, Stein JP, Shi SR, Raghavan D et al (2011) Phase III study of molecularly targeted adjuvant therapy in locally advanced urothelial cancer of the bladder based on p53 status. J Clin Oncol 29:3443–3449
Sui W, Matulay JT, Onyeji IC, Theofanides MC, James MB, RoyChoudhury A et al (2017) Contemporary treatment patterns and outcomes of sarcomatoid bladder cancer. World J Urol 35:1055–1061
Suttmann H, Lehan N, Bohle A, Brandau S (2003) Stimulation of neutrophil granulocytes with Mycobacterium bovis Bacillus Calmette-Guerin induces changes in phenotype and gene expression and inhibits spontaneous apoptosis. Infect Immun 71:4647–4656
Taber A, Christensen E, Lamy P, Nordentoft I, Prip F, Lindskrog SV et al (2020) Molecular correlates of cisplatin-based chemotherapy response in muscle invasive bladder cancer by integrated multi-omics analysis. Nat Commun 11:4858
Takashi M, Wakai K, Hattori T, Ono Y, Ohshima S (2002) Evaluation of multiple recurrence events in superficial bladder cancer patients treated with intravesical

Bacillus Calmette-Guerin therapy using the Andersen-Gill's model. Int Urol Nephrol 34:329–334

Teo MY, Bambury RM, Zabor EC, Jordan E, Al-Ahmadie H, Boyd ME et al (2017) DNA damage response and repair gene alterations are associated with improved survival in patients with platinum-treated advanced urothelial carcinoma. Clin Cancer Res 23:3610–3618

Thalmann GN, Sermier A, Rentsch C, Mohrle K, Cecchini MG, Studer UE (2000) Urinary Interleukin-8 and 18 predict the response of superficial bladder cancer to intravesical therapy with bacillus Calmette-Guerin. J Urol 164:2129–2133

Vaisman A, Varchenko M, Umar A, Kunkel TA, Risinger JI, Barrett JC et al (1998) The role of hMLH1, hMSH3, and hMSH6 defects in cisplatin and oxaliplatin resistance: correlation with replicative bypass of platinum-DNA adducts. Cancer Res 58:3579–3585

Van Allen EM, Mouw KW, Kim P, Iyer G, Wagle N, Al-Ahmadie H et al (2014) Somatic ERCC2 mutations correlate with cisplatin sensitivity in muscle-invasive urothelial carcinoma. Cancer Discov 4:1140–1153

van den Bosch S, Alfred WJ (2011) Long-term cancer-specific survival in patients with high-risk, non-muscle-invasive bladder cancer and tumour progression: a systematic review. Eur Urol 60:493–500

van der Heijden MS, Powles T, Petrylak D, de Wit R, Necchi A, Sternberg CN et al (2022) Predictive biomarkers for survival benefit with ramucirumab in urothelial cancer in the RANGE trial. Nat Commun 13:1878

Vousden KH, Lane DP (2007) p53 in health and disease. Nat Rev Mol Cell Biol 8:275–283

Warrick JI, Hovelson DH, Amin A, Liu CJ, Cani AK, McDaniel AS et al (2015) Tumor evolution and progression in multifocal and paired non-invasive/invasive urothelial carcinoma. Virchows Arch 466:297–311

Watanabe E, Matsuyama H, Matsuda K, Ohmi C, Tei Y, Yoshihiro S et al (2003) Urinary interleukin-2 may predict clinical outcome of intravesical Bacillus Calmette-Guerin immunotherapy for carcinoma in situ of the bladder. Cancer Immunol Immunother 52:481–486

Watanabe J, Nishiyama H, Okubo K, Takahashi T, Toda Y, Habuchi T et al (2004) Clinical evaluation of p53 mutations in urothelial carcinoma by IHC and FASAY. Urology 63:989–993

Williams SB, Kamat AM, Mmeje C, Ye Y, Huang M, Chang DW et al (2017) Genetic variants in the inflammation pathway as predictors of recurrence and progression in non-muscle invasive bladder cancer treated with Bacillus Calmette-Guerin. Oncotarget 8:88782–88791

Wood RD, Araujo SJ, Ariza RR, Batty DP, Biggerstaff M, Evans E et al (2000) DNA damage recognition and nucleotide excision repair in mammalian cells. Cold Spring Harb Symp Quant Biol 65:173–182

Yamada T, Tsuchiya K, Kato S, Kamei S, Taniguchi M, Takeuchi T et al (2010) A pretreatment nomogram predicting recurrence- and progression-free survival for nonmuscle invasive bladder cancer in Japanese patients. Int J Clin Oncol 15:271–279

Yamamoto K, Okamoto A, Isonishi S, Ochiai K, Ohtake Y (2001) Heat shock protein 27 was up-regulated in cisplatin resistant human ovarian tumor cell line and associated with the cisplatin resistance. Cancer Lett 168:173–181

Yang X, Yin H, Zhang Y, Li X, Tong H, Zeng Y et al (2018) Hypoxia-induced autophagy promotes gemcitabine resistance in human bladder cancer cells through hypoxia-inducible factor 1alpha activation. Int J Oncol 53:215–224

Yin M, Joshi M, Meijer RP, Glantz M, Holder S, Harvey HA et al (2016) Neoadjuvant chemotherapy for muscle-invasive bladder cancer: a systematic review and two-step meta-analysis. Oncologist 21:708–715

Yin H, Yang X, Gu W, Liu Y, Li X, Huang X et al (2017) HMGB1-mediated autophagy attenuates gemcitabine-induced apoptosis in bladder cancer cells involving JNK and ERK activation. Oncotarget 8:71642–71656

Yu H, Su J, Xu Y, Kang J, Li H, Zhang L et al (2011) p62/SQSTM1 involved in cisplatin resistance in human ovarian cancer cells by clearing ubiquitinated proteins. Eur J Cancer 47:1585–1594

Zang Z, Lim YK, Chan YH, Raman L, Esuvaranathan K, Chiong E et al (2021) Polymorphism in autophagy gene ATG2B is not associated with bladder cancer recurrence after intravesical Bacillus Calmette-Guerin (BCG) immunotherapy in Asian patients. Urol Oncol 39(238):e1–e7

Zargar H, Espiritu PN, Fairey AS, Mertens LS, Dinney CP, Mir MC et al (2015) Multicenter assessment of neoadjuvant chemotherapy for muscle-invasive bladder cancer. Eur Urol 67:241–249

Zargar H, Zargar-Shoshtari K, Lotan Y, Shah JB, van Rhijn BW, Daneshmand S et al (2016) Final pathological stage after neoadjuvant chemotherapy and radical cystectomy for bladder cancer-does pT0 predict better survival than pTa/Tis/T1? J Urol 195:886–893

Part VII

Therapeutic Application Based on Molecular Insights

21 New Treatment Approaches in Non-Muscle-Invasive Bladder Cancer

Sung Han Kim and Seth P. Lerner

Abstract

Non-muscle-invasive bladder cancer (NMIBC) accounts for two-thirds of all BC cases. NMIBC is further classified into disease subtypes based on the morphological appearance and nuclear grade, probability of response to treatment and progression stratified as low, intermediate, and high risk. In 2018, The US Food and Drug Administration published a guidance document for treatment of BCG-unresponsive NMIBC codifying a registration pathway and rapidly accelerating drug development. In this chapter we discuss these new treatments applied across the spectrum of NMIBC disease states.

Keywords

Bladder cancer · Non-muscle invasive · Intravesical therapy · Targeted treatment · Immunotherapy · Clinical trials

21.1 Introduction

Non-muscle-invasive bladder cancer (NMIBC) comprises approximately 70–80% of all BC cases (Lenis et al. 2020; Richters et al. 2020). The majority are papillary tumors confined to the urothelium (Ta), or tumors with invasion into the subepithelial connective tissue (T1). Carcinoma in situ (CIS) is a high-grade intraepithelial cancer confined to the urothelium and can occur with or without Ta or T1 papillary disease. The recurrence rate of NMIBC is high at 50–70%, and 10–30% of patients exhibit disease progression to either muscle-invasive bladder cancer (MIBC) or metastases (Lenis et al. 2020; Del Giudice et al. 2023). The main goals of NMIBC treatment are to decrease the recurrence rate and prevent disease progression, with long-term durable cure if possible. Prognosis is risk-stratified as low, intermediate, and high specifically regarding progression (Table 21.1) (Sylvester et al. 2021). The Club Urologico Espanol de Tratamiento Oncologico (CUETO; Spanish Urological Oncology Group) showed an interval range for recurrence of 15–61% and progression of 0.2–17% at 1 year after 12 doses of intravesical Bacillus Calmette-Guerin (BCG) and at 5 years

S. H. Kim · S. P. Lerner (✉)
Scott Department of Urology, Dan L Duncan Cancer Center, Baylor College of Medicine Medical Center, Houston, TX, USA
e-mail: slerner@bcm.edu

M. A. Knowles, L. Dyrskjøt (eds.), *Biology of Bladder Cancer*,
https://doi.org/10.1007/978-3-031-68505-7_21

Table 21.1 Differences of risk group classification between EAU, AUA, and NCCN guidelines

Risk group	Low-risk	Intermediate-risk	High-risk
EAU (Burger et al. 2013; Babjuk et al. 2022)	Primary, solitary	All tumors except the low- and high-risk tumors	T1 tumor
	Ta		HG/G3 tumor
	LG/G1		CIS
	<3 cm		Multiple & recurrent and large (≥3 cm) Ta, G1, G2 tumors
	No CIS		
NCCN (Flaig et al. 2022)	LG Ta	HG Ta	All T1 (CIS listed separately)
AUA (Chang et al. 2016)	Small volume	Multifocal and/or large volume LG Ta	HG Ta
	LG Ta	(High risk of recurrence, low risk of progression)	T1 LG and HG
			CIS

EAU, European Association of Urology; AUA, American Urological Association; NCCN, National Comprehensive Cancer Network; LG, low grade; HG, high grade; CIS, carcinoma in situ

31–78% and 0.8–45%, respectively (Fernandez-Gomez et al. 2009). In the European Association of Urology (EAU) NMIBC risk model, the 1- and 5-year progression rates were reported as 0.06–16% and 0.93–40%, including 0.06–0.93% for the low-risk group, 1.0–4.9% for the intermediate risk group, 3.5–9.6% for the high-risk group, and 16–40% for the very high-risk group (Babjuk et al. 2022).

Diagnosis and treatment for NMIBC starts with transurethral resection of the bladder tumor (TURBT) to establish grade and histology, presence and depth of invasion, as well as the complete surgical removal of all visible papillary disease within the bladder (Lenis et al. 2020). To eradicate any intravesical circulating tumor cells or occult papillary tumors, single-dose instillation of Mitomycin-C (MMC) or gemcitabine immediately after TURBT is recommended for suspected low- or intermediate-risk disease. Adjuvant intravesical instillation with chemotherapy (MMC, Gemcitabine, Docetaxel, and others either alone or in combination), or immunotherapy with BCG, is recommended for intermediate- and high-risk disease, respectively. The instillation frequencies and durations are dependent on the risk group. Intravesical BCG instillation includes 6 weeks of induction with 1 year of maintenance weekly for 3 weeks at months 3, 6, and 12 for patients with recurrent intermediate-risk disease following intravesical chemotherapy and maintenance to 3 years for patients with high-risk disease. This approach decreases both the recurrence and progression rates with an initial complete response rate after induction therapy and 3-month maintenance as high as 85% (Lamm et al. 2000) (see also Chap. 5).

Despite advances in TURBT quality, enhanced cystoscopic imaging, and a personalized risk-stratified treatment approach with low-intensity treatment for low-risk and high-intensity treatment for high risk with BCG and maintenance, optimizing the durability of response remains a substantial challenge. The recurring challenge of the global supply of BCG has been another driving force to test alternative treatment approaches (Bandari et al. 2018). For patients treated with adequate BCG who recur with high-grade (HG disease;BCG-unresponsive), new therapeutic agents with novel mechanisms of actions are needed to prevent disease progression to MIBC and reduce the need for radical cystectomy (Golla et al. 2019). In this chapter we provide an overview of ongoing clinical trials assessing the role of innovative immunological and targeted agents in patients with BCG-naïve and BCG-unresponsive NMIBC including immune checkpoint inhibitors (ICI), oncolytic viral gene therapy, immunotherapy, targeted therapy, immune stimulatory therapy, and cell-mediated peptide vaccine therapies as new innovative therapeutic concepts for BC treatment. We also review several novel drug delivery technologies.

21.2 BCG Responsiveness

High-risk NMIBC is a heterogeneous group comprised largely of patients with high-grade urothelial cancer, in which identification of well-defined subgroups with variable prognostic features is important for future clinical trial design (Kamat et al. 2016; Sylvester et al. 2021). Three NMIBC categories are further subcategorized based on responsiveness to prior intravesical BCG therapy: BCG-naïve (no prior intravesical BCG); BCG-exposed (prior BCG within 24 months but not meeting the criteria for BCG-unresponsive); and BCG-unresponsive (Roumiguié et al. 2022). BCG-unresponsive is defined as patients with high-grade NMIBC who have been treated with adequate BCG and are unlikely to benefit from and should not receive further intravesical BCG (Lerner et al. 2015). These are patients with CIS with or without Ta/T1 disease within 12 months of completion of adequate BCG (defined as induction cycle of 5~6 BCG instillations and maintenance cycle of at least 2 cycles of BCG [minimum 5 + 2] or two induction courses of BCG) or patients with Ta/T1 that recur within 6 months of completion of BCG or have persistent stage T1HG disease after a single induction course (Roumiguié et al. 2022). In addition, BCG resistance is defined as either a presence of high-grade Ta or CIS at the 3-month evaluation after BCG induction and delayed relapse after adequate BCG therapy that does not meet the criteria for BCG-unresponsive disease (Bandari et al. 2018).

Radical cystectomy is recommended for patients with BCG-unresponsive NMIBC due to a substantially decreased probability of cancer-specific survival (CSS) if performed at the time of progression to muscle invasive disease (Burger et al. 2013; Flaig et al. 2022). However, the potential negative impact on quality of life and both short- and long-term morbidity associated with radical cystectomy are barriers to the widespread adoption of radical cystectomy and are a powerful motivating force for drug development in these NMIBC disease states. The challenge is to develop therapeutic alternatives with high initial complete response rates that are durable, to enable safe and effective bladder preservation without diminution of survival probability.

21.3 NMIBC Therapy

21.3.1 Immune Checkpoint Inhibitors

Immune checkpoint inhibitors (ICI) target immune checkpoints including the programmed cell death 1 protein (PD-1)/programmed cell death 1 protein-ligand (PDL1) axis, which is involved in immune escape and has been implicated in the process of BCG resistance (Table 21.2) (Mukherjee et al. 2018; Fukumoto et al. 2018) (Table 21.2) (see also Chap. 23). Among patients treated with BCG, 69% of tumors expressed PD-L1 compared to 30% of BCG-naïve patients. In the phase 2 KEYNOTE-057 trial, Pembrolizumab was associated with a 3-month 41% complete response (CR) rate and 19% overall maintained a CR at 12 months among patients with BCG-unresponsive CIS with acceptable toxicity (Balar et al. 2021). This trial supported FDA approval in January 2020 for patients with BCG-unresponsive CIS with or without papillary disease who refuse or are ineligible for radical cystectomy. Pembrolizumab (MK-3475-676, Merck) is currently being tested in combination with BCG for patients with high-risk disease who recur after BCG (NCT03711032/ KEYNOTE-676) (Kamat et al. 2020).

Atezolizumab and Durvalumab are PDL1-targeted monoclonal antibody inhibitors. Atezolizumab which has shown long-term durable remission in patients with metastatic urothelial cancer who are ineligible for cisplatin or after prior platinum therapy has been evaluated as monotherapy for BCG-unresponsive disease in SWOG 1605 (NCT02844816) (Black et al. 2023). The 6-month CR rate in patients with CIS with or without papillary disease was 27% with 56% of these patients maintaining a CR at 12 months (Black et al. 2023). Together with Keynote 057, these two trials support the use of systemic ICI agents targeting PD-L1/PD1 for

Table 21.2 NMIBC clinical trials testing immune-based monoclonal antibodies

Agent or technology	Indication	Mode of action	Number of estimated enrolling participants	Clinical trial number
Zalifrelimab	BCG-unresponsive	Intravesical, anti-CTLA-4 antibody alone or in combination with Imiquimod (UGN-201)	60 patients	Phase 1, NCT05375903
Catumaxomab	Intermediate- and high-risk BCG-naive	Trifunctional Anti-EPCAM × Anti-CD3 antibody	30 patients	Phase 1 CATUNIBLA trial, NCT04819399
Camrelizumab	BCG-unresponsive	Intravesical or IV, anti-PD-1(SHR-1210)	56 patients	Phase 1/2; NCT04706598
Tislelizumab	High-risk BCG-naive	IV, anti-PD-1 + BCG	6 patients	TACBIN-01, NCT04922047
Sasanlimab	High-risk BCG-naive	Subcutaneous, anti-PD-1 monoclonal antibody inhibitor + BCG induction +/– maintenance	1070 patients	Phase 3 CREST trial; NCT04165317
Sasanlimab	BCG-unresponsive	Subcutaneous, anti-PD-1 monoclonal antibody inhibitor	160 patients	Phase 3 CREST trial; NCT04165317
Pembrolizumab	BCG-unresponsive, high-risk BCG-naive	IV, anti-PD-1 + BCG	1405 patients	MK-3475-676, KEYNOTE-676 trial, NCT03711032
Atezolizumab	High-risk, BCG-naive	IV, anti-PD-L1	516 patients for NCT03799835	Phase 3 ALBAN trial, NCT03799835
			40 patients for NCT04134000	Phase 1 BladderGATE trial, NCT04134000
Durvalumab	BCG-unresponsive	IV, anti-PD-L1	55 patients	Phase 1/2 ADAPT-BLADDER trial, NCT03317158

NMIBC, non-muscle invasive bladder cancer; IV, intravenous; PD-1, programmed death receptor-1; PD-L1, programmed death-ligand 1; CTLA-4, anti-cytotoxic T-lymphocyte antigen-4

BCG-unresponsive NMIBC. However, due to the modest durability of the response, trials combining ICI and BCG for patients with BCG-naïve high-risk NMIBC are ongoing (ALBAN, NCT03799835 & BladderGATE, NCT04134000) (Roupret et al. 2019; Castellano et al. 2020). Durvalumab, approved for patients with locally advanced or metastatic BC who have progressed following platinum-based chemotherapy, has been evaluated alone or in combination with BCG or external beam radiation therapy (EBRT) in patients with BCG-relapsing NMIBC (ADAPT-BLADDER; NCT03317158) (Baldini et al. 2019; Hahn 2023). The overall complete response at 12 months was 46%, 73% with durvalumab + BCG, and 33% with durvalumab + EBRT.

Clinical trials testing other PD1 monoclonal antibodies include Camrelizumab, Tislelizumab, and Sasanlimab. Camrelizumab (AiRuiKa™; SHR-1210; Elevar Therapeutics) has shown potent antitumor activity in advanced/metastatic BC after platinum-based chemotherapy in combination with a receptor tyrosine kinase inhibitor (Qu et al. 2022). A Phase 1/2 trial for patients with high-risk BCG-exposed NMIBC has been launched to investigate intravesical or intravenous approaches to administration (NCT04706598) (Boorjian et al. 2020). Tislelizumab (BGB-A317, ®Tileilizhu Dankang Zhusheye) is another anti-human PD-1 monoclonal IgG4 antibody that targets Fc gamma receptors. Its efficacy has been evaluated in phase 1/2 clinical trials of high-risk NMIBC, including CIS (TACBIN-01 and TACBUN-02 trial, NCT04922047) (Markham 2021). Sasanlimab (PF-06801591) is also a subcutaneously delivered monoclonal antibody against PD-1. The phase 3 CFREST trial (NCT04165317) that evaluates the convenience of subcutaneous administration of Sasanlimab plus BCG induction with or without maintenance in 1070 patients with high-risk treatment-naïve NMIBC has completed accrual of 1070 patients (Steinberg et al. 2024). A separate Cohort B enrolled 160 patients with BCG-unresponsive CIS or papillary NMIBC treated with single agent Sasanlimab and is scheduled to report in 2026 (Shore et al. 2022). Many other immune modulators with diverse modes of action targeting different immune cells, surface antigens, and costimulatory molecules (CTLA-4, EpCAM, and CD3) have been evaluated in BCG-unresponsive NMIBC (Ruf et al. 2021). Zalifrelimab (UGN-301; UroGen Pharma Ltd.) is an anti-CTLA-4 antibody that neutralizes the inhibitory effects of CTLA-4 on tumor-specific T-cell immune responses (Kaplon et al. 2020; Lansford et al. 2021). UGN-301 is an intravesical formulation of zalifrelimab prepared with a reverse thermal hydrogel for local intravesical instillation that maximizes drug concentrations in the bladder with a sustained release over 6–12 h, while minimizing significant systemic exposure. It is delivered as a cold viscous liquid that converts to a semi-solid gel at body temperature. UroGen is conducting a Phase 1 dose escalation trial of UGN-301 alone or in combination with UGN-201 (imiquimod) in patients with BCG-unresponsive high-risk disease (NCT05375903) (Lansford et al. 2021). Catumaxomab (Revumab, LintonPharm Co. Ltd) is a trifunctional bispecific monoclonal antibody targeting EpCAM and CD3 that mediates antibody-dependent cellular cytotoxicity against human epithelial tumor cells, including BC (Ruf et al. 2021). The simultaneous recruitment and activation of T cells and accessory cells leads to physiological co-stimulation of T cells and improved tumor cell elimination. A Phase 1 study is designed to investigate the therapeutic potential of intravesical catumaxomab (CATUNIBLA; NCT04819399) (Ruf et al. 2021).

21.3.2 Intravesical Gene Therapy

The concept of intravesical viral-mediated gene therapy was introduced two decades ago, and its application has evolved based on efficacy using selective tumor cell targeting viruses (Sathianathen et al. 2020). There are multiple recombinant intravesical viral therapies including adenoviral rAd-IFNα/Syn3 mediated interferon-alpha (NCT02773849), oncolytic viral CG0070 granulocyte-macrophage colony-stimulating factor (GM-CSF; NCT02365818), and intravesical Cavatak (Coxsackie virus, CVA21) (NCT02316171), and other intravesical non-viral agents such as EG-70 (RIG-1 agonist) (NCT04752722), and Anktiva (IL-15RαFc superagonist, N-803) (NCT03022825) (Packiam et al. 2018; Boorjian et al. 2020, 2021; Steinberg et al. 2023) (Table 21.3).

Nadofaragene firadenovec (NF; also known as rAd-IFNa/Syn3) is a replication-deficient recombinant adenovirus that carries the transgene for human IFN-a2b with antitumor activity in patients with NMIBC (Navai et al. 2016; Boorjian et al. 2021). When combined with the polyamide compound Syn3, which is a surfactant enhancing the viral transduction of the urothelium, intravesical administration of rAd-IFN results in the synthesis and expression of large amounts of IFN-a2b protein. The efficacy of intravesical nadofaragene firadenovec (Adstiladrin®, Instiladrin) was demonstrated in a Phase 3 trial, treating patients with BCG-unresponsive CIS with or without Ta/T1 NMIBC and patients with Ta or T1 high-grade cancers without CIS (Boorjian et al. 2021). Of the 103 patients with CIS, 53.4% showed a CR within 3 months of the first dose, and this response was maintained in 45.5% of 55 patients at 12 months for an overall 12-month durable response (DR) rate of 23%. With an acceptable safety profile, the FDA approved NF in December 2022 for adult patients with high-risk BCG-

Table 21.3 Clinical trials of intravesical gene therapies

Agent or technology	Indication	Mode of action	Number of estimated enrolling participants	Clinical trial number
Intravesical Nadofaragene firadenovec (rAd-IFNa/Syn3)	BCG-unresponsive	Replication-deficient recombinant adenovirus	157 patients	Phase 3, NCT02773849
Intravesical CG0070	BCG-unresponsive NMIBC	Replication-competent oncolytic adenovirus CG0070	110 patients for NCT04452591	Phase 3, BOND-003 trial, NCT04452591
			35 patients for NCT04387461	Phase 2, NCT04387461
Intravesical Cavatak (CVA21)	NMIBC	Intravesical Coxsackievirus A21 (CVA21) with MMC	16 patients	Phase 1, CANON trial, NCT02316171
Intravesical EG-70	BCG-unresponsive high-grade NMIBC	RIG-1 agonist	222 patients	Phase 1/2 LEGEND trial, NCT04752722

NMIBC, non-muscle invasive bladder cancer; RIG-1, retinoic acid-inducible gene I; BCG, Bacillus Calmette-Guérin; MMC, mitomycin-C; Ty21a, live oral typhoid vaccine

unresponsive CIS with or without papillary tumors.

The replication-competent oncolytic adenovirus CG0070 carries the transgene human granulocyte-macrophage colony-stimulating factor (GM-CSF). GM-CSF can present tumor antigens and induce tumor cell lysis. A phase 2 trial reported a 65% CR rate at any time, CRs maintained in 28% at 12 months, and a good safety profile in 65 patients with BCG-unresponsive NMIBC (BOND2 trial, NCT02365818) (Packiam et al. 2018). Of the 45 patients with CIS who refused radical cystectomy, 50% achieved a CR at 6 months, including 58% of patients with pure CIS. Based on these results, the phase 3 clinical trial BOND-003 was designed to confirm its efficacy in patients with or without concomitant high-grade Ta or T1 papillary NMIBC (NCT04452591) (Uchio et al. 2022). Another Phase 2 trial is also testing the combination of CG0070 and intravenous Pembrolizumab for BCG-unresponsive CIS (NCT04387461).

Another investigational viral-based therapy is Cavatak (Coxsackie virus or CVA21; Viralytics) which has a good intravesical safety profile and early signs of response in a clinical phase 1 trial (CANON) (Pandha et al. 2016). EG-70 (enGene) is a novel non-viral gene therapy that encodes two cytosolic pattern recognition receptors named retinoic acid-inducible gene I (RIG-I) agonists. The mechanism of action is based on the stimulation of the innate immune system and activation of the adaptive immune system by releasing cytokines such as interleukin (IL)-12 (Jiang et al. 2023). The intravesical introduction of EG-70 caused tumor regression and elicited effective immunological memory with minimal signs of toxicity. This novel non-viral gene therapy produced a CR rate of 83% at 3 months in evaluable patients with BCG-unresponsive CIS and with or without resected papillary tumors (NCT04752722, LEGEND) (Steinberg et al. 2023).

21.3.3 Cancer Vaccines

There are several types of single or combinational vaccine therapies in development (Table 21.4). These include a recombinant poxviral vector vaccine PANVAC(NCT02015104), two peptide vaccines derived from M phase phosphoprotein 1 (MPHOSPH1), and DEP domain containing 1 (DEPDC1). Others include combination vaccines (rec-MAGE-A3 protein + AS15), the allogeneic cell line vaccine Vesigenurtacel-l (HS-410, NCT02010203), a commercial vaccine

Table 21.4 Clinical trials of cancer vaccines, immunostimulatory agents, antibody drug conjugates, and targeted therapy

Agent or technology	Indication	Mode of action	Number of estimated enrolling participants	Clinical trial number
Cancer vaccines				
Recombinant pox-viral vector vaccine (PANVAC)	High-grade NMIBC	PANVAC with BCG	32 patients	Phase 1, NCT02015104
Intradermal vesigenurtacel-L (HS-104)	NMIBC	Vesigenurtacel-L(HS-104) with intravesical BCG.	104 patients	Phase 1/2, NCT02010203
Typhoid vaccine (Ty21a/Vivotif)	NMIBC	Intravesical Ty21a/Vivotif in patients not requiring BCG	25 patients	Phase 1/2, NCT03421236
S-488210/S-488211 vaccine	NMIBC	Subcutaneous S-488210/S-488211 vaccine with durvalumab (MEDI4736)	64 patients	Phase 1b/2 DURANCE trial, NCT04106115
Other immunostimulatory agents				
ALT-803 (N-803)	BCG-unresponsive NMIBC	Intravesical Bacillus Calmette-Guerin (BCG) in combination with ALT-803 (N-803)	133 patients	Phase 2/3, QUILT-3.032 trial, NCT03022825
ALT-801	BCG-unresponsive NMIBC	ALT-801 combined with gemcitabine	52 patients	Phase 1b/2, NCT01625260
Imiquimod (TMX-101)	CIS NMIBC	Intravesical Imiquimod (TMX-101)	12 patients	Phase 2, NCT01731652
Antibody drug conjugates				
Enfortumab vedotin (EV, Padcev)	Low or intermediate-risk, FGFR3-mutated, BCG-naïve NMIBC	A combined agent of a Nectin-4-directed antibody and microtubule inhibitor	112 patients	Phase 1, NCT 05316155
Intravesical Vicinium™ (VB4-845)	BCG-treated NMIBC	A recombinant fusion protein in *Escherichia coli* (*E. coli*) specific for the epithelial cell adhesion molecule (EpCAM) antigen linked to ETA (252-608)	133 patients	Phase 3 VISTA trial, NCT02449239
Targeted therapy				
Erdafitinib	High-risk, BCG-unresponsive NMIBC	Oral FGFR3 inhibitor	107 patients	Phase 2, NCT04172675
Infigratinib	FGFR3-mutated/ rearranged BCG-unresponsive intermediate-risk Ta NMIBC	Oral FGFR1-3 inhibitor	12 patients	Phase 1 BLASST-3 trial, NCT04972253
Nitroxoline	Various NMIBC cohorts from intermediate to chemorefractory intermediate/ high-risk NMIBC	Oral Methionine Aminopeptidase 2 (MetAP2, APL-1202) inhibitor	41 patients for NCT04498702	Phase 2, NCT04498702
			6 patients for NCT03672240	Phase 1b, NCT03672240
			800 patients for NCT04736394	Phase 3, NCT04736394
			359 patients for NCT04490993	Phase 3, NCT04490993

NMIBC, non-muscle invasive bladder cancer; FGFR, fibroblast growth factor receptor; BCG, Bacillus Calmette-Guérin; Ty21a, live oral typhoid vaccine for typhoid fever (Ty21a, NCT03421236), and a peptide vaccine designated as S-488210/S-488211 (NCT04106115) (Annels et al. 2019; Kokorovic et al. 2022; Steinberg et al. 2023). However, more data is still needed to evaluate their role in treatment for NMIBC including BCG-unresponsive disease.

21.3.4 Other Immunostimulatory Agents

Several cytokines and T-cell receptors have been introduced as potential immunostimulatory agents (Table 21.4). The cytokine IL-15 plays a crucial role in the immune system by modulating the development, maintenance, and function of natural killer and T cells without stimulating regulatory T-cell (Treg) proliferation and inducing T-cell apoptosis (Waldmann 2006; Chang et al. 2022; Chamie et al. 2023). Anktiva™ (ALT-803; ImmunityBio, Inc.) is a novel IL-15RαFc superagonist complex (N-803) consisting of an IL-15 mutant (IL-15N72D) bound to an IL-15 receptor that has longer persistence in lymphoid tissues and more enhanced antitumor activity than native, non-complexed IL-15 (Waldmann et al. 2006; Chang et al. 2022; Han et al. 2011; Rosser et al. 2018; Chen et al. 2022). A Phase 2/3 open-label multicenter trial of patients with BCG-unresponsive CIS with or without Ta/T1 and a separate cohort of Ta/T1 without CIS reported CR rates of 72% in the CIS population and a 12-month disease-free rate of 57% (QUILT-3.032 trial, NCT03022825) (Chamie et al. 2023). This trial showed that ALT-803 plus BCG was safe and well tolerated with no treatment or immune-related adverse events with a cystectomy-free rate of 92% and a 24-month CSS of 99.5%, and recently obtained regulatory approval from the FDA in April 2024. Other immunostimulatory agents, such as the recombinant T-cell Receptor (TCR)-IL-2 fusion protein ALT-801 (Sonpavde et al. 2016) (NCT01625260), the intravesical TLR-agonist imiquimod (TMX-101) (NCT01731652) (Donin et al. 2017; Camargo et al. 2018), sirolimus (rapamycin) (NCT02753309) (Mukherjee et al. 2018), and VAX014 (NCT03854721) (Tsuji et al. 2022) are potential candidates for NMIBC.

Interleukin (IL)-2 is another well-known antineoplastic cytokine growth factor in multiple cancers acting as an immunostimulator and targeting properties on immune effector cells, with limitations of strict half-life time of activation and severe adverse immunologic reactions (Belmont et al. 2006). T-cell receptor (TCR)-IL-2 fusion protein (ALT-801) is a novel antigen recognition molecule with antineoplastic efficacy (Wen et al. 2008). A phase I clinical trial evaluating the safety and activity of intravenous injection of ALT-801, a recombinant humanized TCR-IL-2 fusion protein has been launched in BCG-resistant NMIBC (NCT01625260) (Sonpavde et al. 2016).

Imiquimod, a Toll-like receptor 7 (TLR7) agonist, is a well-known topical agent for basal cell carcinoma and melanoma (Corogeanu et al. 2023). The systemic introduction of TCR7 agonists induces broad immune activation that leads to adverse reactions through innate immune cells such as dendritic cells (DC) and macrophages which present antigens to CD4 and CD8 T cells. However, intravesically targeted delivery of a TLR agonist to the tumor tissues may overcome these adverse effects. A phase 2 trial using a TCR7 agonist named TMX-101 (Vesimune) reported its clinical activity on urinary cytokines from 12 patients with CIS treated intravesically without any severe graded adverse events (NCT01731652) (Donin et al. 2017).

Rapamycin has been found to have a therapeutic role in enhancing BCG vaccine efficacy against tuberculosis and the killing capacity of gammadelta (γδ) T cells (Mukherjee et al. 2018). In a clinical trial of 31 patients with NMIBC including 11 patients treated with placebo, oral administration of rapamycin (0.5 mg low dose encapsulated rapamycin) demonstrated safety and tolerability (12.5% of grade 1 and 2 adverse events) in combination with BCG (NCT02753309). The trial showed that rapamycin enhanced BCG-specific T-cell immunity and boosted urinary cytokines during BCG treatment (26% for placebo vs. 9.6% for rapamycin) (Ji et al. 2021; Mukherjee et al. 2018). They showed the enhancing role of rapamycin for BCG-specific T-cell immunity and boosting of urinary cytokines during BCG treatment. A phase 2 double-blind randomized controlled trial of long-term (1 year) prevention with oral rapamycin (versus placebo) is now recruiting to investigate rapamycin for secondary prevention in patients with diagnosed NMIBC (NCT04375813).

VAX014 is a novel bacterial minicell-based, integrin-targeted oncolytic agent that has been intravesically introduced in the treatment of NMIBC (Tsuji et al. 2022). With a rationale for the clinical investigation of VAX014 and systemic PD-1/PD-L1 blockade in advanced-stage bladder cancer, an orthotopic bladder cancer model showed a significant improvement in tumor clearance rates and the development of protective antitumor immunologic memory. A phase 1 trial has been launched to evaluate its safety and tolerability in NMIBC (NCT03854721)

21.3.5 Antibody Drug Conjugates

Antibody drug conjugates (ADCs) are composed of a monoclonal antibody with the ability to bind to specific tumor antigen and linked to a cytotoxic payload (Table 21.4) (Lattanzi and Rosenberg 2020). Enfortumab vedotin (EV, Padcev) combines a Nectin-4-directed antibody and microtubule inhibitor, which was approved for use in metastatic BC in 2019 by the FDA (André et al. 2022). Intravesical EV has been investigated in high-risk NMIBC including CIS with/without papillary tumors (phase 1 trial, NCT 05014139) (Kamat et al. 2023). Vicinium (oportuzumab monatox, VB4-845) is an epithelial cell adhesion molecule (*EpCAM*) monoclonal antibody protein combined with exotoxin A from *Pseudomonas* (NCT02449239, VISTA trial) (Lattanzi and Rosenberg 2020). The EpCAM surface marker is expressed on urothelial carcinoma plasma membranes, and binding of anti-EpCAM causes receptor-mediated endocytic internalization of the exotoxin, which causes inhibition of protein synthesis (Chehroudi and Black 2020; Boorjian et al. 2021). In a phase 3 trial, Vicinium showed high compliance with 3% of treatment discontinuation due to adverse events and 40% of high CR rate during 3-month follow-up and 96% of 2-year overall survival (OS) rate among 89 patients with CIS. Of the 40% of 3-month CIS responders, a 52% 12-month disease-free survival was observed (Shore et al. 2020). Vicinium, however, did not get FDA approval.

21.3.6 Targeted Therapies

Several targeted agents have been introduced for treatment of NMIBC (Table 21.4). Erdafitinib, a pan-FGFR inhibitor that was approved in 2019 for treatment of metastatic BC, is being compared to intravesical chemotherapy in a phase 2 trial for patients who received BCG and recurred with high-risk NMIBC (NCT04172675) (Romero 2024; Catto et al. 2024). Among the 107 participants recruited, 51 patients with *FGFR3* mutation had better recurrence-free survival rates during 60 months of follow-up (39% vs. 65%, $p < 0.05$) (Steinberg et al. 2020). Infigratinib, a selective oral FGFR1-3 inhibitor, showed a 75% 7-week CR with *FGFR3*-mutated/rearranged BCG-recurrent intermediate-risk Ta NMIBC in a phase 1 clinical trial (NCT04972253, BLASST-3 trial). However, there was an unacceptable toxicity profile, including eye disorders, skin and nail disorders, and elevations in transaminases (Cha et al. 2020). Other FGFR inhibitors (pemigatinib and rogaratinib) are under investigation for safety and antitumor efficacy in recurrent FGFR-mutated/rearranged NMIBC (Sathianathen et al. 2020).

Nitroxoline (APL-1202, Asieris Pharmaceuticals) is a selective methionine aminopeptidase 2 (MetAP2) inhibitor of the STAT3 pathway and has both anti-angiogenic and antitumor activities (Lin et al. 2021). This novel MetAP2 inhibitor had a potential synergistic effect with BCG or epirubicin and was designed as a first-line oral agent for BCG-naïve intermediate-risk NMIBC. (ASCETAIN, phase 3, NCT04736394) (Lin et al. 2021) A phase 2 trial evaluating APL1202 in BCG-unresponsive NMIBC has shown preliminary safety results and activity for Ta or T1 tumors with 1-year recurrence-free-rate of 54.3% (95% CI 37.2–73.2%) (NCT04498702) (Ye et al. 2017; Lin et al. 2021).

21.4 New Potential Technologies

Several novel technologies and drug delivery strategies have been introduced as potential therapies for BC including theragnostic nanotechnology, photodynamic sensitizing materials, and a newly applied antibiotic for BC (Table 21.5).

21.4.1 Nanotechnology

Nanotechnology using gold nanoparticles, photosensitizers, and biological agents can target cancer cells with improved simplicity and speed, and perhaps more specific targeting of cancer cells (Xu et al. 2021). Gold nanoparticles can be used to distinguish between normal and abnormal bladder cells during cystoscopy, and thus provide clinicians with additional evidence for the complete removal of malignant lesions within the bladder. Nanoparticles can be administered intravenously or intravesically by modifying the nan-

Table 21.5 New potential technologies and novel intravesical or intratumoral therapies

Agent or technology	Indication	Mode of action	Number of estimated enrolling participants	Clinical trial number
Nanoparticle				
PLZ4-coated paclitaxel-loaded nanoscale micelle (PPM) from VA Office of Research and Development	Bladder cancer	Nanoparticle for cancer targeting	29 patients	Phase 1, NCT05519241
Photodynamic therapy				
Intravesical photosensitizer TLD-1433	BCG-Unresponsive	Photosensitizer TLD-1433 administration (Ruvidar®) followed by activation with intravesical laser	125 patients	Phase 2, NCT03945162
Novel intravesical/intratumoral therapies				
Intravesical EMDA-Mitomycin-C (FB10)	High-risk NMIBC	Electromotive drug administration (EMDA-MMC)	300 patients	Phase 3, NCT03664869
Intravesical Ty21a	NMIBC (low- or intermediate-risk not requiring BCG)	Bacterial vaccine (Ty21a/Vivotif)	25 patients	Phase 1, NCT03421236
Intravesical TAR-200 and TAR-210	NMIBC with FGFR Mutations or Fusions	Erdafitinib Intravesical Delivery System (TAR-210)	200 patients for TAR-200 92 patients for TAR-210	Phase 2, NCT04640623 fro TAR-200 Phase 1, NCT05316155 for TAR-210
Intratumoral belzupacap sarotalocan (AU-011)	NMIBC	A papillomavirus-like particle drug conjugate	23 patients	phase 1, NCT05483868
Intravesical rapamycin (ABI-009, nab-sirolimus;)	BCG-unresponsive NMIBC	Nanoparticle albumin bound (nab) rapamycin (ABI-009, nab-sirolimus;)	21 patients	phase 1/2, NCT02009332

NMIBC, non-muscle invasive bladder cancer; PPM, paclitaxel-loaded nanosized micelle; PDT, photodynamic therapy; PpIx. Protoporphyrin IX; MMC, Mitomycin-C; BCG, Bacillus Calmette-Guérin; Ty21a, Live Oral Typhoid Vaccine; nab, nanoparticle albumin bound otechnology for optimal delivery to the target. This approach has shown high antitumor efficacy and the potential for combination therapy with phototherapy and targeted therapy (Swain et al. 2016). A phase I clinical trial in 29 patients with BCG-experienced NMIBC was conducted to determine the optimum intravesical dose of PLZ4-coated paclitaxel-loaded nanoscale micelles (PPM), to assess toxicity, and obtain preliminary efficacy data (NCT05519241) (Sun et al. 2022; Farrukh et al. 2023). PLZ4 is a human bladder cancer-specific peptide with specific amino acid sequences that bind to urothelium and has the potential to be used as a guide molecule for chemotherapeutic agents containing PPM to specifically target and deliver paclitaxel to BC cells (Farrukh et al. 2023).

21.4.2 Photodynamic Therapy

Photodynamic therapy comprises transurethral resection followed by fluorescent diagnosis and administration of a photosensitizer and has been used for BC treatment since 1993 (Kustov et al. 2021; Rahman et al. 2023). In 2010, fluorescence cystoscopy using the protoporphyrin derivative IX (hexaminolevulinic acid) was approved by the FDA for the photodynamic diagnosis of NMIBC (Stenzl et al. 2010; Witjes et al. 2010). 5-ALA (aminolevulinic acid) is a precursor of protoporphyrin IX and is also used in photodynamic diagnosis (Sansaloni-Pastor and Lange 2023). Another phase 2, open-label, single-arm, multicenter trial (NCT03945162) includes patients with BCG-unresponsive NMIBC and is evaluating the efficacy of a single intravesical instillation of cytotoxic TLD-1433 (RuvidarTM; Theralase Technologies Inc), which is a potential antineoplastic ruthenium-based coordination complex, generating radical oxygen species and a water-soluble photosensitizer targeting via transferrin receptor with BC selectivity (Kulkarni et al. 2023). Interim results have been reported from a phase 2 trial of intravesical TLD-1433 (0.70 mg/cm^2) activated by the proprietary TLC-3200 Medical Laser System (90 J/cm^2) in 59 BCG-unresponsive NMIBC CIS patients. The 6-, 12-, and 15-month CR rate was 54%, 38%, and 37%, respectively (NCT03945162).

21.5 Novel Intravesical/Intratumoral Therapy

Several novel agents are in Phase 1 and Phase 2 trials using intravesical and intratumoral delivery (Table 21.5)

21.5.1 Intravesical Electromotive Drug Administration (EMDA) for Mitomycin-C (EMDA-MMC) and BCG

The EMDA device (Physionizer® 30, manufactured by Physion®, Medolla, Italy) consists of a generator that emits an electrical current between a specialized 16 Fr catheter that works as an anode and a cathode patch placed on the hypogastrium of the patient (Racioppi et al. 2018). EMDA is used to increase the absorption of intravesical mitomycin-C (MMC; 40 mg diluted in 50 mg of distilled water). A clinical trial compared two adjuvant instillation therapies (MMC administered using EMDA and BCG) for the treatment of high-risk NMIBC (NCT03664869) (Packiam et al. 2019). Results from a prospective trial suggested that sequential EMDA-MMC and BCG treatments may be more effective against NMIBC than BCG therapy alone for the endpoints recurrence, progression, and OS (Arrabal Polo et al. 2023; Zazzara et al. 2023).

21.5.2 Intravesical Ty21a (Vivotif)

A commercial vaccine against typhoid fever called Ty21a/Vivotif has been used for the last 30 years in millions of individuals as a typhoid fever vaccine with a high safety record. Typhoid fever vaccine (Ty21a/Vivotif) administration in a BC orthotopic mouse model was found to be more effective than BCG for inducing tumor regression and survival using intravesical instillation; it is also potentially safer because Ty21a bacteria do not infect/persist in human bladder tissue, in contrast to BCG (Domingos-Pereira et al. 2019). One phase 1 trial tested the safety of intravesical administration of Ty21a and its effect on bladder immunity in patients with NMIBC for whom BCG therapy is not recommended (NCT03421236) (Domingos-Pereira et al. 2019). The generation of antitumor adaptive immunity was identified as a key process underlying Ty21a-mediated treatment efficacy, suggesting its potential as a safe and effective treatment for NMIBC patients.

21.5.3 Intravesical Delivery System (TAR)

The TAR platform (also known as the "pretzel") is a device that is placed within the bladder via a standard cystoscopy and can be loaded with a variety of agents. Drugs are released via osmotic pump for sustained release. TAR-200 is loaded with gemcitabine and is being evaluated as single agent therapy for patients with BCG failure (NCT06211764) and in a randomized trial with or without cetrelimab (anti-PD-1) for BCG-unresponsive disease (NCT04640623). TAR-210 is loaded with erdafitinib, targeting FGFR3, and is being evaluated in a phase 1 study to evaluate the safety and tolerability in patients with NMIBC and MIBC (NCT05316155). Interim results showed that 82% were recurrence-free for 3.7 months median duration of treatment exposure among 18 participants with recurrent, BCG-unresponsive high-risk NMIBC (high-grade Ta/T1; papillary only) who refused or were ineligible for radical cystectomy (Vilaseca et al. 2023).

21.5.4 Intramural Injection of Belzupacap Sarotalocan (AU-011)

Belzupacap sarotalocan (AU-011, Aura Biosciences, Inc.) is a first-in-class virus-like drug conjugate that uses a papillomavirus-like particle drug conjugate. Fast-track designation has been granted for the treatment of patients with NMIBC (Kines et al. 2021). A phase 1 trial for NMIBC is ongoing to evaluate the efficacy and safety of intramural injection with or without intratumoral injection of AU-011 in patients with low-grade tumors to determine safety and preliminary efficacy (NCT05483868) (Wagner et al. 2019; Lerner et al. 2023).

21.5.5 Nanoparticle Albumin-Bound (nab) Rapamycin (ABI-009, nab-Sirolimus)

Inactivation of PTEN promotes BC progression via dysregulation of the mammalian target of rapamycin signaling pathway (mTOR) (Ashrafizadeh et al. 2020). The nanoparticle albumin-bound rapamycin (ABI-009, nab-rapamycin, Celgene Inc, Summit, NJ) has been introduced as an enhancing delivery system of mTOR inhibitor and is suitable for intravenous administration to enhance the efficacy of oral rapamycin (Gradishar et al. 2005). It has better binding affinity to human albumin which accumulates in tumors, making it an ideal candidate for drug delivery (McKiernan et al. 2015). With the advent of nab-rapamycin (ABI-009; Aadi Bioscience, Inc), this hydrophobic agent has been tested for intravesical delivery. A Phase 1/2 clinical trial investigating the safety and efficacy of nab-rapamycin (ABI-009) for BCG-refractory or recurrent NMIBC has completed the Phase 1 portion establishing safety, and the Phase 2 is planned (NCT020093) (Wagner et al. 2019).

21.6 Conclusion

Various new molecular agents such as ICI, targeted agents, antibiotics, vaccines, new therapeutic technologies with gene therapy, photodynamic therapy, and nanomolecule-based therapy, and new technical approaches with artificial intelligence and enhancing delivery system via intravesical/tumoral/systemic administration will elicit a new era for BCG-unresponsive NMIBC. In addition, combinational therapy with different modes of therapeutic agents with better delivery systems will open a more diverse therapeutic regimen in the theragnosis of BCG-unresponsive NMIBC.

Until the completion of ongoing trials of these agents and their combinational therapies, the efficacy of these new modalities and agents in the treatment of BCG-unresponsive NMIBC remains unclear. However, several interim reports from trials have shown promising outcomes for NMIBC, including higher efficacy and good tolerability without severe adverse events, suggesting possible new therapeutic options for patients with NMIBC. These new candidate molecules and technologies will further improve the treatment options for NMIBC for both clinicians and patients.

Funding Disclosure There was no funding support for this article.

Author Contribution Manuscript writing: All authors

Final approval of manuscript: All authors

Author's Disclosures and Potential Conflicts of Interest S. Lerner: Clinical trial support from Aura Bioscience, Endo, FKD, JBL (SWOG), Genentech (SWOG), Merck (Alliance) QED Therapeutics, Vaxiion, Viventia; Consultant/advisory board for Astra Zeneca, Aura Bioscience, BMS, C2iGenomics, Ferring, Incyte, Pfizer/EMD Serono, Protara, Stimit, Vaxiion, Verity; Patent for TCGA classifier; Honoraria from Grand Rounds Urology, UroToday.

SH. Kim: has no conflicts of interest to declare

References

Annels NE, Mansfield D, Arif M, Ballesteros-Merino C, Simpson GR, Denyer M, Sandhu SS, Melcher AA, Harrington KJ, Davies B, Au G, Grose M, Bagwan I, Fox B, Vile R, Mostafid H, Shafren D, Pandha HS (2019) Phase I trial of an ICAM-1-targeted immunotherapeutic-coxsackievirus A21 (CVA21) as an oncolytic agent against non-muscle-invasive bladder cancer. Clin Cancer Res 25(19):5818–5831. https://doi.org/10.1158/1078-0432.CCR-18-4022

Arrabal Polo MÁ, Melgarejo Segura MT, Yáñez Castillo Y, Morales Martínez A, Pareja Vílchez M, Arrabal Martín M (2023) Adjuvant intravesical treatment in patients with intermediate and high-risk non-muscle-invasive bladder cancer with BCG versus MMC applied with COMBAT or EMDA. Results of a prospective study. J Cancer Res Clin Oncol 149(10):7453–7459. https://doi.org/10.1007/s00432-023-04688-0

Ashrafizadeh M, Zarrabi A, Samarghandian S, Najafi M (2020) PTEN: What we know of the function and regulation of this onco-suppressor factor in bladder cancer? Eur J Pharmacol 881:173226. https://doi.org/10.1016/j.ejphar.2020.173226

Babjuk M, Burger M, Capoun O, Cohen D, Compérat EM, Dominguez Escrig JL, Gontero P, Liedberg F, Masson-Lecomte A, Mostafid AH, Palou J, Van Rhijn BWG, Rouprêt M, Shariat SF, Seisen T, Soukup V, Sylvester RJ (2022) European Association of Urology guidelines on non-muscle-invasive bladder cancer (Ta, T1, and carcinoma in situ). Eur Urol 81(1):75–94. https://doi.org/10.1016/j.eururo.2021.08.010

Baldini C, Champiat S, Vuagnat P, Massard C (2019) Durvalumab for the management of urothelial carcinoma: a short review on the emerging data and therapeutic potential. Onco Targets Ther 12:2505–2512. https://doi.org/10.2147/OTT.S141040

Bandari J, Maganty A, MacLeod LC, Davies BJ (2018) Manufacturing and the market: rationalizing the shortage of Bacillus Calmette-Guérin. Eur Urol Focus 4(4):481–484. https://doi.org/10.1016/j.euf.2018.06.018

Belmont HJ, Price-Schiavi S, Liu B, Card KF, Lee H, Han K, Wen J, Tang S, Zhu X, Merrill J, Chavillaz P-A, Wong JL, Rhode PR, Wong HC (2006) Potent antitumor activity of a tumor-specific soluble TCR/IL-2 fusion protein. Clin Immunol 121(1):29–39. https://doi.org/10.1016/j.clim.2006.05.005

Black PC, Tangen CM, Singh P, McConkey DJ, Lucia MS, Lowrance WT, Koshkin VS, Stratton KL, Bivalacqua TJ, Kassouf W, Porten SP, Bangs R, Plets M, Thompson IM, Lerner SP (2023) Phase 2 trial of atezolizumab in Bacillus Calmette-Guérin-unresponsive high-risk non-muscle-invasive bladder cancer: SWOG S1605. Eur Urol. https://doi.org/10.1016/j.eururo.2023.08.004

Boorjian SA, CPN D, SUO Clinical Trials Consortium (2020) Safety and efficacy of intravesical nadofaragene firadenovec for patients with high-grade, BCG-unresponsive nonmuscle invasive bladder cancer (NMIBC): Results from a phase III trial. J Clin Oncol 38(6_suppl):442–442. https://doi.org/10.1200/JCO.2020.38.6_suppl.442

Boorjian SA, Alemozaffar M, Konety BR, Shore ND, Gomella LG, Kamat AM, Bivalacqua TJ, Montgomery JS, Lerner SP, Busby JE, Poch M, Crispen PL, Steinberg GD, Schuckman AK, Downs TM, Svatek RS, Mashni J, Lane BR, Guzzo TJ, Bratslavsky G, Karsh LI, Woods ME, Brown G, Canter D, Luchey A, Lotan Y, Krupski T, Inman BA, Williams MB, Cookson MS, Keegan KA, Andriole GL, Sankin AI, Boyd A, O'Donnell MA, Sawutz D, Philipson R, Coll R, Narayan VM, Treasure FP, Yla-Herttuala S, Parker NR, Dinney CPN (2021) Intravesical nadofaragene firadenovec gene therapy for BCG-unresponsive non-muscle-invasive

bladder cancer: a single-arm, open-label, repeat-dose clinical trial. Lancet Oncol 22(1):107–117. https://doi.org/10.1016/S1470-2045(20)30540-4
Burger M, Oosterlinck W, Konety B, Chang S, Gudjonsson S, Pruthi R, Soloway M, Solsona E, Sved P, Babjuk M, Brausi MA, Cheng C, Comperat E, Dinney C, Otto W, Shah J, Thürof J, Witjes JA (2013) ICUD-EAU international consultation on bladder cancer 2012: non-muscle-invasive urothelial carcinoma of the bladder. Eur Urol 63(1):36–44. https://doi.org/10.1016/j.eururo.2012.08.061
Camargo JA, Passos GR, Ferrari KL, Billis A, Saad MJA, Reis LO (2018) Intravesical immunomodulatory imiquimod enhances Bacillus Calmette-Guérin downregulation of nonmuscle-invasive bladder cancer. Clin Genitourin Cancer 16(3):e587–e593. https://doi.org/10.1016/j.clgc.2017.10.019
Castellano D, De Velasco G, Martin Soberón MC, Carretero-González A, Dueñas M, Paramio J, De La Rosa F, Sanz JL, Guerrero F (2020) Atezolizumab + intravesical BCG (Bacillus Calmette-Guerin) in high-risk non-muscle invasive bladder cancer (NMIBC) patients: Institutional clinical and translational study (BladderGATE). J Clin Oncol 38(6_suppl):TPS598. https://doi.org/10.1200/JCO.2020.38.6_suppl.TPS598
Catto JWF, Tran B, Rouprêt M, Gschwend JE, Loriot Y, Nishiyama H, Redorta JP, Daneshmand S, Hussain SA, Cutuli HJ, Procopio G, Guadalupi V, Vasdev N, Naini V, Crow L, Triantos S, Baig M, Steinberg G, THOR-2 Cohort 1 Investigators (2024) Erdafitinib in BCG-treated high-risk non-muscle-invasive bladder cancer. Ann Oncol 35(1):98–106. https://doi.org/10.1016/j.annonc.2023.09.3116
Cha EK, Iyer G, Funt SA, Regazzi AM, Francis J, Heinemann MH, Ostrovnaya I, Dalbagni G, Bajorin DF, Bochner BH, Rosenberg JE (2020) Marker lesion study of oral FGFR inhibitor BGJ398 in patients with FGFR3-altered intermediate-risk nonmuscle-invasive bladder cancer. J Clin Oncol 38(6_suppl):510. https://doi.org/10.1200/JCO.2020.38.6_suppl.510
Chamie K, Chang SS, Kramolowsky E, Gonzalgo ML, Agarwal PK, Bassett JC, Bjurlin M, Cher ML, Clark W, Cowan BE, David R, Goldfischer E, Guru K, Jalkut MW, Kaffenberger SD, Kaminetsky J, Katz AE, Koo AS, Sexton WJ, Tikhonenkov SN, Trabulsi EJ, Trainer AF, Spilman P, Huang M, Bhar P, Taha SA, Sender L, Reddy S, Soon-Shiong P (2023) IL-15 superagonist NAI in BCG-unresponsive non-muscle-invasive bladder cancer. NEJM Evid 2(1). https://doi.org/10.1056/EVIDoa2200167
Chang SS, Chamie K, Gonzalgo ML, Kramolowsky EV, Sexton WJ, Reddy SK, Bhar P, Huang M, Soon-Shiong P (2022) Positive efficacy and safety phase 3 results in both CIS and papillary cohorts BCG-unresponsive nonmuscle invasive bladder cancer (NMIBC) after IL-15RαFc superagonist N-803 (Anktiva) and BCG infusion. J Clin Oncol 40(6_suppl):431. https://doi.org/10.1200/JCO.2022.40.6_suppl.431
Chang SS, Boorjian SA, Chou R, Clark PE, Daneshmand S, Konety BR, Pruthi R, Quale DZ, Ritch CR, Seigne JD, Skinner EC, Smith ND (2016) Diagnosis and Treatment of Non-Muscle Invasive Bladder Cancer: AUA/SUO Guideline. McKiernan JM.J Urol. 196(4):1021–9. https://doi.org/10.1016/j.juro.2016.06.049. Epub 2016 Jun 16. PMID: 27317986
Chehroudi AC, Black PC (2020) Emerging intravesical therapies for the management of bacillus Calmette–Guérin (BCG)-unresponsive non-muscle-invasive bladder cancer: Charting a path forward. Can Urol Assoc J 14(6). https://doi.org/10.5489/cuaj.6101
Chen W, Liu N, Yuan Y, Zhu M, Hu X, Hu W, Wang S, Wang C, Huang B, Xing D (2022) ALT-803 in the treatment of non-muscle-invasive bladder cancer: Preclinical and clinical evidence and translational potential. Front Immunol 13:1040669. https://doi.org/10.3389/fimmu.2022.1040669
Corogeanu D, Zaki K, Beavil AJ, Arnold JN, Diebold SS (2023) Antibody conjugates for targeted delivery of Toll-like receptor 9 agonist to the tumor tissue. PLoS One 18(3):e0282831. https://doi.org/10.1371/journal.pone.0282831
Del Giudice F, Asero V, Bologna E, Scornajenghi CM, Carino D, Dolci V, Viscuso P, Salciccia S, Sciarra A, D'Andrea D, Pradere B, Moschini M, Mari A, Albisinni S, Krajewski W, Szydełko T, Małkiewicz B, Nowak Ł, Laukhtina E, Gallioli A, Mertens LS, Marcq G, Cimadamore A, Afferi L, Soria F, Mori K, Tully KH, Pichler R, Ferro M, Tataru OS, Autorino R, Crivellaro S, Crocetto F, Busetto GM, Basran S, Eisenberg ML, Chung BI, De Berardinis E (2023) Efficacy of different Bacillus of Calmette-Guérin (BCG) strains on recurrence rates among intermediate/high-risk non-muscle invasive bladder cancers (NMIBCs): single-arm study systematic review, cumulative and network meta-analysis. Cancers 15(7):1937. https://doi.org/10.3390/cancers15071937
Domingos-Pereira S, Sathiyanadan K, La Rosa S, Polák L, Chevalier MF, Martel P, Hojeij R, Derré L, Haefliger J-A, Jichlinski P, Nardelli-Haefliger D (2019) Intravesical Ty21a vaccine promotes dendritic cells and T cell-mediated tumor regression in the MB49 bladder cancer model. Cancer Immunol Res 7(4):621–629. https://doi.org/10.1158/2326-6066.CIR-18-0671
Donin NM, Chamie K, Lenis AT, Pantuck AJ, Reddy M, Kivlin D, Holldack J, Pozzi R, Hakim G, Karsh LI, Lamm DL, Belkoff LH, Belldegrun AS, Holden S, Shore N (2017) A phase 2 study of TMX-101, intravesical imiquimod, for the treatment of carcinoma in situ bladder cancer. Urol Oncol Semin Orig Investig 35(2):39:e1–e39.e7. https://doi.org/10.1016/j.urolonc.2016.09.006
Farrukh H, Zhu Z, Garisto Risco J, Lam KS, Pan C (2023) A phase I dose-escalation clinical trial with PLZ4-coated paclitaxel-loaded micelles (PPM) in patients with recurrent or refractory non-myoinvasive bladder cancer. J Clin Oncol 41(16_suppl):TPS4615. https://doi.org/10.1200/JCO.2023.41.16_suppl.TPS4615

Fernandez-Gomez J, Madero R, Solsona E, Unda M, Martinez-Piñeiro L, Gonzalez M, Portillo J, Ojea A, Pertusa C, Rodriguez-Molina J, Camacho JE, Rabadan M, Astobieta A, Montesinos M, Isorna S, Muntañola P, Gimeno A, Blas M, Martinez-Piñeiro JA (2009) Predicting nonmuscle invasive bladder cancer recurrence and progression in patients treated with Bacillus Calmette-Guerin: the CUETO scoring model. J Urol 182(5):2195–2203. https://doi.org/10.1016/j.juro.2009.07.016

Flaig TW, Spiess PE, Abern M, Agarwal N, Bangs R, Boorjian SA, Buyyounouski MK, Chan K, Chang S, Friedlander T, Greenberg RE, Guru KA, Herr HW, Hoffman-Censits J, Kishan A, Kundu S, Lele SM, Mamtani R, Margulis V, Mian OY, Michalski J, Montgomery JS, Nandagopal L, Pagliaro LC, Parikh M, Patterson A, Plimack ER, Pohar KS, Preston MA, Richards K, Sexton WJ, Siefker-Radtke AO, Tollefson M, Tward J, Wright JL, Dwyer MA, Cassara CJ, Gurski LA (2022) NCCN Guidelines® insights: bladder cancer, version 2.2022: Featured updates to the NCCN Guidelines. J Natl Compr Cancer Netw 20(8):866–878. https://doi.org/10.6004/jnccn.2022.0041

Gradishar WJ, Tjulandin S, Davidson N, Shaw H, Desai N, Bhar P, Hawkins M, O'Shaughnessy J (2005) Phase III trial of nanoparticle albumin-bound paclitaxel compared with polyethylated castor oil-based paclitaxel in women with breast cancer. J Clin Oncol 23:7794–7803

Hahn N (2023) Modern immunotherapy in BCG-unresponsive, BCG-relapsing and high-risk BCG-naive non-muscle invasive urothelial carcinoma of the bladder (ADAPT-BLADDER)

Han KP, Zhu X, Liu B, Jeng E, Kong L, Yovandich JL, Vyas VV, Marcus WD, Chavaillaz PA, Romero CA, Rhode PR, Wong HC (2011) IL-15:IL-15 receptor alpha superagonist complex: high-level co-expression in recombinant mammalian cells, purification and characterization. Cytokine 56:804–810. https://doi.org/10.1016/j.cyto.2011.09.028

Ji N, Mukherjee N, Reyes RM, Gelfond J, Javors M, Meeks JJ, McConkey DJ, Shu ZJ, Ramamurthy C, Dennett R, Curiel TJ, Svatek RS (2021) Rapamycin enhances BCG-specific γδ T cells during intravesical BCG therapy for non-muscle invasive bladder cancer: a randomized, double-blind study. J Immunother Cancer 9(3):e001941. https://doi.org/10.1136/jitc-2020-001941

Jiang Y, Zhang H, Wang J, Chen J, Guo Z, Liu Y, Hua H (2023) Exploiting RIG-I-like receptor pathway for cancer immunotherapy. J Hematol Oncol J Hematol Oncol 16(1):8. https://doi.org/10.1186/s13045-023-01405-9

Kamat AM, Hahn NM, Efstathiou JA, Lerner SP, Malmström P-U, Choi W, Guo CC, Lotan Y, Kassouf W (2016) Bladder cancer. Lancet 388(10061):2796–2810. https://doi.org/10.1016/S0140-6736(16)30512-8

Kamat AM, Shore N, Hahn N, Alanee S, Nishiyama H, Shariat S, Nam K, Kapadia E, Frenkl T, Steinberg G (2020) KEYNOTE-676: Phase III study of BCG and pembrolizumab for persistent/recurrent high-risk NMIBC. Future Oncol 16(10):507–516. https://doi.org/10.2217/fon-2019-0817

Kamat AM, Lotan Y, Roupret M, Steinberg GD, Inman BA, Powles T, Redorta JP, Porten SP, Kulkarni GS, Uchio EM, Gorla SR, Haas GP, Yu Y, Chia YL, Birrenkott M, Kates MR (2023) A first-in-human trial of intravesical enfortumab vedotin (EV), an antibody-drug conjugate (ADC), in patients with non-muscle invasive bladder cancer (NMIBC): Interim results of a phase 1 study (EV-104). J Clin Oncol 41(16_suppl):4596. https://doi.org/10.1200/JCO.2023.41.16_suppl.4596

Kaplon H, Muralidharan M, Schneider Z, Reichert JM (2020) Antibodies to watch in 2020. MAbs 12(1):1703531. https://doi.org/10.1080/19420862.2019.1703531

Kines RC, Thompson CD, Spring S, Li Z, De Los Pinos E, Monks S, Schiller JT (2021) Virus-like particle-drug conjugates induce protective, long-lasting adaptive antitumor immunity in the absence of specifically targeted tumor antigens. Cancer Immunol Res 9(6):693–706. https://doi.org/10.1158/2326-6066.CIR-19-0974

Kokorovic A, Ory J, Saad F (2022) Emerging treatment options for bacillus Calmette–Guérin-unresponsive non-muscle invasive bladder cancer. Curr Opin Support Palliat Care 16(1):48–53. https://doi.org/10.1097/SPC.0000000000000587

Kulkarni GS, Richards KA, Black PC, Rendon RA, Chin J, Shore ND, Jayram G, Kramolowsky EV, Saltzstein D, Agarwal PK, Belkoff L, O'Donnell MA, Kamat AM, Jewett MAS, Lamm DL, DeGruttola V, Mandel A, Dumoulin-White R, Kassouf W (2023) A phase II clinical study of intravesical photo dynamic therapy in patients with BCG-unresponsive NMIBC (interim analysis). J Clin Oncol 41(6_suppl):528. https://doi.org/10.1200/JCO.2023.41.6_suppl.528

Kustov AV, Smirnova NL, Privalov OA, Moryganova TM, Strelnikov AI, Morshnev PK, Koifman OI, Lyubimtsev AV, Kustova TV, Berezin DB (2021) Transurethral resection of non-muscle invasive bladder tumors combined with fluorescence diagnosis and photodynamic therapy with chlorin e6-type photosensitizers. J Clin Med 11(1):233. https://doi.org/10.3390/jcm11010233

Lamm DL, Blumenstein BA, Crissman JD, Montie JE, Gottesman JE, Lowe BA, Sarosdy MF, Bohl RD, Grossman HB, Beck TM, Leimert JT, Crawford ED (2000) Maintenance bacillus Calmette-Guerin immunotherapy for recurrent TA, T1 and carcinoma in situ transitional cell carcinoma of the bladder: a randomized Southwest Oncology Group Study. J Urol 163(4):1124–1129

Lansford H, Lahiri S, Schoenberg M, Seltzer E, UR001 Study Group, Creasy C (2021) A phase 1 dose-escalation study of ugn-301 (zalifrelimab) as monotherapy and in combination with other agents in patients with recurrent non-muscle invasive bladder cancer (NMIBC) SUO 22nd, Poster #189

Lattanzi M, Rosenberg JE (2020) The emerging role of antibody-drug conjugates in urothelial carcinoma. Expert Rev Anticancer Ther 20(7):551–561. https://doi.org/10.1080/14737140.2020.1782201

Lenis AT, Lec PM, Chamie K, Mshs MD (2020) Bladder cancer: a review. JAMA 324(19):1980–1991. https://doi.org/10.1001/jama.2020.17598

Lerner SP, Dinney C, Kamat A, Bivalacqua TJ, Nielsen M, O'Donnell M, Schoenberg MP, Steinberg G (2015) Clarification of bladder cancer disease states following treatment of patients with intravesical BCG. Bladder Cancer 1(1):29–30. https://doi.org/10.3233/BLC-159002

Lerner SP, Bivalacqua T, Kim IY, Murray C, Rich CC, Agarwal PK, Shore ND (2023) A phase 1, open-label trial to evaluate feasibility and safety of intramural injection of belzupacap sarotalocan (AU-011) in non-muscle-invasive bladder cancer (NMIBC). J Clin Oncol 41(6_suppl):TPS596. https://doi.org/10.1200/JCO.2023.41.6_suppl.TPS596

Lin W, Sun J, Sadahira T, Xu N, Wada K, Liu C, Araki M, Xu A, Watanabe M, Nasu Y, Huang P (2021) Discovery and validation of nitroxoline as a novel STAT3 inhibitor in drug-resistant urothelial bladder cancer. Int J Biol Sci 17(12):3255–3267. https://doi.org/10.7150/ijbs.63125

Markham A (2021) Zimberelimab: first approval. Drugs 81(17):2063–2068. https://doi.org/10.1007/s40265-021-01628-5

McKiernan JM, Lascano D, Ahn J, Ghandour R, Pak JS, RoyChoudhury A, Chang S, DeCastro GJ, Desai N (2015) A phase I/II multi-center study of intravesical nanoparticle albumin-bound rapamycin (ABI-009) in the treatment of BCG refractory non-muscle invasive bladder cancer. J Clin Oncol 33(15_suppl):TPS4576. https://doi.org/10.1200/jco.2015.33.15_suppl.tps4576

Mukherjee N, Svatek RS, Mansour AM (2018) Role of immunotherapy in bacillus Calmette–Guérin-unresponsive non-muscle invasive bladder cancer. Urol Oncol Semin Orig Investig 36(3):103–108. https://doi.org/10.1016/j.urolonc.2017.12.020

Navai N, Benedict WF, Zhang G, Abraham A, Ainslie N, Shah JB, Grossman HB, Kamat AM, Dinney CP (2016) Phase 1b trial to evaluate tissue response to a second dose of intravesical recombinant adenoviral interferon alpha2b formulated in Syn3 for failures of Bacillus Calmette-Guerin (BCG) therapy in nonmuscle invasive bladder cancer. Ann Surg Oncol 23(12):4110–4114. https://doi.org/10.1245/s10434-016-5300-6

Packiam VT, Lamm DL, Barocas DA, Trainer A, Fand B, Davis RL, Clark W, Kroeger M, Dumbadze I, Chamie K, Kader AK, Curran D, Gutheil J, Kuan A, Yeung AW, Steinberg GD (2018) An open label, single-arm, phase II multicenter study of the safety and efficacy of CG0070 oncolytic vector regimen in patients with BCG-unresponsive non-muscle-invasive bladder cancer: Interim results. Urol Oncol Semin Orig Investig 36(10):440–447. https://doi.org/10.1016/j.urolonc.2017.07.005

Packiam VT, Werntz RP, Steinberg GD (2019) Current clinical trials in non-muscle-invasive bladder cancer: heightened need in an era of chronic BCG shortage. Curr Urol Rep 20(12):84. https://doi.org/10.1007/s11934-019-0952-y

Pandha HS, Annels N, Arif M, Mostafid H, Sandhu S, Harrington K, Melcher A, Mansfield D, Au G, Grose M, Karpathy R, Shafren D (2016) Phase I/II CANON study: oncolytic immunotherapy for the treatment of non-muscle invasive bladder (NMIBC) cancer using intravesical coxsackievirus A21. Ann Oncol 27:vi361. https://doi.org/10.1093/annonc/mdw378.09

Qu Y-Y, Sun Z, Han W, Zou Q, Xing N, Luo H, Zhang X, He C, Bian X-J, Cai J, Chen C, Wang Q, Ye D-W (2022) Camrelizumab plus famitinib for advanced or metastatic urothelial carcinoma after platinum-based therapy: data from a multicohort phase 2 study. J Immunother Cancer 10(5):e004427. https://doi.org/10.1136/jitc-2021-004427

Racioppi M, Di Gianfrancesco L, Ragonese M, Palermo G, Sacco E, Bassi PF (2018) ElectroMotive drug administration (EMDA) of Mitomycin C as first-line salvage therapy in high risk 'BCG failure' non muscle invasive bladder cancer: 3 years follow-up outcomes. BMC Cancer 18(1):1224. https://doi.org/10.1186/s12885-018-5134-7

Rahman KMM, Giram P, Foster BA, You Y (2023) Photodynamic therapy for bladder cancers, a focused review. Photochem Photobiol 99(2):420–436. https://doi.org/10.1111/php.13726

Richters A, Aben KKH, Kiemeney LALM (2020) The global burden of urinary bladder cancer: an update. World J Urol 38(8):1895–1904. https://doi.org/10.1007/s00345-019-02984-4

Romero D (2024) THOR provides new data on the efficacy of erdafitinib. Nat Rev Clin Oncol 21(1):4. https://doi.org/10.1038/s41571-023-00836-0

Rosser CJ, Nix J, Ferguson L, Hernandez L, Wong HC (2018) Phase Ib trial of ALT-803, an IL-15 superagonist, plus BCG for the treatment of BCG-naïve patients with non-muscle-invasive bladder cancer. J Clin Oncol 36(6_suppl):510. https://doi.org/10.1200/JCO.2018.36.6_suppl.510

Roumiguié M, Kamat AM, Bivalacqua TJ, Lerner SP, Kassouf W, Böhle A, Brausi M, Buckley R, Persad R, Colombel M, Lamm D, Palou-Redorta J, Soloway M, Brothers K, Steinberg G, Lotan Y, Sylvester R, Alfred Witjes J, Black PC (2022) International Bladder Cancer Group consensus statement on clinical trial design for patients with Bacillus Calmette-Guérin-exposed high-risk non-muscle-invasive bladder cancer. Eur Urol 82(1):34–46. https://doi.org/10.1016/j.eururo.2021.12.005

Roupret M, Neuzillet Y, Bertaut A, Pignot G, Houede N, Champiat S, Nénan-Le Ficher S, Chausson M, Loriot Y (2019) ALBAN: An open label, randomized, phase III trial, evaluating efficacy of atezolizumab in addition to one year BCG (bacillus Calmette-Guerin) bladder instillation in BCG-naive patients with high-risk nonmuscle invasive bladder cancer (AFU-GETUG

37). J Clin Oncol 37(15_suppl):TPS4589. https://doi.org/10.1200/JCO.2019.37.15_suppl.TPS4589

Ruf P, Bauer HW, Schoberth A, Kellermann C, Lindhofer H (2021) First time intravesically administered trifunctional antibody catumaxomab in patients with recurrent non-muscle invasive bladder cancer indicates high tolerability and local immunological activity. Cancer Immunol Immunother 70(9):2727–2735. https://doi.org/10.1007/s00262-021-02930-7

Sansaloni-Pastor S, Lange N (2023) Unleashing the potential of 5-Aminolevulinic acid: Unveiling a promising target for cancer diagnosis and treatment beyond photodynamic therapy. J Photochem Photobiol B 247:112771. https://doi.org/10.1016/j.jphotobiol.2023.112771

Sathianathen NJ, Regmi S, Gupta S, Konety BR (2020) Immuno-oncology approaches to salvage treatment for non-muscle invasive bladder cancer. Urol Clin North Am 47(1):103–110. https://doi.org/10.1016/j.ucl.2019.09.012

Shore N, O'Donnell M, Keane T, Jewett MAS, Kulkarni GS, Dickstein R, Wolk F, Dunshee C, Belkoff L, Dillon RL, Cizeau J, Kassouf W (2020) Phase 3 results of vicinium in BCG-unresponsive non-muscle invasive bladder cancer. J Urol 203(Suppl 4):PD03-02. https://doi.org/10.1097/JU.0000000000000823.02

Shore ND, Powles T, Bedke J, Galsky MD, Kopyltsov E, Necchi A, Palou J, Vermette JJ, Randall AE, Pierce KJ, Cesari R, Steinberg GD (2022) A phase 3 study of the subcutaneous programmed cell death protein 1 inhibitor sasanlimab as single agent for patients with bacillus Calmette-Guérin, unresponsive, high-risk, non-muscle invasive bladder cancer: CREST Study Cohort B. J Clin Oncol 40(16_suppl):TPS4614. doi: https://doi.org/10.1200/JCO.2022.40.16_suppl.TPS4614

Sonpavde G, Rosser CJ, Pan C, Parikh RA, Nix J, Gingrich JR, Hernandez L, Huang B-Y, Wong HC (2016) Phase I trial of ALT-801, a first-in-class T-cell receptor (TCR)-interleukin (IL)-2 fusion molecule, plus gemcitabine (G) for Bacillus Calmette Guerin (BCG)-resistant non-muscle-invasive bladder cancer (NMIBC). J Clin Oncol 34(2_suppl):451. https://doi.org/10.1200/jco.2016.34.2_suppl.451

Steinberg GD, Palou-Redorta J, Gschwend JE, Tran B, Loriot Y, Daneshmand S, Roupret M, Santiago-Walker AE, Switzky JC, Major C, Baig M, Xia Q, Catto JW (2020) A randomized phase II study of erdafitinib (ERDA) versus intravesical chemotherapy (IC) in patients with high-risk nonmuscle invasive bladder cancer (HR-NMIBC) with FGFR mutations or fusions, who recurred after Bacillus Calmette-Guérin (BCG) therapy. J Clin Oncol 38(6_suppl):TPS603. https://doi.org/10.1200/JCO.2020.38.6_suppl.TPS603

Steinberg GD, Kalota SJ, Lotan Y, Warner L, Dauphinee S, Mazanet R (2023) Clinical results of a phase 1 study of intravesical EG-70 in patients with BCG-unresponsive NMIBC. J Clin Oncol 41(6_suppl):512. https://doi.org/10.1200/JCO.2023.41.6_suppl.512

Steinberg GD, Shore ND, Redorta JP, Galsky MD, Bedke J, Ku JH, Kretkowski M, Hu H, Penkov K, Vermette JJ, Tarazi JC, Randall AE, Pierce KJ, Saltzstein D, Powles TB (2024) CREST: phase III study of sasanlimab and Bacillus Calmette-Guérin for patients with Bacillus Calmette-Guérin-naïve high-risk non-muscle-invasive bladder cancer. Future Oncol 20(14):891–901. https://doi.org/10.2217/fon-2023-0271. Epub 2024 Jan 8

Stenzl A, Burger M, Fradet Y, Mynderse LA, Soloway MS, Witjes JA, Kriegmair M, Karl A, Shen Y, Grossman HB (2010 Nov) (2010) Hexaminolevulinate guided fluorescence cystoscopy reduces recurrence in patients with nonmuscle invasive bladder cancer. J Urol 184(5):1907–1913. https://doi.org/10.1016/j.juro.2010.06.148

Sun B, Mullapudi SS, Zhang Y, Neoh KG (2022) Glycosylated phospholipid-coated upconversion nanoparticles for bioimaging of non-muscle invasive bladder cancers. Microchim Acta 189(9):349. https://doi.org/10.1007/s00604-022-05411-5

Swain S, Sahu P, Beg S, Babu S (2016) Nanoparticles for cancer targeting: current and future directions. Curr Drug Deliv 13(8):1290–1302. https://doi.org/10.2174/1567201813666160713121122

Sylvester RJ, Rodríguez O, Hernández V, Turturica D, Bauerová L, Bruins HM, Bründl J, Van Der Kwast TH, Brisuda A, Rubio-Briones J, Seles M, Hentschel AE, Kusuma VRM, Huebner N, Cotte J, Mertens LS, Volanis D, Cussenot O, Subiela Henríquez JD, De La Peña E, Pisano F, Pešl M, Van Der Heijden AG, Herdegen S, Zlotta AR, Hacek J, Calatrava A, Mannweiler S, Bosschieter J, Ashabere D, Haitel A, Côté J-F, El Sheikh S, Lunelli L, Algaba F, Alemany I, Soria F, Runneboom W, Breyer J, Nieuwenhuijzen JA, Llorente C, Molinaro L, Hulsbergen-van De Kaa CA, Evert M, Kiemeney LALM, N'Dow J, Plass K, Čapoun O, Soukup V, Dominguez-Escrig JL, Cohen D, Palou J, Gontero P, Burger M, Zigeuner R, Mostafid AH, Shariat SF, Rouprêt M, Compérat EM, Babjuk M, Van Rhijn BWG (2021) European Association of Urology (EAU) Prognostic Factor Risk Groups for Non-muscle-invasive Bladder Cancer (NMIBC) incorporating the WHO 2004/2016 and WHO 1973 classification systems for grade: an update from the EAU NMIBC Guidelines Panel. Eur Urol 79(4):480–488. https://doi.org/10.1016/j.eururo.2020.12.033

Theralase Technologies Inc (2024) Theralase(R) provides update on phase II bladder cancer clinical study. News release. Published online. https://www.biospace.com/article/releases/theralase-r-provides-update-on-phase-ii-bladder-cancer-clinical-study/?s=86. Accessed 15 Jan 2024

Tsuji S, Reil K, Nelson K, Proclivo VH, McGuire KL, Giacalone MJ (2022) Intravesical VAX014 synergizes with PD-L1 blockade to enhance local and systemic control of bladder cancer. Cancer Immunol Res 10(8):978–995. https://doi.org/10.1158/2326-6066.CIR-21-0879

Uchio EM, Lamm DL, Shore ND, Kamat AM, Tyson M, Tran B, Anderson P, Grandi P, Burke JM (2022) A phase 3, single-arm study of CG0070 in subjects with nonmuscle invasive bladder cancer (NMIBC) unresponsive to Bacillus Calmette-Guerin (BCG). J Clin

Oncol 40(6_suppl):TPS598. https://doi.org/10.1200/JCO.2022.40.6_suppl.TPS598

Vilaseca A, Jayram G, Raventos C, Shore ND, Zainfeld D, Kang TW, Ku JH, Meeks J, Rodríguez Faba Ó, Roghmann F, Daneshmand S, Beeharry N, Cost C, Kalota A, Lauring J, Peterson M, Quiroz M, Stone N, Zhu W, Guerrero-Ramos F (2023) First safety and efficacy results of the TAR-210 erdafitinib intravesical delivery system in patients with non-muscle-invasive bladder cancer (NMIBC) with select FGFR alterations. ESMO 2023. Abstract. https://doi.org/10.1016/j.annonc.2023.10.110

Wagner AJ, Ravi V, Ganjoo KN, Van Tine BA, Riedel RF, Chugh R, Cranmer LD, Gordon EM, Hornick JL, Kwiatkowski DJ, Du H, Grigorian B, Schmid AN, Hou S, Harris K, Desai N, Dickson MA (2019) ABI-009 (nab-sirolimus) in advanced malignant perivascular epithelioid cell tumors (PEComa): Preliminary efficacy, safety, and mutational status from AMPECT, an open label phase II registration trial. J Clin Oncol 37(15_suppl):11005. https://doi.org/10.1200/JCO.2019.37.15_suppl.11005

Waldmann TA (2006) The biology of interleukin-2 and interleukin-15: implications for cancer therapy and vaccine design. Nat Rev Immunol 6(8):595–601. https://doi.org/10.1038/nri1901

Wen J, Zhu X, Liu B, You L, Kong L, Lee H, Han K, Wong JL, Rhode PR, Wong HC (2008) Targeting activity of a TCR/IL-2 fusion protein against established tumors. Cancer Immunol Immunother 57(12):1781–1794. https://doi.org/10.1007/s00262-008-0504-7

Witjes JA, Redorta JP, Jacqmin D, Sofras F, Malmström PU, Riedl C, Jocham D, Conti G, Montorsi F, Arentsen HC, Zaak D, Mostafid AH, Babjuk M (2010) Hexaminolevulinate-guided fluorescence cystoscopy in the diagnosis and follow-up of patients with non-muscle-invasive bladder cancer: review of the evidence and recommendations. Eur Urol 57(4):607–614. https://doi.org/10.1016/j.eururo.2010.01.025

Xu Y, Luo C, Wang J, Chen L, Chen J, Chen T, Zeng Q (2021) Application of nanotechnology in the diagnosis and treatment of bladder cancer. J Nanobiotechnol 19(1):393. https://doi.org/10.1186/s12951-021-01104-y

Ye D, Yao X, Wang G, Pu J, Yao X, Zhou F, Qi J, Ye Z, Xie L, Chen J et al (2017) An oral methionine aminopeptidase II inhibitor for high-risk non-muscle invasive bladder cancer relapsed after intravesical therapies: Update of a phase II trial. J Clin Oncol 35:303. https://doi.org/10.1200/JCO.2017.35.6_suppl.303

Zazzara M, Nazaraj A, Scarcia M, Cardo G, Carando R, Ludovico GM (2023) Electromotive drug administration of mitomycin C (EMDA/MMC) versus intravesical immunotherapy with Bacillus Calmette-Guérin (BCG) in intermediate and high risk non-muscle invasive bladder cancer. Urol Int 107(1):64–71. https://doi.org/10.1159/000520630. Epub 2021 Dec 21

22 New Treatment Approaches in Muscle-Invasive Bladder Cancer

Aditi Gupta and Jonathan E. Rosenberg

Abstract

Muscle-invasive bladder cancer (MIBC) constitutes 25% of newly diagnosed cases of bladder cancer per year. Muscle invasive disease remains a poor prognostic factor due to the presence of occult metastases and about 50% of patients have disease recurrence within 2 years of definitive local therapy. The treatment of MIBC has not changed significantly in over 20 years. Radical cystectomy with pelvic lymph node dissection remains the gold standard as definitive therapy for muscle-invasive bladder cancer and cisplatin-based neoadjuvant chemotherapy is the standard of care. Trimodality therapy, consisting of maximal surgical resection followed by concurrent chemoradiation, is an alternative curative approach for select patients who are poor surgical candidates. Adjuvant treatment is recommended for patients with high-risk disease or lymph node involvement. Although the current standard of care is with cisplatin-based regimens, numerous studies are underway evaluating perioperative combinations that may challenge this treatment paradigm. Building from the metastatic disease setting, immune checkpoint inhibitors and novel targeted therapies are being evaluated alone and in combination with chemotherapy for neoadjuvant management of MIBC. Furthermore, identification of biomarkers based on somatic alterations in DNA damage repair genes may predict response to cisplatin-based neoadjuvant chemotherapy and are being validated in prospective studies. In this chapter, we review data in support of the current recommendations for neoadjuvant, definitive local and adjuvant treatment, and discuss ongoing studies in each of these areas and their impact on clinical practice.

Keywords

Neoadjuvant chemotherapy · Immune checkpoint inhibitors · Antibody–drug conjugates · Radical cystectomy · Trimodality therapy

The treatment of muscle-invasive bladder cancer (MIBC) has not changed significantly in over 20 years. Radical cystectomy remains the gold standard as definitive therapy. While between 60 and 75% of patients are cured with radical surgery,

A. Gupta
Department of Medicine, Memorial Sloan Kettering Cancer Center, New York, NY, USA

J. E. Rosenberg (✉)
Genitourinary Oncology Service, Memorial Sloan Kettering Cancer Center, New York, NY, USA

Weill Cornell Medical College, New York, NY, USA
e-mail: rosenbj1@mskcc.org

M. A. Knowles, L. Dyrskjøt (eds.), *Biology of Bladder Cancer*,
https://doi.org/10.1007/978-3-031-68505-7_22

surgical complication rates, and readmissions may approach 30%, even in high-volume centers. Alternatively, trimodality therapy with transurethral resection, chemotherapy, and radiation is an appropriate option for many patients (see Chap. 6). Despite definitive local therapy, about half of patients with muscle-invasive bladder cancer (MIBC) involving the muscularis propria (≥T2) develop metastatic disease within 2 years of diagnosis and often succumb to their disease.

22.1 Radical Cystectomy Versus Bladder-Preserving Approach

Following neoadjuvant treatment with cisplatin-based chemotherapy, patients are directed toward curative intent treatment. Radical cystectomy (RC) and urinary diversion remain the standard of care for non-metastatic MIBC (T2–T4a, cN0M0), as endorsed by multidisciplinary society guidelines (Chang et al. 2017). For patients with significant comorbidities for which RC poses a major risk or for patients who desire to retain their bladder, trimodality therapy (TMT) with bladder-preserving strategies combined with concurrent radiation therapy (RT) and radiosensitizing chemotherapy can be considered as an alternative. This treatment decision is largely guided by appropriate patient selection and patient/physician preference as no randomized control trials have been published comparing the oncological outcomes of patients treated with RC compared to TMT.

RC is a major surgical procedure that not only involves removal of the bladder, but also adjacent organs and lymph nodes. In men, RC involves a cystoprostatectomy with removal of the bladder, prostate, and seminal vesicles. In women, the procedure involves a cystectomy and possible removal of the uterus, fallopian tubes, ovaries, and anterior vaginal wall to achieve the best oncologic outcome (Chang et al. 2017; Aminoltejari and Black 2020). For pathologically organ-confined pT2 disease, RC may cure the majority of patients. For those with locoregionally spread pT3 disease, RC can cure 50–60% of patients and 20–30% of patients with pT4 low-volume lymph node-positive disease (Aragon-Ching et al. 2018). Given the considerable morbidity and mortality associated with this surgery, patients are recommended to undergo RC at high-volume centers experienced in treating high-acuity complex surgical cases.

In addition to RC, a thorough pelvic lymph node dissection (LND) is critical to accurate staging and prognosis. Current guidelines recommend concurrent bilateral pelvic lymphadenectomy at the time of any surgery with curative intent, but there is still much debate about the optimal extent of lymph node resection to maximize tumor control. Consensus recommendations are to evaluate a minimum of 12 lymph nodes (Chang et al. 2017). Retrospective studies have found that extended lymph node dissection to the level of the aortic bifurcation, as opposed to standard dissection that is bound by the bifurcation of the common iliac artery, is associated with improved recurrence-free survival (Dhar et al. 2008) and all-cause bladder cancer-specific mortality (Sanderson et al. 2006; Chang et al. 2017). A further extensive resection did not lead to improved outcomes. The Southwest Oncology Group trial SWOG S1011 recently evaluated the benefit of an extended over a standard lymph node dissection. This phase III trial randomized patients with cT2-T4a N0-2 disease undergoing radical cystectomy to either a standard bilateral pelvic LND or extended LND up to at least the aortic bifurcation. The primary endpoint was disease-free survival. Six hundred and eighteen patients were randomized and median follow-up was 6.1 years in both arms. While patients undergoing extended LND had higher pathologic *N* stage, there was no difference in disease-free survival (HR 1.10, 95% CI 0.87–1.42; $p = 0.82$) or overall survival (HR 1.15, 95% CI 0.89–1.48; $p = 0.87$) between the groups. Extended LND was associated with increased grade 3–4 AEs (16% versus 8%) and higher perioperative mortality (16 deaths within 90 days of RC in extended LND arm versus 9 deaths in standard LND arm) (Lerner et al. 2023). The lack of benefit seen with extended LND could also be attributed to the fact that patients who intraoperatively were found to be *N*+ were excluded from randomization. Such censoring of patients with clinically occult disease led the study to be underpowered to identify the added benefit of extended LND in this patient population. Given the potential for increased surgical complications, an extended node dissection is not uniformly recommended for all patients (Chang et al. 2017; Aragon-Ching et al. 2018).

Robotic-assisted cystectomy is becoming increasingly more common, and it is estimated that about 25% of RCs in the USA are performed robotically. Based on results from three major randomized studies, complication rates, hospital stays, and pathological outcomes are similar between open and robotic approaches to RC (Parekh et al. 2018; Bochner et al. 2015; Khan et al. 2016). The RAZOR trial, the largest study to date that randomized 302 patients to open versus robotic RC, demonstrated non-inferiority of a robotic approach with respect to 2-year progression-free survival (robotic RC 72.3% [95% CI 64.3–78.8] versus open 71.6% [95% CI, 63.6–78.2]) (Parekh et al. 2018). A Cochrane review analyzed the results from five randomized control trials comprising 541 patients and found no difference in oncological outcomes or risk of major complications between robotic versus open RC (Rai et al. 2019). While a robotic platform can improve the precision of surgery and can offer future technological enhancements, its high cost without clear benefit must be considered.

As many patients with MIBC are older than 65 years and often have significant comorbidities that make them poor surgical candidates, trimodality therapy (TMT) offers an alternative bladder-sparing approach. TMT consists of maximal transurethral resection of bladder tumor (TURBT) followed by external beam radiotherapy (EBRT) with concurrent sensitizing chemotherapy (chemoRT). Established by Radiation Therapy Oncology Group (RTOG) trials, TMT utilizes once- or twice-daily radiation targeting the bladder, distal ureter, and proximal urethra (including the prostate), with concurrent cisplatin-based chemotherapy combined with either 5-fluorouracil (5-FU) (RTOG 9506) (Kaufman et al. 2000) or paclitaxel (RTOG 9906) (Kaufman et al. 2009). RTOG 0233 compared 5-FU with cisplatin to paclitaxel with cisplatin with concurrent radiation in patients with T2 disease and found that both regimens resulted in similar rates of complete response (CR) and 5-year overall survival. As candidates for TMT may have contraindications to cisplatin, other concurrent chemotherapy regimens have been evaluated. The BC2001 trial tested the combination of 5-FU with mitomycin-C with concurrent radiotherapy and showed a 67% rate of locoregional disease-free survival at 2 years and improved 5-year overall survival of 48% (95% CI, 40–55) with impressive tolerability, compared to radiotherapy alone (James et al. 2012). Another phase II study established the efficacy of concurrent weekly gemcitabine during radiotherapy and showed an 88% cystoscopic response rate, and a 3-year overall survival of 75% (Choudhury et al. 2011). Twice-weekly low-dose gemcitabine with daily radiation was recently compared to a regimen of twice-daily radiation with 5-FU and cisplatin RTOG 0712, which showed that both regimens resulted in distant metastasis-free survival at 3 years of >75% (84% with gemcitabine regimen versus 78% with 5-FU/cisplatin) (Coen et al. 2019). While a direct comparison of the effect of different radiation fractionation schedules cannot be made given different chemotherapy regimens, daily radiation is often more convenient for patients, and hypofractionated approaches are becoming standard. Based on these studies, concurrent radiochemotherapy with 5-FU/cisplatin, 5-FU/mitomycin, and low-dose gemcitabine can be considered and should be tailored based on patient preferences and contraindications for cisplatin-based regimens.

Additional therapies are also being considered in combination with traditional chemoRT in TMT. The additive benefit of immune checkpoint inhibition is being evaluated in an ongoing SWOG/NRG phase III study (NCT03775265) in which patients with localized MIBC who refuse or are unfit for RC are randomized to chemoRT with or without atezolizumab. Atezolizumab is given every 3 weeks for a total of 6 months in the absence of disease progression or major toxicity.

The primary endpoint is bladder intact event-free survival (BI-EFS) measured up to 5 years (Singh et al. 2020).

Appropriate patient selection is critical to achieving optimal results with selective bladder preservation. The CR rate for patients with T2–T4a disease treated with TMT is approximately 70% (Mak et al. 2014). Analysis of patients achieving a complete response on pooled RTOG studies helps identify ideal candidates for TMT and define exclusion criteria. Factors that impact the likelihood of achieving a CR following TMT and should be considered when guiding patients include completeness of transurethral resection of bladder tumor (TURBT), tumor stage, presence of hydronephrosis (blockage of the kidney or ureter), multifocality of disease, and carcinoma in situ (CIS). A pooled analysis of six RTOG studies found that a visibly complete TURBT was associated with a significantly higher rate of CR (Mak et al. 2014) and Rödel et al. similarly showed that completeness of resection after initial TURBT is an independent predictor of CR (Rödel et al. 2002). Thus, a visibly complete TURBT is ideal; a less than complete TURBT is not an absolute contraindication to TMT as numerous trials have demonstrated acceptable CR rates without a complete resection. With regard to tumor stage, pooled analysis of RTOG studies confirmed that T stage did not predict the likelihood of CR to TMT (Mak et al. 2014), and increasing T stage has reproducibly been shown to be associated with reduced long-term survival after TMT (Rödel et al. 2002; Efstathiou et al. 2012). Tumor-related hydronephrosis has been established as an exclusion criterion for TMT. RTOG 8903 found that the presence of hydronephrosis was associated with reduced CR (38% vs. 64%) and decreased 5-year survival (33% vs. 54%) (Shahab 1999). Similarly, RTOG 8802 found that hydronephrosis was the only factor to be significantly associated with distant metastases and death (Tester et al. 1996). Patients with tumor-related hydronephrosis are poor candidates for bladder preservation and it is frequently seen as an absolute contraindication for selective bladder-preserving approaches. Next, multifocal disease is thought to be a predictive factor for decreased response to TMT. While multifocality may not predict lower rates of CR, it is associated with higher rates of local relapse and therefore TMT is not recommended for those with diffuse multifocal disease (Rödel et al. 2002). Similarly, the presence of extensive CIS has been associated with lower rates of CR to radiation alone and combination TMT (Fung et al. 1991). European societies suggest that the presence of extensive CIS be considered a relative and not an absolute contraindication to TMT since CIS affects risk of recurrence after TMT and not overall survival (Milosevic et al. 2007; EAU Guidelines 2024). Lastly, prostatic urethral invasion is not a contraindication to bladder preservation therapy if it is amenable to visibly complete resection. European guidelines recommend prostatic urethral biopsies in cases of bladder neck tumors as part of pre-treatment evaluation (Witjes et al. 2023). In addition to these considerations, patient compliance and motivation can be key to matching patients to optimal therapy either with TMT or with RC and ultimately identifying early recurrences for consideration of salvage therapies. Table 22.1 summarizes the recommendations regarding ideal and poor candidates for bladder-preserving approaches.

Due to poor accrual and patient difficulty with accepting randomization to surgery, there are no completed randomized controlled trials comparing oncological outcomes with TMT versus RC. Numerous retrospective studies and meta-analyses have been completed to guide treatment decisions. While each study has different nuances, they globally show that both approaches have similar rates of overall survival and disease-free survival in appropriately selected patients. The largest and most recent retrospective analysis by Zlotta et al. used propensity scores to analyze differences in survival outcomes between 837 patients who underwent RC and 282 who received TMT. After matching for numerous variables, the study found that there was no difference in 5-year metastasis-free survival (74% of RC versus 75% with TMT) or 5-year cancer-specific survival (81% with RC versus 84% with TMT). Overall survival favored TMT with HR 0.70 (95% CI 0.53–0.92, $p = 0.010$) (Zlotta et al.

Table 22.1 Patient characteristics to consider for selective bladder preservation therapy

Ideal	Relative contraindications	Absolute contraindications
• No hydronephrosis • Absence of CIS • Visibly complete TURBT • Unifocal tumor • Willingness to undergo regular surveillance • No prior pelvic radiotherapy	• Diffuse CIS • Multifocal tumor • Incomplete TURBT • Lymph node positive • Prostatic stromal invasion	• Advancing T stage • Tumor-related hydronephrosis • Prior pelvic radiation therapy • Not a candidate for chemotherapy

2023). These results suggest that TMT and RC provide similar oncological outcomes and TMT should be offered to suitable patients with MIBC regardless of their eligibility for surgery.

Despite recommendations for either RC or TMT for non-metastatic MIBC, about 50% of MIBC patients in the USA receive no definitive therapy (Park and Jeong 2018). This could be attributed to advanced age or comorbid conditions of patients or lack of understanding regarding either approach. Unfortunately, many patients are not good candidates for radical cystectomy due to comorbid conditions. These patients should be considered for chemoradiation regardless of the above-noted optimal patient characteristics, as otherwise, they would not receive treatment. As all data published to date shows similar outcomes between RC and TMT, clinicians must inform patients of curative approaches to guide patient-centered decision-making in MIBC management.

22.2 Neoadjuvant Treatment

22.2.1 Neoadjuvant Chemotherapy

Muscle invasive disease remains a poor prognostic factor due to occult micrometastases. This results in relapse following definitive local therapy in many patients. This has led to the widespread incorporation of systemic therapy into the treatment paradigm to reduce the risk of metastatic disease following resection or radiation. Neoadjuvant chemotherapy has been established as the gold standard based on two randomized phase III trials. SWOG 8710 enrolled 317 patients randomized to radical cystectomy, or three cycles of methotrexate, vinblastine, doxorubicin, and cisplatin (MVAC) followed by radical cystectomy. The use of chemotherapy prior to surgery led to a median survival of 77 months, compared to 46 months with surgery alone (two-sided $p = 0.06$). Neoadjuvant chemotherapy was associated with a higher pathologic complete response rate (38% versus 15%), a 14% improvement in 5-year survival, and a 25% reduction in the overall risk of death. Surgical complication rates were not significantly increased with neoadjuvant chemotherapy (Grossman et al. 2003). EORTC 30894 randomized patients with MIBC to either definitive local therapy (radiation or radical cystectomy) or cisplatin, methotrexate, and vinblastine (CMV) followed by definitive local therapy. This trial randomized 976 patients and showed that neoadjuvant therapy led to a 16% reduction in risk of death (HR 0.84, 95% CI 0.72–0.99; $p = 0.037$) (International Collaboration of Trialists et al. 2011). A recent meta-analysis in 2020 comparing 17 studies that evaluated platinum-based neoadjuvant regimens against locoregional treatment alone found an improvement in overall survival in the group that received neoadjuvant chemotherapy followed by radical cystectomy (HR 0.82, 95% CI 0.71–0.95, $p = 0.009$) (Hamid et al. 2020). Based on these results, platinum-based combination neoadjuvant chemotherapy has been recommended as the standard of care for MIBC.

Several single-arm phase II studies tested dose-dense chemotherapy regimens as neoadjuvant therapy. In metastatic urothelial cancer, dose-dense chemotherapy (given every 2 weeks instead of every 4 weeks with higher doses of cisplatin and doxorubicin per cycle) might be associated with superior long-term outcomes (Sternberg et al. 2005). Two phase II studies tested dose-dense MVAC (ddMVAC) chemotherapy. In one study, three cycles of chemotherapy were administered prior to radical cystectomy in 44 patients with MIBC. This was associated with a 38% pathologic complete response rate, and 52% pathologic downstaging to non-muscle invasive disease (Plimack et al. 2014). The other study enrolled 39 patients treated with four cycles prior to cystectomy, and resulted in 26% having a pathologic complete response, and 49% downstaged to less than T2 disease (Choueiri et al. 2014).

Multiple retrospective analyses have evaluated the doublet chemotherapy regimen gemcitabine and cisplatin as neoadjuvant therapy. One study by Dash et al. retrospectively evaluated neoadjuvant gemcitabine/cisplatin in 42 patients prior to radical cystectomy. This analysis found that four cycles of neoadjuvant gemcitabine/cisplatin achieved pathologic complete response in 26% of patients and downstaged 36% of patients to <T2 disease, rates similar to those achieved with MVAC and with significantly decreased toxicity (Dash et al. 2008).

To compare different neoadjuvant regimens, the phase III VESPER study compared the efficacy of gemcitabine/cisplatin against ddMVAC in the preoperative setting. This study randomized 437 patients to receive either four cycles of gemcitabine/cisplatin or six cycles of ddMVAC as perioperative therapy (either neoadjuvant or adjuvant). The trial found that rates of pathologic complete response (42% versus 36%, $p = 0.021$) were higher in the ddMVAC group. The primary analysis of the study found that 3-year progression-free survival (PFS) was higher in the group that received ddMVAC (64% versus 56%, HR 0.77 [0.57–1.02], $p = 0.066$), but the trial did not meet the pre-specified threshold for statistical significance. When looking only at the neoadjuvant group, PFS at 3 years was significantly higher in the ddMVAC arm (66% vs. 56%, HR = 0.70 [95% CI, 0.51–0.96], $p = 0.025$). Treatment with ddMVAC was associated with higher toxicity, especially higher rates of severe hematological ($p < 0.001$) and gastrointestinal ($p = 0.003$) complications (Pfister et al. 2022). Notably, this trial did not enroll any patients aged over 70 years, and used a duration of neoadjuvant therapy (six cycles of ddMVAC) that is difficult to achieve in practice (only 60% of patients could complete this course). Secondary endpoints of the study included time to progression and overall survival. Time to progression at 3 years was extended in the ddMVAC arm (69% vs. 58%, HR = 0.68 [95% CI, 0.50–0.93], $p = 0.014$) and this postponement of progression was more pronounced in the neoadjuvant arm (3 year rate: 71% vs. 59%, HR = 0.62 [95% CI, 0.44–0.85], $p = 0.005$). Survival data at 5 years is still maturing but the current estimates with 40 months of median follow-up are in favor of ddMVAC (HR = 0.74 [95% CI, 0.47–0.92]) (Pfister et al. 2022). These data support the use of ddMVAC as neoadjuvant therapy in appropriately selected patients, although the appropriate duration of treatment remains unclear, and may not be generalizable to all cisplatin-eligible patients, particularly older patients and those with multiple comorbidities.

22.2.2 Neoadjuvant Immunotherapy

Immune checkpoint inhibition (ICI) with monoclonal antibodies directed against various immunoregulatory targets have become another pillar of bladder cancer treatment (see also Chap. 23). Approximately half of the patients are ineligible to receive cisplatin, mostly due to chronic kidney disease (creatinine clearance <60 mL/min), peripheral neuropathy, hearing loss, New York Heart Association (NYHA) class ≥III heart failure, and poor performance status Eastern Cooperative Oncology Group (ECOG) >1. ICIs have been tested as a treatment option for cisplatin-ineligible patients in the neoadjuvant setting. Most of the existing literature is based on single-arm phase II studies, as detailed below.

The first study to evaluate the antitumor response of preoperative ICI involved 12 patients treated with ipilimumab, an anti-cytotoxic T-lymphocyte antigen 4 (CTLA-4) monoclonal antibody. This small trial not only established the safety of presurgical ICI as most drug-related adverse events consisted of grade 1/2 toxicities, but also demonstrated that immune responses can be monitored in the preoperative setting as potential biomarkers of response (Carthon et al. 2010). Two single-arm phase II studies established the activity of a single-agent neoadjuvant targeting of the PD-1 pathway in urothelial carcinoma, either via inhibition of the receptor programmed cell death protein 1 (PD-1) or its ligand programmed cell death-ligand 1 (PD-L1). The PURE-01 trial assessed the activity of pembrolizumab, a monoclonal antibody against PD-1, in 50 patients with MIBC prior to radical cystectomy. Patients were enrolled regardless of cisplatin eligibility (92% of patients were cisplatin-eligible) and PD-L1 positivity was defined as ≥10% by combined positive score (CPS). Pembrolizumab (200 mg) was administered every 3 weeks for 3 cycles and patients underwent radical cystectomy within 1–3 weeks after their last dose. The primary endpoint for the study was pathologic complete response (pCR), which was defined as pT0 at surgery. Neoadjuvant pembrolizumab yielded an overall pCR rate of 42%, with 54% downstaging to non-muscle invasive disease. Of note, in those patients with a PD-L1 CPS ≥10% the rate of pCR was 54.3%, compared to 13.3% in patients with PD-L1 CPS <10. Such high response rates must be considered along with the fact that 67% of the patient population had a PD-L1 Combined Positive Score (CPS) score ≥10%, an outlier compared to other studies. Treatment was well tolerated with only 6% of patients experiencing grade ≥3 adverse events (Necchi et al. 2018). Updated survival outcomes after a median follow-up of 3 years from PURE-01 shows that event-free survival and OS were 74.4% [95% CI, 67.8–81.7] and 83.8% (95% CI, 77.8–90.2) in the intention-to-treat (ITT) population. Responses were graded based on pathological outcomes with higher recurrence-free survival (RFS) rates in patients achieving a complete pathologic response (lack of any residual tumor; ypT0N0; RFS 96.3%; "y" denotes post-treatment) compared to those with ypT1N0 (RFS 96.1%), ypT2-4N0 (RFS 74.9%) and lowest RFS rates for those with $ypT_{any}N1$-3 responses (RFS 58.3%). Regarding biomarker analysis, PD-L1 CPS showed a correlation with event-free survival (HR, 0.96; 95% CI, 0.95–0.98; $p = 0.001$) (Basile et al. 2022). These data confirmed the sustained clinical benefit of single-agent ICI prior to radical cystectomy.

The ABACUS study was another single-arm phase II trial that evaluated neoadjuvant atezolizumab, a monoclonal antibody targeting PD-L1, in 95 patients prior to surgery. Contrary to the PURE-01 trial, all patients were ineligible for or refused cisplatin-based therapy. Prior to radical cystectomy, patients received atezolizumab 1200 mg every 3 weeks for two cycles. PD-L1 positivity was defined as ≥5% on immune cells and the primary endpoint was pCR. The rates of pCR and downstaging to non-muscle invasive disease in the overall population were 31% and 39%, respectively. pCR was 37% in patients who were PD-L1 positive. Treatment-related grade 3–4 toxicities occurred in 12% of patients and grade 3–4 surgical complications in 31% of cases (Powles et al. 2019).

Given non-redundant pathways in immune regulation, ICI combination with anti-PD-1 and anti-CTLA-4 blockade has been evaluated in recent studies. The NABUCCO trial examined ipilimumab (anti-CTLA-4) plus nivolumab (anti-PD-1) as a combination neoadjuvant immunotherapy for 24 patients with stage II urothelial cancer. In this single-arm feasibility study, patients were administered ipilimumab 3 mg/kg on Day 1, then ipilimumab 3 mg/kg plus nivolumab 1 mg/kg on Day 22, and then nivolumab 3 mg/kg on Day 43. The primary endpoint was feasibility to resect within 12 weeks from the start of treatment and pCR was evaluated as a secondary endpoint. A total of 23 (96%) patients underwent surgery within 12 weeks, with 11 (46%) patients achieving a pCR and 14 (58%) patients having no remaining invasive disease (pCR or pTisN0/pTaN0). In patients who were PD-L1 positive, defined as CPS score >10%, the pCR rate was 73%. However, 55% of patients experienced grade 3–4 immune-related adverse events (irAEs) (van Dijk et al. 2020).

Two studies have recently evaluated the combination of dual PD-L1 and CTLA-4 blockade. The DUTRENEO study was a phase II study that compared a combination of durvalumab (anti-PD-L1) plus tremelimumab (anti-CTLA-4) versus neoadjuvant chemotherapy in cisplatin-eligible patients. Patients were stratified as having immunologically "hot" or "cold" tumors based on the tumor immune score devised by NanoString Technologies. Patients with "hot" tumors were randomized to receive three cycles of combination ICI or standard cisplatin-based chemotherapy, while patients with "cold" tumors received cisplatin-based neoadjuvant treatment. Patients with "hot tumors" received either durvalumab/tremelimumab, with 37.5% (8/22) achieving pCR, or cisplatin-based neoadjuvant therapy, with comparable pCR rate of 34.8% (8/23). In the "cold" arm patients were only treated with cisplatin-based regimens and as many as 68.8% (11/16) of patients achieved pCR. There were more PD-L1 low tumors in the "cold" arm (Grande et al. 2020). A similar trial from MD Anderson Cancer Center evaluated a combination of durvalumab and tremelimumab in patients with high-risk MIBC (defined as having lymphovascular invasion, hydronephrosis, T3b disease, or variant histology) prior to cystectomy who were ineligible for neoadjuvant cisplatin. Of the 21 patients who underwent cystectomy, 9 (43%) had a pCR and 14 (67%) had downstaging of disease. Five patients developed grade 3 immune-related toxicities and 2 patients experienced >30 days delay in their surgery (Gao et al. 2019). A summary of neoadjuvant ICI trials discussed is detailed in Table 22.2.

22.2.3 Neoadjuvant Chemotherapy + Immunotherapy

As chemotherapy can elicit tumor-specific immune responses via induction of immunogenic cell death, the combination of traditional chemotherapy with immunotherapy has been extensively investigated. While many studies are currently ongoing, initial outcomes from published studies show promising preliminary results, although no randomized comparisons have been reported yet.

BLASST-1, a phase II, single-arm study, evaluated the efficacy and safety of neoadjuvant nivolumab (anti-PD-1) with gemcitabine/cisplatin for MIBC (cT2-T4a, $N \leq 1$, M0). Patients were treated with four cycles of gemcitabine/cisplatin with concurrent nivolumab every 21 days, followed by surgery within 8 weeks of last treatment. Pathologic response, defined as ≤pT1N0, was seen in 65.8% of patients (27/41) with a favorable safety profile. The overall rate of grade 3–4 adverse events (AE) was 20% and immune-related AEs were seen in three patients (Gupta et al. 2020). Similarly, two studies have evaluated the safety and efficacy of neoadjuvant gemcitabine/cisplatin with another anti-PD-1 immunotherapy, pembrolizumab. HCRN GU14-188 is a phase I/II trial in which patients were divided into cisplatin-eligible, treated with gemcitabine/cisplatin, or ineligible, treated with gemcitabine alone. Both cohorts received 5 doses of neoadjuvant pembrolizumab. In the cisplatin-eligible cohort, pathologic response (≤pT1N0) and pCR were seen in 61.1% and 44.4% of patients, respectively. The 36-month relapse-free survival was 63% with overall survival of 82% (Hoimes et al. 2020). In the cisplatin-ineligible cohort pathologic response rate was 53%, with 41% of patients achieving pCR. Eighteen months relapse-free survival was 65.1% and 36-month overall survival was 65.7% (Brown et al. 2023). A similar phase II study by Rose et al. demonstrated the efficacy of neoadjuvant pembrolizumab in combination with gemcitabine and split-dose cisplatin in MIBC patients eligible for radical cystectomy. Patients received pembrolizumab 200 mg IV on day 1, split-dose cisplatin 25 mg/m^2 on Days 1 and 8 and gemcitabine 1000 mg/m^2 on Days 1 and 8 every 21 days for four cycles. The primary endpoint was pathological downstaging (<pT2N0), with 22/39 (56%) patients achieving downstaging of disease and 14/39 (36%) experiencing a pCR after a median of four cycles of therapy. Seventy-four percent of patients experienced grade 3 or higher treatment-related AEs, with one patient developing new-onset type 1 diabetes mellitus with ketoacidosis (Rose et al. 2021). These studies indicate that neoadjuvant chemotherapy in combination with single-agent ICI is safe and results in pathologic downstaging rates of ~50–60%, numerically higher than that achieved with neoadjuvant chemotherapy alone.

Table 22.2 Published clinical trials of neoadjuvant immunotherapy for MIBC

Trial name	NCT	Number of patients	Regimen	pCR (pT0) rates (%)	Downstaging (<pT2) (%)	*N*+ (%)
Ipilimumab		12	Ipilimumab	–	67	8.3
PURE-01	NCT02736266	50	Pembrolizumab	42	54	20
ABACUS	NCT02662309	95	Atezolizumab	31	39	–
NABUCCO	NCT03387761	24	Ipilimumab + nivolumab	46	58	33
DUTRENEO	NCT02812420	24	Durvalumab + tremelimumab	37.5	57.5	21
MDACC	NCT02812420	21	Durvalumab + tremelimumab	43	14	–

Table 22.3 Published clinical trials of neoadjuvant chemoimmunotherapy for MIBC

Trial name	NCT	Number of patients	Regimen	pCR (pT0) rates (%)	Downstaging (<pT2) (%)	*N*+ (%)
BLASST-1	NCT03294304	41	Nivolumab + gem/cis	34	66	–
SAKK 06/17	NCT03406650	61	Durvalumab + gem/cis	30	63	13
HCRN GU14-188	NCT02365766	43	Pembrolizumab + gem/cis	44	61	14
MSKCC	NCT02989584	39	Atezolizumab + gem/cis	41	69	18

Two clinical trials have evaluated a combination of anti-PDL1 ICI with chemotherapy. SAKK 6/17 tested durvalumab plus gemcitabine/cisplatin in patients with operable MIBC (cT2-T4a cN0-1) followed by adjuvant durvalumab. Treatment consisted of four cycles of neoadjuvant gemcitabine/cisplatin in combination with four cycles of durvalumab given every 3 weeks followed by resection. Durvalumab was continued after surgery for ten cycles dosed every 4 weeks. Data for the primary endpoint, event-free survival at 2 years, has not matured yet. Pathologic response, a secondary endpoint, was observed in 60% of patients, with 18 (34%) achieving pCR. Grade 3 irAEs occurred in 7 (12%) patients related to durvalumab (Cathomas et al. 2021). Another multicenter, single-arm phase II study evaluated atezolizumab (anti-PD-L1) in combination with gemcitabine/cisplatin. Eligible patients with cT2-T4aN0M0 MIBC received a dose of atezolizumab, followed 2 weeks later by atezolizumab plus gemcitabine/cisplatin every 21 days for four cycles. Patients received one additional dose of atezolizumab 3 weeks later prior to radical cystectomy. The primary end point was non-muscle-invasive downstaging to <pT2N0, which was met in 27 (69%) patients, including 16 (41%) pT0N0. No patient with <pT2N0 relapsed with a median follow-up of 16.5 months (Funt et al. 2022). Acceptable safety and tolerability were seen in both studies. Grade 3 irAEs occurred in 5 (11%) patients related to atezolizumab (Funt et al. 2022).

The relative contribution of immune checkpoint blockade in combination with neoadjuvant cisplatin-based regimens remains unclear. A summary of the published neoadjuvant chemoimmunotherapy trials discussed is detailed in Table 22.3.

22.2.4 Neoadjuvant Antibody-Drug Conjugates

Antibody–drug conjugates (ADC) represent a novel therapeutic class that can selectively deliver cytotoxic chemotherapy to cancer cells. Enfortumab Vedotin (EV) is an ADC that targets

Nectin-4, which is highly expressed in urothelial cancer (Rosenberg et al. 2020). EV was first evaluated in patients with metastatic or locally advanced urothelial cancer (UC) following progression on prior platinum-based chemotherapy and PD-1/PD-L1 treatment. The phase III study EV-301 showed an overall response rate (ORR 40.6% vs. 17.9%; $p < 0.001$) and a survival advantage (HR, 0.70; CI 0.56–0.89; $p = 0.001$) over traditional chemotherapy (Powles et al. 2021). Based on these results, EV gained FDA approval for the treatment of platinum- and ICI refractory advanced/metastatic UC patients, and is now being evaluated in the neoadjuvant setting.

Several studies are underway to evaluate the efficacy of neoadjuvant EV alone and in combination with ICI in MIBC. Analysis from cohort H of EV-103, a large ongoing multi-cohort phase Ib/II study (NCT03288545) evaluating EV and combination EV plus pembrolizumab in early and late-stage disease, showed promising activity of neoadjuvant EV monotherapy in cisplatin-ineligible MIBC patients. Patients were treated with three cycles of neoadjuvant EV and evaluated based on the primary endpoint of pCR (ypT0N0). Of 22 patients who were treated, 36.4% had a pCR and 50% of patients had pathological downstaging of disease (yp T0, Tis, Ta, T1, N0). Median event-free survival (EFS) has not been reached and the EFS rate at 12 months was 76.4% (CI, 52.2-89.4). While no surgeries were delayed due to EV administration, 18.2% of patients had grade ≥3 treatment-related adverse events (fatigue, alopecia, and altered taste), and several grade 5 events were observed (Flaig et al. 2023).

Based on a remarkable objective response rate (ORR) of 64.5% (CI, 52.7–75.1) in cohort K of EV-103, which evaluated combination EV/pembrolizumab as first-line treatment for locally advanced/metastatic cisplatin-ineligible MIBC patients (O'Donnell et al. 2023), multiple trials are ongoing to establish the antitumor efficacy of this combination in the neoadjuvant setting. A single-arm phase II study is exploring the efficacy of combination EV/pembrolizumab as preoperative therapy in patients with locally advanced/lymph node-positive disease, with the primary endpoint of pCR (NCT05239624). Similarly, EV-303 and EV-304 are ongoing randomized phase III studies testing neoadjuvant combination EV/pembrolizumab. EV-303 (NCT03924895) will evaluate the efficacy and safety of perioperative pembrolizumab alone or in combination with EV compared to radical cystectomy with pelvic lymph node dissection in cisplatin-ineligible MIBC patients. The study will assess dual primary endpoints of pCR and event-free survival (Necchi et al. 2023). EV-304 (NCT04700124) will compare neoadjuvant EV/pembrolizumab versus standard-of-care gemcitabine/cisplatin in cisplatin-eligible MIBC patients. EV-304 will determine whether a combination ADC/ICI is superior to traditional chemotherapy by analyzing the co-primary endpoints of pCR and event-free survival (Hoimes et al. 2021). Another trial, VOLGA (NCT04960709), is underway to evaluate whether dual ICI treatment in combination with EV produces superior outcomes. This international randomized phase III trial hypothesizes that preoperative EV in combination with PD-L1 and CTLA-4 inhibition can downstage disease before cystectomy and improve EFS. Patients will be randomized into three arms to receive three cycles of neoadjuvant therapy followed by adjuvant ICI: arm 1 will be treated with neoadjuvant durvalumab (anti-PD-L1), tremelimumab (anti-CTLA-3) and EV followed by adjuvant durvalumab/tremelimumab, arm 2 will receive neoadjuvant durvalumab/EV followed by adjuvant durvalumab, and arm 3 will receive adjuvant nivolumab in high-risk patients or no adjuvant treatment. Efficacy will be assessed by the same endpoints (Powles et al. 2022). These studies and others aim to challenge the current treatment paradigm of neoadjuvant cisplatin-based chemotherapy. An abundance of choice between combinations ICI with other targeted therapies offers hope for neoadjuvant strategies beyond conventional chemotherapy. Table 22.4 provides a list of a few of the ongoing neoadjuvant studies evaluating ICI in combination with other targeted therapies.

Table 22.4 Ongoing combination studies of ICI and other therapies in neoadjuvant MIBC

Trial name	NCT	Phase	Regimen	Primary endpoint
ICI + ADC				
EV-ECLIPSE	NCT05239624	II	EV + pembrolizumab prior to RC	pCR
EV-303	NCT03924895	III	EV + pembrolizumab prior to RC	EFS
EV-304	NCT04700124	III	EV + pembrolizumab versus gem/cis	pCR and EFS
VOLGA	NCT04960709	III	Arm 1: durvalumab + tremelimumab + EV → RC → durvalumab + tremelimumab Arm 2: durvalumab + EV → RC → durvalumab Arm 3: RC → +/– nivolumab	pCR and EFS
ICI + targeted therapy				
BLASST-2	NCT03773666	I	Durvalumab +/– Oleclumab	Feasibility
Johns Hopkins	NCT02845323	II	Nivolumab +/– Urelumab	Tumor-infiltrating CD8+ T cell density at cystectomy
PrE0807	NCT03532451	I	Nivolumab +/– Lirilumab	Number of participants with treatment-related adverse events as assessed by CTCAE V5.0
NEODURVARIB	NCT03534492	II	Durvalumab + Olaparib	pCR
ICI + chemotherapy				
RETAIN 2	NCT04506554	II	AMVAC + nivolumab	Two-year metastasis-free survival
NEMIO	NCT03549715	I/II	Durvalumab + ddMVAC +/– tremelimumab	pCR and grade ≥3 treatment-related toxicity rate

22.2.5 Biomarker Directed Therapy

With the advent of tumor genomic profiling, biomarkers of response to neoadjuvant chemotherapy have been identified and are prospectively being validated to guide treatment decisions following initial therapy. SWOG S1314 attempted to utilize a predictive gene expression model to generate a co-expression extrapolation (COXEN) score that would predict outcomes to either neoadjuvant gem/cis or ddMVAC. Of the 82 patients treated with gem/cis and 85 patients treated with ddMVAC, the proportion of pCR was comparable at 30% and 28% ($p = 0.75$), respectively, as well as the rate of pathological downstaging (40% in gem/cis versus 47% in ddMVAC, $p = 0.27$). In comparison to VESPER, all patients received 3–4 cycles of chemotherapy. The primary endpoint to evaluate treatment-specific COXEN scores as predictive of pCR or pathological downstaging was not met in either the gem/cis or ddMVAC groups. While this biomarker failed to identify responders, delayed or abandoned cystectomies and lack of sufficient patients who received protocol-defined chemotherapy limited the statistical power of the trial to detect the intended effect (Flaig et al. 2021).

Fibroblast Growth Factor Receptors (FGFRs) have recently emerged as targetable oncogenic drivers of bladder cancer. In particular, *FGFR3* gene rearrangements are common in bladder cancer. *FGFR3* mutations and fusions have been detected in 10–20% of MIBC patients, while FGFR3 overexpression has been reported in 40–50% of MIBC cases (Tomlinson et al. 2007). *FGFR3* activating genomic alterations were also detected more frequently in "luminal-papillary" UC subtypes, as identified by TCGA (Cancer Genome Atlas Research Network 2014). A recent study interrogated the AACR Project GENIE database, which contains >3000 samples from patients diagnosed with bladder cancer, and found that *FGFR3* mutations were mutually exclusive with mutations in *TP53* and *RB1*, but not with others, such as *ERBB2* and *KRAS* (Ascione et al. 2023). These findings suggest that selective tyrosine kinase inhibitors (TKI) may be an effective therapeutic approach for the treatment of *FGFR3* mutated MIBC. In 2019, the FDA granted accelerated approval to erdafitinib, a selective pan-FGFR TKI, for the treatment of locally advanced or metastatic bladder cancer with FGFR alterations following progression on two prior therapies (including an anti-PD-1/PD-L1) (Loriot et al. 2019). Erdafitnib gained full approval in 2024 for use in *FGFR3* mutated metastatic UC following the results of the phase III THOR study (NCT03390504), which demonstrated an improved OS of erdafitnib over chemotherapy (12.1% versus 7.8%; HR 0.64, $p = 0.005$) (Loriot et al. 2023). In MIBC, continuous intravesical delivery with the TAR-210 device is evaluating safety and efficacy. This "pretzel" shaped device provides local, continuous release of erdafitnib within the bladder and is being tested in a phase I study of recurrent non-MIBC and MIBC with *FGFR3/2* alterations (NCT05316155). Cohort 4 of this study will enroll cisplatin-ineligible patients with cT2–T3a MIBC pending radical cystectomy who were not treated with neoadjuvant therapy. The primary endpoint is safety and secondary endpoints include pharmacokinetics and response assessments (Vilaseca et al. 2023).

22.3 Adjuvant Treatment

22.3.1 Adjuvant Chemotherapy

While radical cystectomy and pelvic lymph node dissection can be curative in a substantial number of patients with localized MIBC, locoregional or distant disease recurrence postoperatively portends poor outcomes. For locally advanced MIBC, including those with pT3–T4 or lymph node involvement, the 5-year recurrence-free survival is 35–60% and overall survival is 25–50% (Stein et al. 2001; Sternberg et al. 2013). These low survival outcomes in locally advanced MIBC are thought to be due to occult micrometastases perioperatively that cannot be detected on imaging and often result in distant recurrences. Even though neoadjuvant cisplatin-based regimens have level 1 evidence in MIBC, due to an absolute survival increase of 5–7% and an increase in median survival of 3 years (Advanced Bladder Cancer Meta-analysis Collaboration 2003; Grossman et al. 2003), in many countries immediate cystectomy is preferred. As stage and lymph node status are known prognostic factors for progression and survival, patients at highest risk of recurrence can then be selected postoperatively for adjuvant treatment. Given the observed benefit of neoadjuvant therapy (Advanced Bladder Cancer Meta-analysis Collaboration 2003; Grossman et al. 2003), the survival advantage of adjuvant chemotherapy with cisplatin-based regimens was investigated and showed an improvement in outcomes. However, due to limitations in early studies, there is no consensus regarding which adjuvant regimens should be used clinically.

Initial studies evaluating adjuvant chemotherapy were plagued by issues in design and execution. An early study by Skinner et al. evaluated adjuvant cisplatin, doxorubicin, and cyclophosphamide after radical cystectomy and reported a delay in time to progression ($p = 0.001$) and increase in median survival of 1.9 years. However, the study failed to obey randomization and investigators modified the chemotherapy regimen being evaluated, rendering its data questionable (Skinner et al. 1991). Torti et al tested the utility of adjuvant MVAC following radical cystectomy. However, the study was closed early after only 55 patients were accrued, and no statistically significant impact on overall survival was identified (Freiha et al. 1996). As MIBC patients receiving adjuvant therapy are often elderly with comorbid conditions, overall survival can be confounded by death from other causes. Given the promising initial results seen with adjuvant cytotoxic therapy, additional studies were conducted and included disease-free survival (DFS) as a primary endpoint to capture the survival benefit of adjuvant treatment more accurately.

The Spanish Oncology Genito-Urinary Group 99/01 trial was one of the first randomized studies to demonstrate a survival advantage to adjuvant cisplatin-based chemotherapy. The study evaluated 4 cycles of paclitaxel, gemcitabine, cisplatin versus observation in patients with resected high-risk MIBC (pT3–4 and/or node-positive disease). While the study prematurely closed due to poor recruitment and was relatively underpowered, it did demonstrate an improvement in overall survival (HR 0.38; 95% CI 0.22–0.65; $p < 0.0009$) with a median follow-up of 30 months. This trial has only been reported in abstract form and the small sample size limits the robustness of these conclusions (Paz-Ares et al. 2010). Similarly, an Italian, phase III randomized clinical trial evaluating two different schedules of gemcitabine/cisplatin versus observation following cystectomy closed early due to slow accrual and then failed to show an improvement in overall survival ($p = 0.24$, HR 1.29, 95% CI 0.84–1.99] or disease-free survival ($p = 0.70$, HR 1.08, 95% CI 0.73–1.59) (Cognetti et al. 2012). A large phase III EORTC study 30994 that randomized 284 patients with pT3–T4 or node-positive disease after radical cystectomy demonstrated an improvement in progression-free survival (PFS). The study did not allow for neoadjuvant therapy. Patients were randomized to either immediate adjuvant cisplatin-based chemotherapy within 90 days of cystectomy or six cycles of deferred chemotherapy at relapse. However, this study like its predecessors was closed early due to poor accrual after 284 of the planned 660 patients had been included. After a median follow-up of 7 years, there was a trend toward an improvement in overall survival between immediate versus deferred adjuvant chemotherapy, although it did not meet statistical significance (HR 0.78; 95% CI 0.56–1.08; $p = 0.13$). The study did find that immediate treatment following surgery significantly prolonged 5-year PFS (HR 0.54, 95% CI 0.4–0.73, $p < 0.0001$). Exploratory analyses suggest that immediate adjuvant chemotherapy might lengthen survival in patients without lymph node involvement (5-year overall survival was 79.5% versus 59%, HR 0.37; 95% CI 0.16–0.83; $p = 0.012$), and not those with nodal involvement, which is counterintuitive to the expected results (Sternberg et al. 2015). Lastly, the POUT study was a phase III study that randomized patients with upper tract urothelial carcinoma to surveillance or four cycles of adjuvant platinum-based chemotherapy following surgical resection. The primary endpoint was 3-year DFS and the study closed early due to the impressive observed benefit. Updated results show an improved DFS with HR 0.48 (95% CI 0.33–0.71; $p = 0.0003$), but without overall survival benefit (HR 0.72, 95% CI 0.47–1.08; $p = 0.26$) (Birtle et al. 2020, 2021).

To extract meaningful data from the multitude of studies that have tested the utility of adjuvant chemotherapy, several systematic reviews and meta-analyses were conducted. Most recently, two large-scale meta-analyses have been published. In 2017, Kim et al. completed a meta-analysis using 11 randomized controlled trials comprising 1546 patients that evaluated adjuvant chemotherapy. Using a pairwise analysis to compare studies that used cystectomy followed by chemotherapy versus surgery alone, their meta-analysis showed a significantly improved PFS (HR 0.64; 95% CI, 0.49–0.85) and overall survival (HR 0.79; 95% CI, 0.68–0.92) with the use of adjuvant chemotherapy. Further, the study showed that the combination gemcitabine/cisplatin/paclitaxel was the only adjuvant regimen associated with significant improvement in both PFS (HR 0.38; 95% CI, 0.25–0.58) and overall survival (HR 0.38; 95% CI 0.22–0.65) (Kim et al. 2017). The most recent meta-analysis by the Advanced Bladder Cancer Meta-analysis Collaborators Group found similar results. Analysis of ten randomized control trials, comprising 1183 participants, found that cisplatin-based adjuvant chemotherapy demonstrated an overall survival benefit (HR 0.82, 95% CI 0.70–0.96, $p = 0.02$). This translates into an absolute improvement in survival of 6% at 5 years (increasing from 50 to 56%) and a 9% absolute benefit when adjusted for age, sex, tumor stage, and lymph node involvement. Adjuvant chemotherapy also improved recurrence-free survival (HR = 0.71, 95% CI = 0.60–0.83, $p < 0.001$) and metastasis-free survival (HR = 0.79, 95% CI = 0.65–0.95, $p = 0.01$) with absolute improvement in survival of 11% and 8%, respectively (Advanced Bladder Cancer Meta-analysis Collaborators Group 2022). Critics of this work have noted that the meta-analysis included heterogenous studies with poor accrual across a wide time frame.

While these large-scale database analyses suggest a survival advantage to adjuvant cisplatin-based chemotherapy, prospective randomized trials are needed to validate these findings and establish the optimal adjuvant regimen in MIBC patients. Given the varying results, National

Comprehensive Cancer Network (NCCN) guidelines currently recommend the use of adjuvant cisplatin-based regimens for patients with high-risk disease (pT3–T4, node positive, lymphovascular invasion) who did not receive neoadjuvant treatment.

22.3.2 Adjuvant Immunotherapy

Based on the conflicting data available for adjuvant chemotherapy and the challenges in timely administration of cisplatin-based regimens to patients recovering from surgery, the efficacy of ICI was assessed in the adjuvant setting.

Checkmate 274 was a randomized, double blind, phase III study that enrolled patients with high-risk MIBC after radical cystectomy to either nivolumab, administered every 2 weeks for up to 1 year, or placebo. The trial allowed patients to receive neoadjuvant cisplatin-based chemotherapy before randomization. The study defined patients with a high risk of recurrence as pT3–T3a or pN+ if they did not receive adjuvant cisplatin-based therapy and ypT2–T4a or ypN+ for patients who received neoadjuvant cisplatin. The primary endpoints were disease-free survival in all patients and in those with PD-L1 ≥ 1%. Following a median follow-up of 21 months in 709 patients, median disease-free survival was 20.8 months in the nivolumab arm (95% CI, 16.5–27.6) and 10.8 months in the placebo arm (95% CI, 8.3–13.9). At 6 months, 74.9% of nivolumab-treated patients and 60.3% of placebo-treated patients were alive and disease free (HR for disease recurrence or death 0.70, 98.2% CI 0.55–0.90; $p < 0.001$). Among the PD-L1-positive population, 74.5% of nivolumab-treated and 55.7% of placebo-treated patients were alive and disease free (hazard ratio for disease recurrence or death, 0.55; 98.72% CI, 0.35–0.85; $p < 0.001$). The benefit in disease-free survival with nivolumab was noted to be independent of PD-L1 status, nodal involvement, or use of neoadjuvant chemotherapy. As expected, grade 3 or higher treatment-related AEs occurred more frequently in the treatment arm (17.9% versus 7.2%) (Bajorin et al. 2021). Based on the results of this study, the FDA granted accelerated approval to nivolumab for the adjuvant therapy of MIBC at high risk of recurrence, irrespective of PD-L1 status. Overall survival data from this study are still maturing.

Adjuvant anti-PD-L1 treatment has also been evaluated. IMvigor010 was an open label, randomized, phase III study that evaluated adjuvant atezolizumab in patients with high-risk MIBC following radical surgery. Similar to the Checkmate 274 study, IMvigor010 allowed patients to receive neoadjuvant chemotherapy prior to enrolling and high-risk patients were defined as ypT2–T4a or ypN+ following neoadjuvant therapy or pT3–T4a or pN+ if no neoadjuvant therapy was administered. Patients were randomized to either atezolizumab given every 3 weeks for up to 1 year or observation. The primary endpoint was disease-free survival. The study enrolled 809 patients and median follow-up was 21.9 months. This study did not meet its primary endpoint as median disease-free survival was 19.4 months (95% CI 15.9–24.8) with atezolizumab and 16.6 months (95% CI 11.2–24.8) with observation (HR for disease recurrence or death 0.89, 95% CI 0.74–1.08; $p = 0.24$). In pre-specified subgroup analyses, PD-L1 status, primary malignancy stage, and lymph node involvement were not significantly associated with benefit from atezolizumab. The lack of treatment efficacy of atezolizumab, compared to nivolumab in Checkmate 274, could be attributed in part to the high rate of censoring in the observation arm and adverse events in the treatment arm leading to discontinuation. Twenty-point 5% of patients in the observation arm were censored due to withdrawal of consent, protocol violation/noncompliance, or loss to follow-up versus 8.2% in the treatment arm. Serious adverse events were noted in 31% of the atezolizumab arm, of which 39% of patients discontinued treatment, compared to 18% in the observation arm, of whom 44% of patients discontinued treatment (Bellmunt et al. 2021). Higher rates of withdrawal from the observation arm may lead to informative censoring where patients who come off study may have a greater likelihood of recurrence. This would lead to better DFS observed in the observation arm than would occur if all patients had been followed to document recurrence and may explain the lack of benefit seen in IMvigor010 as opposed to Checkmate 274 (Martini et al. 2022).

Several trials are currently underway to investigate the use of adjuvant ICI, a setting in which the benefit of adjuvant platinum-based chemotherapy is unclear. The AMBASSADOR study (NCT03244384) is a randomized phase III trial of pembrolizumab versus observation in patients with muscle invasive or locally advanced UC following surgery that is currently ongoing. Similar to previous trials, enrollment criteria include previous neoadjuvant therapy with ≥ pT2 and/or pN+ at surgery or in patients who are cisplatin-ineligible/refused adjuvant cisplatin have ≥ pT3 and/or pN+ at surgery. Patients were randomized to receive pembrolizumab every 3 weeks for 1 year or observation. The dual primary endpoints are disease-free survival (DFS) and overall survival. Numerous correlative studies are also planned (Apolo et al. 2019). At a pre-specified interim analysis, the study showed an improvement in DFS of 15 months with pembrolizumab compared to observation (HR 0.69; 95% CI 0.55–0.87; $p = 0.0013$). The trial's other dual primary endpoint of OS did not reach statistical significance at this time (The ASCO Post Staff 2024). Table 22.5 provides a list of additional ongoing studies evaluating the benefit of adjuvant ICI alone and in combination with other therapies.

Table 22.5 Ongoing studies of adjuvant ICI in MIBC

Trial name	NCT	Phase	Regimen	Primary endpoint
AMBASSADOR	NCT03244384	III	Arm A: Pembrolizumab Arm B: Observation	DFS and OS
IMvigor011	NCT04660344	III	Arm A: Atezolizumab in ctDNA-positive patients B: Observation in ctDNA-positive patients	DFS
PCR-MIB	NCT02662062	II	Single-arm pembrolizumab + concurrent cisplatin/radiation	Number of patients with grade 3 or 4 acute toxicities
KEYNOTE-992	NCT04241185	III	Arm A: pembrolizumab + chemotherapy (cisplatin or 5-FU or mitomycin) + RT (conventional or hypofractionated) Arm B: placebo + chemotherapy (cisplatin or 5-FU or mitomycin) + RT (conventional or hypofractionated)	Bladder intact EFS
DUART	NCT04249362	II	Cohort A: standard RT (prior to study entry) → durvalumab Cohort B: palliative RT (prior to study entry) → durvalumab	Safety/toxicity
ENERGIZE	NCT03661320	III	Arm A: gem/cis → RC → No adjuvant therapy Arm B: nivolumab + placebo + gem/cis → RC → nivolumab + placebo Arm C: nivolumab + IDO-inhibitor + gem/cis → RC → nivolumab + IDO-inhibitor	pCR and EFS
NIAGARA	NCT03732677	III	Arm A: durvalumab + gem/cis → RC → durvalumab Arm B: gem/cis → RC → No adjuvant therapy	pCR and EFS
KEYNOTE-866	NCT03924856	III	Arm A: pembrolizumab + gem/cis → RC → pembrolizumab Arm B: placebo + gem/cis → RC → placebo	EFS
SWOG 1806	NCT03775265	III	Arm I: RT + chemotherapy (gemcitabine, cisplatin, 5-FU, or mitomycin) Arm II: RT + chemotherapy (gemcitabine, cisplatin, 5-FU, or mitomycin) + atezolizumab	Bladder intact EFS

22.3.3 Adjuvant Antibody-Drug Conjugates

With the observed efficacy of Enfortumab vedotin (EV) in patients with locally advanced or metastatic urothelial cancer, numerous trials are currently evaluating EV as perioperative therapy in patients with MIBC. Cohort L of EV-103 (NCT03288545) is evaluating EV monotherapy in cisplatin-ineligible MIBC patients as perioperative therapy in which patients will receive three cycles of neoadjuvant EV and six cycles of adjuvant EV following radical cystectomy. The primary endpoint is pCR per central pathology review (Hoimes et al. 2022). Similarly, given the antitumor activity of EV in combination with pembrolizumab in patients with metastatic disease, this treatment paradigm is being investigated as perioperative management in two phase II studies, EV-303 (NCT03924895) and EV-304 (NCT04700124). Arm C of EV-303 will evaluate the efficacy and safety of perioperative EV and pembrolizumab followed by radical surgery in cisplatin-ineligible patients; EV-304 will compare perioperative EV and pembrolizumab to standard of care neoadjuvant gemcitabine/cisplatin. The primary endpoints for both studies are pCR and event-free survival (Hoimes et al. 2021).

When these studies (and others listed in Table 22.2) report their results, the management for perioperative treatment may shift to incorporate novel approaches.

22.4 Divergent Differentiation and Histological Subtypes

While the majority of conducted studies focus on the most common histologic subtype of bladder cancer, urothelial (transitional cell) carcinoma, at least 10–25% of bladder tumors harbor less common histological subtypes (Chalasani et al. 2009). These rare subtypes can offer unique diagnostic and therapeutic challenges as many trials typically exclude patients with greater than 50% rare histology. With the exception of squamous and glandular differentiation, having a rare subtype is generally considered an adverse risk feature. Although any single subtype is relatively rare, together they represent a significant subset of patients and must be considered in the optimal clinical management of patients with MIBC. Rare histologies can impact two critical treatment paradigms in MIBC: consideration of radiation therapy over radical cystectomy and utility of neoadjuvant chemotherapy.

Due to a lack of evidence, radical cystectomy is still recommended over radiation therapy for rare histological subtypes, other than small cell or squamous/glandular differentiation. A retrospective analysis from Massachusetts General Hospital investigating trimodality therapy in patients with rare subtypes found that less common histologies did not correlate with outcomes. In the series of 303 patients treated, 66 had an alternate subtype with 50 patients with squamous/glandular differentiation and 16 with other forms. Complete response rates after induction trimodality therapy did not differ between patients with pure and less common subtypes of urothelial carcinoma (Krasnow et al. 2017). These data suggest that patients with largely squamous or glandular components may have a similar prognosis with trimodality therapy as patients with urothelial histology.

A secondary analysis of the landmark Southwest Oncology Group 8710 trial found that patients with squamous and/or glandular differentiation benefit from neoadjuvant cisplatin-based chemotherapy. This study was a randomized trial of neoadjuvant MVAC followed by cystectomy versus cystectomy alone for treatment of locally advanced bladder cancer. Of the 295 patients randomized, 59 had tumors of non-urothelial subtypes, the vast majority of which were squamous and glandular histologies. The study found a survival benefit from neoadjuvant platinum-based chemotherapy in patients with rare histologies (HR 0.46, 95% CI 0.25–0.87; $p = 0.02$) (Scosyrev et al. 2011). Patients with squamous and glandular histology should not be excluded from receiving neoadjuvant platinum-based chemotherapy prior to radical cystectomy.

Small cell histology represents another well-characterized subtype and treatment algorithms for small cell carcinoma of the bladder are derived from the thoracic literature. As small cell carcinoma of the lung is highly chemosensitive, chemotherapy with cisplatin/etoposide is the mainstay of treatment of lung cancer and has been adopted in bladder cancer. The treatment paradigm for small cell bladder cancer is therefore primary chemotherapy with cisplatin (or carboplatin)/etoposide followed by radical surgery, or concurrent chemoradiation with cisplatin (or carboplatin) and etoposide. As small cell carcinoma metastasizes early and has a propensity to spread to the brain and bones, staging should include head imaging and a bone scan. There is not yet compelling evidence to suggest prophylactic whole-brain radiation, as is the standard in small cell carcinoma of the lung.

As treatment for MIBC advances, additional studies are needed to evaluate the benefit of novel therapies in rare subtypes. PURE-01, a single-arm study that investigated neoadjuvant pembrolizumab, included patients with less common subtypes and provides an indication into the relative benefit of immunotherapy in this patient population. Thirty-four of 114 patients had a component of rare histology and 19 had >50% rare subtype. A broad spectrum of subtypes was included, with squamous differentiation representing the majority. pCR was seen in 39% of patients with pure urothelial carcinoma, 53% of patients if a rare subtype included ≤50% of the tumor and 16% of patients if a rare subtype represented >50% of the tumor. Similarly, downstaging to ≤ypT1N0 was observed in 56% of pure urothelial carcinoma, 67% of patients if a rare subtype represented ≤50% of the tumor, and 42% of patients if a rare subtype represented >50% of the tumor. However, responses were only observed in patients with squamous differentiation or lymphoepithelioma-like subtype, with no responses seen in patients with other subtypes. Patients with squamous or lymphoepithelioma-like subtypes may display immunotherapy sensitivity due to their enrichment of cases with high tumor mutational burden and CPS scores (Necchi et al. 2020). Further studies are required to explore the role of immunotherapy in rare subtypes.

22.5 Summary

Treatment of MIBC is evolving rapidly. At this time, cisplatin-based chemotherapy with dose-dense MVAC or gemcitabine/cisplatin remains the standard of care in MIBC for patients who are candidates for neoadjuvant treatment. Radical cystectomy with pelvic lymph node dissection is the current recommendation for curative intent therapy; however, a bladder-sparing approach with trimodality therapy can be considered in appropriate patients. Adjuvant chemotherapy is frequently administered in cases of high-risk disease following cystectomy. Adjuvant immunotherapy is indicated in the USA after neoadjuvant chemotherapy for residual invasive or node-positive disease or in cases of extra-vesical disease without prior chemotherapy. Multiple studies are underway to challenge this paradigm to incorporate perioperative combinations of chemotherapy, immunotherapy, and antibody-drug conjugates.

As dramatic advances are made with novel therapies in the management of metastatic bladder cancer, many trials are now evaluating these treatments in earlier settings to increase the number of patients who may derive benefit and potential cure. We are encouraged by these ongoing studies that are exploring new perioperative approaches to the treatment of MIBC.

References

Advanced Bladder Cancer Meta-analysis Collaboration (2003) Neoadjuvant chemotherapy in invasive bladder cancer: a systematic review and meta-analysis. Lancet 361:1927–1934

Advanced Bladder Cancer Meta-analysis Collaborators Group (2022) Adjuvant chemotherapy for muscle-invasive bladder cancer: a systematic review and meta-analysis of individual participant data from randomised controlled trials. Eur Urol 81:50–61

Aminoltejari K, Black PC (2020) Radical cystectomy: a review of techniques, developments and controversies. Transl Androl Urol 9:3073–3081

Apolo AB, Rosenberg JE, Kim WY, Chen RC, Sonpavde G, Srinivas S, Mortazavi A, Watt C, Mallek M, Graap K, Diaz C, Odegaard M, Ballman KV, Morris MJ (2019) Alliance A031501: Phase III randomized adjuvant study of MK-3475 (pembrolizumab) in muscle-invasive and locally advanced urothelial carcinoma (MIBC) (AMBASSADOR) versus observation. J Clin Oncol 37:TPS504

Aragon-Ching JB, Werntz RP, Zietman AL, Steinberg GD (2018) Multidisciplinary management of muscle-invasive bladder cancer: current challenges and future directions. Am Soc Clin Oncol Educ Book 38:307–318

Ascione CM, Napolitano F, Esposito D, Servetto A, Belli S, Santaniello A, Scagliarini S, Crocetto F, Bianco R, Formisano L (2023) Role of FGFR3 in bladder cancer: Treatment landscape and future challenges. Cancer Treat Rev 115:102530

Bajorin DF, Witjes JA, Gschwend JE, Schenker M, Valderrama BP, Tomita Y, Bamias A, Lebret T, Shariat SF, Park SH, Ye D, Agerbaek M, Enting D, McDermott R, Gajate P, Peer A, Milowsky MI, Nosov A, Neif Antonio J Jr, Tupikowski K, Toms L, Fischer BS, Qureshi A, Collette S, Unsal-Kacmaz K, Broughton E, Zardavas D, Koon HB, Galsky MD (2021) Adjuvant nivolumab versus placebo in muscle-invasive urothelial carcinoma. N Engl J Med 384:2102–2114

Basile G, Bandini M, Gibb EA, Ross JS, Raggi D, Marandino L, Costa de Padua T, Crupi E, Colombo R, Colecchia M, Luciano R, Nocera L, Moschini M, Briganti A, Montorsi F, Necchi A (2022) Neoadjuvant pembrolizumab and radical cystectomy in patients with muscle-invasive urothelial bladder cancer: 3-year median follow-up update of PURE-01 trial. Clin Cancer Res 28:5107–5114

Bellmunt J, Hussain M, Gschwend JE, Albers P, Oudard S, Castellano D, Daneshmand S, Nishiyama H, Majchrowicz M, Degaonkar V, Shi Y, Mariathasan S, Grivas P, Drakaki A, O'Donnell PH, Rosenberg JE, Geynisman DM, Petrylak DP, Hoffman-Censits J, Bedke J, Kalebasty AR, Zakharia Y, van der Heijden MS, Sternberg CN, Davarpanah NN, Powles T, IMvigor010 Study Group (2021) Adjuvant atezolizumab versus observation in muscle-invasive urothelial carcinoma (IMvigor010): a multicentre, open-label, randomised, phase 3 trial. Lancet Oncol 22:525–537

Birtle A, Johnson M, Chester J, Jones R, Dolling D, Bryan RT, Harris C, Winterbottom A, Blacker A, Catto JWF, Chakraborti P, Donovan JL, Elliott PA, French A, Jagdev S, Jenkins B, Keeley FX Jr, Kockelbergh R, Powles T, Wagstaff J, Wilson C, Todd R, Lewis R, Hall E (2020) Adjuvant chemotherapy in upper tract urothelial carcinoma (the POUT trial): a phase 3, open-label, randomised controlled trial. Lancet 395:1268–1277

Birtle AJ, Chester JD, Jones RJ, Jenkins B, Johnson M, Catto JWF, Powles T, Bryan RT, Blacker A, Chakraborti PR, Jagdev S, Wagstaff J, Tolentino A, Webster L, Lewis R, Hall E (2021) Updated outcomes of POUT: A phase III randomized trial of perioperative chemotherapy versus surveillance in upper tract urothelial cancer (UTUC). J Clin Oncol 39:455

Bochner BH, Dalbagni G, Sjoberg DD, Silberstein J, Keren Paz GE, Donat SM, Coleman JA, Mathew S, Vickers A, Schnorr GC, Feuerstein MA, Rapkin B, Parra RO, Herr HW, Laudone VP (2015) Comparing open radical cystectomy and robot-assisted laparoscopic radical cystectomy: a randomized clinical trial. Eur Urol 67:1042–1050

Brown J, Kaimakliotis HZ, Kelly WK, Ammons V, Picus J, Walling R, Hashemi-Sadraei N, Pingfu Fu, Margevicius SP, Adra N, Garcia JA, McKay RR, Hoimes CJ (2023) HCRN GU14-188: Phase Ib/II study of neoadjuvant pembrolizumab and chemotherapy for T2-4aN0M0 urothelial cancer. J Clin Oncol 41:448–448

Cancer Genome Atlas Research Network (2014) Comprehensive molecular characterization of urothelial bladder carcinoma. Nature 507:315–322

Carthon BC, Wolchok JD, Yuan J, Kamat A, Ng Tang DS, Sun J, Ku G, Troncoso P, Logothetis CJ, Allison JP, Sharma P (2010) Preoperative CTLA-4 blockade: tolerability and immune monitoring in the setting of a presurgical clinical trial. Clin Cancer Res 16:2861–2871

Cathomas R, Rothschild S, Hayoz S, Spahn M, Schardt J, Seiler R, Erdmann A, Aeppli S, Mach N, Strebel R, Hadaschik BA, Berthold DR, Pless M, Zihler D, Schmid M, Schneider M, Maniecka Z, Petrausch U (2021) Safety and efficacy of perioperative cisplatin/gemcitabine (cis/gem) and durvalumab (durva) for operable muscle-invasive urothelial carcinoma (MIUC): SAKK 06/17. J Clin Oncol 39:430–430

Chalasani V, Chin JL, Izawa JI (2009) Histologic variants of urothelial bladder cancer and nonurothelial histology in bladder cancer. Can Urol Assoc J 3:S193–S198

Chang SS, Bochner BH, Chou R, Dreicer R, Kamat AM, Lerner SP, Lotan Y, Meeks JJ, Michalski JM, Morgan TM, Quale DZ, Rosenberg JE, Zietman AL, Holzbeierlein JM (2017) Treatment of non-metastatic muscle-invasive bladder cancer: AUA/ASCO/ASTRO/SUO guideline. J Urol 198:552–559

Choudhury A, Swindell R, Logue JP, Anthony Elliott P, Livsey JE, Wise M, Symonds P, Wylie JP, Ramani V, Sangar V, Lyons J, Bottomley I, McCaul D, Clarke NW, Kiltie AE, Cowan RA (2011) Phase II study of conformal hypofractionated radiotherapy with concurrent gemcitabine in muscle-invasive bladder cancer. J Clin Oncol 29:733–738

Choueiri TK, Jacobus S, Bellmunt J, Qu A, Appleman LJ, Tretter C, Bubley GJ, Stack EC, Signoretti S, Walsh M, Steele G, Hirsch M, Sweeney CJ, Taplin ME, Kibel AS, Krajewski KM, Kantoff PW, Ross RW, Rosenberg JE (2014) Neoadjuvant dose-dense methotrexate, vinblastine, doxorubicin, and cisplatin with pegfilgrastim support in muscle-invasive urothelial cancer: pathologic, radiologic, and biomarker correlates. J Clin Oncol 32:1889–1894

Coen JJ, Zhang P, Saylor PJ, Lee CT, Wu CL, Parker W, Lautenschlaeger T, Zietman AL, Efstathiou JA, Jani AB, Kucuk O, Souhami L, Rodgers JP, Sandler HM, Shipley WU (2019) Bladder preservation with twice-a-day radiation plus fluorouracil/cisplatin or once daily radiation plus gemcitabine for muscle-invasive bladder cancer: NRG/RTOG 0712-a randomized phase II trial. J Clin Oncol 37:44–51

Cognetti F, Ruggeri EM, Felici A, Gallucci M, Muto G, Pollera CF, Massidda B, Rubagotti A, Giannarelli D, Boccardo F, Group Study (2012) Adjuvant chemotherapy with cisplatin and gemcitabine versus chemotherapy at relapse in patients with muscle-invasive bladder cancer submitted to radical cystectomy: an Italian, multicenter, randomized phase III trial. Ann Oncol 23:695–700

Dash A, Pettus JA 4th, Herr HW, Bochner BH, Dalbagni G, Donat SM, Russo P, Boyle MG, Milowsky MI, Bajorin DF (2008) A role for neoadjuvant gemcitabine plus cisplatin in muscle-invasive urothelial carcinoma of the bladder: a retrospective experience. Cancer 113:2471–2477

Dhar NB, Klein EA, Reuther AM, Thalmann GN, Madersbacher S, Studer UE (2008) Outcome after radical cystectomy with limited or extended pelvic lymph node dissection. J Urol 179:873–878. Discussion 78

EAU Guidelines (2024) Edn. presented at the EAU annual congress Paris 2024. ISBN 978-94-92671-23-3

Efstathiou JA, Spiegel DY, Shipley WU, Heney NM, Kaufman DS, Niemierko A, Coen JJ, Skowronski RY, Paly JJ, McGovern FJ, Zietman AL (2012) Long-term outcomes of selective bladder preservation by combined-modality therapy for invasive bladder cancer: the MGH experience. Eur Urol 61:705–711

Flaig TW, Tangen CM, Daneshmand S, Alva A, Lerner SP, Lucia MS, McConkey DJ, Theodorescu D, Goldkorn A, Milowsky MI, Bangs R, MacVicar GR, Bastos BR, Fowles JS, Gustafson DL, Plets M, Thompson IM Jr (2021) A randomized phase II study of coexpression extrapolation (COXEN) with neoadjuvant chemotherapy for bladder cancer (SWOG S1314; NCT02177695). Clin Cancer Res 27:2435–2441

Flaig TW, Rosenberg JE, Hoimes CJ, O'Donnell PH, Mar N, Gourdin TS, Henry S, Bilen MA, George S, Barata PC, Srinivas S, Rao SK, Assikis VJ, Burgess EF, Ramamurthy C, Haas GP, Lukas JJ, Mildiner-Earley S, Yao Y, Petrylak DP (2023) Study EV-103: neoadjuvant treatment with enfortumab vedotin monotherapy in cisplatin-ineligible patients (pts) with muscle invasive bladder cancer (MIBC): Updated results for Cohort H. J Clin Oncol 41:4595

Freiha F, Reese J, Torti FM (1996) A randomized trial of radical cystectomy versus radical cystectomy plus cisplatin, vinblastine and methotrexate chemotherapy for muscle invasive bladder cancer. J Urol 155:495–499. Discussion 99–500

Fung CY, Shipley WU, Young RH, Griffin PP, Convery KM, Kaufman DS, Althausen AF, Heney NM, Prout GR Jr (1991) Prognostic factors in invasive bladder carcinoma in a prospective trial of preoperative adjuvant chemotherapy and radiotherapy. J Clin Oncol 9:1533–1542

Funt SA, Lattanzi M, Whiting K, Al-Ahmadie H, Quinlan C, Teo MY, Lee CH, Aggen D, Zimmerman D, McHugh D, Apollo A, Durdin TD, Truong H, Kamradt J, Khalil M, Lash B, Ostrovnaya I, McCoy AS, Hettich G, Regazzi A, Jihad M, Ratna N, Boswell A, Francese K, Yang Y, Folefac E, Herr HW, Donat SM, Pietzak E, Cha EK, Donahue TF, Goh AC, Huang WC, Bajorin DF, Iyer G, Bochner BH, Balar AV, Mortazavi A, Rosenberg JE (2022) Neoadjuvant atezolizumab with gemcitabine and cisplatin in patients with muscle-invasive bladder cancer: a multicenter, single-arm, phase II trial. J Clin Oncol 40:1312–1322

Gao J, Siefker-Radtke AO, Navai N, Campbell MT, Tidwell RS, Guo C, Kamat AM, Matin SF, Araujo JC, Shah AY, Msaouel P, Blando JM, Vence LM, Duan F, Basu S, Singh S, Zhao H, Allison JP, Dinney CPN, Sharma P (2019) A pilot presurgical study evaluating anti-PD-L1 durvalumab (durva) plus anti-CTLA-4 tremelimumab (treme) in patients (pts) with high-risk muscle-invasive bladder carcinoma (MIBC) who are ineligible for cisplatin-based neoadjuvant chemotherapy (NAC). J Clin Oncol 37:4551

Grande E, Guerrero F, Puente J, Galante I, Duran I, Dominguez M, Gordoa TA, Burgos J, Font A, Pinto A, Alvarez-Maestro M, Reig O, Maroto J, del Muro XG, Galvan P, Garcia JF, Malats N, Prat A, Real FX, Castellano D (2020) DUTRENEO trial: A randomized phase II trial of DUrvalumab and TREmelimumab versus chemotherapy as a NEOadjuvant approach to muscle-invasive urothelial bladder cancer (MIBC) patients (pts) prospectively selected by an interferon (INF)-gamma immune signature. J Clin Oncol 38:5012

Grossman HB, Natale RB, Tangen CM, Speights VO, Vogelzang NJ, Trump DL, deVere White RW, Sarosdy MF, Wood DP Jr, Raghavan D, Crawford ED (2003) Neoadjuvant chemotherapy plus cystectomy compared with cystectomy alone for locally advanced bladder cancer. N Engl J Med 349:859–866

Gupta S, Sonpavde G, Weight CJ, McGregor BA, Gupta S, Maughan BL, Wei XX, Gibb E, Thyagarajan B, Einstein DJ, Dechet CB, Lowrance WT, Murugan PJ, Kilbridge KL, Agarwal N, Davicioni E, Eckstein M, Mossanen M, Preston MA, Konety BR (2020) Results from BLASST-1 (Bladder Cancer Signal Seeking Trial) of nivolumab, gemcitabine, and cisplatin in muscle invasive bladder cancer (MIBC) undergoing cystectomy. J Clin Oncol 38:439

Hamid A, Ridwan FR, Parikesit D, Widia F, Mochtar CA, Umbas R (2020) Meta-analysis of neoadjuvant chemotherapy compared to radical cystectomy alone in improving overall survival of muscle-invasive bladder cancer patients. BMC Urol 20:158

Hoimes CJ, Adra N, Fleming MT, Kaimakliotis HZ, Picus J, Smith ZL, Walling R, Trabulsi EJ, Hoffman-Censits JH, Koch MO, Cary C, Abouassaly R, Eitman C, Pingfu F, Goolamier G, Calaway AC, Ponsky LE, Kelly WK (2020) Phase Ib/II neoadjuvant (N-) pembrolizumab (P) and chemotherapy for locally advanced urothelial cancer (laUC): Final results from the cisplatin (C)-eligible cohort of HCRN GU14-188. J Clin Oncol 38:5047

Hoimes CJ, Bedke J, Loriot Y, Nishiyama H, Fang X, Kataria RS, Moreno BH, Galsky MD (2021) KEYNOTE-B15/EV-304: Randomized phase 3 study of perioperative enfortumab vedotin plus pembrolizumab versus chemotherapy in cisplatin-eligible patients with muscle-invasive bladder cancer (MIBC). J Clin Oncol 39:TPS4587

Hoimes CJ, Flaig TW, Srinivas S, Mar N, Petrylak DP, O'Donnell PH, Bilen MA, Sasse C, Yao Y, Birrenkott M, Rosenberg JE (2022) Study EV-103 cohort L: Evaluating perioperative enfortumab vedotin monotherapy in cis-ineligible muscle invasive bladder cancer (MIBC) (trial in progress). J Clin Oncol 40:TPS587

International Collaboration of Trialists, Party Medical Research Council Advanced Bladder Cancer Working, Research European Organisation for, Group Treatment of Cancer Genito-Urinary Tract Cancer, Group Australian Bladder Cancer Study, Group National Cancer Institute of Canada Clinical Trials, Finnbladder, Group Norwegian Bladder Cancer Study, Group Club Urologico Espanol de Tratamiento Oncologico, Griffiths G, Hall R, Sylvester R, Raghavan D, Parmar MK (2011) International phase III trial assessing neoadjuvant cisplatin, methotrexate, and vinblastine chemotherapy for muscle-invasive bladder cancer: long-term results of the BA06 30894 trial. J Clin Oncol 29:2171–2177

James ND, Hussain SA, Hall E, Jenkins P, Tremlett J, Rawlings C, Crundwell M, Sizer B, Sreenivasan T, Hendron C, Lewis R, Waters R, Huddart RA, BC2001 Investigators (2012) Radiotherapy with or without chemotherapy in muscle-invasive bladder cancer. N Engl J Med 366:1477–1488

Kaufman DS, Winter KA, Shipley WU, Heney NM, Chetner MP, Souhami L, Zlotecki RA, Sause WT, True LD (2000) The initial results in muscle-invading bladder cancer of RTOG 95-06: phase I/II trial of transurethral surgery plus radiation therapy with concurrent cisplatin and 5-fluorouracil followed by selective bladder preservation or cystectomy depending on the initial response. Oncologist 5:471–476

Kaufman DS, Winter KA, Shipley WU, Heney NM, Wallace HJ 3rd, Toonkel LM, Zietman AL, Tanguay S, Sandler HM (2009) Phase I-II RTOG study (99-06) of patients with muscle-invasive bladder cancer undergoing transurethral surgery, paclitaxel, cisplatin, and twice-daily radiotherapy followed by selective bladder preservation or radical cystectomy and adjuvant chemotherapy. Urology 73:833–837

Khan MS, Gan C, Ahmed K, Ismail AF, Watkins J, Summers JA, Peacock JL, Rimington P, Dasgupta P (2016) A single-centre early phase randomised controlled three-arm trial of open, robotic, and laparoscopic radical cystectomy (CORAL). Eur Urol 69:613–621

Kim HS, Jeong CW, Kwak C, Kim HH, Ku JH (2017) Adjuvant chemotherapy for muscle-invasive bladder cancer: a systematic review and network meta-analysis of randomized clinical trials. Oncotarget 8:81204–81214

Krasnow RE, Drumm M, Roberts HJ, Niemierko A, Wu CL, Wu S, Zhang J, Heney NM, Wszolek MF, Blute ML, Feldman AS, Lee RJ, Zietman AL, Shipley WU, Efstathiou JA (2017) Clinical outcomes of patients with histologic variants of urothelial cancer treated with trimodality bladder-sparing therapy. Eur Urol 72:54–60

Lerner SP, Tangen C, Svatek RS, Daneshmand S, Pohar KS, Skinner EC, Schuckman AK, Sagalowsky AI, Smith ND, Kamat AM, Kassouf W, Plets M, Bangs R, Koppie TM, Alva AS, La Rosa FG, Pal SK, Kibel AS, Canter D, Thompson IM (2023) SWOG S1011: A phase III surgical trial to evaluate the benefit of a standard versus an extended lymphadenectomy performed at time of radical cystectomy for muscle invasive urothelial cancer. J Clin Oncol 41:4508

Loriot Y, Necchi A, Park SH, Garcia-Donas J, Huddart R, Burgess E, Fleming M, Rezazadeh A, Mellado B, Varlamov S, Joshi M, Duran I, Tagawa ST, Zakharia Y, Zhong B, Stuyckens K, Santiago-Walker A, De Porre P, O'Hagan A, Avadhani A, Siefker-Radtke AO, B. L. C. Study Group (2019) Erdafitinib in locally advanced or metastatic urothelial carcinoma. N Engl J Med 381:338–348

Loriot Y, Matsubara N, Park SH, Huddart RA, Burgess EF, Houede N, Banek S, Guadalupi V, Ku JH, Valderrama BP, Tran B, Triantos S, Kean Y, Akapame S, Deprince K, Mukhopadhyay S, Stone NL, Siefker-Radtke AO, Thor Cohort 1 Investigators (2023) Erdafitinib or chemotherapy in advanced or metastatic urothelial carcinoma. N Engl J Med 389:1961–1971

Mak RH, Hunt D, Shipley WU, Efstathiou JA, Tester WJ, Hagan MP, Kaufman DS, Heney NM, Zietman AL (2014) Long-term outcomes in patients with muscle-invasive bladder cancer after selective bladder-preserving combined-modality therapy: a pooled analysis of Radiation Therapy Oncology Group protocols 8802, 8903, 9506, 9706, 9906, and 0233. J Clin Oncol 32:3801–3809

Martini A, Yu M, Raggi D, Joshi H, Fallara G, Montorsi F, Necchi A, Galsky MD (2022) Adjuvant immunotherapy in patients with high-risk muscle-invasive urothelial carcinoma: The potential impact of informative censoring. Cancer 128:2892–2897

Milosevic M, Gospodarowicz M, Zietman A, Abbas F, Haustermans K, Moonen L, Rodel C, Schoenberg M, Shipley W (2007) Radiotherapy for bladder cancer. Urology 69:80–92

Necchi A, Anichini A, Raggi D, Briganti A, Massa S, Luciano R, Colecchia M, Giannatempo P, Mortarini R, Bianchi M, Fare E, Monopoli F, Colombo R, Gallina A, Salonia A, Messina A, Ali SM, Madison R, Ross JS, Chung JH, Salvioni R, Mariani L, Montorsi F (2018) Pembrolizumab as neoadjuvant therapy before radical cystectomy in patients with muscle-invasive urothelial bladder carcinoma (PURE-01): an open-label, single-arm, phase II study. J Clin Oncol 36:3353–3360

Necchi A, Raggi D, Gallina A, Madison R, Colecchia M, Luciano R, Montironi R, Giannatempo P, Fare E, Pederzoli F, Bandini M, Bianchi M, Colombo R, Gandaglia G, Fossati N, Marandino L, Capitanio U, Deho F, Ali SM, Chung JH, Ross JS, Salonia A, Briganti A, Montorsi F (2020) Updated results of

PURE-01 with preliminary activity of neoadjuvant pembrolizumab in patients with muscle-invasive bladder carcinoma with variant histologies. Eur Urol 77:439–446

Necchi A, Bedke J, Galsky MD, Shore ND, Plimack ER, Xylinas E, Jia C, Hennika T, Moreno BH, Witjes AA (2023) Phase 3 KEYNOTE-905/EV-303: Perioperative pembrolizumab (pembro) or pembro + enfortumab vedotin (EV) for muscle-invasive bladder cancer (MIBC). J Clin Oncol 41:TPS585

O'Donnell PH, Milowsky MI, Petrylak DP, Hoimes CJ, Flaig TW, Mar N, Moon HH, Friedlander TW, McKay RR, Bilen MA, Srinivas S, Burgess EF, Ramamurthy C, George S, Geynisman DM, Bracarda S, Borchiellini D, Geoffrois L, Maroto Rey JP, Ferrario C, Carret AS, Yu Y, Guseva M, Homet Moreno B, Rosenberg JE (2023) Enfortumab vedotin with or without pembrolizumab in cisplatin-ineligible patients with previously untreated locally advanced or metastatic urothelial cancer. J Clin Oncol 41:4107–4117

Parekh DJ, Reis IM, Castle EP, Gonzalgo ML, Woods ME, Svatek RS, Weizer AZ, Konety BR, Tollefson M, Krupski TL, Smith ND, Shabsigh A, Barocas DA, Quek ML, Dash A, Kibel AS, Shemanski L, Pruthi RS, Montgomery JS, Weight CJ, Sharp DS, Chang SS, Cookson MS, Gupta GN, Gorbonos A, Uchio EM, Skinner E, Venkatramani V, Soodana-Prakash N, Kendrick K, Smith JA Jr, Thompson IM (2018) Robot-assisted radical cystectomy versus open radical cystectomy in patients with bladder cancer (RAZOR): an open-label, randomised, phase 3, non-inferiority trial. Lancet 391:2525–2536

Park J, Jeong H (2018) Morbidity, mortality, and survival for radical cystectomy. In: Ku JH (ed) Bladder cancer. Elsevier

Paz-Ares LG, Solsona E, Esteban E, Saez A, Gonzalez-Larriba J, Anton A, Hevia M, de la Rosa F, Guillem V, Bellmunt J (2010) Randomized phase III trial comparing adjuvant paclitaxel/gemcitabine/cisplatin (PGC) to observation in patients with resected invasive bladder cancer: Results of the Spanish Oncology Genitourinary Group (SOGUG) 99/01 study. J Clin Oncol 28:LBA4518

Pfister C, Gravis G, Flechon A, Chevreau C, Mahammedi H, Laguerre B, Guillot A, Joly F, Soulie M, Allory Y, Harter V, Culine S, Vesper Trial Investigators (2022) Dose-dense methotrexate, vinblastine, doxorubicin, and cisplatin or gemcitabine and cisplatin as perioperative chemotherapy for patients with nonmetastatic muscle-invasive bladder cancer: results of the GETUG-AFU V05 VESPER trial. J Clin Oncol 40:2013–2022

Plimack ER, Hoffman-Censits JH, Viterbo R, Trabulsi EJ, Ross EA, Greenberg RE, Chen DY, Lallas CD, Wong YN, Lin J, Kutikov A, Dotan E, Brennan TA, Palma N, Dulaimi E, Mehrazin R, Boorjian SA, Kelly WK, Uzzo RG, Hudes GR (2014) Accelerated methotrexate, vinblastine, doxorubicin, and cisplatin is safe, effective, and efficient neoadjuvant treatment for muscle-invasive bladder cancer: results of a multicenter phase II study with molecular correlates of response and toxicity. J Clin Oncol 32:1895–1901

Powles T, Kockx M, Rodriguez-Vida A, Duran I, Crabb SJ, Van Der Heijden MS, Szabados B, Pous AF, Gravis G, Herranz UA, Protheroe A, Ravaud A, Maillet D, Mendez MJ, Suarez C, Linch M, Prendergast A, van Dam PJ, Stanoeva D, Daelemans S, Mariathasan S, Tea JS, Mousa K, Banchereau R, Castellano D (2019) Clinical efficacy and biomarker analysis of neoadjuvant atezolizumab in operable urothelial carcinoma in the ABACUS trial. Nat Med 25:1706–1714

Powles T, Rosenberg JE, Sonpavde GP, Loriot Y, Duran I, Lee JL, Matsubara N, Vulsteke C, Castellano D, Wu C, Campbell M, Matsangou M, Petrylak DP (2021) Enfortumab vedotin in previously treated advanced urothelial carcinoma. N Engl J Med 384:1125–1135

Powles T, Drakaki A, Teoh JY-C, Grande E, Fontes-Sousa M, Porta C, Esther W, Goluboff ET, Ho S, Hois S, Gupta AK, Catto JWF (2022) A phase 3, randomized, open-label, multicenter, global study of the efficacy and safety of durvalumab (D) + tremelimumab (T) + enfortumab vedotin (EV) or D + EV for neoadjuvant treatment in cisplatin-ineligible muscle-invasive bladder cancer (MIBC) (VOLGA). J Clin Oncol 40:TPS579

Rai BP, Bondad J, Vasdev N, Adshead J, Lane T, Ahmed K, Khan MS, Dasgupta P, Guru K, Chlosta PL, Aboumarzouk OM (2019) Robotic versus open radical cystectomy for bladder cancer in adults. Cochrane Database Syst Rev 4:CD011903

Rödel C, Grabenbauer GG, Kühn R, Papadopoulos T, Dunst J, Meyer M, Schrott KM, Sauer R (2002) Combined-modality treatment and selective organ preservation in invasive bladder cancer: long-term results. J Clin Oncol 20:3061–3071

Rose TL, Harrison MR, Deal AM, Ramalingam S, Whang YE, Brower B, Dunn M, Osterman CK, Heiling HM, Bjurlin MA, Smith AB, Nielsen ME, Tan H-J, Wallen E, Woods ME, George D, Zhang T, Drier A, Kim WY, Milowsky MI (2021) Phase II study of gemcitabine and split-dose cisplatin plus pembrolizumab as neoadjuvant therapy before radical cystectomy in patients with muscle-invasive bladder cancer. J Clin Oncol 39:3140–3148

Rosenberg J, Sridhar SS, Zhang J, Smith D, Ruether D, Flaig TW, Baranda J, Lang J, Plimack ER, Sangha R, Heath EI, Merchan J, Quinn DI, Srinivas S, Milowsky M, Wu C, Gartner EM, Zuo P, Melhem-Bertrandt A, Petrylak DP (2020) EV-101: a phase I study of single-agent enfortumab vedotin in patients with nectin-4-positive solid tumors, including metastatic urothelial carcinoma. J Clin Oncol 38:1041–1049

Sanderson KM, Skinner D, Stein JP (2006) The prognostic and staging value of lymph node dissection in the treatment of invasive bladder cancer. Nat Clin Pract Urol 3:485–494

Scosyrev E, Ely BW, Messing EM, Speights VO, Grossman HB, Wood DP, de Vere White RW, Vogelzang NJ, Trump DL, Natale RB, Tangen CM, Crawford ED, Thompson IM (2011) Do mixed histological features affect survival benefit from neoadjuvant platinum-based combination chemotherapy in patients with locally advanced bladder cancer? A secondary analysis of Southwest Oncology Group-Directed Intergroup Study (S8710). BJU Int 108:693–699

Shahab N (1999) Bladder preservation trial: Radiation Therapy Oncology Group 89-03. J Clin Oncol 17:1327–1328

Singh P, Tangen C, Efstathiou JA, Lerner SP, Jhavar SG, Hahn NM, Costello BA, Sridhar SS, Weliang D, Meeks JJ, Faltas BM, Grivas P, Feng FY, Chen RC, Morgans AK, Gupta A, Bangs RC, Winter KA, Vogelzang NJ, Thompson IM (2020) INTACT: Phase III randomized trial of concurrent chemoradiotherapy with or without atezolizumab in localized muscle invasive bladder cancer—SWOG/NRG1806. J Clin Oncol 38:TPS586

Skinner DG, Daniels JR, Russell CA, Lieskovsky G, Boyd SD, Nichols P, Kern W, Sakamoto J, Krailo M, Groshen S (1991) The role of adjuvant chemotherapy following cystectomy for invasive bladder cancer: a prospective comparative trial. J Urol 145:459–464. Discussion 64–7

Stein JP, Lieskovsky G, Cote R, Groshen S, Feng AC, Boyd S, Skinner E, Bochner B, Thangathurai D, Mikhail M, Raghavan D, Skinner DG (2001) Radical cystectomy in the treatment of invasive bladder cancer: long-term results in 1,054 patients. J Clin Oncol 19:666–675

Sternberg CN, de Mulder PHM, Schornagel JH, Theodore C, Fossa SD, van Oosterom AT, Witjes F, Spina M, van Groeningen CJ, de Balincourt C, Collette L (2005) Seven year update of an EORTC phase III trial of high dose intensity M-VAC chemotherapy and G-CSF versus classic M-VAC in advanced urothelial tract tumors. J Clin Oncol 23:4528

Sternberg CN, Bellmunt J, Sonpavde G, Siefker-Radtke AO, Stadler WM, Bajorin DF, Dreicer R, George DJ, Milowsky MI, Theodorescu D, Vaughn DJ, Galsky MD, Soloway MS, Quinn DI, Cancer International Consultation on Urologic Disease-European Association of Urology Consultation on Bladder (2013) ICUD-EAU international consultation on bladder cancer 2012: chemotherapy for urothelial carcinoma-neoadjuvant and adjuvant settings. Eur Urol 63:58–66

Sternberg CN, Skoneczna I, Kerst JM, Albers P, Fossa SD, Agerbaek M, Dumez H, de Santis M, Theodore C, Leahy MG, Chester JD, Verbaeys A, Daugaard G, Wood L, Witjes JA, de Wit R, Geoffrois L, Sengelov L, Thalmann G, Charpentier D, Rolland F, Mignot L, Sundar S, Symonds P, Graham J, Joly F, Marreaud S, Collette L, Sylvester R, Research European Organisation for, Group Treatment of Cancer Genito-Urinary Cancers, Urogenitales Groupe d'Etude des Tumeurs, Group National Cancer Research Institute Bladder Cancer Study, Group National Cancer Institute of Canada Clinical Trials, and Oncology German Association of Urologic (2015) Immediate versus deferred chemotherapy after radical cystectomy in patients with pT3-pT4 or N+ M0 urothelial carcinoma of the bladder (EORTC 30994): an intergroup, open-label, randomised phase 3 trial. Lancet Oncol 16:76–86

Tester W, Caplan R, Heaney J, Venner P, Whittington R, Byhardt R, True L, Shipley W (1996) Neoadjuvant combined modality program with selective organ preservation for invasive bladder cancer: results of Radiation Therapy Oncology Group phase II trial 8802. J Clin Oncol 14:119–126

The ASCO Post Staff (2024) AMBASSADOR: pembrolizumab in muscle-invasive and locally advanced urothelial carcinoma. https://ascopost.com/news/january-2024/ambassador-pembrolizumab-in-muscle-invasive-and-locally-advanced-urothelial-carcinoma/#:~:text=AMBASSADOR%20(A031501)%20is%20a%20randomized,and%20locally%20advanced%20urothelial%20carcinoma

Tomlinson DC, Baldo O, Harnden P, Knowles MA (2007) FGFR3 protein expression and its relationship to mutation status and prognostic variables in bladder cancer. J Pathol 213:91–98

van Dijk N, Gil-Jimenez A, Silina K, Hendricksen K, Smit LA, de Feijter JM, van Montfoort ML, van Rooijen C, Peters D, Broeks A, van der Poel HG, Bruining A, Lubeck Y, Sikorska K, Boellaard TN, Kvistborg P, Vis DJ, Hooijberg E, Schumacher TN, van den Broek M, Wessels LFA, Blank CU, van Rhijn BW, van der Heijden MS (2020) Preoperative ipilimumab plus nivolumab in locoregionally advanced urothelial cancer: the NABUCCO trial. Nat Med 26:1839–1844

Vilaseca A, Guerrero F, Zainfeld D, Shore ND, Faba OR, Meijer RP, Witjes JA, Mcree AJ, Kalota A, Stone NL, Lauring JD, Zhu W, Beeharry N, O'Dondi LA, Jayram G (2023) Safety and efficacy of the erdafitinib (erda) intravesical delivery system, TAR-210, in patients (pts) with non-muscle-invasive bladder cancer (NMIBC) or muscle-invasive bladder cancer (MIBC) harboring select FGFR mutations or fusions: Phase 1 first-in-human study. J Clin Oncol 41(6, suppl):TPS583

Witjes JA, Bruins HM, Carrion A, Cathomas R, Comperat E, Efstathiou JA, Fietkau R, Gakis G, Lorch A, Martini A, Mertens LS, Meijer RP, Milowsky MI, Neuzillet Y, Panebianco V, Redlef J, Rink M, Rouanne M, Thalmann GN, Saebjornsen S, Veskimae E, van der Heijden AG (2023) European Association of Urology guidelines on muscle-invasive and metastatic bladder cancer: summary of the 2023 guidelines. Eur Urol 85:17–31

Zlotta AR, Ballas LK, Niemierko A, Lajkosz K, Kuk C, Miranda G, Drumm M, Mari A, Thio E, Fleshner NE, Kulkarni GS, Jewett MAS, Bristow RG, Catton C, Berlin A, Sridhar SS, Schuckman A, Feldman AS, Wszolek M, Dahl DM, Lee RJ, Saylor PJ, Michaelson MD, Miyamoto DT, Zietman A, Shipley W, Chung P, Daneshmand S, Efstathiou JA (2023) Radical cystectomy versus trimodality therapy for muscle-invasive bladder cancer: a multi-institutional propensity score matched and weighted analysis. Lancet Oncol 24:669–681

Targeting the Immune Checkpoint in Bladder Cancer

23

Chiara Mercinelli, Valentina Tateo, Emanuele Crupi, Antonio Cigliola, and Andrea Necchi

Abstract

The introduction of immune checkpoint inhibitors (ICIs) has revolutionized the therapeutic landscape of urothelial cancer (UC). Many treatment approaches in different settings are being investigated to harness the immune system. Novel combination strategies are emerging with promising results, offering potential synergistic effects and improved treatment outcomes. However, challenges persist, particularly regarding identifying patients who most benefit from these therapeutic strategies. While some patients experience significant improvements in response and survival, the clinical benefit remains uncertain in some scenarios. In this context, tumor-associated biomarkers hold promise in guiding personalized treatment approaches. By analyzing different biomarkers such as genomic profiles, tumor mutational burden, mutation spectrum, and tumor-associated biomarkers such as PD-1/PD-L1 expression, several groups have tried to stratify patients based on their likelihood of responding to immunotherapy. Moreover, the emergence of liquid biomarkers offers unprecedented opportunities for real-time monitoring of treatment response and disease progression. However, the lack of standardization and the presence of conflicting results in biomarker assessments pose significant challenges. Further prospective trials are warranted to identify reliable biomarkers, and standardization of methodology is necessary to ensure its consistency and accuracy.

This chapter explores various facets of immunotherapy in UC, shedding light on the current therapeutic targets within the immune-checkpoint cascade, tumor-associated biomarkers either tissue- or liquid-based. Additionally, we present the emerging data on immunotherapy strategies' efficacy in UC with variant histologies. Lastly, we explore novel immunotherapy combinations, such as IO-FGFRi and IO-ADCs.

Chiara Mercinelli, Valentina Tateo, Emanuele Crupi and Antonio Cigliola contributed equally with all other contributors.

C. Mercinelli
Department of Medical Oncology, IRCCS San Raffaele Hospital, Milan, Italy

Medical Oncology Unit 2, Azienda Ospedaliero-Universitaria Pisana, Pisa, Italy

V. Tateo · A. Cigliola
Department of Medical Oncology, IRCCS San Raffaele Hospital, Milan, Italy

E. Crupi
Vita-Salute San Raffaele University, Milan, Italy

A. Necchi (✉)
Department of Medical Oncology, IRCCS San Raffaele Hospital, Milan, Italy

Vita-Salute San Raffaele University, Milan, Italy
e-mail: necchi.andrea@hsr.it

M. A. Knowles, L. Dyrskjøt (eds.), *Biology of Bladder Cancer*,
https://doi.org/10.1007/978-3-031-68505-7_23

Keywords

Immune checkpoints · Immunotherapy · Bladder cancer · Biomarkers · ctDNA · Variant histologies · Immunotherapy combinations

23.1 Introduction

The immune system serves the vital roles of immune surveillance, defense, and regulation. Its remarkable ability to discern between "self" and "non-self" enables it to neutralize potential threats to the body.

It is commonly divided into two cooperative defense systems: innate immunity, also known as non-specific immunity, which is responsible for dealing with microorganisms and does not require prior antigen exposure to be active, and acquired immunity, also called specific for its ability to tailor the immune response to different types of invaders. Acquired immunity has an immunological memory, which means that it requires initial exposure to the antigen to be fully effective and takes time to be activated after first contact with a new invader, but in subsequent exposures responds very quickly. These systems act through different cells, including macrophages, neutrophils, dendritic cells (DCs), mast cells, eosinophils, basophils, and natural killer (NK) cells for innate immunity, and B- and T-lymphocytes for acquired immunity.

Cluster of differentiation-8 (CD8+) cytotoxic T-cells are immune cells that are particularly effective at mediating antitumor immune responses. These cells can recognize tumor-specific antigens presented by major histocompatibility complex (MHC) class I molecules and, after appropriate stimulation, mediate tumor cell death. Antigen-presenting cells (APCs) also provide co-stimulatory signals, which consist of surface receptors and cytokines. CD4+ T-helper cells play a crucial role in adaptive immunity, aiding the activity of other immune cells by releasing cytokines. Like all T-cells, they express a T-Cell Receptor (TCR)–CD3 complex, which in the case of CD4+ cells have a high affinity for MHC class II molecules. APCs express MHC-II on their surface, and their interaction with CD4+ TCR is essential for activation of the immune adaptive response.

Tumor cells can avoid immune destruction by several mechanisms, such as evading immune recognition by downregulating MHC I proteins and through promoting a tolerant immune microenvironment. The latter can be obtained via upregulation of immune checkpoint molecules, which are the "gatekeepers" of immune responses, playing a crucial role in preventing excessive immune reactions and maintaining immune homeostasis. More and more checkpoints have been identified and studied in cancer in the past decade, including the negative regulatory molecules cytotoxic T-lymphocyte associated protein 4 (CTLA-4 or CD152) and programmed death 1 (PD-1 or CD279). On chronic tumor antigen exposure, T-cells can become "exhausted," which itself leads to checkpoint upregulation.

In recent years, the advent of drugs capable of modulating the immune response through the inhibition of immune checkpoint proteins has completely changed the treatment landscape of many tumor types and improved disease outcomes, making these compounds key players in current clinical practice. The mechanisms of action of the main checkpoints studied as current or possible targets of immunotherapeutic agents are addressed in the following paragraphs and summarized in Fig. 23.1.

A full list of clinical trials testing ICIs in UC in different disease settings is reported in Tables 23.1 and 23.2.

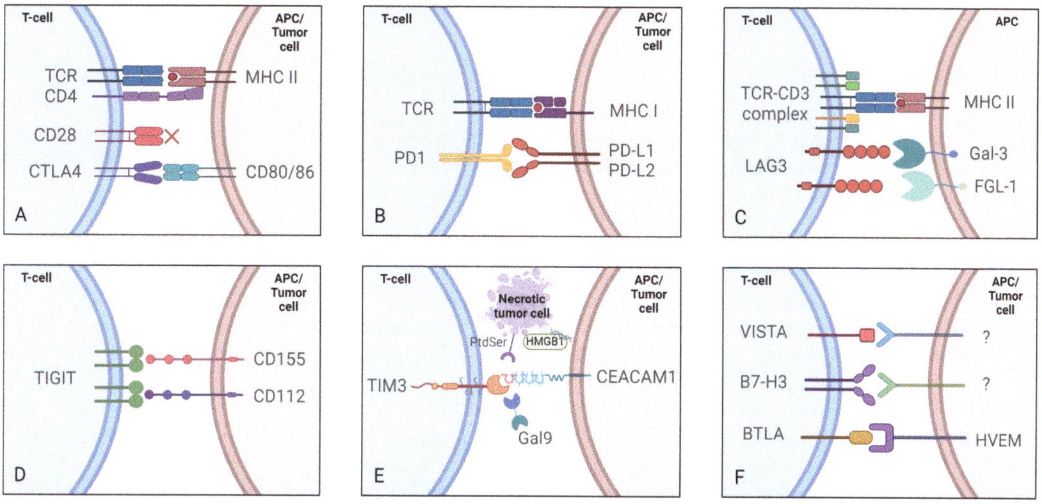

Fig. 23.1 Summary of the mechanisms of action of the main immune checkpoints. Immune checkpoints are sophisticated gatekeepers tasked with maintaining the balance between immunity and tolerance, in order to maintain immune homeostasis. The image illustrates the intricate mechanism of action of immune checkpoint proteins, which are expressed on the surface of of T-cells. The main proteins involved are: CTLA-4 (**a**); PD-1/PD-L1 (**b**); LAG-3 (**c**); TIGIT (**d**); TIM-3 (**e**); and VISTA, B7-H3, and BTLA (**f**). Immune checkpoint inhibitors (ICIs) work by blocking the interaction between checkpoint proteins and their ligands, freeing the immune system to activate against cancer cells. Created with Biorender.com

23.2 Current Therapeutic Targets in the Immune-Checkpoint Cascade

23.2.1 CTLA-4

CTLA-4, also known as CD-125, is a member of the immunoglobulin superfamily that downregulates the immune system by inhibiting T-cell functions (Kolar et al. 2009). CTLA-4 is induced on activated T-cells and mediates immunosuppression by competing with the T-cell co-stimulatory receptor CD-28 (Hossen et al. 2023). Both these receptors bind B7-1 (CD80) and B7-2 (CD86), two integral membrane proteins located on antigen-presenting cells (APCs), mediating opposite feedback for T-cell activation, in order to coordinate the strength of the immune response (Seidel et al. 2018).

Due to its stronger affinity for CD80 and CD86, CTLA-4 limits CD-28-mediated signalling during antigen presentation. It can also remove CD80 and CD86 from the surface of APCs, reducing availability of these stimulatory receptors to other CD28-expressing T-cells (Qureshi et al. 2011). Without CD28 signal, the interaction is biologically interpreted as non-pathogenic or self, inducing the development of immune tolerance.

The humanized CTLA-4 antibody ipilimumab was the first available immune checkpoint inhibitor (ICI), leading to a revolution in clinical cancer care (Hodi et al. 2010).

23.2.2 PD-1

PD-1, also known as CD279, is one of the best-known immune checkpoint proteins, primarily involved in inhibitory immune signalling and adaptive response regulation. It was first described in 1992 by Ishida et al., during their studies on T-cell death (Ishida et al. 1992).

PD-1 is a transmembrane glycoprotein belonging to the CD28/CTLA4 family that negatively regulates T-cells during long-term antigen exposure, as in cancers or chronic viral infections. Most T-cells do not express PD-1 constitutively, but they can be induced to do so upon stimulation through the TCR or exposure to

Table 23.1 Summary of ongoing clinical trials in the panorama of urothelial carcinoma, involving drugs directed against PD-1/PD-L1

Trial ID/name	Title	Trial design	Treatment strategy	Status
ANTI-PD-1: Pembrolizumab—localized disease				
NCT05072600	A pilot study of pembrolizumab monotherapy as maintenance therapy in MIBC patients who received bladder-preserving trimodally therapy and achieved CR	Phase 2, single group assignment, open label	Pembrolizumab (anti-PD-1)	Recruiting
NCT05535218 (SURE-02)	An open-label, single-arm, phase 2 study of perioperative pembrolizumab plus sacituzumab govitecan for patients with MIBC who cannot receive or refuse cisplatin-based chemotherapy	Phase 2, single group assignment, open label	Pembrolizumab (anti-PD-1) Sacituzumab Govitecan (ADC anti-Trop2)	Recruiting
NCT04241185 (MK-3475-992/ KEYNOTE-992)	Phase 3, randomized, double-blind, placebo-controlled clinical trial to study the efficacy and safety of pembrolizumab in combination with CRT versus CRT alone in participants with MIBC	Phase 3, randomized, parallel assignment, blinded	Pembrolizumab (anti-PD-1) Radiation therapy Cisplatin 5-FU MMC Gemcitabine	Recruiting
NCT03504163	Phase 2 study of pembrolizumab and BCG as first-line treatment for high-risk T1 NMIBC and high-grade NMI-UTUCC	Phase 2, non-randomized, parallel assignment, open label	Pembrolizumab (anti-PD-1) BCG	Recruiting
NCT05879653	A phase 2, open-label, multi-institutional study to evaluate the efficacy of induction therapy with pembrolizumab and EV followed by radiation therapy with pembrolizumab in patients with MIBC who are unfit for or refuse radical cystectomy	Phase 2, single group assignment, open label	Pembrolizumab (anti-PD-1) EV (ADC anti-nectin-4) radiation therapy	Recruiting
NCT05406713	Neoadjuvant pembrolizumab in patients with muscle-invasive bladder cancer with selective bladder sparing	Phase 2, single group assignment, open label	Pembrolizumab (anti-PD-1)	Recruiting
NCT03924895 (KEYNOTE-905/ EV-303)	Randomized phase 3 study evaluating cystectomy with perioperative pembrolizumab and cystectomy with perioperative enfortumab vedotin and pembrolizumab versus cystectomy alone in participants who are cisplatin-ineligible or decline cisplatin with MIBC	Phase 3, randomized, parallel assignment, open label	Pembrolizumab (anti-PD-1) EV (ADC anti-Nectin-4)	Recruiting
NCT02690558	Phase 2 single-arm study of gemcitabine and cisplatin plus pembrolizumab as neoadjuvant therapy prior to radical cystectomy in patients with MIBC	Phase 2, single-group assignment, open label	Pembrolizumab (anti-PD-1) Gemcitabine Cisplatin	Active, not recruiting

(continued)

Table 23.1 (continued)

Trial ID/name	Title	Trial design	Treatment strategy	Status
NCT03924856 (MK-3475-866/ KEYNOTE-866)	Phase 3, randomized, double-blind study to evaluate perioperative pembrolizumab (MK-3475) + neoadjuvant chemotherapy versus perioperative placebo + neoadjuvant chemotherapy in cisplatin-eligible participants with MIBC	Phase 3, randomized, parallel assignment, blinded	Pembrolizumab (anti-PD-1) Gemcitabine Cisplatin	Recruiting
NCT04700124 (MK-3475-B15/ KEYNOTE-B15/ EV-304)	Phase 3, randomized, open-label study to evaluate perioperative enfortumab vedotin plus pembrolizumab (MK-3475) versus neoadjuvant gemcitabine and cisplatin in cisplatin-eligible participants with MIBC	Phase 3, randomized, parallel assignment, open label	Pembrolizumab (anti-PD-1) EV (ADC anti-Nectin-4) Gemcitabine Cisplatin	Recruiting
NCT03711032 (MK-3475-676/ KEYNOTE-676)	Phase 3, randomized, comparator-controlled clinical trial to study the efficacy and safety of pembrolizumab in combination with BCG in participants with high-risk NMIBC persistent or recurrent following BCG induction or naïve to BCG treatment	Phase 3, randomized, parallel assignment, open label	Pembrolizumab (anti-PD-1) BCG	Recruiting
NCT05239624 (EV-ECLIPSE)	Enfortumab vedotin in combination with pembrolizumab for locally advanced and/or node-positive urothelial carcinoma prior to surgery	Phase 2, single group assignment, open label	Pembrolizumab (anti-PD-1) EV (ADC anti-Nectin-4)	Recruiting
NCT03244384 (AMBASSADOR)	Phase 3 randomized adjuvant study of pembrolizumab in muScle invaSive and locAlly aDvanced urOthelial caRcinoma versus observation	Phase 3, randomized, parallel assignment, open label	Pembrolizumab (anti-PD-1)	Active, not recruiting
ANTI-PD-1: Pembrolizumab—locally advanced unresectable or metastatic disease				
NCT03534804 (PemCab)	Cabozantinib plus pembrolizumab as first-line therapy for cisplatin-ineligible advanced urothelial carcinoma	Phase 2, single group assignment, non-randomized, open label	Pembrolizumab (anti-PD-1) Cabozantinib (anti-VEGR)	Active, not recruiting
NCT03236935	Phase 1b Trial of L-NMMA in combination with pembrolizumab in patients with solid tumors	Phase 1, single-group assignment, open label	Pembrolizumab (anti-PD-1) L-NMMA (pan-nitric oxide synthase inhibitor)	Active, not recruiting
NCT03854474	A pilot study of tazemetostat and pembrolizumab (MK-3475) in advanced urothelial carcinoma	Phase 1/2, single group assignment, open label	Pembrolizumab (anti-PD-1) Tazemetostat (EZH2 inhibitor)	Active, not recruiting
NCT04879329	A phase 2 multi-cohort, open-label, multi-center clinical study evaluating the efficacy and safety of disitamab vedotin (RC48-ADC) alone or in combination with pembrolizumab in subjects with locally advanced unresectable or metastatic urothelial carcinoma that expresses HER2	Phase 2, randomized, parallel assignment, open label	Pembrolizumab (anti-PD-1) Disitamab vedotin (ADC anti-HER2)	Recruiting

(continued)

Table 23.1 (continued)

Trial ID/name	Title	Trial design	Treatment strategy	Status
NCT05911295	An open-label, randomized, controlled phase 3 study of disitamab vedotin in combination with pembrolizumab versus chemotherapy in subjects with previously untreated locally advanced or metastatic urothelial carcinoma that expresses HER2 (IHC 1+ and greater)	Phase 3, randomized, parallel assignment, open label	Pembrolizumab (anti-PD-1) Disitamab Vedotin (ADC anti-HER2) Gemcitabine Cisplatin Carboplatin	Recruiting
ANTI-PD-1: Nivolumab				
NCT04876313 (NURE-Combo)	An open-label, single-arm, phase 2 study of neoadjuvant nivolumab and nab-paclitaxel before radical cystectomy for patients with muscle-invasive bladder cancer	Phase 2, single group assignment, open label	Nivolumab (anti-PD-1) Nab-Paclitaxel	Active, not recruiting
NCT03558087	Neoadjuvant gemcitabine, cisplatin, plus nivolumab in patients with muscle-invasive bladder cancer with selective bladder sparing	Phase 2, single group assignment, open label	Nivolumab (anti-PD-1) Gemcitabine Cisplatin	Active, not recruiting
NCT03171025 (NEXT)	A phase 2 open-label single-arm study of adjuvant nivolumab following chemoradiation in localized MIBC	Phase 2, single group assignment, open label	Nivolumab (anti-PD-1)	Active, not recruiting
NCT05203913 (CNN-BC)	Efficacy and safety of the combination of cisplatin plus nab-paclitaxel and nivolumab with radiotherapy after maximal tumor resection in non-metastatic MIBC	Phase 2, single group assignment, open label	Nivolumab (anti-PD-1) Nab-Paclitaxel Cisplatin	Recruiting
NCT02845323	Randomized phase 2 study of neoadjuvant nivolumab with and without urelumab in cisplatin-ineligible or CRT-refusing patients with MIBC of the bladder	Phase 2, parallel assignment, open label	Nivolumab (anti-PD-1) Urelumab (CD137 agonist)	Active, not recruiting
ANTI-PD-1: Cetrelimab				
NCT04640623 (SunRISe-1)	Phase 2b clinical study evaluating efficacy and safety of TAR-200 in combination with cetrelimab, TAR-200 alone, or cetrelimab alone in participants with high-risk NMIBC unresponsive to intravesical BCG who are ineligible for or elected not to undergo radical cystectomy	Phase 2, randomized, parallel assignment, open label	Cetrelimab (anti-PD-1) TAR200 (Gemcitabine-Releasing Intravesical System)	Recruiting
NCT04658862 (SunRISe-2)	Phase 3, multi-center, randomized study evaluating efficacy of TAR-200 in combination with cetrelimab versus concurrent chemoradiotherapy in participants with MIBC of the bladder who are not receiving radical cystectomy	Phase 3, randomized, parallel assignment, open label	Cetrelimab (anti-PD-1) TAR200 CRT	Recruiting
NCT05714202 (SunRISe-3)	Phase 3, open-label, multi-center, randomized study evaluating the efficacy and safety of TAR-200 in combination with cetrelimab or TAR-200 alone versus intravesical BCG in participants with BCG-naïve high-risk NMIBC	Phase 3, randomized, parallel assignment, open label	Cetrelimab (anti-PD-1) TAR200	Recruiting

(continued)

Table 23.1 (continued)

Trial ID/name	Title	Trial design	Treatment strategy	Status
NCT04919512 (SunRISe-4)	A phase 2, open-label, multi-center, randomized study of TAR-200 in combination with cetrelimab and cetrelimab alone in participants with MIBC who are scheduled for radical cystectomy and are ineligible for or refusing platinum-based neoadjuvant chemotherapy	Phase 2, randomized, parallel assignment, open label	Cetrelimab (anti-PD-1) TAR200	Recruiting
Other anti-PD-1				
NCT05975307 (BCIRT-01)	Single-arm, phase 2 clinical trial to treat muscle-invasive bladder cancer with induction chemotherapy plus anti-PD-1 therapy followed by radiotherapy plus concurrent anti-PD-1 therapy	Phase 2, single-group assignment, open label	Toripalimab (anti-PD-1) Gemcitabin Cisplatin Carboplatin Radiation therapy	Recruiting
NCT04861584 (GZZJU-2021NB)	Phase 2 study of neoadjuvant toripalimab with gemcitabine-cisplatin in subjects with T2-4aN0M0 bladder cancer	Phase 2, single group assignment, open label	Toripalimab (anti-PD-1) Gemcitabin Cisplatin	Recruiting
NCT05241340 (RAD-VACCINE)	Phase 2 clinical trial of neoadjuvant sasanlimab and stereotactic body radiation therapy as an in situ vaccine for cisplatin-ineligible muscle-invasive bladder cancer	Phase 2, single group assignment, open label	Sasanlimab (anti-PD-1) Radiation therapy	Recruiting
NCT04779151 (NIRADO)	Open-label phase 2 basket trial exploring the efficacy and safety of the combination of niraparib and dostarlimab in patients with DNA repair-deficient or platinum-sensitive solid tumors	Phase 2, non-randomized, parallel assignment, open label	Dostarlimab (anti-PD-1) Niraparib (PARPi)	Recruiting
ANTI-PD-L1: Atezolizumab				
NCT03697850 (BladderSpar)	Phase 2 study of maintenance anti-PD-L1 treatment with atezolizumab after chemoradiotherapy for MIBC patients not eligible for radical cystectomy: bladder sparing	Phase 2, single group assignment, open label	Atezolizumab (anti-PD-L1)	Active, not recruiting
NCT04289779	A phase 2 study of cabozantinib in combination with atezolizumab as neoadjuvant treatment for MIBC	Phase 2, single group assignment, open label	Atezolizumab (anti-PD-L1) Cabozantinib (anti-VEGFR)	Recruiting
NCT02989584	A pilot safety study and single-arm phase 2 study of gemcitabine and cisplatin with atezolizumab in patients with metastatic and MIBC, respectively	Phase 1/2, single group assignment, open label	Atezolizumab (anti-PD-L1) Gemcitabine Cisplatin	Active, not recruiting
NCT04660344 (IMvigor 011)	A phase 3, double-blind, multi-center, randomized study of atezolizumab (anti-PD-L1 antibody) versus placebo as adjuvant therapy in patients with high-risk MIBC who are ctDNA positive following cystectomy	Phase 3, randomized, parallel assignment, blinded	Atezolizumab (anti-PD-L1)	Recruiting

(continued)

Table 23.1 (continued)

Trial ID/name	Title	Trial design	Treatment strategy	Status
NCT04630730	Intravesical recombinant BCG followed by perioperative chemo-immunotherapy for patients with MIBC. A multi-center, single-arm phase 2 trial	Phase 2, single group assignment, open label	Atezolizumab (anti-PD-L1) Gemcitabine Cisplatin	Recruiting
NCT03775265	Phase 3 randomized trial of concurrent chemoradiotherapy with or without atezolizumab in localized MIBC	Phase 3, randomized, parallel assignment, open label	Atezolizumab (anti-PD-L1) Cisplatin 5FU Gemcitabine	Recruiting
ANTI-PD-L1: Durvalumab				
NCT04543110 (RADIANT)	Neoadjuvant immune-modulating radiation with durvalumab (MEDI4736) prior to radical cystectomy in patients with MIBC	Phase 2, single group assignment, open label	Durvalumab (anti-PD-L1) Radiation therapy	Recruiting
NCT05943106 (PATAPSCO)	A phase 3b open-label, single-arm, multi-center, US study of BCG administered in combination with durvalumab in adult BCG-naïve, high-risk NMIBC participants	Phase 3, single group assignment, open label	Durvalumab (anti-PD-L1) BCG	Recruiting
NCT03732677 (NIAGARA)	A phase 3, randomized, open-label, multi-center, global study to determine the efficacy and safety of durvalumab in combination with gemcitabine+cisplatin for neoadjuvant treatment followed by durvalumab alone for adjuvant treatment in patients with MIBC	Phase 3, randomized, parallel assignment, open label	Durvalumab (anti-PD-L1) Cisplatin Gemcitabine	Active, not recruiting
NCT05137262	Durvalumab and standard chemotherapy for the treatment of lymph node-positive bladder cancer	Phase 2, randomized, single group assignment, open label	Durvalumab (anti-PD-L1) Cisplatin Methotrexate Vinblastine Doxorubicin Hydrochloride	Recruiting
ANTI-PD-L1: Avelumab				
NCT03674424 (AURA)	Avelumab as neoadjuvant therapy in subjects with urothelial MIBC	Phase 2, randomized, parallel assignment, open label	Avelumab (anti-PD-L1) Cisplatin + Gemcitabine dd-MVAC Paclitaxel + Gemcitabine	Recruiting
NCT05092958 (MAIN-CAV)	Phase 3 randomized trial of maintenance cabozantinib and avelumab vs maintenance avelumab after first-line platinum-based chemotherapy in patients with metastatic urothelial cancer	Phase 3, randomized, parallel assignment, open label	Avelumab (anti-PD-L1) Cabozantinib	Recruiting

Abbreviations: MIBC, muscle-invasive bladder cancer; ADC, antibody–drug conjugate; Trop-2, trophoblast surface antigen 2; BCG, Bacillus Calmette–Guérin; CRT, chemoradiation therapy; MMC, mitomycin C; NMIBC, non-muscle-invasive bladder cancer; NMI-UTUCC, non-muscle-invasive upper tract urothelial cell carcinoma; EV, enfortumab vedotin; VEGFR, vascular endothelial growth factor receptor; EZH2, enhancer of zeste homolog 2; HER2, human epidermal growth factor receptor-2; IHC, immunohistochemistry; PARPi, poly (ADP-ribose) polymerase inhibitors; dd-MVAC, dose dense Methotrexate + vinblastine + cisplatin + doxorubicin

Table 23.2 Summary of ongoing clinical trials in the panorama of urothelial carcinoma, involving drugs directed against CTLA-4, LAG3, TIGIT, TIM3, GDF-15, VISTA, B7-H3, and BTLA, eventually associated with anti-PD-(L)1

Trial ID	Title	Trial design	Treatment strategy	Status
NCT03520491 (CA209-9DJ)	A pilot study to evaluate the safety of neoadjuvant nivolumab alone or in combination with ipilimumab for cisplatin-ineligible patients with MIBC	Phase 2, non-randomized, sequential assignment, open label	Ipilimumab (anti-CTLA4) Nivolumab (anti-PD-1)	Recruiting
NCT04863885	Phase 1/2 study of ipilimumab plus nivolumab (IPI-NIVO) combined with sacituzumab govitecan (SG)as first-line treatment for cisplatin-ineligible metastatic urothelial carcinoma	Phase 1/2, non-randomized, sequential assignment, open label	Ipilimumab (anti-CTLA4) Nivolumab (anti-PD-1) Sacituzumab govitecan (ADC anti-Trop2)	Active, not recruiting
NCT05180799	A phase 1/2 study of BA3071 as monotherapy and in combination with a PD-1 blocking antibody in patients with advanced solid tumors	Phase 1/2, non-randomized, open-label	BA3071 (anti-CTLA4) Nivolumab (anti-PD-1) Pembrolizumab (anti-PD-1)	Recruiting
NCT03601455	Phase 2 study of radiation therapy and anti-PD-L1 checkpoint inhibitor (durvalumab) with or without anti-CTLA-4 inhibition (tremelimumab) in patients with unresectable, locally advanced, or metastatic urothelial bladder cancer that are ineligible or refusing chemotherapy	Phase 2, randomized, open label	Radiation therapy Durvalumab (anti-PD-L1) Tremelimumab (anti-CTLA-4)	Active, not recruiting
NCT02812420	A pilot pre-surgical study evaluating anti-PD-L1 antibody (Durvalumab) plus anti-CTLA-4 (tremelimumab) in patients with muscle-invasive, high-risk urothelial carcinoma who are ineligible for cisplatin-based neoadjuvant chemotherapy	Phase 1, single group assignment, open label	Durvalumab (anti-PD-L1) Tremelimumab (anti-CTLA-4)	Active, not recruiting
NCT04960709 (VOLGA)	Phase 3 randomized, open-label, multi-center study to determine the efficacy and safety of durvalumab in combination with tremelimumab and enfortumab vedotin or durvalumab in combination with enfortumab vedotin for perioperative treatment in patients ineligible for cisplatin or who refuse cisplatin undergoing radical cystectomy for MIBC	Phase 3, randomized, parallel assignment, open label	Durvalumab (anti-PD-L1) Tremelimumab (anti-CTLA-4) Enfortumab Vedotin (ADC anti-Nectin4)	Recruiting
NCT04940299	A phase 2 study to assess the safety and efficacy of tocilizumab in combination with ipilimumab and nivolumab in patients with advanced melanoma, non-small cell lung cancer, or urothelial carcinoma	Phase 2, randomized, open label	Ipilimumab (anti-CTLA-4) Nivolumab (anti-PD-1) Tocilizumab (anti IL-6R)	Active, not recruiting

(continued)

Table 23.2 (continued)

Trial ID	Title	Trial design	Treatment strategy	Status
NCT02496208	A phase 1 study of cabozantinib plus nivolumab (CaboNivo) alone or in combination with ipilimumab (CaboNivoIpi) in patients with advanced/metastatic urothelial carcinoma and other genitourinary tumors	Phase 1, non-randomized, parallel assignment, open label	Cabozantinib S-malate Ipilimumab (anti-CTLA-4) Nivolumab (anti-PD-1)	Active, not recruiting
NCT04606472	Phase I clinical study to evaluate the safety, tolerability, pharmacokinetic characteristics, and preliminary efficacy of SI-B003, a PD-1/CTLA-4 bispecific antibody, in patients with advanced solid tumors	Phase 1, sequential assignment, open label	SI-B003 (bispecific antibody anti-PD-1 and CTLA4)	Recruiting
NCT04388852	DS3201 with ipilimumab in patients with metastatic aggressive variant prostate (AVPC), urothelial (UC), and renal cell (RCC) carcinomas	Phase 1, single group assignment, open label	Ipilimumab (anti-CTLA4) Valemetostat (EZH1/2 inhibitor)	Recruiting
NCT04140526 (PRESERVE-001)	Safety, pharmacokinetics (PK), and efficacy of ONC-392 as a single agent and in combination with pembrolizumab in advanced solid tumors and NSCLC: an open-label phase 1A/1B study	Phase 1/2, non-randomized, sequential assignment, open label	ONC-392 (anti-CTLA4) Pembrolizumab (anti PD-1)	Recruiting
NCT06237920 (TURANDORELA)	A phase 2 trial in stage II–IIIa urothelial cancer randomizing pre-operative nivolumab with or without relatlimab	Phase 2, randomized, parallel assignment, open label	Nivolumab (anti-PD-1) Relatlimab (anti-LAG3)	Recruiting
NCT05645692 (BO44157)	A phase 2, randomized, multi-center, open-label, controlled study of tobemstomig alone or in combination with tiragolumab versus atezolizumab in patients with previously untreated locally advanced or metastatic urothelial cancer who are ineligible for platinum-containing chemotherapy	Phase 2, randomized, open-label, multi-center	Atezolizumab (anti-PD-L1) Tobemstomig (bispecific antibody anti-PD-1 and LAG3) Tiragolumab (anti-TIGIT)	Recruiting

(continued)

Table 23.2 (continued)

Trial ID	Title	Trial design	Treatment strategy	Status
NCT03869190 (MORPHEUS-UC)	A phase 1b/2, open-label, multi-center, randomized umbrella study evaluating the efficacy and safety of multiple immunotherapy-based treatments and combinations in patients with urothelial carcinoma	Phase 1/2, randomized, parallel assignment, open label	Atezolizumab (anti-PD-L1) Enfortumab Vedotin (ADC anti-Nectin4) Niraparib (PARPi) Magrolimab (CD47 inhibitor) Tiragolumab (anti-TIGIT) Sacituzumab Govitecan (ADC anti-Trop2) Tocilizumab (anti IL-6R) Cisplatin Gemcitabine	Recruiting
NCT04586244 (OPTIMUS)	An open-label, randomized, phase 2, umbrella study to investigate the biological rationale of various neoadjuvant therapies for participants with muscle-invasive urothelial carcinoma of the bladder who are cisplatin-ineligible or refuse cisplatin therapy and undergoing radical cystectomy	Phase 2, randomized, open-label, multi-center	Retifanlimab (anti-PD-1) Epacadostat (anti-IDO1) INCAGN02385 (anti-LAG3) INCAGN02390 (anti-TIM3)	Terminated
NCT02625961 (MK-3475-057/ KEYNOTE-057)	A phase 2 clinical trial to study the efficacy and safety of pembrolizumab and pembrolizumab in combination with other investigational agents in subjects with high-risk nmibc unresponsive to BCG therapy	Phase 2, randomized, parallel assignment, open label	Pembrolizumab (anti-PD-1) Pembrolizumab/ vibostolimab (anti-TIGIT) coformulation Favezelimab/ pembrolizumab coformulation (anti-LAG3)	Recruiting
NCT05007106 (MK-7684A-005/ KEYVIBE-005)	Multi-center, open-label, phase 2 basket study of MK-7684A, a co-formation of vibostolimab (MK-7684) With pembrolizumab (MK-3475), with or without other anticancer therapies in participants with selected solid tumors	Phase 2, randomized, parallel assignment, open label	Pembrolizumab/ vibostolimab (anti-TIGIT) coformulation Lenvatinib (multiple TKI-Ri) Various ChT regimens	Recruiting
NCT05394337	Neoadjuvant PD-1 plus TIGIT blockade in patients with cisplatin-ineligible operable high-risk urothelial carcinoma	Phase 1/2, non-randomized, single group assignment, single blinded (participant)	Atezolizumab (anti-PD-L1) Tiragolumab (anti-TIGIT)	Recruiting

(continued)

Table 23.2 (continued)

Trial ID	Title	Trial design	Treatment strategy	Status
NCT05327530 (JAVELIN Bladder Medley)	A phase 2, multi-center, randomized, open label, parallel-arm, umbrella study of avelumab (MSB0010718C) in combination with other AntiTumor agents as a maintenance treatment in participants with locally advanced or metastatic urothelial carcinoma whose disease did not progress with first-line platinum-containing chemotherapy	Phase 3, randomized, parallel assignment, open label	Avelumab (anti PD-L1) Sacituzumab Govitecan (ADC anti-Trop2) M6223 (anti-TIGIT) NKTR-255 (recombinant human IL-15)	Recruiting
NCT06059547	A multi-center phase 2 study of neoadjuvant immunotherapy in combination with the anti-GDF-15 antibody visugromab (CTL-002) for the treatment of muscle-invasive bladder	Phase 2, non-randomized, parallel assignment, single-blinded (participant)	Nivolumab (anti-PD-1) Visugromab (CTL-002; anti-GDF-15)	Recruiting
NCT05864144	Phase 1/2, open-label study evaluating the safety, tolerability, pharmacokinetics, pharmacodynamics, and efficacy of SNS-101 (anti-VISTA) as monotherapy and in combination with cemiplimab in patients with advanced solid tumors	Phase 1/2, non-randomized, sequential assignment, open label	SNS-101 (anti-VISTA) Cemiplimab (anti-PD-L1)	Recruiting
NCT02628535	Phase 1, first-in-human, open label, dose-escalation study of MGD009, a humanized B7-H3 x CD3 dual-affinity retargeting (DART) protein in patients with unresectable or metastatic B7-H3-expressing neoplasms	Phase 1, single-group assignment, open label	Orlotamab (Humanized B7-H3 x CD3 DART protein)	Terminated
NCT04773951	Phase 1 clinical study to evaluate the safety, tolerability, and pharmacokinetics of recombinant humanized monoclonal antibody specific to B- and T-lymphocyte attenuator, BTLA (JS004) injection in patients with advanced solid tumors	Phase 1, single-group assignment, open label	JS004 (anti-BTLA) Toripalimab (anti-PD-1)	Recruiting

Abbreviations: CTLA-4, cytotoxic T-lymphocyte antigen 4; PD-1, programmed cell death protein 1; PD-L1, programmed death-ligand 1; LAG3, lymphocyte activation gene 3; TIGIT, T-cell immunoreceptor with Ig and ITIM domains; TIM3, T-cell immunoglobulin and mucin domain 3; GDF-15, growth/differentiation factor 15; VISTA, V-domain immunoglobulin suppressor of T-cell activation; BTLA, B and T-lymphocyte attenuator; MIBC, muscle-invasive bladder cancer; NMIBC, non-muscle-invasive bladder cancer; BCG, Bacillus Calmette–Guérin; IL-6 R, interleukin-6 receptor; EZH1/2, enhancer of zeste homolog 1/2; NSCLC, non-small cell lung cancer; ADC, antibody–drug conjugate; Trop-2, Trophoblast surface antigen 2; DART, dual-affinity retargeting; TKI-Ri, tyrosine kinase receptor inhibitor

cytokines such as IL-2, IL-7, IL-15, IL-21, and TGF-β (Seidel et al. 2018).

PD-1 ligands are Programmed Death-Ligand 1 (PD-L1, also known as B7-H1 or CD274) and Ligand 2 (PD-L2, also known as B7-DC or CD273), two transmembrane glycoproteins that are constitutively expressed or can be induced in a variety of lymphoid and non-lymphoid tissues (Seidel et al. 2018; Okazaki et al. 2007). In particular, PD-L1 is expressed on various non-hematopoietic tissues, whereas PD-L2 is expressed only on antigen-presenting cells in lymphoid tissues or chronic inflammatory environments, and is rarely detected in non-lymphoid organs under normal conditions. Interferon γ (IFN-γ) is the main trigger known to cause PD-L1 and PD-L2 upregulation (Brown et al. 2003).

After the binding of PD-1, CD28, and TCR with their ligands, respectively, PD-L1 or PD-L2, CD80 or CD86, and MHC class I or II, the Src kinase Lck (P56Lck) bound on the intracellular tail of CD4 and CD8, phosphorylates tyrosine residues of PD-1 and CD28. PD-1 carries an immunoreceptor tyrosine-based inhibitory motif (ITIM) and an immunoreceptor tyrosine-based switch motif (ITSM) on its intracellular tail (Okazaki et al. 2007). Phosphorylation of ITSM causes recruitment of the Src homology region 2 domain-containing phosphatase 2 (SHP-2); simultaneously, the phosphorylated tail of CD28 recruits phosphatidylinositol 3-kinase (PI-3K) and growth factor receptor-bound protein 2 (Grb2).

SHP-2 association with PD-1 decreases dephosphorylation of the cytoplasmic tail of CD28 and of the CD3 chain, therefore preventing the recruitment of further downstream signalling factors associated with these molecules. By disrupting signalling of CD28 via PI-3K and Grb2, PD-1 leads to decreased signalling in pathways important for cytokine production, such as IL-2, IFN-γ, and tumor necrosis factor-α (TNF-α), and cell cycle progression.

In the absence of its ligands, PD-1 is not recruited to the immune synapse and cannot interfere with activation signalling (Chemnitz et al. 2004). PD-1 can be dephosphorylated by SHP-2 itself via a negative self-feedback mechanism. A variety of tumor cells has been demonstrated to express PD-L1 and to upregulate it in response to IFN-γ. Several anti-PD-1/PD-L1 inhibitors have been developed and have now replaced chemotherapy in various tumor types.

23.2.3 LAG-3

In recent years, lymphocyte activation gene-3 (LAG-3 or CD223) was identified as a checkpoint suppressing the antitumor function of T-cells (Chocarro et al. 2021), with an activity comparable to CTLA-4 and PD-1. It is a cell surface molecule expressed on several immune cells, including CD4+ and CD8+ T-cells, and can be upregulated under various types of antigen stimulation. Its expression on the cell surface requires T-cell activation, and it is upregulated by cytokines such as IL-2 (Annunziato et al. 1996). LAG-3 protein expression directly correlates with IFN-γ production, and inversely correlates with IL-4 levels (Annunziato et al. 1996).

LAG-3 physically associates with the TCR:CD3 complex on T-cells, leading to downregulation of TCR signal transduction, causing termination of cell proliferation and cytokine secretion in response to CD3 signalling (Hannier et al. 1998). LAG-3 binds MHC class II molecules with higher affinity than CD4, contributing to escape of cancer cells from apoptosis. Furthermore, this bond facilitates recruitment of CD4 T-cells, but with a reduction of the CD8 T-cell response (Donia et al. 2015).

Until recently, immunosuppression caused by LAG-3 was thought to be mediated primarily via MHC-II. However, other LAG-3 ligands have been identified, suggesting that LAG-3 does not function only by disrupting CD4:MHC-II interactions. These ligands are galectin-3 (Gal-3), a galactose-binding lectin, and the liver-secreted fibrinogen-like protein 1 (FGL1), a member of the fibrinogen family. Both molecules when bound to LAG-3 cause negative modulation of T-cell activation (Kashio et al. 2003; Wang et al. 2019a). FGL1 expression is induced by IL-6 and often upregulated in several cancer types. It was demonstrated that elevated FGL1 levels were associated with worse prognosis and anti-PD-1 therapy resistance (Wang et al. 2019a), suggesting a possible synergistic role of FGL1/LAG3 targeting in combination with anti-PD-1/PD-L1.

Recently the first-in-class human IgG4 anti-LAG3 called Relatlimab was tested in a large phase 2/3 trial in combination with the anti-PD-1 Nivolumab, demonstrating an advantage in terms of median progression-free survival (PFS) compared to Nivolumab alone in patients with previously untreated metastatic or unresectable melanoma (Tawbi et al. 2022).

23.2.4 TIGIT

T-cell immunoreceptor with immunoglobulin and ITIM domain (TIGIT) is a promising new target for cancer immunotherapy which is upregulated by immune cells, including activated T-cells, natural killer cells, and regulatory T-cells. TIGIT is part of a co-stimulatory network that involves multiple inhibitory receptors, a competing co-stimulatory receptor (DNAM-1/CD226) and two ligands: CD155 (Poliovirus receptor or PVR) and CD112 (PVRL2, nectin-2) (Chauvin et al. 2020). Recent findings demonstrated that TIGIT also binds nectin-4 (Reches et al. 2020), but we still know little about the immunological implications of this link.

In cancer, TIGIT was found to be co-expressed with PD-1 on tumor antigen-specific CD8+ T-cells and CD8+ tumor-infiltrating lymphocytes (TILs); it is also co-expressed with other immune checkpoints such as LAG-3 and TIM-3, on exhausted T-cells. Several mechanisms of TIGIT inhibition of T-cells in the tumor microenvironment (TME) have been revealed.

Among its ligands, the one with which TIGIT has the greatest affinity is CD155. CD155 is involved in cell-cell adhesion, and normally it is expressed on monocytes, dendritic cells (DCs), fibroblasts, and endothelial cells. It has been found to be overexpressed in several cancer types, where it promotes tumor cell growth and migration (Takai et al. 2003).

By virtue of its link with CD155, TIGIT delivers intracellular inhibitory signals that act on TCR, reducing its expression and signalling. TIGIT/CD155 on APCs induces IL-10 expression and decreases IL-12 production, which leads to inhibition of T-cells. Moreover, TIGIT competes with CD226, reducing its co-stimulator activity on T-cells (Ge et al. 2021).

In light of these data, the combination of anti-PD-1/PD-L1 and anti-TIGIT is extremely promising; many clinical trials are already testing this strategy.

23.2.5 TIM-3

Discovered in 2002 (Monney et al. 2002), the T-cell immunoglobulin and mucin domain containing-3 (TIM-3) was initially found to be expressed on the surface of CD4+ Th1 and CD8+ T cytotoxic 1 (Tc1) cells and has since been found on other immune cells, such as macrophages, dendritic cells, and monocytes (Zhao et al. 2021). It is a transmembrane protein that binds to different ligands on immune cells to cause signal transduction: galectin-9 (Gal-9) (Li et al. 2012), high mobility group box 1 (HMGB1) (Tang et al. 2012), phosphatidylserine (PtdSer) (DeKruyff et al. 2010), and carcinoembryonic antigen cell adhesion molecule 1 (Ceacam-1) (Huang et al. 2015). The mechanisms by which TIM-3 and its ligands determine immune tolerance are not yet fully understood.

Gal-9 was the first ligand identified. It binds TIM-3 with higher affinity than other galectins, and this bond determines T-helper type 1 (Th1) cell apoptosis (Zhu et al. 2005), probably due to calcium flow into the intracellular area of Th1 mediated by Gal-9 (Kashio et al. 2003). Gal-9/TIM-3 interaction also induces the death of the effectors of Th1 cells and mediates T-cell exhaustion.

HMGB1 is a DNA-binding protein that plays a key role in inflammation, immune response, and genome stability. Tumor-infiltrating DCs highly express TIM-3 protein, which competes with the nucleic acid released by tumor cells to bind to HMGB1. Through this link, nucleic acids cannot enter endosomes and consequently they cannot stimulate the innate immune response further (Tang et al. 2012).

The interaction of TIM-3 and PtdSer helps to clear apoptotic bodies and promote the cross-presentation of dendritic cells (DCs). Signals sent by PtdSer on apoptotic cells to promptly activate cell phagocytosis are essential to maintain tolerance and prevent autoimmunity.

Finally, Ceacam-1 binds TIM-3 to form a heterodimer, promoting the stable expression of TIM-3 on the surface of immune cells. Interactions between Ceacam-1 and TIM-3 determine the tolerance-inducing function of TIM-3 (Huang et al. 2015).

Many in vivo studies have shown evidence of synergy of anti-PD-1 and anti-TIM3, which is why this combination is currently undergoing clinical trials.

23.2.6 GDF-15

The growth-differentiation factor 15 (GDF-15), also named macrophage inhibitory cytokine-1 (MIC-1), is a stress-induced cytokine, a member of the transforming growth factor β (TGF-β) family.

It is abundant primarily in the placenta, where T-cells are functionally inhibited due to the need for tolerance to neoantigens, which is essential during pregnancy. Normally it has a low constitutive expression in most healthy somatic tissues but can be upregulated in response to stress-related proteins, such as IL-1β, IL-2, TNF-α, and macrophage colony-stimulating factor-1 (MCSF-1) (Adela et al. 2015). Elevated GDF-15 levels in cancer patients have been reported frequently, which seems to correlate with a worse outcome, absence of T-cell infiltration, and altered T-cell priming (Weide et al. 2016; Zhou et al. 2013). In a recent study, Haake et al. better clarified the mechanism of action of GDF-15 (Haake et al. 2023). Based on in vitro pharmacological studies, mouse models, and analyses of human melanoma patients, they demonstrated that GDF-15 impaired leukocyte function associated antigen-1 (LFA-1)/β2-integrin-mediated adhesion of T-cells to activated endothelial cells, which is essential for adhesion to, rolling on and transmigration across the endothelial barrier.

For these reasons, GDF-15 inhibition results in improved T-cell infiltration of tumor-draining lymph nodes. This blockade also improves the efficacy of immune checkpoint blockade in mouse tumor models expressing GDF-15, making it a possible synergistic target for immunotherapy.

23.2.7 VISTA, B7-H3, BTLA, and Siglec-15

In addition to the most well-known checkpoints discussed above, new promising targets are emerging (Qin et al. 2019).

V-domain Ig suppressor of T-cell activation (VISTA) is a potent negative regulator of T-cell function that is expressed in hematopoietic cells, whose levels are elevated in the tumor microenvironment (Lines et al. 2014). It is also known as PD-1 homolog (PD-1H). VISTA suppresses proliferation of T-cells but not B-cells and induces Foxp3 expression (Tagliamento et al. 2021).

B7-H3 or CD276, is a transmembrane glycoprotein, involved in the inhibition of T-cells (Chapoval et al. 2001; Prasad et al. 2004; Suh et al. 2003). It was first described to be a co-stimulator of CD4 and CD8 T-cell response and IFN-γ production (Chapoval et al. 2001). Its ligand has not yet been identified, but given the different functions identified, it is possible that B7-H3 binds different ligands with distinct immunomodulatory activity (Kontos et al. 2021).

B- and T-lymphocyte attenuator (BTLA) or CD272 belongs to the CD28 superfamily, and binds herpesvirus entry mediator (HVEM), a member of the tumor necrosis factor receptor (TNFR) superfamily (Ning et al. 2021; Sedy et al. 2005). BTLA was found to be overexpressed in TILs, and could provide both inhibitory and stimulatory signals to T-cells (Murphy et al. 2010).

Sialic acid-binding immunoglobulin (Ig)-like lectin 15 (Siglec-15), a transmembrane protein first described in 2019, has recently emerged as a modulator of immune responses that can be expressed by tumor-associated macrophages (TAMs) (Wang et al. 2019b; Lenza et al. 2023). By binding to its ligands, Siglec-15 induces antigen T-cell response suppression. Its expression is mutually exclusive with B7-H1.

23.3 Tumor-Associated Biomarkers of Immunotherapy Benefit

23.3.1 General Considerations

In recent years, immunotherapy has emerged as a pivotal component in the treatment of advanced urothelial carcinoma (UC), occupying a central role in therapeutic strategies. In the near future, applications of immunotherapy in UC will probably expand to involve localized disease, based on the results already available, and, hopefully, on the awaited results of many ongoing trials. However, despite the growing effort in immunotherapy investigation in UC, there is still insufficient understanding of the predictive factors for immunotherapy benefit, with consequent difficulties in the identification of patients who will respond to immunotherapy or will present primary resistance. The identification of reliable predictive biomarkers is necessary to lead immuno-oncology toward precision medicine, in order to offer a tailored treatment to each patient, according to their tumor and microenvironment characteristics.

Immunotherapy trials in UC have investigated various tissue biomarkers, already studied in other cancers, such as PD-L1 expression, tumor mutational burden (TMB), mutational spectrum, gene expression profile (GEP), and quantification and quality assessment of the immune infiltrate. There are many critical issues hindering biomarker development in UC and other cancers; however, the most relevant are: (1) poor biomarker analyses in various studies; (2) non-uniform assessment of the same biomarker across different trials; (3) discordant results about the predictive role of a specific biomarker in different clinical settings; and (4) discordant results on the predictive role of a specific biomarker in the same clinical setting with different drugs. These problems reveal the need for a more precise co-design of biomarkers and drugs, taking into account different disease settings. Disease setting is an important consideration since tumor and microenvironment biology undergo changes from localized to advanced disease and before and after therapy. That implies that there will be different responses to treatments and different expression and predictive values of biomarkers across disease phases. Neoadjuvant/perioperative trials are the best opportunity to investigate predictive biomarkers since they allow a dynamic analysis of biomarkers, before (biopsy of the treatment-naïve primary cancer) and after therapies (surgical specimen). On the other hand, trials in advanced disease provide less clean data since the available tissues may not be representative of the tumor and its microenvironment at the moment of trial intervention (e.g., biopsy or surgical specimen from localized phase or before other therapy lines).

23.3.2 Principal Tissue Biomarkers Investigated in UC

23.3.2.1 PD-L1

PD-L1 is the most intuitive biomarker for targeting the PD-1/PD-L1 axis and it has been explored extensively as a tissue biomarker in cancer. The detailed biological role of PD-L1 has been described above (Sect. 23.2.2). Tumor expression of PD-L1 in human cancer varies widely across different histologies but also within a given histology, depending on individual reports. Variations of PD-L1 expression within one tumor type depend on many factors, including the disease setting (localized vs advanced, untreated vs treated), the assay used to test PD-L1 expression, and the selected cutoff value to define positivity (Davis and Patel 2019; Patel et al. 2015). For UC, PD-L1 expression in localized disease ranges from 20 to 70% (Necchi et al. 2018; Powles et al. 2019; van Dijk et al. 2020; Faraj et al. 2015), while in advanced disease the incidence of positive PD-L1 expression varies from 30 to 65% (Bellmunt et al. 2017; Patel et al. 2018; Powles et al. 2018, 2020a; Massard et al. 2016; Sharma et al. 2017; Balar et al. 2017a, b). As previously stated, analytic variables influence the wide range of PD-L1 positivity, but they also produce discordant results on their predictive value. There are various immunohistochemistry (IHC) assays to test PD-L1, four of which have been approved as companion diagnostics by the US Food and Drug Administration (FDA) with specific indications for cancer type, drug, and therapeutic line (FDA n.d.): Ventana PD-L1 (SP142), Ventana PD-L1 (SP263), Dako PD-L1 IHC 22C3 pharmDx, and Dako PD-L1 IHC 28-8 pharmDx. PD-L1 IHC expression can be assessed on tumor cells (TC), tumor-associated immune cells (IC) or both (combined positive score—CPS), and different cutoffs have been established to determine test positivity. The interchangeability of these tests is not yet clearly defined, but available data suggest a higher concordance among assays when tested on TC rather than IC (Prince et al. 2021). Moreover, when PD-L1 expression is assessed on TC and/or IC, highly discordant results are obtained using the same assay (Galsky et al.

2023). Looking at the predictive value of PD-L1 expression across multiple studies of immunotherapy, it is clear that tumor PD-L1 IHC expression is not the unique determinant of which cancer will respond to anti-PD-1/PD-L1 inhibitors, since some patients with a high PD-L1 expression do not benefit from immunotherapy while others with low expression do (Davis and Patel 2019; Patel et al. 2015; Gibney et al. 2016). Indeed, besides analytical problems, there are other biological issues affecting the efficacy of immunotherapy, given the many pathways involved in the cancer-immune system interface (Chen et al. 2013). In UC, available data from clinical trials confirm this statement, with some relevant exceptions.

In the neoadjuvant trial PURE-01, PD-L1 expression assessed with the Dako PD-L1 IHC 22C3 pharmDx assay and scored using the CPS, was predictive of immunotherapy benefit. A significantly higher pathological complete response (pCR) rate was obtained in the cystectomy specimen after pre-operative pembrolizumab in patients with tumors expressing PD-L1 CPS ≥ 10 at diagnosis, compared to those with a CPS < 10 (54.3 vs. 13.3%; $p = 0.011$). Moreover, event-free survival (EFS) at a median follow-up of 36 months was significantly correlated with PD-L1 value (3 years EFS: 59.7 vs. 76.7 vs. 89.8% in low, intermediate, and high CPS tertiles, respectively; $p = 0.001$). Additionally, a non-statistically significant increase in PD-L1 CPS in the surgical specimen of patients with high-risk residual disease (≥pT2) was observed after neoadjuvant pembrolizumab, which could reflect the existence of a resistance mechanism (Necchi et al. 2018; Basile et al. 2022). In the NABUCCO trial (neoadjuvant nivolumab plus ipilimumab) the pCR rate was higher in patients with PD-L1 CPS ≥10 (assessed with the same assay used in the PURE-01 trial), but the difference was not statistically significant (73 vs. 33%; $p = 0.15$) (van Dijk et al. 2020). On the contrary, non-significant differences in outcome were observed between patients with positive (≥ 5% IC) and negative PD-L1 expression, tested with the Ventana PD-L1 (SP142) assay on IC in the neoadjuvant atezolizumab ABACUS trial (Powles et al. 2019; Szabados et al. 2022). PD-L1 expression in the CheckMate 274 trial was first prospectively assessed on TC with the Dako PD-L1 IHC 28-8 pharmDx assay, revealing a benefit from adjuvant nivolumab in both the intention-to-treat (ITT) and PD-L1 ≥ 1% population, with an exploratory subgroup analysis showing a non-statistically significant benefit trend also in the PD-L1 negative group (Bajorin et al. 2021). Subsequently, PD-L1 expression was scored by CPS. The number of PD-L1 CPS ≥ 1% was higher than PD-L1 TC ≥ 1, because some tumors defined as PD-L1 negative by TC were positive when defined by CPS; survival benefit was observed in patients with PD-L1 CPS ≥ 1%, TC ≥ 1%, and TC <1%, but not in the PD-L1 CPS < 1% subpopulation (however this subgroup accounted for only 11% of the population so the sample is too small for accurate conclusions) (Galsky et al. 2023). In the negative IMvigor010 trial of adjuvant atezolizumab, PD-L1 expression was evaluated with the Ventana PD-L1 (SP142) assay on IC (IC0 <1%, IC1 1-<5%, IC2/3 ≥5%). PD-L1 expression was not predictive of atezolizumab benefit, since no survival differences were observed among IC0, IC1, and IC2/3 subpopulations treated with adjuvant immunotherapy. However, a prognostic role for PD-L1 expression was observed, with a longer disease-free survival (DFS) in the IC2/3 subgroup, independent of treatment group (atezolizumab vs observation) (Bellmunt et al. 2021).

Highly discordant results on the predictive value of PD-L1 expression have been reported in metastatic disease, from first-line therapy trials Keynote-052, Keynote-361, IMvigor210, IMvigor130, and DANUBE trials. Regarding pembrolizumab studies (22C3 pharmDx assay—CPS), PD-L1 with a CPS cutoff ≥10% seems to present predictive value in cisplatin-ineligible patients in Keynote-052, although some patients with low or absent PD-L1 also showed a response (Balar et al. 2017b). This trend was confirmed in Keynote-361, in which cisplatin-unfit patients with CPS ≥10% presented the highest, but not statistically significant, survival benefit from pembrolizumab in comparison to carboplatin-based chemotherapy (HR 0.82; 95% CI

0.57–1.17) (Powles et al. 2021a). In the atezolizumab trials (Ventana sp142 assay—IC), PD-L1 did not enrich for responses in IMvigor210 but seemed to have a predictive value in IMvigor130, since only patients with tumors with PD-L1 IC2/3 experienced a survival benefit from atezolizumab compared to chemotherapy. However, this data also did not reach statistical significance (HR 0,68; 95% CI 0.43–1.08) (Balar et al. 2017a; Galsky et al. 2020a). In the DANUBE trial (Ventana sp263 assay—TC and/or IC), PD-L1 expression seems to show the same trend of enhanced efficacy across treatment groups but is not sufficient alone to select patients. This is in contrast with the previous results of Study 1108 in pretreated patients, in which high PD-L1 expression was clearly predictive of durvalumab benefit (Massard et al. 2016; Powles et al. 2020b). In the maintenance trial JAVELIN Bladder 100 (Ventana sp263 assay—TC and/or IC), PD-L1 expression correlated with a better prognosis. Moreover, PD-L1 positive tumors received greater benefit from avelumab maintenance, but a significant benefit was seen also in the PD-L1 negative population, as already observed in the JAVELIN Solid Tumors trial (73-10 PharmDx assay—TC) of avelumab in pretreated patients (Patel et al. 2018; Powles et al. 2020a).

In trials of more advanced therapy lines, the predictive role of PD-L1 remains unclear. In the IMvigor211 trial (Ventana sp142 assay—IC), a favorable prognostic role for PD-L1, but no predictive value was observed (Powles et al. 2018). Similarly, no predictive role for PD-L1 was observed in Keynote-045 (22C3 pharmDx assay—CPS) and Checkmate 275 (28-8 PharmDx assay—TC) (Bellmunt et al. 2017; Sharma et al. 2017).

23.3.2.2 Tumor Mutational Burden (TMB)

TMB, expressed as the number of mutations per megabase DNA (mut/Mb), represents the frequency of somatic mutations in a tumor genome. TMB can be assessed with whole-exome sequencing (WES), which routinely records only non-synonymous mutations, or with other technologies such as the comprehensive genomic profiling (CGP) assay (FoundationOne CDx—324 genes), already approved by the FDA, which includes synonymous and non-synonymous mutations, and also short insertions/deletions (indels) in intronic regions. Highly mutated tumors are associated with high neoantigen production, and this is the rational basis for why TMB could be a good biomarker for immunotherapy benefit. Indeed, pembrolizumab received accelerated FDA approval for patients with advanced solid tumors, pretreated or without valid alternative treatments, with a TMB ≥10 mut/Mb, based on the results of the analysis of the cohorts of patients with high TMB (TMB-H) enrolled in the KEYNOTE-158 study. Although the FDA used a cutoff of ≥10 mut/Mb for approving TMB as a tumor-agnostic biomarker, the optimal cutoff is still debated (Marabelle et al. 2020; Tateo et al. 2023). TMB has been investigated in some clinical trials of immunotherapy in UC, especially in neoadjuvant trials.

The PURE-01 trial has explored several biomarkers, including TMB, assessed with FoundationOne CDx. Median TMB was 11.4 mut/Mb, with no evidence of microsatellite unstable tumors. No correlation between PD-L1 expression and TMB was observed. There was a significant ($p = 0.022$) nonlinear association between TMB and pathologic complete response (pCR) response after neoadjuvant pembrolizumab, and a predictive cutoff was set at ≥15 mut/Mb. A significant reduction in TMB (5.7 vs. 11.4 mut/Mb; $p = 0.002$) was observed in the surgical specimen of patients with high-risk residual disease after neoadjuvant pembrolizumab, and this could be due to a potential resistance mechanism of tumor cells to immunotherapy (possibly immune evasion through selection of less antigenic clones). Baseline TMB also correlated with survival: 3-year EFS was 71.8% in patients with low TMB, 63.0% in those with intermediate TMB and 87.3% in patients with TMB-H ($p = 0.001$) (Necchi et al. 2018; Basile et al. 2022). In the NABUCCO trial, TMB was assessed by WES, and a trend toward a higher TMB was observed in patients achieving pCR after ipilimumab plus nivolumab neoadjuvant therapy compared with patients without a complete response to treatment ($p = 0.056$) (van Dijk et al. 2020). Finally, in the ABACUS trial, TMB assessment was performed with FoundationOne CDx, with a baseline median TMB of 10.09 mut/Mb. Unexpectedly, no enrichment in pCR was observed in the TMB-H (≥10 mut/Mb) tumors. Moreover, there was no significant correlation between TMB and relapse (relative risk—RR = 0.80; 95% CI 0.38–1.7, $p = 0.54$). No modifications in post-treatment TMB were observed in the surgical specimens (Powles et al. 2019).

In the metastatic setting, TMB, using FoundationOne CDx, was investigated in the IMvigor210 trial, showing that in responder patients TMB was significantly higher than in non-responders, also with a positive association with survival (Balar et al. 2017a).

23.3.2.3 Gene Expression Profiling (GEP)

GEP refers to analysis of the transcriptome or of a pattern of genes expressed in specific cells or conditions, representative of specific biological functions. GEP has already been investigated in many cancers and the expression of genes involved in immune response mechanisms could be a promising biomarker for immunotherapy efficacy (Cristescu et al. 2018). Using quantitative polymerase chain reaction, a GEP of 22 "immune-associated" genes was performed in the PURE-01 trial. Additionally, the expression of another six genes potentially involved in innate resistance to anti-PD-1 therapy (CCL2, CCL7, CCL8, IL10, VEGFA, and VEGFC) was investigated. Gene expression analysis showed that in patients with a pCR after neoadjuvant pembrolizumab, the expression in the pre-therapy tissue of 18 of the 22 "immune-associated" genes was significantly higher compared to patients with a post-therapy high-risk residual disease. Involved genes were those of the interferon-gamma pathway, antigen presentation, CD8+ T-cells and T-cell functional differentiation markers, chemokines and chemokine receptors, inhibitory receptors and ligands, and IDO1. In post-therapy surgical specimens with high-risk residual disease, an overall increase in expression of all genes analyzed was observed, including those associated with innate resistance to immunotherapy, probably representing expression of immune-mediated adaptive resistance mechanisms (Necchi et al. 2018). A larger immune expression signature, Immune190, which analyzed the expression of 190 immune-associated genes, was then performed in the PURE-01 study, showing a significant association with pathological response and outcome (Necchi et al. 2020a). GEP was also investigated in the NABUCCO trial, in particular a TGF-β-related expression signature, an INF-γ signature, a tumor inflammation signature (TIS), and the CD8+ T-cell effector signature. An increase in expression of genes of the TGF-β signature was observed at baseline in patients with a non-complete response compared to those who achieved a complete response after neoadjuvant immunotherapy, confirming the role of this gene signature in cancer immune resistance. No differences in the other expression signatures were observed between complete responders and non-complete responders. In a multiplex immunofluorescence analysis, no correlation was observed between baseline CD8+ T-cell density and response to ipilimumab plus nivolumab, with an identical complete response rate in both the lowest and highest CD8+ cell density quartiles. Other performed analyses were: B-cell-related gene expression, which was noticed to be upregulated at baseline in non-responders, suggesting an immunosuppressive activity of intratumoral B-cells and tertiary lymphoid structure (TLS)-related gene expression, which was increased with therapy, in particular in patients who achieved a complete response. These observations were coherent with multiplex immunofluorescence analysis, which revealed a numerical increase of B-cells in non-responding tumors and an induction of TLS in responding tumors (van Dijk et al. 2020). Contrasting results were reported in the ABACUS trial. There was just a non-significant trend in the increment of TGF-β signature expression in non-responders with an excluded immune phenotype, compared to immune inflamed phenotype tumors. Preexisting T-cell immunity was correlated with response, since pCR rate was significantly higher in tumors with baseline high infiltration of CD8+ cells (40 vs. 20%; $p < 0.05$). This observation was confirmed with the eight-gene cytotoxic T-cell transcriptional signature (tGE8), which was significantly increased in responders compared to other patients ($p < 0.01$) (Powles et al. 2019). GEP analysis has also been performed in metastatic disease. In the IMvigor210 trial, the six-gene T-cell effector signature was not significantly associated with response (Balar et al. 2017a), while in the Checkmate275 trial higher values of the 25-gene INF-γ signature were associated with response to nivolumab ($p = 0.0003$) and higher PD-L1 expression. Moreover, tumors of nivolumab responders expressed higher levels of a 12-chemokine signature (Sharma et al. 2017).

GEP has been widely used to identify molecular subtypes in tumors, with likely prognostic and therapeutic implications. In MIBC, several key molecular classifications have been published, including the Lund molecular taxonomy, The Cancer Genome Atlas (TCGA) classification, a Genomic Subtyping Classifier (GSC), and a Consensus Molecular Classification. These classifications show some partial overlaps among the defined molecular subtypes (see Chap. 14) (Robertson et al. 2017; Seiler et al. 2017; Kamoun et al. 2020; Sjödahl et al. 2012). The role of molecular classifications in predicting the benefit of ICIs has been tested in the PURE-01, ABACUS, IMvigor210, and Checkmate275 trials. In PURE-01, tumors were classified according to the consensus model, with a good correspondence with TCGA and GSC models. There were no significant differences in responses across different molecular subtypes, however, basal-type tumors had higher response rates. The highest major response rates were seen for Ba/Sq and LumU according to the Consensus classification, and for "claudin-low" in GSC classification, but without reaching statistical significance (Necchi et al. 2020a). In the ABACUS trial, molecular subgroups were identified by the Lund taxonomy. Interestingly, it was observed that the majority of tumors had undergone a taxonomy change after therapy. In particular, tumors with the best responses almost all switched to "infiltrated" subtype after therapy (Powles et al. 2019).

In the IMvigor210 trial, tumors were subtyped according to TCGA classification. Responses were observed across all subtypes but were most frequent in the "luminal II" subtype (Balar et al. 2017a). In the Checkmate275 trial molecular subtyping was again performed according to TCGA classification, but the highest proportion of responses was seen in the "basal 1" subgroup (Sharma et al. 2017).

23.3.2.4 Other Analyses on Immune Infiltrate

Quantification and characterization of tumor immune infiltrate could provide important information regarding response to immunotherapy. In addition to GEP of immune signatures and IHC quantification of immune infiltrate, described above, other IHC analyses have been performed, specifically in the ABACUS trial. The quality of the immune infiltrate was explored with dual staining for CD8 and GZMB (a surrogate marker of activated CD8+ cells). Notably, dual staining was high in responding tumors with an inflamed phenotype, while relapsing inflamed tumors showed low levels of CD8+ and GZMB+ cells (87 vs. 30%; $p < 0.05$). Another important IHC biomarker investigated was fibroblast activation protein (FAP), which is a surrogate marker for cancer-associated fibroblasts and TGF-β-induced microenvironment. After therapy, FAP remained high in non-responders, while decreased in responders ($p < 0.001$), showing that FAP expression was linked to treatment resistance. Overall, these data show that the quality of the immune infiltrate and the stromal component of the tumor microenvironment have a relevant role in response to immunotherapy and can predict outcomes (Powles et al. 2019).

23.3.2.5 Single-Gene Aberrations

Several genes, such as DNA damage repair (DDR) genes, *FGF3, RB1, PBRM1*, and other cell cycle genes, with possible implications in immunotherapy response, have been investigated in UC, particularly in these neoadjuvant trials that conducted extensive biomarker analysis. In PURE-01, DDR gene mutations correlated with pCR, but they were also associated with TMB, so probably the predictive value is linked to the consequent TMB-H status. *RB1* mutations, when adjusted for TMB interaction, also lost significance. *PBRM1* seemed to correlate with pCR, but it was not significant after multiple hypothesis testing, probably due to the small sample size (Necchi et al. 2018). In the NABUCCO trial, DDR genes were assessed, with evidence of enrichment of complete responses in tumors with DDR mutations ($p = 0.03$) (van Dijk et al. 2020). Finally, in the ABACUS trial, amplification of *FGF3, FGF19*, and *CCND1*, was observed in responding tumors, while there was no association between cell cycle genes and DDR gene mutations and outcomes (Powles et al. 2019).

23.4 Liquid Biomarkers and Immunotherapy

Traditional cancer diagnostic methods have relied heavily on invasive tissue biopsies. However, these procedures may result in complications, discomfort to the patient, and limitations in obtaining representative tumor samples. In recent years, liquid biopsy has emerged as a promising alternative in this context (Fig. 23.2) (Serrano et al. 2020) (see also Chap. 19).

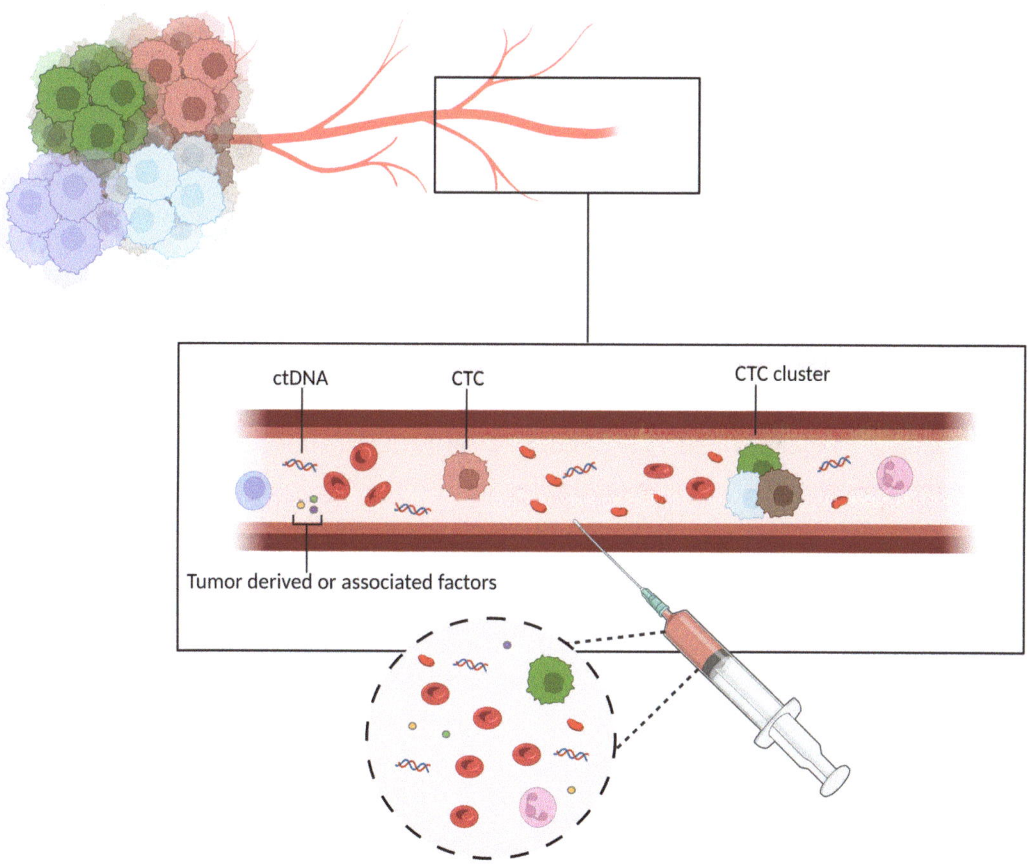

Fig. 23.2 Liquid biopsy concept. Liquid biopsy stands as a revolutionary minimally invasive diagnostic technique, useful in the detection of genetic alterations and cancer-associated biomarkers. It involves the collection of bodily fluids like blood or urine from the patient. Once collected, various techniques such as polymerase chain reaction (PCR), next-generation sequencing (NGS), or digital PCR are employed to analyze the genetic material and circulating biomarkers within the sample. This figure shows how liquid biopsy is performed. Abbreviations: CtDNA, circulating tumor DNA; CTC, circulating tumor cell. Created with Biorender.com

23.4.1 ctDNA

Recently, a Systematic Review was published, summarizing the prognostic and predictive role of ctDNA in the perioperative setting of UC (Crupi et al. 2024). The ABACUS trial was a phase 2 trial that investigated two cycles of atezolizumab before cystectomy in patients with muscle-invasive UC unwilling or ineligible to receive neoadjuvant cisplatin-based chemotherapy. In this trial, ctDNA analysis was performed using Natera's Signatera assay, a highly sensitive and personalized molecular residual disease (MRD) assay custom-built on the unique mutation signature of each patient's tumor (Powles et al. 2019). The presence of ctDNA before treatment correlated with disease status and response. Patients who cleared ctDNA after neoadjuvant atezolizumab showed a complete pathological response at surgery. The detection of ctDNA post-neoadjuvant treatment correlated with lymph node involvement and tumor stage at cystectomy. No relapses were observed in ctDNA-negative patients at baseline and after neoadjuvant therapy. In contrast, patients who were ctDNA positive after surgery had a higher recurrence rate than negative patients (Relapse-free survival [RFS], HR 78.22 CI 95% 8.64–707.73, $p < 0.001$) (Powles et al. 2021a).

Recently, updated results of exploratory biomarker analysis of the ABACUS trial were presented. Two definitions of ctDNA response were used: ctDNA clearance and a 50% or greater reduction in ctDNA variant allele frequency (VAF). The results were then correlated with the pathological complete response rate at cystectomy and relapse-free survival. There was no association between VAF reduction of 50 or 75% and pathologic complete response ($p = 0.24$) (Young et al. 2024).

In the IMVIGOR010 phase 3 trial, ctDNA analysis using the same assay was conducted on high-risk UC patients treated with adjuvant atezolizumab (Bellmunt et al. 2021; Powles et al. 2021b). CtDNA-positive patients had a higher risk of recurrence, while ctDNA-negative patients had improved disease-free survival (DFS HR = 3.36 95% CI: 2.44–4.62) and overall survival (OS). Similar findings were observed for ctDNA clearance during adjuvant treatment, which was associated with improved outcomes (DFS HR = 0.26 (95% CI: 0.12–0.56), $p = 0.0014$; median DFS: not reached, OS HR = 0.14, 95% CI: 0.03–0.59). Patients with ctDNA+ persistent after two cycles of atezolizumab had a higher risk for disease progression and recurrence than ctDNA-negative patients (observation arm DFS HR = 8.65(95% CI: 5.67–13.18; $p < 0.0001$) (Powles et al. 2021b). Based on the encouraging outcomes of the IMvigor010 post-hoc analysis, IMvigor 011 was initiated to evaluate the effectiveness of adjuvant atezolizumab in 495 patients with ctDNA-positive, high-risk MIBC after radical cystectomy.

In the phase 1B NABUCCO trial, different dosing regimens of ipilimumab-ninolumab were evaluated in the neoadjuvant setting of locoregionally advanced MIBC, including patients with lymph node-positive disease (cT3-4aN0M0 or cT1-4aN1-3M0). CtDNA analysis demonstrated that undetectable plasma ctDNA after neoadjuvant treatment correlated with pathological complete response (HR: 4.0; 95% CI: 4.9–416.5) in the bladder and PFS (HR: 10.4; 95% CI: 2.9–37.5) (van Dijk et al. 2020).

POLARIS-03 was a multi-center, open-label, single-arm, phase 2 clinical trial to evaluate the safety and efficacy of toripalimab (anti-PD-1) in chemotherapy-refractory metastatic UC (mUC). The study utilized serial plasma specimens and the PredicineATLAS liquid biopsy assay to detect somatic variants and determine cancer cell fraction (CCF) alongside low-pass whole genome sequencing for copy number abnormality (CNA) scores. Baseline CCF or CNA showed limited predictive value, but early ctDNA response after one cycle (at week 8) correlated with toripalimab efficacy and patient survival. Moreover, dynamic changes in CCF and CNA reflected disease status, aligning with radiographic assessments (Zang et al. 2023).

These studies support the feasibility and effectiveness of longitudinal ctDNA profiling as a biomarker for immunotherapy response in UC, indicating its potential for clinical use in treatment stratification and monitoring.

23.4.2 Role of Circulating Cytokines

Several cytokines have been identified as potential prognostic and predictive biomarkers with relevance to immunotherapy of UC. Transforming Growth Factor-Beta (TGF-β) signalling is a multifunctional, highly conserved, and complex pathway involved in several cancer hallmarks (David and Massagué 2018). Dysregulated TGF-β signalling contributes to UC's tumor growth, invasion, and metastasis. Moreover, it is linked to immunosuppressive effects within the tumor microenvironment (Benjamin and Lyou 2021).

A recent study included a group of 51 patients who underwent radical cystectomy for MIBC or intravesical immuno- and/or chemotherapy for refractory carcinoma in situ (CIS), Ta, or T1 NMIBC. Pre-operative plasma levels of TGF-β were measured, and their correlation with pathologic features and clinical outcomes was assessed. Patients with metastases to distant or regional lymph nodes showed higher pre-operative plasma TGF-β levels than those with NMIBC (non-metastatic Tis, Ta, or T1 UC) and healthy individuals. Elevated TGF-β levels correlated with lymphovascular invasion, lymph node metastases, disease recurrence, and disease-specific survival. In patients with MIBC, TGF-β levels were associated with disease recurrence and cancer-specific mortality (Shahrokh et al. 2001).

Promising results have been shown in recent preclinical and phase 1 studies that combine TGF-β pathway inhibitors with immunotherapy agents in UC. By blocking TGF-β-mediated immunosuppression, these combination approaches enhance antitumor immune responses and improve treatment outcomes for UC patients. There are currently several small-molecule inhibitors and monoclonal antibodies targeting the TGF-β pathway. Most of these agents were first studied as monotherapies and are now being studied in combination therapy with ICIs for several tumor types, including UC (Benjamin and Lyou 2021; Mariathasan et al. 2018).

High levels of pro-inflammatory cytokines, such as interleukin-6 (IL-6), Interleukin-8 (IL-8), and tumor necrosis factor-alpha (TNF-α), have been associated with poorer prognosis and aggressive tumor behavior. On the other hand, elevated levels of immune-stimulatory cytokines, like interferon-gamma (IFN-γ), have shown positive associations with immunotherapy response.

In pre-clinical models, combined blockade of PD-L1 and the IL-6 receptor (IL6R) caused synergistic regression of large established tumors and substantially improved antitumor $CD8^+$ cytotoxic T-lymphocyte (CTL) responses compared with anti-PD-L1 alone. Circulating CTLs from cancer patients with high plasma IL-6 display a repressed functional profile based on single-cell RNA sequencing, and IL-6-STAT3 signalling inhibits classical cytotoxic differentiation of CTLs in vitro (Huseni et al. 2023). In the IMvigor210 and IMvigor211 trials, plasma IL-6 was elevated compared to healthy controls and associated with poor OS in multivariate survival analysis. C-reactive protein, triggered by IL-6 during the acute phase response, was found to have a similar association with plasma IL-6 and a poor overall survival rate (Powles et al. 2018; Balar et al. 2017a; Rosenberg et al. 2016).

A phase 1b/2 clinical trial evaluated the intravesical administration of autologous IFN-γ-activated macrophages (MAK) in patients with NMIBC. Monitoring of the patients showed that urinary IL-8, GM-CSF, and IL-18 were increased following MAK instillations, providing evidence of a local immunostimulant signature (Pagès et al. 2002). A study evaluated circulating serum cytokine profiles in 41 NMIBC patients before and after intravesical combination immunotherapy with Bacillus Calmette-Guerin (BCG) plus interferon-α2b (IFN-α2b). Before therapy, T-Helper (Th) 1 cells, cytokines like IL-2 and TNF-α were reduced, while IL-4, IL-6, and IL-10 typically associated with Th2 response were enhanced compared to controls. Following immunotherapy, there was a shift in cytokine profiles toward an increase in Th1-associated cytokines (IFN-γ, IL-2, TNF-α) and a decrease in Th2-associated cytokines (IL-4, IL-10), suggesting a restoration of immune balance, with a strengthened Th1 response, usually related to mediation of cellular immunity, macrophage activation, antibody-dependent cytotoxicity and suppression of the dominant Th2 status, which are generally associated with anti-inflammatory responses. This shift indicates a more favorable immune environment for combating cancer progression, as Th1 responses are typically associated with antitumor immunity and cytotoxic activity (Agarwal et al. 2010).

Emerging evidence suggests that high expression of IL-8 in myeloid cells is linked to suppression of tumor antigen presentation. Elevated levels of IL-8 in the bloodstream and increased IL-8 gene expression in peripheral blood mononuclear cells have been associated with reduced efficacy of atezolizumab in patients with metastatic UC. Furthermore, fluctuations in IL-8 levels during treatment could be used as a biomarker of response (Yuen et al. 2020). Interestingly, in another study, IL-8 urinary levels were greater in subjects with UC than in healthy subjects and those with successfully treated UC. IL-8 levels increased with stage. According to these findings, the authors suggested that reducing urinary IL-8 levels after treatment with BCG or mitomycin C may reflect a decrease in UC cells and/or other cells that produce IL-8 (Sheryka et al. 2003).

In intermediate or high-risk NMIBC treated with BCG, a serial panel assessment of urinary cytokine levels was performed. Changes in a combination of cytokines were the most accurate predictor of recurrence, although increases in single cytokines also showed a correlation with recurrence. A nomogram was created based on the levels of nine inducible cytokines found in urine (IL-2, IL-6, IL-8, IL-18, IL-1ra, TRAIL, IFN-γ, IL-12 [p70], and TNF-α) to determine the chances of recurrence with 85.5% accuracy (CI 95% 77.9–93.1%) (Kamat et al. 2016). Another study conducted on patients with CIS treated with BCG showed a significantly higher urinary level of IL-2, IL-6, IL-8, IL-10, and TNF-alpha in the responder group than in the non-responder group (Watanabe et al. 2003).

23.4.3 Circulating Immune Cell Profiles and Extracellular Vesicles

Circulating immune cell profiles, particularly the assessment of T-cell subsets, have emerged as potential predictors of response to immunotherapy in UC. T-cells play a crucial role in antitumor immune responses, and their functional status and distribution can influence treatment outcomes. In different cancer types, a high ratio of effector T-cells to regulatory T-cells (Tregs) has been associated with improved response to immune checkpoint inhibitors (ICIs). Monitoring changes in circulating T-cell subsets during immunotherapy can provide valuable information about treatment response and guide therapeutic strategies (Wang et al. 2020).

In a recent study, a high frequency of CD57 was observed in neoantigen-specific CD8 T and bulk CD8 T-cells in patients with metastatic UC responding to atezolizumab. Single-cell RNA sequencing analysis identified a clonally expanded cluster enriched within $CD57^+$ CD8 T-cells in responding patients. Responders had higher expression of genes associated with cytotoxicity, activation, and tissue-resident memory markers. Additionally, the T-cell receptors (TCRs) of CD57+ CD8 T-cells had more significant overlap with the TCR repertoire of tumor-infiltrating T-cells compared to CD57–CD8 T-cells (Fehlings et al. 2022).

The NCT02108652 trial evaluated the efficacy of atezolizumab in locally advanced or metastatic UC (Fidelle et al. 2023). In a cohort of 24 patients, pre-treatment, and longitudinal post-treatment assessments of peripheral $CD8^+$ T-cells were conducted. The results showed that after 3 weeks of treatment, patients with disease control had peripheral tumor neoantigen-reactive CD8+ T-cells characterized by a PD-1+ Ki67+ effector phenotype and higher CD39 levels compared to virus-antigen-reactive CD8+ T-cells and bulk CD8+ T-cells (Holm et al. 2022). According to these findings and a growing body of literature, ICIs seem to rapidly induce an immunological T-cell response in the peripheral blood and suggest that early-stage neoantigen-reactive CD8+

T-cell expansion and activation are associated with response to ICI in patients with metastatic UC.

Extracellular vesicles (EVs), including exosomes and microvesicles, are small membrane-bound structures released by cells into the extracellular space. They carry a cargo of proteins, nucleic acids, lipids, and other bioactive molecules that can be transferred to recipient cells, influencing their behavior and function. There is increasing evidence that intercellular communication and the involvement of extracellular vesicles (EVs) play an important role in various disease processes. In bladder cancer, EVs have emerged as a novel and intriguing mediator contributing to tumor progression and therapeutic responses. EVs derived from tumor cells can reflect the unique molecular profile of the tumor. Additionally, EVs released by immune cells can modulate the tumor microenvironment, promoting or suppressing antitumor immune responses.

In a recent study, serum samples were collected from 20 healthy donors, 50 patients with localized UC, and 31 patients with mUC who had undergone pembrolizumab treatment. Given the growing body of evidence that gut and urinary microbiota could modulate immune response (Fidelle et al. 2023; Drobner et al. 2023) and that components of cancer-specific microflora have also been reported in the bloodstream but with unclear implications, the correlation of EV-derived blood microflora information and tumor immunological status was evaluated. The authors found that patients with lower levels of peripheral EVs carrying Firmicutes phylum bacteria DNA had a higher infiltration of T-cells in tumor tissues, along with increased expression of activation markers on their surface. On the contrary, all patients with higher levels of EVs carrying Firmicutes DNA abundance had disease progression without any clinical response ($p = 0.026$) and significantly inferior prognosis for pembrolizumab therapy ($p = 0.035$) (Jingushi et al. 2022).

Despite their potential benefits, EVs are not commonly utilized in clinical practice due to the complexity of biological samples, the presence of other physiological extracellular vesicles, and the absence of cost-effective and precise methods for isolation and detection. Thus, more sensitive platforms should be developed to assist in the search for UC-specific EVs.

23.4.4 Urinary PD-L1 as a Surrogate for Tissue-Based Assays

As previously mentioned, urine is a rich source of potential biomarkers that can reflect the molecular traits and dynamic changes in bladder tumors (Rose et al. 2023). One advantage of utilizing urine when dealing with UC is its proximity to the tumor. This allows direct capture of shed tumor-derived components and a reflection of the tumor microenvironment.

For instance, immune-related proteins, including immune checkpoint molecules (e.g., PD-L1), cytokines, and chemokines, can be detected in urine samples and may help to indicate immunotherapy response or resistance. Changes in the expression levels of these biomarkers during treatment can provide valuable information about treatment efficacy. However, their role in the disease remains a topic of debate and controversy due to conflicting findings and interpretations from various studies. On one hand, PD-L1 expression in UC patients has been associated with poor prognosis and aggressive tumor behavior. Conversely, PD-L1 expression has also been associated with favorable outcomes in specific scenarios (Balar et al. 2017a). As discussed above, PD-L1's role as a predictive biomarker through tissue-based studies is unclear, and as an alternative or additional source of information, urine analysis has been assessed in pre- and post-operative samples.

A recent study compared PD-L1 protein levels in pre-operative urine samples from UC patients with PD-L1 expression in post-operative pathological sections. The authors found that urinary PD-L1 levels were comparable to PD-L1 tissue expression. Additionally, elevated levels of PD-L1 in urine were associated with more advanced stages of muscle-invasive bladder cancer (MIBC) and a worse prognosis (Bellmunt et al. 2015).

In another study, PD-L1 levels were assessed through the Enzyme-Linked ImmunoSorbent Assay (ELISA) in urine and serum samples taken from 132 patients with UC. This was then compared to 51 control patients who had hematuria. Soluble PD-L1 was detected in almost 100% of the serum samples and around 35% of the urine samples. No significant difference in serum levels of PD-L1 between cases and controls was found ($p = 0.61$); however, patients with MIBC had significantly higher PD-L1 levels than patients with NMIBC ($p = 0.004$). Moreover, patients with a high-grade tumor had significantly higher levels of PD-L1 compared to those with a low-grade tumor ($p = 0.006$). A survival analysis revealed that patients with PD-L1 levels above the median (94.0 pg/mL) had a shorter overall survival time (19.6 months) compared to those with levels below the median value (26.4 months, $p < 0.05$). No correlation was found between serum PD-L1 and urinary PD-L1 levels ($p = 0.22$). Patients with UC had significantly higher levels of PD-L1 in urine than healthy controls ($p = 0.038$). Additionally, the frequency of PD-L1 detection tended to be higher in cases than controls ($p = 0.07$). There was no significant correlation between the levels of PD-L1 in urine and the stage and grade of the tumor (low vs. high, p-values of 0.09 and 0.09, respectively). However, patients diagnosed with metastatic disease or who developed distant metastases during follow-up had higher levels of urinary PD-L1 compared to patients without metastatic disease, with a p-value of 0.05 (Vikerfors et al. 2021).

In another study, PD-L1 levels in pre-operative urine samples from 138 UC patients ($n = 90$ NMIBC, $n = 26$ MIBC, $n = 22$ UTUC) were evaluated through ELISA. Urinary PD-L1 was detected in 77 of 138 individuals (55.8%). When stratifying according to pathology results (NMIBC, MIBC, upper tract UC [UTUC]), no statistical differences in urine PD-L1 levels were observed among the groups (UTUC vs. NMIBC: $p = 0.105$; UTUC vs. MIBC $p = 0.924$, NMIBC vs. MIBC $p = 0.080$). When NMIBC patients were classified into high- and low-risk groups based on American Urological Association (AUA) risk groups, there was also no significant difference in urine PD-L1 levels ($p = 0.223$). Patients who had undergone intravenous chemotherapy had higher urinary PD-L1 levels than others ($p = 0.048$). To investigate the feasibility of replacing tissue PD-L1 with urinary PD-L1 levels in bladder UC, the correlation between them was analyzed. The results showed a significant correlation between the two ($p < 0.0001$). In the survival analysis of bladder cancer patients, the participants were divided into two groups based on their urinary PD-L1 levels—high PD-L1 group and low PD-L1 group. The median value was used to determine the cutoff point. No significant differences in overall survival (OS) between the two groups was found. Univariate analysis revealed that an increase in urinary PD-L1 is a risk factor for predicting recurrence outcomes in MIBC, with 110% higher odds of recurrence for every one-unit increase in uPD-L1 ($p = 0.048$) (Ma et al. 2023).

The concordance of PD-L1 expression between paired surgical resection specimens (SRSs) and urine cell blocks (UCBs) was studied in a retrospective cohort of 58 UTUC patients (Cohort 1) and then in a prospective cohort of 12 UTUC patients (Cohort 2). In Cohort 1 concordance between paired surgical resection specimens (SRSs) and urine cell blocks (UCBs) was found to be 94.4%. To determine the best criteria for positive PD-L1 expression in UCBs, the authors analyzed PD-L1 expression as a continuous variable. They found that PD-L1 expression < 10% and > 10% of tumor cells in UCBs were the best predictors of negative and positive expression in SRSs, respectively. The samples showed a high agreement rate of 98.1%. In cohort 2, PD-L1 expression in UCBs was obtained before neoadjuvant ICI immunotherapy. At the 10% cutoff for PD-L1 expression, the best response predictive value was found to be 83.3% in PD-L1-positive patients, while the non-response predictive value was found to be 50% in PD-L1-negative patients (Chen et al. 2023).

In conclusion, liquid biopsy represents a groundbreaking approach to non-invasive cancer detection and monitoring, providing real-time insights into tumor biology, treatment response, and resistance. Combining information from liquid biomarkers with traditional clinical parameters could enhance patient stratification for immunotherapy. However, challenges related to standardization, validation, technical limitations, and ethical considerations must be addressed before widespread implementation. Prospective larger studies are warranted to validate the growing body of evidence on a larger scale.

23.5 Immunotherapy Response in Histological Subtypes and Urothelial Carcinoma with Divergent Differentiation

Most urinary tract cancers are histologically categorized as pure urothelial carcinoma (PUC) (Moch et al. 2022). However, UC has various histological morphologies, either single (pure subtype) or combined subtypes.

The 2022 World Health Organization (WHO) classification refined the criteria for defining urothelial carcinoma subtypes and those with divergent differentiation based on pathological features (Netto et al. 2022). Subtypes include micropapillary, sarcomatoid, plasmacytoid, nested, lymphoepithelioma-like, and some other rarities. Urothelial carcinoma with divergent differentiation includes tumors with pure squamous, glandular, trophoblastic, or Müllerian differentiation (for more detail see Chaps. 4 and 15).

The most common forms of differentiation of urothelial carcinoma apart from pure urothelial are squamous cell-like features, detected in ~20% of advanced UC, and more rarely glandular features (Netto et al. 2022). Patients whose tumors are predominantly characterized by these histologies, often experience an aggressive clinical course, with the exception of the non-urothelial neuroendocrine subtype, which exhibits distinct sensitivity to chemotherapy (Siefker-Radtke et al. 2009). Patients with predominant subtypes or mixed features are not included in the majority of clinical trials, and data regarding effectiveness of chemotherapy and immunotherapy are limited, highlighting an urgent unmet medical need. A study examining the impact of chemotherapy in patients with unresectable or metastatic UC revealed that those with a subtype experienced notably poorer progression-free survival (PFS; 6.1 versus 3.8 months, $p = 0.004$) and overall survival (OS; median OS 11.3 vs. 15.9 months, $p = 0.007$) compared to patients with pure UC (PUC) (Hsieh et al. 2015). However, contrasting studies have indicated that the response to neoadjuvant cisplatin-based chemotherapy or trimodal bladder-sparing therapy was not affected by the presence of a histological subtype or mixed histological features (Scosyrev et al. 2011; Krasnow et al. 2017).

23.5.1 Immunotherapy Response of Urothelial Subtypes or Those with Mixed Histological Features in the Advanced/Metastatic Setting

The introduction of ICIs has dramatically changed the treatment landscape for advanced and metastatic UC, particularly with avelumab, as maintenance after response to first-line platinum (PT)-based chemotherapy (Powles et al. 2020a), and with pembrolizumab, as second-line treatment after progression following PT-based chemotherapy (Bellmunt et al. 2017). The lack of clarity concerning the response to chemotherapy among subtypes or tumors with mixed features is even more pronounced with immunotherapy. The efficacy of immunotherapy in such patients has rarely been reported and is yet to be fully elucidated (Miller et al. 2020; Kobayashi et al. 2022). In 2020, a retrospective analysis was conducted on 519 patients with advanced urothelial carcinoma (aUC) who received several kinds of ICIs, aimed at understanding the impact of histological subtypes on ICI treatment response and exploring potential biomarkers for predicting response (Miller et al. 2020). The results showed that the histological subtype did not significantly affect the overall response rate (ORR, 28% for PUC vs. 29% for subtypes, p 0.90), PFS (4.1 months for PUC 5.2 months for subtypes, p 0.43), or OS (11.0 months for PUC vs. 10.1 months for subtypes, p 0.6) in patients treated with ICI, except for those with neuroendocrine (NE) features, who had shorter OS (4.6 months, 9 patients, HR 2.75, 95% CI 1.40–5.40, *p* 0.09). In this study, mixed histology in upper tract tumors was also associated with shorter OS compared to PUC (Miller et al. 2020). These results suggested that histological subtype may not be a reliable biomarker for ICI response in aUC, except for tumors with NE features, which are characterized by poor long-term outcomes. The knowledge that not all immunotherapies act in the same way or produce identical immunological effects prompted the initiation of studies concentrating on specific types of ICI. No studies have evaluated the efficacy of avelumab on histological subtypes, while for pembrolizumab two retrospective studies have evaluated this. In the retrospective analysis by Kobayashi et al. on 755 patients with advanced chemo-resistant UC who received pembrolizumab, they compared the clinical outcomes of patients with a subtype or mixed features with those of patients with PUC (Kobayashi et al. 2022). Overall, patients with a subtype or mixed features had similar objective response rates (ORR, 24.5% vs. 17.3%, $p = 0.098$) and disease control rates (DCR, 36.7% vs. 30.2%, $p = 0.195$). Among the different types of histology, the most common, those with squamous differentiation, showed no significant difference in clinical outcomes compared to PUC or other non-squamous histologies. The patients with sarcomatoid subtype (2.5%) had significantly better objective response rate (ORR) (36.8%, $p = 0.031$), DCR (52.6%, $p = 0.032$), and OS (HR 0.37, 95% CI 0.15-0.90; $p = 0.023$) compared to patients with PUC. A recent retrospective study evaluated the efficacy of pembrolizumab in patients with advanced UC and upper urinary tract cancer based on histological subtypes (Minato et al. 2022). In this study, authors compared the therapeutic response and survival outcomes in patients with PUC and other UC subtypes treated with pembrolizumab after platinum-based chemotherapy. The results showed that patients with other UC subtypes had significantly better ORR (59.1% vs. 29.6%, $p = 0.014$) and comparable DCR (68.2% vs. 49.4%, $p = 0.150$) compared to those with PUC. However, there were no significant differences between the PUC and subtype groups with respect to PFS (median 5.0 months vs. 10.4 months, $p = 0.222$) or OS (median 13.5 months vs. 23.8 months, $p = 0.497$). These results suggest that pembrolizumab may be an effective treatment option for patients with non-PUC subtypes and that certain histologic features, such as squamous differentiation, may respond particularly well to this therapy. Overall, while histological subtype may not be a reliable biomarker for ICI response in advanced UC, these findings provide valuable insights into potential treatment efficacy for specific subtypes/differentiation states, such as those with sarcomatoid and squamous differentiation, and warrant further investigation and consideration in clinical decision-making.

23.5.2 Immunotherapy Response of Urothelial Subtypes or Those with Mixed Histological Features in the Neoadjuvant Setting

The current understanding of neoadjuvant immunotherapy's effects on histological subtypes is limited, both because these patients are usually not included in clinical trials and because the results of these trials are relatively recent. The only published study focusing on subtypes or mixed histology in this setting is with neoadjuvant pembrolizumab. On the basis of the exciting results of the PURE-1 study, which demonstrated a pathological complete response (pCR) rate of 37% in cT2-4N0M0 cisplatin-fit patients (Necchi et al. 2018), Necchi et al. evaluated patients with a predominant subtype or mixed histology enrolled in the trial (Necchi et al. 2020b). The authors observed that tumor responses were significantly heterogeneous, depending primarily on tumor biomarkers rather than histological features (Necchi et al. 2020b). Patients with squamous cell carcinoma ($n = 7$) and lymphoepithelioma-like ($n = 3$) tumors exhibited immunotherapy sensitivity due to their enrichment in elevated TMB and high PD-L1 expression. In contrast, other histologies such as adenocarcinoma, demonstrated poor sensitivity to single-agent immune checkpoint inhibition. The study suggests that combination therapies may offer potential opportunities for these tumors and highlights the significance of patient selection through biomarkers for future advancements of immune checkpoint inhibitor use in MIBC. However, it is important to acknowledge the study's limitations, such as the small sample size within each histological subgroup and the preliminary nature of the data.

In conclusion, the increasing prominence of ICIs in this setting and the scarcity of data regarding the role of immunotherapy on urothelial subtypes highlight the necessity to further focus studies on neoadjuvant immunotherapy, with a specific emphasis on these histologies.

23.5.3 Future Perspectives

The knowledge that the presence of histological subtypes, or mixed histology cases of UC can potentially provide guidance toward a more targeted treatment approach, has led to several phase 2 trials focusing on them. In the metastatic setting, the use of the combination of durvalumab with the multi-tyrosine kinase inhibitor cabozantinib in patients with UC, including those with a subtype or cases with another component, showed promising results in safety and preliminary activity in the phase 2 study ARCADIA (NCT03824691) (Marandino et al. 2021). More robust data from an increased sample size and completion of the study are needed to establish the effectiveness in such cases. Other ongoing phase 2 trials in advanced and metastatic disease are evaluating the combination of enfortumab vedotin (EV) and pembrolizumab (NCT05756569) and the combination of anti-PD-1 and anti-CTLA-4 with nivolumab and ipilimumab (NCT03333616). In the neoadjuvant setting, an ongoing phase 2 trial (NCT03912818) is investigating the side effects of durvalumab combined with chemotherapy before surgery in patients with UC with different subtypes. These trials represent critical efforts to explore the role of immunotherapy in addressing different histologies of UC. By focusing on specific histological subtypes, researchers aspire to develop more targeted and effective treatment approaches for patients with these challenging and less understood forms of bladder cancer.

23.6 Novel Immunotherapy Combinations

The significant progress in the ICI treatment landscape of UC within neoadjuvant, adjuvant, and metastatic settings, and the significant results obtained with antibody–drug conjugates (ADCs) and fibroblast growth factor receptor (FGFR) inhibitors in advanced disease, have suggested innovative strategies to further enhance therapeutic outcomes. Recently, the potential benefits of combining immunotherapy with FGFR inhibitors and ADCs have been investigated (see also Chap. 22).

FGFR inhibitors have emerged as a promising avenue in the treatment of urothelial carcinoma as dysregulation of FGFR signalling pathways is implicated in the development and progression of UC (Peng et al. 2022; Siefker-Radtke et al. 2022; Loriot et al. 2023). Furthermore, FGFR alterations seem to influence the response to immunotherapy, making FGFR inhibitors—ICI combinations an interesting therapeutic option (Rezazadeh et al. 2020; Kim et al. 2020).

The integration of ADCs into the therapeutic armamentarium holds the potential to further improve treatment efficacy. These innovative agents combine the specificity of monoclonal antibodies with the cytotoxic effects of chemotherapeutic agents, to deliver potent anti-cancer drugs directly to tumor cells. The most important ADCs in the treatment of UC are Enfortumab Vedotin (EV), an anti-Nectin-4 monoclonal antibody (mAb) coupled with the microtubule-disrupting agent monomethyl auristatin E (MMAE) (Hoffman-Censits et al. 2021; Powles et al. 2021c), and Sacituzumab Govitecan (SG), an anti-Trop-2 mAb linked with the topoisomerase inhibitor SN-38 (Tagawa et al. 2021). Beyond Nectin-4 and Trop-2, there are multiple other promising targets that are under evaluation in ongoing trials, such as Human Epidermal Growth Factor Receptor 2 (HER-2) and SLIT And NTRK Like Family Member-6 (SLITRK6). Indeed, results are awaited from other ADCs such as trastuzumab Deruxtecan, which combines an anti-HER2 mAb with a potent topoisomerase-I inhibitor (de Padua et al. 2022).

The most significant data and ongoing trials with the combinations of ICIs-FGFR inhibitors and ICIs-ADCs are described below.

23.6.1 Immunotherapy–Fibroblast Growth Factor Receptor Inhibitors

Urothelial cancers harboring FGFR aberrations (e.g., mutations, amplifications, and fusions) have traditionally exhibited limited responses to immunotherapy. Data from Santiago-Walker et al. highlighted that median overall survival (OS) in FGFR+ patients was notably lower than in FGFR–patients, suggesting an unmet need for effective treatment strategies (Kim et al. 2020). This was confirmed by a retrospective study which indicated that FGFR+ patients undergoing anti-PD-L1 therapy exhibited lower overall response rates (ORR) and disease control rates than FGFR–patients (Rezazadeh et al. 2020). Therefore, recent clinical trials have been exploring novel combinations with immunotherapy to address these challenges, with a particular focus on targeting FGFR aberrations and augmenting immune responses.

Preliminary data from the FIGHT-205 trial pave the way for a new frontline strategy. In this phase 2 study, the combination of the FGFR1-3 inhibitor Pemigatinib with pembrolizumab in first line for cisplatin-ineligible UC patients with *FGFR3* mutations or rearrangements significantly enhanced outcomes (Galsky et al. 2020b).

On the basis of an encouraging preclinical study in a mouse model of lung cancer with *FGFR2* and *TP53* mutations showing notable improvements in overall survival (OS) with the combination of erdafitinib with immune checkpoint inhibitors (ICI) (Palakurthi et al. 2019), the NORSE trial is currently evaluating this FGFR inhibitor with the PD-1 inhibitor Cetrelimab in metastatic or locally advanced UC (NCT03473743).

Other phase 1b-2 studies are investigating the combination of atezolizumab with the FGFR inhibitors erdafitinib (NCT05564416), derazantinib (NCT04045613), and rogaratinib (NCT03473756, FORT-2) in patients with advanced UC with *FGFR2/3* mutations. Furthermore, futibatinib-pembrolizumab synergy is being explored in a phase 2 trial for advanced UC (NCT04601857) and the FGFR inhibitor AZD4547-Tislelizumab combination is also under investigation in the NCT05775874 trial. As these trials unfold, they signify a shift toward personalized and synergistic treatments for UC, setting the stage for potentially groundbreaking approaches that could redefine the treatment landscape for patients with FGFR genetic aberrations.

23.6.2 Immunotherapy–Antibody–Drug Conjugates

In the dynamic landscape of cancer therapeutics, a particularly auspicious trajectory has emerged through the amalgamation of ICIs and ADCs. For the combinations involving EV, the most interesting results derive from the EV 103 trial, a multicohort phase 1–2 study evaluating EV as monotherapy or in combination with various anticancer therapies in the first- and second-line setting of mUC. Preliminary results of the cohort evaluating pembrolizumab associated with EV as first-line treatment in 45 platinum-ineligible mUC showed an ORR of 73.3% (95% CI: 58.1–85.4), including 17.8% CR and 57.8% PR, with a median duration of response (DOR) of 25.6 months (95% CI: 8.3–not reached) (Rosenberg et al. 2020). The updated data with 24.9 months of follow-up showed a median PFS of 12.3 months (95% CI: 8.0–not reached) and a median OS of 26.1 months (95% CI: 15.74–not reached), with a 2-year OS of 56.3% (95% CI: 39.8–69.9) (Friedlander et al. 2021). The ongoing phase 3 trial EV-302 is currently testing this combination vs. standard platinum-based chemotherapy in patients with locally advanced or mUC in first line, including patients eligible for platinum-based regimens (NCT04223856).

The TROPHY-U-01 trial introduces another fascinating dimension to the ICI-ADC paradigm by elucidating the potential of the combination of SG and pembrolizumab, specifically in the context of disease progression post platinum-based chemotherapy. Encouraging interim results come from Cohort 3 of the trial testing SG in combination with pembrolizumab after progression on platinum-based chemotherapy. After a median follow-up of 5.8 months, among 41 patients, the ORR was 34% (95% CI, 20.1–50.6; 1 CR; 13 PR) with a median time to response of 2.0 months (95% CI, 1.3–2.8). The 6-month PFS rate was 47%, and no new safety signals were identified (Grivas et al. 2022). Cohorts 4 and 5 of the TROPHY-U-01 trial are aimed at evaluating SG in combination with cisplatin or with cisplatin and avelumab, followed by maintenance avelumab therapy as first-line therapy in patients with mUC who are eligible to receive cisplatin-based chemotherapy (Tagawa et al. 2022).

Finally, other multiple combination strategies are under evaluation with SG, ICI, or PARP inhibitors (NCT03869190; NCT03992131). Preliminary results of a phase 1b/2 trial testing disitamab vedotin (DV) (targeting HER2) in combination with toripalimab, an anti-PD-1 monoclonal antibody, showed an ORR of 75% and DCR of 95%, with 15% of CR. Interestingly, the response rates were higher according to HER2 expression (HER2 3+ 100%; HER2 2+ 77.8%; HER2 1+ 66.7%; HER2 negative 50%) (Zhou et al. 2022). A phase 3 trial will test this combination in first-line treatment in patients with HER2-positive mUC, compared with platinum-based chemotherapy (NCT05302284).

Finally, a phase 1b study is evaluating trastuzumab deruxtecan, a HER2-targeted ADC, in association with nivolumab in treating centrally confirmed HER2-expressing mUC after previous platinum-based chemotherapy. The ORR in cohort 3 (IHC 2+/3+; high expression) was 36.7% (95% CI, 19.9–56.1) with 13.3% CR, 23.3% PR, and median DOR was 13.1 months (95% CI, 4.1–NE) (Galsky et al. 2022).

23.7 Conclusions

Investigation of ICIs and drugs targeting new pathways has revolutionized cancer treatment, improving patient outcomes across various malignancies. In recent years, immunotherapy has become an essential treatment in advanced UC, with potential extension to the localized disease context soon. However, understanding predictive factors for immunotherapy benefit remains challenging, but improvement of drug-biomarker co-development is fundamental for precision medicine.

Tissue biomarkers investigated in UC, such as PD-L1, TMB, and GEP hold promise for guiding immunotherapy in UC, although they present many limitations, with discordant evidence on their predictive value for immunotherapy benefit across several trials. Circulating biomarkers, particularly ctDNA, hold significant potential for non-invasive and real-time monitoring of treatment response and recurrence risk, but further evidence from prospective studies is warranted to translate liquid biopsy-based approaches into routine clinical practice.

Regarding the use of immunotherapy in urothelial carcinoma subtypes and tumors with mixed histology, studies are limited but suggest potential efficacy, especially in tumors with squamous differentiation. Ongoing trials focusing on such tumors aim to develop more targeted treatment approaches. Several innovative combination therapies are under investigation, with trials combining ICIs with targeted therapies, such as FGFR inhibitors, or ADCs, potentially reshaping UC therapy in the future.

References

Adela R et al (2015) GDF-15 as a target and biomarker for diabetes and cardiovascular diseases: A translational prospective. J Diabetes Res 2015:490842. https://doi.org/10.1155/2015/490842

Agarwal A et al (2010) Serum Th1 and Th2 cytokine balance in patients of superficial transitional cell carcinoma of bladder pre-and post-intravesical combination immunotherapy. Immunopharmacol Immunotoxicol 32(2):348–356. https://doi.org/10.3109/08923970903300151

Annunziato F et al (1996) Expression and release of LAG-3-encoded protein by human CD4 + T cells are associated with IFN-γ production. FASEB J 10(7):769–776. https://doi.org/10.1096/fasebj.10.7.8635694

Bajorin DF et al (2021) Adjuvant nivolumab versus placebo in muscle-invasive urothelial carcinoma. N Engl J Med 384(22):2102–2114. https://doi.org/10.1056/nejmoa2034442

Balar AV et al (2017a) Atezolizumab as first-line treatment in cisplatin-ineligible patients with locally advanced and metastatic urothelial carcinoma: a single-arm, multicentre, phase 2 trial. Lancet 389(10064):67–76. https://doi.org/10.1016/S0140-6736(16)32455-2

Balar AV et al (2017b) First-line pembrolizumab in cisplatin-ineligible patients with locally advanced and unresectable or metastatic urothelial cancer (KEYNOTE-052): a multicentre, single-arm, phase 2 study. Lancet Oncol 18(11):1483–1492. https://doi.org/10.1016/S1470-2045(17)30616-2

Basile G et al (2022) Neoadjuvant pembrolizumab and radical cystectomy in patients with muscle-invasive urothelial bladder cancer: 3-year median follow-up update of PURE-01 Trial. Clin Cancer Res 28(23):5107–5114. https://doi.org/10.1158/1078-0432.CCR-22-2158

Bellmunt J et al (2015) Association of PD-L1 expression on tumor-infiltrating mononuclear cells and overall survival in patients with urothelial carcinoma. Ann Oncol 26(4):812–817. https://doi.org/10.1093/annonc/mdv009

Bellmunt J et al (2017) Pembrolizumab as second-line therapy for advanced urothelial carcinoma. N Engl J Med 376(11):1015–1026. https://doi.org/10.1056/nejmoa1613683

Bellmunt J et al (2021) Adjuvant atezolizumab versus observation in muscle-invasive urothelial carcinoma (IMvigor010): a multicentre, open-label, randomised, phase 3 trial. Lancet Oncol 22(4):525–537. https://doi.org/10.1016/S1470-2045(21)00004-8

Benjamin DJ, Lyou Y (2021) Advances in immunotherapy and the TGF-β resistance pathway in metastatic bladder cancer. Cancers (Basel) 13(22):5724. https://doi.org/10.3390/cancers13225724

Brown JA et al (2003) Blockade of programmed death-1 ligands on dendritic cells enhances T cell activation and cytokine production. J Immunol 170(3):1257–1266. https://doi.org/10.4049/jimmunol.170.3.1257

Chapoval AI et al (2001) B7-H3: A costimulatory molecule for T cell activation and IFN-γ production. Nat Immunol 2(3):269–274. https://doi.org/10.1038/85339

Chauvin JM et al (2020) TIGIT in cancer immunotherapy. J Immunother Cancer 8(2):e000957. https://doi.org/10.1136/jitc-2020-000957

Chemnitz JM et al (2004) SHP-1 and SHP-2 associate with immunoreceptor tyrosine-based switch motif of programmed death 1 upon primary human T cell stimulation, but only receptor ligation prevents T cell activation. J Immunol 173(2):945–954. https://doi.org/10.4049/jimmunol.173.2.945

Chen DS et al (2013) Oncology meets immunology: The cancer-immunity cycle. Immunity 39(1):1–10. https://doi.org/10.1016/j.immuni.2013.07.012

Chen Y et al (2023) Cutoff values of PD-L1 expression in urinary cytology samples for predicting response to immune checkpoint inhibitor therapy in upper urinary tract urothelial carcinoma. Cancer Cytopathol 131(3):179–187. https://doi.org/10.1002/cncy.22661

Chocarro L et al (2021) Understanding lag-3 signaling. Int J Mol Sci 22(10):5282. https://doi.org/10.3390/ijms22105282

Cristescu R et al (2018) Pan-tumor genomic biomarkers for PD-1 checkpoint blockade-based immunotherapy. Science 362(6411):eaar3593. https://doi.org/10.1126/science.aar3593

Crupi E et al (2024) Circulating tumor DNA as a predictive and prognostic biomarker in the perioperative treatment of muscle-invasive bladder cancer: a systematic review. Eur Urol Oncol 7(1):44–52. https://doi.org/10.1016/j.euo.2023.05.012

David CJ, Massagué J (2018) Contextual determinants of TGFβ action in development, immunity and cancer. Nat Rev Mol Cell Biol 19(7):419–435. https://doi.org/10.1038/s41580-018-0007-0

Davis AA, Patel VG (2019) The role of PD-L1 expression as a predictive biomarker: An analysis of all US food and drug administration (FDA) approvals of immune checkpoint inhibitors. J Immunother Cancer 7(1):1–8. https://doi.org/10.1186/s40425-019-0768-9

DeKruyff RH et al (2010) T cell/transmembrane, Ig, and mucin-3 allelic variants differentially recognize phosphatidylserine and mediate phagocytosis of apoptotic cells. J Immunol 184(4):1918–1930. https://doi.org/10.4049/jimmunol.0903059

de Padua TC et al (2022) Efficacy and toxicity of antibody-drug conjugates in the treatment of metastatic urothelial cancer: A scoping review. Urol Oncol 40(10):413–423. https://doi.org/10.1016/j.urolonc.2022.07.006

Donia M et al (2015) Aberrant expression of MHC class II in melanoma attracts inflammatory tumor-specific CD4+T-cells, which dampen CD8+T-cell antitumor reactivity. Cancer Res 75(18):3747–3759. https://doi.org/10.1158/0008-5472.CAN-14-2956

Drobner JC et al (2023) Examining the role of microbiota-centered interventions in cancer therapeutics: applications for urothelial carcinoma. Technol Cancer Res Treat 22:15330338231164196. https://doi.org/10.1177/15330338231164196

Faraj SF et al (2015) Assessment of tumoral PD-L1 expression and intratumoral CD8+ T cells in urothelial carcinoma. Urology 85(3):703.e1–703.e6. https://doi.org/10.1016/j.urology.2014.10.020

FDA (n.d.) List of cleared or approved companion diagnostic devices (in vitro and imaging tools). https://www.fda.gov/medical-devices/in-vitro-diagnostics/list-cleared-or-approved-companion-diagnostic-devices-in-vitro-and-imaging-tools

Fehlings M et al (2022) Single-cell analysis reveals clonally expanded tumor-associated CD57 +CD8 T cells are enriched in the periphery of patients with metastatic urothelial cancer responding to PD-L1 blockade. J Immunother Cancer 10(8):e004759. https://doi.org/10.1136/jitc-2022-004759

Fidelle M et al (2023) A microbiota-modulated checkpoint directs immunosuppressive intestinal T cells into cancers. Science 380(6649):eabo2296. https://doi.org/10.1126/science.abo2296

Friedlander TW et al (2021) Study EV-103: Update on durability results and long term outcome of enfortumab vedotin + pembrolizumab in first line locally advanced or metastatic urothelial carcinoma (la/mUC). J Clin Oncol 39(15_suppl):4528. https://doi.org/10.1200/jco.2021.39.15_suppl.4528

Galsky MD et al (2020a) Atezolizumab with or without chemotherapy in metastatic urothelial cancer (IMvigor130): a multicentre, randomised, placebo-controlled phase 3 trial. Lancet 395(10236):1547–1557. https://doi.org/10.1016/S0140-6736(20)30230-0

Galsky MD et al (2020b) FIGHT-205: Phase II study of first-line pemigatinib (PEMI) plus pembrolizumab (PEMBRO) versus PEMI alone versus standard of care (SOC) for cisplatin (CIS)—Ineligible urothelial carcinoma (UC) with FGFR3 mutation or rearrangement. J Clin Oncol 38(6_suppl):TPS592. https://doi.org/10.1200/jco.2020.38.6_suppl.tps592

Galsky MD et al (2022) Primary analysis from DS8201-A-U105: A phase 1b, two-part, open-label study of trastuzumab deruxtecan (T DXd) with nivolumab (nivo) in patients (pts) with HER2-expressing urothelial carcinoma (UC). J Clin Oncol 40(6_suppl):438. https://doi.org/10.1200/jco.2022.40.6_suppl.438

Galsky MD et al (2023) Disease-free survival analysis for patients with high-risk muscle-invasive urothelial carcinoma from the randomized CheckMate 274 Trial by PD-L1 combined positive score and tumor cell score. Eur Urol 83(5):432–440. https://doi.org/10.1016/j.eururo.2023.01.016

Ge Z et al (2021) TIGIT, the next step towards successful combination immune checkpoint therapy in cancer. Front Immunol 12:699895. https://doi.org/10.3389/fimmu.2021.699895

Gibney GT et al (2016) Predictive biomarkers for checkpoint inhibitor-based immunotherapy. Lancet Oncol 17(12):e542–e551. https://doi.org/10.1016/S1470-2045(16)30406-5

Grivas P et al (2022) TROPHY-U-01 Cohort 3: Sacituzumab govitecan (SG) in combination with pembrolizumab (Pembro) in patients (pts) with metastatic urothelial cancer (mUC) who progressed after platinum (PLT)-based regimens. J Clin Oncol 40(6_suppl):434. https://doi.org/10.1200/jco.2022.40.6_suppl.434

Haake M et al (2023) Tumor-derived GDF-15 blocks LFA-1 dependent T cell recruitment and suppresses responses to anti-PD-1 treatment. Nat Commun 14(1):4253. https://doi.org/10.1038/s41467-023-39817-3

Hannier S et al (1998) CD3/TCR complex-associated lymphocyte activation gene-3 molecules inhibit CD3/TCR signaling. J Immunol 161(8):4058–4065. https://doi.org/10.4049/jimmunol.161.8.4058

Hodi FS et al (2010) Improved survival with ipilimumab in patients with metastatic melanoma. N Engl J Med 363(8):711–723. https://doi.org/10.1056/nejmoa1003466

Hoffman-Censits JH et al (2021) Expression of nectin-4 in Bladder urothelial carcinoma, in morphologic variants, and nonurothelial histotypes. Appl Immunohistochem Mol Morphol 29(8):619–625. https://doi.org/10.1097/PAI.0000000000000938

Holm JS et al (2022) Neoantigen-specific CD8 T cell responses in the peripheral blood following PD-L1 blockade might predict therapy outcome in metastatic urothelial carcinoma. Nat Commun 13(1):1935. https://doi.org/10.1038/s41467-022-29342-0

Hossen MM et al (2023) Current understanding of CTLA-4: from mechanism to autoimmune diseases. Front Immunol 14:1198365. https://doi.org/10.3389/fimmu.2023.1198365

Hsieh MC et al (2015) The prognostic impact of histopathological variants in patients with advanced urothelial carcinoma. PLoS One 10(6):e0129268. https://doi.org/10.1371/journal.pone.0129268

Huang YH et al (2015) CEACAM1 regulates TIM-3-mediated tolerance and exhaustion. Nature 517(7534):386–390. https://doi.org/10.1038/nature13848

Huseni MA et al (2023) CD8+ T cell-intrinsic IL-6 signaling promotes resistance to anti-PD-L1 immunotherapy. Cell Rep Med 4(1):100878. https://doi.org/10.1016/j.xcrm.2022.100878

Ishida Y et al (1992) Induced expression of PD-1, a novel member of the immunoglobulin gene superfamily, upon programmed cell death. EMBO J 11(11):3887–3895. https://doi.org/10.1002/j.1460-2075.1992.tb05481.x

Jingushi K et al (2022) Circulating extracellular vesicles carrying Firmicutes reflective of the local immune status may predict clinical response to pembrolizumab in urothelial carcinoma patients. Cancer Immunol Immunother 71(12):2999–3011. https://doi.org/10.1007/s00262-022-03213-5

Kamat AM et al (2016) Cytokine panel for response to intravesical therapy (CyPRIT): nomogram of changes in urinary cytokine levels predicts patient response to Bacillus Calmette-Guérin. Eur Urol 69(2):197–200. https://doi.org/10.1016/j.eururo.2015.06.023

Kamoun A et al (2020) A consensus molecular classification of muscle-invasive bladder cancer. Eur Urol 77(4):420–433. https://doi.org/10.1016/j.eururo.2019.09.006

Kashio Y et al (2003) Galectin-9 induces apoptosis through the calcium-calpain-caspase-1 pathway. J

Immunol 170(7):3631–3636. https://doi.org/10.4049/jimmunol.170.7.3631

Kim WY et al (2020) Predictive value of fibroblast growth factor receptor (FGFR) alterations on anti-PD-(L)1 treatment outcomes in patients (Pts) with advanced urothelial cancer (UC): Pooled analysis of real-world data. J Clin Oncol 37(7_suppl):419. https://doi.org/10.1200/jco.2020.38.6_suppl.493

Kobayashi M et al (2022) Impact of histological variants on outcomes in patients with urothelial carcinoma treated with pembrolizumab: a propensity score matching analysis. BJU Int 130(2):226–234. https://doi.org/10.1111/bju.15510

Kolar P et al (2009 Jan) CTLA-4 (CD152) controls homeostasis and suppressive capacity of regulatory T cells in mice. Arthritis Rheum 60(1):123–132. https://doi.org/10.1002/art.24181

Kontos F et al (2021) B7-H3: An attractive target for antibody-based immunotherapy. Clin Cancer Res 27(5):1227–1235. https://doi.org/10.1158/1078-0432.CCR-20-2584

Krasnow RE et al (2017) Clinical outcomes of patients with histologic variants of urothelial cancer treated with trimodality bladder-sparing therapy. Eur Urol 72(1):54–60. https://doi.org/10.1016/j.eururo.2016.12.002

Lenza MP et al (2023) Structural insights into Siglec-15 reveal glycosylation dependency for its interaction with T cells through integrin CD11b. Nat Commun 14(1):3496. https://doi.org/10.1038/s41467-023-39119-8

Li H et al (2012) Tim-3/galectin-9 signaling pathway mediates T-cell dysfunction and predicts poor prognosis in patients with hepatitis B virus-associated hepatocellular carcinoma. Hepatology 56(4):1342–1351. https://doi.org/10.1002/hep.25777

Lines JL et al (2014) VISTA is an immune checkpoint molecule for human T cells. Cancer Res 74(7):1924–1932. https://doi.org/10.1158/0008-5472.CAN-13-1504

Loriot Y et al (2023) Phase 3 THOR study: Results of erdafitinib (erda) versus chemotherapy (chemo) in patients (pts) with advanced or metastatic urothelial cancer (mUC) with select fibroblast growth factor receptor alterations. J Clin Oncol 41(17_suppl)

Ma J et al (2023) Urine PD-L1 is a tumor tissue candidate substitute and is associated with poor survival in muscle-invasive bladder cancer patients. Int Immunopharmacol 114:109535. https://doi.org/10.1016/j.intimp.2022.109535

Marabelle A et al (2020) Association of tumour mutational burden with outcomes in patients with advanced solid tumours treated with pembrolizumab: prospective biomarker analysis of the multicohort, open-label, phase 2 KEYNOTE-158 study. Lancet Oncol 21(10):1353–1365. https://doi.org/10.1016/S1470-2045(20)30445-9

Marandino L et al (2021) Cabozantinib plus durvalumab in patients with advanced urothelial carcinoma after platinum chemotherapy: safety and preliminary activity of the open-label, single-arm, phase 2 ARCADIA trial. Clin Genitourin Cancer 19(5):457–465. https://doi.org/10.1016/j.clgc.2021.04.001

Mariathasan S et al (2018) TGFβ attenuates tumour response to PD-L1 blockade by contributing to exclusion of T cells. Nature 554(7693):544–548. https://doi.org/10.1038/nature25501

Massard C et al (2016) Safety and efficacy of durvalumab (MEDI4736), an anti-programmed cell death ligand-1 immune checkpoint inhibitor, in patients with advanced urothelial bladder cancer. J Clin Oncol 34(26):3119–3125. https://doi.org/10.1200/JCO.2016.67.9761

Miller NJ et al (2020) Histological subtypes and response to PD-1/PD-L1 blockade in advanced urothelial cancer: a retrospective study. J Urol 204(1):63–70. https://doi.org/10.1097/JU.0000000000000761

Minato A et al (2022) Efficacy of pembrolizumab in patients with variant urothelial carcinoma: a multicenter retrospective study. Clin Genitourin Cancer 20(5):499.e1–499.e8. https://doi.org/10.1016/j.clgc.2022.05.001

Moch H et al (2022) The 2022 World Health Organization classification of tumours of the urinary system and male genital organs—part A: renal, penile, and testicular tumours. Eur Urol 82(5):458–468. https://doi.org/10.1016/j.eururo.2022.06.016

Monney L et al (2002) Th1-specific cell surface protein Tim-3 regulates macrophage activation and severity of an autoimmune disease. Nature 415(6871):536–541. https://doi.org/10.1038/415536a

Murphy TL et al (2010) Slow down and survive: Enigmatic immunoregulation by BTLA and HVEM. Annu Rev Immunol 28:389–411. https://doi.org/10.1146/annurev-immunol-030409-101202

Necchi A et al (2018) Pembrolizumab as neoadjuvant therapy before radical cystectomy in patients with muscle-invasive urothelial bladder carcinoma (PURE-01): an open-label, single-arm, phase II study. J Clin Oncol 36(34):3353–3360. https://doi.org/10.1200/JCO.18.01148

Necchi A et al (2020a) Impact of molecular subtyping and immune infiltration on pathological response and outcome following neoadjuvant pembrolizumab in muscle-invasive bladder cancer [formula presented]. Eur Urol 77(6):701–710. https://doi.org/10.1016/j.eururo.2020.02.028

Necchi A et al (2020b) Updated results of PURE-01 with preliminary activity of neoadjuvant pembrolizumab in patients with muscle-invasive bladder carcinoma with variant histologies. Eur Urol 77(4):439–446. https://doi.org/10.1016/j.eururo.2019.10.026

Netto GJ et al (2022) The 2022 World Health Organization classification of tumors of the urinary system and male genital organs—part B: prostate and urinary tract tumors. Eur Urol 82(5):469–482. https://doi.org/10.1016/j.eururo.2022.07.002

Ning Z et al (2021) Roles of BTLA in immunity and immune disorders. Front Immunol 12:654960. https://doi.org/10.3389/fimmu.2021.654960

Okazaki T et al (2007) PD-1 and PD-1 ligands: From discovery to clinical application. Int Immunol 19(7):813–824. https://doi.org/10.1093/intimm/dxm057

Pagès F et al (2002) Local immunostimulation induced by intravesical administration of autologous interferon-gamma-activated macrophages in patients with superficial bladder cancer. Clin Exp Immunol 127(2):303–309. https://doi.org/10.1046/j.1365-2249.2002.01766.x

Palakurthi S et al (2019) The combined effect of fgfr inhibition and PD-1 blockade promotes tumor-intrinsic induction of antitumor immunity. Cancer Immunol Res 7(9):1457–1471. https://doi.org/10.1158/2326-6066.CIR-18-0595

Patel SP et al (2015) PD-L1 expression as a predictive biomarker in cancer immunotherapy. Mol Cancer Ther 14(4):847–856. https://doi.org/10.1158/1535-7163.MCT-14-0983

Patel MR et al (2018) Avelumab in metastatic urothelial carcinoma after platinum failure (JAVELIN Solid Tumor): pooled results from two expansion cohorts of an open-label, phase 1 trial. Lancet Oncol 19(1):51–64. https://doi.org/10.1016/S1470-2045(17)30900-2

Peng J, Sridhar S, Siefker-Radtke AO, Selvarajah S, Jiang DM (2022) Targeting the FGFR pathway in urothelial carcinoma: the future is now. Curr Treat Options Oncol 23(9). https://doi.org/10.1007/s11864-022-01009-4

Powles T et al (2018) Atezolizumab versus chemotherapy in patients with platinum-treated locally advanced or metastatic urothelial carcinoma (IMvigor211): a multicentre, open-label, phase 3 randomised controlled trial. Lancet 391(10122):748–757. https://doi.org/10.1016/S0140-6736(17)33297-X

Powles T et al (2019) Clinical efficacy and biomarker analysis of neoadjuvant atezolizumab in operable urothelial carcinoma in the ABACUS trial. Nat Med 25(11):1706–1714. https://doi.org/10.1038/s41591-019-0628-7

Powles T et al (2020a) Avelumab maintenance therapy for advanced or metastatic urothelial carcinoma. N Engl J Med 383(13):1218–1230. https://doi.org/10.1056/nejmoa2002788

Powles T et al (2020b) Durvalumab alone and durvalumab plus tremelimumab versus chemotherapy in previously untreated patients with unresectable, locally advanced or metastatic urothelial carcinoma (DANUBE): a randomised, open-label, multicentre, phase 3 trial. Lancet Oncol 21(12):1574–1588. https://doi.org/10.1016/S1470-2045(20)30541-6

Powles T et al (2021a) Pembrolizumab alone or combined with chemotherapy versus chemotherapy as first-line therapy for advanced urothelial carcinoma (KEYNOTE-361): a randomised, open-label, phase 3 trial. Lancet Oncol 22(7):931–945. https://doi.org/10.1016/S1470-2045(21)00152-2

Powles T et al (2021b) ctDNA guiding adjuvant immunotherapy in urothelial carcinoma. Nature 595(7867):432–437. https://doi.org/10.1038/s41586-021-03642-9

Powles T et al (2021c) Enfortumab vedotin in previously treated advanced urothelial carcinoma. N Engl J Med 384(12):1125–1135. https://doi.org/10.1056/nejmoa2035807

Prasad DVR et al (2004) Murine B7-H3 is a negative regulator of T cells. J Immunol 173(4):2500–2506. https://doi.org/10.4049/jimmunol.173.4.2500

Prince EA et al (2021) Analytical concordance of PD-L1 assays utilizing antibodies from FDA-approved diagnostics in advanced cancers: a systematic literature review. JCO Precis Oncol 5:953–973. https://doi.org/10.1200/PO.20.00412

Qin S et al (2019) Novel immune checkpoint targets: Moving beyond PD-1 and CTLA-4. Mol Cancer 18(1):155. https://doi.org/10.1186/s12943-019-1091-2

Qureshi OS et al (2011) Trans-endocytosis of CD80 and CD86: A molecular basis for the cell-extrinsic function of CTLA-4. Science (1979) 332(6029):600–603. https://doi.org/10.1126/science.1202947

Reches A et al (2020) Nectin4 is a novel TIGIT ligand which combines checkpoint inhibition and tumor specificity. J Immunother Cancer 8(1):e000266. https://doi.org/10.1136/jitc-2019-000266

Rezazadeh A et al (2020) An observational study of outcomes of patients (pts) with advanced urothelial carcinoma (UC) after anti-programmed death-(Ligand) 1 (PD-[L]1) therapy by fibroblast growth factor receptor gene alteration (FGFRa) status. Ann Oncol 31(suppl 4):S586–S587. Abstract 757P. https://doi.org/10.1016/j.annonc.2020.08.829

Robertson AG et al (2017) Comprehensive molecular characterization of muscle-invasive bladder cancer. Cell 171(3):540–556.e25. https://doi.org/10.1016/j.cell.2017.09.007

Rose KM et al (2023) Circulating and urinary tumour DNA in urothelial carcinoma — upper tract, lower tract and metastatic disease. Nat Rev Urol 20(7):452. https://doi.org/10.1038/s41585-023-00725-2

Rosenberg JE et al (2016) Atezolizumab in patients with locally advanced and metastatic urothelial carcinoma who have progressed following treatment with platinum-based chemotherapy: A single-arm, multicentre, phase 2 trial. Lancet 387(10031):1909–1920. https://doi.org/10.1016/S0140-6736(16)00561-4

Rosenberg JE et al (2020) Study EV-103: preliminary durability results of enfortumab vedotin plus pembrolizumab for locally advanced or metastatic urothelial carcinoma. J Clin Oncol 38(6_suppl):441. https://doi.org/10.1200/jco.2020.38.6_suppl.441

Scosyrev E et al (2011) Do mixed histological features affect survival benefit from neoadjuvant platinum-based combination chemotherapy in patients with locally advanced bladder cancer? A secondary analysis of Southwest Oncology Group-Directed Intergroup Study (S8710). BJU Int 108(5):693–699. https://doi.org/10.1111/j.1464-410X.2010.09900.x

Sedy JR et al (2005) B and T lymphocyte attenuator regulates T cell activation through interaction with herpesvirus entry mediator. Nat Immunol 6(1):90–98. https://doi.org/10.1038/ni1144

Seidel JA et al (2018) Anti-PD-1 and anti-CTLA-4 therapies in cancer: Mechanisms of action, efficacy, and limitations. Front Oncol 28:86. https://doi.org/10.3389/fonc.2018.00086

Seiler R et al (2017) Impact of molecular subtypes in muscle-invasive bladder cancer on predicting response and survival after neoadjuvant chemotherapy. Eur Urol 72(4):544–554. https://doi.org/10.1016/j.eururo.2017.03.030

Serrano MJ et al (2020) Precision prevention and cancer interception: The new challenges of liquid biopsy. Cancer Discov 10(11):1635–1644. https://doi.org/10.1158/2159-8290.CD-20-0466

Shahrokh F et al (2001) Preoperative plasma levels of transforming growth factor beta1 (TGF-β1) strongly predict progression in patients undergoing radical prostatectomy. JCO 19(11):2856–2864. https://doi.org/10.1200/JCO.2001.19.11.2856

Sharma P et al (2017) Nivolumab in metastatic urothelial carcinoma after platinum therapy (CheckMate 275): a multicentre, single-arm, phase 2 trial. Lancet Oncol 18(3):312–322. https://doi.org/10.1016/S1470-2045(17)30065-7

Sheryka E et al (2003) Urinary interleukin-8 levels are elevated in subjects with transitional cell carcinoma. Urology 62(1):162–166. https://doi.org/10.1016/S0090-4295(03)00134-1

Siefker-Radtke AO et al (2009) Phase II clinical trial of neoadjuvant alternating doublet chemotherapy with ifosfamide/doxorubicin and etoposide/cisplatin in small-cell urothelial cancer. J Clin Oncol 27(16):2592–2597. https://doi.org/10.1200/JCO.2008.19.0256

Siefker-Radtke AO et al (2022) Efficacy and safety of erdafitinib in patients with locally advanced or metastatic urothelial carcinoma: long-term follow-up of a phase 2 study. Lancet Oncol 23(9):1269–1287. https://doi.org/10.1016/S1470-2045(21)00660-4

Sjödahl G et al (2012) A molecular taxonomy for urothelial carcinoma. Clin Cancer Res 18(12):3377–3386. https://doi.org/10.1158/1078-0432.CCR-12-0077-T

Suh WK et al (2003) The B7 family member B7-H3 preferentially down-regulates T helper type 1-mediated immune responses. Nat Immunol 4(9):899–906. https://doi.org/10.1038/ni967

Szabados B et al (2022) Final results of neoadjuvant atezolizumab in cisplatin-ineligible patients with muscle-invasive urothelial cancer of the bladder. Eur Urol 82(2):212–222. https://doi.org/10.1016/j.eururo.2022.04.013

Tagawa ST et al (2021) TROPHY-U-01: a phase II open-label study of sacituzumab govitecan in patients with metastatic urothelial carcinoma progressing after platinum-based chemotherapy and checkpoint inhibitors. J Clin Oncol 39(22):2474–2485. https://doi.org/10.1200/JCO.20.03489

Tagawa ST et al (2022) TROPHY-U-01 cohort 4: Sacituzumab govitecan (SG) in combination with cisplatin (Cis) in platinum (PLT)-naïve patients (pts) with metastatic urothelial cancer (mUC). J Clin Oncol 40(6_suppl):TPS581. https://doi.org/10.1200/jco.2022.40.6_suppl.tps581

Tagliamento M et al (2021) Vista: A promising target for cancer immunotherapy? Immunotargets Ther 10:185–200. https://doi.org/10.2147/ITT.S260429

Takai Y et al (2003) Nectins and nectin-like molecules: Roles in cell adhesion, migration, and polarization. Cancer Sci 94(8):655–667. https://doi.org/10.1111/j.1349-7006.2003.tb01499.x

Tang D et al (2012) Tumor immunity times out: TIM-3 and HMGB1. Nat Immunol 13(9):808–810. https://doi.org/10.1038/ni.2396

Tateo V et al (2023) Agnostic approvals in oncology: getting the right drug to the right patient with the right genomics. Pharmaceuticals (Basel) 16(4):614. https://doi.org/10.3390/ph16040614

Tawbi HA et al (2022) Relatlimab and nivolumab versus nivolumab in untreated advanced melanoma. N Engl J Med 386(1):24–34. https://doi.org/10.1056/nejmoa2109970

van Dijk N et al (2020) Preoperative ipilimumab plus nivolumab in locoregionally advanced urothelial cancer: the NABUCCO trial. Nat Med 26(12):1839–1844. https://doi.org/10.1038/s41591-020-1085-z

Vikerfors A et al (2021) Soluble PD-L1 in serum and urine in urinary bladder cancer patients. Cancers (Basel) 13(22):5841. https://doi.org/10.3390/cancers13225841

Wang J et al (2019a) Fibrinogen-like protein 1 is a major immune inhibitory ligand of LAG-3. Cell 176(1–2):334–347.e12. https://doi.org/10.1016/j.cell.2018.11.010

Wang J et al (2019b) Siglec-15 as an immune suppressor and potential target for normalization cancer immunotherapy. Nat Med 25(4):656–666. https://doi.org/10.1038/s41591-019-0374-x

Wang Y et al (2020) Immune-related signature predicts the prognosis and immunotherapy benefit in bladder cancer. Cancer Med 9(20):7729–7741. https://doi.org/10.1002/cam4.3400

Watanabe E et al (2003) Urinary interleukin-2 may predict clinical outcome of intravesical bacillus Calmette-Guérin immunotherapy for carcinoma in situ of the bladder. Cancer Immunol Immunother 52(8):481–486. https://doi.org/10.1007/s00262-003-0384-9

Weide B et al (2016) High GDF-15 serum levels independently correlate with poorer overall survival of patients with tumor-free stage III and unresectable stage IV melanoma. J Invest Dermatol 136(12):2444–2452. https://doi.org/10.1016/j.jid.2016.07.016

Young MN et al (2024) Predictive value of dynamic changes in ctDNA and baseline biomarkers with neoadjuvant atezolizumab in operable urothelial carcinoma in the ABACUS trial. JCO 42(4_suppl)

Yuen KC et al (2020) High systemic and tumor-associated IL-8 correlates with reduced clinical benefit of PD-L1 blockade. Nat Med 26(5):693–698. https://doi.org/10.1038/s41591-020-0860-1

Zang J et al (2023) Integrated longitudinal circulating tumor DNA profiling predicts immunotherapy response of metastatic urothelial carcinoma in the POLARIS-03 trial. J Pathol 261(2):198–209. https://doi.org/10.1002/path.6166

Zhao L et al (2021) TIM-3: An update on immunotherapy. Int Immunopharmacol 99:107933. https://doi.org/10.1016/j.intimp.2021.107933

Zhou Z et al (2013) Growth differentiation factor-15 suppresses maturation and function of dendritic cells and inhibits tumor-specific immune response. PLoS One 8(11):e78618. https://doi.org/10.1371/journal.pone.0078618

Zhou L et al (2022) Study RC48-C014: Preliminary results of RC48-ADC combined with toripalimab in patients with locally advanced or metastatic urothelial carcinoma. J Clin Oncol 40(6_suppl):515. https://doi.org/10.1200/jco.2022.40.6_suppl.515

Zhu C et al (2005) The Tim-3 ligand galectin-9 negatively regulates T helper type 1 immunity. Nat Immunol 6(12):1245–1252. https://doi.org/10.1038/ni1271

Part VIII

Future Directions in Bladder Cancer Research

Future Directions in Bladder Cancer Research and Clinical Implications

24

Margaret A. Knowles and Lars Dyrskjøt

Abstract

This chapter discusses how the understanding of bladder cancer biology and the search for appropriate biomarkers has changed with the development of new omics tools and assays. It discusses where current understanding is most likely to have impact in the clinic and highlights remaining key questions and challenges for future research.

Keywords

Biomarkers · Molecular profiling · Therapeutic strategies · Clinical trials

Two decades ago, little was known about the biology of bladder cancer despite its high incidence and prevalence, and limited progress had been made in therapy over many years. Although many patients with non-muscle-invasive bladder cancer (NMIBC) enjoyed good outcomes, there was a dismal outlook for patients with muscle-invasive bladder cancer (MIBC). This situation is surprising given the high economic burden of this disease, which incurs the highest lifetime treatment cost per patient of all cancers (Joyce et al. 2023). One reason that progress had lagged behind that in other cancers was a critical lack of funding for research. For this reason, bladder cancer has often been termed a "cinderella" cancer (Boormans and Zwarthoff 2016).

Although there is still a major discrepancy in funding compared to other cancers, the past two decades have seen an explosion of information about the biology of the disease and a burgeoning literature. Limited funding requires prioritization of effort and indeed much of the recent work described here, has focussed on key unanswered research questions identified following consultation with patient and public involvement representatives and healthcare professionals (Bessa et al. 2019).

24.1 Where Is Understanding of Disease Biology Likely to Have an Impact in the Clinic?

Impact may be through the identification of biomarkers for disease detection, differential diagnosis, prognosis, or prediction of therapeutic response. Certainly, characterization of the

M. A. Knowles (✉)
Division of Molecular Medicine, Leeds Institute of Medical Research at St James's, St James's University Hospital, Leeds, UK
e-mail: m.a.knowles@leeds.ac.uk

L. Dyrskjøt
Department of Clinical Medicine, Aarhus University, Aarhus, Denmark

Department of Molecular Medicine, Aarhus University Hospital, Aarhus, Denmark

M. A. Knowles, L. Dyrskjøt (eds.), *Biology of Bladder Cancer*,
https://doi.org/10.1007/978-3-031-68505-7_24

bladder cancer genome, transcriptome, and methylome has yielded a profusion of biomarkers, many of which show great promise. Urine- and blood-based tests offer non-invasive methods for application at diagnosis, for detection of disease recurrence during disease monitoring and assessment of therapeutic response and relapse. Further work in this area must now focus on validation of the utility of these assays and biomarkers through clinical trials. Some biomarker-guided clinical trials are already ongoing with a focus on NMIBC surveillance using urine tests, and detection of minimal residual disease in MIBC using blood tests. Some biomarkers may also have application in imaging, which may allow identification of metastatic sites and influence treatment choices. The risk of developing bladder cancer in relation to sex, race, lifestyle, genetic, and environmental factors is now clear and some of these tests may be applicable to screening for early detection in high-risk populations.

Improved biological understanding may also identify novel therapies. Specific targets are already suggested by molecular profiling efforts. However, it is likely that the distinct clinical behavior and molecular profiles of NMIBC and MIBC will dictate different approaches. Even where the same target gene is present in both disease states, localized rather than systemic approaches are required for NMIBC. Already innovative approaches are making use of the confined and protected intravesical environment to deliver localized therapy. A promising target is FGFR3, systemic targeting of which shows efficacy in some patients with advanced disease. The results of localized targeting of FGFR3 in NMIBC where mutations of *FGFR3* are so common will be of great interest. Similarly, mutations that affect DNA repair capacity may drive therapeutic vulnerabilities, particularly in MIBC, for example to cisplatin-based chemotherapy or PARP inhibitors.

One of the exciting developments during the past decade has been the introduction of systemic immunotherapy approaches and the characterization of the immune landscape of bladder tumors. This has transformed the treatment options and outcomes for many patients and has led to a profusion of clinical trials. Furthermore, the recent use of antibody–drug conjugates in combination with immunotherapy, has demonstrated significant improvements in patient survival.

Transcriptional subtyping identifies the underlying disease biology and has been demonstrated to be associated with, e.g., chemo- and immunotherapy response. Importantly, there are already ongoing clinical trials that test the clinical potential of guiding chemo- and immunotherapy based on subtype information. The readout of these first proof-of-concept trials may provide important information about the prognostic (and predictive) value of the subtypes—and their clinical usefulness.

24.2 What Remain as the Key Unanswered Questions and How Can the Limited Funding Available for Research Be Prioritized?

One area of interest is in the prediction of risks of disease development and disease progression. Further research into the causes and risk factors for tumor development may lead to prevention strategies and monitoring of those at highest risk. Careful risk stratification of NMIBC in order to maintain conservative treatment (local resection and single dose of intravesical chemotherapy) for all except patients at high risk of progression has long been a goal. While current tools based on clinicopathologic characteristics show good performance in determining high risk (e.g., those with large tumors, multifocal disease, presence of CIS, and high grade) objective molecular markers may help to improve risk assessment, particularly in patients currently scored as at intermediate risk. Similarly, in MIBC more objective markers may determine whether to give NAC prior to cystectomy. Much of the current molecular information has shown that patient outcomes can be related to specific mutations or transcriptional subtypes, but although such features may allow patients to be divided into sub-populations with different outcomes, none yet provide robust risk prediction for individual patients.

A second area of interest is prediction of response to current standard-of-care treatments such as BCG treatment in NMIBC and cisplatin-based regimens in MIBC and advanced disease. Transcriptional subtyping according to treatment response is already providing exciting information in this area that may shape therapeutic strategies in the future. However, results are still not robust across studies and need to be replicated in larger prospective cohorts. It is essential that we learn more about disease biology to better understand treatment response and identify biomarkers for guiding treatment with novel drug combinations. Many new treatments are also associated with significant adverse effects—and importantly also high costs to healthcare systems.

Another important aspect to consider is the patient's immune system capacity. The focus has largely been on the tumor microenvironment and immune cell contexture there. However, increasing evidence points to the relevance of investigating how "healthy" the immune system is in the individual patient, and taking a more comprehensive approach to understand tumor–host interactions. Increased understanding of immunology may also pave the way for example, development of novel cancer vaccines.

The transcriptional profiles of large numbers of MIBC have contributed to the consensus classification and large numbers of profiles of NMIBC are available for the generation of a similar consensus. It is debatable whether further bulk tumor transcriptional profiling will improve understanding. However, integration of genomic, transcriptomic, and methylation data has not yet been explored in detail and is predicted to provide additional granularity. Integration of germline variants associated with risk and prognosis may also add valuable information as may consideration of patients' race and sex. As current datasets do not have all such information, additional profiling will be needed for this purpose. Currently, little is known about non-coding DNA in bladder tumors and it is predicted that further analysis of regulatory elements and other non-coding sequences using whole genome sequence data may also improve understanding. Ultimately, for all classification systems, clinical utility of subtype assignment in predicting therapeutic response or prognosis remains to be validated through clinical trials and comparisons made with performance of simpler, single gene, or biomarker panels.

A major confounding factor in interpreting molecular data is intra-tumor heterogeneity. To date, all molecular profiling has used bulk tumor samples and it has become clear that RNA analysis of different individual regions of a tumor or immunohistochemistry can identify multiple expression subtypes within the same tumor. This is most prevalent in MIBC, where complex subclonal evolution can present many difficulties in interpretation. In predicting prognosis or assessing relevant therapies, identification of the most important drivers of tumor phenotype, key therapeutic targets, and components of highest risk will be critical. Single cell analysis may help to elucidate this but methods to interpret and apply such knowledge remain to be developed.

While biological understanding has improved dramatically in recent years and key genes involved in bladder cancer development are now known, there remains a large gap in our knowledge of the function of many of these genes and how and when they play a role during disease pathogenesis. For example, many chromatin regulator genes are implicated but knowledge of how they influence phenotype is only in its infancy. As the vast majority of bladder tumors of all grades and stages carry mutations in such genes, further understanding and assessment of the potential role of drugs targeting these genes are needed. Current trials of epidrugs may help to define key areas on which to focus.

Having defined so many key players in bladder cancer development, it is now crucial that relevant preclinical functional studies are carried out. These may involve both in vitro work with normal urothelial cells, tumor cell lines, and tumor-derived organoids and work with animal models. Ordering of events during disease pathogenesis is critical and must be tested using such approaches.

Artificial intelligence (AI) has great potential to contribute to interpretation of large datasets and ultimately to clinical decision-making. This includes interpretation and classification of tissue and cytology images at the time of diagnosis and of cystoscopic, radiographic, and other clinical images. AI may also be used to improve performance of current clinicopathologic assessment of risks of recurrence and progression by inclusion of molecular features. There are also potential applications in prediction of therapeutic response. To date, the ability of AI to help in interpretation of the huge molecular datasets now collected for bladder cancer is largely untapped.

Our purpose in compiling this book was to provide a current view of biological understanding and how this is now translating into clinical impact. Understanding has improved dramatically and there is now an explosion of rationally designed clinical trials that are predicated on this burgeoning pool of information. The next few years will see the outcome of the many trials described in this book that are testing hypotheses related to tumor biology. This should allow the development of rational combinations of chemo-, radio-, immuno-, and targeted therapies for indications dictated by tumor biology, to provide personalized treatment. Dramatic advances have been made and the outlook for patients with bladder cancer is now extremely promising.

References

Bessa A, Maclennan S, Enting D, Bryan R, Josephs D, Hughes S, Amery S, Khan MS, Malde S, Nair R, Cahill F, Wylie H, Thurairaja R, Chatterton K, Kinsella N, Haggstrom C, Van Hemelrijck M (2019) Consensus in bladder cancer research priorities between patients and healthcare professionals using a four-stage modified Delphi method. Eur Urol 76:258–259

Boormans JL, Zwarthoff EC (2016) Limited funds for bladder cancer research and what can we do about it. Bladder Cancer 2:49–51

Joyce DD, Sharma V, Williams SB (2023) Cost-effectiveness and economic impact of bladder cancer management: an updated review of the literature. Pharmacoeconomics 41:751–769

MIX
Papier aus verantwortungsvollen Quellen
Paper from responsible sources
FSC® C105338

If you have any concerns about our products,
you can contact us on
ProductSafety@springernature.com

In case Publisher is established outside the EU,
the EU authorized representative is:
Springer Nature Customer Service Center GmbH
Europaplatz 3, 69115 Heidelberg, Germany

Printed by Libri Plureos GmbH
in Hamburg, Germany